Pharmacology of Pain

Mission Statement of IASP Press®

IASP brings together scientists, clinicians, health care providers, and policy makers to stimulate and support the study of pain and to translate that knowledge into improved pain relief worldwide. IASP Press publishes timely, high-quality, and reasonably priced books relating to pain research and treatment.

Pharmacology of Pain

Editors

Pierre Beaulieu, MD, PhD
Departments of Anesthesiology and Pharmacology, University of Montreal, Montreal, Quebec, Canada

David Lussier, MD, FRCP(C)
Geriatric Institute, University of Montreal; Division of Geriatric Medicine and Alan-Edwards Centre for Research on Pain, McGill University, Montreal, Quebec, Canada

Frank Porreca, PhD
Professor of Pharmacology and Anesthesiology, University of Arizona, Tucson, Arizona, USA

Anthony H. Dickenson, PhD, FMedSci
Department of Pharmacology, University College London, London, United Kingdom

IASP PRESS® ◆ SEATTLE

Library of Congress Cataloging-in-Publication Data

Pharmacology of pain / editors, Pierre Beaulieu ... [et al.].
p. ; cm.
Includes bibliographical references and index.
Summary: "This book provides a complete review of the pharmacology of pain, including mechanisms of drug actions, clinical aspects of drug use, and new developments. It describes the different systems involved in the perception, transmission, and modulation of pain and discusses the available options for pharmacological treatment of pain"--Provided by publisher.
ISBN 978-0-931092-78-7 (alk. paper)
1. Analgesics. 2. Pain. I. Beaulieu, Pierre, 1958- II. International Association for the Study of Pain.
[DNLM: 1. Analgesics--pharmacology. 2. Pain--drug therapy. QV 95 P5365 2010]
RM319.P43 2010
615'.783--dc22
2009047451

Published by:
IASP Press®
International Association for the Study of Pain
111 Queen Anne Ave N, Suite 501
Seattle, WA 98109-4955, USA
Fax: 206-283-9403
www.iasp-pain.org

Printed in the United States of America

Contents

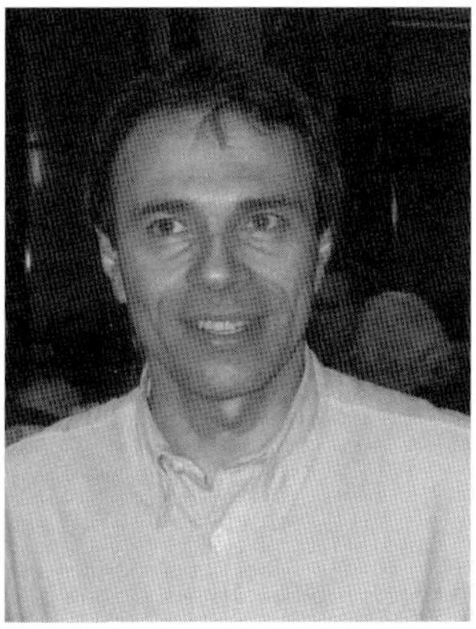

Pierre Beaulieu, MD, PhD, FRCA, is Associate Professor of Pharmacology and Anesthesiology at the University of Montreal, Quebec, Canada. He received his MD at the University of Bordeaux, France, trained in anesthesiology in London, United Kingdom, and received his PhD in pharmacology in Montreal. He holds a clinical research scholarship from the Quebec Health Research Funding agency and is a member of the Quebec Pain Research Network. His research concentrates on the pharmacology of cannabinoids in the treatment of pain through the modulation of the endocannabinoid system. His group has also developed an animal model of neuropathic pain targeted at the saphenous nerve for the study of mechanisms of neuropathic pain.

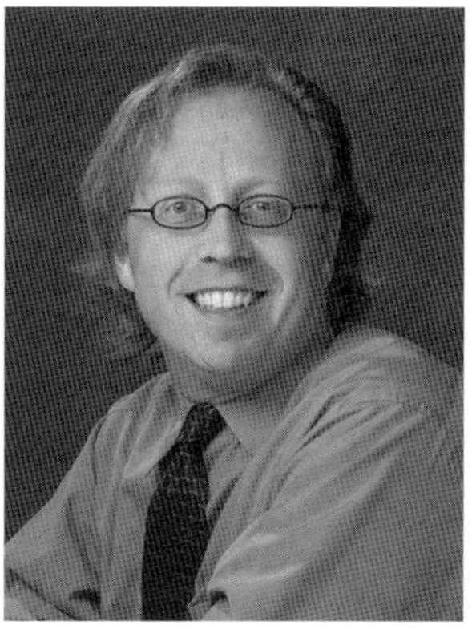

David Lussier, MD, obtained his medical degree from the University of Montreal, Canada, and later completed a residency in internal medicine and a fellowship in geriatric medicine. He completed a three-year training in pain medicine and palliative care at Beth Israel Medical Center, New York. He is now Associate Professor at University of Montreal and Adjunct Professor at McGill University, Montreal, and a member of McGill's Alan-Edwards Center for Research on Pain. He is also a practicing physician at the University of Montreal Geriatric Institute and the McGill University Health Center, where he has developed pain clinics especially devoted to older patients. Dr. Lussier's research interests include pharmacology of analgesics and new approaches to manage pain, with a special focus on older persons. He has written several review articles and book chapters on the treatment of pain in older patients and in patients with cancer, as well as on adjuvant analgesics. He has lectured at numerous conferences, both at national and international levels. Dr. Lussier is the founding chairman of a Special Interest Group of the International Association for the Study on Pain, on pain in older persons.

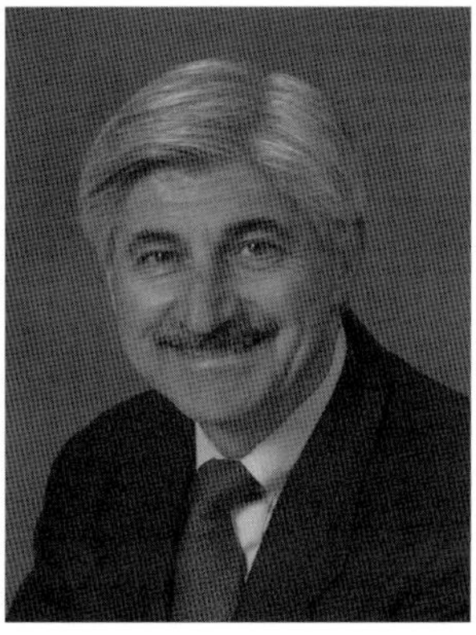

Frank Porreca, PhD, is Professor of Pharmacology and Anesthesiology at the University of Arizona, Tucson, Arizona, USA. He is a member of the Arizona Cancer Center at the University of Arizona. He received his MS in biomedical engineering at Drexel University, Philadelphia, and his PhD in pharmacology at Temple University, Philadelphia. He is Pharmacology Section Editor of PAIN, journal of the International Association for the Study of Pain, and Co-Executive Editor-in-Chief of Life Sciences. Dr. Porreca has received numerous honors and awards, including the F.W. Kerr Award of the American Pain Society in 2000. His current research includes mechanisms of neuropathic and other chronic pains, headache pain, opioid-induced hyperalgesia, and new modalities for treatment of pain and drug abuse. He has a particular interest in descending pain modulatory circuits and reward.

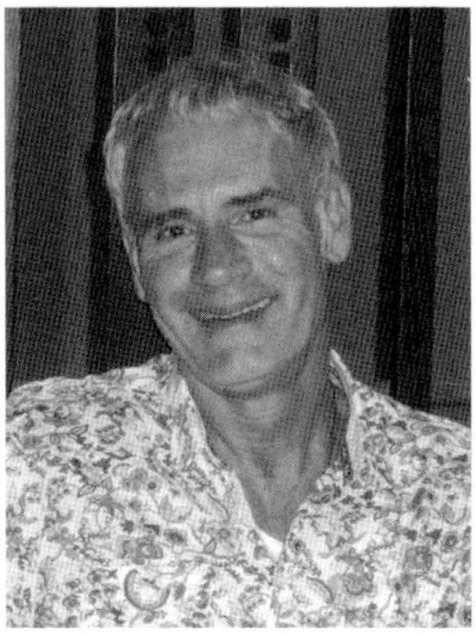

Anthony Dickenson, PhD, FMedSci, is Professor of Neuropharmacology in the Department of Pharmacology at University College, London, United Kingdom. He gained his PhD at the National Institute for Medical Research, London, has held posts in Paris, California, and Sweden, and was appointed to the Department of Pharmacology at University College in 1983. His research interests are pharmacology of the brain, including the mechanisms of pain and how pain can be controlled in both normal and pathophysiological conditions, and how to translate basic science to the patient.

Prof. Dickenson was a member of the Council of the International Association for the Study of Pain for 6 years and was an associate editor for the journal Pain. He has authored more than 250 refereed publications due to his outstanding and motivated research team and has made many media appearances. He is a founding and continuing member of the Wellcome Trust-funded London Pain Consortium. Prof. Dickenson has given plenary lectures at the World Congress on Pain, the American Pain Society, the European Pain Congress, the Canadian Pain Society, the Belgium Pain Society, ASEAPS, the Scandinavian Pain Society, the British Pain Society (of which he is an Honorary Member), the Thailand Pain Society, the Irish Pain Society, the Singapore Pain Society, the Australian Pain Society, the New Zealand Pain Society, and many other international and national meetings. He has also spoken at the Royal Institution and to general practitioners and schools on pain.

Contributing Authors

Ralf Baron, Dr med *Department of Neurological Pain Research and Therapy, Neurological Clinic, University Hospital Schleswig Holstein, Campus Kiel, and Department of Physiology, Christian-Albrechts University of Kiel, Kiel, Germany*

Pierre Beaulieu, MD, PhD, FRCA *Departments of Anesthesiology and Pharmacology, University of Montreal, Montreal, Quebec, Canada*

Jean-Louis Beneytout, PhD *Laboratory of Biochemistry and Molecular Biology, Faculty of Pharmacy, University of Limoges, Limoges, France*

Sylvie Bourgoin, PhD *Faculty of Medicine, Pierre et Marie Curie-Paris University, INSERM/CPN U894, Paris, France*

Stephen C. Brown, MD *Department of Anaesthesia and Pain Medicine, Divisional Centre of Pain Management and Pain Research, Hospital for Sick Children; Department of Anesthesia, University of Toronto, Toronto, Ontario, Canada*

Eduardo Bruera, MD *Department of Symptom Control and Palliative Care, MD Anderson Cancer Center, Houston, Texas, USA*

Geoffrey Burnstock, PhD *Autonomic Neuroscience Centre, Royal Free and University College Medical School, London, United Kingdom*

Andrew C. Charles, MD *Hatos Center for Neuropharmacology and Department of Neurology, UCLA, Los Angeles, California, USA*

Gehoon Chung, DDS *National Research Laboratory for Pain, Dental Research Institute, and Department of Physiology, School of Dentistry, Seoul National University, Seoul, Korea*

Ulises Coffeen, MSc *Ramón de la Fuente National Institute of Psychiatry, Neuroscience Division, Mexico City, Mexico*

Maxine G.J. de la Cruz, MD *Department of Symptom Control and Palliative Care, MD Anderson Cancer Center, Houston, Texas, USA*

Theodore Cummins, PhD *Department of Pharmacology and Toxicology, Stark Neurosciences Research Institute, Indiana University School of Medicine, Indianapolis, Indiana, USA*

Andre Dray, PhD *AstraZeneca R&D, Montreal, Quebec, Canada*

Ronald Dubner, DDS, PhD *Department of Neural and Pain Sciences, Dental School, and Program in Neuroscience, University of Maryland, Baltimore, Maryland, USA*

Alain Eschalier, MD, PhD *INSERM, Unit 766, Faculties of Medicine and Pharmacy; Laboratory of Medical Pharmacology, Faculty of Medicine, Clermont University; Pharmacology Service, Clermont-Ferrand University Hospital Center, G. Montpied Hospital, Clermont-Ferrand, France*

Christopher J. Evans, MPH, PhD *Hatos Center for Neuropharmacology and Department of Psychiatry and Biobehavioral Sciences, UCLA, Los Angeles, California, USA*

Luiz F. Ferrari, PhD *Department of Pharmacology, Faculty of Medicine of Ribeirão Preto, University of São Paulo, Ribeirão Preto, Brazil*

Sérgio H. Ferreira, MD *Department of Pharmacology, Faculty of Medicine of Ribeirão Preto, University of São Paulo, Ribeirão Preto, Brazil*

Philippe Goffaux, PhD *Faculty of Medicine, University of Sherbrooke, Sherbrooke, Quebec, Canada*

Josée Guindon, PhD *Neuroscience and Behavior Program, Psychology Department, University of Georgia, Athens, Georgia, USA*

Michel Hamon, PhD *Faculty of Medicine, Pierre et Marie Curie-Paris University, INSERM/CPN U894, Paris, France*

Per T. Hansson, MD, DMSci, DDS *Departments of Molecular Medicine and Surgery, Clinical Pain Research, and Neurosurgery, Pain Center, Karolinska Institute/Karolinska University Hospital, Stockholm, Sweden*

Andrea G. Hohmann, PhD *Neuroscience and Behavior Program, Psychology Department, University of Georgia, Athens, Georgia, USA*

Orlando Jaimes, *Chem Ramón de la Fuente National Institute of Psychiatry, Neuroscience Division, Mexico City, Mexico*

Wilfrid Jänig, Dr med *Department of Neurological Pain Research and Therapy, Neurological Clinic, University Hospital Schleswig Holstein, Campus Kiel, and Department of Physiology, Christian-Albrechts University of Kiel, Kiel, Germany*

Sung Jun Jung, MD, PhD *Department of Physiology, College of Medicine, Kangwon National University, Chunchon, Korea*

Valérie Kayser, PhD *Faculty of Medicine, Pierre et Marie Curie-Paris University, INSERM/CPN U894, Paris, France*

Wing-Fai Kwan, MD *Department of Anesthesiology, Harbor-UCLA Medical Center, University of California at Los Angeles, Los Angeles, California, USA*

Daniel Le Bars, DVM, DSci *Team "Pain," INSERM UMRS 975, CNRS UMR 7225, and Faculty of Medicine, Pierre and Marie Curie University, Paris, France*

Michel Le Moal, MD, DrSci *Neurocenter Magendie, INSERM U862, Victor Segalen University, and François Magendie Institute, Bordeaux, France*

Guillaume Léonard, MSc *Faculty of Medicine, University of Sherbrooke, Sherbrooke, Quebec, Canada*

Alberto López-Avila, MD, PhD *Ramón de la Fuente National Institute of Psychiatry, Neuroscience Division, Mexico City, Mexico*

David Lussier, MD, FRCP(C) *Geriatric Institute, University of Montreal; Division of Geriatric Medicine and Alan-Edwards Centre for Research on Pain, McGill University, Montreal, Quebec, Canada*

Yao-Ying Ma, MD, PhD *Hatos Center for Neuropharmacology and Department of Psychiatry and Biobehavioral Sciences, UCLA, Los Angeles, California, USA*

Christophe Mallet, PhD *INSERM, Unit 766, Faculties of Medicine and Pharmacy; Laboratory of Medical Pharmacology, Faculty of Medicine, Clermont University, Clermont-Ferrand, France*

Serge Marchand, PhD *Department of Neurosurgery, Faculty of Medicine, University of Sherbrooke, Sherbrooke, Quebec, Canada*

Juan Carlos Marvizon, PhD *Hatos Center for Neuropharmacology and Department of Medicine, UCLA, Los Angeles, California, USA*

John S. McDonald, MD *Departments of Anesthesiology and Obstetrics and Gynecology, David Geffen School of Medicine, University of California at Los Angeles, Los Angeles, California, USA*

Patricia A. McGrath, PhD *Department of Psychology, York University; Department of Anaesthesia and Pain Medicine, Hospital for Sick Children; Department of Anesthesia, University of Toronto, Toronto, Ontario, Canada*

Stephen B. McMahon, PhD *London Pain Consortium, Wolfson CARD, King's College London, Guy's Campus, London SE1 1UL*

Benoît Michot, PhD *Faculty of Medicine, Pierre et Marie Curie-Paris University, INSERM/CPN U894, Paris, France*

Jeffrey S. Mogil, PhD *Department of Psychology and Alan Edwards Centre for Research on Pain, McGill University, Montreal, Quebec, Canada*

Seog Bae Oh, DDS, PhD *National Research Laboratory for Pain, Dental Research Institute, and Department of Physiology, School of Dentistry, Seoul National University, Seoul, Korea*

J. Manuel Ortega-Legaspi, MD *Ramón de la Fuente National Institute of Psychiatry, Neuroscience Division, Mexico City, Mexico*

Francisco Pellicer, MD, PhD *Ramón de la Fuente National Institute of Psychiatry, Neuroscience Division, Mexico City, Mexico*

Martin N. Perkins, PhD *AstraZeneca R&D, Montreal, Quebec, Canada*

Gisèle Pickering, MD, PhD *Clinical Pharmacology Department, University Hospital, Clermont Ferrand, France*

Léon Plaghki, MD, PhD *Physical Medicine Service, Catholic University of Louvain, Brussels, Belgium*

Wiliam A. Prado, PhD *Department of Pharmacology, Faculty of Medicine of Ribeirão Preto, University of São Paulo, Ribeirão Preto, Brazil*

Pierre Rainville, PhD *Faculty of Dentistry, University of Montreal, Montreal, Quebec, Canada*

Ke Ren, MD, PhD *Department of Neural and Pain Sciences, Dental School, and Program in Neuroscience, University of Maryland, Baltimore, Maryland, USA*

Jana Sawynok, PhD *Department of Pharmacology, Dalhousie University, Halifax, Nova Scotia, Canada*

Frédérique Servin, MD *Department of Anesthesiology, Bichat Hospital, Paris, France*

Guy Simonnet, PhD *University Victor Segalen, Bordeaux, France*

Claudia Sommer, MD *Department of Neurology, University of Würzburg, Würzburg, Germany*

Amelia A. Staniland, PhD *Wolfson Centre for Age-Related Diseases, King's College, London, United Kingdom*

Anna Taddio, PhD *Leslie Dan Faculty of Pharmacy, University of Toronto, Toronto, Ontario, Canada*

Pascale Vergne-Salle, MD, PhD *Department of Rheumatology and Pain Medicine, Dupuytren University Hospital Center, Limoges, France*

Florent Viguier, PhD *Faculty of Medicine, Pierre et Marie Curie-Paris University, INSERM/CPN U894, Paris, France*

Jean-Sébastien Walczak, PhD *Anesthesia Research Unit, Faculty of Medicine, Faculty of Dentistry, and Alan Edwards Center for Research on Pain, McGill University, Montreal, Quebec, Canada*

Wendy Walwyn, PhD *Hatos Center for Neuropharmacology and Department of Psychiatry and Biobehavioral Sciences, UCLA, Los Angeles, California, USA*

Stephen G. Waxman, MD, PhD *Department of Neurology and Center for Neuroscience and Regeneration Research, Yale University School of Medicine, New Haven, Connecticut, USA; Rehabilitation Research Center, VA Connecticut Healthcare System, West Haven, Connecticut, USA*

Fletcher White, PhD *Departments of Cell Biology, Neurobiology and Anatomy, and Anesthesiology, Loyola University, Chicago, Illinois, USA*

Preface

From the use of opium poppy extracts by the Egyptians millennia ago to the development of novel analgesics, our knowledge of the pharmacology of pain has evolved considerably. Most of this improved knowledge has occurred in the past few decades. Previously, analgesics were still mainly derived from extracts of the willow and the poppy. Improved understanding of the mechanisms of pain at cellular, molecular, and synaptic levels has allowed the development of analgesics acting on new targets, providing new hope for better pain management and improved quality of life in millions of patients worldwide.

This rapid evolution of knowledge was the inspiration for this book. The most recent book on the topic was edited by Dickenson, Besson, and Appleton in 1997. This older book did not even mention some of the mechanisms of pain and analgesia to which entire chapters of *Pharmacology of Pain* are devoted. In fact, the vast majority of studies cited as references in our book were published in the past 10 years. These studies include breakthrough work on the role played by glia in the pathophysiology of pain, the modulation of pain signals by descending facilitation and inhibition, and the importance of the transient receptor potential family of receptors, the cannabinoid system, neuropeptides, and cytokines. Our understanding of placebo analgesia has also evolved tremendously; what was recently often still interpreted as a sign of malingering is now known to be mediated by several neurochemical and neurophysiological mechanisms. New classes of analgesics have also been developed since 1997. Apart from tricyclic antidepressants, none of the analgesics recommended as first-line therapy for neuropathic pain (gabapentinoids, duloxetine, and topical lidocaine) were available at that time. We therefore felt that a new book was badly needed to fill a gap in the literature—a book that would offer a comprehensive review of the pharmacology of pain that would be useful for basic scientists, clinical researchers, clinicians, and other health professionals.

Each chapter provides a detailed review of the current state of knowledge on a specific topic and offers a framework for considering future developments on that topic. Chapter 2 presented a particular challenge, but we felt it was a very important chapter to include because it provides a conceptual framework for the rest of the book in offering a taxonomy of analgesic drugs. In addition to several chapters on diverse mechanisms of pain transmission and analgesic targets, we thought it important to include a section on clinical pharmacology of pain, guiding clinicians on the pharmacological management of pain in different patient populations.

In preparing this book, we faced two main challenges. The first was to cover a very broad area but still provide detailed information on each topic without exceeding a reasonable number of pages. The second challenge we encountered was to provide reviews that would still be timely after the book was published, given the rapid evolution of knowledge in this field. We are confident that we have succeeded in meeting both challenges, mainly because all chapters were authored by leading experts on the topic covered. We are very fortunate that we were able to include so many world-renowned experts on the pharmacology of pain in a single book. We therefore extend our gratitude to all those who agreed to take up the challenge of providing this state-of-the-art review of such rapidly evolving fields. Our gratitude also goes to Elizabeth Endres and all the IASP Press staff, for their help and copy editing of all the manuscripts, several written by authors for whom English is not their first language. Finally, we would like to thank Dr. Catherine Bushnell, Editor-in-Chief of IASP Press, for her guidance throughout the process.

Pierre Beaulieu, MD, PhD
David Lussier, MD, FRCP(C)
Frank Porreca, PhD
Anthony H. Dickenson, PhD, FMedSci

Part I

Background

1

Applied Pain Neurophysiology

Serge Marchand

Department of Neurosurgery, Faculty of Medicine, University of Sherbrooke, Sherbrooke, Quebec, Canada

Pain is a dynamic phenomenon. Nociceptive signals are modulated at all levels of the peripheral and central nervous systems. Current scientific concepts regarding pain mechanisms take into account genetic and environmental factors, which will influence the development of persistent pain. Moreover, the maintenance of chronic pain is not only the result of continued and increased nociceptive activity, mostly arising at the peripheral site of pathology, but also depends on additional changes within the central nervous system (CNS), such as an increase of excitatory or reduction of inhibitory endogenous pain modulation mechanisms. This plasticity speaks to the nervous system's ability to adapt and change.

Multiple endogenous excitatory and inhibitory mechanisms have been identified [58]. This chapter will introduce the scientific basis for the understanding of pain mechanisms and will highlight the importance of endogenous excitatory and inhibitory controls in the CNS. These innate control systems have an impact on the evolution of chronic pain. They may be manipulated to alter the pain process and therefore have implications regarding treatment. Understanding the neurophysiological mechanisms involved in the development and maintenance of pain will help the clinician to devise a more effective treatment plan guided by pathophysiological dysfunction.

The Somatosensory System

The somatosensory system can be divided into four distinct modalities: touch, proprioception, temperature, and nociception. Each of these modalities has its own receptors, fibers, and pathways. This division was introduced in relation to the specificity theory that was first introduced by Descartes [20] and refined on the basis of modern physiology by

Pharmacology of Pain
edited by Pierre Beaulieu, David Lussier, Frank Porreca, and Anthony H. Dickenson
IASP Press, Seattle, © 2010

Müller [59] and Frey [28], who proposed that the somatosensory system could be divided according to specific receptors for tactile, hot, cold, and pain receptors. Inspired by the Müller and Frey postulates, researchers have established exclusive relationships between the sensory modalities and peripheral afferents, such as the role of Aδ and C fibers and the specialization of the spinothalamic tract with regard to nociceptive afferents.

The physiological basis for the specialization of these afferents and higher centers is that the sensory and affective components of the pain experience are integrated by different structures [10]. Even today, the specificity theory is confirmed by the identification of specific receptors, fibers, pathways, and CNS structures that are responsible for our perception of these somatosensory modalities. However, the pain mechanisms involved in different conditions, such as the increasing perception of pain with repetitive nociceptive stimuli (temporal summation) or with a larger surface area of stimulation (spatial summation), or even in some chronic pain conditions, make it clear that the specificity theory alone cannot explain the complexity of pain.

The pattern theory, introduced by Goldscheider [34], suggested that not only the type of fiber but also the pattern of impulses in the nervous system can modulate pain perception. Based on this theory, it is easier to understand that a thermal stimulus can pass from a warm perception to burning hot if the stimulation persists at the same temperature (temporal summation) or is presented on a larger surface area (spatial summation).

Before becoming a pain perception, the nociceptive signal will go through four distinct processes that can be identified as transduction, transmission, modulation, and perception. Transduction refers to the process by which the energy of the mechanical, thermal, or chemical stimulus is transposed as electrophysiological activity in the primary nociceptive afferents. Transmission refers to the transport of the electrophysiological signal from the periphery to the spinal cord, from the spinal cord to the brainstem and thalamus, and finally to the cortex. Modulation occurs at all the levels of the CNS and will result in an increase or a decrease of neuronal activity. As described in the following sections, both excitatory and inhibitory mechanisms can play a role in chronic pain conditions. Perception is the final process, when the cortical regions responsible for the sensory and affective components of pain process the complex integration of the different aspects implicated in the pain experience.

The evolution from a purely linear concept of the nociceptive pathways to a more circular model where patterns of impulses modulate our perception has played a major role in our growing understanding of the factors implicated in the development and persistence of some pain conditions.

From Nociception to Pain

A good way to understand the physiology of pain is to follow the nociceptive signal pathways from the periphery to the brain, with an emphasis on the integration and modulation of the nociceptive signal at different steps within the CNS (Fig. 1).

Mechanical, chemical, or thermal nociceptive stimulation will recruit peripheral nociceptors that conduct the nociceptive signal in the primary somatosensory neuron to the dorsal horn of the spinal cord. In the dorsal horn, the primary afferent neuron will make a synaptic contact with the secondary or projection neuron. Secondary neurons from the spinothalamic (lateral) and spinoreticular (medial) tracts will immediately cross in the spinal cord and send afferent projections to higher centers. A large proportion of afferents will make a second synapse in the lateral and medial nuclei of the thalamus, which subsequently make synaptic contact with tertiary neurons. It is important to emphasize that the secondary neurons may also synapse with neurons in different nuclei of the brainstem, including the periaqueductal gray (PAG) and the nucleus raphe magnus (NRM), areas involved in descending endogenous pain modulation. Tertiary neurons from the thalamus send afferents to the primary and secondary somatosensory cortices (S1 and

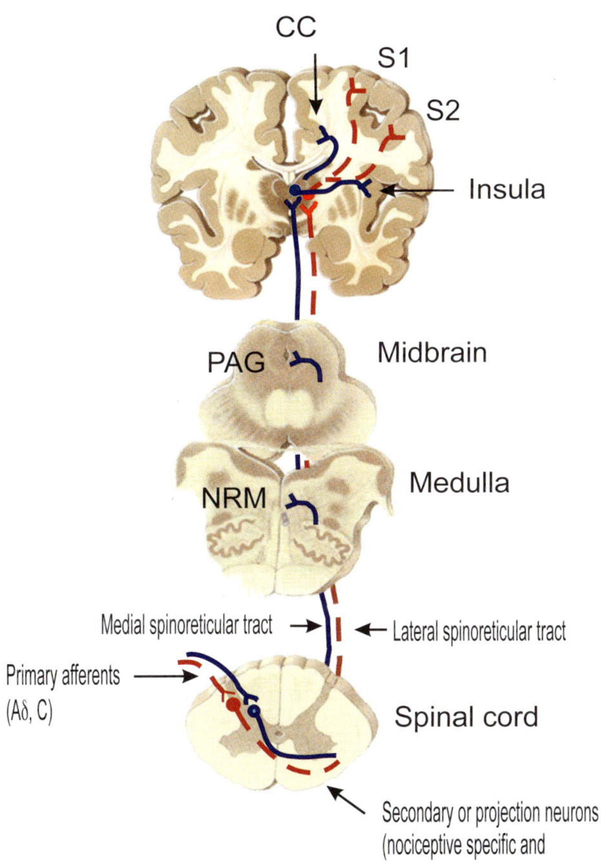

Fig. 1. The nociceptive pathways from the periphery will conduct to the brain after two synaptic relays. The Aδ and C fibers will make their first synapse with the projection neurons in the dorsal horn of the spinal cord. The secondary neurons will decussate immediately in the spinal cord and conduct to the thalamic nuclei where they will make the second synaptic contact. The tertiary neurons will finally project to the somatosensory cortices (S1, S2) for the sensory-discriminative component of pain and to limbic structures—anterior cingulate cortex (ACC) and insula—for the motivational component of pain. PAG = periaqueductal gray; NRM = nucleus raphe magnus.

S2). The S1 and S2 cortices are involved in the sensory quality of pain, which includes its location, duration, and intensity. Tertiary neurons also project to limbic structures, including the anterior cingulate cortex (ACC) and the insula, which are involved in the affective or emotional component of pain. The various synaptic contacts with excitatory and inhibitory neurons at all levels of the CNS are important integration regions that are the target of most pharmacological approaches.

The Periphery: Nociceptors

An injury that causes a potential risk to the organism will activate free nerve endings that respond to nociceptive stimulation. Most of these nociceptors are polymodal and will respond to different modalities including mechanical, thermal, and chemical stimuli [57]. The nociceptors are responsible for the transduction and transmission of the nociceptive signal. However, there is no nociceptive receptor per se, only unmyelinated free nerve endings in the skin, muscle, articulation, fascia, and viscera. To be characterized as a nociceptor, two conditions are needed: (1) a response proportional to the intensity of the stimulation and (2) a higher threshold than that of the innocuous thermal and mechanical receptors [57].

A nociceptive stimulus will initiate a cascade of events. Pronociceptive inflammatory molecules will be released into the periphery and will produce peripheral hyperalgesia. These molecules originate from various blood cells (mastocytes, polymorphonuclear cells, and platelets), which produce bradykinins, prostaglandins, histamine, serotonin, and adenosine triphosphate, and also from immune cells, which produce interleukins, interferons, and tumor necrosis factors [9,54]. Substance P and calcitonin gene-related peptide (CGRP), which act as neurotransmitters in the CNS, are also released into the periphery, where they act as proinflammatory factors, favoring neurogenic inflammation [54]. There is also a class of silent nociceptors that will only be activated when sensitized in an inflammatory environment. The inflammatory activation of the C fibers containing silent nociceptors may contribute to spatial summation at central synapses and hence to hyperalgesia [75]. Recordings from the peripheral nociceptors in humans using microneurography have established a good correlation between the frequency of discharge of the nociceptors and the perceived intensity of pain [85].

Primary Hyperalgesia: Hyperactivity of Peripheral Nociceptors

Injured tissues will release various pronociceptive substances, such as potassium, prostaglandins, histamine, and bradykinins, and will also invoke an immune response. These inflammatory and immune factors will sensitize the nociceptive receptors directly within the lesion and in the surrounding neurons [9]. Primary hyperalgesia that follows the release of these factors may be measured as a lowered pain threshold in and around the lesion. Several mechanisms are implicated in primary hyperalgesia, including the sensitization of the nociceptors, the expansion of the receptive field, and the loss of central inhibition in the primary zone [57].

Sensory Afferents from the Periphery to the Spinal Cord

Afferent fibers originating in the periphery fall into three groups, namely Aβ, Aδ, and C fibers. The Aβ fibers are large myelinated fibers that conduct at high speed and usually transmit non-nociceptive signals (Fig. 2). They do, however, also participate in pain modulation, as will be explained below. Two other classes of fibers, the myelinated Aδ fibers and the thin unmyelinated C fibers, mainly transmit nociceptive messages.

Myelination and increasing size of a nerve fiber facilitate the speed of conduction of the stimulus. The Aδ fibers conduct the signal relatively rapidly from the periphery to the spinal cord. Because of this rapid conduction velocity, they are responsible for the sharp localization of pain and for the rapid spinal response, which can be measured in the laboratory as the nociceptive reflex. In contrast, the C fibers, with their slow conducting velocity, will mediate a dull, aching pain, known as "second pain." Let us examine the characteristics of these fibers in more detail.

Aβ Fibers

The Aβ fibers are principally involved in the conduction of non-nociceptive input such as vibration, movement, or light touch. They are large, myelinated fibers with a rapid conduction velocity (35 to 75 m/s). The stimulation of Aβ fibers will also recruit inhibitory interneurons in the substantia gelatinosa of the dorsal horn of the spinal cord, which will inhibit nociceptive input at the same spinal segment. This mechanism is one of the

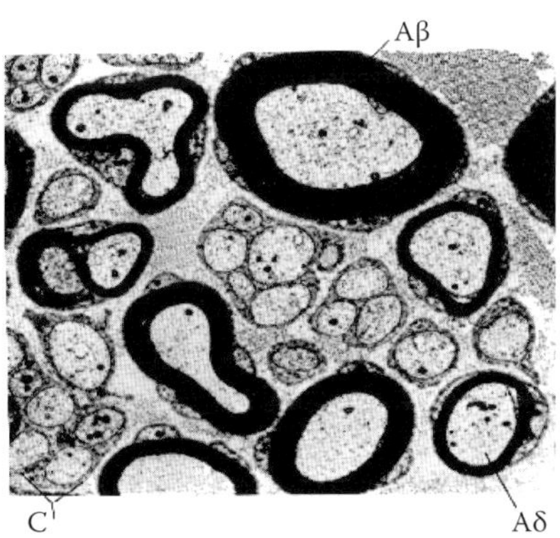

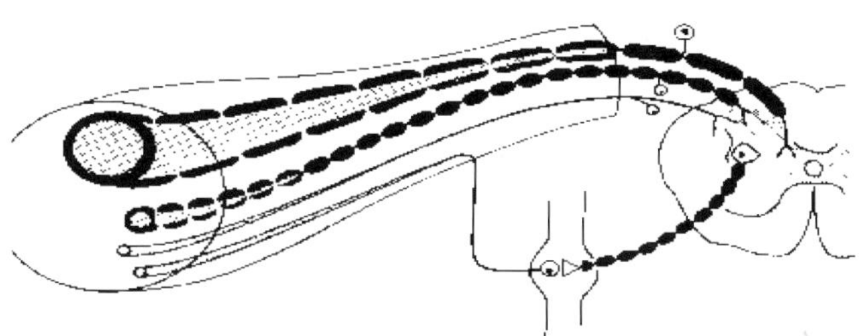

	Aβ	Aδ	C
Diameter	6 to 12 μm Myelinated	1 to 5 μm Myelinated	0.2 to 1.5 μm Unmyelinated
Conduction	35 to 75 m/s	5 to 30 m/s	0.5 to 2 m/s
Role	Light touch, proprioception	Temperature, nociception (mechanical, thermal)	Nociception (mechanical, thermal, and chemical)

Fig. 2. The nociceptive afferent fibers can be separated according to their physical characteristics and conduction velocity. On this nerve section, where the myelin has been stained in black, we can see the large myelinated Aβ fibers, the smaller and myelinated Aδ fibers, and the unmyelinated C fibers. As we can see in the table, conduction velocity will increase with the diameter and thickness of the myelin sheath.

fundamental components of the gate control theory, whereby an innocuous stimulus will reduce nociceptive input from the same region [56]. Besides playing a dynamic inhibitory role when recruited, the Aβ fibers seem also to play a tonic inhibitory role in nociceptive input. Blocking the input from these large fibers will result in an increased response to nociceptive stimuli [64].

Aδ Fibers

The Aδ fibers are relatively large myelinated fibers that conduct more slowly than the Aβ fibers, but faster (5 to 30 m/s) than the C fibers. They represent the majority of the myelinated fibers. Two types of Aδ fibers exist, categorized according to the specificity of their responses to different stimulation [9]: (1) the mechanonociceptors respond preferentially to intense and potentially harmful mechanical stimulation; and (2) the polymodal Aδ fibers respond to mechanical, thermal, and chemical stimulation. However, mechanonociceptors will also increase their discharge after intense thermal stimulation, which is one of the mechanisms of hyperalgesia. Because of their rapid conduction velocity, the Aδ fibers are responsible for the sensation of "first pain," a rapid, pinprick-like, sharp, and transient sensation.

C Fibers

Because of their small caliber and lack of myelin, the C fibers conduct relatively slowly (0.5 to 2 m/s). They represent three-quarters of the sensory afferent input and are mostly recruited by nociceptive stimulation. Because of their slow conduction velocity, they are responsible for second pain, a dull, diffuse sensation. However, they are also involved in non-nociceptive somatosensory information such as the sensation of itch (pruritus) [78], and paradoxically, in the perception of pleasant touch, as documented in a patient with a rare disease linked to a deafferentation of the myelinated sensory fibers [60].

First and Second Pain

The differences in conduction velocity between the Aδ and C fibers can be appreciated by isolating the sensations of first and second pain (Fig. 3). Following brief nociceptive stimulation, the Aδ fibers will rapidly transmit a brief and acute pinprick-like sensation perceived to be precisely located at the point of stimulation. It is this precision and fast conduction that will result in the nociceptive withdrawal reflex. Following this activity, C fibers will transmit their information, with a relatively long delay (100 milliseconds to 1 second depending on the stimulus location). This second sensory input results in a deep, more diffuse pain sensation.

It is possible to isolate first and second pain in the laboratory. Using a blood pressure cuff, we can temporarily block trophic factors present in the blood from reaching the nerves, resulting in a reduction of nerve conduction. The first fibers that will show reduced activity are those with the largest diameter, including the Aδ fibers. This experimental model allows the activity of C fibers to be isolated and independently studied. Following this procedure, a nociceptive stimulus—whether hot, cold, or mechanical—will be perceived with a certain delay as a deeper pain sensation.

The application of capsaicin, a hot pepper extract, will produce a burning sensation due to the activation of the vanilloid receptors on the C fibers. However, at higher doses, C fibers will be blocked as a result of a specific action on ionic calcium channels, with resulting isolation of the Aδ fibers at the skin surface. This time, the same nociceptive sensation will be perceived as a sharp pinprick-like sensation without the second burning pain sensation.

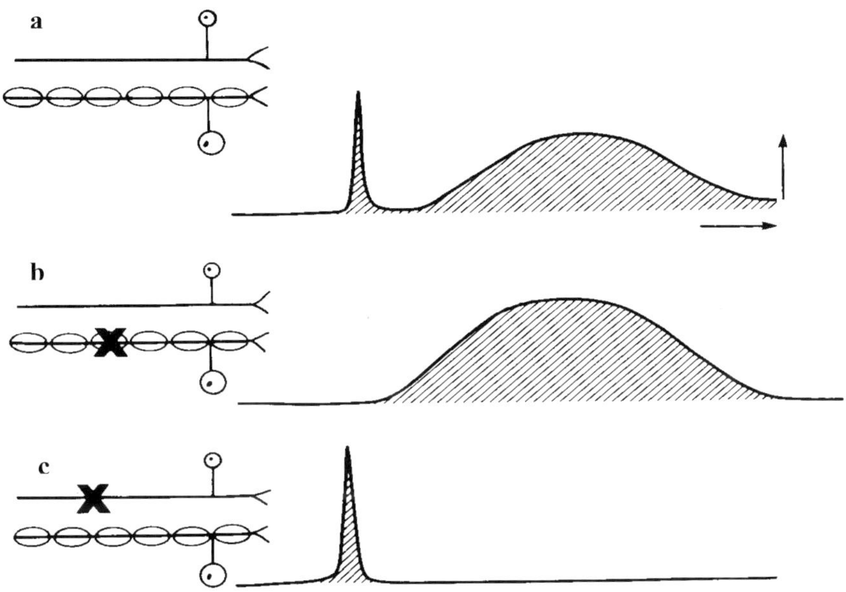

Fig. 3. Because of the differences in conduction velocity between the relatively rapid Aδ and slow C fibers, nociceptive stimulation will induce a first pain having the characteristics of a localized and sharp pinprick sensation related to the fast action of the Aδ fibers, and a second slower and more diffuse burning perception related to the slower activity of the C fibers (a). Using a blood pressure cuff, we can temporarily block the activity of the fibers with the largest diameter, including the Aδ fibers (b). This process allows the activity of C fibers to be isolated and independently studied. A nociceptive stimulus will only be conducted by the C fibers and will be perceived as a diffuse burning sensation independently of the stimulation type (b). If we block the activity of the small C fibers by using capsaicin, only the sharp pinprick perception will persist (c).

Visceral Nociceptors

As for the somatosensory system, the visceral nociceptors play a protective role, informing the CNS of a potential danger and thus prompting an adaptive response. Even if our visceral system did not have nociceptive reflexes comparable to the rapid withdrawal of a limb from a noxious event, different responses such as vomiting or avoidance could be regarded as the protective reflexes that accompany visceral pain.

It is not clear if visceral nociceptive information is relayed from specific nociceptors or if nociception depends on the activity of receptors that normally respond to innocuous stimuli. However, Aδ and C fibers have been identified in the heart, pleura, abdominal cavity, gallbladder, and testicles, and they play a role in nociceptive signaling [11]. Non-neuronal epithelial and visceral elements act as nociceptive messengers [12]. For example, they are responsible for the gradual sensation of fullness changing to a painful sensation when the bladder becomes overly full.

The visceral system is a very sophisticated sensory system that comprises the concomitant activity of two extrinsic innervations, vagal and spinal, as well as numerous intrinsic neurons [41]. For example, the intestinal tract has a neuronal system known as the brain-gut axis that operates independently but also interacts with the rest of the CNS. Several visceral pain syndromes, such as irritable bowel syndrome, present no clear lesion or dysregulation of the painful organ. Better knowledge of the brain-gut axis, which seems to play an important role in these syndromes, may help us to understand the interaction between external events such as a stressful situation and an effect on the painful symptoms [39].

As is the case for somatic pain, chronic visceral pain is related to both peripheral and central sensitization. Excitatory and inhibitory descending spinal pathways are also implicated in the visceral system, suggesting an important central influence on visceral sensitivity. Accordingly, some types of chronic visceral pain present the characteristics of neuropathic pain. Finally, the autonomic nervous system's influence on visceral sensitivity may help explain the role of emotions on the modulation of visceral pain [41].

Another particularity of visceral pain is its referred presentation to the somatosensory system. A classical example is myocardial infarction, which will produce a dull pain in the left arm. Frequently, visceral pain will be located far from the sick organ, which may lead to a wrong diagnosis [6,69]. A kidney problem could in some cases mimic classical low back pain. Therefore, it is important to consider a possible visceral problem, even when the clinical signs indicate a somatosensory problem.

Somatovisceral and Viscerosomatic Reflexes

Another important aspect to consider is the interactions, direct or indirect, between the visceral and somatosensory systems. For example, we know that a somatic pain, such as catching one's finger in the car door, would produce visceral reactions such as heart acceleration and even nausea. These somatovisceral [74] and viscerosomatic [5] reflexes can have important clinical effects. The treatment of pain associated with irritable bowel syndrome reduces both visceral pain and pain radiating to the legs [89]. The reverse effect can also occur—reduction of visceral pain with a somatic treatment. Menstrual pain (dysmenorrhea) or esophageal pain can be treated with transcutaneous electrical nerve stimulation (TENS), suggesting that the somatic stimulation has a somatovisceral reflex effect on the visceral pain [13,51]. Understanding the interaction between the somatic and visceral systems is important for a better appreciation of various pain conditions and their treatments.

Secondary Neurons in the Spinal Cord

When recruited, the Aδ and C fibers transport their signal to the spinal cord, where they have their first synaptic contact with secondary neurons that are principally located in the superficial zones of the dorsal horn (laminae I, II) and lamina V [84]. Both nociceptive and non-nociceptive afferents to the spinal cord will also make synaptic contact with an important network of inhibitory and excitatory interneurons that modulate the nociceptive signal before the secondary neuron projects to higher centers. We can divide the secondary neurons into two classes: nociceptive-specific neurons and wide-dynamic-range (WDR) neurons [57,83].

Nociceptive-Specific Neurons

As indicated by their name, nociceptive-specific neurons respond only to nociceptive stimulation. They can be divided in two subclasses depending on whether they are recruited by Aδ fibers or by a combination of Aδ and C fibers.

Wide-Dynamic-Range Neurons

WDR neurons respond gradually to stimuli ranging from innocuous to nociceptive. Their capacity to respond to both innocuous and nociceptive stimuli is related to the fact that they receive input from Aδ and C fibers, and also from Aβ fibers. The receptive field of WDR neurons is dynamic, as the name implies, and changes in conditions of persistent pain. Animal studies have shown that inflammatory pain will have multiple effects on the function of WDR neurons. Changes in their receptive fields, in the permeability of their membrane to ion exchange, and in their discharge frequency all suggest that these neurons play a substantial role in the chronicity of pain [45].

Excitatory Mechanisms

Secondary Hyperalgesia

Secondary hyperalgesia is a phenomenon that refers to sensitization that occurs within the CNS [83]. Repeated recruitment of C fibers after an injury will produce central sensitization by changing the response properties of the membrane of secondary neurons (Fig. 4). This change will result in an increase in firing rate, a phenomenon known as wind-up [101]. The high-frequency recruitment of C fibers, either by increased repetitive stimuli or by tonic stimulation [35], will then induce an increase in perceived pain, even if the intensity of the stimulation remains constant (Fig. 4a,b). This central sensitization at the spinal level sometimes lasts for only a few minutes, but it can also persist for hours and even days [99]. The prolonged activation of *N*-methyl-D-aspartate (NMDA) receptors will induce the transcription of rapidly expressed genes (*c-fos, c-jun*), resulting in sensitization of nociceptors. This neuronal plasticity of the secondary neuron will result in the reduced recruitment threshold or the spontaneous activity of these neurons in the spinal cord and can produce hyperalgesic and allodynic responses that may persist even after the healing of the injury. To address the impact of sensitization, an aggressive and early treatment plan to reduce pain will help in preventing ongoing chronic pain.

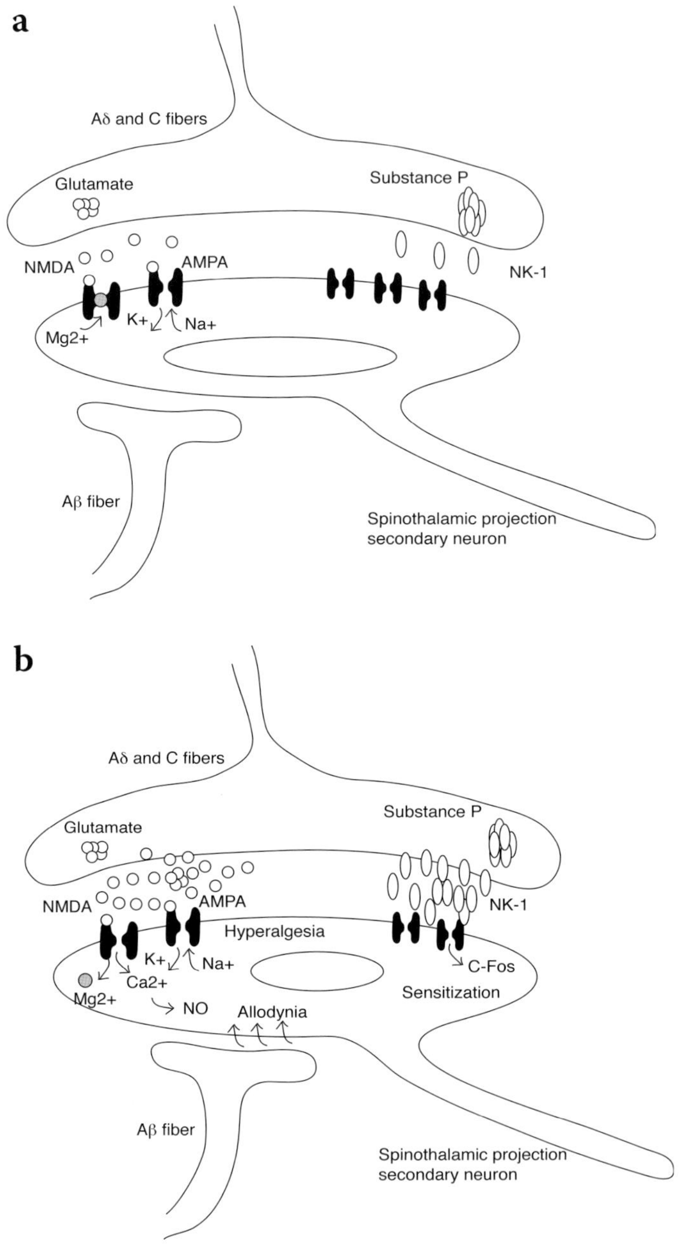

Fig. 4. Central sensitization occurs when the secondary neurons of the spinal cord change their discharge frequency following a sustained recruitment from the primary nociceptive afferents. (a) In this schematic representation, we can see that an acute discharge from the nociceptive primary afferents (C fibers) will induce the release of peptides (substance P, calcitonin gene-related peptide [CGRP]), and glutamate, which in turn will recruit the neurokinin-1 (NK1) and AMPA receptors. (b) A sustained discharge will recruit the NMDA receptors and produce a sensitization of the secondary neurons that will now discharge at a higher frequency when recruited by nociceptive (hyperalgesia) and non-nociceptive stimulation (allodynia). This phenomenon is generally transitory but may persist over a long time and participate in pain chronicity.

Temporal Summation

The temporal summation paradigm is a good illustration of the importance of signal conduction in Aδ and C fibers [66]. In this paradigm, pain perception is compared with repeated stimulations at the same intensity but at different rates. The rationale is that a high frequency of stimulation will produce a temporal summation of C-fiber activity, as a result of the relatively slow conduction of these fibers. This temporal summation increases the perceived intensity of the second pain, related to C-fiber activity, without changing the perception of the first pain, subserved by Aδ fibers [90]. The accumulation of nociceptive activity will produce a transient change in the excitability of the spinal cord second neuron, or wind-up, that may lead to central sensitization. Wind-up, a transient effect related to the frequency of discharge from the primary neuron, is different from central sensitization, however [99].

Central sensitization refers to a phenomenon in which the membrane permeability of the second neuron changes and responds at higher frequency when recruited by nociceptive (hyperalgesia) and non-nociceptive primary input (allodynia). Central sensitization is defined as an increase in excitability and spontaneous discharge at the dorsal horn neurons, along with an associated increase in the receptive field for these neurons. This phenomenon will principally affect the WDR neurons from the dorsal horn and is dependent on the activity of the NMDA receptors [24,102]. Central sensitization may persist for prolonged periods after termination of stimulation and has an important effect on the persistence of pain.

Spatial Summation

Another important phenomenon in the CNS is spatial summation. The stimulation of a large territory will recruit more nociceptors than when a smaller area is stimulated and will result in more intense pain perception. However, increasing the surface area that is stimulated recruits both excitatory and inhibitory mechanisms and may cause paradoxical responses in some situations in which the stimulation of a larger territory will trigger more inhibition, resulting in a reduction of pain perception [53].

Clinical Implications of Temporal and Spatial Summation

It is possible to study the relative role of dysfunction in endogenous pain excitatory and inhibitory mechanisms in certain chronic pain conditions using tests of temporal [80] and spatial summation [40]. We have examined the spatial summation paradigm in patients with fibromyalgia, and observed no differences in pain perception between the increasing and decreasing nociceptive area, suggesting a deficit of endogenous pain modulation. Interestingly, this deficit was not present in patients with low back pain, suggesting that the deficit in endogenous pain modulation is not present in all chronic pain conditions [40]. A chronic pain condition may therefore be related to either hyperactivity of nociceptive activity or conversely to hypoactivity of endogenous pain inhibitory mechanisms at different levels of the CNS. Exploring the role of dysfunction of excitatory and inhibitory mechanisms in different patient populations will help to better characterize the underlying deficit and optimize treatment choices.

Loss of Inhibition in the Spinal Cord: Clinical Implications

It is important to keep in mind the importance of the inhibitory interneurons in the spinal cord that will reduce nociceptive activity pre- and postsynaptically. Various neurotransmitters are implicated, such as glycine, adenosine, and enkephalin, but it is γ-aminobutyric acid (GABA) that plays the most prominent role in reducing the nociceptive signal. Peripheral nerve injury would reduce inhibitory GABAergic current due to the loss of GABAergic neurons, which may play a role in disinhibition in neurogenic pain [101]. Moreover, GABA is a powerful inhibitory neurotransmitter that will, under normal conditions, hyperpolarize the postsynaptic neuron. However, after nerve injury, an increase in cholecystokinin (CCK), the transporter of K^+ and Cl^-, which is normally found at low levels in the intact animal, will change the membrane properties to a point where GABA release would produce a depolarization of the neuron, changing from inhibitory to excitatory [15].

Another example of the importance of understanding the dynamic mechanisms of the interaction between excitatory and inhibitory neurotransmitters is opioid hyperalgesia. Opioids are the gold standard of analgesics. However, in some conditions, opioids may produce hyperalgesia. Several mechanisms have been proposed to explain this paradoxical response, including the sensitization of pronociceptive receptors by the activation of NMDA and CCK receptors and the blockade of endogenous inhibitory mechanisms [52,103]. From a pharmacological point of view, these proposed mechanisms shed some light on strange clinical observations, such as pain augmentation following the use of a strong opioid analgesic (see Chapter 18 by Simonnet et al.).

The Role of Glial Cells

During the last century, all efforts to understand the CNS mechanisms implicated in pain were focused on neurons. We are just beginning to realize that glial cells not only support and protect the neurons, but also play a major active role in several CNS processes, including pain transmission [19]. The role of astrocytes [38] and microglia [81] has been well documented in the development and persistence of pain, especially in models of neuropathic pain. In normal conditions, glial cells seem to play a limited role in pain, with few or no effects on pain threshold [81]. However, after an injury, microglia become reactive. Activation of microglia in the dorsal horn is concomitant with the development of neuropathic pain [87]. Microglia release several factors that are pronociceptive and are mediated through a complex signaling system involving cytokines [101]. Interestingly, there are several microglia-targeting drugs that can be developed based on the results from animal research [81,93,101]. Thus, we can no longer focus on the neurophysiology of pain without taking into account the major role of the glial cells and their potential roles in the development and treatment of pain.

Pain Pathways from the Spine to the Superior Centers

Secondary neurons travel to superior centers by two main pathways—the spinothalamic tract, which sends afferents to the lateral nuclei of the thalamus; and the spinoreticular tract, with afferents to the medial thalamus and nuclei of the brainstem, including the NRM and the PAG, two nuclei involved in descending pain modulation [26]. However, the medial dorsal cord lemniscal pathway, mostly associated with non-nociceptive afferents, also conducts nociceptive afferent signals from the viscera [61,62].

Sensory Spinothalamic Tract

The spinothalamic tract comprises the lateral part of sensory input and projects directly to the lateral nuclei of the ventrobasal thalamus (the ventral posterior lateral [VPL] and ventral posterior median [VPM] nuclei). The projection neurons from the spinothalamic tract originate primarily from laminae I and IV–VI of the spinal cord [97] and project to the contralateral nuclei of the thalamus.

Fibers of the spinothalamic tract conduct rapidly, and projection neurons have relatively small receptive fields, directed toward regions of the thalamus and somatosensory cortex that have a defined somatotopic representation. The spinothalamic tract has all the characteristics of a sensory pathway transmitting nociceptive afferent signals [96].

Affective Spinoreticular Tract

Most afferents from the spinoreticular tract are from deep laminae VII and VIII of the spinal cord and project to the medial nuclei of the thalamus as well as to structures of the brainstem involved in pain modulation, including the PAG and NRM [96]. Unlike the spinothalamic tract, the spinoreticular tract projects to neurons that have large receptive fields that may cover wide areas of the body, and it plays a role in pain memory and in the affective component of pain [96].

Thalamic Organization

Secondary neurons from the spinal cord send their afferent fibers to the thalamic nuclei. The thalamic nociceptive neurons are localized in two groups of nuclei: the ventrobasal (VPL and VPM) and centromedian nuclei. The ventrobasal complex principally receives the afferents from the spinothalamic tract and projects their tertiary neurons to the primary and secondary somatosensory cortices (S1, S2). The centromedian neurons, receiving most of their afferents from the spinoreticular tract, project to structures of the limbic system. This simplified description of the thalamus projections suggests that the sensory and motivational components of pain are organized early in the CNS.

Moreover, the thalamus also plays a role in certain chronic pain conditions. Upon stimulation of specific nuclei of the thalamus, patients have experienced memory recall of the sensory and affective components of a previous pain that had long since disappeared. This phenomenon suggests that some thalamic neurons may conserve a past painful experience that can be masked by a circuitry of inhibitory interneurons [48]. It is therefore plausible that a localized stroke in the thalamus may destroy tonic inhibitory circuitry and unmask nociceptive activity, leading to the well-recognized thalamic pain syndrome.

The Brain and Pain

Pain can only be experienced when nociceptive afferents reach the cortex. It is for this reason that the term "nociception" is used to describe the signal following a lesion, whereas "pain" is a complex perception requiring activity in higher centers.

A complex network of cortical structures is activated during pain perception. Similar to the thalamic nuclei, the cortex can be represented in a simplified way by subdivision into structures involved in either the sensory or the affective components of pain. Brain imaging has demonstrated four cortical structures important for the perception of pain [14,82]: the primary somatosensory cortex (S1) in the postcentral circumvolution of the parietal lobe, the secondary somatosensory cortex (S2) in the parietal operculum, the ACC above the corpus callosum circumvolution, and the insular cortex (IC) under the temporal and frontal lobes at the level of the Sylvian fissure. The first two structures (S1 and S2) are mainly involved in the sensory-discriminative aspect of pain, whereas the ACC and IC are associated with the affective component.

The prefrontal cortex plays a major role in pain perception and pain modulation. One important aspect related to the prefrontal cortex is the perception of control over a painful event. In an experimental setup, controllable pain is characterized by an increased activity in the right part of the ventrolateral prefrontal cortex (VLPFC) [95]. The VLPFC plays an active role in pain modulation, because increased activity in this region is negatively correlated with perceived pain intensity. Interestingly, this inhibitory mechanism seems to be related to a cortical modulation implicated in reducing attention to pain [50]. Patients with chronic pain show a decrease of gray matter density in the VLPFC, suggesting impairment of an endogenous pain inhibition mechanism in the prefrontal cortex [3].

Most brain imaging studies report an activation of the sensory and affective brain structures following a nociceptive stimulus, demonstrating that pain perception is a complex experience with emotions, cognitive factors, and previous experience playing an important role. It can therefore be understood why the clinician should address both the physical and emotional aspects of pain.

Endogenous Pain Modulation Mechanisms

Because pain is a dynamic phenomenon, the nociceptive signal will be modulated at multiple levels of the CNS before pain is fully perceived. Because of the dynamic and plastic characteristics of the nervous system, pain perception, especially in a chronic pain condition, will change over time, depending on different factors. Pain perception is the final outcome of complex mechanisms that modulate the nociceptive afferent signal. As described above, the modulation of the nociceptive signal starts at the periphery and involves several

CNS structures including excitatory and inhibitory mechanisms from the brainstem, the autonomic nervous system, and the cortical structures responsible for the emotional and cognitive aspects of pain perception [36].

Based on knowledge of the neurophysiology of pain, we can conclude that the development and maintenance of chronic pain depend on several factors. Persistent pain can arise from the activity of nociceptive afferents, but it can also be related to a reduction of endogenous inhibition or an augmentation of endogenous excitatory mechanisms. The literature on central sensitization supports the importance of endogenous pain excitatory circuitry in the development and maintenance of pain. The excitatory and inhibitory roles played by different structures of the brainstem have been well documented [26].

Endogenous Excitatory Mechanisms

Primary afferents are normally activated by nociceptive stimuli that can potentially induce an injury and by pronociceptive activation triggered by the inflammatory response.

Spinal Excitatory Mechanisms

As previously described, excitatory mechanisms can induce central sensitization at the spinal level, defined as an increase in the excitability and spontaneous discharge of the nociceptive spinal neurons, an augmentation of the receptive field, and an accentuated response of spinal neurons to nociceptive input (hyperalgesia) and non-nociceptive input (allodynia). Central sensitization depends on the activation of the NMDA receptors of the spinal neurons, which are activated by a sustained release of glutamate [24,98,100]. The neurophysiological and neurochemical mechanisms involved in central sensitization are responsible for modification of the spinal nociceptive circuitry and contribute to the maintenance of pain (Fig. 4a,b).

Descending Excitatory Mechanisms

It is now well documented that several supraspinal excitatory and inhibitory mechanisms play a major role in pain perception and most probably in certain chronic pain conditions [1]. The work of Fields describing activation of "ON" cells and inhibition of "OFF" cells in the brainstem during nociceptive activity has demonstrated the importance of excitatory mechanisms in amplifying the nociceptive response [27].

Recent studies have also demonstrated that certain physiological conditions, such as nociceptive hyperactivity, may change the usual neuronal response to specific neurotransmitters. A particular example is the hyperalgesic effect, mentioned above, that can be observed in some patients using opioid medications, mostly at higher doses [76]. Therefore, drugs with opioid activity may under certain circumstances produce a completely opposite effect and enhance pain by producing a hyperalgesic response [18,76]. The same is also true for GABA, which has been clearly identified as an inhibitory neurotransmitter, but in certain conditions may cause hyperpolarization of neurons, as described above [15]. These observations support the concept of pain as a dynamic phenomenon. An understanding of these complex mechanisms can help explain the clinical variability in treatment response in patients with chronic pain.

Endogenous Inhibitory Mechanisms

In order to better understand the role of endogenous pain inhibitory mechanisms in the development and treatment of pain, we should appreciate three levels of modulation in the CNS (Fig. 5): (1) spinal mechanisms producing localized analgesia, (2) descending inhibitory mechanisms from the brainstem producing diffuse inhibition, and (3) superior center effects that will either modulate descending mechanisms or change the perception of pain by reinterpreting the nociceptive signal.

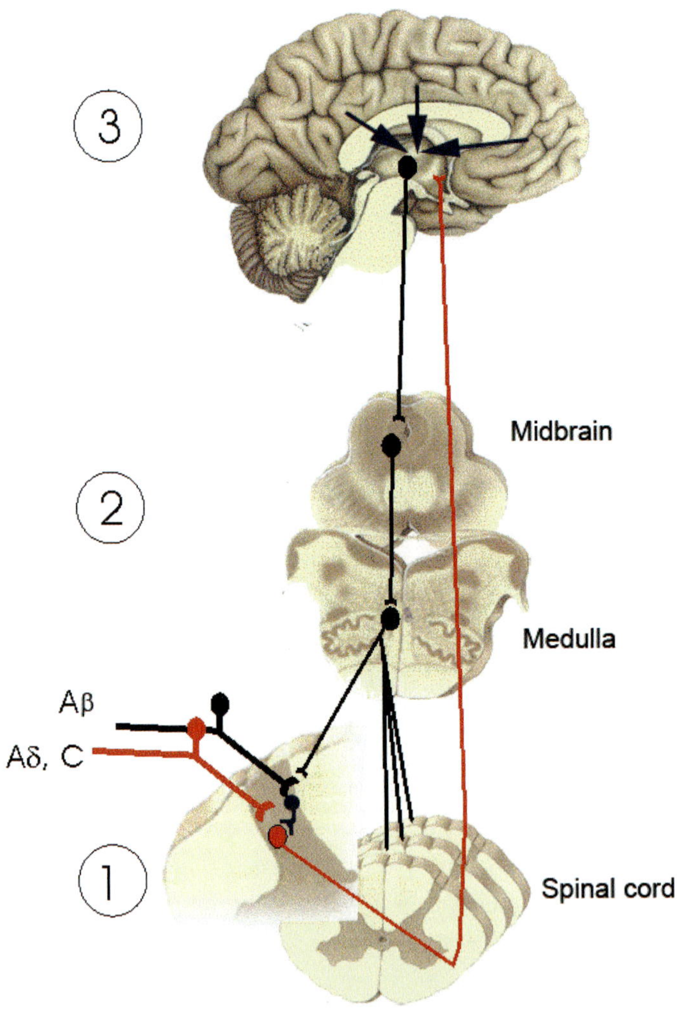

Fig. 5. A schematic representation of the main three levels of endogenous pain modulation: (1) spinal inhibitory mechanisms, (2) inhibitory mechanisms descending from the brainstem, and (3) inhibitory mechanisms descending from higher centers. As described in the text, better understanding of these mechanisms helps in developing a mechanistic approach for the treatment of certain chronic pain conditions that are related to a deficit of these mechanisms.

Spinal Inhibitory Mechanisms

Since the proposal of the gate control theory by Melzack and Wall [56], the modulation of nociceptive afferents at entry into the spinal cord has been well documented. This input may be increased or decreased at the level of the spinal cord. The gate control theory hypothesizes that, among other mechanisms, selective activation of non-nociceptive afferent Aβ fibers will recruit inhibitory interneurons in the substantia gelatinosa of the posterior spinal cord, producing a localized analgesia and decreasing pain perception. In contrast, in certain neuropathic pain conditions, the nociceptive secondary projection neurons will be recruited at high frequency to transmit a pain signal following an innocuous stimulation (a phenomenon known as allodynia), as well as increased pain perception. Certain pain conditions may also result from a reduced efficacy of tonic inhibitory controls within the spinal cord [58,86].

Diffuse Noxious Inhibitory Controls

A few years after the gate control theory was proposed, Reynolds demonstrated that stimulation of the PAG produced a strong inhibition [70]. The role of the rostroventral medulla in the modulation of pain has since been well documented [26]. Regions such as the PAG and the NRM have been identified as important serotoninergic and noradrenergic descending inhibitory pathways. These inhibitory pathways recruit enkephalinergic interneurons in the spinal cord to produce the analgesic response.

We had to wait until the end of the 1970s before a model known as diffuse noxious inhibitory controls (DNIC) was proposed [46,47]. This model is based on the observation that a localized nociceptive stimulation can produce a diffuse analgesic effect over the rest of the body, an analgesic approach known as counterirritation. In the DNIC model, Le Bars and his colleagues proposed that a nociceptive stimulus will send input to superior centers, but will also send afferents to the PAG and NRM of the brainstem, recruiting inhibitory output at multiple levels of the spinal cord [46,47].

Animal studies demonstrate that a lesion of the dorsolateral funiculus, the main descending inhibitory pathway, will produce hyperalgesia, suggesting a role for tonic descending inhibition under normal conditions [1,17,94]. Certain clinical conditions are related to reduced endogenous inhibition. For example, the low concentration of serotonin and norepinephrine in the cerebrospinal fluid of patients with fibromyalgia [72] suggests a deficit of DNIC, as confirmed by increasing evidence from other studies [40,42,44,79].

Documenting the role of descending inhibitory mechanisms will help us to better understand certain chronic pain conditions, such as fibromyalgia. It will also help us understand the mechanism of action of pharmacological approaches such as the use of antidepressants in chronic pain conditions.

Superior Control Centers

There has been increasing appreciation of the role of supraspinal centers in pain and pain modulation. Several cortical regions receive input from the spinothalamic tract and interact to produce the multidimensional experience of pain perception [65]. The use of brain imaging techniques has shown robust activation of certain cortical regions, including the primary and secondary somatosensory cortices, related to the sensory aspect of pain, and the ACC and IC, implicated in the affective component of the pain experience [2].

There is no doubt that cognitive manipulations such as distraction, hypnosis, and expectation influence pain perception [2]. Hypnosis has been demonstrated to change both the sensory and affective components of pain perception. Subjects given the same nociceptive stimulus perceive both the intensity and unpleasantness of pain differently depending on the suggestion given [67]. Using positron emission tomography (PET) to obtain brain activity images, researchers have determined that the activity of the primary somatosensory cortex is proportional to the perceived intensity of pain [37], whereas cingulate cortex activity reflects the unpleasantness of pain [68]. These data confirm that a simple suggestion can change the brain activity related to pain perception.

In a recent study, we were able to demonstrate that manipulating the expectation related to an analgesic procedure can totally reverse the analgesic effect of endogenous pain modulation and alter the related pain experience. After hearing the suggestion that a procedure that is normally analgesic would produce more pain, subjects indeed reported more pain. Therefore, suggestion was able to totally block the administered analgesic effect. Suggestion was also able to reverse both the inhibition of the spinal nociceptive reflex (RIII) and the inhibition of brain activity, as measured by somatosensory evoked potentials [33]. These results support the idea that cognitive information can modulate the efficacy of endogenous pain modulation and emphasize the importance of the patient's expectations regarding analgesia. This area will be addressed in the chapter on placebo mechanisms (see Chapter 20 by Goffaux et al.).

Pharmacology of Endogenous Modulation

Based on our knowledge of pain neurophysiology mechanisms, we can adapt the pharmacological treatment of pain by either reducing excitatory mechanisms or increasing the activity of inhibitory mechanisms. (See Chapter 2 by Lussier and Beaulieu for a taxonomy of analgesics.) The first goal is to identify the mechanisms of the patient's pain.

For acute nociceptive pain, depending on the nature of the injury, topical or systemic anti-inflammatory and analgesic agents (NSAIDs or coxibs) or other analgesics (e.g., ion channels blockers) would be primarily indicated [55]. However, even if nociceptive activity is clearly identified to be peripheral and inflammatory, central sensitization may also have occurred, leading to neuropathic pain [73]. Pharmacological approaches for the treatment of neuropathic pain aim to reverse or reduce the hyperactivity of the nociceptive neurons. Commonly used agents include anticonvulsants, antiarrhythmics, antidepressants, opioids, and even NMDA-receptor antagonists (e.g., ketamine) [104].

Functional neuropathic pain is a subcategory of neuropathic pain occurring in the absence of a defined anatomic lesion within the nervous system, but rather representing a dysfunction of pain modulation mechanisms. This type of pain may occur as a result of central activation of endogenous excitatory systems that will amplify the nociceptive signal or may result from a dysfunction of endogenous inhibitory mechanisms [36,58].

An example of central hyperactivity is the thalamic syndrome (a type of poststroke pain) following a lesion of thalamic nuclei as a result of a cerebral event. This lesion will produce hyperactivity of thalamic neurons that are normally inhibited by a complex interneuronal network. A small lesion within the thalamus may result in intense pain over a large body area, frequently involving almost half of the body. In contrast, another pain syndrome, fibromyalgia, may be at least partly explained by a deficit of descending endogenous pain inhibitory mechanisms [40]. In this condition, the hyperalgesia is related to lack of inhibition rather than just hyperactivity of the nociceptive neurons.

Therefore, strategies for the treatment of functional neuropathic pain will be focused either on reduction of nociceptive hyperactivity or on activation of endogenous inhibition. Anticonvulsants or gabapentinoids [25] will reduce sensory input by their effect on ion channels in hyperactive nociceptive neurons, whereas antidepressant medications will augment inhibition by their effect on serotoninergic and noradrenergic systems [21].

Risk Factors for Developing Chronic Pain

Understanding factors other than the primary disease process that are involved in the development and maintenance of pain will help prevent a chronic pain state. Three factors have been proposed to play a role in the chronicity of pain: (1) individual predisposition, (2) environmental factors, and (3) psychological factors. Paying attention to these elements will facilitate the management of patients with chronic pain.

Individual Predisposition to Chronic Pain

Individual predisposition refers to the acquired or innate characteristics that will influence a person's predisposition to pain. Under this category are the roles of gender and sex, age, and endogenous pain modulation responses.

Gender and Sex

Chronic pain syndromes affect women more frequently than men. The reason for women's greater predisposition to chronic pain is likely to be multifactorial, with sex hormones probably playing an important role. Animal research supports differential responses between the sexes and supports the effect of sex hormones on pain experience. For instance, females show greater nociceptive responses than males to the same stimulus, but this difference disappears after gonadectomy [29]. Moreover, if gonadectomized rats receive replacement hormones of the opposite sex—females receiving testosterone and males receiving estrogen and progesterone—they demonstrate nociceptive behavior attributable to their sex hormone status [30]. Interestingly, this influence of sex hormones seems also to be true in humans, because the difference in response to pain between men and women appears only after puberty and disappears after menopause/andropause [71,91].

Age

Although we know that an increase in the prevalence of chronic pain among older individuals is partly due to the progressive musculoskeletal degeneration that accompanies aging, a decline in the efficacy of endogenous pain control systems may also contribute to the high prevalence of pain in the elderly. Studies have shown a deficit of endogenous mechanisms with aging [22,92] and also a significant decrease of DNIC that can occur as early as 50 years of age [43]. This reduction in endogenous pain control with age probably contributes to the higher prevalence of chronic pain in the older population.

Endogenous Pain Modulation Responses

The efficiency of the endogenous inhibitory system, which can be measured by DNIC, has been shown to be a good predictor for the development of chronic pain. More effective inhibitory control was correlated with less clinical pain [23]. The finding of a deficit of DNIC in fibromyalgia, but not in low back pain [40], also supports the role of DNIC in chronic pain, but indicates that it may be specific to certain pathologies.

Genetic Predisposition

There is increasing evidence that some individuals are more prone than others to the development of chronic pain. Genetic predisposition to the development of pain and to the response to pain treatments is now well documented in the literature [7,77] (see Chapter 19 by Mogil). This genetic predisposition helps explain the differences among individuals regarding the development of chronic pain following an injury. The persistence of pain after an injury, which at times may be without objective pathology, such as occurs in whiplash-associated disorder, may be influenced by genetic factors. The same applies for certain treatments. Clinicians recognize that different patients respond differently to individual analgesic medications with regard to both efficacy and side-effect profile.

Environmental Factors

External stressors such as a history of previous pain [88] or abuse [49] are also good predictors of the development of chronic pain. For instance, it has been demonstrated that children born prematurely, receiving painful clinical interventions, will be more sensitive to pain later in life [8,32]. The mechanisms by which these children may be sensitized to pain can be partly explained by deficits in pain inhibitory mechanisms. We have recently reported that children born prematurely and exposed to repeated painful clinical procedures will demonstrate a deficit of DNIC when tested in later childhood [32].

Psychological Factors

Finally, psychological factors such as anxiety, depression, and catastrophizing are also important predictors of pain chronicity [4,16,31,63]. Psychological factors will not only predict one's reactions to a pain experience or one's ability to cope with the pain, but will also affect the evolution of the chronic pain symptoms. The treatment of pain should always take into consideration the role of psychological factors as an important predictor of pain chronicity.

Conclusion

In this chapter, we have described the complexity of the neurophysiological basis of the pain phenomenon and explained mechanisms involved in the development and maintenance of pain conditions. This knowledge is a strong foundation on which to develop a therapeutic guide for the treatment of pain. Although there is commonality in the nociceptive pathways of our patients, each individual will respond differently to pain as a result of differences in genetic and environmental background. This variability in perception of pain and response to pain may lead to physician bias or even misinterpretation of an individual patient's symptoms. Keeping in mind the heterogeneity of the pain response and the unique characteristics of an individual patient will lead to better patient care. Understanding the neurophysiological mechanisms underlying the development and maintenance of pain will help focus treatments more effectively against the specific abnormality causing pain. The science of pain provides an opportunity to address pain from a mechanistic approach with the objective of reinforcing inhibitory mechanisms or reducing the hyperactivity of nociceptive responses.

References

[1] Abbott FV, Hong Y, Franklin KB. The effect of lesions of the dorsolateral funiculus on formalin pain and morphine analgesia: a dose-response analysis. Pain 1996;65:17–23.

[2] Apkarian AV, Bushnell MC, Treede RD, Zubieta JK. Human brain mechanisms of pain perception and regulation in health and disease. Eur J Pain 2005;9:463–84.

[3] Apkarian AV, Sosa Y, Sonty S, Levy RM, Harden RN, Parrish TB, Gitelman DR. Chronic back pain is associated with decreased prefrontal and thalamic gray matter density. J Neurosci 2004;24:10410–5.

[4] Auerbach SM, Laskin DM, Frantsve LM, Orr T. Depression, pain, exposure to stressful life events, and long-term outcomes in temporomandibular disorder patients. J Oral Maxillofac Surg 2001;59:628–3.

[5] Beal MC. Viscerosomatic reflexes: a review. J Am Osteopath Assoc 1985;85:786–801.

[6] Bielefeldt K, Christianson JA, Davis BM. Basic and clinical aspects of visceral sensation: transmission in the CNS. Neurogastroenterol Motil 2005;17:488–99.

[7] Buskila D. Genetics of chronic pain states. Best Pract Res Clin Rheumatol 2007;21:535–47.

[8] Buskila D, Neumann L, Zmora E, Feldman M, Bolotin A, Press J. Pain sensitivity in prematurely born adolescents. Arch Pediatr Adolesc Med 2003;157:1079–82.

[9] Byers MR, Bonica JJ, Loeser JD. Peripheral pain mechanisms and nociceptor plasticity. In: Bonica's management of pain. New York: Lippincott Williams & Wilkins; 2001. p. 26–72.

[10] Casey KL, Bushnell MC. Pain imaging. Progress in pain research and management, Vol. 18. Seattle: IASP Press; 2000.

[11] Cervero F, Jänig W. Visceral nociceptors: a new world order. Trends Neurosci 1992;15:374–8.

[12] Cervero F, Laird JM. Understanding the signaling and transmission of visceral nociceptive events. J Neurobiol 2004;61:45–54.

[13] Chang FY, Chey WY, Ouyang A. Effect of transcutaneous nerve stimulation on esophageal function in normal subjects-evidence for a somatovisceral reflex. Am J Chin Med 1996;24:185–92.

[14] Coghill RC, Talbot JD, Evans AC, Meyer E, Gjedde A, Bushnell MC, Duncan GH. Distributed processing of pain and vibration by the human brain. J Neurosci 1994;14:4095–108.

[15] Coull JA, Boudreau D, Bachand K, Prescott SA, Nault F, Sik A, De Koninck P, De Koninck Y. Trans-synaptic shift in anion gradient in spinal lamina I neurons as a mechanism of neuropathic pain. Nature 2003;424:938–42.

[16] Currie SR, Wang J. Chronic back pain and major depression in the general Canadian population. Pain 2004;107:54–60.

[17] Davies JE, Marsden CA, Roberts MH. Hyperalgesia and the reduction of monoamines resulting from lesions of the dorsolateral funiculus. Brain Res 1983;261:59–68.

[18] Davis MP, Shaiova LA, Angst MS. When opioids cause pain. J Clin Oncol 2007;25:4497–8.

[19] De Leo JA, Sorkin LS, Watkins LR. Immune and glial regulation of pain. Seattle: IASP Press; 2007. p. 443.
[20] Descartes R. Traité de l'homme. In: Descartes R. Oeuvres et lettres. Gallimard: Bibliothèque de la Pléiade; 1644. p. 803–73.
[21] Dickenson AH, Ghandehari J. Anti-convulsants and anti-depressants. Handb Exp Pharmacol 2007;177:145–77.
[22] Edwards RR, Fillingim RB, Ness TJ. Age-related differences in endogenous pain modulation: a comparison of diffuse noxious inhibitory controls in healthy older and younger adults. Pain 2003;101:155–65.
[23] Edwards RR, Ness TJ, Weigent DA, Fillingim RB. Individual differences in diffuse noxious inhibitory controls (DNIC): association with clinical variables. Pain 2003;106:427–37.
[24] Eide PK. Wind-up and the NMDA receptor complex from a clinical perspective. Eur J Pain 2000;4:5–15.
[25] Field MJ, Cox PJ, Stott E, Melrose H, Offord J, Su TZ, Bramwell S, Corradini L, England S, Winks J, et al. Identification of the alpha2-delta-1 subunit of voltage-dependent calcium channels as a molecular target for pain mediating the analgesic actions of pregabalin. Proc Natl Acad Sci USA 2006.103:17537–42.
[26] Fields HL, Basbaum A, Heinrich RL. Central nervous system mechanisms of pain modulation. In: McMahon SB, Koltzenburg M, editors. Wall and Melzack's textbook of pain. Philadelphia: Elsevier; 2006. p. 125–42.
[27] Fields HL, Malick A, Burstein R. Dorsal horn projection targets of ON and OFF cells in the rostral ventromedial medulla. J Neurophysiol 1995;74:1742–59.
[28] Frey MV. Treatise on the sensory functions of the human skin. In: Handwerker HO, editor. Classical German contributions to pain research. Deutsche Gesellschaft zum Studium des Schmerzes; 1897. p. 69–132.
[29] Gaumond I, Arsenault P, Marchand S. The role of sex hormones on formalin-induced nociceptive responses. Brain Res 2002;958:139–45.
[30] Gaumond I, Arsenault P, Marchand S. Specificity of female and male sex hormones on excitatory and inhibitory phases of formalin-induced nociceptive responses. Brain Res 2005;1052:105–11.
[31] Gauthier N, Sullivan M J, Adams H, Stanish WD, Thibault P. Investigating risk factors for chronicity: the importance of distinguishing between return-to-work status and self-report measures of disability. J Occup Environ Med 2006;48:312–8.
[32] Goffaux P, Lafrenaye S, Morin M, Patural H, Demers G, Marchand S. Preterm births: can neonatal pain alter the development of endogenous gating systems? Eur J Pain 2008;12:945–51.
[33] Goffaux P, Redmond WJ, Rainville P, Marchand S. Descending analgesia: when the spine echoes what the brain expects. Pain 2007;130:137–43.
[34] Goldscheider A. The specific energy of the sensory nerves of the skin, In: Handwerker HO, editor. Classical German contributions to pain research. Deutsche Gesellschaft zum Studium des Schmerzes; 1884. p. 47–69.
[35] Granot M, Granovsky Y, Sprecher E, Nir RR, Yarnitsky D. Contact heat-evoked temporal summation: tonic versus repetitive-phasic stimulation. Pain 2006;122:295–305.
[36] Heinricher MM, Tavares I, Leith JL, Lumb BM. Descending control of nociception: specificity, recruitment and plasticity. Brain Res Rev 2009;60:214–25.
[37] Hofbauer RK, Rainville P, Duncan GH, Bushnell MC. Cortical representation of the sensory dimension of pain. J Neurophysiol 2001;86:402–11.
[38] Ji RR, Kawasaki Y, Zhuang ZY, Wen YR, Decosterd I. Possible role of spinal astrocytes in maintaining chronic pain sensitization: review of current evidence with focus on bFGF/JNK pathway. Neuron Glia Biol 2006;2:259–69.
[39] Jones MP, Dilley JB, Drossman D, Crowell MD. Brain-gut connections in functional GI disorders: anatomic and physiologic relationships. Neurogastroenterol Motil 2006;18:91–103.
[40] Julien N, Goffaux P, Arsenault P, Marchand S. Widespread pain in fibromyalgia is related to a deficit of endogenous pain inhibition. Pain 2005;114:295–302.
[41] Knowles CH, Aziz Q. Basic and clinical aspects of gastrointestinal pain. Pain 2009;141:191–209.
[42] Kosek E, Hansson P. Modulatory influence on somatosensory perception from vibration and heterotopic noxious conditioning stimulation (HNCS) in fibromyalgia patients and healthy subjects. Pain 1997;70:41–51.
[43] Lariviere M, Goffaux P, Marchand S, Julien N. Changes in pain perception and descending inhibitory controls start at middle age in healthy adults. Clin J Pain 2007;23:506–10.
[44] Lautenbacher S, Rollman GB. Possible deficiencies of pain modulation in fibromyalgia. Clin J Pain 1997;13:189–96.
[45] Le Bars D. The whole body receptive field of dorsal horn multireceptive neurones. Brain Res Brain Res Rev 2002;40:29–44.
[46] Le Bars D, Dickenson AH, Besson JM. Diffuse noxious inhibitory controls (DNIC). 1. Effects on dorsal horn convergent neurones in the rat. Pain 1979;6:283–304.
[47] Le Bars D, Dickenson AH, Besson JM. Diffuse noxious inhibitory controls (DNIC). II. Lack of effect on non-convergent neurones, supraspinal involvement and theoretical implications. Pain 1979;6:305–27.
[48] Lenz FA, Gracely RH, Romanoski AJ, Hope EJ, Rowland LH, Dougherty PM. Stimulation in the human somatosensory thalamus can reproduce both the affective and sensory dimensions of previously experienced pain. Nat Med 1995;1:910–3.
[49] Linton SJ. A population-based study of the relationship between sexual abuse and back pain: establishing a link. Pain 1997;73:47–53.
[50] Lorenz J, Minoshima S, Casey KL. Keeping pain out of mind: the role of the dorsolateral prefrontal cortex in pain modulation. Brain 2003;126:1079–91.
[51] Lundeberg T, Bondesson L, Lundstrom V. Relief of primary dysmenorrhea by transcutaneous electrical nerve stimulation. Acta Obstet Gynecol Scand 1985;64:491–7.
[52] Mao J. Opioid-induced abnormal pain sensitivity: implications in clinical opioid therapy. Pain 2002;100:213–7.
[53] Marchand S, Arsenault P. Spatial summation for pain perception: interaction of inhibitory and excitatory mechanisms. Pain 2002;95:201–6.

[54] McMahon SB, Bennet DLH, Bevan S. Inflammatory mediators and modulators of pain. In: McMahon SB, Koltzenburg M, editors. Wall and Melzack's textbook of pain. Philadelphia: Elsevier; 2006. p. 49–72.
[55] McQuay HJ, Moore A, McMahon SB, Koltzenburg M. NSAIDs and coxibs: clinical use. In: Wall and Melzack's textbook of pain. Edinburgh: Elsevier Churchill Livingston; 2006. p. 471–80.
[56] Melzack R, Wall PD. Pain mechanisms: a new theory. Science 1965;150:971–9.
[57] Meyer RA, Ringkamp M, Campbell JN, Raja SN. Peripheral mechanisms of nociception. In: McMahon SB, Koltzenburg M, editors. Wall and Melzack's textbook of pain. Philadelphia: Elsevier; 2006. p. 3–34.
[58] Millan MJ. Descending control of pain. Prog Neurobiol 2002;66:355–474.
[59] Müller J. On the sense of feeling. In: Handwerker HO, editor. Classical German contributions to pain research. Deutsche Gesellschaft zum Studium des Schmerzes; 1837. p. 27–47.
[60] Olausson H, Lamarre Y, Backlund H, Morin C, Wallin BG, Starck G, Ekholm S, Strigo I, Worsley K, Vallbo AB, Bushnell MC. Unmyelinated tactile afferents signal touch and project to insular cortex. Nat Neurosci 2002;5:900–4.
[61] Palecek J, Paleckova V, Willis WD. Fos expression in spinothalamic and postsynaptic dorsal column neurons following noxious visceral and cutaneous stimuli. Pain 2003;104:249–57.
[62] Palecek J, Willis WD. The dorsal column pathway facilitates visceromotor responses to colorectal distention after colon inflammation in rats. Pain 2003;104:501–7.
[63] Pincus T, Burton AK, Vogel S, Field AP. A systematic review of psychological factors as predictors of chronicity/disability in prospective cohorts of low back pain. Spine 2002;27:E109–20.
[64] Price DD. Psychological mechanisms of pain and analgesia, Progress in pain research and management, Vol. 15. Seattle: IASP Press; 1999.
[65] Price DD. Psychological and neural mechanisms of the affective dimension of pain. Science 2000;288:1769–72.
[66] Price DD, Dubner R. Mechanisms of first and second pain in the peripheral and central nervous systems. J Invest Dermatol 1977;69:167–71.
[67] Rainville P, Carrier B, Hofbauer RK, Bushnell MC, Duncan GH. Dissociation of sensory and affective dimensions of pain using hypnotic modulation. Pain 1999;82:159–71.
[68] Rainville P, Duncan GH, Price DD, Carrier B, Bushnell MC. Pain affect encoded in human anterior cingulate but not somatosensory cortex. Science 1997;277:968–71.
[69] Raj PP. Visceral pain. Agri 2004;16:7–20.
[70] Reynolds DV. Surgery in the rat during electrical analgesia. Science 1969;164:444–5.
[71] Robinson JE, Short RV. Changes in breast sensitivity at puberty, during the menstrual cycle, and at parturition. BMJ 1977;1:1188–91.
[72] Russell IJ. Neurochemical pathogenesis of fibromyalgia. Z Rheumatol 1998;57:63–6.
[73] Samad TA, Moore KA, Sapirstein A, Billet S, Allchorne A, Poole S, Bonventre JV, Woolf CJ. Interleukin-1beta-mediated induction of Cox-2 in the CNS contributes to inflammatory pain hypersensitivity. Nature 2001;410:471–5.
[74] Sato A. Somatovisceral reflexes. J Manipulative Physiol Ther 1995;18:597–602.
[75] Schmidt R, Schmelz M, Forster C, Ringkamp M, Torebjork E, Handwerker H. Novel classes of responsive and unresponsive C nociceptors in human skin. J Neurosci 1995;15:333–41.
[76] Simonnet G, Rivat C. Opioid-induced hyperalgesia: abnormal or normal pain? NeuroReport 2003;14:1–7.
[77] Stamer UM, Stuber F. Genetic factors in pain and its treatment. Curr Opin Anaesthesiol 2007;20:478–84.
[78] Stander S, Steinhoff M, Schmelz M, Weisshaar E, Metze D, Luger T. Neurophysiology of pruritus: cutaneous elicitation of itch. Arch Dermatol 2003;139:1463–70.
[79] Staud R, Robinson ME, Vierck CJ, Price DD. Diffuse noxious inhibitory controls (DNIC) attenuate temporal summation of second pain in normal males but not in normal females or fibromyalgia patients. Pain 2003;1012:167–74.
[80] Staud R, Vierck CJ, Cannon RL, Mauderli AP, Price DD. Abnormal sensitization and temporal summation of second pain (wind-up) in patients with fibromyalgia syndrome. Pain 2001;91:165–75.
[81] Suter MR, Wen YR, Decosterd I, Ji RR. Do glial cells control pain? Neuron Glia Biol 2007;3:255–68.
[82] Talbot JD, Marrett S, Evans AC, Meyer E, Bushnell MC, Duncan GH. Multiple representations of pain in human cerebral cortex. Science 1991;251:1355–8.
[83] Terman GW, Bonica JJ, Loeser JD. Spinal mechanisms and their modulation. In: Bonica's management of pain. New York: Lippincott Williams & Wilkins; 2001. p. 73–152.
[84] Todd AJ, Koerber HR, McMahon SB, Koltzenburg M. Neuroanatomical substrate of spinal nociception. In: McMahon SB, Koltzenburg M, editors. Wall and Melzack's textbook of pain. Philadelphia: Elsevier; 2006. p. 73–90.
[85] Torebjork HE, Lamotte RH, Robinson CJ. Peripheral neural correlates of magnitude of cutaneous pain and hyperalgesia: simultaneous recordings in humans of sensory judgments of pain and evoked responses in nociceptors with C-fibers. J Neurophysiol 1984;51:325–39.
[86] Traub RJ. Spinal modulation of the induction of central sensitization. Brain Res 1997;778:34–42.
[87] Tsuda M, Inoue K, Salter MW. Neuropathic pain and spinal microglia: a big problem from molecules in "small" glia. Trends Neurosci 2005;28:101–7.
[88] Turner JA, Dworkin SF. Screening for psychosocial risk factors in patients with chronic orofacial pain: recent advances. J Am Dent Assoc 2004;135:1119–25.
[89] Verne GN, Robinson ME, Vase L, Price DD. Reversal of visceral and cutaneous hyperalgesia by local rectal anesthesia in irritable bowel syndrome (IBS) patients. Pain 2003;105:223–30.
[90] Vierck CJ Jr, Cannon RL, Fry G, Maixner W, Whitsel BL. Characteristics of temporal summation of second pain sensations elicited by brief contact of glabrous skin by a preheated thermode. J Neurophysiol 1997;78:992–1002.
[91] Von Korff M, Dworkin SF, Le Resche L, Kruger A. An epidemiologic comparison of pain complaints. Pain 1988;32:173–83.

[92] Washington LL, Gibson SJ, Helme RD. Age-related differences in the endogenous analgesic response to repeated cold water immersion in human volunteers. Pain 2000;89:89–96.
[93] Watkins LR, Maier SF. Glia: a novel drug discovery target for clinical pain. Nat Rev Drug Discov 2003;2:973–85.
[94] Wei F, Dubner R, Ren K. Nucleus reticularis gigantocellularis and nucleus raphe magnus in the brain stem exert opposite effects on behavioral hyperalgesia and spinal Fos protein expression after peripheral inflammation. Pain 1999;80:127–41.
[95] Wiech K, Ploner M, Tracey I. Neurocognitive aspects of pain perception. Trends Cogn Sci 2008;12:306–13.
[96] Willis WD. Nociceptive pathways: anatomy and physiology of nociceptive ascending pathways. Philos Trans R Soc Lond B Biol Sci 1985;308:253–70.
[97] Willis WD, Basset EG, Beers RF. Physiology of dorsal horn and spinal cord pathways related to pain. In: Mechanisms of pain and analgesic compounds. New York: Raven Press; 1979. p. 143–56.
[98] Woolf CJ. Generation of acute pain: central mechanisms. Br Med Bull 1991;47:523–33.
[99] Woolf CJ. Windup and central sensitization are not equivalent. Pain 1996;66:105–8.
[100] Woolf CJ, Salter MW. Neuronal plasticity: increasing the gain in pain. Science 2000;288:1765–9.
[101] Woolf CJ, Salter MW. Plasticity and pain: role of the dorsal horn. In: McMahon SB, Koltzenburg M, editors. Wall and Melzack's textbook of pain. Philadelphia: Elsevier; 2006. p. 91–105.
[102] Woolf CJ, Thompson SW. The induction and maintenance of central sensitization is dependent on N-methyl-D-aspartic acid receptor activation; implications for the treatment of post-injury pain hypersensitivity states. Pain 1991;44:293–9.
[103] Xu XJ, Colpaert F, Wiesenfeld-Hallin Z. Opioid hyperalgesia and tolerance versus 5-HT1A receptor-mediated inverse tolerance. Trends Pharmacol Sci 2003;24:634–9.
[104] Yaksh TL, Chaplan SR. Physiology and pharmacology of neuropathic pain. Anesthesiol Clin North America 1997;15:335–52.

Correspondence to: Serge Marchand, PhD, Department of Neurosurgery, Faculty of Medicine, University of Sherbrooke, CRC-CHUS, 3001, 12e Avenue Nord, Sherbrooke, Quebec, Canada J1H 5N4. Email: serge.marchand@usherbrooke.ca.

Toward a Rational Taxonomy of Analgesic Drugs

2

David Lussier[a,b,c] and Pierre Beaulieu[d]

[a]Alan-Edwards Centre for Research on Pain and [b]Division of Geriatric Medicine, Department of Medicine, McGill University, Montreal, Quebec, Canada; [c]Geriatric Institute and [d]Departments of Anesthesiology and Pharmacology, CHUM, University of Montreal, Montreal, Quebec, Canada

History of Analgesics

Analgesic drugs (from the Greek "an" [without] and "algos" [pain]) have been used for millennia. As early as 3400 BCE, the opium poppy was cultivated by the Egyptians, Sumerians, Babylonians, and Assyrians, and there are reports of extracts from cannabis being used in the same period. Hippocrates can be credited for the first description of an analgesic, the Hippocratic Corpus, a multiherbal source of pain relief. He also used salicin powder, made from the leaves and bark of the willow tree, to treat headache, fever, and pain, as well as opium, the first narcotic used to treat pain.

While opium and willow tree extracts have been used in several civilizations throughout history, the modern history of analgesics really started in the 19th century, with the development of morphine and acetylsalicylic acid. At the beginning of the 19th century, an alkaloid compound was isolated from the resinous gum secreted by the opium poppy (*Papaver somniferum*) by a young German pharmacist's assistant, Friedrich Wilhelm Adam Sertürner. He named the compound morphine (after Morpheus, the Greek god of dreams), for its tendency to induce sleep. Reports of his experiments, as well as a French publication on morphine's analgesic and hypnotic activities, stimulated interest from the medical community and led to its commercial availability by the mid-1820s. Morphine was produced by a few pharmaceutical companies, including a new company

Pharmacology of Pain
edited by Pierre Beaulieu, David Lussier, Frank Porreca, and Anthony H. Dickenson
IASP Press, Seattle, © 2010

founded by Heinrich Emanuel Merck. By the 1850s, morphine had become standard treatment for perioperative and postoperative analgesia. Physicians became aware of the drug's addictive potential two decades later, which stimulated interest in the development of less addictive molecules and led to the discovery of a more potent narcotic, diacetylmorphine, in 1874, by German chemist Felix Hoffman. Marketed in 1898 under the name "heroin" (because of its "heroic" ability to relieve pain), the new drug was withdrawn in 1913 when it became obvious that it was even more addictive than morphine.

While trying to find a treatment for "ague" (symptoms of intermittent fever, pain, and fatigue associated with malaria) that would be less expensive than the standard treatment (Peruvian bark, with quinine as its active ingredient), the Englishman Edward Stone discovered in 1773 that extracts from the bark of white willow (*Salix alba*) could relieve the fever associated with the disease, without curing it. Starting at the beginning of the 19th century, experiments progressively led to more pure and potent extracts of white willow, culminating in 1838 with the isolation of a potent extract, named salicylic acid. From then on, salicylates were widely used to relieve pain, fever, and inflammation, but their gastric toxicity limited their use and stimulated research for less irritating compounds. Acetylsalicylic acid was first synthesized in 1853, and different methods were used for its synthesis until Hoffman (the chemist who developed heroin) found the best method in 1897, in which salicylic acid is refluxed with acetic anhydride. Two years later, in 1899, the drug was commercialized by Bayer under the name Aspirin.

Acetaminophen (paracetamol) was first synthesized in 1877 at Johns Hopkins University, and was used on patients in 1887. It was discarded a few years later because of reports suggesting that it caused methemoglobinemia, and replaced by another aniline derivative, phenacetin. In the late 1940s, several studies denied its association with methemoglobinemia and showed that phenacetin was actually metabolized to acetaminophen. The commercialization of acetaminophen began in 1953, quickly followed by the withdrawal of phenacetin due its renal and hematological toxicities.

Nitrous oxide, the first anesthetic, was first produced by the English chemist Joseph Priestley in 1772. Towards the end of the century, Humphrey Davy concluded from his experiments that breathing it could relieve toothache, for which it was first used in 1848. Despite Davy's objections, the gas was commonly called "laughter gas" because it was often used as a source of amusement and entertainment.

Most of the other classes of analgesics were developed in the first half of the 20th century. Phenytoin, the first anticonvulsant used as an analgesic, was synthesized in 1908 and was first used to treat seizures in 1938. Imipramine, the first tricyclic antidepressant, was commercialized in the 1950s, and other tricyclics soon followed. Lidocaine was developed in 1943 and ketamine in 1962.

The limits of the anti-inflammatory activity of acetylsalicylic acid were noted, and the first steroid-based drug, cortisone, was developed in 1948. Ibuprofen, the first nonsteroidal anti-inflammatory drug (NSAID), was discovered in 1960 and commercialized in 1969.

The past two decades are mostly remarkable for the discovery of the cyclooxygenase 2 (COX-2) enzyme by Daniel Simmons (at Brigham Young University) in 1988 and the subsequent development of selective COX-2 inhibitors, and for the development of new types of analgesics for neuropathic pain, mainly the gabapentinoids (gabapentin and pregabalin) and the norepinephrine and serotonin reuptake inhibitor duloxetine.

It is interesting to note that the basic approach to analgesia, which had not changed since the days of Hippocrates, has recently evolved. Although the analgesics we depend on for many types of pain associated with tissue damage are still composed of derivatives of the willow bark (NSAIDs) and the opium poppy (opioids), drugs for neuropathic pain now have their own indication. The greatest advancements accomplished by modern medicine are related to the development of these "nontraditional" or "adjuvant" analgesics, which now include several different classes of drugs primarily used for an indication other than pain. The analgesic properties of these drugs have become more and more well known, and their use as analgesics has increased, sometimes exceeding their primary indication. As reviewed by Dray and Perkins in Chapter 17, several new drugs are in development, most of them in early stages of research, which target novel pain pathways.

Currently Existing Classifications of Analgesics

Taxonomy is the science and practice of classification [3], or a method of organizing content into ordered groups or categories, according to a predetermined system, providing a conceptual framework for discussion, analysis, or information retrieval [7]. Categories and subcategories should be mutually exclusive, unambiguous, and comprehensive. The taxonomy should be simple, easy to remember, and easy to use [7].

Establishing a classification or taxonomy of analgesics is surely not an easy task, due to the complexity of the pain experience, the variety of classes of drugs used for pain treatment, and the ever-evolving understanding of pain mechanisms and treatment. Analgesics can be categorized based on different criteria. The currently existing classifications are based either on severity of pain (e.g., World Health Organization), type of pain (e.g., postoperative pain, neuropathic pain, cancer pain), therapeutic classes of analgesics (e.g., antidepressants, anticonvulsants), mechanisms of action, or a combination of different criteria.

World Health Organization Classification

The World Health Organization (WHO) established the basis of treatment for cancer pain, which has been extrapolated to noncancer pain, with the WHO pain ladder [9]. The pain ladder is a stepwise approach to the use of analgesics depending on pain severity (see Chapter 25 by Servin). Nonopioid analgesics (acetaminophen or NSAIDs) are recommended for mild pain, whereas "weak" opioids (hydrocodone, codeine, low-dose oxycodone, or propoxyphene) are recommended for moderate pain and "strong" opioids (morphine, hydromorphone, high-dose oxycodone, fentanyl, or methadone) are recommended for severe pain. Additional drugs ("adjuvants") should be used "to calm fears and anxiety."

There are several problems with this classification. The distinction between "weak" and "strong" opioids is somewhat arbitrary because opioid response is dose-dependent rather than drug-dependent. Of course, nowadays, adjuvant analgesics are not reserved for the treatment of fear and anxiety because several of them possess analgesic properties, and several of these drugs are now the primary treatments for neuropathic pain.

The WHO has proposed another classification, in which analgesics are categorized as either nonopioids, opioids, coanalgesics (antidepressants, anticonvulsants, ketamine, and local anesthetics), or adjuvants (steroids, muscle relaxants [diazepam, baclofen], and bisphosphonates) [8].

International Association for the Study of Pain Classification

In its *Core Curriculum for Professional Education in Pain,* the International Association for the Study of Pain (IASP) outlines the pharmacological treatment of pain, dividing analgesics into the following categories: opioids, antipyretics (NSAIDs, acetaminophen, and phenazone derivatives), antidepressants, anticonvulsants, and "miscellaneous." The latter category includes neuroleptics, antihistamines, analeptics, corticosteroids, muscle relaxants and antispasticity drugs, *N*-methyl-D-aspartate (NMDA) antagonists, local anesthetics and membrane-stabilizing drugs, sympatholytics, baclofen, cannabinoids, drugs modifying the serotoninergic pathways, and topical agents [6].

Classification Based on Clinical Efficacy

The most common classification, derived from the WHO pain ladder, divides pain treatment into "analgesics" (nonopioids and opioids) and "adjuvant analgesics." This classification is taught in medical schools and is found in most textbooks. Adjuvant analgesics can be further divided based on their clinical efficacy and original therapeutic class: multipurpose (antidepressants, corticosteroids, α_2-adrenergic agonists, and neuroleptics), neuropathic pain (anticonvulsants, sodium channel blockers, NMDA-receptor blockers, cannabinoids, and miscellaneous drugs [baclofen, calcitonin, drugs used for sympathetically maintained pain, and anticholinesterase]), bone pain (calcitonin, bisphosphonates, and radiopharmaceuticals), musculoskeletal pain ("muscle relaxants"), and topical analgesics (capsaicin, local anesthetics, tricyclics, and NSAIDs) [4].

Classification Based on Pain Mechanisms

A few mechanistic approaches to pain treatment have been proposed. In 2008, Marchand [5] concluded a review of the physiology of pain mechanisms by suggesting that treatment could be aimed at either reducing excitatory mechanisms or enhancing inhibitory activity, depending on the mechanisms of pain involved in a particular case. Pain mechanisms can be divided into nociceptive (somatic, visceral, or inflammatory pain) and neuropathic (complex regional pain syndromes, peripheral and central neuropathic pain, spinal cord injury, functional pain, etc.), where there is a lesion or disease of the nerves. Optimal pain treatment can be selected based on a patient's pain categorization. Nociceptive pain could be treated by reducing inflammation (NSAIDs), by blocking the activity of the nerve fibers (e.g., ion channel blockers), or by using agents that act on C-fiber receptors (e.g., capsaicin). In fact, with the exception of central pain syndromes, virtually all pain is reduced by blockade of afferent inputs. If there is hyperactivity of the spinal neurons following sensitization of the central nervous system, either primarily or secondarily following chronic pain (see Chapter 1 by Marchand), anticonvulsants, local anesthetics, or NMDA antagonists can be used to reduce the hyperactivity. Antidepressants with serotoninergic and noradrenergic properties act to produce alterations in descending modulation, and additionally many of these drugs also bind to sodium channels, probably inhibiting afferent drive as well.

Classifications Based on Pain Mechanism Molecular Targets

Other mechanistic classifications are based on both the pain mechanism and the molecular targets of the analgesics. Costigan and Woolf [2] have divided pain mechanisms into peripheral sensitization, ectopic discharge, sympathetically maintained pain, central sensitization, and reduced inhibition/increased transmission. In addition to currently available drugs, they have included drugs under development. Analgesics modulating peripheral sensitization act either on the transient receptor potential vanilloid 1 (capsaicin) receptor (TRPV1), block tetrodotoxin-resistant voltage-gated sodium channels, or are antagonists of nerve growth factors (NGF) or NGF-tyrosine kinase receptors, bradykinin, or serotonin. Modulators of ectopic discharge are sodium channel blockers (carbamazepine, lamotrigine, mexiletine, or lidocaine) or potassium channel activators. Drugs reducing sympathetically maintained pain act on the α_1-adrenergic receptors (phentolamine or guanethidine). Modulators of central sensitization are mainly NMDA antagonists and COX-2 selective inhibitors, as well as experimental agents. Finally, analgesics modulating the inhibitory and excitatory pathways are opioids, gabapentinoids, clonidine, tricyclic antidepressants, γ-aminobutyric acid (GABA) agonists, and cannabinoid CB_2-receptor agonists.

Beydoun and Backonja [1] have taken the mechanistic classification one step further by categorizing analgesics for neuropathic pain (antineuralgics) based on their mechanism of action and subcategorizing them according to their molecular targets. They suggest that antineuralgics work at different levels of the development of neuropathic pain. They are modulators of either peripheral sensitization, central sensitization, or descending inhibition. The modulators of peripheral sensitization act on the sodium channels in the peripheral nervous system, by preventing the generation of spontaneous ectopic discharges. This group of drugs includes several anticonvulsants (carbamazepine, oxcarbazepine, phenytoin, topiramate, and lamotrigine), the local anesthetic lidocaine and the antiarrhythmic mexiletine, and tricyclic antidepressants. The modulators of descending inhibition reduce the reuptake of biogenic amines, either serotonin (selective serotonin reuptake inhibitors), norepinephrine (the secondary amines subgroup of tricyclic antidepressants), or both (norepinephrine and serotonin reuptake inhibitors, the tertiary amines subgroup of tricyclic antidepressants, and tramadol). In this classification, opioids are considered as modulators of descending inhibition because the activation of supraspinal opioid receptors switches descending pathways to an inhibitory function. Opioids, however, also have very clear direct spinal actions where they reduce neurotransmitter release from afferent terminals and act postsynaptically on spinal neurons. By reducing spinal excitability, they attenuate ascending signals to the brain and so indirectly alter descending controls as well as reducing the sensory experience. Finally, the modulators of central sensitization are either calcium channel blockers (gabapentinoids), sodium channel blockers (oxcarbazepine, lamotrigine), or NMDA-receptor antagonists (ketamine, dextromethorphan, memantine, and methadone—an opioid with potential non-opioid actions). Since this classification is based on molecular targets, antineuralgic agents that act on several neurotransmitters are classified under several categories. For example, oxcarbazepine and lamotrigine are categorized as modulators of both peripheral and central sensitization, and tricyclic antidepressants are modulators of peripheral sensitization and descending inhibition.

Finally, in Chapter 18 of this book, Simonnet and Le Moal outline the importance of central sensitization and hypersensitivity in the pathogenesis of pain, and they suggest that preventing these phenomena is crucial for adequate pain treatment. They propose that analgesics be classified based on their hyperalgesic properties: (1) specific antinociceptive drugs (e.g., acetaminophen), (2) analgesics with hyperalgesic properties (e.g., opioids), (3) antihyperalgesics (e.g., NMDA-receptor antagonists), and (4) analgesics with antihyperalgesic properties (e.g., gabapentinoids, nitrous oxide, and COX-2 inhibitors).

Comparison of Currently Existing Classifications

A comparison of the currently existing classifications of analgesics (Table I) shows the considerable progress since the WHO and IASP classifications, made possible by better understanding of the pain mechanisms. Although they use different terms, the mechanistic classifications are very similar, especially those proposed by Costigan and Woolf [2] and Beydoun and Backonja [1]. These two classifications are restricted, however, to the use of drugs to treat neuropathic pain, and they do not discuss antinociceptive agents. Simonnet and Le Moal offer a novel approach, based on modulation of hyperalgesia, but their classification is not comprehensive. Tricyclic antidepressants, for example, are not included in any category, and the classification contains drugs that are analgesic in one context but antihyperalgesic or even hyperalgesic in others.

Proposed Taxonomy

The proposed taxonomy (Table II) is similar to the currently available mechanistic classifications, with a few significant differences. It has been developed following a few general and specific principles:

1) It should fulfill the criteria for a "good taxonomy" [7]: it should be simple, easy to remember, and easy to use; categories and subcategories should be mutually exclusive, unambiguous, and comprehensive.

2) Classifications based on clinical efficacy, as suggested by Lussier and Portenoy [4], are subject to considerable change over time, as basic and clinical researchers provide evidence for analgesic efficacy in other types of pain. For example, gabapentinoids are usually categorized as "adjuvants for neuropathic pain," but there is increasing evidence that they can be effective in postoperative pain or nociceptive pain with central sensitization. The term "antineuralgics" therefore does not reflect their clinical efficacy.

3) The terms "adjuvant analgesic" and "coanalgesic" are obsolete. An "adjuvant drug" is defined as "a substance added to a drug to aid its action" [3]. This is the definition used by the WHO classification, which makes the distinction between "coanalgesics" (anticonvulsants and antidepressants) and "adjuvant medicine" (steroids, muscle relaxants, and bisphosphonates). An "adjuvant analgesic" has been defined as "any drug that has a primary indication other than pain, but is analgesic in some painful conditions" [4]. Most drugs currently considered to be "adjuvant analgesics" do not correspond to these definitions. Several of them are often used alone (e.g., gabapentinoids or tricyclics for neuropathic pain), and pain is a primary indication for some (e.g., pregabalin). We therefore propose that these drugs, which have shown analgesic properties, should be categorized as "analgesics."

4) Given that drugs previously referred to as "adjuvant analgesics" are now being considered "analgesics," the term "nonopioid analgesics" is not appropriate because several types of analgesics do not have any opioid activity. Acetaminophen and NSAIDs should therefore be classified as "nonopioid antinociceptive analgesics."

5) Categorizing drugs under their therapeutic class (e.g., antidepressants or anticonvulsants) should be avoided because it might imply that: (i) all drugs from the class have analgesic properties, and (ii) all drugs from a same class have similar mechanisms of analgesia. None of these statements is true.

6) Some drugs exert their analgesic activity via several mechanisms of action. When one mechanism is generally accepted as the most important one, it has been categorized under that mechanism. For example, tricyclics have been shown to be sodium channel modulators, but this is not known to contribute to their analgesic action, which is likely mostly due to their modulation of the descending inhibitory pathways, hence their inclusion under the latter category, similarly to Costigan and Woolf [2]. However, the analgesic activity of tramadol and tapentadol is mediated both by their inhibition of serotonin and norepinephrine reuptake and by their opioid agonist properties. The taxonomy reflects this dual mechanism.

7) While only currently clinically used drugs have been included in the proposed taxonomy, investigational drugs can easily be added, based on their mechanisms of analgesia.

The description of the mechanisms of analgesic activity of each drug or class of drug is beyond the scope of this chapter and is presented in Section II of the book. Table III, however, presents a summary of analgesics used for different pain syndromes, along with their molecular targets.

Table I
Comparison of existing classifications of analgesics and proposition of a new taxonomy

Drug	WHO	IASP	Lussier and Portenoy	Marchand	Costigan and Woolf	Beydoun and Backonja	Simonnet and Le Moal	Proposed Taxonomy
Acetaminophen	Nonopioids	Antipyretics	Nonopioids	Nociceptive somatic			Specific antinociceptive	Antinociceptive
α_2-adrenergic agonists			Multipurpose adjuvants		↓ inhibition/ ↑ transmission	Descending inhibition		Descending modulation
Analeptics		Miscellaneous						
Anticholinesterase			Neuropathic pain					
Anticonvulsants	Coanalgesics	Anticonvulsants	Neuropathic pain	Neurogenic				
Antidepressants	Coanalgesics	Antidepressants	Multipurpose adjuvants	Neurogenic				
Antihistamines		Miscellaneous						
Baclofen	Adjuvants	Miscellaneous	Neuropathic pain					
Bisphosphonates	Adjuvants		Bone pain					Other
Calcitonin			Neuropathic pain; bone pain					Other
Cannabinoids		Miscellaneous	Neuropathic pain	Neurogenic functional				Antinociceptive
Capsaicin		Topical	Topical		Peripheral sensitization			Peripheral transmission/ sensitization
Carbamazepine	Coanalgesics	Anticonvulsants	Neuropathic pain	Neurogenic	Ectopic discharge	Peripheral sensitization		Peripheral transmission/ sensitization
Corticosteroids	Adjuvants	Miscellaneous	Multipurpose adjuvants	Nociceptive somatic; nociceptive inflammatory				

Gabapentinoids	Coanalgesics	Anticonvulsants	Neuropathic pain	Neurogenic	↓ inhibition/ ↑ transmission	Central sensitization	Antihyperalgesic properties	Antihyperalgesic
Lamotrigine	Coanalgesics	Anticonvulsants	Neuropathic pain	Neurogenic	Ectopic discharge	Peripheral sensitization; central sensitization		Antihyperalgesic
Levetiracetam	Coanalgesics	Anticonvulsants	Neuropathic pain	Neurogenic		Central sensitization		Antihyperalgesic
Local anesthetics	Coanalgesics	Miscellaneous	Topical		Peripheral sensitization	Peripheral sensitization		Peripheral transmission/ sensitization
Muscle relaxants	Adjuvants	Miscellaneous	Musculoskeletal pain					
Neuroleptics		Miscellaneous	Multipurpose adjuvants					
Nitrous oxide							Antihyperalgesic properties	Antihyperalgesic
NMDA antagonists		Miscellaneous	Neuropathic pain		Central sensitization	Central sensitization	Antihyperalgesic	Antihyperalgesic
NSAIDs	Nonopioids	Antipyretics	Non-opioids	Nociceptive inflammatory			Antihyperalgesic properties (some)	Antinociceptive
SNRIs	Coanalgesics	Antidepressants	Multipurpose adjuvants	Neurogenic		Descending inhibition		Descending modulation
Opioids	Opioids	Opioids	Opioids	Nociceptive somatic; neurogenic	↓ inhibition/ ↑ transmission	Descending inhibition	Hyperalgesic properties	Antinociceptive
Oxcarbazepine	Coanalgesics	Anticonvulsants	Neuropathic pain	Neurogenic		Peripheral sensitization; central sensitization		Peripheral transmission/ sensitization

(Table I continues on next page)

Table I
Continued

Drug	WHO	IASP	Lussier and Portenoy	Marchand	Costigan and Woolf	Beydoun and Backonja	Simonnet and Le Moal	Proposed Taxonomy
Sodium channel blockers								Peripheral transmission/ sensitization
SSRIs	Coanalgesics	Antidepressants	Multipurpose adjuvants	Neurogenic		Descending inhibition		Descending modulation
Sympatholytics		Miscellaneous	Neuropathic pain		Sympathetically maintained pain			
Topical analgesics		Topical	Topical					Peripheral transmission/ sensitization
Topiramate	Coanalgesics	Anticonvulsants	Neuropathic pain	Neurogenic		Peripheral sensitization		Peripheral sensitization
Tramadol						Descending inhibition		Mixed: antinociceptive and descending modulation
Tricyclics	Coanalgesics	Antidepressants	Multipurpose adjuvants	Neurogenic	↓ inhibition/ ↑ transmission	Peripheral sensitization; descending inhibition		Descending modulation

Abbreviations and symbols: IASP = International Association for the Study of Pain; NMDA= *N*-methyl-D-aspartate; NSAIDs= nonsteroidal anti-inflammatory drugs; SNRIs= serotonin-norepinephrine (noradrenaline) reuptake inhibitors; SSRIs= selective serotonin reuptake inhibitors; WHO = World Health Organization; ↓ decrease; ↑ = increase.

Table II
Proposed taxonomy of analgesics

Proposed taxonomy of analgesics
Antinociceptive Analgesics
Nonopioids
Acetaminophen (paracetamol)
NSAIDs
Opioids
Cannabinoids
Antihyperalgesics
NMDA antagonists
Gabapentinoids (gabapentin, pregabalin)
Levetiracetam
Lamotrigine
Nefopam
Nitrous oxide
Coxibs
Modulators of Descending Inhibition or Excitation
Tricyclic antidepressants
SNRIs
SSRIs
α_2-adrenergic agonists
Modulators of Peripheral Transmission/Sensitization
Local anesthetics
Carbamazepine
Oxcarbazepine
Topiramate
Capsaicin
Mixed: Antinociceptive Analgesics and Modulators of Descending Inhibition or Excitation
Tramadol
Tapentadol
Other
Calcitonin
Bisphosphonates

Abbreviations: Coxibs = selective cyclooxygenase-2 inhibitors; NMDA = *N*-methyl-D-aspartate; NSAIDs = nonsteroidal anti-inflammatory drugs; SNRIs = serotonin-norepinephrine reuptake inhibitors; SSRIs = selective serotonin reuptake inhibitors.

Table III

Analgesics used for different pain syndromes, with their molecular targets

Pain Syndrome	Symptoms/Localization	Mechanisms	Drug Targets	Analgesics (Commercially Available and *Experimental**)
Somatic pain	Acute pain: skin, muscle, tendon, fascia	Mechanical (trauma, fracture, dislocation, sprain), thermal (burns, frostbite), chemical injury (acid, base)	Prostaglandins Opioid receptors Voltage-gated Na^+ and Ca^{2+} channels NMDA receptors (if there is opioid-induced hyperalgesia) Neuropeptides (substance P, CGRP, galanin, etc.)	Acetaminophen NSAIDs Opioids Local anesthetics Ketamine Gabapentinoids *NK_1 antagonists* *CGRP-receptor antagonists*
Inflammatory pain	Diffuse pain, spontaneous pain, hyperalgesia, allodynia, edema: musculoskeletal tissue	Inflammation of tissue (inflammatory mediators)	TRPV1 Prostaglandins NGF/TrkA Bradykinin Serotonin (5-HT) CB_2 receptors	NSAIDs Steroids Capsaicin *NGF antagonists* *Bradykinin antagonists* *Serotonin antagonists* *CB_2 agonists*
Visceral pain	Diffuse pain, cramps, poor localization, autonomic nervous system involvement, referred pain: bladder, gastrointestinal tract, heart, other visceral organs	Visceral distension, ischemia, referred pain theories	Prostaglandins Opioid receptors Adrenoreceptors	NSAIDs Opioids $5\text{-}HT_3$-receptor antagonists Gabapentinoids Antidepressants *$5\text{-}HT_4$ receptor agonists* *κ-opioid receptor agonists: fedotozine* *Probiotics* *α_2- and β_3-adrenoceptor agonists* *CRF1-receptor antagonists* *TRP-channel antagonists* *Protease-activated receptor type 2 (PAR2)* *CRF2-receptor agonists*

Chronic pain neuropathic pain other chronic pain syndromes (e.g., low back pain)	Spontaneous pain (lancinating, burning pain, shock-like pain), paroxysmal pain, allodynia, hyperalgesia: central nervous system (trigeminal neuralgia), peripheral nerves (diabetic and postherpetic neuralgia), spinal cord injury, etc.	Central and peripheral lesions of the sensory system, ectopic discharges (altered Na^+ channels expression), sympathetically maintained pain, central sensitization	Voltage-gated Na^+ and Ca^{2+} channels Descending modulatory mechanisms in serotoninergic and adrenergic neurotransmission in the spinal cord α-adrenergic receptors NMDA receptors Cannabinoid receptors	Anticonvulsants Antidepressants Topical, intravenous local anesthetics Opioids Other anticonvulsants, antidepressants Cannabinoids Ketamine Marijuana, THC Phentolamine Guanethidine blocks
Cancer pain	Could be a combination of acute, neuropathic, visceral pain depending on the state of the disease: all organs, bone metastasis	All of the above mechanisms possible, as well as the mass effect of the tumor, bone changes	Voltage-gated Na^+ and Ca^{2+} channels Descending modulatory mechanisms in serotoninergic and adrenergic neurotransmission in the spinal cord α-adrenergic receptors NMDA receptors Cannabinoid receptors	Acetaminophen NSAIDs Opioids Local anesthetics Gabapentinoids Antidepressants Ketamine α_2-adrenoceptor agonists Marijuana, THC Bisphosphonates Calcitonin Radiotherapy
Migraine	Abnormal perception of otherwise normal circumstances, such as pain without evidence of primary nociceptive activation, and light and sound sensitivity without change in ambient stimuli: central nervous system	The disturbance in the brain is of the subcortical aminergic sensory modulatory systems; it probably includes brainstem, hypothalamic, and thalamic changes	Serotonin ($5\text{-}HT_1$) receptors CGRP receptors	Triptans, dihydroergotamine CGRP receptor antagonists *TRPV1 antagonists* *Prostaglandin E_4-receptor antagonists* *Serotonin $5\text{-}HT_{1F}$-receptor agonists* *Nitric oxide synthase inhibitors*

Abbreviations: CB = cannabinoid; CGRP = calcitonin gene-related peptide; CRF = corticotropin-releasing factor; 5-HT = 5-hydroxytryptamine; NGF = nerve growth factor; NMDA = *N*-methyl-D-aspartate; NSAIDs = nonsteroidal anti-inflammatory drugs; THC = tetrahydrocannabinol; TrkA = tyrosine kinase A; TRP = transient receptor potential.

* Experimental drugs are italicized.

Conclusion

Analgesics have been used since ancient times, and until recently, the most popular and effective drugs have been mainly based on extracts of the willow and the poppy. However, improved understanding of mechanisms of pain at cellular, synaptic, and molecular levels has opened a new area of drug development. Mechanisms that were not known before could lead to the emergence of new drug targets. Therefore, a rethinking of the classification of current analgesics was necessary. The taxonomy of analgesics has been addressed in the past by numerous authors and international organizations. However, no taxonomy has been completely satisfactory due to various reasons discussed in the previous section. More specifically, the words "adjuvants" and "coanalgesics" should now be avoided, and drugs should be classified according to a mechanistic pattern that will evolve with the discovery of new analgesics. Such a new and simple classification is proposed in this chapter.

References

[1] Beydoun A, Backonja MM. Mechanistic stratification of antineuralgic agents. J Pain Symptom Manage 2003;25:S18–S30.
[2] Costigan M, Woolf CJ. Pain: molecular mechanisms. J Pain 2000;1(Suppl 1):35–44.
[3] Dictionary.com. Available at: www.dictionary.com. Accessed July 31, 2009.
[4] Lussier D, Portenoy RK. Adjuvant analgesics in pain management. In: Hanks G, Cherny N, Christakis N, Fallon M, Kaasa S, Portenoy RK, editors. Oxford textbook of palliative medicine, 4th edition. Oxford: Oxford University Press; in press.
[5] Marchand S. The physiology of pain mechanisms: from the periphery to the brain. Rheum Dis Clin North Am 2008;34:285–309.
[6] Pilowsky, I. An outline curriculum on pain for medical schools. Pain 1988;33:1–2.
[7] Technology management strategies for the midmarket CIO. Available at: www.searchcio-midmarket.techtarget.com. Accessed July 31, 2009.
[8] World Health Organization. Treatment guidelines on pain related to cancer, HIV and other progressive life-threatening illnesses in adults. Adopted in WHO Steering Group on Pain Guidelines, October 14, 2008.
[9] World Health Organization. WHO's pain ladder. Available at: www.who.int/cancer/palliative/painladder/en/. Accessed July 31, 2009.

Correspondence to: Pierre Beaulieu, MD, PhD, Departments of Pharmacology and Anesthesiology, CHUM-University of Montreal, 3840 rue St-Urbain, Montreal, Quebec, Canada H2W 1T8. Email: pierre.beaulieu@umontreal.ca.

Part II

Specific Pharmacological Pain Targets

Targeting the Cyclooxygenase Pathway

3

Pascale Vergne-Salle[a] and Jean-Louis Beneytout[b]

[a]Department of Rheumatology and Pain Medicine, Dupuytren University Hospital Center, Limoges, France; [b]Laboratory of Biochemistry and Molecular Biology, Faculty of Pharmacy, University of Limoges, Limoges Cedex, France

The COX Pathway

Traditional nonsteroidal anti-inflammatory drugs (NSAIDs) are widely used to treat pain and inflammation. They act through inhibition of the two isoforms of cyclooxygenase (COX): COX-1 and COX-2. The long-term use of NSAIDs is limited by serious gastrointestinal (GI) side effects. Inhibitors selective for the type 2 isozyme were developed to minimize these complications. However, the role of selective COX-2 inhibitors in medical practice became controversial when evidence emerged that their use is associated with increased cardiovascular risk. A similar, but much lower, risk probably exists with traditional nonselective NSAIDs. Therefore, treatment of pain must take into account the GI and cardiovascular risk factors of individual patients.

Prostanoids

The more important prostaglandins, known as the "2-series" prostaglandins, belong to the eicosanoid family of oxygenated C20 polyunsaturated fatty acids. Cyclooxygenases, also known as prostaglandin endoperoxide H synthases, are enzymes that catalyze the insertion of two molecules of oxygen into polyunsaturated fatty acids. The major precursor of 2-series prostaglandins, arachidonic acid, is metabolized first into prostaglandin G_2 (PGG_2), and then into PGH_2, which is converted in a cell-specific manner to the

Pharmacology of Pain
edited by Pierre Beaulieu, David Lussier, Frank Porreca, and Anthony H. Dickenson
IASP Press, Seattle, © 2010

prostaglandin isoforms PGE_2, PGD_2, $PGF_{2\alpha}$, PGI_2, or thromboxane A_2 (TXA_2), which are called prostanoids (Fig. 1).

Prostanoids exert most of their action through membrane receptors. For example, four PGE_2 receptors have been identified and named EP1, EP2, EP3, and EP4. The EP1 receptor is associated with intracellular calcium mobilization, whereas EP2, EP3, and EP4 are G-protein-coupled receptors. EP2 and EP4 are linked to stimulation of adenylate cyclase via a stimulating G protein, and EP3 is linked to inhibition of adenylate cyclase via an inhibiting G protein.

Most studies of prostanoids have focused on the role of PGE_2 in inflammation, immune responses, and pain. Although the various prostanoids may have different effects, it is well known that activation of COX enzymes increases inflammation and pain and that NSAIDs and selective COX-2 inhibitors have anti-inflammatory and analgesic effects.

Phospholipase A_2

Arachidonic acid is a C20 polyunsaturated fatty acid that is located in the cell membrane. It is released from membrane phospholipids by hydrolysis of the sn-2 bond by phospholipase A_2 (PLA_2) enzymes and then oxygenated by cyclooxygenases. PLA_2 activity determines the amount of arachidonic acid that will be metabolized into prostaglandins.

There are three main classes of PLA_2 enzymes: secreted PLA_2 ($sPLA_2$), intracellular calcium-independent PLA_2 ($iPLA_2$), and cytosolic PLA_2 ($cPLA_2$) [58]. Calcium is

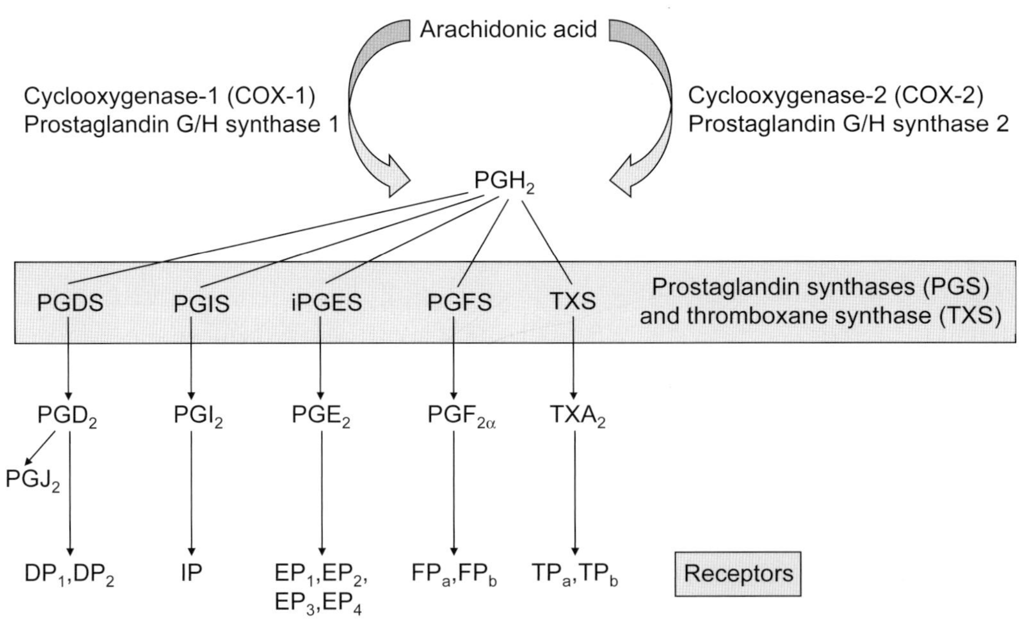

Fig. 1. Arachidonic acid is catalyzed to prostaglandin G_2 (PGG_2, not shown) and PGH_2 by the activity of cyclooxygenase enzymes. Then PGH_2 is converted to prostaglandin D_2, I_2, E_2, $F_{2\alpha}$ and thromboxanes (TXS) by prostaglandin and thromboxane synthases. These biologically active products bind to prostanoid receptors to produce contrasting biological effects.

required for $sPLA_2$ to exert its enzymatic function, whereas it is not necessary for $iPLA_2$ to be active, but in some cells, it seems to upregulate its activity [36,53].

Only one form of $cPLA_2$, known as $cPLA_{2\alpha}$, appears to have as a primary function the release of arachidonic acid from membrane phospholipids for prostanoid production. This enzyme, found in the majority of cells, shows a high specificity for the sn-2 position of arachidonic acid in phospholipids. The translocation of $cPLA_{2\alpha}$ from the cytosol to the nuclear envelope or to the endoplasmic reticulum is upregulated in the presence of increased intracellular calcium concentration or by phosphorylation of serines (505, 515, and 727) in its catalytic domain by mitogen-activated protein kinase (MAPK) and calcium-calmodulin kinase [54].

Two COX Isoforms

Each COX enzyme contains three domains: an N-terminal epidermal growth factor domain, a helical membrane-binding domain, and a catalytic domain at the C-terminus. The catalytic domain is constituted by two active sites, mechanistically linked but not adjacent to the cyclooxygenase and the peroxidase sites [27]. Arachidonic acid enters the catalytic domain, where it is cyclized and oxidized to PGG_2 (with a 15-hydroperoxy group) prior to being reduced to PGH_2 (reduction of the 15-hydroperoxy group) (Fig. 2).

The two isoforms of COX, COX-1 and COX-2, have 60% sequence identity and have similar catalytic mechanisms and similar K_M and V_{max} for arachidonic acid (i.e., maximum rate of enzyme-catalyzed reaction according to the Michaelis-Menten equation). COX-1 is called a constitutive enzyme because its expression is induced throughout the life of cells. COX-1 mRNA and protein are stable, and COX-1 protein levels are relatively constant. COX-1 is distributed throughout the body and has functions involving cell homeostasis such as platelet functions, cytoprotection in the GI tract, and renal perfusion.

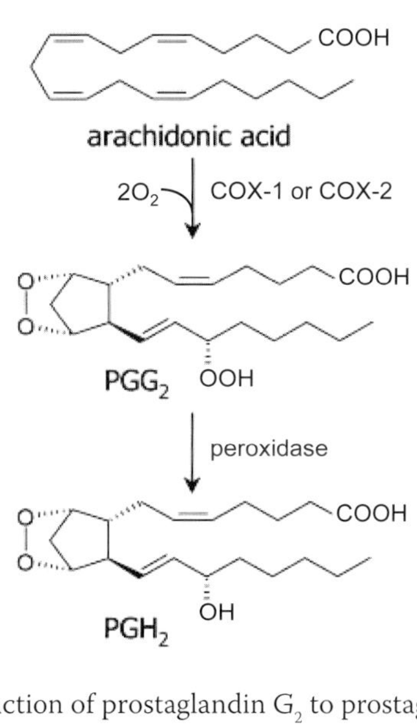

Fig. 2. Reduction of prostaglandin G_2 to prostaglandin H_2.

In contrast, COX-2 mRNA and COX-2 protein have shorter half-lives, and COX-2 protein is only present transiently during inflammation, pain, or cancer. COX-2 is thus considered an inducible enzyme. However, there are many exceptions: for example, COX-1 is inducible in the kidneys and liver under inflammatory conditions [25,28], and COX-2 is constitutively expressed in the blood vessels, kidneys, and central nervous system (CNS) [80].

Important differences are found in the promoter region of the two genes [3,72]. The promoter region of the COX-1 gene lacks the TATA box and CAAT box, causing COX-1 to be a constitutive enzyme in the majority of cells; however, the presence of two Sp1 motifs in the promoter region allows COX-1 to be induced in some cell lines by binding to Sp-1.

On the contrary, the COX-2 promoter region contains many transcriptional regulatory sequences such as a TATA box, two AP-2 sites, three Sp-1 sites, two NF-κB sites, and a CRE motif. Therefore, COX-2 gene expression can be induced by numerous growth factors and cytokines [78]. COX-2 can be upregulated during inflammation by pro-inflammatory cytokines such as interleukin-1β (IL-1β) and tumor necrosis factor-α (TNF-α); IL-1β is a major inducer of COX-2 in the CNS under inflammatory conditions [51]. Moreover, NF-κB and p38 MAPK pathways seem to play a role in the induction of COX-2 [3].

COX-1 protein is located in cells of the endoplasmic reticulum and in nuclear membranes, whereas COX-2 protein is found more often in nuclear membranes than in the endoplasmic reticulum.

In cells only expressing COX-1, prostaglandin synthesis begins a few seconds after treatment with classical stimuli such as hormones that bind to specific receptors, causing mobilization of intracellular calcium that activates $cPLA_{2\alpha}$ and induces the release of arachidonic acid and prostaglandin synthesis.

In the same cells, after other stimuli, some prostaglandins begin to appear later (45 minutes after stimulation) and continue to appear for several hours. This "late" phase involves a coordinated induction of $cPLA_{2\alpha}$ and COX-2, but because COX-2 degrades rapidly, COX-2 protein is present only transiently in these cells [54].

Despite their well-known beneficial effects, these compounds have side effects such as GI toxicity and nephrotoxicity due to the inhibition of physiological prostaglandin formation, and much work has been done to develop drugs that are better tolerated. The COX-2-selective inhibitors cause fewer GI side effects than NSAIDs, but in 2000, it was reported that these compounds could present unforeseen side effects, such as a higher risk of cardiovascular events. These results have prompted researchers to work on other targets such as prostaglandin synthases and prostanoid receptors.

Prostaglandin Synthases

PGH_2 has no significant biological properties. It serves as a substrate for enzymes that produce the prostanoids PGE_2, PGD_2, $PGF_{2\alpha}$, PGI_2, and TXA_2. PGE_2 is the most abundant prostaglandin in the human body, and PGE_2 synthase (PGES) enzymes have received the most research attention. The synthesis of PGE_2 is catalyzed by three different enzymes: a cytosolic PGE_2 synthase (cPGES) and two membrane-bound PGE_2 synthases, mPGES-1 and mPGES-2. Of these enzymes, both cPGES and mPGES are constitutively expressed; cPGES is associated with COX-1 and mPGSE-2 with COX-1 and COX-2. The mPGES-1 form is an inducible enzyme that is associated with COX-2 [63].

Much research has focused on mPGES-1, which belongs to the family of membrane-associated proteins involved in eicosanoids and glutathione metabolism. It requires glutathione as a cofactor for its activity and is located in the nuclear membrane. It is constitutively expressed in many tissues at low levels but is also induced in response to inflammatory stimuli such as IL-1β. mPGES-1 preferentially couples with COX-2 to increase the production of PGE_2 in inflammation, osteogenesis, and cancer [52]. mPGES-1 and COX-2 are coinduced by IL-1β, which acts by stimulating the extracellular signal-regulated kinase (ERK) pathway, one of the MAPK pathways.

The New Lipid Mediators in the Resolution of Inflammation

Lipoxins and Aspirin-Triggered 15-Epi-Lipoxins

Lipoxygenases (LOXs) constitute a family of lipid-peroxidizing enzymes capable of oxygenating polyunsaturated fatty acids to their corresponding hydroperoxy derivatives. In mammals, LOXs are classified with respect to their positional specificity of arachidonic acid oxygenation into 5-, 8-, 12-, and 15-lipoxygenases.

Lipoxins are "lipoxygenase interaction" products that are synthesized from arachidonic acid via the successive action of two different LOXs during cellular interactions to give specific trihydroxy-eicosatetraenoic acids: lipoxin A_4 (5S,6R,15S-trihydoxy-eicosatetraenoic acid) and lipoxin B_4 (5S,14R,15S-trihydoxy-eicosatetraenoic acid). Lipoxins are formed in vivo; they display anti-inflammatory effects and stimulate the resolution of inflammation (Fig. 3) [67].

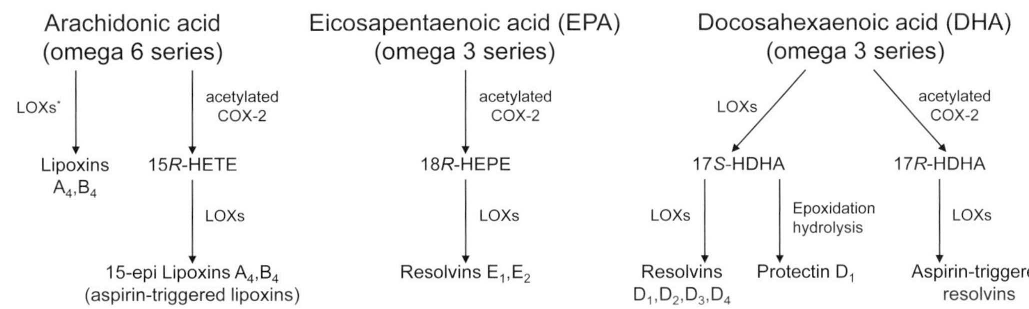

Fig. 3. New anti-inflammatory lipid mediators. LOX: lipoxygenase; 15*R*-HETE: 15*R*-hydroxyeicosatetraenoic acid; COX-2: cyclooxygenase-2; 18*R*-HEPE: 18*R*-hydroxyeicosapentaenoic; 17*S*-HDHA: 17*S*-hydroxydocosahexaenoic acid; 17*R*-HDHA: 17*R*-hydroxydocosahexaenoic acid; lipoxin A_4: 5*S*,6*R*,15*S*-trihydroxyeicosatetraenoic acid; lipoxin B_4: 5*S*,14*R*,15*S*-trihydroxyeicosatetraenoic acid; resolvin E_1: 5*S*,12*R*,18*R*-trihydroxyeicosapentaenoic acid; resolvin E_2: 5*S*,18-dihydroxyeicosapentaenoic acid; resolvin D_1: 7*S*,8*R*,17*S*-trihydroxydocosahexaenoic acid; aspirin-triggered resolvin D_1: 7*S*,8*R*,17*R*-trihydroxydocosahexaenoic acid; protectin D_1: 10*R*,17*S*-dihydroxydocosahexaenoic acid.

Aspirin has long been known to be an inhibitor of COX function, but this effect does not explain all of its pharmacological actions. When aspirin binds to cyclooxygenases, it inactivates them through acetylation of an active site, especially the serine 530 site. However, the acetylated form of COX-2 (aspirin-COX-2) is still active and is able to convert arachidonic acid to 15R-hydroxyeicosatetraenoic acid, which is then metabolized by a 5-lipoxygenase into a compound that is metabolized into two aspirin-triggered lipoxins, 15-epi-lipoxin A_4 and 15-epi-lipoxin B_4. Aspirin-triggered lipoxins share the potent anti-inflammatory effects of lipoxins [67].

The Bioactive Compounds Derived from Omega-3 Polyunsaturated Fatty Acids

Resolvins are a family of mediators recently discovered in inflammatory exudates in murine systems. The E-series resolvins are generated from eicosapentaenoic acid, an omega-3 fatty acid. This compound is metabolized by aspirin-COX-2 to 18R-hydroxyeicosapentaenoic acid, which is converted to resolvin E1 (5S,12R,18R-trihydroxy-eicosapentaenoic acid) by a leukocyte 5-lipoxygenase and to resolvin E2 (5S,18-dihydroxyeicosapentaenoic acid) by a human recombinant 5-lipoxygenase (Fig. 3). Resolvin E1 interacts selectively with two distinct G-protein-coupled receptors to reduce and promote resolution of inflammation [68].

The 17D-series resolvins are formed from docosahexaenoic acid, another omega-3 fatty acid, which is found at high concentrations in the brain and the retina. The action of at least two LOXs generates epoxide intermediates that are reduced to the 17S-resolvin D series. Resolvin D1 is also known as 7S,8R,17S-trihydroxydocosahexaenoic acid.

From docosahexaenoic acid, aspirin-COX-2 generates 17R-hydroxydocosahexaenoic acid, which is metabolized by LOXs to the 17R-resolvin D series (aspirin-triggered resolvin D). These compounds have anti-inflammatory properties and protective effects in some injuries. For example, researchers reported that they stopped migration of human and murine neutrophiles [66] and had protective effects against kidney injury in mice [14].

Docosahexaenoic acid is also metabolized into a 17S-HDHA via a lipoxygenase mechanism which is converted, after epoxidation and hydrolysis, into a 10R,17S-dihydroxydocosahexaenoic acid that is named protectin D1. This compound shows protective actions in corneal epithelial cells and can help prevent retinopathy.

All these compounds deriving from eicosapentaenoic acid and docosahexaenoic acid have anti-inflammatory and resolving properties and act in a cell-type-specific manner. Thus, these new lipid mediators may have therapeutic potential in pain and inflammation management.

Mechanisms of Action of COX-1 and COX-2 Inhibitors

The sequences of the active sites of COX-1 and COX-2 are highly conserved, but the 3D structures are significantly different. Indeed, the mutation of some amino acids results in a larger active site with a new cavity called a "side pocket." This "side pocket" is used by COX-2 selective inhibitors. The phenylsulfonamide group of SC-558 (a close analogue of celecoxib) interacts with the residues Arg513, His90 and Phe518 in the "side pocket" [38].

The COX inhibitors can be classified into five types. Aspirin is the only type that irreversibly inactivates both COX-1 and COX-2 by acetylating the serine 530 residue of the active site. The second type, including ibuprofen and mefenamate, consists of reversible, competitive inhibitors of COX-1 and COX-2, which compete with substrate for the active cyclooxygenase sites. The third group, including indomethacin and flurbiprofen, induces a slow, time-dependent inhibition of both isoforms. The fourth group induces a weak, time-dependent binding, as shown by naproxen and oxicams. The fifth group is represented by COX-2 inhibitors or coxibs, which bind tightly to COX-2 in a time-dependent manner [20].

Selective and Nonselective Nonsteroidal Anti-Inflammatory Drugs

Nonsteroidal anti-inflammatory drugs (NSAIDs) are among the most widely used drugs worldwide and are especially valued for their analgesic and anti-inflammatory properties. NSAIDs are the medications most commonly used to treat arthritic and inflammatory conditions as well as acute and chronic pain. They exert their major therapeutic effects by inhibiting COX, which is a key enzyme for prostanoid synthesis, as described above. In addition, they decrease the production of PGE_2 and PGI_2, that sensitize sensory fibers to painful stimuli. Researchers hypothesized that the inhibition of inducible COX-2 suppresses production of prostaglandins (especially PGE_2, which mediates inflammation and pain), whereas inhibition of constitutive COX-1 decreases the prostanoids involved in the maintenance of homeostasis (integrity of GI mucosa, platelet aggregation, and kidney function). The COX-2 strategy suggested that a drug with selectivity for COX-2 would have anti-inflammatory effects with fewer or none of the typical GI side effects of nonselective NSAIDs (ns-NSAIDs). Selective inhibitors of COX-2 (coxibs) were developed, such as celecoxib and rofecoxib, which had efficacy similar to that of traditional ns-NSAIDs in multiple phase II and III clinical trials [73]. However, data from long-term placebo-controlled chemoprevention trials indicate an increased rate of thrombotic cardiovascular (CV) adverse events compared with placebo.

These data triggered substantial debate about the GI benefits and the CV risk with coxibs in particular and with NSAIDs in general. The most important clinical question for patients with chronic rheumatic disease who require the use of a NSAID involves how to weigh the overall benefit/risk ratio of NSAID treatment.

Classification of COX Inhibitors

The biochemical selectivity of COX inhibitors toward COX-2 is currently assessed using human whole blood assays [10]. These assays are based on the measurement of PGE_2

production in response to lipopolysaccharides added to heparinized blood samples for 24 hours, which reflects the induction of COX-2 in circulating monocytes [60]. The parallel measurement of thromboxane B_2 production during blood clotting is used as an index of platelet COX-1 activity. Assessment of IC_{50} values (the concentration of the drug required to inhibit COX activity by 50%) for COX-1 and COX-2 and the calculation of the COX-1/COX-2 IC_{50} ratio for different NSAIDs leads to the conclusion that the biochemical selectivity of COX inhibitors is a continuous variable. Thus, it is difficult to fix a COX-1/COX-2 IC_{50} ratio value that separates nonselective from selective NSAIDs. However, for agents such as ibuprofen or ketoprofen and naproxen, such data are adequate to classify them as ns-NSAIDs. In contrast, the cluster of COX-2 inhibitors should include some traditional NSAIDs such as meloxicam, nimesulide, and diclofenac, as well as the coxibs. Among coxibs, there is a wide IC_{50} ratio, ranging from 30 for celecoxib to 433 for lumiracoxib, with the ratio for valdecoxib, rofecoxib, and etoricoxib falling between these values [77].

Evaluation of the Gastrointestinal Toxicity of NSAIDs

Gastrointestinal complications related to NSAID therapy are the most prevalent category of adverse drug reactions. Indeed, in a systematic review of case-control and cohort studies, the relative risk of upper GI tract bleeding/perforation after exposure to NSAIDs was 3.8 (95% CI = 3.6–4.1) [31]. In a meta-analysis by Ofman et al. [56], the pooled odds ratio of perforations, ulcers, and bleeds was 5.36 for the 16 randomized, placebo-controlled clinical trials, 2.7 for the 9 cohort studies, and 3 for the 23 case-control studies. The risk of GI ulcers and ulcer complications with ns-NSAIDs is 2–4%, is constant over time, and can be detected as early on as the first week of use [45]. Many of the risk factors for upper GI bleeding in patients taking NSAIDs are well defined. The predominant risk factors are previous ulcer history and older age (Table I).

Table I
Risk factors for gastrointestinal complications in patients taking nonsteroidal anti-inflammatory drugs (NSAIDs)

Patient-Related Risk Factors
Age >65 years
Previous history of ulcer
Helicobacter pylori infection
Concomitant severe comorbidities
Treatment-Related Risk Factors
NSAID dose
Combination of two NSAIDs
Concomitant use of aspirin
Concomitant use of corticosteroids
Concomitant use of anticoagulants and antiplatelet agents

A study undertaken in Spain investigated 50,114 GI bleeding episodes and found that 18,191 GI complications and 1,022 deaths could be attributed to the use of aspirin or other NSAIDs. The overall mortality rate was estimated as 1.5 cases per 10,000 patients taking aspirin or NSAIDs, a lower rate than those reported in previous studies in the United Kingdom and United States, probably because of the rise in the use of proton-pump inhibitors [43].

Do Coxibs Have a Clear Gastrointestinal Safety Advantage?

The Celecoxib Long-term Arthritis Safety Study (CLASS) was a double-blind, randomized controlled trial (RCT) of celecoxib (400 mg, twice daily) versus ibuprofen (800 mg, 3 times daily) or diclofenac (75 mg, twice daily) in 8,059 patients suffering from osteoarthritis (OA) or rheumatoid arthritis (RA) [69]. Twenty percent of participants were also taking low-dose aspirin. Fifty-seven percent of participants received treatment for 6 months. Celecoxib, at dosages greater than those indicated clinically, was associated with a lower incidence of ulcer complications compared with ns-NSAIDs (annualized incidence rate: 0.44% vs. 1.27%, respectively, $P = 0.04$). These results apply only to participants who were not taking aspirin. However, the long-term outcome of CLASS (a 12-month analysis) that was subsequently presented at hearings of the U.S. Food and Drug Administration (FDA) failed to confirm a significant advantage of celecoxib over the comparators.

In the Vioxx Gastrointestinal Outcomes Research (VIGOR) study, 8,076 patients with RA were randomly assigned to receive 50 mg per day of rofecoxib or 500 mg of naproxen twice daily [5]. During a median follow-up of 9 months, the rate of confirmed GI events (symptomatic upper GI ulcers and ulcer complications) was lower with rofecoxib compared to naproxen (2.1 versus 4.5 per 100 patient-years respectively; $P < 0.001$). The results were identical concerning ulcer perforation, obstruction, and bleeding (0.6 versus 1.4 per 100 patient-years; $P = 0.005$). However, unlike the CLASS study, patients receiving treatment with aspirin were excluded from this study. This fact probably explains in part the difference in GI safety findings for the two coxibs.

A second generation of coxibs has been developed that includes valdecoxib, parecoxib, etoricoxib, and lumiracoxib. The Therapeutic Arthritis Research and Gastrointestinal Event Trial (TARGET) aimed to assess the GI and CV safety of lumiracoxib compared with two ns-NSAIDs [64]. A population of 18,325 patients with OA was randomized to lumiracoxib (400 mg/d), naproxen (500 mg twice daily), or ibuprofen (800 mg 3 times daily) for 52 weeks, with stratification for low-dose aspirin use and age. Reductions in ulcer complications (perforation, obstruction, and bleeding) were significant in patients not taking aspirin and in the overall population, but not in those taking aspirin. Clearly, the co-administration of aspirin reduced the safety advantage of coxibs over that of ns-NSAIDs.

More recently, the Multinational Etoricoxib and Diclofenac Arthritis Long-term (MEDAL) program has pooled the results of three double-blind randomized comparisons of etoricoxib (60 or 90 mg/d) and diclofenac (150 mg/d) in 34,701 patients with OA or RA.

Low-dose aspirin and gastroprotective agents were permitted. Although uncomplicated GI adverse events and the rate of discontinuations due to GI adverse events were reduced with etoricoxib, the incidence of complicated ulcers, perforation, and bleeding did not differ significantly between the groups [2,35,42].

Garcia Rodriguez et al. [19] conducted a nested case-control study using the Health Improvement Network Database to evaluate the GI safety of coxibs in the general population. They identified 1,561 cases of upper GI complications associated with current use of ns-NSAIDs or coxibs between 2000 and 2005. The results indicated that ns-NSAIDs are associated with an overall three- to fourfold increase risk of GI complications, with an adjusted relative risk of 3.7 (95% CI: 3.1–4.3). Coxibs presented a better upper-GI safety profile than ns-NSAIDs, with a relative risk (RR) of 2.6 (95% CI: 1.9–3.6). The use of aspirin abolished completely the GI safety advantage of coxibs over ns-NSAIDs. The risk of GI complications was clearly determined by the daily dose of the individual agent and was higher with ketoprofen (RR: 5.4), indomethacin (RR: 7.2), and naproxen (RR: 8.1).

Serious lower GI events occurred at a rate of 0.9% per year in patients with RA taking naproxen, accounting for nearly 40% of the serious GI events observed in these patients. Serious lower-GI events were 54% lower with the use of rofecoxib [40]. In capsule endoscopic studies, celecoxib led to a significant reduction in lower bowel lesions compared with the combination of naproxen with a proton-pump inhibitor [22].

The Cochrane systematic review on GI safety of coxibs demonstrated a clear advantage of coxibs over NSAIDs, with a 60% relative risk reduction in clinically important ulcer complications [62]. There is good evidence that coxibs cause minimal gastroduodenal endoscopic damage [29,39]. The extent to which the endoscopic findings translate into clinical benefits remains unclear.

However, these data call for some remarks: (1) coxibs are not devoid of GI adverse events; (2) coxibs clearly decrease GI adverse events, but to an extent that is difficult to evaluate because the results differ with the patient's characteristics and NSAID comparators; and (3) we do not know if coxibs should be preferred over the combination of an ns-NSAID with a proton-pump inhibitor.

Cardiovascular Risk of Coxibs and Nonselective NSAIDs

The VIGOR trial in 8,076 patients with RA raised the first concerns about the risk of acute cardiac events associated with rofecoxib. The results showed that rofecoxib was associated with 5 times as many myocardial infarctions than was naproxen [5,76]. These findings were interpreted as being due to: (1) the inclusion of patients (4% of the study population) with a high risk of myocardial infarction who were not taking aspirin; (2) a cardioprotective effect of naproxen; (3) a deleterious effect of high-dose rofecoxib; or (4) a combination of these factors.

There are several mechanisms whereby NSAIDs can increase CV events in high-risk patients, such as an increase in blood pressure, as well as sodium retention due to the renal effects of COX inhibition. The other hypothesis is an imbalance between PGI_2 (a vasodilator and inhibitor of platelet aggregation produced by the endothelium via the COX-2 enzyme) and TXA_2 (a potent vasoconstrictor and prothrombotic prostaglandin produced by COX-1) (Fig. 4) [47]. Therefore, the selective COX-2 inhibitors could be responsible for the imbalance by inhibiting PGI_2 synthesis while not affecting TXA_2 production [26]. In contrast to aspirin, which irreversibly inhibits the production of TXA_2, the ns-NSAIDs are reversible inhibitors of platelet COX-1 with various potencies. Most ns-NSAIDs do not induce a sustained inhibition of platelet aggregation. One exception may be naproxen, which has a longer half-life [8].

Rofecoxib was withdrawn from the market by Merck in September 2004 when the APPROVe trial of rofecoxib (25 mg/d) versus placebo for polyp prevention showed a twofold increase in the number of CV events (myocardial infarctions and ischemic cerebrovascular events) [6]. The risk of thrombotic events became apparent after 18 months of rofecoxib treatment. This risk did not appear to be significantly influenced by baseline or subsequent use of low-dose aspirin. There was also an increased frequency of investigator-reported events such as hypertension, edema, and congestive heart failure, which occurred much earlier (at approximately 5 months).

A review of the CLASS study with celecoxib found no significant difference between treatment groups concerning the incidence of myocardial infarction. However, in contrast to the VIGOR study, the two comparator agents in CLASS—diclofenac and ibuprofen—have only weak platelet effects, and patients were allowed to take aspirin for CV protection.

The 3-year Adenoma Prevention with Celecoxib (APC) trial comparing celecoxib with placebo for prevention of colon adenoma was stopped early because of a significantly high number of CV events with celecoxib 400 mg and 200 mg twice daily [75]. A second placebo-controlled study (Prevention of Spontaneous Adenoma Polyps, PreSAP) with a

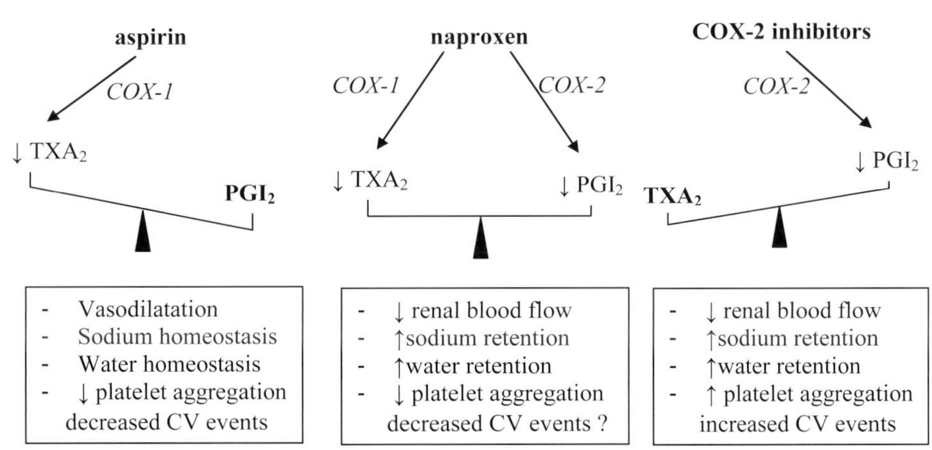

Fig. 4. Schematic representation of the balance between thromboxane A_2 (TXA_2) and prostacyclin (PGI_2) production after either low-dose aspirin, high-dose naproxen, or selective COX-2 inhibition, and the mechanisms implicated in modulation of cardiovascular (CV) events. Reprinted from [47].

comparable study design did not show any increased CV risk with celecoxib 400 mg daily after a similar mean treatment period (33 months). The placebo-controlled, three-arm Alzheimer's Disease Anti-inflammatory Prevention Trial (ADAPT) included 2400 volunteer subjects who were treated with naproxen or celecoxib (200 mg b.i.d.) and was stopped before the end. Surprisingly, in this study, it was the naproxen group that showed a significant increase in CV risk compared with placebo. The celecoxib group showed no abnormal findings [4].

Two studies with parecoxib in patients undergoing coronary artery bypass surgery suggested an increase in myocardial infarction compared with placebo [55,57]. But these studies included patients who were placed on a cardiac bypass pump and were taking aspirin postoperatively. Moreover, the events described included intraoperative myocardial infarctions that preceded the drug's administration. In April 2005, the manufacturer agreed to suspend the use of parecoxib/valdecoxib in Europe and the United States [30].

In the TARGET study, no significant difference was recorded in the composite CV endpoint (myocardial infarction, stroke, and CV death) between lumiracoxib and either ibuprofen or naproxen, irrespective of aspirin use [15]. However, the incidence of myocardial infarction fell with naproxen compared with lumiracoxib and rose with ibuprofen when compared with lumiracoxib, although the differences were not significant. Moreover, this study was underpowered to address the CV question and was not designed to establish the difference in CV risk among the treatment groups. The MEDAL (Multinational Etoricoxib and Diclofenac Arthritis Long Term) program was designed to assess the relative CV risk of etoricoxib versus diclofenac [7]. The investigators pooled data from three randomized double-blind trials in which patients with OA (n = 24913) or RA (n = 9787) were randomly assigned to etoricoxib (60 or 90 mg/d) or diclofenac (150 mg/d) (the MEDAL study, EDGE study, and EDGE II study). Patients with CV and GI risk factors were enrolled. When it was indicated, low-dose aspirin and gastroprotective agent were prescribed. Average treatment duration was 18 months. The results showed no discernible difference between etoricoxib and diclofenac. Indeed, the rates of thrombotic CV events were 1.24 and 1.30 per 100 patient-years for etoricoxib and diclofenac, respectively, and the hazard ratio was 0.95 (95% CI 0.81–1.11). The subgroup analyses showed that the presence of CV risk factors and the use of aspirin did not affect the results. However, congestive heart failure and edema were more frequent with the high dose of etoricoxib (90 mg/d) compared with diclofenac. Discontinuations due to hypertension were more frequent with both doses of etoricoxib than with diclofenac.

As described by FitzGerald [16], these results support the hypothesis that the CV risk from NSAIDs results from suppression of COX-2-derived PGI_2 and PGE_2. When the comparison spans a wide range of COX selectivity, a significant difference is observed among the CV events and even among complicated GI events, as in the VIGOR trial, in the studies comparing etoricoxib and naproxen, and in the TARGET substudy comparing lumiracoxib and naproxen. Conversely, comparison across a narrower spectrum of selectivity for COX-2, as in the MEDAL program (etoricoxib vs. diclofenac), fails to detect any difference in thrombotic events and also in complicated GI events.

Kearney et al. [33] published a meta-analysis of 138 randomized trials that compared coxibs with placebo or with an ns-NSAID to evaluate the risk of CV events. The results showed that coxibs were associated with a moderate increase in the risk of CV events, as were high-dose regimens of ibuprofen (2400 mg/d) and diclofenac (150 mg/d), but not high-dose naproxen (1000 mg/d). However, this meta-analysis was influenced by the largest studies—CLASS, VIGOR, and TARGET—and did not include the results of the MEDAL program. In a systematic review of the observational studies (case-control or cohort design), McGettigan et al. [48] confirmed the findings from randomized trials regarding the risk of CV events with rofecoxib, noting that the risk is dose-related and is observed during the first 30 days of treatment. These authors suggested that celecoxib in standardly used doses (up to 200 mg/d) may not increase the risk. Among ns-NSAIDs, naproxen, piroxicam, and ibuprofen had a relative risk close to 1. In contrast with previous hypothesis, the use of naproxen was not associated with any reduction in risk. Of more concern, diclofenac, an older NSAID, had the highest risk, which confirms the results of previous meta-analyses [32,33]. Diclofenac is one of the NSAIDs with the greatest COX-2 selectivity, whereas naproxen is the most potent inhibitor of COX-1. These observations suggest that relative COX-1/COX-2 inhibition may be important for cardiovascular risk.

Recently, Scott et al. [65] evaluated the available published evidence by undertaking a systematic review of the risk of myocardial infarction with coxibs and ns-NSAIDs in observational studies and with coxibs in RCTs in colonic adenoma and in arthritis. The overall risk of myocardial infarction appeared to be small or nonexistent with standard doses of most ns-NSAIDs and most coxibs. Rofecoxib showed a significant increase in the risk of myocardial infarction, and diclofenac showed a possible risk. The analysis of RCTs showed more myocardial infarctions with coxibs but fewer serious GI events. The MEDAL program, which found no difference in the risk of myocardial infarction between etoricoxib and diclofenac, was not included in this review. However, the interpretation of the MEDAL results depends on the assessment of risk with diclofenac, which is increased compared with the other ns-NSAIDs in the two systematic reviews described above.

The Association between Aspirin and NSAIDs

Low-dose aspirin is one of the main therapeutic strategies for the secondary prevention of myocardial infarction and stroke and is often recommended for the primary prevention of CV events in high-risk patients [49]. Aspirin acts as an irreversible inhibitor of COX-1, with antiplatelet effects that reduce thrombotic events. Therefore, a combination of aspirin and NSAIDs may decrease the CV risk potentially induced by NSAIDs. However, both aspirin and NSAIDs bind to the same active site on COX; in theory, therefore, a pharmacodynamic interaction between the agents may exist. Catella-Lawson et al. [11] showed that ibuprofen—but not rofecoxib, diclofenac, or acetaminophen—inhibited the antiplatelet effect of aspirin if taken before aspirin. Capone et al. [9] subsequently demonstrated another interaction between naproxen and aspirin, resulting in time-dependent inhibition of platelet aggregation.

Data from RCTs with coxibs do not show whether or not low-dose aspirin is cardioprotective because the numbers of participants are small, and those taking aspirin have a higher CV risk [76]. In the MEDAL program, there was no difference between etoricoxib and diclofenac in terms of CV events, and the subgroup analysis showed that the use of low-dose aspirin did not affect the results [7]. In the meta-analysis of 138 RCTs that compared coxibs with placebo or coxibs with ns-NSAIDs, there was no evidence that aspirin modifies the risk of CV events with coxibs [33].

A large cohort study showed that concomitant aspirin reduced the risk of CV events when given with rofecoxib and abolished the risk when given with celecoxib, meloxicam, or indomethacin, but this was not the case with ibuprofen [70,71]. The FDA published a warning in September 2006 against the use of ibuprofen with aspirin. However, the multiple observational studies, reviewed by Corman et al. [12], gave contradictory results such as those mentioned above, and their conclusions should be interpreted with caution. In the cohort study of McDonald [46], the combined use of aspirin and ibuprofen is associated with a higher risk of mortality from any cause or from CV events compared with the use of aspirin alone. A subgroup analysis of the Physician's Health Study suggested an interaction between aspirin and NSAIDs, with nearly 3 times the risk of myocardial infarction in patients using NSAIDs frequently [37]. However, this study included several limitations such as the self-reported use of NSAIDs. Another observational study included Medicare patients who were hospitalized for myocardial infarction and were prescribed aspirin at discharge [13]. The primary outcome was mortality within the first year after discharge, which was similar in the group with aspirin plus ibuprofen and in the group with aspirin plus other NSAIDs compared with the aspirin-only group. In contrast to the previous results, a matched cohort study showed a reduction in the incidence of myocardial infarction in patients taking concomitant aspirin and ibuprofen compared with those taking aspirin alone [59]. However, this study design also had significant limitations.

Kimmel et al. [34] conducted a case-control study in patients who had experienced their first nonfatal myocardial infarction. Exposure to the study drug was defined as any use within 1 week before the onset of symptoms of myocardial infarction or within 1 week of telephone contact for control patients. Among patients taking aspirin, NSAID use was associated with a reduction in risk of myocardial infarction in the unadjusted model, but not in the adjusted model for confounders. A secondary stratified analysis showed that aspirin did not reduce the risk of myocardial infarction in patients taking NSAIDs, making the results contradictory. In summary, in the absence of clinical RCTs, it is difficult to determine the potential advantage or appropriateness of concomitant use of aspirin and NSAIDs.

Are the GI Benefits of Coxibs Conserved with the Use of Concomitant Low-Dose Aspirin?

Some studies indicate that the GI benefits of coxibs are canceled out by concomitant aspirin use. In the CLASS study [69], the aspirin subgroup assigned to celecoxib had nonsignificant reductions in the number of symptomatic ulcers and ulcer complications [21]. In the APC study, GI events were more common among subjects taking celecoxib plus aspirin than among those taking placebo plus aspirin, whereas the overall results were in favor of celecoxib compared to placebo [74]. In another study, patients with OA received 81 mg enteric-coated aspirin alone or aspirin plus rofecoxib versus placebo or ibuprofen, and endoscopies were performed at 6 and 12 weeks. The rate of ulcers was similar between the rofecoxib plus aspirin group and the ibuprofen group, and both were higher than those of the placebo and aspirin-only groups [41]. In a case-control study in Spain including 2,777 consecutive hospitalized patients with endoscopy-proven GI bleeding, low-dose aspirin increased the risk of GI events with both ns-NSAIDs and coxibs [44].

On the contrary, in the larger MEDAL program, the 35% of patients taking aspirin plus etoricoxib had fewer uncomplicated GI events compared to patients on diclofenac plus aspirin [42]. In a meta-analysis of celecoxib trials, celecoxib was associated with a reduction of endoscopically detected gastroduodenal ulcers compared to ns-NSAIDs, irrespective of aspirin use [50]. In a large trial, patients taking 81 or 325 mg of aspirin received naproxen plus a proton-pump inhibitor (PPI), celecoxib, or placebo [24]. The occurrence of ulcers detected by endoscopy at 12 weeks did not differ between the group taking celecoxib and the group taking naproxen plus a PPI, irrespective of dose of aspirin. One additional endoscopy study gave the same results [23]. In a retrospective case-control study in elderly patients hospitalized for GI perforation or hemorrhage and taking low-dose aspirin associated with coxibs or ns-NSAIDs, a combination of aspirin plus coxibs (celecoxib or rofecoxib) reduced GI events by about 50% compared with a combination of aspirin plus ns-NSAIDs [61].

Overall, the coxibs seem to conserve their GI benefits when used in combination with low-dose aspirin. However, studies with contradictory results, such as those studies of Laine [41] and Lanas [44], make it difficult to draw a definite conclusion on this topic.

Use of Nonsteroidal Anti-Inflammatory Drugs: Recommendations

Advice from Regulatory Authorities

The U.S. FDA and the European Agency for the Evaluation of Medicine Products (EMEA) have formulated guidelines on the prescribing of coxibs. All COX-2 inhibitors are contraindicated in patients with ischemic heart disease or stroke. Clinicians must exercise caution when prescribing COX-2 inhibitors for patients with risk factors for heart disease, such as hypertension, hyperlipidemia, diabetes, and smoking, as well as for patients with peripheral arterial disease. Moreover, the FDA has determined that there are significant CV risks with all NSAIDs, whereas the EMEA concluded that coxibs present only specific risks.

Recommendations of the American Heart Association

The scientific statement from the American Heart Association (AHA) suggests a stepped-care approach to management of patients with musculoskeletal symptoms, as shown in Fig. 5. Initial treatment should focus on nonpharmacological approaches [1]. When choosing any medication, the prescriber should try the least risky medication first, with escalation only if the medication is ineffective. The AHA recommends starting with acetaminophen or aspirin, or even with opioid medications, for short-term pain relief. When these medications are ineffective, the next step could be an ns-NSAID, with naproxen as the preferred choice. Subsequent steps involve prescription of drugs with increasing degrees of COX-2-inhibitory activity, ultimately concluding with the coxibs. In patients with a risk of GI bleeding, a PPI may diminish that risk in those who require low-dose aspirin. If an NSAID is required, it may be reasonable to consider a COX-2 inhibitor. In patients at risk for CV events, prudence dictates extra caution in the use of COX-2 inhibitors. Renal function and blood pressure should be monitored. In patients using aspirin for cardioprotection, ibuprofen would reduce the protective effect of aspirin.

It is the first step of these recommendations that presents the greatest area of controversy. FitzGerald argues that there is little randomized evidence (among the drugs cited in the first step) on which to base a choice of drug with respect to either efficacy or unwanted effects [16]. Tolerance of opioids under chronic dosing conditions is not well known, and the GI profile of acetaminophen may resemble that of ns-NSAIDs [18].

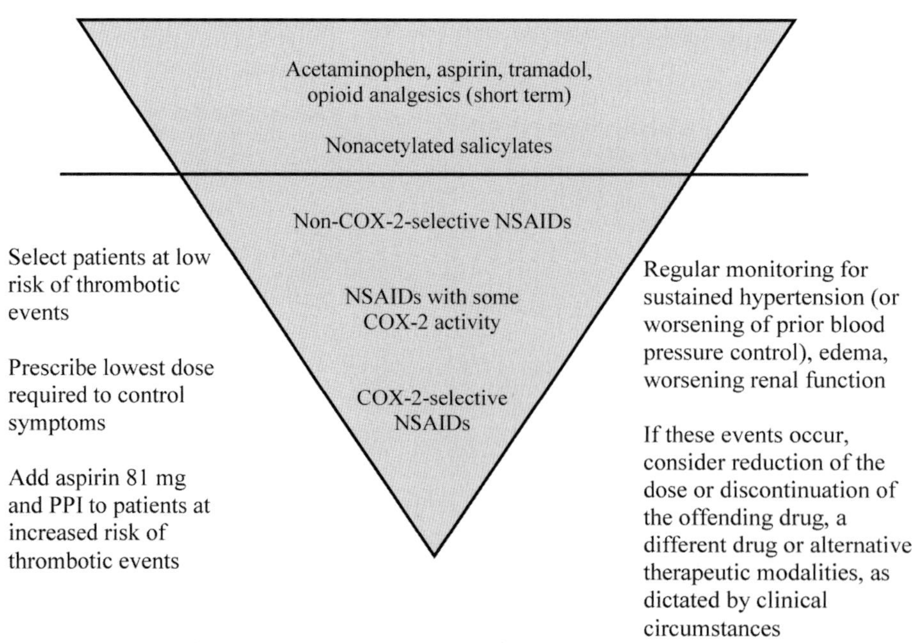

Fig. 5. "Stepped-care" approach to the management of musculoskeletal symptoms recommended by the American Heart Association [1]. PPI = proton pump inhibitor.

Recommendations of the Third Canadian Consensus Conference and Bolten

The recommendations of the third Canadian Consensus Conference [79] and those of Bolten [4] are less restrictive about the prescription of coxibs. Indeed, coxibs could be prescribed to patients with elevated GI risk and without CV risk, and a combination of a coxib and a PPI could be proposed for patients taking aspirin with or without an elevated GI risk (Table II) [79]. According to Bolten's recommendations, if there is a CV risk (patients taking aspirin) without a GI risk, an ns-NSAID (with or without a PPI) should be preferred to a coxib plus a PPI [4].

Table II
Guidelines for the use of nonsteroidal anti-inflammatory drugs (NSAIDs)

Aspirin Use	No Elevated GI Risk	Elevated GI Risk*
Not taking aspirin	ns-NSAID alone	Coxib or ns-NSAID + PPI
Taking aspirin	ns-NSAID + PPI or coxib + PPI	Coxib + PPI or ns-NSAID + PPI

Source: The third Canadian consensus conference [79].
Abbreviations: Coxib = selective COX-2 inhibitor; GI = gastrointestinal; ns-NSAID = nonselective NSAID; PPI = proton pump inhibitor.
* A patient aged 65 or over would be considered to have an elevated GI risk.

Recommendations of the American College of Rheumatology

Very recently, the American College of Rheumatology (ACR) published recommendations for the use of NSAIDs [73]. Among these recommendations, those concerning the toxicity of selective and nonselective NSAIDs are as follows. If a patient is taking aspirin for cardioprotective benefit, then selective NSAIDs and ns-NSAIDs should be avoided. If an NSAID is prescribed, then a PPI or misoprostol should be added to the regimen. A patient who is at moderate to high risk of a future CV event, is taking low-dose aspirin for cardioprotection, and needs continuous treatment of arthritis pain should be managed initially with acetaminophen or naproxen. Selective NSAIDs and other ns-NSAIDs have been associated with an increased CV risk. If the patient and provider agree to use an NSAID for arthritis pain relief and the patient is taking aspirin for CV prevention, then continuous use of ibuprofen should be avoided because the drug interaction reduces aspirin's cardioprotective benefit. If a patient and provider agree to use an NSAID for arthritis pain relief, and the patient has risk factors for GI bleeding, then the patient should be treated concomitantly with either misoprostol or a PPI. These recommendations are summarized in Table III.

Table III
Summary of the recommendations on the use of nonselective nonsteroidal anti-inflammatory drugs (ns-NSAIDs) and selective COX-2 inhibitors (coxibs)

Cardiovascular Risk Status	Low GI Risk (0 Risk Factors)	Moderate GI Risk (1–2 Risk Factors)	High GI Risk (≥3 Risk Factors or Aspirin Use)	Very High GI Risk (Prior Serious GI Complications)
No cardiovascular risk	ns-NSAIDs	ns-NSAIDs + PPI or M or coxibs	*Only if necessary:* coxib + PPI or M	Avoid all NSAIDs
Cardiovascular risk (hypertension, hyper-lipidemia, diabetes, smoking, peripheral arterial disease); aspirin use	ns-NSAIDs (naproxen) + PPI or M; short-term use; avoid ibuprofen	ns-NSAIDs (naproxen) + PPI or M; short-term use; avoid ibuprofen	*Only if necessary*: ns-NSAIDs (naproxen) + PPI or M; short-term use; avoid ibuprofen	Avoid all NSAIDs
Previous stroke; ischemic heart disease; heart failure	*Only if necessary*: ns-NSAIDs (naproxen) + PPI or M; short-term use; avoid coxibs	*Only if necessary*: ns-NSAIDs (naproxen)+ PPI or M; short-term use; avoid coxibs	Avoid all NSAIDs	Avoid all NSAIDs

Abbreviations: GI = gastrointestinal; M = misoprostol; PPI = proton pump inhibitor.

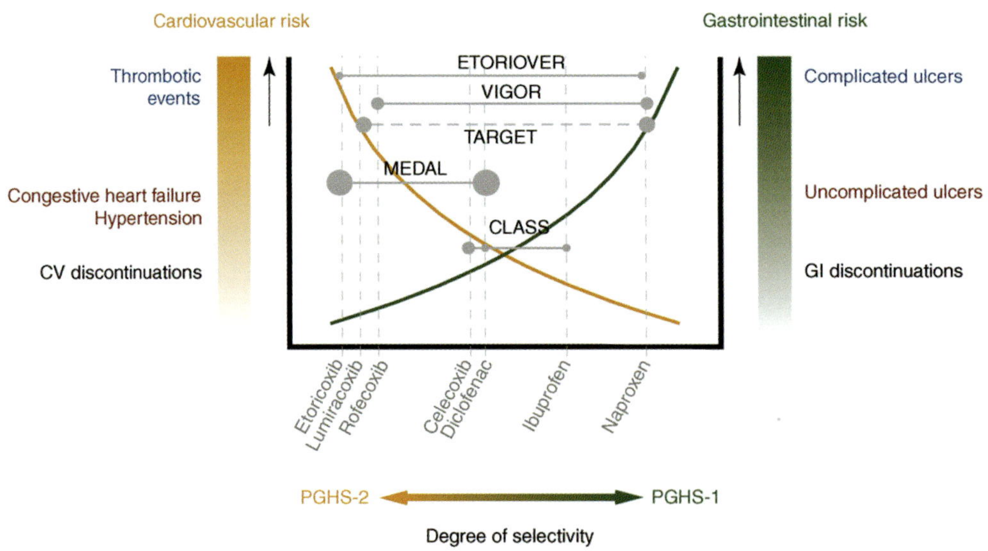

Fig. 6. Increasing degrees of selectivity for COX-2 are associated with augmented cardiovascular (CV) risk, whereas increasing degrees of selectivity for COX-1 are associated with augmented gastrointestinal (GI) risk. The relative size of the circles indicates the variation in sample sizes among the trials. ETORIOVER = overview of phase II and phase III trials of etoricoxib; VIGOR = Vioxx Gastrointestinal Outcomes Research study; TARGET = Therapeutic Arthritis Research and Gastrointestinal Event Trial; MEDAL = Multinational Etoricoxib and Diclofenac Arthritis Long-term program; CLASS = Celecoxib Long-term Arthritis Safety Study. Reprinted from [16].

Conclusion

On the whole, it appears that coxibs have a more favorable upper- and lower-GI safety profile than do ns-NSAIDs. However, coxibs cause myocardial infarction dose-dependently, and all NSAIDs seem to increase weakly the risk of myocardial infarction and thrombosis, with the probable exception of naproxen. The degree of CV risk is correlated with COX-2 selectivity, but also with variables such as dosing, frequency of administration, half-life, duration of treatment, cumulative exposure, and individual susceptibility [17]. Increasing degrees of selectivity for COX-2 seem to be associated with augmented CV risk, while increasing degrees of selectivity for COX-1 are associated with greater GI risk (Fig. 6). For treatment of pain and inflammation, NSAIDs should preferably be used for short periods, at a low dose and with an individualized and periodically reassessed prescription in order to balance the risks and benefits. Coxibs should be the first choice for patients with a previous history of severe GI events and a low CV risk, whereas ns-NSAIDs should be reserved for patients with a low GI risk. Patients with a high CV risk should continue receiving a low-dose aspirin, knowing that its coadministration with a coxib removes the GI benefits of the coxib and that coadministration with an ns-NSAID will increase the risk of GI toxicity and may lead to pharmacological interactions blunting the effect of aspirin, such as those described with ibuprofen. In patients with a history of GI complications and cardiovascular disease, there is insufficient evidence to guide decision making on NSAIDs. Moreover, there is no doubt that both ns-NSAIDs and coxibs substantially enhance the risk of increased blood pressure, sodium retention, and heart failure, all of which should be monitored.

References

[1] Antman EM, Bennett JS, Daugherty A, Furberg C, Roberts H, Taubert KA. Use of nonsteroidal anti-inflammatory drugs: an update for clinicians. A scientific statement from the American Heart Association. Circulation 2007;115:1634–42.

[2] Baraf HS, Fuentealba C, Greenwald M, Brzezicki J, O'Brien K, Soffer B, Polis A, Bird S, Kaur A, Curtis SP, et al. Gastrointestinal side effects of etoricoxib in patients with osteoarthritis: results of the etoricoxib versus diclofenac sodium gastrointestinal tolerability and effectiveness (EDGE) trial. J Rheumatol 2007;34:408–20.

[3] Bingham S, Beswick PJ, Blum DE, Gray NM, Chessell IP. The role of cyclooxygenase pathway in nociception and pain. Semin Cell Dev Biol 2006;17:544–54.

[4] Bolten WW. Problem of the atherothrombotic potential of non-steroidal anti-inflammatory drugs. Ann Rheum Dis 2006;65:7–13.

[5] Bombardier C, Laine L, Reicin A, Shapiro D, Burgos-Vargas R, Davis B, Day R, Ferraz MB, Hawkey CJ, Hochberg MC, et al. Comparison of upper gastrointestinal toxicity of rofecoxib and naproxen in patients with rheumatoid arthritis. N Engl J Med 2000;343:1520–8.

[6] Bresalier RS, Sandler RS, Quan H, Bolognese JA, Oxenius B, Horgan K, Lines C, Riddell R, Morton D, et al.; Adenomatous Polyp Prevention on Vioxx (APPROVe) Trial Investigators. Cardiovascular events associated with rofecoxib in a colorectal adenoma chemoprevention trial. N Engl J Med 2005;352:1092–102.

[7] Cannon CP, Curtis SP, FitzGerald GA, Krum H, Kaur A, Bolognese JA, Reicin AS, Bombardier C, Weinblatt ME, van der Heijde D, et al. Cardiovascular outcomes with etoricoxib and diclofenac in patients with osteoarthritis and rheumatoid arthritis in the Multinational Etoricoxib and Diclofenac Arthritis Long-term (MEDAL) programme: a randomized comparison. Lancet 2006;368:1771–81.

[8] Capone ML, Tacconelli S, Sciulli MG, Grana M, Ricciotti E, Minuz P, et al. Clinical pharmacology of platelet, monocyte, and vascular cyclooxygenase inhibition by naproxen and low-dose aspirin in healthy subjects. Circulation 2004;109:1468–71.

[9] Capone ML, Sciulli MG, Tacconelli S, Grana M, Ricciotti E, Renda G, et al. Pharmacodynamic interaction of naproxen with low-dose aspirin in healthy subjects. J Am Coll Cardiol 2005;45:1295–1301.

[10] Capone ML, Tacconelli S, Di Francesco L, Sacchetti A, Sciulli MG, Patrignani P. Pharmacodynamic of cyclooxygenase inhibitors in humans. Prostaglandins Other Lipid Mediat 2007;82:85–94.
[11] Catella-Lawson F, Reilly MP, Kapoor SC, Cucchiara AJ, DeMarco S, Tournier B, Vyas SN, FitzGerald GA. Cyclooxygenase inhibitors and the antiplatelet effects of aspirin. N Engl J Med 2001;345:1809–17.
[12] Corman SL, Fedutes BA, Ansani NT. Impact of nonsteroidal anti-inflammatory drugs on the cardioprotective effects of aspirin. Ann Pharmacother 2005;39:1073–9.
[13] Curtis JP, Wang Y, Portnay EL, Masoudi FA, Havranek EP, Krumholz HM. Aspirin, ibuprofen, and mortality after myocardial infarction: retrospective cohort study. BMJ 2003;327:1322–3.
[14] Duffield JS, Hong S, Vaidya VS, Lu Y, Fredman G, Serhan CN, Bonventre JV. Resolvin D series and protectin D1 mitigate acute kidney injury. J Immunol 2006;177:5902–11.
[15] Farkouh ME, Kirshner H, Harrington RA, Ruland S, Verheugt FW, Schnitzer TJ, Burmester GR, Mysler E, Hochberg MC, Doherty M, et al. Comparison of lumiracoxib with naproxen and ibuprofen in the Therapeutic Arthritis Research and Gastrointestinal Event Trial (TARGET), cardiovascular outcomes: randomized controlled trial. Lancet 2004;364:675–84.
[16] FitzGerald GA. COX-2 in play at the AHA and the FDA. Trends Pharmacol Sci 2007;28:303–7.
[17] Fries S, Grosser T, Price TS, Lawson JA, Kapoor S, DeMarco S, Pletcher MT, Wiltshire T, FitzGerald GA. Marked interindividual variability in the response to selective inhibitors of cyclooxygenase-2. Gastroenterology 2006;130:55–64.
[18] Garcia Rodriguez LA, Hernandez Diaz S. Relative risk of upper gastrointestinal complications among users of acetaminophen and non-steroidal anti-inflammatory drugs. Epidemiology 2001;12:570–6.
[19] Garcia Rodriguez LA, Barreales Tolosa L. Risk of upper gastrointestinal complications among users of traditional NSAIDs and coxibs in the general population. Gastroenterology 2007;132:498–506.
[20] Gierse JK, Koboldt, Walker MC, Seibert K, Isakson PC. Kinetics basis for selective inhibition of cyclooxygenases. Biochem J 1999;339:607–14.
[21] Goldstein JL. Gastrointestinal event rates in the CLASS study: 6-month vs long-term follow-up analyses. Gastroenterology 2002;122:A469.
[22] Goldstein JL, Eisen GM, Lewis B, Gralnek IM, Zlotnick S, Fort JG. Video capsule endoscopy to prospectively assess small bowel injury with celecoxib, naproxen plus omeprazole, and placebo. Clin Gastroenterol Hepatol 2005;3:133–41.
[23] Goldstein JL, Lowry SC, Lanza FL, Schwartz HI, Dodge WE. The impact of low-dose aspirin on endoscopic gastric and duodenal ulcer rates in users of a non-selective non-steroidal anti-inflammatory drug or a cyclo-oxygenase-2-selective inhibitor. Aliment Pharmacol Ther 2006;23:1489–98.
[24] Goldstein JL, Cryer B, Amer F, Hunt B. Celecoxib plus aspirin versus naproxen and lansoprazole plus aspirin: a randomized, double-blind, endoscopic trial. Clin Gastroenterol Hepatol 2007;5:1167–74.
[25] Graupera M, March S, Engel P, Rodes J, Bosh J, Garcia-Pagan JC. Sinusoidal endothelial COX-1-derived prostanoids modulate the hepatic vascular tone of cirrhotic rat livers. Am J Physiol Gastrointest Liver Physiol 2005;288:G763–70.
[26] Grosser T, Fries S, FitzGerald GA. Biological basis for the cardiovascular consequences of COX-2 inhibition: therapeutic challenges and opportunities. J Clin Invest 2006;116:4–15.
[27] Gupta K, Selinsky BS, Kaub CJ, Katz AK, Loll PJ. The 2.0 a resolution crystal structure of prostaglandin H2 synthase-1: structural insights into an unusual peroxidase. J Mol Biol 2004;335:503–18.
[28] Hartner A, Pahl A, Brune K, Goppelt-Struebe M. Upregulation of cyclooxygenase-1 and the PGE2 receptor EP2 in rat and human mesangioproliferative glomerulonephritis. Inflamm Res 2000;49:345–54.
[29] Hawkey CJ, Simon T, Beaulieu A; Rofecoxib Osteoarthritis Endoscopy Multinational Study Group. Comparison of the effect of rofecoxib (a cyclooxygenase-2 specific inhibitor), ibuprofen, and placebo on the gastroduodenal mucosa of patients with osteoarthritis. Arthritis Rheum 2000;43:370–7.
[30] Hawkey CJ. COX-2 chronology. Gut 2005;54:1509–14.
[31] Hernandez-Diaz S, Rodriguez LA. Association between nonsteroidal anti-inflammatory drugs and upper gastrointestinal tract bleeding/perforation: an overview of epidemiologic studies published in the 1990s. Arch Intern Med 2000;160:2093–9.
[32] Hernandez-Diaz S, Varas-Lorenzo C, Garcia Rodriguez LA. Non-steroidal anti-inflammatory drugs and the risk of acute myocardial infarction. Basic Clin Pharmacol Toxicol 2006;98:266–74.
[33] Kearney PM, Baigent C, Godwin J, Halls H, Emberson JR, Patrono C. Do selective cyclo-oxygenase-2 inhibitors and traditional non-steroidal anti-inflammatory drugs increase the risk of atherothrombosis? Meta-analysis of randomized trials. BMJ 2006;332:1302–8.
[34] Kimmel SE, Berlin JA, Reilly M, Jaskowiak J, Kishel L, Chittams J, Strom BL. The effects of non-selective non-aspirin non-steroidal anti-inflammatory medications on the risk of nonfatal myocardial infarction and their interaction with aspirin. J Am Coll Cardiol 2004;43:985–90.
[35] Krueger K, Lino L, Dore R, Radominski S, Zhang Y, Kaur A, Simpson R, Curtis S. Gastrointestinal tolerability of etoricoxib in rheumatoid arthritis patients: results of the etoricoxib vs diclofenac sodium gastrointestinal tolerability and effectiveness trial (EDGE-II). Ann Rheum Dis 2008;67:315–22.
[36] Kudo I, Murakami M. Phospholipases A2 enzymes. Prostaglandins Other Lipid Mediat 2002;68–69:3–58.
[37] Kurth T, Glynn RJ, Walker AM, Chan KA, Buring JE, Hennekens CH, Gaziano JM. Inhibition of clinical benefits of aspirin on first myocardial infarction by nonsteroidal anti-inflammatory drugs. Circulation 2003;108:1191–5.
[38] Kurumbail RG, Stevens AM, Gierse JK, McDonald JJ, Stegeman RA, Pak JY, Gildehaus D, Miyashiro JM, Penning TD, Seibert K, et al. Structural basis for selective inhibition of cyclooxygenase-2 by anti-inflammatory agents. Nature 1996;384: 644–8.
[39] Laine L, Harper S, Simon T, Bath R, Johanson J, Schwartz H, Stern S, Quan H, Bolognese J; Rofecoxib Osteoarthritis Endoscopy Study Group. A randomized trial comparing the effect of rofecoxib, a cyclooxygenase 2-specific inhibitor, with that of ibuprofen on the gastroduodenal mucosa of patients with osteoarthritis. Gastroenterology 1999;117:776–83.

[40] Laine L, Connors LG, Reicin A, Hawkey CJ, Burgos-Vargas R, Schnitzer TJ, Yu Q, Bombardier C. Serious lower gastrointestinal clinical events with nonselective NSAID or coxib use. Gastroenterology 2003;124:288–92.
[41] Laine L, Maller ES, Yu C, Quan H, Simon T. Ulcer formation with low-dose enteric-coated aspirin and the effect of COX-2 selective inhibition: a double-blind trial. Gastroenterology 2004;127:395–402.
[42] Laine L, Curtis SP, Cryer B, Kaur A, Cannon CP; MEDAL Steering Committee. Assessment of upper GI safety of etoricoxib in patients with osteoarthritis and rheumatoid arthritis in the Multinational Etoricoxib and Diclofenac Arthritis Long-term (MEDAL) programme: a randomized comparison. Lancet 2007;369:465–73.
[43] Lanas A, Perez-Aisa MA, Feu F, Ponce J, Saperas E, Santolaria S, Rodrigo L, Balanzo J, Bajador E, et al.; Investigators of the Asociación Española de Gastroenterología (AEG). A nationwide study of mortality associated with hospital admission due to severe gastrointestinal events and those associated with nonsteroidal antiinflammatory drug use. Am J Gastroenterol 2005;100:1685–93.
[44] Lanas A, García-Rodríguez LA, Arroyo MT, Gomollón F, Feu F, González-Pérez A, Zapata E, Bástida G, Rodrigo L, Santolaria S, et al. Risk of upper gastrointestinal ulcer bleeding associated selective COX-2 inhibitors, traditional non-aspirin NSAIDs, aspirin, and combinations. Gut 2006;55:1731–8.
[45] MacDonald TM, Morant SV, Robinson GC, et al. Association of upper gastrointestinal toxicity of non-steroidal anti-inflammatory drugs with continued exposure: cohort study. BMJ 1997;315:1333–7.
[46] MacDonald TM, Wei L. Effect of ibuprofen on cardioprotective effect of aspirin. Lancet 2003;36:573–4.
[47] Maillard M, Burnier M. Comparative cardiovascular safety of traditional nonsteroidal anti-inflammatory drugs. Expert Opin Drug Saf 2006;5:83–94.
[48] McGettigan P, Henry D. Cardiovascular risk and inhibition of cyclooxygenase. A systematic review of the observational studies of selective and nonselective inhibitors of cyclooxygenase 2. JAMA 2006;296:E1–11.
[49] Miller MC, Lucas BD, Papademetriou V, Elhabyan AK. Aspirin under fire: aspirin use in the primary prevention of coronary heart disease. Pharmacotherapy 2005;25:847–61.
[50] Moore RA, Derry S, Makinson GT, McQuay HJ. Tolerability and adverse events in clinical trials of celecoxib in osteoarthritis and rheumatoid arthritis: systematic review and meta analysis of information from company clinical reports. Arthritis Res Ther 2005;5:R644–55.
[51] Morita I. Distinct functions of COX-1 and COX-2. Prostaglandins Other Lipid Mediat 2002;68–9:165–175.
[52] Murakami M, Naraba H, Tanioka T, Semmyo N, Nakatani Y, Kojima F, Ikeda T, Fueki M, Ueno A, Oh S, Kudo I. Regulation of prostaglandin E2 biosynthesis by inducible membrane-associated prostaglandin E2 synthase that acts in concert with cyclooxygenase-2. J Biol Chem 2003;275:32783–92.
[53] Murakami M, Kudo I. Recent advances in molecular biology and physiology of the prostaglandin E2-biosynthetic pathway. Prog Lipid Res 2004;43:3–35.
[54] Muthalif MM, Hefner Y, Canaan S, Harper J, Zhou H, Parmentier JH, Aebersold R, Gelb MH, Malik KU. Functional interaction of calcium/calmodulin-dependent protein kinase II and cytosolic phospholipase A2. J Biol Chem 2001;276:39653–60.
[55] Nussmeier NA, Whelton AA, Brown MT, Langford RM, Hoeft A, Parlow JL, Boyce SW, Verburg KM. Complications of the COX-2 inhibitors parecoxib and valdecoxib after cardiac surgery. N Engl J Med 2005;352:1081–91.
[56] Ofman JJ, MacLean CH, Straus WL, Morton SC, Berger ML, Roth EA, Shekelle P. A metaanalysis of severe upper gastrointestinal complications of nonsteroidal anti-inflammatory drugs. J Rheumatol 2002;29:804–12.
[57] Ott E, Nussmeier NA, Duke PC, Feneck RO, Alston RP, Snabes MC, Hubbard RC, Hsu PH; The Multicenter Study of Perioperative Ischemia (McSPI) Research Group; Ischemia Research and Education Foundation (IREF) Investigators. Efficacy and safety of cyclooxygenase-2 inhibitors parecoxib and valdecoxib in patients undergoing coronary artery bypass surgery. J Thorac Cardiovasc Surg 2003;125:1481–92.
[58] Park JY, Pillinger MH, Abramson SB. Prostaglandin E2 synthesis and secretion: the role of PGE2 synthases. Clin Immunol 2006;119:229–40.
[59] Patel TH, Goldberg KC. Use of aspirin and ibuprofen compared with aspirin alone and the risk of myocardial infarction. Arch Intern Med 2004;164:852–6.
[60] Patrignani P, Panara MR, Greco A, Fusco O, Natoli C, Iacobelli S, Cipollone F, Ganci A, Créminon C, Maclouf J, et al. Biochemical and pharmacological characterization of the cyclooxygenase activity of human blood prostaglandin endoperoxide synthases. J Pharmacol Exp Ther 1994;271:1705–12.
[61] Rahme E, Bardou M, Dasgupta K, Toubouti Y, Ghosn J, Barkun AN. Hospitalization for gastrointestinal bleeding associated with non-steroidal anti-inflammatory drugs among elderly patients using low-dose aspirin: a retrospective cohort study. Rheumatology 2006;46:256–72.
[62] Rostom A, Muir K, Dubé C, Jolicoeur E, Boucher M, Joyce J, Tugwell P, Wells GW. Gastrointestinal safety of cyclooxygenase-2 inhibitors: a Cochrane Collaboration Systematic Review. Clin Gastroenterol Hepatol 2007;5:818–28.
[63] Samuelsson B, Morgenstern R, Jackobson PJ. Membrane prostaglandin E synthase-1: a novel therapeutic target. Pharmacol Rev 2007;59:207–24.
[64] Farkouh ME, Kirshner H, Harrington RA, Ruland S, Verheugt FW, Schnitzer TJ, Burmester GR, Mysler E, Hochberg MC, Doherty M, et al. Comparison of lumiracoxib with naproxen and ibuprofen in the Therapeutic Arthritis Research and Gastrointestinal Event Trial (TARGET), reduction in ulcer complications: randomized controlled trial. Lancet 2004;364:665–74.
[65] Scott PA, Kingsley GH, Smith CM, Choy EH, Scott DL. Non-steroidal anti-inflammatory drugs and myocardial infarctions: comparative systematic review of evidence from observational studies and randomized controlled trials. Ann Rheum Dis 2007;66:1296–304.
[66] Serhan CN, Hong S, Gronert K, Colgan SP, Devchand PR, Mirick G, Moussignac RL. Resolvins: a family of bioactive products of omega-3 fatty acid transformation circuits initiated by aspirin treatment that counter proinflammation signals. J Exp Med 2002;196:1025–37.

[67] Serhan CN. Lipoxins and aspirin-triggered 15-epi-lipoxins are the first lipid mediators on endogenous anti-inflammation and resolution. Prostaglandins Leukot Essent Fatty Acids 2005;73:141–62.
[68] Serhan CN, Chiang N. Endogenous pro-resolving and anti-inflammatory lipid mediators: a new pharmacologic genus. Br J Pharmacol 2008;153:S200–15.
[69] Silverstein FE, Faich G, Goldstein JL, Simon LS, Pincus T, Whelton A, Makuch R, Eisen G, Agrawal NM, Stenson WF, et al. Gastrointestinal toxicity with celecoxib vs nonsteroidal anti-inflammatory drugs for osteoarthritis and rheumatoid arthritis. The CLASS study: a randomized controlled trial. JAMA 2000;13:1247–55.
[70] Singh G, Mithal A, Triadafilopoulos G. Both selective COX-2 inhibitors and non-selective NSAIDs increase the risk of acute myocardial infarction in patients with arthritis: selectivity is with the patient, not the drug class. Ann Rheum Dis 2005;64:S85–6.
[71] Singh G, Graham D, Wang H, Mithal A, Triadafilopoulos G. Concomitant aspirin use reduces the risk of acute myocardial infarction in users of cyclooxygenase-2 selective and some non-selective nonsteroidal anti-inflammatory drugs. Ann Rheum Dis 2006;65:S61.
[72] Smith WL. Nutritionally essential fatty acids and biologically indispensable cyclooxygenase. Trends Biochem Sci 2007;33:27–37.
[73] Desai SP, Solomon DH, Abramson SB, Buckley L, Crofford LJ, Cush JC, Lovell DJ, Saag KG; The American College of Rheumatology Ad Hoc Group on Use of Selective and Nonselective Nonsteroidal Anti-inflammatory Drugs. Recommendations for use of selective and nonselective nonsteroidal anti-inflammatory drugs: an American College of Rheumatology white paper. Arthritis Rheum 2008;59:1058–73.
[74] Solomon SD, McMurray JJ, Pfeffer MA, Wittes J, Fowler R, Finn P, Anderson WF, Zauber A, Hawk E, Bertagnolli M; Adenoma Prevention with Celecoxib (APC) Study Investigators. Cardiovascular risk associated with celecoxib in a clinical trial for colorectal adenoma prevention. N Engl J Med 2005;352:1071–80.
[75] Solomon SD, Pfeffer MA, McMurray JJ, Fowler R, Finn P, Levin B, Eagle C, Hawk E, Lechuga M, Zauber AG, et al.; The APC and PreSAP Trial Investigators. Effect of celecoxib on cardiovascular events and blood pressure in two trials for the prevention of colorectal adenomas. Circulation 2006;114:1028–35.
[76] Strand V. Are COX-2 inhibitors preferable to non-selective non-steroidal anti-inflammatory drugs in patients with risk of cardiovascular events taking low-dose aspirin? Lancet 2007;370:2138–51.
[77] Tacconelli S, Capone ML, Sciulli MG, Ricciotti E, Patrignani P. The selectivity of novel COX-2 inhibitors in human whole blood assays of COX-isozyme activity. Curr Med Res Opin 2002;18:503–11.
[78] Tanabe T, Tohnai N. Cyclooxygenase isozymes and their gene structures and expression. Prostaglandins Other Lipid Mediat 2002;68–69:95–114.
[79] Tannenbaum H, Bombardier C, Davis P, Russell AS; The Third Canadian Consensus Conference Group. An evidence-based approach to prescribing nonsteroidal anti-inflammatory drugs. Third Canadian Consensus Conference. J Rheumatol 2006;33:140–57.
[80] Warner TD, Mitchell JA. Cyclooxygenases: new forms, new inhibitors and lessons from the clinic. FASEB J 2004;18:790–804.

Correspondence to: Pascale Vergne-Salle, MD, PhD, Service de Rhumatologie et Unité d'évaluation et de traitement de la douleur, CHU Dupuytren, 2 avenue Martin Luther King, 87042 Limoges, France. Tel: 33 5 55 05 64 69; fax: 33 5 55 05 68 89; email: pascale.vergne-salle@chu-limoges.fr.

Pharmacology and Mechanism of Action of Acetaminophen

4

Christophe Mallet[a,b] and Alain Eschalier[a,b,c]

[a]INSERM, Unit 766, Faculties of Medicine and Pharmacy, Clermont-Ferrand, France; [b]Laboratory of Medical Pharmacology, Faculty of Medicine, Clermont University, Clermont-Ferrand, France; [c]Pharmacology Service, Clermont-Ferrand University Hospital Center, G. Montpied Hospital, Clermont-Ferrand, France

Analgesic and antipyretic properties and superior tolerance make acetaminophen (also known as paracetamol) appropriate for widespread use in patients (including children, the elderly, and pregnant women). Yet despite many years of use worldwide and numerous studies, acetaminophen still jealously guards the secret of its mechanism of action. This analgesic is still a topic of conflict among research laboratories on many points: Does it have a central or peripheral action? What is its toxicity? What endogenous systems (opioidergic, serotoninergic?) or targets (COX-3?) are involved?

History

The story of acetaminophen began in 1886 with a medical error at the University of Strasbourg, France. Professor Kussmaul, from the Department of Medicine, asked two assistants, Cahn and Hepp, to prescribe naphthalene to a patient with intestinal parasites. The treatment had little effect on the parasites, but the patient's strong fever decreased. Because of a mistake made at the pharmacy, this patient had in fact been treated with acetanilide instead of naphthalene. The antipyretic property of acetanilide had just been discovered.

The publication of this property of acetanilide encouraged a chemist from the Bayer firm, Harmon Northrop Morse, to synthesize several derivatives of this molecule, including acetaminophen and phenacetin [103]. In 1893, Joseph von Mering introduced

Pharmacology of Pain
edited by Pierre Beaulieu, David Lussier, Frank Porreca, and Anthony H. Dickenson
IASP Press, Seattle, © 2010

the use of these two compounds in the clinic [164]. The following year, Hinsberg and Treupel [69] showed that acetaminophen was just as effective an antipyretic as antipyrine and phenacetin. Unfortunately, due to some clinical reports, they became convinced that acetaminophen was much more nephrotoxic than phenacetin [69]. Thus, acetaminophen fell into disuse for many years.

It was only after more than 60 years and a few cases of lethal renal insufficiency due to phenacetin that the "providential rediscovery" of acetaminophen was hailed. Indeed, studies by Brodie and Axelrod showed that, in patients, phenacetin was metabolized into *p*-phenetidin, responsible for its toxic effects on the kidney, and into acetaminophen [26]. At the same time, another team showed that acetaminophen is the major metabolite of acetanilide and phenacetin [154,155]. In addition, from 1948 to the mid-50s, the effectiveness of acetaminophen was confirmed in various pain models and numerous clinical trials [50]. Its tolerance, particularly with regard to renal function, seemed excellent, and its popularity began to grow. In 1950, acetaminophen was marketed to the United States in combination with aspirin and caffeine under the name of Triogesic. One year later, it was withdrawn from the market, suspected of causing agranulocytosis, although this fear was unfounded. In 1955, the Food and Drug Administration (FDA) allowed acetaminophen to be put back on the market in the United States. Acetaminophen (called paracetamol) was introduced in Great Britain and Australia in 1956. In France, acetaminophen appeared in 1957 combined with an antihistamine compound for use in children, and in 1961 acetaminophen began to be used in adults.

Therapeutic Use

The analgesic efficacy of acetaminophen was highlighted early on [50]. It has been used for mild to moderate pain [69]. However, acetaminophen has limited efficacy after major surgery [5,113] and has been found less effective compared to nonsteroidal anti-inflammatory drugs (NSAIDs) in some studies [81,142]. It provides enhanced (though moderate) analgesia when combined with NSAIDs, codeine, or dextropropoxyphene [77,142].

Several studies indicate that acetaminophen provides rapid pain relief for acute pain (postoperative pain, including dental extraction) [e.g. 11,101,142]. In these conditions, acetaminophen has morphine-sparing properties [68,82,113]. However, this effect has been questioned [5,29], pointing to potential bias in some studies. For example, the reduction in morphine requirement, although statistically significant, is modest (weaker than with NSAIDs [49]) and does not yield a significant difference in the incidence of opioid-induced side effects. Moreover, the morphine-sparing effect of acetaminophen seems to depend on the intensity of the postoperative pain [5].

Several studies support the efficacy of orally administered acetaminophen in relieving migraine pain [e.g., 117,131] and in lessening the functional disability, photophobia, and phonophobia associated with migraine [92]. However, intravenous acetaminophen is not superior to placebo in relieving pain in severe migraine attacks. [88].

In osteoarthritis, most studies [e.g., 161,168] show that acetaminophen provides effective pain relief, although it seems less effective than NSAIDs (for review, see [108]). Despite the relative superiority of NSAIDs over acetaminophen, the latter drug is recommended in first-line therapy to relieve pain in several clinical guidelines, such as those of the American College of Rheumatology [3] or the European League of Associations of Rheumatology [75], based on its higher safety profile.

Several clinical guidelines from around the world recommend acetaminophen as part of the first line of care for patients with low back pain [80]. However, a recent systematic review of randomized controlled trials performed to assess the efficacy of acetaminophen in the treatment of pain and disability in patients with nonspecific low back pain concluded that there is still insufficient evidence to determine the drug's effectiveness [44].

Acetaminophen is considered to be ineffective in neuropathic pain. However, it has been studied in combination with other analgesics such as tramadol [53] and codeine [111], with the combination being found effective. Acetaminophen is also effective in animal models of neuropathic pain [58].

In addition to its analgesic effect, acetaminophen is also widely used for its antipyretic effect because it has a better tolerability than NSAIDs, including aspirin [66,116]. However, some studies and meta-analyses would show superior efficacy of ibuprofen over acetaminophen for the relief of fever [58,66,116]. Recently, a study in children showed that a combination of acetaminophen and ibuprofen reduced fever more quickly and for a longer duration compared to acetaminophen alone (but not compared to ibuprofen alone) [66].

Acetaminophen is usually used orally in various preparations, but it is also widely used intravenously, especially for the management of postoperative pain. In this context, acetaminophen is either diluted in water (10 mg/mL) or, due to its low hydrosolubility, as a prodrug (propacetamol) that is soluble in water (1 g of the prodrug corresponds to 0.5 g of acetaminophen). Propacetamol metabolizes very quickly into acetaminophen and induces a rapid analgesic effect. Nurses and doctors must be cautious when they use this prodrug because of a risk of sensitization; a specific protocol has therefore been proposed for its use.

Finally, although experts have not reached consensus [9,10,63], several clinical studies show a correlation between the analgesic efficiency of acetaminophen and its concentration in plasma, with better efficacy for a dose of 2 g than for 1 g [76,120].

Pharmacokinetics

Absorption and Distribution

Absorption of oral acetaminophen involves passive diffusion with a first-order kinetic [9,33] linked to its physicochemical properties (weak base, pKa 9.5). Absorption occurs in the intestine (70%) and in the stomach and colon (30%). The rate of absorption is rapid, independent of the dose (Table I); it is influenced by gastric emptying and the type of pharmaceutical preparation. The T_{max} (time needed to reach the maximum plasma concentration) is between 15–60 minutes and 2–3 hours, depending on the pharmaceutical preparation and route of administration [10,33]. Bioavailability is dose-dependent [138], ranging from 63% to 89% after a single oral dose [33].

Acetaminophen is rapidly and uniformly distributed in the tissues [33], and protein binding is low (10%), which translates into a significant volume of distribution (0.8 to 1.4 L/kg in adults) [33,138]. Its passage through the blood-brain barrier is quite fast, and the concentrations found in the cerebrospinal fluid are similar to plasma concentrations [9].

Elimination

Acetaminophen is metabolized by the liver, and only 2–5% is excreted unchanged in the urine (Fig. 1). The first-pass metabolism in the liver depends on the dose and number of administrations [10,33]. Ninety percent of acetaminophen is metabolized by two major routes: glucuroconjugation (glucuronic acid) and sulfoconjugation (sulfuric acid); these routes rapidly reach saturation at doses higher than therapeutic doses [100,138]. Within 24 hours, 90% of the dose administered is excreted in the urine, mainly in the glucuroconjugated (60–80%) and sulfoconjugated forms (20–30%) [157] (Table I, Fig. 1).

Approximately 4% of acetaminophen is catabolized by cytochrome P450 [99,125] into NAPQI (*N*-acetyl-para-benzoquinone imine) [15], which is rapidly reduced by glutathione and excreted in the urine after conjugation to cysteine and mercapturic acid [130,137]. Cytochrome P450 2E1 (CYP2E1) is considered the major isoform involved in this metabolism in humans [112,137], but other cytochromes are also involved: CYP1A2, CYP2A6, CYP3A4 and CYP2D6 [112,130,137]. In acetaminophen overdose, sulfo- and glucuroconjugation systems are saturated, producing a massive accumulation of NAPQI [100,130,138] (see the section on hepatotoxicity below).

The total clearance of acetaminophen at therapeutic doses in healthy subjects is around 3 to 5 mL/min/kg, while clearance of derivatives is 7 and 9 mL/min/kg for glucuro- and sulfoconjugates, respectively [130]. The plasma half-life is about 2 hours [33] (Table I).

Pharmacodynamics

In 1971, John Vane showed that NSAIDs work by inhibiting the synthesis of prostaglandins [162]. The following year, in collaboration with Flower he proposed that acetaminophen acts preferentially on central cyclooxygenases (COX) [51]. Since this date, involvement of other systems and other targets have emerged, making the mechanisms of the analgesic action of this compound more complex and still unresolved.

Involvement of Cyclooxygenases in the Analgesic Action of Acetaminophen

Some authors have deepened this hypothesis by studying the effect of acetaminophen in vitro with purified COX. In most cases, acetaminophen is shown to be a weak inhibitor or activator of COX [158]. In cell culture, inhibition of COX by acetaminophen was observed in microglial cells [60]; platelets and leukocytes [150]; brain slices or homogenate [51]; endothelial cell culture from the human umbilical vein [25]; whole blood [165]; and tissue samples of aorta, lung, heart, and blood [166].

These cellular models have also been used to try to distinguish the involvement of COX-1 and COX-2 but again, data from the literature are contradictory. In fact, it appears that inhibition of acetaminophen on COX-1 or COX-2 or both would be dependent on cell type and experimental conditions [158].

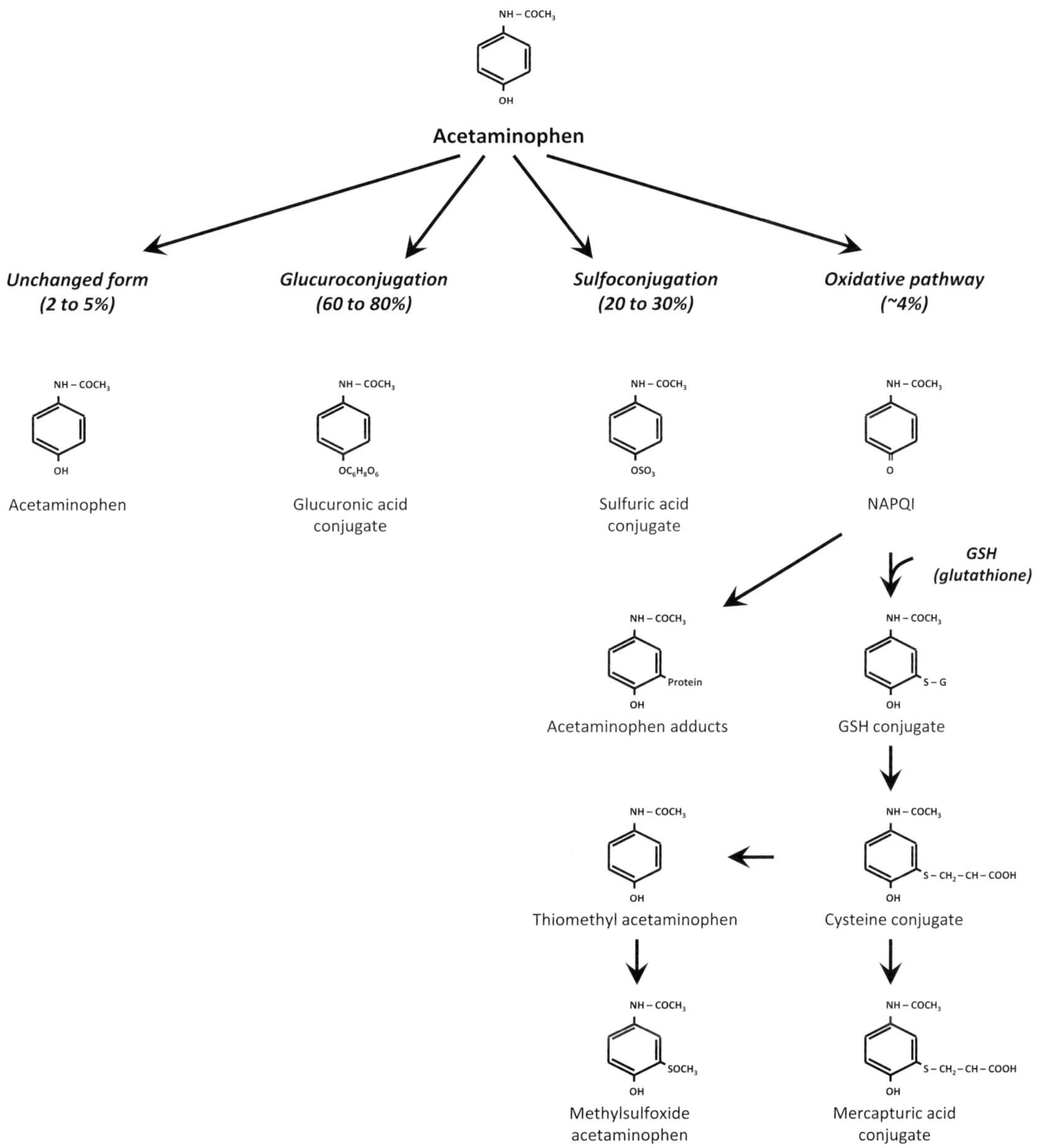

Fig. 1. Metabolism of acetaminophen in the liver after administration of therapeutic doses. GSH, glutathione; NAPQI, *N*-acetyl-para-benzoquinone imine. Adapted from Clissold [33].

Table I
Pharmacokinetics of acetaminophen (paracetamol)

Variable	Absorption/Distribution
T_{max} (time to maximum plasma concentration)	15 minutes (effervescent form) 30–60 minutes (other oral forms) 2–3 hours (suppository)
C_{max} (maximum plasma concentration)	5–23 mg/L (0.03–0.15 mmol/L)
Volume of distribution	0.8–1.4 L/kg
Protein binding ratio	10%
Bioavailability	0.63–0.89
Liver metabolism	
Sulfoconjugated form	20–30%
Glucuroconjugated form	60–80%
Renal excretion	
Elimination half-life ($t_{1/2}$)	1.5–3 hours
Total clearance	3–5 mL/minute/kg

Source: Adapted from Bannwarth and Pehourcq [10] and Clissold [33].

The prostaglandin E_2 (PGE_2) assay can provide direct evidence of the involvement of COX in the effect of acetaminophen. In cats, acetaminophen reduces prostaglandins in the cerebrospinal fluid simultaneously with its antipyretic action [48]. In addition, acetaminophen inhibits the release of PGE_2 in the dorsal horn of the spinal cord induced by the formalin test in rats and reduces the animals' pain behavior [104]. However, it does not inhibit the secretion of urinary PGE_2, $PGF_{1\alpha}$, or $PGF_{2\alpha}$, indicating that the synthesis of prostaglandins is not affected [104]. In mice, Ayoub et al. [7] show that acetaminophen reduced the number of abdominal writhings and the release of PGE_2 induced by intraperitoneal (i.p.) injection of iloprost (a PGI_2 analog) in central nervous system tissue but not in peripheral tissue. This effect is identical in genetically modified COX-$2^{-/-}$ mice, but is not found in COX-$1^{-/-}$ mice. Indeed, in COX-$1^{-/-}$ mice subjected to the abdominal writhing test, acetaminophen had no analgesic property and did not reduce PGE_2 production [7].

Clinical studies have shown that acetaminophen does not reduce inflammation in patients with rheumatoid arthritis [21]. In addition, concentrations of PGE_2 in the synovial fluid of patients with rheumatoid arthritis are not modified by acetaminophen treatment [141,152]. However, acetaminophen, orally administered at a dose of 500 mg, reduced the synthesis of prostacyclin, as measured by the inactive urinary metabolite, the 2,3-dinor-6-keto-$PGF_{1\alpha}$, in healthy volunteers without affecting the excretion rates of the urinary metabolite of thromboxane, the 2,3-dinor-TXB_2 [61]. The excretion of the urinary metabolite of PGE_2 is reduced in volunteers receiving 3 g of acetaminophen on each of two consecutive days [17]. Several studies have shown that acetaminophen reduces inflamed tissue after dental surgery [e.g., 20,153]. A microdialysis study in patients treated with 1 g of acetaminophen after surgical removal of the third molar revealed that the drug reduced the production of PGE_2, but not TXB_2, in the inflamed tissue compared to placebo [87]. However, no causal relationship between decrease of PGE_2 levels and analgesia has been described.

An ex vivo study, measuring the level of PGE_2 induced by lipopolysaccharide after inactivation of COX-1 (reflecting the activity of COX-2) and the level of coagulation induced by TXB_2 (reflecting the activity of COX-1), was conducted on blood samples of volunteers who received 1 g of acetaminophen orally [70]. Acetaminophen reduced COX-2 activity by 80% and COX-1 activity by 56% [70]. The inhibition of 56% of COX-1 activity is not sufficient to suppress platelet function, which would require inhibition of COX-1 by more than 95% [70].

In animal studies, an indirect way to investigate the interaction of a compound with the metabolism of prostaglandins is to measure the possible anti-inflammatory action of this compound. Various in vivo studies conducted to determine the ability of acetaminophen to induce an anti-inflammatory effect have led to divergent results. Seegers et al. [151] measured an anti-inflammatory effect of acetaminophen in a model of edema induced by carrageenan in the rat paw. This result was confirmed by other authors in the same or other models of inflammation [e.g., 140,163,167]. However, several groups have not observed any anti-inflammatory effect of acetaminophen in the carrageenan model or in other models of inflammation [e.g., 3,16,22,51,89].

Several hypotheses have been advanced to explain the molecular mechanism of inhibition of COX by acetaminophen: (1) Competition of acetaminophen with arachidonic acid on the active site of COX [38]. (2) Inhibition by NAPQI (*N*-acetyl-p-benzoquinone imine) [65]. This hypothesis has not been verified [148]. (3) Inhibition of a COX isoform in the central nervous system, commonly known as COX-3 [32]. COX-3, discovered in the canine brain, corresponds to COX-1 and the retained intron 1 (90 bp in dogs) [32]. This hypothesis was supported by experimental data that explain the antinociceptive and antipyretic actions of acetaminophen in this way [6,7]. However, a year after COX-3 was discovered, its existence was questioned. Studies reported that intron 1 of COX-1 was 94 and 98 bp in humans and in mice, respectively, leading to a frameshift and a premature stop codon [149]. Indeed, in mouse and rat, COX-3 mRNA encodes a protein that has a completely different amino acid sequence than that of the known COX isoforms. Researchers have concluded that COX-3 exists in vivo in multiple tissues but does not have any COX activity [78,156]. (4) Reduction of COX in an inactive form by inhibition of a peroxide tone [25,110,148]. (5) Inhibition of COX by AM404, another metabolite of acetaminophen [62,71]. Taken together, the published data have led us to conclude that there is no convincing evidence about the contribution of COX to the analgesic action of acetaminophen.

Involvement of the Serotoninergic System in the Analgesic Action of Acetaminophen

An interaction between the serotoninergic system and the analgesic effect of acetaminophen was first described by Hole's team in 1991 [159]. These authors showed that the action of acetaminophen was reduced after lesion of the serotoninergic bulbospinal pathway by 5,6-dihydroxytryptamine but not after lesion of the noradrenergic bulbospinal pathway by 6-hydroxydopamine. Later, these results were confirmed by Pini et al. [123], who reported that global depletion of central serotonin (5-HT) synthesis by *p*-chlorophenylalanine reduced the analgesic effect of acetaminophen.

Our team has demonstrated the involvement of spinal 5-HT receptors in the antinociceptive effect of acetaminophen. Intrathecal (i.t.) administration of different 5-HT receptor antagonists reduced the analgesic effect of acetaminophen [2,22–24,35,114]. Moreover, we demonstrated that the analgesic action of acetaminophen involves different 5-HT receptors depending of the nature of the stimulus. For example, i.t. administration of the 5-HT_{1A} receptor antagonist, WAY-100635, suppressed the analgesic effect of acetaminophen in rats subjected to the formalin test (a chemical stimulus) but not to the paw pressure test (a mechanical stimulus), whereas tropisetron, a nonspecific 5-HT_3-receptor antagonist, had the opposite effect. In a study to investigate the involvement of 5-HT_3 receptors, we showed that an antisense approach targeting these receptors failed to reduce the analgesic effect of acetaminophen, demonstrating the involvement of a spinal tropisetron-sensitive, non-5-HT_3-receptor-mediated effect [91].

The fact that acetaminophen affects different targets depending on the stimulus applied could be explained by the differential efficacy and power of 5-HT relative to different noxious tests [12] (see Chapter 9 by Kayser et al.). The nature of the stimulus may contribute to the different actions of the antagonists. A given stimulus could involve different neural pathways, offering an opportunity for a subtype of serotonin receptors to play a stimulus-dependent role.

Acetaminophen does not directly bind to 5-HT receptors [114]. Thus, a 5-HT mobilization mechanism and augmentation of this system has been hypothesized. Indeed, studies have revealed that acetaminophen dose-dependently increases tissue concentrations of 5-HT in the cortex, hypothalamus, striatum, hippocampus, and brainstem [35,123,124]. A release of 5-HT was also detected on depolarized neurons from slices of cortex and hippocampus previously treated with acetaminophen [35]. Moreover, an acute treatment with acetaminophen decreased the number of 5-HT_{2A} receptors in the cortex and brainstem [123,147]. This result was interpreted as a compensatory negative feedback response to an increased level of 5-HT. Indeed, the same phenomenon was observed in rats treated with a 5-HT_2-receptor agonist [41].

We have also shown that, in different pain tests, the involvement of 5-HT receptors is the same for 5-HT and acetaminophen [23]. This finding provides additional evidence that acetaminophen strengthens the serotonin bulbospinal pathway and mobilizes spinal 5-HT to exert its analgesic effect.

Another study focused on cellular events occurring in the spinal cord after activation of 5-HT_{1A} receptors in rats subjected to the formalin test and treated with acetaminophen (Fig. 2B). Observations included a phosphorylation of ERK-1; an increase of transcript and protein levels of low-affinity neurotrophin receptor, insulin-like growth factor-1

(IGF-1) receptor alpha subunit, and growth hormone receptor; and a reduced amount of somatostatin 3 receptor (sst3R) mRNA [24].

Recently, our team has shown the involvement of the serotoninergic system in the effect of acetaminophen in humans. Pickering et al. [119] showed that the administration of tropisetron (5 mg, i.v.) or granisetron (3 mg, i.v.) in a clinical pain model induced by electrical stimulation suppressed the analgesic effect of acetaminophen (1 g, p.o.). The

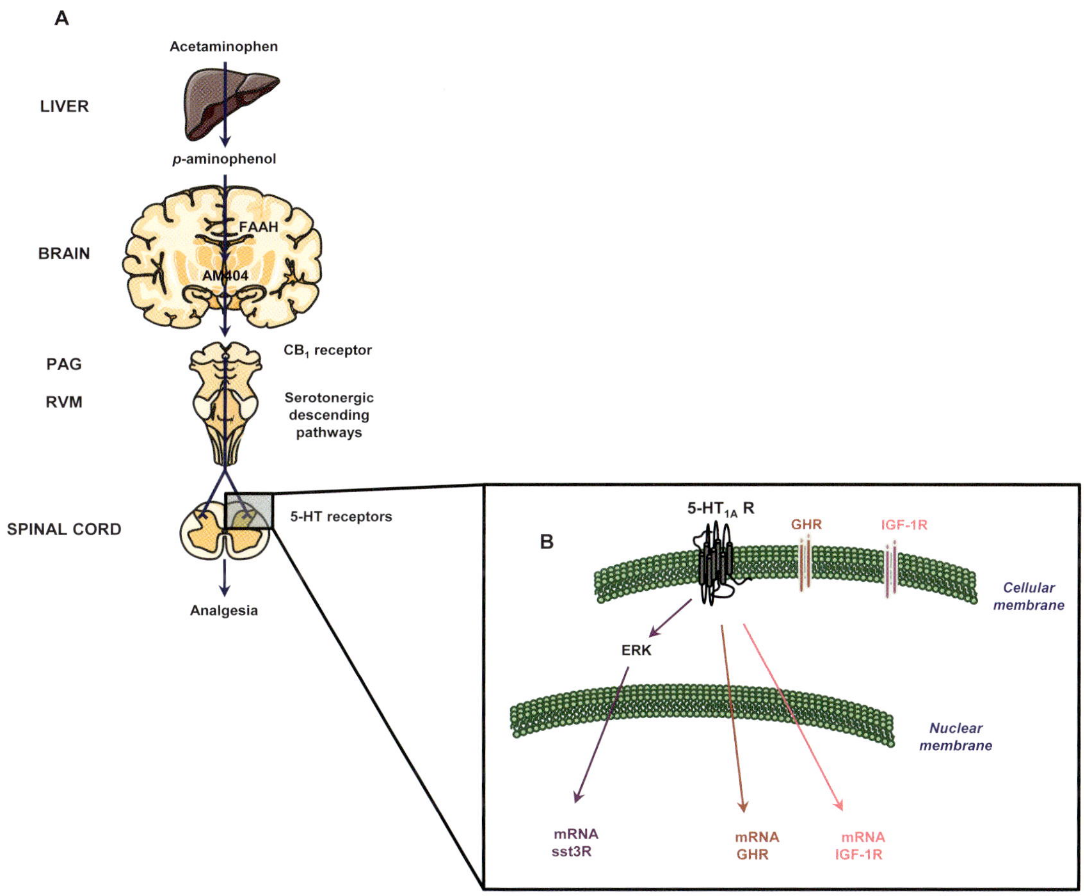

Fig. 2. Sequence of events suspected to be involved in the antinociceptive activity of acetaminophen after an oral administration. (A) Acetaminophen is deacetylated into *p*-aminophenol in the liver, and then metabolized into AM404 by fatty acid amide hydrolase (FAAH) in the brain. AM404 reinforces the activity of the supraspinal endocannabinoid system through CB_1 receptors, which in turn reinforce the activity of serotoninergic descending pathways. Spinal release of serotonin (5-HT) stimulates either the $5\text{-}HT_{3/4}$ receptors in a mechanical pain test or the $5\text{-}HT_{1A}$ receptors in a chemical pain test to inhibit the transmission of noxious stimuli and therefore produce antinociception. (B) Molecular events downstream of the $5\text{-}HT_{1A}$ receptor occurring in the spinal cord after acetaminophen administration in rats subjected to a chemical pain test. These events rely on an activation of the extracellular regulated kinase (ERK)1/2 pathway, a downregulation of somatostatin 3 (sst3R) mRNA, and an upregulation of protein expression such as growth hormone (GH) and insulin-like growth factor-1 (IGF-1) receptors, which are demonstrated to be involved in the antinociceptive effect of acetaminophen. GHR, growth hormone receptor; IGF-1R, insulin-like growth factor-1 receptor; PAG, periaqueductal gray; RVM, rostroventral medulla. Adapted from Mallet et al. [96] and Bonnefont et al. [24].

removal of this analgesic effect by tropisetron (5 mg, i.v.) was confirmed in another human study showing a reinforcement of inhibitory bulbospinal controls by acetaminophen, an effect that was inhibited by tropisetron [118].

Involvement of the Endocannabinoid System in the Analgesic Action of Acetaminophen

The team of Högestätt and Zygmunt [71] first suggested the possibility of an interaction between the endocannabinoid system and acetaminophen. They showed that after administration of $[^2H_4]$acetaminophen in rats, radioactive *p*-aminophenol (a metabolite of acetaminophen) and AM404 were detected in the brain. AM404 is a compound created by the FAAH (fatty acid amide hydrolase)-dependent conjugation of *p*-aminophenol with arachidonic acid. AM404 is also found in small amounts in the spinal cord, but not in the liver or blood, while *p*-aminophenol is present in all tissues, including the liver, where its concentrations are the highest. These authors also showed that AM404 formation after an i.p. administration of acetaminophen was suppressed in rats treated with PMSF, a nonselective FAAH inhibitor, or in $FAAH^{-/-}$ mice. The incubation of *p*-aminophenol in brain homogenates led to a FAAH-dependent AM404 synthesis, while very high levels of acetaminophen are needed to create detectable levels of AM404. All these data suggest that acetaminophen is deacetylated in the liver into *p*-aminophenol, which in turn is combined with arachidonic acid by FAAH in the brain to form AM404, a compound that (1) reinforces the activity of the endocannabinoid system through both the inhibition of cellular reuptake and the reduction of degradation of anandamide (via inhibition of FAAH), (2) activates the vanilloid receptor TRPV1 [170], and (3) inhibits COX [71].

A subsequent study in rats subjected to the hotplate test showed that pretreatment with a cannabinoid (CB_1) receptor antagonist prevented the antinociceptive effect of acetaminophen [109]. However, the high doses used in this study were questioned [96]. Another study showed that the antiallodynic and antihyperalgesic effects of locally administered acetaminophen in the paw of neuropathic rats involved peripheral CB_1 and CB_2 receptors [40]. However, no involvement of CB_1 receptors in the effect of acetaminophen was found in mice subjected to the phenylbenzoquinone-induced abdominal writhing test [64].

In line with the work of Högestätt et al. [71] previously described, we have recently demonstrated that FAAH and CB_1 receptors are involved in the analgesic action of acetaminophen [96]. Indeed, the pharmacological inhibition of FAAH or the pharmacological and genetical inactivation of the cannabinoid receptor CB_1 abolished the antinociceptive effect of acetaminophen in several pain tests [96].

Moreover, a link between the endocannabinoid and the serotoninergic systems emerged in this study. As previously shown for acetaminophen, the antinociceptive activity of arachidonyl-2'-chloroethylamide (ACEA), a CB_1-receptor agonist, was inhibited by a lesion of the bulbospinal serotoninergic pathways or by the i.t. injection of 5-HT_{1A}- and 5-HT_3-receptors antagonist, depending on the type of noxious stimulus [96]. Thus, we now propose a novel concept of the mechanism of the antinociceptive action of acetaminophen as a prodrug, involving the following sequence: (1) hepatic deacetylation into *p*-aminophenol; (2) central FAAH-dependent metabolism of *p*-aminophenol into AM404; (3) indirect involvement of CB_1 receptors by this metabolite; (4) endocannabinoid-dependent reinforcement of the serotoninergic bulbospinal pathways; and (5) involvement of spinal pain-suppressing serotoninergic receptors (Fig. 2A). However, further studies are needed to elucidate different steps in this sequence.

Involvement of Other Systems in the Analgesic Action of Acetaminophen

The Opioidergic System

The involvement of the opioidergic system in the analgesic action of acetaminophen was first described by Pini et al. [124]. Several subsequent studies have moved toward the same conclusions [e.g., 28,134,147]. However, other authors did not find any evidence to support an opioidergic mechanism. Indeed, naloxone did not inhibit the effect of acetaminophen, as evaluated by electrophysiological approaches [30] or using behavioral nociceptive tests with electrical [73], chemical [18], or mechanical stimulation [114].

Nitric Oxide Synthase

Investigators have demonstrated that the analgesic effect of acetaminophen is suppressed by i.t. administration of L-arginine, the substrate of nitric oxide synthase (NOS) [19], suggesting an inhibitory effect of NOS by acetaminophen. In parallel with these data, it is interesting to note that NOS inhibitors increased and prolonged acetaminophen's antinociceptive effect [27,28]. In macrophages, acetaminophen dose-dependently inhibited NO release as well as the expression of inducible NOS (iNOS) and interferon-γ induced by lipopolysaccharide [146].

It seems that the inhibition of expression of iNOS by acetaminophen is due to the binding inhibition of the transcription factor nuclear factor-κB on the promoter of iNOS [146]. In addition, on murine spinal cord slices, acetaminophen inhibited the synthesis of NO induced by glutamate and glycine [57]. These data are called into question by other studies showing that acetaminophen has no effect on the activity of NOS [132].

The Adrenergic System

Studies on the involvement of this system have led to contradictory results. Jensen et al. [73] showed that the antinociceptive effect of i.t. acetaminophen in rabbits was abolished by i.t. administration of yohimbine, a specific α_2-adrenergic receptor antagonist. Later, Pinardi et al. [121] studied the involvement of this receptor in mice subjected to the tail-flick test. Yohimbine did not significantly reduce antinociception induced by acetaminophen, but prazosin (a specific α_1-adrenergic receptor antagonist), and phenoxybenzamine (a nonspecific α_1- and α_2-adrenergic receptor antagonist) did reduce its effect [121].

In a test of abdominal writhing induced by acetylcholine bromide in mice, Raffa et al. [133] showed a synergistic effect of phentolamine (α_1-blocker) administered i.t. on the analgesic effect of acetaminophen administered by the same route [133]. In the same study, coadministration in the spinal cord of acetaminophen and antagonists (prazosin, yohimbine) or of an agonist (azepexole) of α-adrenergic receptors had no effect on the antinociceptive effect of acetaminophen [133].

Other rat studies have questioned the involvement of the adrenergic system, because neither a lesion of the descending noradrenergic pathway [159] nor a systemic administration of yohimbine [27,114] affected the antinociceptive effect of acetaminophen in the formalin test and the pressure test, respectively.

The Cholinergic System

The involvement of the cholinergic system in the analgesic action of acetaminophen was suggested by Miranda et al. [98]. These authors found that in mice subjected to the abdominal writhing test induced by acetic acid, the antinociceptive effect of acetaminophen (administered i.p. or i.t.) was potentiated by an i.t. or i.p. injection of neostigmine, an acetylcholinesterase inhibitor. The following year, the same group demonstrated that systemic administration of atropine, a nonselective antagonist of muscarinic cholinergic receptors, reversed the antinociceptive effect of acetaminophen in mice submitted to the tail-flick test [122]. Moreover, in this study, a central cholinergic depletion induced by an intracerebroventricular injection of hemicholinium-3 abolished the effect of acetaminophen [122].

The synergistic effect of neostigmine [98] and the antagonistic effect of atropine [122] on acetaminophen action could be interpreted as a supraspinal modulation leading to the release of acetylcholine in the spinal cord. This hypothesis is supported by the existence of several subtypes of muscarinic receptors in the dorsal horn of the spinal cord and by the analgesic effect of cholinergic agonists administered i.t. [46]. However, Abelson et al. [1] have shown that acetaminophen (administered subcutaneously) inhibited the release of acetylcholine in the spinal cord.

Antipyretic Action of Acetaminophen

It is commonly accepted that the antipyretic effect of acetaminophen involves the inhibition of COX [4,25,48,51,104]. Indeed, Ayoub et al. [6] showed a correlation between the hypothermic response of acetaminophen and reduced PGE_2 in the brain. In addition, this team showed that COX-$1^{-/-}$ mice treated with acetaminophen had reduced hypothermia compared to wild-type mice or COX-$2^{-/-}$ mice. They argued that this result would suggest an involvement of COX-3 isoform [6]. However, a recent study demonstrated that the COX-3 hypothesis was "irrelevant" with regard to the antipyretic or hypothermic effect of acetaminophen [90].

Adverse Effects/Toxicity

Hepatotoxicity

At therapeutic doses, acetaminophen is safe for the liver (for review see [84]). The hepatotoxicity of acetaminophen mainly appears in cases of acute poisoning, whether accidental or deliberate [126]. The problem of hepatotoxicity is of concern because acetaminophen poisoning is the most common cause of acute liver failure in the United States and Great

Britain [43,86], and acetaminophen overdose is the leading cause for calls to poison control centers in Australia [39]. Each year, acetaminophen overdose is the major cause for more than 56,000 emergency room visits, 2,600 hospitalizations, and an estimated 458 deaths due to acute liver failure in the United States [86]. Overdose occurs after ingestion of more than 8 to 10 g for adults and 125 mg/kg in children. A "nomogram" was performed to correlate the plasma concentrations of acetaminophen and the risk of hepatotoxicity in order to improve the prognosis of acute poisoning [128].

After an overdose of acetaminophen, the glucuroconjugation and sulfoconjugation pathways (previously described) become saturated, shifting acetaminophen into the cytochrome CYP pathway [100,138]. The elevated level of the toxic NAPQI metabolite extensively depletes hepatocellular glutathione [144] and covalently binds to mitochondrial proteins [105]. The precise biochemical mechanism of cell necrosis is not fully understood, but many lines of evidence suggest multicellular events, summarized as follows (for reviews, see [72,84,139]). Covalent binding to mitochondrial proteins may be responsible for the initial mitochondrial dysfunction. This dysfunction, associated with ATP depletion, extensive DNA fragmentation, alteration of the calcium homeostasis, and modification of intracellular proteins, contributes to the development of oncotic necrotic cell death in the liver after acetaminophen overdose.

Researchers have investigated acetaminophen protein adducts (combination of NAPQI with liver proteins) of acetaminophen as specific markers of the drug's liver toxicity [43]. These adducts are specifically detectable in cases of liver failure without overdose [43]. This finding is particularly interesting with regard to situations in which there is a risk of liver damage at therapeutic doses (alcohol consumption, malnutrition, or use in children or older adults) or in an idiosyncratic reaction.

N-acetylcysteine (NAC), available since 1974, is the antidote for acetaminophen poisoning [128]. It works by regenerating stocks of mitochondrial and cytoplasmic glutathione, but it can also repair oxidative damage caused by NAPQI, either directly or by generating glutathione [67]. NAC is most effective when administered to patients within 8 to 10 hours after acetaminophen ingestion [145]. Adverse effects of NAC may include anaphylactic reactions, nausea, vomiting, and diarrhea.

Renal Toxicity

Numerous epidemiological, experimental, and clinical studies demonstrate that acetaminophen, in normal use, even for long periods, would not induce specific nephrotoxicity [59,129]. However, overdose of acetaminophen can cause severe kidney necrosis in humans and animals [52,79]. This renal toxicity could involve NAPQI, which would share the same toxic mechanism as that previously described in the liver [99]. Another mechanism could involve *p*-aminophenol obtained after deacetylation of acetaminophen. Indeed, this biotransformation has been demonstrated in the kidneys [31], and *p*-aminophenol has long been known as a powerfully nephrotoxic compound [14] with relatively low hepatotoxicity [36]. It appears that deacetylation [106] is involved in the nephrotoxicity of acetaminophen in rats. Acetaminophen and *p*-aminophenol induce identical kidney damage and lead to a reduced concentration of renal glutathione [107].

Gastrotoxicity

Several epidemiological studies show that acetaminophen has excellent digestive tolerance [74,102]. However, two studies have shown a correlation between acetaminophen use and an increased risk of gastrointestinal adverse effects [55,135], but these data have been criticized [8,37]. Clinical and preclinical studies have shown that acetaminophen was not only weakly "aggressive" to the gastroduodenal mucosa [136] but also had a protective role for the gastric mucosa against injury induced by acetylsalicylic acid, alcohol, and stress.

Hemotoxicity

Acetaminophen has good hematological tolerability and does not alter hemostasis. Rare disorders of blood cells have been attributed to acetaminophen, including thrombocytopenia and agranulocytosis.

Other Side Effects

Allergic reactions are rare with acetaminophen, although the occurrence of anaphylactic shock has been reported [54]. Other reports of rare side effects have not clearly demonstrated that acetaminophen was responsible. These reports include facilitation of asthma attacks, Stevens-Johnson syndrome, acute pancreatitis when acetaminophen is used in combination with codeine, chronic active hepatitis, granulomatous hepatitis, rectal ulceration with rectal administration, vascular purpura, and rhabdomyolysis.

Consumer Safety Considerations and Contraindications

Drug Interactions

Some studies suggest that acetaminophen may potentiate the effect of anticoagulants, thus increasing the risk of bleeding in patients receiving both drugs [56,160]. However, all these studies must be interpreted with caution because of methodological bias: retrospective studies, unsatisfactory assessment of coagulation, low numbers of patients, and high doses of acetaminophen that do not reflect normal therapeutic use [95]. In addition, differences in study protocols may explain the differing results. This effect is a matter of debate dating back 40 years because some studies do not show any potentiation of anticoagulants [47]. In 2005, a prospective double-blind placebo study showed that acetaminophen (4 g/day, p.o.) induced a significant increase in INR (anticoagulant effect expressed as the international normalized ratio) in patients receiving stabilized warfarin treatment [94]. The following year, the same team confirmed their results and studied the biological process causing the potentiation [93]. It could involve the cytochrome P450 enzymes leading to an increased plasma level of warfarin [95,160]. However, this hypothesis seems unlikely because, in response to acetaminophen, plasma concentration of warfarin remains constant while the INR increases [56]. The other assumption is the interaction of acetaminophen or its metabolites with enzymes involved in the synthesis of clotting factors dependent on vitamin K, which could potentiate the anticoagulant response generated by warfarin. Indeed, a recent study showed that patients receiving a stabilized oral treatment of warfarin and acetaminophen (4 g/day, p.o.) had an increased INR and decreased plasma vitamin K-dependent clotting factors II, VII, IX, and X [93].

Liver Failure

In patients with liver failure, acetaminophen, at therapeutic dose, has an increased half-life time but does not seem to cause further liver damage [13].

Renal Failure

In patients with renal failure who are taking acetaminophen at therapeutic doses, the plasma half-life of its sulfo- and glucuroconjugated metabolites is increased [97]. Despite some controversial cases showing an increased risk of renal failure [52,115], acetaminophen is the non-opioid analgesic of choice in these patients. A maximum dose of 3 g daily (1 g three times a day) is recommended in these patients.

Alcohol-Related Toxicity

Numerous studies have reported that acetaminophen hepatotoxicity is potentiated in patients with chronic alcoholism [e.g., 34,169]. Because of the high doses, methodological bias, or lack of accuracy of these studies, other authors have questioned these data [42,86,143]. Some studies do not show increased hepatotoxicity [83,127]. In animals, chronic administration of ethanol induced acetaminophen hepatotoxicity. However, human studies have found no increase of toxic metabolites of acetaminophen in subjects with chronic alcoholism [85]. It is clear that acetaminophen toxicity in individuals with alcoholism is complex and that further studies remain to be carried out.

Conclusion

While acetaminophen is an old drug, widely used all over the world, this chapter shows that it remains a mystery and that research studies are still needed to understand both the mechanism of its therapeutic effects and its hepatotoxicity. However, data summarized in this chapter provide a new profile of the analgesic action of acetaminophen, which seems to be a prodrug involving a complex network including various metabolites and different endogenous systems of neuromediation. This complexity leads us to predict that acetaminophen will not cease to surprise us. We think that a better understanding of acetaminophen's mechanism of action will highlight molecular targets that will lead to novel analgesics with better efficacy.

References

[1] Abelson KS, Kommalage M, Hoglund AU. Spinal cholinergic involvement after treatment with aspirin and paracetamol in rats. Neurosci Lett 2004;368:116–20.

[2] Alloui A, Chassaing C, Schmidt J, Ardid D, Dubray C, Cloarec A, Eschalier A. Paracetamol exerts a spinal, tropisetron-reversible, antinociceptive effect in an inflammatory pain model in rats. Eur J Pharmacol 2002;443:71–7.

[3] American College of Rheumatology. Recommendations for the medical management of osteoarthritis of the hip and knee: 2000 update. American College of Rheumatology Subcommittee on Osteoarthritis Guidelines. Arthritis Rheum 2000;43:1905–15.

[4] Aronoff DM, Neilson EG. Antipyretics: mechanisms of action and clinical use in fever suppression. Am J Med 2001;111:304–15.

[5] Aubrun F, Kalfon F, Mottet P, Bellanger A, Langeron O, Coriat P, Riou B. Adjunctive analgesia with intravenous propacetamol does not reduce morphine-related adverse effects. Br J Anaesth 2003;90:314–9.

[6] Ayoub SS, Botting RM, Goorha S, Colville-Nash PR, Willoughby DA, Ballou LR. Acetaminophen-induced hypothermia in mice is mediated by a prostaglandin endoperoxide synthase 1 gene-derived protein. Proc Natl Acad Sci USA 2004;101:11165–9.

[7] Ayoub SS, Colville-Nash PR, Willoughby DA, Botting RM. The involvement of a cyclooxygenase 1 gene-derived protein in the antinociceptive action of paracetamol in mice. Eur J Pharmacol 2006;538:57–65.

[8] Bannwarth B. Gastrointestinal safety of paracetamol: is there any cause for concern? Expert Opin Drug Saf 2004;3:269–72.

[9] Bannwarth B, Netter P, Lapicque F, Gillet P, Pere P, Boccard E, Royer RJ, Gaucher A. Plasma and cerebrospinal fluid concentrations of paracetamol after a single intravenous dose of propacetamol. Br J Clin Pharmacol 1992;34:79–81.

[10] Bannwarth B, Pehourcq F. Pharmacologic basis for using paracetamol: pharmacokinetic and pharmacodynamic issues. Drugs 2003;63:5–13.

[11] Barden J, Edwards J, Moore A, McQuay H. Single dose oral paracetamol (acetaminophen) for postoperative pain. Cochrane Database Syst Rev 2004;CD004602.

[12] Bardin L, Bardin M, Lavarenne J, Eschalier A. Effect of intrathecal serotonin on nociception in rats: influence of the pain test used. Exp Brain Res 1997;113:81–7.

[13] Benson GD, Koff RS, Tolman KG. The therapeutic use of acetaminophen in patients with liver disease. Am J Ther 2005;12:133–41.

[14] Bernheim F, Bernheim ML. The action of P-Aminophenol on tissue oxidations. Science 1937;86:197.

[15] Bessems JG, Vermeulen NP. Paracetamol (acetaminophen)-induced toxicity: molecular and biochemical mechanisms, analogues and protective approaches. Crit Rev Toxicol 2001;31:55–138.

[16] Bianchi M, Panerai AE. The dose-related effects of paracetamol on hyperalgesia and nociception in the rat. Br J Pharmacol 1996;117:130–2.

[17] Bippi H, Frolich JC. Effects of acetylsalicylic acid and paracetamol alone and in combination on prostanoid synthesis in man. Br J Clin Pharmacol 1990;29:305–10.

[18] Bjorkman R. Central antinociceptive effects of non-steroidal anti-inflammatory drugs and paracetamol. Experimental studies in the rat. Acta Anaesthesiol Scand Suppl 1995;103:1–44.

[19] Bjorkman R, Hallman KM, Hedner J, Hedner T, Henning M. Acetaminophen blocks spinal hyperalgesia induced by NMDA and substance P. Pain 1994;57:259–64.

[20] Bjornsson GA, Haanaes HR, Skoglund LA. A randomized, double-blind crossover trial of paracetamol 1000 mg four times daily vs ibuprofen 600 mg: effect on swelling and other postoperative events after third molar surgery. Br J Clin Pharmacol 2003;55:405–12.

[21] Boardman PL, Hart FD. Clinical measurement of the anti-inflammatory effects of salicylates in rheumatoid arthritis. Br Med J 1967;4:264–8.

[22] Bonnefont J, Alloui A, Chapuy E, Clottes E, Eschalier A. Orally administered paracetamol does not act locally in the rat formalin test: evidence for a supraspinal, serotonin-dependent antinociceptive mechanism. Anesthesiology 2003;99:976–81.

[23] Bonnefont J, Chapuy E, Clottes E, Alloui A, Eschalier A. Spinal 5-HT1A receptors differentially influence nociceptive processing according to the nature of the noxious stimulus in rats: effect of WAY-100635 on the antinociceptive activities of paracetamol, venlafaxine and 5-HT. Pain 2005;114:482–90.

[24] Bonnefont J, Daulhac L, Etienne M, Chapuy E, Mallet C, Ouchchane L, Deval C, Courade JP, Ferrara M, Eschalier A, Clottes E. Acetaminophen recruits spinal p42/p44 MAPKs and GH/IGF-1 receptors to produce analgesia via the serotonergic system. Mol Pharmacol 2007;71:407–15.

[25] Boutaud O, Aronoff DM, Richardson JH, Marnett LJ, Oates JA. Determinants of the cellular specificity of acetaminophen as an inhibitor of prostaglandin H_2 synthases. Proc Natl Acad Sci USA 2002;99:7130–5.

[26] Brodie BB, Axelrod AE. The fate of acetophenetidin (phenacetin) in man and methods for the estimation of acetophenetidin and its metabolites in biological material. J Pharmacol Exp Ther 1949;97:58–67.

[27] Bujalska M. Effect of cyclooxygenase and NO synthase inhibitors administered centrally on antinociceptive action of acetaminophen (Part II). Pol J Pharmacol 2003;55:1001–11.

[28] Bujalska M. Effect of nonselective and selective opioid receptors antagonists on antinociceptive action of acetaminophen [part III]. Pol J Pharmacol 2004;56:539–45.

[29] Cakan T, Inan N, Culhaoglu S, Bakkal K, Basar H. Intravenous paracetamol improves the quality of postoperative analgesia but does not decrease narcotic requirements. J Neurosurg Anesthesiol 2008;20:169–73.

[30] Carlsson KH, Jurna I. Central analgesic effect of paracetamol manifested by depression of nociceptive activity in thalamic neurones of the rat. Neurosci Lett 1987;77:339–43.

[31] Carpenter HM, Mudge GH. Acetaminophen nephrotoxicity: studies on renal acetylation and deacetylation. J Pharmacol Exp Ther 1981;218:161–7.

[32] Chandrasekharan NV, Dai H, Roos KL, Evanson NK, Tomsik J, Elton TS, Simmons DL. COX-3, a cyclooxygenase-1 variant inhibited by acetaminophen and other analgesic/antipyretic drugs: cloning, structure, and expression. Proc Natl Acad Sci USA 2002;99:13926–31.

[33] Clissold SP. Paracetamol and phenacetin. Drugs 1986;4:46–59.

[34] Collins C, Starmer GA. A review of the hepatotoxicity of paracetamol at therapeutic or near-therapeutic dose levels, with particular reference to alcohol abusers. Drug Alcohol Rev 1995;14:63–79.

[35] Courade JP, Caussade F, Martin K, Besse D, Delchambre C, Hanoun N, Hamon M, Eschalier A, Cloarec A. Effects of acetaminophen on monoaminergic systems in the rat central nervous system. Naunyn Schmiedebergs Arch Pharmacol 2001;364:534–7.

[36] Crowe CA, Yong AC, Calder IC, Ham KN, Tange JD. The nephrotoxicity of p-aminophenol. I. The effect on microsomal cytochromes, glutathione and covalent binding in kidney and liver. Chem Biol Interact 1979;27:235–43.

[37] Cryer BL. Acetaminophen not associated with gastrointestinal toxicity: comment on the article by Rahme et al. Arthritis Rheum 2003;48:2074–5; author reply 2075–7.

[38] Cushman DW, Cheung HS. Effect of substrate concentration on inhibition of prostaglandin synthetase of bull seminal vesicles by anti-inflammatory drugs and fenamic acid analogs. Biochim Biophys Acta 1976;424:449–59.

[39] Daly FF, Fountain JS, Murray L, Graudins A, Buckley NA. Guidelines for the management of paracetamol poisoning in Australia and New Zealand: explanation and elaboration. A consensus statement from clinical toxicologists consulting to the Australasian poisons information centres. Med J Aust 2008;188:296–301.

[40] Dani M, Guindon J, Lambert C, Beaulieu P. The local antinociceptive effects of paracetamol in neuropathic pain are mediated by cannabinoid receptors. Eur J Pharmacol 2007;573:214–5.

[41] Darmani NA, Martin BR, Glennon RA. Behavioral evidence for differential adaptation of the serotonergic system after acute and chronic treatment with (+/−)-1-(2,5-dimethoxy-4-iodophenyl)-2-aminopropane (DOI) or ketanserin. J Pharmacol Exp Ther 1992;262:692–8.

[42] Dart RC, Kuffner EK, Rumack BH. Treatment of pain or fever with paracetamol (acetaminophen) in the alcoholic patient: a systematic review. Am J Ther 2000;7:123–34.

[43] Davern TJ 2nd, James LP, Hinson JA, Polson J, Larson AM, Fontana RJ, Lalani E, Munoz S, Shakil AO, Lee WM; Acute Liver Failure Study Group. Measurement of serum acetaminophen-protein adducts in patients with acute liver failure. Gastroenterology 2006;130:687–94.

[44] Davies RA, Maher CG, Hancock MJ. A systematic review of paracetamol for non-specific low back pain. Eur Spine J 2008.

[45] Depre M, van Hecken A, Verbesselt R, Tjandra-Maga TB, Gerin M, de Schepper PJ. Tolerance and pharmacokinetics of propacetamol, a paracetamol formulation for intravenous use. Fundam Clin Pharmacol 1992;6:259–62.

[46] Eisenach JC. Muscarinic-mediated analgesia. Life Sci 1999;64:549–54.

[47] Fattinger K, Frisullo R, Masche U, Braunschweig S, Meier PJ, Roos M. No clinically relevant drug interaction between paracetamol and phenprocoumon based on a pharmacoepidemiological cohort study in medical inpatients. Eur J Clin Pharmacol 2002;57:863–7.

[48] Feldberg W, Gupta KP. Pyrogen fever and prostaglandin-like activity in cerebrospinal fluid. J Physiol 1973;228:41–53.

[49] Fletcher D, Negre I, Barbin C, Francois A, Carreres C, Falgueirettes C, Barboteu A, Samii K. Postoperative analgesia with i.v. propacetamol and ketoprofen combination after disc surgery. Can J Anaesth 1997;44:479–85.

[50] Flinn FB, Brodie BB. The effect on the pain threshold of N-acetyl p-aminophenol, a product derived in the body from acetanilide. J Pharmacol Exp Ther 1948;76–7.

[51] Flower RJ, Vane JR. Inhibition of prostaglandin synthetase in brain explains the anti-pyretic activity of paracetamol (4-acetamidophenol). Nature 1972;240:410–1.

[52] Fored CM, Ejerblad E, Lindblad P, Fryzek JP, Dickman PW, Signorello LB, Lipworth L, Elinder CG, Blot WJ, McLaughlin JK, et al. Acetaminophen, aspirin, and chronic renal failure. N Engl J Med 2001;345:1801–8.

[53] Freeman R, Raskin P, Hewitt DJ, Vorsanger GJ, Jordan DM, Xiang J, Rosenthal NR; CAPSS-237 Study Group. Randomized study of tramadol/acetaminophen versus placebo in painful diabetic peripheral neuropathy. Curr Med Res Opin 2007;23:147–61.

[54] Freie HMP. Antipyretic analgesics. In: Dukes MNG, Aronson JK, editors. Meyler's side effects of drugs: an encyclopedia of adverse reactions and interactions, 14th ed. Amsterdam: Elsevier; 2000. p. 231–46.

[55] Garcia Rodriguez LA, Hernandez-Diaz S. Relative risk of upper gastrointestinal complications among users of acetaminophen and nonsteroidal anti-inflammatory drugs. Epidemiology 2001;12:570–6.

[56] Gebauer MG, Nyfort-Hansen K, Henschke PJ, Gallus AS. Warfarin and acetaminophen interaction. Pharmacotherapy 2003;23:109–12.

[57] Godfrey L, Bailey I, Toms NJ, Clarke GD, Kitchen I, Hourani SM. Paracetamol inhibits nitric oxide synthesis in murine spinal cord slices. Eur J Pharmacol 2007;562:68–71.

[58] Goldman RD, Ko K, Linett LJ, Scolnik D. Antipyretic efficacy and safety of ibuprofen and acetaminophen in children. Ann Pharmacother 2004;38:146–50.

[59] Grafova VN, Reshetniak VK, Kukushkin ML, Smirnova VS, Zinkevich VA. [Effects of paracetamol and naproxen on pain syndromes of various genesis]. Eksp Klin Farmakol 2001;64:14–8.

[60] Graham GG, Graham RI, Day RO. Comparative analgesia, cardiovascular and renal effects of celecoxib, rofecoxib and acetaminophen (paracetamol). Curr Pharm Des 2002;8:1063–75.

[60] Greco A, Ajmone-Cat MA, Nicolini A, Sciulli MG, Minghetti L. Paracetamol effectively reduces prostaglandin E2 synthesis in brain macrophages by inhibiting enzymatic activity of cyclooxygenase but not phospholipase and prostaglandin E synthase. J Neurosci Res 2003;71:844–52.
[61] Green K, Drvota V, Vesterqvist O. Pronounced reduction of in vivo prostacyclin synthesis in humans by acetaminophen (paracetamol). Prostaglandins 1989;37:311–5.
[62] Guhring H, Hamza M, Sergejeva M, Ates M, Kotalla CE, Ledent C, Brune K. A role for endocannabinoids in indomethacin-induced spinal antinociception. Eur J Pharmacol 2002;454:153–63.
[63] Hahn TW, Mogensen T, Lund C, Jacobsen LS, Hjortsoe NC, Rasmussen SN, Rasmussen M. Analgesic effect of i.v. paracetamol: possible ceiling effect of paracetamol in postoperative pain. Acta Anaesthesiol Scand 2003;47:138–45.
[64] Haller VL, Cichewicz DL, Welch SP. Non-cannabinoid CB1, non-cannabinoid CB2 antinociceptive effects of several novel compounds in the PPQ stretch test in mice. Eur J Pharmacol 2006;546:60–8.
[65] Harvison PJ, Egan RW, Gale PH, Christian GD, Hill BS, Nelson SD. Acetaminophen and analogs as cosubstrates and inhibitors of prostaglandin H synthase. Chem Biol Interact 1988;64:251–66.
[66] Hay AD, Costelloe C, Redmond NM, Montgomery AA, Fletcher M, Hollinghurst S, Peters TJ. Paracetamol plus ibuprofen for the treatment of fever in children (PITCH): randomised controlled trial. BMJ 2008;337:a1302.
[67] Heard KJ. Acetylcysteine for acetaminophen poisoning. N Engl J Med 2008;359:285–92.
[68] Hernandez-Palazon J, Tortosa JA, Martinez-Lage JF, Perez-Flores D. Intravenous administration of propacetamol reduces morphine consumption after spinal fusion surgery. Anesth Analg 2001;92:1473–6.
[69] Hinsberg O, Treupel G. Ueber die physiologische Wirkung des p-Aminophenols und einiger Derivate desselben. Naunyn Schmiedebergs Arch Exp Pathol Pharmakol 1894;33:216–50.
[70] Hinz B, Cheremina O, Brune K. Acetaminophen (paracetamol) is a selective cyclooxygenase-2 inhibitor in man. FASEB J 2007.
[71] Högestätt ED, Jonsson BA, Ermund A, Andersson DA, Bjork H, Alexander JP, Cravatt BF, Basbaum AI, Zygmunt PM. Conversion of acetaminophen to the bioactive N-acylphenolamine AM404 via fatty acid amide hydrolase-dependent arachidonic acid conjugation in the nervous system. J Biol Chem 2005;280:31405–12.
[72] Jaeschke H, Bajt ML. Intracellular signaling mechanisms of acetaminophen-induced liver cell death. Toxicol Sci 2006;89:31–41.
[73] Jensen FM, Dahl JB, Frigast C. Direct spinal effect of intrathecal acetaminophen on visceral noxious stimulation in rabbits. Acta Anaesthesiol Scand 1992;36:837–41.
[74] Jerussi TP, Caubet JF, McCray JE, Handley DA. Clinical endoscopic evaluation of the gastroduodenal tolerance to (R)-ketoprofen, (R)-flurbiprofen, racemic ketoprofen, and paracetamol: a randomized, single-blind, placebo-controlled trial. J Clin Pharmacol 1998;38:19S–24S.
[75] Jordan KM, Arden NK, Doherty M, Bannwarth B, Bijlsma JW, Dieppe P, Gunther K, Hauselmann H, Herrero-Beaumont G, Kaklamanis P, et al. EULAR Recommendations 2003: an evidence based approach to the management of knee osteoarthritis: Report of a Task Force of the Standing Committee for International Clinical Studies Including Therapeutic Trials (ESCISIT). Ann Rheum Dis 2003;62:1145–55.
[76] Juhl GI, Norholt SE, Tonnesen E, Hiesse-Provost O, Jensen TS. Analgesic efficacy and safety of intravenous paracetamol (acetaminophen) administered as a 2 g starting dose following third molar surgery. Eur J Pain 2006;10:371–7.
[77] Kehlet H, Werner MU. Role of paracetamol in the acute pain management. Drugs 2003;63:15–22.
[78] Kis B, Snipes JA, Gaspar T, Lenzser G, Tulbert CD, Busija DW. Cloning of cyclooxygenase-1b (putative COX-3) in mouse. Inflamm Res 2006;55:274–8.
[79] Kleinman JG, Breitenfield RV, Roth DA. Acute renal failure associated with acetaminophen ingestion: report of a case and review of the literature. Clin Nephrol 1980;14:201–5.
[80] Koes BW, van Tulder MW, Ostelo R, Kim Burton A, Waddell G. Clinical guidelines for the management of low back pain in primary care: an international comparison. Spine 2001;26:2504–13; discussion 2513–4.
[81] Kokki H, Homan E, Tuovinen K, Purhonen S. Perioperative treatment with i.v. ketoprofen reduces pain and vomiting in children after strabismus surgery. Acta Anaesthesiol Scand 1999;43:13–8.
[82] Korpela R, Korvenoja P, Meretoja OA. Morphine-sparing effect of acetaminophen in pediatric day-case surgery. Anesthesiology 1999;91:442–7.
[83] Kuffner EK, Dart RC, Bogdan GM, Hill RE, Casper E, Darton L. Effect of maximal daily doses of acetaminophen on the liver of alcoholic patients: a randomized, double-blind, placebo-controlled trial. Arch Intern Med 2001;161:2247–52.
[84] Larson AM. Acetaminophen hepatotoxicity. Clin Liver Dis 2007;11:525–48, vi.
[85] Lauterburg BH, Velez ME. Glutathione deficiency in alcoholics: risk factor for paracetamol hepatotoxicity. Gut 1988;29:1153–7.
[86] Lee WM. Acetaminophen and the U.S. Acute Liver Failure Study Group: lowering the risks of hepatic failure. Hepatology 2004;40:6–9.
[87] Lee YS, Kim H, Brahim JS, Rowan J, Lee G, Dionne RA. Acetaminophen selectively suppresses peripheral prostaglandin E2 release and increases COX-2 gene expression in a clinical model of acute inflammation. Pain 2007;129:279–86.
[88] Leinisch E, Evers S, Kaempfe N, Kraemer C, Sostak P, Jurgens T, Straube A, May A. Evaluation of the efficacy of intravenous acetaminophen in the treatment of acute migraine attacks: a double-blind, placebo-controlled parallel group multicenter study. Pain 2005;117:396–400.
[89] Lewis AJ, Nelson DJ, Sugrue MF. On the ability of prostaglandin E1, and arachidonic acid to modulate experimentally induced oedema in the rat paw. Br J Pharmacol 1975;55:51–6.
[90] Li S, Dou W, Tang Y, Goorha S, Ballou LR, Blatteis CM. Acetaminophen: antipyretic or hypothermic in mice? In either case, PGHS-1b (COX-3) is irrelevant. Prostaglandins Other Lipid Mediat 2008;85:89–99.

[91] Libert F, Bonnefont J, Bourinet E, Doucet E, Alloui A, Hamon M, Nargeot J, Eschalier A. Acetaminophen: a central analgesic drug that involves a spinal tropisetron-sensitive, non-5-HT_3 receptor-mediated effect. Mol Pharmacol 2004;66:728–34.
[92] Lipton RB, Baggish JS, Stewart WF, Codispoti JR, Fu M. Efficacy and safety of acetaminophen in the treatment of migraine: results of a randomized, double-blind, placebo-controlled, population-based study. Arch Intern Med 2000;160:3486–92.
[93] Mahé I, Bertrand N, Drouet L, Bal Dit Sollier C, Simoneau G, Mazoyer E, Caulin C, Bergmann JF. Interaction between paracetamol and warfarin in patients: a double-blind, placebo-controlled, randomized study. Haematologica 2006;91:1621–7.
[94] Mahé I, Bertrand N, Drouet L, Simoneau G, Mazoyer E, Bal dit Sollier C, Caulin C, Bergmann JF. Paracetamol: a haemorrhagic risk factor in patients on warfarin. Br J Clin Pharmacol 2005;59:371–4.
[95] Mahe I, Caulin C, Bergmann JF. Does paracetamol potentiate the effects of oral anticoagulants? A literature review. Drug Saf 2004;27:325–33.
[96] Mallet C, Daulhac L, Bonnefont J, Ledent C, Etienne M, Chapuy E, Libert F, Eschalier A. Endocannabinoid and serotonergic systems are needed for acetaminophen-induced analgesia. Pain 2008;139:190–200.
[97] Martin U, Temple RM, Winney RJ, Prescott LF. The disposition of paracetamol and the accumulation of its glucuronide and sulphate conjugates during multiple dosing in patients with chronic renal failure. Eur J Clin Pharmacol 1991;41:43–6.
[98] Miranda HF, Sierralta F, Pinardi G. Neostigmine interactions with non steroidal anti-inflammatory drugs. Br J Pharmacol 2002;135:1591–7.
[99] Mitchell JR, Jollow DJ, Potter WZ, Davis DC, Gillette JR, Brodie BB. Acetaminophen-induced hepatic necrosis. I. Role of drug metabolism. J Pharmacol Exp Ther 1973;187:185–94.
[100] Mitchell JR, Jollow DJ, Potter WZ, Gillette JR, Brodie BB. Acetaminophen-induced hepatic necrosis. IV. Protective role of glutathione. J Pharmacol Exp Ther 1973;187:211–7.
[101] Moore A, Collins S, Carroll D, McQuay H. Paracetamol with and without codeine in acute pain: a quantitative systematic review. Pain 1997;70:193–201.
[102] Moore N, Charlesworth A, Van Ganse E, LeParc JM, Jones JK, Wall R, Schneid H, Verrière F. Risk factors for adverse events in analgesic drug users: results from the PAIN study. Pharmacoepidemiol Drug Saf 2003;12:601–10.
[103] Morse HN. Ueber eine neue Darstellungsmethode der Acetylamidophenole. Ber Deutscher Chem Ges 1878;232–3.
[104] Muth-Selbach US, Tegeder I, Brune K, Geisslinger G. Acetaminophen inhibits spinal prostaglandin E2 release after peripheral noxious stimulation. Anesthesiology 1999;91:231–9.
[105] Nelson SD. Molecular mechanisms of the hepatotoxicity caused by acetaminophen. Semin Liver Dis 1990;10:267–78.
[106] Newton JF, Kuo CH, DeShone GM, Hoefle D, Bernstein J, Hook JB. The role of p-aminophenol in acetaminophen-induced nephrotoxicity: effect of bis(p-nitrophenyl) phosphate on acetaminophen and p-aminophenol nephrotoxicity and metabolism in Fischer 344 rats. Toxicol Appl Pharmacol 1985;81:416–30.
[107] Newton JF, Yoshimoto M, Bernstein J, Rush GF, Hook JB. Acetaminophen nephrotoxicity in the rat. II. Strain differences in nephrotoxicity and metabolism of p-aminophenol, a metabolite of acetaminophen. Toxicol Appl Pharmacol 1983;69:307–18.
[108] Nikles CJ, Yelland M, Del Mar C, Wilkinson D. The role of paracetamol in chronic pain: an evidence-based approach. Am J Ther 2005;12:80–91.
[109] Ottani A, Leone S, Sandrini M, Ferrari A, Bertolini A. The analgesic activity of paracetamol is prevented by the blockade of cannabinoid CB1 receptors. Eur J Pharmacol 2006;531:280–1.
[110] Ouellet M, Percival MD. Mechanism of acetaminophen inhibition of cyclooxygenase isoforms. Arch Biochem Biophys 2001;387:273–80.
[111] Palangio M, Damask MJ, Morris E, Doyle RT Jr, Jiang JG, Landau CJ, de Padova A. Combination hydrocodone and ibuprofen versus combination codeine and acetaminophen for the treatment of chronic pain. Clin Ther 2000;22:879–92.
[112] Patten CJ, Thomas PE, Guy RL, Lee M, Gonzalez FJ, Guengerich FP, Yang CS. Cytochrome P450 enzymes involved in acetaminophen activation by rat and human liver microsomes and their kinetics. Chem Res Toxicol 1993;6:511–8.
[113] Peduto VA, Ballabio M, Stefanini S. Efficacy of propacetamol in the treatment of postoperative pain. Morphine-sparing effect in orthopedic surgery. Italian Collaborative Group on Propacetamol. Acta Anaesthesiol Scand 1998;42:293–8.
[114] Pelissier T, Alloui A, Caussade F, Dubray C, Cloarec A, Lavarenne J, Eschalier A. Paracetamol exerts a spinal antinociceptive effect involving an indirect interaction with 5-hydroxytryptamine3 receptors: in vivo and in vitro evidence. J Pharmacol Exp Ther 1996;278:8–14.
[115] Perneger TV, Whelton PK, Klag MJ. Risk of kidney failure associated with the use of acetaminophen, aspirin, and nonsteroidal antiinflammatory drugs. N Engl J Med 1994;331:1675–9.
[116] Perrott DA, Piira T, Goodenough B, Champion GD. Efficacy and safety of acetaminophen vs ibuprofen for treating children's pain or fever: a meta-analysis. Arch Pediatr Adolesc Med 2004;158:521–6.
[117] Pfaffenrath V, Scherzer S. Analgesics and NSAIDs in the treatment of the acute migraine attack. Cephalalgia 1995;15:14–20.
[118] Pickering G, Esteve V, Loriot MA, Eschalier A, Dubray C. Acetaminophen reinforces descending inhibitory pain pathways. Clin Pharmacol Ther 2008;84:47–51.
[119] Pickering G, Loriot MA, Libert F, Eschalier A, Beaune P, Dubray C. Analgesic effect of acetaminophen in humans: first evidence of a central serotonergic mechanism. Clin Pharmacol Ther 2006;79:371–8.
[120] Piguet V, Desmeules J, Dayer P. Lack of acetaminophen ceiling effect on R-III nociceptive flexion reflex. Eur J Clin Pharmacol 1998;53:321–4.

[121] Pinardi G, Sierralta F, Miranda HF. Adrenergic mechanisms in antinociceptive effects of non steroidal anti-inflammatory drugs in acute thermal nociception in mice. Inflamm Res 2002;51:219–22.
[122] Pinardi G, Sierralta F, Miranda HF. Atropine reverses the antinociception of nonsteroidal anti-inflammatory drugs in the tail-flick test of mice. Pharmacol Biochem Behav 2003;74:603–8.
[123] Pini LA, Sandrini M, Vitale G. The antinociceptive action of paracetamol is associated with changes in the serotonergic system in the rat brain. Eur J Pharmacol 1996;308:31–40.
[124] Pini LA, Vitale G, Ottani A, Sandrini M. Naloxone-reversible antinociception by paracetamol in the rat. J Pharmacol Exp Ther 1997;280:934–40.
[125] Potter WZ, Davis DC, Mitchell JR, Jollow DJ, Gillette JR, Brodie BB. Acetaminophen-induced hepatic necrosis. 3. Cytochrome P-450-mediated covalent binding in vitro. J Pharmacol Exp Ther 1973;187:203–10.
[126] Prescott LF. Therapeutic misadventure with paracetamol: fact or fiction? Am J Ther 2000;7:99–114.
[127] Prescott LF, Critchley JA. Drug interactions affecting analgesic toxicity. Am J Med 1983;75:113–6.
[128] Prescott LF, Newton RW, Swainson CP, Wright N, Forrest AR, Matthew H. Successful treatment of severe paracetamol overdosage with cysteamine. Lancet 1974;1:588–92.
[129] Prescott WR. General toxicity. In: Taylor, Francis, editors. Paracetamol (acetaminophen). A critical bibliographic review, 2nd ed. 2001. p. 297–323.
[130] Prescott LF. Pharmacokinetics of paracetamol. In: Prescott LF. Paracetamol (acetaminophen). A critical bibliographic review, 2nd ed. London: Taylor and Francis; 2001. p. 189–223.
[131] Prior MJ, Cooper KM, May LG, Bowen DL. Efficacy and safety of acetaminophen and naproxen in the treatment of tension-type headache. A randomized, double-blind, placebo-controlled trial. Cephalalgia 2002;22:740–8.
[132] Raffa RB. Acetaminophen and metabolite: lack of effect on nitric oxide synthase (constitutive or inducible). Headache 2002;42:237–8.
[133] Raffa RB, Stone DJ Jr, Tallarida RJ. Unexpected and pronounced antinociceptive synergy between spinal acetaminophen (paracetamol) and phentolamine. Eur J Pharmacol 2001;412:R1–2.
[134] Raffa RB, Walker EA, Sterious SN. Opioid receptors and acetaminophen (paracetamol). Eur J Pharmacol 2004;503:209–10.
[135] Rahme E, Pettitt D, LeLorier J. Determinants and sequelae associated with utilization of acetaminophen versus traditional nonsteroidal antiinflammatory drugs in an elderly population. Arthritis Rheum 2002;46:3046–54.
[136] Rainsford KD, Roberts SC, Brown S. Ibuprofen and paracetamol: relative safety in non-prescription dosages. J Pharm Pharmacol 1997;49:345–76.
[137] Raucy JL, Lasker JM, Lieber CS, Black M. Acetaminophen activation by human liver cytochromes P450IIE1 and P450IA2. Arch Biochem Biophys 1989;271:270–83.
[138] Rawlins MD, Henderson DB, Hijab AR. Pharmacokinetics of paracetamol (acetaminophen) after intravenous and oral administration. Eur J Clin Pharmacol 1977;11:283–6.
[139] Reid AB, Kurten RC, McCullough SS, Brock RW, Hinson JA. Mechanisms of acetaminophen-induced hepatotoxicity: role of oxidative stress and mitochondrial permeability transition in freshly isolated mouse hepatocytes. J Pharmacol Exp Ther 2005;312:509–16.
[140] Robak J, Kostka-Trabka E, Duniec Z. The influence of three prostaglandin biosynthesis stimulators on carrageenin-induced edema of rat paw. Biochem Pharmacol 1980;29:1863–5.
[141] Robinson DR, McGuire MB, Bastian D, Kantrowitz F, Levine L. The effects of anti-inflammatory drugs on prostaglandin production by rheumatoid synovial tissue. Prostaglandins Med 1978;1:461–77.
[142] Romsing J, Moiniche S, Dahl JB. Rectal and parenteral paracetamol, and paracetamol in combination with NSAIDs, for postoperative analgesia. Br J Anaesth 2002;88:215–26.
[143] Rumack BH. Acetaminophen misconceptions. Hepatology 2004;40:10–5.
[144] Rumack BH, Matthew H. Acetaminophen poisoning and toxicity. Pediatrics 1975;55:871–6.
[145] Rumack BH, Peterson RC, Koch GG, Amara IA. Acetaminophen overdose. 662 cases with evaluation of oral acetylcysteine treatment. Arch Intern Med 1981;141:380–5.
[146] Ryu YS, Lee JH, Seok JH, Hong JH, Lee YS, Lim JH, Kim YM, Hur GM. Acetaminophen inhibits iNOS gene expression in RAW 264.7 macrophages: differential regulation of NF-kappaB by acetaminophen and salicylates. Biochem Biophys Res Commun 2000;272:758–64.
[147] Sandrini M, Vitale G, Ruggieri V, Pini LA. Effect of acute and repeated administration of paracetamol on opioidergic and serotonergic systems in rats. Inflamm Res 2007;56:139–42.
[148] Schildknecht S, Daiber A, Ghisla S, Cohen RA, Bachschmid MM. Acetaminophen inhibits prostanoid synthesis by scavenging the PGHS-activator peroxynitrite. FASEB J 2008;22:215–24.
[149] Schwab JM, Beiter T, Linder JU, Laufer S, Schulz JE, Meyermann R, Schluesener HJ. COX-3: a virtual pain target in humans? FASEB J 2003;17:2174–5.
[150] Sciulli MG, Seta F, Tacconelli S, Capone ML, Ricciotti E, Pistritto G, Patrignani P. Effects of acetaminophen on constitutive and inducible prostanoid biosynthesis in human blood cells. Br J Pharmacol 2003;138:634–41.
[151] Seegers AJ, Jager LP, Zandberg P, van Noordwijk J. The anti-inflammatory, analgesic and antipyretic activities of non-narcotic analgesic drug mixtures in rats. Arch Int Pharmacodyn Ther 1981;251:237–54.
[152] Seppala E, Laitinen O, Vapaatalo H. Comparative study on the effects of acetylsalicylic acid, indomethacin and paracetamol on metabolites of arachidonic acid in plasma, serum and urine in man. Int J Clin Pharmacol Res 1983;3:265–9.
[153] Skoglund LA, Eidsaunet W, Pettersen N. The anti-oedematous efficacy of oxindanac equals that of paracetamol in acute postoperative inflammation; are weak cyclooxygenase inhibitors more effective than strong inhibitors? Int J Clin Pharmacol Res 1989;9:371–5.

[154] Smith JN, Williams RT. Studies in detoxication: 16. The metabolism of acetanilide in the rabbit. Biochem J 1948;42:538–44.
[155] Smith JN, Williams RT. Studies in detoxication. 22. The metabolism of phenacetin (p-ethoxyacetanilide) in the rabbit and a further observation on acetanilide metabolism. Biochem J 1949;44:239–42.
[156] Snipes JA, Kis B, Shelness GS, Hewett JA, Busija DW. Cloning and characterization of cyclooxygenase-1b (putative cyclooxygenase-3) in rat. J Pharmacol Exp Ther 2005;313:668–76.
[157] Steventon GB, Mitchell SC, Waring RH. Human metabolism of paracetamol (acetaminophen) at different dose levels. Drug Metabol Drug Interact 1996;13:111–7.
[158] Swierkosz TA, Jordan L, McBride M, McGough K, Devlin J, Botting RM. Actions of paracetamol on cyclooxygenases in tissue and cell homogenates of mouse and rabbit. Med Sci Monit 2002;8:BR496–503.
[159] Tjolsen A, Lund A, Hole K. Antinociceptive effect of paracetamol in rats is partly dependent on spinal serotonergic systems. Eur J Pharmacol 1991;193:193–201.
[160] Toes MJ, Jones AL, Prescott L. Drug interactions with paracetamol. Am J Ther 2005;12:56–66.
[161] Towheed TE, Judd MJ, Hochberg MC, Wells G. Acetaminophen for osteoarthritis. Cochrane Database Syst Rev 2003;CD004257.
[162] Vane JR. Inhibition of prostaglandin synthesis as a mechanism of action for aspirin-like drugs. Nat New Biol 1971;231:232–5.
[163] Vinegar R, Truax JF, Selph JL. Quantitative comparison of the analgesic and anti-inflammatory activities of aspirin, phenacetin and acetaminophen in rodents. Eur J Pharmacol 1976;37:23–30.
[164] Von Mering J. Beitrage zur kenntniss der Antipyretica. Ther Monatsschr 1893;577–87.
[165] Warner TD, Giuliano F, Vojnovic I, Bukasa A, Mitchell JA, Vane JR. Nonsteroid drug selectivities for cyclo-oxygenase-1 rather than cyclo-oxygenase-2 are associated with human gastrointestinal toxicity: a full in vitro analysis. Proc Natl Acad Sci USA 1999;96:7563–8.
[166] Warner TD, Vojnovic I, Giuliano F, Jimenez R, Bishop-Bailey D, Mitchell JA. Cyclooxygenases 1, 2, and 3 and the production of prostaglandin I2: investigating the activities of acetaminophen and cyclooxygenase-2-selective inhibitors in rat tissues. J Pharmacol Exp Ther 2004;310:642–7.
[167] Wong S, Gardocki JF. Anti-inflammatory and antiarthritic evaluation of acetaminophen and its potentiation of tolmetin. J Pharmacol Exp Ther 1983;226:625–32.
[168] Zhang W, Jones A, Doherty M. Does paracetamol (acetaminophen) reduce the pain of osteoarthritis? A meta-analysis of randomised controlled trials. Ann Rheum Dis 2004;63:901–7.
[169] Zimmerman HJ, Maddrey WC. Acetaminophen (paracetamol) hepatotoxicity with regular intake of alcohol: analysis of instances of therapeutic misadventure. Hepatology 1995;22:767–73.
[170] Zygmunt PM, Chuang H, Movahed P, Julius D, Högestätt ED. The anandamide transport inhibitor AM404 activates vanilloid receptors. Eur J Pharmacol 2000;396:39–42.

Correspondence to: Alain Eschalier, INSERM, U766, Facultés de Médecine et de Pharmacie, 28 Place Henri Dunant, B.P. 38, F-63001 Clermont-Ferrand Cedex 01, France. Tel: +33 4 73 17 82 32; fax: +33 4 73 27 71 62; email: alain.eschalier@u-clermont1.fr.

5 Pharmacology of the Opioid System

Juan Carlos Marvizon,[a,b] Yao-Ying Ma,[a,c] Andrew C. Charles,[a,d] Wendy Walwyn,[a,c] and Christopher J. Evans[a,c]

[a]*Hatos Center for Neuropharmacology and Departments of* [b]*Medicine,* [c]*Psychiatry and Biobehavioral Sciences, and* [d]*Neurology, UCLA, Los Angeles, California, USA*

Opioids play a central role in nociception. Endogenous opioids modulate the experience of pain, and opioid therapeutics are a mainstay for the clinical management of acute and chronic pain. In spite of such widespread use, current opioid therapeutics are not beneficial in all types of pain, and they can result in unfavorable side effects. The balance between beneficial and adverse effects may be affected by how different opioid treatments signal through their targeted receptors. Recent advances in the understanding of opioid receptor pharmacology provide some insight into these different signaling pathways. This knowledge has led to the development of novel approaches that target these pathways aiming to optimize the treatment of pain by opioids. In this chapter, we will first describe the different components of the opioid system, emphasizing the aspects that remain controversial. We will then cover current understanding on how and where opioid systems control and influence pain. The treatment protocols used by clinicians and their concerns will then be addressed. Finally, we will describe several emerging concepts that may, in the future, change how opioid systems will be manipulated to better modulate and control pain.

Molecular Targets for Opioid Drugs

The opioid receptor family consists of four receptors: μ (also named the mu, MOP, or OP_3 receptor or MOR), δ (also named the delta, DOP, or OP_1 receptor or DOR), κ (also named the kappa, KOP, or OP_2 receptor or KOR), and opioid-like receptor 1 (ORL1 receptor, also named the nociceptin, NOP, orphanin FQ, N/OFQ, or OP_4 receptor). The family of opioid receptors is activated by endogenous peptide ligands and possibly by endogenous morphinans (Fig. 1). Updated information on the pharmacology of these receptors can be obtained from the International Union of Basic and Clinical Pharmacology website (http://www.iuphar.org). All four opioid receptors are widely, but differentially, distributed throughout the central and peripheral nervous systems as well as in endocrine and immune cells, so there should be little surprise that drugs modulating their activity can induce a variety of physiological and behavioral effects. Prior reviews have detailed the complexity of opioid signaling cascades, for example, Law et al. [66], so this aspect will not be a major emphasis of this chapter. In brief, most opioid receptors couple to inhibitory G proteins (G_i and G_o) to inhibit neuronal depolarization. This inhibitory action on peripheral and central neurons is the fundamental mechanism by which opioid analgesia is accomplished. Exactly where in the central nervous system (CNS) opioids mediate analgesia is difficult to determine given the wide distribution of the opioid receptor family and the differences in the route and type of opiate administered. However, the analgesia induced by different opioid receptors has been better defined from studies of mice lacking a specific opioid receptors [32,45].

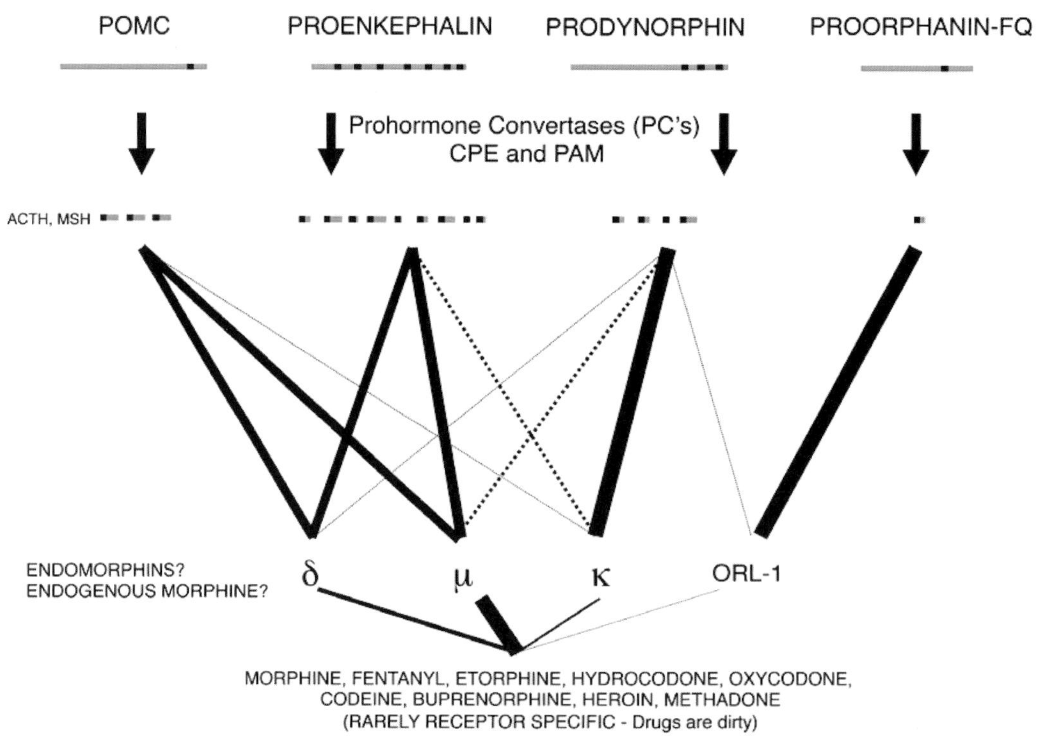

Fig. 1. Opioid peptide precursor proteins proopiomelanocortin (POMC), proenkephalin, prodynorphin, and pro-orphanin-FQ give rise to multiple peptide ligands following enzymatic processing in secretory vesicles. The relative affinity of precursor products for the different receptors is indicated by the thickness of the connecting lines. Dashed connecting lines indicate affinity for receptors but no implicated endogenous interactions. ACTH = adrenocorticotropic hormone, CPE = carboxypeptidase E, MSH = melanocyte-stimulating hormone, PAM = peptidylglycine alpha-amidating monooxygenase.

Mu-Opioid Receptors

In mice, μ-receptors are indisputably the receptors for inducing the analgesic effects of morphine in assays such as the hot plate and tail-flick assays. In μ-knockout mice lacking exon 2, the analgesic effects of morphine-6-glucuronide, morphine-6-ethereal sulfate, and endomorphin-2 are eliminated [71]. However, exon 1 knockout mice show a slightly different phenotype, with morphine-6-glucuronide and heroin analgesia retained [108]. This observation, together with a series of antisense studies, has led to a large body of work showing considerable μ-receptor heterogeneity as a result of alternative splice variants [95]. The μ-receptor genomic locus is complex; 25 splice variants have been identified from the mouse gene controlled by two promoters, 8 splice variants from the rat gene, and 11 splice variants from the human gene. However, the interspecies conservation of many of these alternatively spliced protein products is low, and sequence differences are substantial between human and rodent transcripts and even between mouse and rat transcripts. The lack of conservation and low transcript levels have called into question the significance of these differentially spliced receptor transcripts. One argument in favor of significance was that intense immunostaining of some of these products is suggestive of low mRNA level but high expression of protein levels. However, in the study that led to this hypothesis, focusing on MOR-1C, the antiserum mapping was accomplished in rats using an antiserum made to the mouse sequence, which has less than 20% identity [1]. Adequate controls for antibody specificity for the MOR-1C antiserum and many other opioid receptor antibodies have been questionable, and in a number of instances immunostaining data have misled the G-protein-coupled receptor (GPCR) field. Indeed, in one study from our own laboratory, conducted to map the CNS distribution of ORL-1 receptors using a monoclonal antibody, the results were misleading and subsequently proven incorrect because identical staining patterns were observed in wild-type and ORL-1 knockout mice [4]. In summary, the importance of μ-receptor splice variants has yet to be definitively demonstrated. Although antisense studies have indicated differential agonist activities at the different splice variant receptors, definitive genetic studies are required to validate these findings.

Delta, Kappa, and ORL-1 Receptors

Since opioid drugs are rarely specific for one opioid receptor, the adverse or beneficial side effects of opioid analgesics may be attributable to their interaction with other opioid receptors. However, μ-opioid receptors appear to mediate the prominent actions of most clinically used opioid drugs, while the other members of the opioid receptor family can modulate nociception either directly or indirectly via modulation of μ-mediated effects. The direct analgesic efficacy achieved via activation of κ- or δ-receptors is meager unless there is coactivation of other pathways or systems, such as externalization of the δ receptors to the cell membrane following μ-receptor activation [15]. In the case of ORL1 receptors, central activation negates the analgesic effects of activation of classical opioid receptors [85], and thus the ORL1 receptor system has been labeled as an anti-opioid system. This finding may have clinical significance; for instance, buprenorphine agonist activity at ORL1 receptors compromises buprenorphine's analgesic efficacy via activation of μ-receptors [73]. Table I summarizes the actions of different opioid receptors on nociception.

Table I
Actions of different opioid receptors on nociception, drawn from studies in rodents, including receptor knockout (KO) animals

Receptor	Agonist Actions	Antagonist Actions
μ	Analgesia (Sys, i.c.v.), good efficacy for most pain modalities, but questionable for inflammatory or neuropathic pain. *Respiratory depression, constipation, reward, immune system perturbation, increased locomotion.*	Hyperalgesia (KO). *Aversion (antagonist Sys, i.c.v.): reduced reward from alcohol, THC, and nicotine (KO); reduced attachment behavior (KO).*
δ	Analgesia, but weak or absent unless externalization is triggered (e.g., by morphine or chronic inflammation). *Seizures, antidepressant/anxiolytic, altered gut motility.*	Hyperalgesia in a chronic inflammatory pain model (KO); morphine analgesic tolerance is reduced (KO). *Increases anxiety, alcohol consumption, and depression (KO).*
κ	Analgesia is weak and assessment potentially confounded by hallucinogenic and catatonic activity. *Aversion, catatonia, hallucinations, hyperthermia, blockade of pruritus; water dieresis.*	Antagonists block stress-induced analgesia; enhances sensitivity to chemical visceral pain (KO). *Blocks stress-induced immobility and cocaine relapse (KO).*
ORL-1	Blocks opioid analgesia and stress-induced analgesia (i.c.v.); analgesic (i.t.). *Anxiolytic, impairs aspects of learning and memory (KO).*	Hyperalgesia following chronic nociceptive stimulation (KO). *Hearing-adaptive responses; enhances aspects of learning and memory; antidepressant (KO).*

Note: Information primarily from the International Union of Basic and Clinical Pharmacology (www.iuphar.org). In italics are actions that would be considered side reactions to nociception but may interact with nociceptive processing.
Abbreviations: i.c.v. = intraventricular administration, i.t. = intrathecal administration, KO = phenotype most convincingly based upon receptor knockout mice, Sys = systemic administration, THC = tetrahydrocannabinol.

"Atypical" Opioid Receptors

Apart from the "classical" opioid GPCRs, a considerable literature suggests the existence of atypical effectors for endogenous opioid peptides [137]. For example, *N*-methyl-D-aspartate (NMDA) receptors can be modulated by dynorphins, possibly via the NMDA/glycine-B site. Met-enkephalin has been termed the "opioid growth factor" (OGF), which acts in both neural and non-neural tissues to control development, cellular renewal, anti-tumorigenesis, wound healing, and angiogenesis [142]. The OGF receptor, which has no sequence homology to the classical opioid receptors, is present in both glia and neurons.

This receptor is reported to potently bind Met-enkephalin, but not dynorphins, and is stereospecifically blocked by naloxone. Once bound, the receptors are apparently transported to the nucleus to modulate DNA synthesis. If Met-enkephalin is indeed an important activation ligand for this receptor, mice lacking proenkephalin and those lacking OGF should have phenotypes in common. However, OGF-receptor knockout mice have yet to be generated to enable assessment of any phenotype overlap.

Receptor Oligomers

While there are only three classical opioid receptors, there is now evidence for homo-oligomers and hetero-oligomers of these receptors, changing their pharmacology and signaling profiles [48]. For example, there are interactions between the μ-receptor and other GPCRs such as the cannabinoid CB1 and α_{2a} adrenergic receptors, which confer novel signaling profiles and trafficking properties to both receptors. The pharmacological profiles of relevant opioid receptor oligomers have yet to be clarified, but this intriguing new area of opioid pharmacology promises to provide more selective opioid-receptor-targeted therapeutics. However, the extent of oligomerization in native tissues is unknown. Furthermore, the recent crystallization of the adrenergic receptor does not suggest that oligomerization is required, although technical methodologies for crystallization may have precluded identification of oligomeric forms [64].

Opioid Ligands

Endogenous Opioids

The classical opioid receptors (μ-, δ-, and κ-receptors) are activated by endogenous opioid peptides, of which there are close to 30 [128]. The endogenous opioid peptides derive from processing of three opioid protein precursors: proenkephalin, prodynorphin, and proopiomelanocortin (POMC). Through a process involving specific endoproteases and prohormone convertases, in combination with carboxypeptidase-B activity to cleave C-terminal basic residues, the endogenous opioid peptides are carved out from their protein precursors (see Fig. 1). Action of a peptidylglycine alpha-amidating monooxygenase converts peptides with a C-terminal glycine to generate a C-terminal amide for two endogenous opioid peptides, which prevents extracellular degradation by carboxypeptidases that are prevalent in the extracellular environment. The peptide ligand for the ORL1 receptor has a separate precursor, pro-orphanin FQ or pro-nociceptin, which has a similar structure to the classical opioid precursors. A focus of much prior research has been to determine whether one opioid precursor protein is dedicated to generating ligands for one receptor type. Each precursor can certainly give rise to peptides with affinity for all three classical opioid receptors [128], and furthermore, similar phenotypes are observed in opioid receptor and opioid precursor knockout mice. For example, prodynorphin and κ-receptor knockout mice give the same phenotype in several stress-induced relapse models [83].

Proenkephalin and μ-knockout mice give the same phenotype in multiple assays, including naloxone aversion [109] and various rewarding paradigms of abusive drugs [30].

Whether morphine and endomorphins [141] are endogenous ligands for opioid receptors in mammals remains controversial. In the case of endogenous morphine, questions of metabolic origin of the detected morphine-like immunoreactivity or mass spectrometry peaks have been the focus of much research. Initial studies were clouded by presumed contamination by alkaloid opiates of glassware/apparatus used to isolate the tissue [132]. More recent evidence appears more convincing [115], although questions remain regarding morphine storage and regulation of activity, given morphine's ability to traverse membranes. In the case of endomorphins, no synthetic route has been identified thus far, either via DNA or otherwise, and much identification since the initial isolation relies on antisera of questionable selectivity. Furthermore, the endomorphins have been slated as the endogenous ligands for the μ-opioid receptor, yet the fact that the phenotype of the μ-receptor knockout mice often parallels that of proenkephalin knockouts strongly suggests that peptides derived from this opioid precursor are endogenous μ-ligands.

Exogenous Opioids

Opioid drugs comprise a chemically diverse group of compounds that differ in many pharmacological and physical properties, including hydrophobicity; metabolic stability; opioid receptor selectivity; receptor on/off rates; receptor efficacy as agonists, antagonists, and inverse agonists; and interaction with receptors other than members of the opioid GPCRs. The morphinans, defined as drugs based upon the structure of the opium poppy-derived alkaloids, thebaine, codeine, and morphine, are the most clinically used opioid pharmaceuticals. Morphinans include the partial agonists oxycodone, hydrocodone, morphine, codeine, and diacetylmorphine (heroin); the oripavines buprenorphine and etorphine (semisynthetic agonists derived from thebaine); and the antagonists naloxone and naltrexone. Fentanyl and related pharmaceutical derivatives such as remifentanil are more μ-selective than the morphinans, with fast on and off actions making them preferred analgesics during surgery and childbirth. Methadone, a drug sometimes used as an analgesic, is also selective for μ-receptors as opposed to other opioid receptors, yet it has a slow on/off action, at least in humans.

Over the years it has become evident that opioid pharmaceuticals are rarely specific, and new targets for these compounds regularly come to light. For example, many opioid drugs have high affinity for 5-HT_{3A} and nicotinic receptor channels, and methadone and dynorphins modulate NMDA receptors [137]. Naltrexone and naloxone appear to have high affinity for filamin A, a protein postulated to interact with and modulate μ-opioid receptors [126]. The toll-like receptor 4 appears to mediate the activation of glia by morphine, leading to the production of nitric oxide and pro-inflammatory cytokines. The resulting hyperalgesia opposes the analgesic effects of morphine and is proposed to contribute to tolerance and morphine-induced anti-analgesia [54]. As discussed previously, many opioid peptides and alkaloids have affinity for the opioid growth factor (OGF) receptor [142]. Given the emerging heterogeneity of receptors and proteins that interact with opioid drugs, a careful study of different opioid therapeutics for treatment of different pain modalities is clearly warranted.

Mechanisms of Opioid Analgesia

Peripheral Analgesia and the Immune System

Immune-Derived Opioid Peptides in Inflammation

Although transcript analyses suggest that all opioid and orphanin-FQ/nociceptin precursors are expressed in cells of the immune system, POMC and proenkephalin-derived peptides have been studied most extensively. POMC expression has been demonstrated in leukocytes from a wide variety of species (reviewed by Machelska and Stein [75]). Preproenkephalin mRNA and the enzymes required for post-translational processing are found in mammalian T and B cells, macrophages, and mast cells [120]. Immune-derived opioid peptides are proposed to play a pivotal role in the modulation of inflammatory pain, an area reviewed previously [75]. POMC and proenkephalin mRNA and the peptides β-endorphin and Met-enkephalin are found in circulating lymphocytes and cells derived from lymph nodes of rats with and without hindpaw inflammation [13,14], as well as in resident inflammatory cells [14,116]. The migration of β-endorphin-expressing leukocytes from the circulating blood into inflamed tissues starts with the attachment of these cells to the vascular endothelium, guided by L (leucocyte), P (platelet), and E (endothelial) selectins [87]. The migration of β-endorphin-containing leukocytes into the inflamed tissues can be blocked by fucoidin, a selectin blocker [74].

Opioid Receptors in Peripheral Nerves

Opioid receptors synthesized in the dorsal root ganglia (DRG) may be activated by immune-derived opioid peptides. Indeed, peripheral μ-receptor function increases following inflammation [75] as a result of enhanced receptor transport to the periphery, elevated pH [5], and enhanced primary afferent sprouting within the inflamed tissue [138]. Very recently, Hao et al. found that herpes simplex virus (HSV)-mediated endomorphin-2 expression via a synthetic endomorphin gene in DRG neurons attenuated neuropathic pain. This analgesic effect was reversed by naloxone methiodide, a blood-brain-barrier-impermeable naloxone derivative, injected intraperitoneally or intrathecally [51]. Together, these observations suggest that the access of opioid ligands to opioid receptors on primary afferent neurons is greatly enhanced in inflamed tissues, providing a primary site for opioid modulation of nociception (Fig. 2).

Spinal Cord and Brainstem Circuits Controlling Opioid Analgesia

Opioid Receptors in the Spinal Cord

Neurons of the dorsal horn express all classical and atypical opioid receptors. It is not surprising therefore that opioid receptors, particularly μ-receptors, mediate analgesia in the spinal cord (reviewed by Yaksh [139]). The μ-receptors are expressed in lamina II neurons, which are mostly small islet or stalked cells with dendrites oriented in a rostrocaudal direction and axons projecting to laminae I or III–V [34,80]. Most of these μ-containing interneurons do not express γ-aminobutyric acid (GABA) and are therefore considered excitatory [59]. It is likely that μ-activation inhibits these cells, thus preventing the passage of nociceptive information through the polysynaptic nociceptive pathway (Fig. 2). To determine the contribution of the μ-receptors expressed in dorsal horn neurons to thermal analgesia, Kline and Wiley [63] used dermorphin-saporin to eliminate the majority of

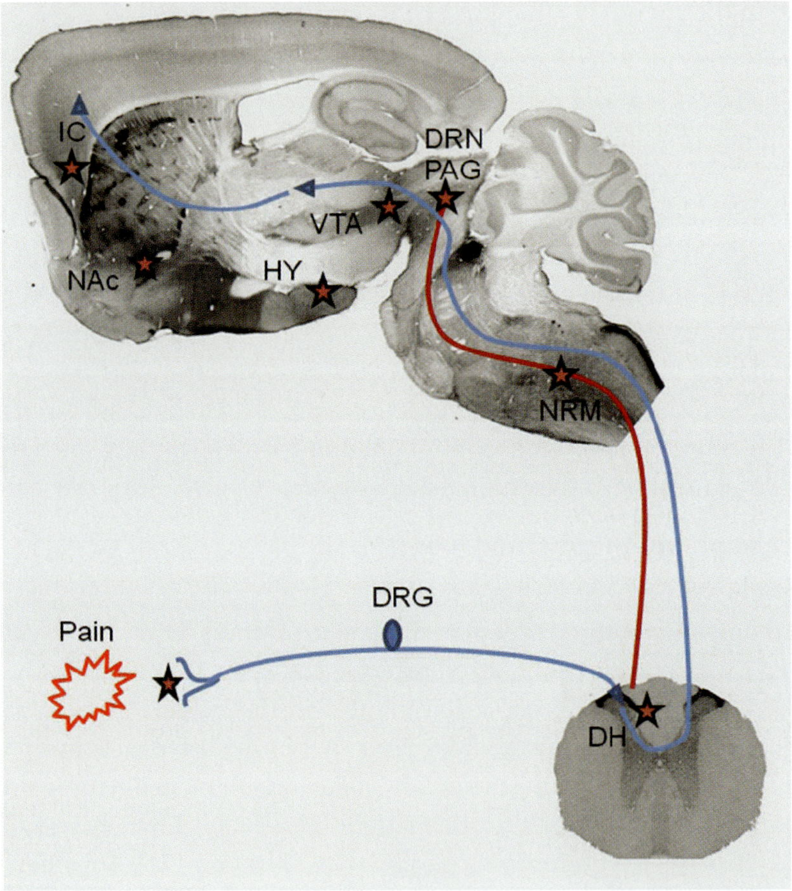

Fig. 2. Mu-opioid agonists, injected in specific regions of the central nervous system (CNS), produce antinociception. This figure shows the distribution of μ-opioid receptors (identified by well-characterized rabbit μ-opioid receptor antisera) in mouse brain and spinal cord and a schematic representation of the major ascending and descending pain pathways. The brain sagittal section is close to the midline (bregma 1.1–1.4), and the spinal cord section is from the thoracic region. Stars and named brain regions represent areas where local injection of μ-opioid agonists produces antinociception. Blue = the ascending spinothalamic tract containing first-, second-, and third-order neurons. Red = the descending modulatory pathway that originates in the cortex (cortical pathway not depicted here) and projects to the PAG, rostroventral medulla, and dorsal horn. Abbreviations: DH = dorsal horn, DRG = dorsal root ganglia, DRN = dorsal raphe nucleus, HY = hypothalamus, IC = insular cortex, NAc = nucleus accumbens, NRM = nucleus raphe magnus, PAG = periaqueductal gray, VTA = ventral tegmental area.

these cells. This procedure reduced the antinociceptive effect of morphine, indicating that μ-expressing dorsal horn neurons do indeed contribute to opioid analgesia. The ORL1, or nociceptin receptor [86] is present in the spinal cord [88], where it has complex effects: low doses of orphanin FQ/nociceptin produce spontaneous pain [105], whereas high doses are analgesic.

Opioid Peptides in the Dorsal Horn

Opioid peptides in the dorsal horn are those encoded by the preproenkephalin and preprodynorphin genes and are expressed in different dorsal horn neurons [31]. Endorphins are not present in the dorsal horn [119], although they are found in the area around the central canal and in the ventral horn. It has been suggested that endomorphins are present in primary afferents, based on the observation that antibodies against endomorphin labeled substance P-containing primary afferent terminals [79,100]. However, anti-endomorphin antibodies did not label DRG neurons [107]. Moreover, endomorphins are not co-released with substance P by capsaicin, NMDA, or dorsal root stimulation [113], suggesting that they do not have a functional role in the dorsal horn. Another peptide found in the dorsal horn is orphanin FQ/nociceptin, the endogenous ligand for ORL1 (NOP_1) receptors.

Both enkephalins and dynorphins are highly susceptible to cleavage by three peptidases: aminopeptidases (E.C. 3.4.11), dipeptidyl carboxypeptidase (E.C. 3.4.15.1), and neutral endopeptidase (E.C. 3.4.24.11) [93]. Because of this, the analgesia produced by intrathecal enkephalin or dynorphin increases substantially upon co-injection of peptidase inhibitors [21,62]. Some peptidase inhibitors are being developed as analgesics. For example, RB 101, a prodrug that generates inhibitors of aminopeptidase and neutral endopeptidase [89,90], produced analgesia in the hot plate, writhing, and tail-flick tests after systemic administration. Remarkably, RB 101 does not appear to induce tolerance or physical dependence [91].

Release of Opioid Peptides

It is unlikely that opioids act in a classic synaptic manner, that is, by binding to receptors across the synaptic cleft. Instead, the presence of opioid receptors in the soma and dendritic tree of dorsal horn neurons suggests that opioids act by volume transmission [44].

Adrenergic α_{2C} receptors, found in enkephalin-containing glutamatergic terminals [94,117], inhibit opioid release [22]. This inhibition does not appear to lead to hyperalgesia, since α_{2C} receptors contribute to the analgesic effect of norepinephrine [36]. It may serve to shut down opioid release when the descending adrenergic system is active. 5-HT_{1A} serotonin receptors also inhibit opioid release in the spinal cord [111]. NMDA receptors inhibit opioid release from spinal cord slices [114]. This inhibition is based on a functional coupling between NMDA receptors and Ca^{2+}-sensitive large-conductance (maxi-K) potassium channels. Ca^{2+} influx through the NMDA receptors causes the opening of the maxi-K channels, which in turn leads to inhibition of neuronal firing. Accordingly, maxi-K channel blockers reversed the inhibition by NMDA, and a maxi-K channel opener inhibited opioid release. Enkephalin release may also be inhibited by $GABA_B$ [18] and δ-receptors [28], and may be facilitated by cholecystokinin (CCK) and neuropeptide FF, which suppress the inhibition by δ-receptors [82]. However, another study found that opioid release was not affected by CCK, $GABA_B$ receptors, or δ-receptors [111].

Given that primary afferents do not contain enkephalins and are not an important source of dynorphins, the main sources of opioids in the dorsal horn are interneurons and supraspinal axons. It has been suggested that opioids are primarily released from intrinsic dorsal horn neurons [31,52]. Electrical stimulation of the dorsal root does not induce any μ-receptor internalization in dorsal horn neurons [113], confirming that opioids are not released from primary afferents or from second-order neurons. In contrast, chemical [23,112] or electrical [113] stimulation of the dorsal horn produces abundant μ-receptor internalization. However, it is possible that these stimuli release opioids from supraspinal axons. Indeed, opioid immunoreactivity occurs in fibers in the dorsolateral funiculus [113], an area that contains axons of supraspinal origin [67]. Another possibility is that opioid release from dorsal horn neurons is driven by descending axons making excitatory synapses with them.

Brainstem Control of Opioid Release in the Spinal Cord

The release of opioids in the spinal cord is the last step of a series of neuronal circuits that modulate pain signals according to the neurophysiological state of the animal. These neural circuits are modulated by opioids at almost every synaptic step. The best characterized of these circuits is a descending pathway linking the dorsal raphe nucleus (DRN), the periaqueductal gray (PAG), the nucleus raphe magnus (NRM), and the dorsal horn of the spinal cord (Fig. 2) [38,81]. The role of these regions in analgesia mediated by spinal opioids has been elucidated in studies following three basic experimental approaches: (1) analgesia induced by stimulation of specific brain regions, (2) spinal opioid release induced by noxious stimuli, and (3) stress-induced analgesia.

Analgesia, or an equivalent decrease in the response of dorsal horn neurons to noxious stimuli, can be induced by stimulating the NRM [143] or the PAG [11]. The fact that this analgesia can be eliminated by spinal application of opioid antagonists shows that it is mediated by opioid release in the spinal cord. However, descending adrenergic and serotonergic pathways also participate in pain inhibition [12,57], and the relative role of each of these neurotransmitter systems is still controversial. For example, one group [2] reported that analgesia produced by stimulating the PAG or the NRM could be blocked by adrenergic and serotonin antagonists but not by opioid antagonists.

Opioid release in the spinal cord is also evoked by noxious stimuli, both acute [19,67] and chronic [7]. Some studies have used sciatic nerve stimulation to mimic noxious signals. As explained above, the opioids are not released directly from the primary afferents or even by second-order neurons. Whether their release is driven by intraspinal circuits or involves supraspinal signals is still a matter of debate. For example, Hutchinson et al. [55] reported that the release of dynorphin A in the cat spinal cord was abolished by spinal transection, indicating that it is driven supraspinally. In contrast, Yaksh and Elde

[140] showed that Met-enkephalin release in the cat spinal cord was unaffected by cold block of the spinal cord, and they therefore concluded that it is not mediated supraspinally.

A third way to investigate supraspinal mechanisms that inhibit pain is to study stress-induced analgesia (SIA). That stress inhibits pain has been known for some time. Studies performed during the 1970s and 80s identified many stressors that produce analgesia, including thermal challenge, restraint, hypoglycemia, social defeat, and electric shock [118]. A key issue in these studies was to determine whether the analgesia was mediated by opioids. This determination was made by assessing whether SIA was blocked by opioid antagonists or was cross-tolerant with morphine. Initial studies seemed to show that the involvement of opioids in SIA depended on the properties of the stressor. For example, Liebeskind's group [118] found that the analgesia was opioid-mediated when induced by intermittent footshock or by continuous footshock of short duration or low intensity, but not by continuous, intense footshock. SIA mediated by opioid release in the spinal cord was driven by a descending pathway originating in the NRM and the adjacent nucleus reticularis paragigantocellularis [127]. Importantly, opioid release was caused by stress and not directly by the footshock, because classical conditioning to the footshock produced opioid-mediated analgesia through the same pathway [127].

The PAG activates the NRM and the adjacent nucleus reticularis paragigantocellularis through neurons releasing excitatory amino acids. The NRM has two characteristic neuronal populations, termed ON and OFF cells, which project to the spinal cord and modulate pain [38,81]. These cells have been studied using rat "tail-flick" responses to radiant heat. The ON cells are activated by noxious stimuli and show a sudden increase in firing just before the tail-flick reflex. In contrast, OFF cells respond to noxious stimuli by a pause in firing that occurs before the tail-flick response. Nociceptive transmission in the dorsal horn is inhibited by OFF cells and facilitated by ON cells. Other cells in the NRM, including spinally projecting serotonergic neurons, do not participate in the tail-flick response and are called neutral cells. This somewhat simplistic classification has been challenged recently, and may not reflect the response of the NRM to all types of noxious stimuli. However, it serves to outline the neuronal architecture of the NRM [38]. ON cells and OFF cells inhibit each other. Enkephalinergic interneurons inhibit the ON cells, which appear to have μ-opioid receptors, and this action leads to disinhibition of the OFF cells. This process is thought to mediate the analgesic effect of opioids in the brainstem.

Opioid Analgesia in the Reward Pathways and Cortex

Analgesia of Reward Expectancy and the Midbrain

The mesostriatal system in the midbrain serves a vital and fundamental role in mediating responses to natural rewards and drugs of abuse. In the mesolimbic system, dopaminergic neurons originating from the ventral tegmental area project to the nucleus accumbens (NAc) [136]. The analgesic effect of reward expectancy was first reported by Dum and

Herz in 1984. In this study, rats were conditioned on an unheated hot plate with either regular laboratory chow or chocolate-covered waffled candy. Then rats were simply placed on a heated hot plate, and those expecting candy demonstrated analgesia. The analgesia was completely blocked by a low dose of naloxone (1 mg/kg), which had no visible effect upon the paw-lick latencies of chow-fed rats. This study suggests that activation of endogenous opioid systems by reward expectancy can modulate nociceptive systems [33].

The analgesic effect of reward expectancy is poorly understood, although there is evidence that the mesostriatal circuit mediating drug and food rewards is involved [37]. Microinjection of the opioid receptor antagonist, naloxone, into the NAc suppressed the antinociceptive effects of reward expectancy [46]. Microinjection of opioids into the mesolimbic circuit produces both reward and analgesia (Fig. 2). These studies link the mechanisms of analgesia to those of reward and implicate mesostriatal dopaminergic neurons in the modulation of nociception [37].

Placebo-Induced Analgesia and Opioid Circuits in the Cortex

Robust placebo effects have been observed in regulating nociception. An initial study of the neurochemical mechanism of placebo analgesia was published in 1978 by Levine at al. The authors demonstrated that the placebo analgesia effect on dental postoperative pain was attenuated by naloxone [69]. Subsequently, using [^{11}C] carfentanil positron emission tomography (PET) imaging, Zubieta et al. [145] demonstrated that sustained pain induced a regional release of endogenous opioids interacting with μ-opioid receptors in various cortical and subcortical brain regions. The regions implicated in opioid release included the anterior cingulate cortex (ACC), prefrontal cortex (PFC), insular cortex, amygdala, thalamus, and NAc, regions coincident with those activated by administration of exogenous opioid drugs [99]. In a follow-up study, patients with sustained pain who had been treated with or without placebo were assessed, and [^{11}C] carfentanil PET imaging showed a significant placebo-induced activation of μ-mediated neurotransmission in the rostral ACC (rACC), the dorsolateral prefrontal cortex (DLPFC), and the insular cortex [144]. These findings provide neurochemical evidence that placebo analgesia can involve activation of endogenous μ-opioid systems in brain areas associated with reward circuitry.

Further insight into the psychological and neural mechanisms that mediate placebo analgesia comes from functional magnetic resonance imaging (fMRI) experiments [123]. Placebo manipulations were found to decrease neural activity in pain-responsive regions of the brain, such as the thalamus, somatosensory cortex, insula, and ACC. The magnitude of this neural decrease correlated with the reduction in reported pain. During the anticipation phase, or "belief" in analgesic efficacy, placebo modulates the activity of the brain regions known to be involved in generating and maintaining expectations of pain relief, such as the PFC (the DLPFC in particular), the orbitofrontal cortex (OFC), and the ACC. In addition, increased neural activity seen within the PAG correlated positively with the DLPFC and OFC activation. Given that the PAG projects upward to the telencephalon as well as downward to the descending pathways that control pain and the endogenous opioid system, these results suggest that opioid systems may be modulated by prefrontal cortically driven expectations of analgesia [8].

PET studies measuring regional cerebral blood flow (rCBF) have also contributed to understanding the neural mechanisms of placebo analgesia. Concomitant nociceptive responses and rCBF were measured during heat pain with placebo treatment or a fast-acting opioid (remifentanil). Increases of rCBF in the OFC, rACC, and brainstem were found irrespective of the treatment [99]. In a later experiment, a validated sham acupuncture procedure was used to explore the brain network involved in placebo analgesia [65]. The authors found that placebo-expectant acupuncture treatment can produce a detectable placebo analgesic effect. A negative correlation was found between subjective pain ratings and activity in the bilateral lateral/orbital prefrontal cortex, rACC, cerebellum, right fusiform, parahippocampus, and pons, indicating that the more powerful the placebo analgesia, the stronger the activity in these brain regions [65]. The discrepancy of these results from those of Wager et al. [123]—who found a placebo-induced blood-oxygen-level-dependent signal signal decrease in the ACC, insular cortex, and thalamus during pain—is not clear, but it may be attributable to the differences in pain modality or in the mechanisms of placebo induction, or to an intrinsic variability of the placebo response [70]. Zubieta and colleagues recently also demonstrated that levels of expectation of analgesia ("belief" in analgesic efficacy) and the subjective experience of pain influence the activation of endogenous opioid neurotransmission during the introduction of a placebo [146].

Clinical Perspectives

Opioid medications are a primary modality for the treatment of acute pain, and an important therapeutic option for cancer pain. In these settings, their benefit is certain, and supported by extensive evidence [42,72]. But their optimal role in the treatment of chronic pain is less clear [6,43,78,97]. Opioid analgesics may have reduced efficacy in the setting of chronic pain, and their chronic use may be associated with a variety of significant adverse effects involving multiple organ systems, often complicated by tolerance, dependence, and addiction. In addition, opioid analgesics have the potential to produce an adverse change in the experience of the same pain that the medications were originally used to treat [92]. The pain may become more constant, more severe, and less responsive to any therapy than it was prior to the therapy. The therapeutic use of opioids therefore requires an ongoing assessment of the beneficial versus adverse effects, particularly in the setting of chronic pain. And while the use of opioid analgesics for the treatment of pain is steadily increasing with time, for many clinical situations there is little information to guide decisions about which patients are the most likely to benefit from this therapy. Understanding the pharmacological and physiological mechanisms of the therapeutic versus deleterious effects of opioid medications is therefore critical to advancing our ability to treat pain.

Pain is commonly classified as somatic, visceral, or neuropathic. In this classification scheme, somatic pain involves skin, muscles, bones, and connective tissue; visceral pain originates from organs or their surrounding tissue; and neuropathic pain is generated primarily by peripheral or central nerves. However, there may be considerable overlap between these different types of pain, and there are multiple types of pain that may not be easily classified in this way (e.g., headache). The burning, electrical, or shooting sensations typical of neuropathic pain, along with the associated hyperalgesia and allodynia, are commonly considered to be less responsive to opioid analgesia. Migraine headache may also be less responsive to opioid analgesia than other types of pain [106]. Nonetheless, opioids may have a place in the therapeutic management of some patients with neuropathic pain or headache, particularly when used acutely, and it is not possible to determine whether a patient is an appropriate candidate for opioid therapy based on simplistic classification of pain type [58]. Again, there is a clear need for better evidence to guide clinicians regarding the specific types of pain for which the use of opioid analgesics is appropriate or contraindicated.

Clinical Differences between Opioid Analgesics

The majority of currently used opioid medications are believed to exert their therapeutic effects by acting as agonists at the μ-receptor. However, there may be considerable variability in the therapeutic and adverse effects of the same opioid medication in different individuals [103]. These differences may become particularly apparent when a patient switches from one opioid analgesic to another. Opioid conversion tables that describe equianalgesic doses of different medications are widely published and are commonly used as guides for switching a patient from one analgesic agent to another [96]. However, clinical experience regarding analgesic and adverse effects with such a change in medication often varies widely from what would be expected based on these tables [96]. In addition, for a given individual in whom the efficacy of one opioid medication decreases over time, changing to an equivalent dose of a different medication with an apparently similar mechanism of action may result in much improved pain relief. The advantages of this type of "rotation" of opioid medications is supported by some small clinical trials [131,135]. The observation that rotation helps maintain clinical effectiveness of opiate therapeutics reveals incomplete cross-tolerance that may be attributed to activation of slightly different populations of receptors due to different properties (receptor selectivity, metabolism, hydrophobicity, etc.) or activation of different signaling pathways. Initial clinical studies also indicate that simultaneous use of combinations of different opioid agonists may be more effective and have reduced adverse effects as compared to those with individual medication [110]. There is also some evidence, from both animal and human studies, to suggest that giving a low dose of the opioid receptor antagonist naltrexone along with an opioid analgesic may improve the therapeutic response [25,50,101]. All of these clinical observations emphasize the fact that there are important distinctions between different opioid analgesics that mediate different clinical responses.

Gender Differences in Opioid Analgesia

The distinctive responses of different individuals to different opioid medications may involve genetic factors, environmental factors, or gender. As explained in previous sections of the chapter, genetic variations in opioid receptors, transporters, and metabolizing enzymes in different individuals may have a significant impact on the efficacy and adverse effects of opioid analgesics. Gender may also play a role, through both chromosomal and hormonal mechanisms. There are conflicting reports regarding the different potential roles of gender in the response to opioid analgesics. Some clinical studies indicate that women consume less morphine in the postoperative setting while achieving similar or lower post-surgical pain ratings [24], and that κ-opioids produce a greater analgesic effect in women than in men [47]. Other studies indicate that women require more morphine than men in order to achieve comparable levels of analgesia [17]. Still other clinical and experimental studies indicate no differences in the analgesic effects of μ-receptor selective opioids in women versus men, but suggest that women more commonly experience adverse effects [39,49]. These highly variable results may depend on the pain model and clinical setting and on the specific opioid analgesics that are used. Regardless of the potential causes for gender differences in responses to opioids, it is interesting to note that epidemiological studies indicate that women have a significantly higher use of prescription opioid analgesics in the outpatient setting as compared with men [53,134]. A better understanding of the role of genetics and gender in the response to opioid analgesics will lead to more selective and effective use of these medications in specific patients.

Adverse Effects and Strategies to Minimize Them

The acute adverse effects of opioids include pruritis (itching), impairment of gastric motility, nausea, urinary retention, sedation, and respiratory depression. Each of these effects appears to be related to direct activation of μ-receptors, either in the CNS or in the periphery. These adverse events may limit the clinical use of opioid analgesia, and so strategies are being developed to suppress them, while maintaining the analgesic effects. For side effects that involve peripheral opioid receptors (nausea and vomiting, constipation), one such strategy is to use peripheral opioid receptor antagonists that do not enter the CNS, such as methylnaltrexone and alvimopan [130]. Alternatively, the medications can be delivered directly into the CNS via implanted pumps, which as a result of significant technological advances are much smaller and more accurate than they were in the past [50,104]. Conversely, in situations in which peripheral opioid receptors are therapeutic targets and activation of central opioid receptors is primarily responsible for side effects (sedation and respiratory depression), opioid analgesics whose action is restricted to the periphery are being developed [110]. Finally, ultra-short-acting opioids may be particularly useful in the critical care or surgical settings, where greater temporal control over medication levels may be important to enable rapid reversal of respiratory depression or sedation [133].

Tolerance and Addiction

Many clinicians are reluctant to prescribe opioid analgesics because of concerns regarding tolerance, dependence, and addiction. However, growing evidence suggests that tolerance that results in progressively increasing doses of opioids over time may not be as significant an issue for most patients as has been generally perceived. A number of studies regarding the chronic use of opioids indicate that in many clinical situations, dose escalation over time is a relatively infrequent problem [56,76,104]. While some studies indicate that addiction and aberrant medication-taking behaviors may be a relatively common problem in patients taking chronic opioids for pain [78], other studies indicate that the problem is relatively infrequent [40,76,92]. A previous history of substance abuse and mental disorders may represent specific risk factors for the development of addiction, such that screening for these risk factors could further reduce the occurrence of addiction in patients who are treated with opioid analgesics for acute or chronic pain [35,41].

Opioid-Induced Hyperalgesia

While concern regarding dose escalation and addiction with opioid analgesic therapy for pain patients is waning somewhat, there is at the same time a growing recognition that the phenomenon of opioid-induced hyperalgesia (OIH) may be a highly significant problem [3,20]. Strictly speaking, tolerance is a shift in the dose-response curve, which can result from desensitization of opioid-regulated circuitry or opponent processes that are triggered by opioid treatments. OIH involves a paradoxical sensitization to nociceptive stimuli, resulting in increased pain that may be similar to or different from the original pain for which the treatment was initiated [27,84,102]. Particularly in patients with OIH, reducing rather than increasing the dose of the opioid analgesic may be advisable in situations where pain is increased on a given dose, an approach that is supported by some reports [122].

The physiological changes responsible for OIH may occur at the level of the peripheral nociceptive afferents, in the dorsal horn of the spinal cord (or trigeminal nucleus caudalis), or in descending centers responsible for modulation of pain such as the rostral ventromedial medulla [6,84]. Several lines of evidence point to a role for glutamate-receptor-mediated signaling in both OIH and tolerance [77,84]. Simultaneous administration of glutamate receptor antagonists may therefore be of benefit in the setting of OIH. Rotation of different opioid medications, or the combination of a low dose opioid receptor antagonist along with an opioid receptor agonist may also help to reduce OIH.

Effects of Opioids on Outcomes in Pain Patients

Ongoing epidemiological studies are continuing to provide new information about the beneficial versus deleterious effects of opioids, especially in the setting of chronic pain. A study examining patients with back pain found that early use of high doses of opioid analgesics for acute low back pain was associated with higher rates of disability, greater overall medical costs, and more likelihood of eventual surgery [129]. While the severity of the pain must be considered as a factor that influenced the early dosing of opioid analgesics, such studies raise the possibility that treatment with opioids early in the course of therapy for low back pain may have an adverse impact on eventual outcome. Another condition in which use of opioid analgesics may lead to an adverse outcome is headache. Growing evidence shows that chronic therapy with opioid analgesics may be a primary factor in the transformation of migraine from an episodic, manageable disorder to a chronic daily headache that is unresponsive to therapy [9,106]. Multiple studies evaluating the use of opioids for chronic pain in general also suggest that chronic opioid use is associated with poor outcome based on a variety of measures [6,43,58]. Decisions regarding opioid therapy for headache, back pain, and other chronic pain conditions may therefore be quite complex, and there are currently no straightforward guidelines. Should a source of substantial short-term relief of pain be withheld on the basis of concern regarding adverse long-term outcome? Should the duration of opioid analgesic therapy be limited in order to improve outcomes? Are specific opioid medications or medication combinations less likely to cause adverse outcomes? These are just a few of the multiple important questions that need to be addressed by basic and clinical science in order for clinicians to be able to most effectively manage pain with opioid medications.

Emerging Concepts in Opioid Pharmacology

Clinical studies have identified several issues that confound the action of opioid treatments. Although tolerance has over the years been a major research focus, diminution of drug efficacy itself is not of paramount concern to physicians. Opponent processes (adaptations opposing the acute opioid actions) that are evident during withdrawal and that may contribute to tolerance can be problematic in the clinic, however. One such process relevant to pain treatment is hyperalgesia. Another issue of major concern is the addictive nature of the opioid drugs. This section will target recent research addressing these key clinical issues.

Opioid Drugs with Reduced Deleterious Side Effects

Addiction and misuse of opioid analgesics is a growing concern that is not restricted to those with pain conditions. Disturbing statistics such as approximately 10% of 12th graders using Vicodin (a trademarked oral formulation of hydrocodone and acetaminophen) illicitly in 2006, and 2.1% of adults using a pain medication illicitly during the month before a U.S. survey by the Substance Abuse and Mental Health Services Association in 2006, are clear indicators that opioid therapeutic abuse is rampant [29]. Rodent studies have identified several systems beside opioid receptors that appear to mediate opioid drug-induced reward behaviors. These include systems involving the CB1 cannabinoid receptor, an abundant CNS receptor activated by cannabinoids, and the NK1 receptor, a G_s-protein-coupled receptor activated by substance P and other neurokinins. In animals lacking CB1 or NK1 receptors, morphine reward behavior is much diminished (for review, see [10]). This finding raises the possibility of combining μ-opioid drugs with either CB1 antagonists (such as rimonabant) or NK1 antagonists in order to reduce the μ-mediated rewarding effects while retaining analgesic efficacy. The result would of course be the "holy grail" for opioid research—an opioid analgesic without rewarding effects. Unfortunately, recent data have implicated the CB1 antagonist rimonabant in suicidal behaviors. Rimonabant is an inverse agonist that blocks constitutive activity of CB1 receptors, and neutral antagonists that are now being developed might be less prone to triggering dysphoric states.

More hopeful is the potential for modulation of μ-opioid-mediated effects by blockade of NK1 receptors. The lack of NK1 receptors not only diminishes morphine reward but also appears to block hyperalgesia induced by chronic opioid treatment [61]. The combination of an NK1 blockade with opioid medication thus has the potential of increasing opioid efficacy during chronic treatments with blunted reward. This drug combination has not to our knowledge been assessed in the clinic.

A third alternative is to limit opioid-induced glial activation, a process that suppresses the analgesic effect of morphine and contributes to tolerance and withdrawal. Although as yet untested, one possibility would be to co-administer with opioid agonists stereospecific opioid isomers of naltrexone, which bind nonclassical opioid receptors present on glia but not classical opioid receptors, or inhibit glial activation by cytokine inhibition.

The blockade of non-opioid systems mediating deleterious opioid-mediated actions is one future possibility for improving opioid medications. A second possibility is improving the drugs themselves to optimize interaction with μ-receptors for promoting analgesia. It has become clear that opioid receptors trigger numerous different signaling cascades and that signaling, as well as trafficking of opioid receptors, is dependent upon the agonist activating the receptor (reviewed by Kieffer and Evans [60]). The concept of GPCRs has changed markedly during the past decade such that the receptors are now viewed as components of receptor complexes with multiple associated proteins. Such complexes include other GPCRs forming homomeric or heteromeric aggregates, the heterotrimeric G proteins, and several other proteins regulated by receptor occupation such as G-protein receptor kinases, other kinases such as protein kinase C, β_1 and β_2 arrestins, and—in the case of μ receptors—calmodulin. It is becoming very clear that receptor complex composition can be radically modified by ligand interaction with the receptor and that as a result the signaling and trafficking profiles of different opioid receptor agonists can be variable. Future research will seek optimal signaling and trafficking cascades for analgesic responses while hoping to silence some of the signaling pathways leading to the deleterious side effects of the opioid drugs.

Modulation of Opioid Receptor Surface Levels

Opioid receptor trafficking plays an important role in regulating the ability of opioid drugs to modulate cellular activity. Most studies have focused on agonist- and antagonist-regulated opioid receptor trafficking of surface receptors [121] and on the ability for agonists to differentially induce receptor internalization. The issues of internalization and tolerance have been the central theme, but it is clear that ligands that efficaciously internalize μ-opioid receptors as well as those that internalize poorly cause desensitization at a cellular level and tolerance at a behavioral level. These issues have been addressed fully in recent reviews [26,60]. More recent studies have revealed more intricate mechanisms of ligand-dependent and -independent trafficking. A particularly intriguing regulatory mechanism involves ligand stabilization of receptor protein conformation in the endoplasmic reticulum that prevents digestion by the proteosome and promotes maturation of receptor protein in the cells [68,98]. This stabilization can be induced by selective agonist and antagonists that traverse the cell membrane. The possibility that surface receptor number could be upregulated to make more receptors available for cellular regulation via either constitutive activity or activation by endogenous or exogenous agonists is a particularly exciting concept.

Mechanisms of upregulation of surface opioid receptors besides ligand promotion of receptor maturation have also been described and are the subject of a thorough recent review by Cahill et al. [15]. Several studies have demonstrated a μ-mediated upregulation of δ-receptors in response to chronic morphine. Additionally, inflammation also appears to upregulate surface δ-receptors [16]. Externalization is in some cases attributable to triggering release of an intracellular vesicular pool of δ-receptors via μ- or δ-receptor signaling, but other studies have implicated μ-receptors as inhibitory of δ-receptor function with DRG cells from μ-receptor knockout animals showing enhanced δ-receptor function [125]. The upregulation of surface, bioavailable δ-receptors presents an intriguing therapeutic target for types of pain, such as chronic inflammatory pain and neuropathic pain, that are poorly treated by μ-agonists. However, an issue confounding δ-ligands as effective drugs is the propensity for agonists to induce internalization, which results in receptor targeting to lysosomes and degradation. It will be difficult to envisage effective δ-agonist treatments unless this degradative trafficking can be eluded and the important confound of δ-receptor activation triggering seizures is fully resolved.

In a recent study, our group demonstrated that β-arrestin-2 is required for internalization of constitutively active μ-opioid receptors from the surface of DRG cells [124]. Thus, in β-arrestin-2 knockout mice there is increased constitutive activity on the surface of DRG neurons, which correlates with a μ-mediated analgesic phenotype in some pain assays. Interestingly, cSrc activity is also required for this internalization of constitutively active μ-receptors. Given this observation, blockade specifically of the arrestin 2-cSrc involvement in μ-receptor trafficking could provide a therapeutic target by upregulation of surface μ-receptors that are constitutively active and require no ligand activation for functionality. The possibility of allosteric regulators or neutral antagonists that disrupt arrestin interactions yet retain constitutive activity would present intriguing new opioid drugs.

Conclusion

An increased understanding of endogenous opioid systems is identifying new therapeutic targets for the treatment of pain and helping to optimize the use of currently available opioid analgesics. Despite this progress, however, advances in the clinical management of pain have been incremental, and the abuse of prescription opioids continues to increase. No treatment-transforming opioid medications have been developed, and there are no clear guidelines for the appropriate use of opioid analgesics in patients with a variety of pain conditions, including back pain, headache, and neuropathic pain. The future holds significant promise, however, for translational research and a more informed and effective use of opioids for the clinical management of pain.

References

[1] Abbadie C, Pan YX, Pasternak GW. Differential distribution in rat brain of mu opioid receptor carboxy terminal splice variants MOR-1C-like and MOR-1-like immunoreactivity: evidence for region-specific processing. J Comp Neurol 2000;419:244–56.
[2] Aimone LD, Jones SL, Gebhart GF. Stimulation-produced descending inhibition from the periaqueductal gray and nucleus raphe magnus in the rat: mediation by spinal monoamines but not opioids. Pain 1987;31:123–36.
[3] Angst MS, Clark D. Opioid-induced hyperalgesia: a qualitative systematic review. Anesthesiology 2006;104:570–87.
[4] Anton B, Fein J, To T, Li X, Silberstein L, Evans CJ. Immunohistochemical localization of ORL-1 in the central nervous system of the rat. J Comp Neurol 1996;368:229–51.
[5] Antonijevic I, Mousa SA, Schafer M, Stein C. Perineurial defect and peripheral opioid analgesia in inflammation. J Neurosci 1995;15:165–72.
[6] Ballantyne JC, Shin NS. Efficacy of opioids for chronic pain: a review of the evidence. Clin J Pain 2008;24:469–78.
[7] Ballet S, Mauborgne A, Hamon M, Cesselin F, Collin E. Altered opioid-mediated control of the spinal release of dynorphin and Met-enkephalin in polyarthritic rats. Synapse 2000;37:262–72.
[8] Benedetti F, Mayberg HS, Wager TD, Stohler CS, Zubieta JK. Neurobiological mechanisms of the placebo effect. J Neurosci 2005;25:10390–402.
[9] Bigal ME, Lipton RB. Excessive acute migraine medication use and migraine progression. Neurology 2008;71:1821–8.
[10] Bryant CD, Zaki PA, Carroll FI, Evans CJ. Opioids and addiction: emerging pharmaceutical strategies for reducing reward and opponent processes. Clin Neurosci Res 2005;5:103–15.
[11] Budai D, Fields HL. Endogenous opioid peptides acting at mu-opioid receptors in the dorsal horn contribute to midbrain modulation of spinal nociceptive neurons. J Neurophysiol 1998;79:677–87.
[12] Budai D, Harasawa I, Fields HL. Midbrain periaqueductal gray (PAG) inhibits nociceptive inputs to sacral dorsal horn nociceptive neurons through $alpha_2$-adrenergic receptors. J Neurophysiol 1998;80:2244–54.
[13] Cabot PJ, Carter L, Gaiddon C, Zhang Q, Schafer M, Loeffler JP, Stein C. Immune cell-derived beta-endorphin. Production, release, and control of inflammatory pain in rats. J Clin Invest 1997;100:142–8.
[14] Cabot PJ, Carter L, Schafer M, Stein C. Methionine-enkephalin-and dynorphin A-release from immune cells and control of inflammatory pain. Pain 2001;93:207–12.
[15] Cahill CM, Holdridge SV, Morinville A. Trafficking of delta-opioid receptors and other G-protein-coupled receptors: implications for pain and analgesia. Trends Pharmacol Sci 2007;28:23–31.
[16] Cahill CM, Morinville A, Hoffert C, O'Donnell D, Beaudet A. Up-regulation and trafficking of delta opioid receptor in a model of chronic inflammation: implications for pain control. Pain 2003;101:199–208.
[17] Cepeda MS, Carr DB. Women experience more pain and require more morphine than men to achieve a similar degree of analgesia. Anesth Analg 2003;97:1464–8.
[18] Cesselin F, Bourgoin S, Artaud F, Hamon M. Basic and regulatory mechanisms of in vitro release of Met-enkephalin from the dorsal zone of the rat spinal cord. J Neurochem 1984;43:763–74.
[19] Cesselin F, Bourgoin S, Clot AM, Hamon M, Le Bars D. Segmental release of Met-enkephalin-like material from the spinal-cord of rats, elicited by noxious thermal stimuli. Brain Res 1989;484:71–7.
[20] Chang G, Chen L, Mao J. Opioid tolerance and hyperalgesia. Med Clin North Am 2007;91:199–211.
[21] Chen W, Song B, Lao L, Perez OA, Marvizon JC. Intrathecal enkephalin requires inhibition of peptidases to produce analgesia and mu-opioid receptor internalization in dorsal horn neurons. Soc Neurosci Abstracts 2006;32:643.18.
[22] Chen W, Song B, Marvizon JC. Inhibition of opioid release in the rat spinal cord by α_{2C} adrenergic receptors. Neuropharmacology 2008;54:944–53.
[23] Chen W, Song B, Zhang G, Marvizon JC. Effects of veratridine and high potassium on μ-opioid receptor internalization in the rat spinal cord: stimulation of opioid release versus inhibition of internalization. J Neurosci Methods 2008;170:285–93.

[24] Chia YY, Chow LH, Hung CC, Liu K, Ger LP, Wang PN. Gender and pain upon movement are associated with the requirements for postoperative patient-controlled iv analgesia: a prospective survey of 2,298 Chinese patients. Can J Anaesth 2002;49:249–55.

[25] Chindalore VL, Craven RA, Yu KP, Butera PG, Burns LH, Friedmann N. Adding ultralow-dose naltrexone to oxycodone enhances and prolongs analgesia: a randomized, controlled trial of Oxytrex. J Pain 2005;6:392–9.

[26] Christie MJ. Cellular neuroadaptations to chronic opioids: tolerance, withdrawal and addiction. Br J Pharmacol 2008;154:384–96.

[27] Chu LF, Clark DJ, Angst MS. Opioid tolerance and hyperalgesia in chronic pain patients after one month of oral morphine therapy: a preliminary prospective study. J Pain 2006;7:43–8.

[28] Collin E, Mauborgne A, Bourgoin S, Benoliel JJ, Hamon M, Cesselin F. Morphine reduces the release of Met-enkephalin-like material from the rat spinal cord in vivo by acting at delta opioid receptors. Neuropeptides 1994;27:75–83.

[29] Compton WM, Volkow ND. Major increases in opioid analgesic abuse in the United States: concerns and strategies. Drug Alcohol Depend 2006;81:103–7.

[30] Contet C, Kieffer BL, Befort K. Mu opioid receptor: a gateway to drug addiction. Curr Opin Neurobiol 2004;14:370–8.

[31] Cruz L, Basbaum AI. Multiple opioid peptides and the modulation of pain: immunohistochemical analysis of dynorphin and enkephalin in the trigeminal nucleus caudalis and spinal cord of the cat. J Comp Neurol 1985;240:331–48.

[32] Dierich A, Kieffer BL. Knockout mouse models in pain research. Methods Mol Med 2004;99:269–99.

[33] Dum J, Herz A. Endorphinergic modulation of neural reward systems indicated by behavioral changes. Pharmacol Biochem Behav 1984;21:259–66.

[34] Eckert WA III, McNaughton KK, Light AR. Morphology and axonal arborization of rat spinal inner lamina II neurons hyperpolarized by mu-opioid-selective agonists. J Comp Neurol 2003;458:240–56.

[35] Edlund MJ, Steffick D, Hudson T, Harris KM, Sullivan M. Risk factors for clinically recognized opioid abuse and dependence among veterans using opioids for chronic non-cancer pain. Pain 2007;129:355–62.

[36] Fairbanks CA, Stone LS, Kitto KF, Nguyen HO, Posthumus IJ, Wilcox GL. $Alpha_{2C}$-adrenergic receptors mediate spinal analgesia and adrenergic-opioid synergy. J Pharmacol Exp Ther 2002;300:282–90.

[37] Fields HL. Understanding how opioids contribute to reward and analgesia. Reg Anesth Pain Med 2007;32:242–6.

[38] Fields HL, Heinricher MM, Mason P. Neurotransmitters in nociceptive modulatory circuits. Annu Rev Neurosci 1991;14:219–45.

[39] Fillingim RB, Ness TJ, Glover TL, Campbell CM, Hastie BA, Price DD, Staud R. Morphine responses and experimental pain: sex differences in side effects and cardiovascular responses but not analgesia. J Pain 2005;6:116–24.

[40] Fishbain DA. Pharmacotherapeutic management of breakthrough pain in patients with chronic persistent pain. Am J Manag Care 2008;14:S123–8.

[41] Fleming MF, Davis J, Passik SD. Reported lifetime aberrant drug-taking behaviors are predictive of current substance use and mental health problems in primary care patients. Pain Med 2008.

[42] Franco M, Alessandra C, Marco L, Luca A, Anna M, Antonella P, Giampiero P, Paolo M, Giustino V. Use of strong opioids in advanced cancer pain: a randomized trial. J Pain Symptom Manage 2004;27:409–16.

[43] Furlan AD, Sandoval JA, Mailis-Gagnon A, Tunks E. Opioids for chronic noncancer pain: a meta-analysis of effectiveness and side effects. CMAJ 2006;174:1589–94.

[44] Fuxe K, Agnati LF. Two principal modes of electrochemical communication in the brain: volume versus wiring transmission. In: Volume transmission in the brain. New York: Raven Press; 1978. p. 1–9.

[45] Gaveriaux-Ruff C, Kieffer BL. Opioid receptor genes inactivated in mice: the highlights. Neuropeptides 2002;36:62–71.

[46] Gear RW, Aley KO, Levine JD. Pain-induced analgesia mediated by mesolimbic reward circuits. J Neurosci 1999;19:7175–81.

[47] Gear RW, Miaskowski C, Gordon NC, Paul SM, Heller PH, Levine JD. Kappa-opioids produce significantly greater analgesia in women than in men. Nat Med 1996;2:1248–50.

[48] Gomes I, Filipovska J, Jordan BA, Devi LA. Oligomerization of opioid receptors. Methods 2002;27:358–65.

[49] Gordon NC, Gear RW, Heller PH, Paul S, Miaskowski C, Levine JD. Enhancement of morphine analgesia by the $GABA_B$ agonist baclofen. Neuroscience 1995;69:345–9.

[50] Hamann S, Sloan P. Oral naltrexone to enhance analgesia in patients receiving continuous intrathecal morphine for chronic pain: a randomized, double-blind, prospective pilot study. J Opioid Manag 2007;3:137–44.

[51] Hao S, Wolfe D, Glorioso JC, Mata M, Fink DJ. Effects of transgene-mediated endomorphin-2 in inflammatory pain. Eur J Pain 2009;13:380–6.

[52] Harlan RE, Shivers BD, Romano GJ, Howells RD, Pfaff DW. Localization of preproenkephalin mRNA in the rat brain and spinal cord by in situ hybridization. J Comp Neurol 1987;258:159–84.

[53] Hudson TJ, Edlund MJ, Steffick DE, Tripathi SP, Sullivan MD. Epidemiology of regular prescribed opioid use: results from a national, population-based survey. J Pain Symptom Manage 2008;36:280–8.

[54] Hutchinson MR, Bland ST, Johnson KW, Rice KC, Maier SF, Watkins LR. Opioid-induced glial activation: mechanisms of activation and implications for opioid analgesia, dependence, and reward. ScientificWorldJournal 2007;7:98–111.

[55] Hutchison WD, Morton CR, Terenius L. Dynorphin A: in vivo release in the spinal cord of the cat. Brain Res 1990;532:299–306.

[56] Jensen MK, Thomsen AB, Højsted J. 10-year follow-up of chronic non-malignant pain patients: opioid use, health-related quality of life and health care utilization. Eur J Pain 2006;10:423–33.

[57] Jensen TS, Yaksh TL. Spinal monoamine and opiate systems partly mediate the antinociceptive effects produced by glutamate at brainstem sites. Brain Res 1984;321:287–97.

[58] Kalso E, Edwards JE, Moore RA, McQuay HJ. Opioids in chronic non-cancer pain: systematic review of efficacy and safety. Pain 2004;112:372–80.

[59] Kemp T, Spike RC, Watt C, Todd AJ. The mu-opioid receptor (MOR1) is mainly restricted to neurons that do not contain GABA or glycine in the superficial dorsal horn of the rat spinal cord. Neuroscience 1996;75:1231–8.

[60] Kieffer BL, Evans CJ. Opioid receptors: from binding sites to visible molecules in vivo. Neuropharmacology 2009;56:205–12.

[61] King T, Gardell LR, Wang R, Vardanyan A, Ossipov MH, Malan TP Jr, Vanderah TW, Hunt SP, Hruby VJ, Lai J, Porreca F. Role of NK-1 neurotransmission in opioid-induced hyperalgesia. Pain 2005;116:276–88.

[62] Kishioka S, Miyamoto Y, Fukunaga Y, Nishida S, Yamamoto H. Effects of a mixture of peptidase inhibitors (amastatin, captopril and phosphoramidon) on Met-enkephalin-, beta-endorphin-, dynorphin$_{1-13}$- and electroacupuncture-induced antinociception in rats. Jpn J Pharmacol 1994;66:337–45.

[63] Kline RH, Wiley RG. Spinal mu-opioid receptor-expressing dorsal horn neurons: role in nociception and morphine antinociception. J Neurosci 2008;28:904–13.

[64] Kobilka B, Schertler GF. New G-protein-coupled receptor crystal structures: insights and limitations. Trends Pharmacol Sci 2008;29:79–83.

[65] Kong J, Gollub RL, Rosman IS, Webb JM, Vangel MG, Kirsch I, Kaptchuk TJ. Brain activity associated with expectancy-enhanced placebo analgesia as measured by functional magnetic resonance imaging. J Neurosci 2006;26:381–8.

[66] Law PY, Erickson LJ, El Kouhen R, Dicker L, Solberg J, Wang W, Miller E, Burd AL, Loh HH. Receptor density and recycling affect the rate of agonist-induced desensitization of mu-opioid receptor. Mol Pharmacol 2000;58:388–98.

[67] Le Bars D, Bourgoin S, Villanueva L, Clot AM, Hamon M, Cesselin F. Involvement of the dorsolateral funiculi in the spinal release of Met-enkephalin-like material triggered by heterosegmental noxious mechanical stimuli. Brain Res 1987;412:190–5.

[68] Leskela TT, Markkanen PM, Pietila EM, Tuusa JT, Petaja-Repo UE. Opioid receptor pharmacological chaperones act by binding and stabilizing newly synthesized receptors in the endoplasmic reticulum. J Biol Chem 2007;282:23171–83.

[69] Levine JD, Gordon NC, Fields HL. The mechanism of placebo analgesia. Lancet 1978;2:654–7.

[70] Lidstone SC, Stoessl AJ. Understanding the placebo effect: contributions from neuroimaging. Mol Imaging Biol 2007;9:176–85.

[71] Loh HH, Liu HC, Cavalli A, Yang W, Chen YF, Wei LN. Mu opioid receptor knockout in mice: effects on ligand-induced analgesia and morphine lethality. Brain Res Mol Brain Res 1998;54:321–6.

[72] Lorenz KA, Lynn J, Dy SM, Shugarman LR, Wilkinson A, Mularski RA, Morton SC, Hughes RG, Hilton LK, Maglione M, et al. Evidence for improving palliative care at the end of life: a systematic review. Ann Intern Med 2008;148:147–59.

[73] Lutfy K, Eitan S, Bryant CD, Yang YC, Saliminejad N, Walwyn W, Kieffer BL, Takeshima H, Carroll FI, Maidment NT, et al. Buprenorphine-induced antinociception is mediated by mu-opioid receptors and compromised by concomitant activation of opioid receptor-like receptors. J Neurosci 2003;23:10331–7.

[74] Machelska H, Cabot PJ, Mousa SA, Zhang Q, Stein C. Pain control in inflammation governed by selectins. Nat Med 1998;4:1425–8.

[75] Machelska H, Stein C. Immune mechanisms in pain control. Anesth Analg 2002;95:1002–8.

[76] Mahowald ML, Singh JA, Majeski P. Opioid use by patients in an orthopedics spine clinic. Arthritis Rheum 2005;52:312–21.

[77] Mao J, Sung B, Ji RR, Lim G. Chronic morphine induces downregulation of spinal glutamate transporters: implications in morphine tolerance and abnormal pain sensitivity. J Neurosci 2002;22:8312–23.

[78] Martell BA, O'Connor PG, Kerns RD, Becker WC, Morales KH, Kosten TR, Fiellin DA. Systematic review: opioid treatment for chronic back pain: prevalence, efficacy, and association with addiction. Ann Intern Med 2007;146:116–27.

[79] Martin-Schild S, Gerall AA, Kastin AJ, Zadina JE. Endomorphin-2 is an endogenous opioid in primary sensory afferent fibers. Peptides 1998;19:1783–9.

[80] Marvizon JC, Grady EF, Waszak-McGee J, Mayer EA. Internalization of μ-opioid receptors in rat spinal cord slices. NeuroReport 1999;10:2329–34.

[81] Mason P. Central mechanisms of pain modulation. Curr Opin Neurobiol 1999;9:436–41.

[82] Mauborgne A, Bourgoin S, Polienor H, Roumy M, Simonnet G, Zajac JM, Cesselin F. The neuropeptide FF analogue, 1DMe, acts as a functional opioid autoreceptor antagonist in the rat spinal cord. Eur J Pharmacol 2001;430:273–6.

[83] McLaughlin JP, Marton-Popovici M, Chavkin C. Kappa opioid receptor antagonism and prodynorphin gene disruption block stress-induced behavioral responses. J Neurosci 2003;23:5674–83.

[84] Mitra S. Opioid-induced hyperalgesia: pathophysiology and clinical implications. J Opioid Manag 2008;4:123–30.

[85] Mogil JS, Grisel JE, Reinscheid RK, Civelli O, Belknap JK, Grandy DK. Orphanin FQ is a functional anti-opioid peptide. Neuroscience 1996;75:333–7.

[86] Mogil JS, Pasternak GW. The molecular and behavioral pharmacology of the orphanin FQ/nociceptin peptide and receptor family. Pharmacol Rev 2001;53:381–415.

[87] Mousa SA, Machelska H, Schafer M, Stein C. Co-expression of beta-endorphin with adhesion molecules in a model of inflammatory pain. J Neuroimmunol 2000;108:160–70.

[88] Neal CR Jr, Mansour A, Reinscheid R, Nothacker HP, Civelli O, Akil H, Watson SJ Jr. Opioid receptor-like (ORL1) receptor distribution in the rat central nervous system: comparison of ORL1 receptor mRNA expression with ^{125}I-[^{14}Tyr]-orphanin FQ binding. J Comp Neurol 1999;412:563–605.

[89] Noble F, Smadja C, Valverde O, Maldonado R, Coric P, Turcaud S, Fournie-Zaluski MC, Roques BP. Pain-suppressive effects on various nociceptive stimuli (thermal, chemical, electrical and inflammatory) of the first orally active enkephalin-metabolizing enzyme inhibitor RB 120. Pain 1997;73:383–91.

[90] Noble F, Soleilhac JM, Soroca-Lucas E, Turcaud S, Fournie-Zaluski MC, Roques BP. Inhibition of the enkephalin-metabolizing enzymes by the first systemically active mixed inhibitor prodrug RB 101 induces potent analgesic responses in mice and rats. J Pharmacol Exp Ther 1992;261:181–90.

[91] Noble F, Turcaud S, Fournie-Zaluski MC, Roques BP. Repeated systemic administration of the mixed inhibitor of enkephalin-degrading enzymes, RB101, does not induce either antinociceptive tolerance or cross-tolerance with morphine. Eur J Pharmacol 1992;223:83–9.
[92] Noble M, Tregear SJ, Treadwell JR, Schoelles K. Long-term opioid therapy for chronic noncancer pain: a systematic review and meta-analysis of efficacy and safety. J Pain Symptom Manage 2008;35:214–28.
[93] Numata H, Hiranuma T, Oka T. Inactivation of dynorphin$_{1-8}$ in isolated preparations by three peptidases. Jpn J Pharmacol 1988;47:417–23.
[94] Olave MJ, Maxwell DJ. An investigation of neurones that possess the alpha 2C-adrenergic receptor in the rat dorsal horn. Neuroscience 2002;115:31–40.
[95] Pasternak GW. Multiple opiate receptors: deja vu all over again. Neuropharmacology 2004;47:312–23.
[96] Patanwala AE, Duby J, Waters D, Erstad BL. Opioid conversions in acute care. Ann Pharmacother 2007;41:255–66.
[97] Pergolizzi J, Boger RH, Budd K, Dahan A, Erdine S, Hans G, Kress HG, Langford R, Likar R, Raffa RB, Sacerdote P. Opioids and the management of chronic severe pain in the elderly: consensus statement of an International Expert Panel with focus on the six clinically most often used World Health Organization step III opioids (buprenorphine, fentanyl, hydromorphone, methadone, morphine, oxycodone). Pain Pract 2008;8:287–313.
[98] Petaja-Repo UE, Hogue M, Bhalla S, Laperriere A, Morello JP, Bouvier M. Ligands act as pharmacological chaperones and increase the efficiency of delta opioid receptor maturation. EMBO J 2002;21:1628–37.
[99] Petrovic P, Kalso E, Petersson KM, Ingvar M. Placebo and opioid analgesia: imaging a shared neuronal network. Science 2002;295:1737–40.
[100] Pierce TL, Grahek MD, Wessendorf MW. Immunoreactivity for endomorphin-2 occurs in primary afferents in rats and monkey. NeuroReport 1998;9:385–9.
[101] Powell KJ, Abul-Husn NS, Jhamandas A, Olmstead MC, Beninger RJ, Jhamandas K. Paradoxical effects of the opioid antagonist naltrexone on morphine analgesia, tolerance, and reward in rats. J Pharmacol Exp Ther 2002;300:588–96.
[102] Reznikov I, Pud D, Eisenberg E. Oral opioid administration and hyperalgesia in patients with cancer or chronic nonmalignant pain. Br J Clin Pharmacol 2005;60:311–8.
[103] Riley JL 3rd, Hastie BA. Individual differences in opioid efficacy for chronic noncancer pain. Clin J Pain 2008;24:509–20.
[104] Roberts LJ, Finch PM, Goucke CR, Price LM. Outcome of intrathecal opioids in chronic non-cancer pain. Eur J Pain 2001;5:353–61.
[105] Sakurada T, Katsuyama S, Sakurada S, Inoue M, Tan-No K, Kisara K, Sakurada C, Ueda H, Sasaki J. Nociceptin-induced scratching, biting and licking in mice: involvement of spinal NK1 receptors. Br J Pharmacol 1999;127:1712–8.
[106] Saper JR, Lake AE 3rd. Continuous opioid therapy (COT) is rarely advisable for refractory chronic daily headache: limited efficacy, risks, and proposed guidelines. Headache 2008;48:838–49.
[107] Schreff M, Schulz S, Wiborny D, Heollt V. Immunofluorescent identification of endomorphin-2-containing nerve fibers and terminals in the rat brain and spinal cord. NeuroReport 1998;9:1031–4.
[108] Schuller AGP, King MA, Zhang JW, Bolan E, Pan YX, Morgan DJ, Chang A, Czick ME, Unterwald EM, Pasternak GW, et al. Retention of heroin and morphine-6 beta-glucuronide analgesia in a new line of mice lacking exon 1 of MOR-1. Nat Neurosci 1999;2:151–6.
[109] Skoubis PD, Matthes HW, Walwyn WM, Kieffer BL, Maidment NT. Naloxone fails to produce conditioned place aversion in mu-opioid receptor knock-out mice. Neuroscience 2001;106:757–63.
[110] Smith HS. Peripherally-acting opioids. Pain Physician 2008;11:S121–32.
[111] Song B, Chen W, Marvizon JC. Inhibition of opioid release in the rat spinal cord by serotonin 5-HT$_{1A}$ receptors. Brain Res 2007;1158:57–62.
[112] Song B, Marvizon JC. Peptidases prevent μ-opioid receptor internalization in dorsal horn neurons by endogenously released opioids. J Neurosci 2003;23:1847–58.
[113] Song B, Marvizon JCG. Dorsal horn neurons firing at high frequency, but not primary afferents, release opioid peptides that produce μ-opioid receptor internalization in the rat spinal cord. J Neurosci 2003;23:9171–84.
[114] Song B, Marvizon JCG. NMDA receptors and large conductance calcium-sensitive potassium channels inhibit the release of opioid peptides that induce μ-opioid receptor internalization in the rat spinal cord. Neuroscience 2005;136:549–62.
[115] Stefano GB, Cadet P, Kream RM, Zhu W. The presence of endogenous morphine signaling in animals. Neurochem Res 2008;33:1933–9.
[116] Stein C, Hassan AH, Przewlocki R, Gramsch C, Peter K, Herz A. Opioids from immunocytes interact with receptors on sensory nerves to inhibit nociception in inflammation. Proc Natl Acad Sci USA 1990;87:5935–9.
[117] Stone LS, Broberger C, Vulchanova L, Wilcox GL, Hokfelt T, Riedl MS, Elde R. Differential distribution of alpha$_{2A}$ and alpha$_{2C}$ adrenergic receptor immunoreactivity in the rat spinal cord. J Neurosci 1998;18:5928–37.
[118] Terman GW, Lewis JW, Liebeskind JC. Two opioid forms of stress analgesia: studies of tolerance and cross-tolerance. Brain Res 1986;368:101–6.
[119] Tsou K, Khachaturian H, Akil H, Watson SJ. Immunocytochemical localization of pro-opiomelanocortin-derived peptides in the adult rat spinal cord. Brain Res 1986;378:28–35.
[120] Vindrola O, Mayer AM, Citera G, Spitzer JA, Espinoza LR. Prohormone convertases PC2 and PC3 in rat neutrophils and macrophages. Parallel changes with proenkephalin-derived peptides induced by LPS in vivo. Neuropeptides 1994;27:235–44.
[121] von Zastrow M, Svingos A, Haberstock-Debic H, Evans C. Regulated endocytosis of opioid receptors: cellular mechanisms and proposed roles in physiological adaptation to opiate drugs. Curr Opin Neurobiol 2003;13:348–53.
[122] Vorobeychik Y, Chen L, Bush MC, Mao J. Improved opioid analgesic effect following opioid dose reduction. Pain Med 2008;9:724–7.

[123] Wager TD, Rilling JK, Smith EE, Sokolik A, Casey KL, Davidson RJ, Kosslyn SM, Rose RM, Cohen JD. Placebo-induced changes in FMRI in the anticipation and experience of pain. Science 2004;303:1162–7.
[124] Walwyn W, Evans CJ, Hales TG. Beta-arrestin2 and c-Src regulate the constitutive activity and recycling of mu opioid receptors in dorsal root ganglion neurons. J Neurosci 2007;27:5092–104.
[125] Walwyn W, Maidment NT, Sanders M, Evans CJ, Kieffer BL, Hales TG. Induction of delta opioid receptor function by up-regulation of membrane receptors in mouse primary afferent neurons. Mol Pharmacol 2005;68:1688–98.
[126] Wang HY, Frankfurt M, Burns LH. High-affinity naloxone binding to filamin a prevents mu opioid receptor-Gs coupling underlying opioid tolerance and dependence. PLoS One 2008;3:e1554.
[127] Watkins LR, Young EG, Kinscheck IB, Mayer DJ. The neural basis of footshock analgesia: the role of specific ventral medullary nuclei. Brain Res 1983;276:305–15.
[128] Weber E, Evans CJ, Barchas JD. Multiple endogenous ligands for opioid receptors. Trends Neurosci 1983;6:333–6.
[129] Webster BS, Verma SK, Gatchel RJ. Relationship between early opioid prescribing for acute occupational low back pain and disability duration, medical costs, subsequent surgery and late opioid use. Spine 2007;32:2127–32.
[130] Webster L, Jansen JP, Peppin J, Lasko B, Irving G, Morlion B, Snidow J, Pierce A, Mortensen E, Kleoudis C, Carter E. Alvimopan, a peripherally acting mu-opioid receptor (PAM-OR) antagonist for the treatment of opioid-induced bowel dysfunction: results from a randomized, double-blind, placebo-controlled, dose-finding study in subjects taking opioids for chronic non-cancer pain. Pain 2008;137:428–40.
[131] Weinstein SM, Shi M, Buckley BJ, Kwarcinski MA. Multicenter, open-label, prospective evaluation of the conversion from previous opioid analgesics to extended-release hydromorphone hydrochloride administered every 24 hours to patients with persistent moderate to severe pain. Clin Ther 2006;28:86–98.
[132] Weitz CJ, Lowney LI, Faull KF, Feistner G, Goldstein A. Morphine and codeine from mammalian brain. Proc Natl Acad Sci USA 1986;83:9784–8.
[133] Wilhelm W, Kreuer S. The place for short-acting opioids: special emphasis on remifentanil. Crit Care 2008;12:S5.
[134] Williams RE, Sampson TJ, Kalilani L, Wurzelmann JI, Janning SW. Epidemiology of opioid pharmacy claims in the United States. J Opioid Manag 2008;4:145–52.
[135] Wirz S, Wartenberg HC, Elsen C, Wittmann M, Diederichs M, Nadstawek J. Managing cancer pain and symptoms of outpatients by rotation t sustained-release hydromorphone: a prospective clinical trial. Clin J Pain 2006;22:770–5.
[136] Wise RA. Brain reward circuitry: insights from unsensed incentives. Neuron 2002;36:229–40.
[137] Wollemann M, Benyhe S. Non-opioid actions of opioid peptides. Life Sci 2004;75:257–70.
[138] Woolf CJ, Ma QP, Allchorne A, Poole S. Peripheral cell types contributing to the hyperalgesic action of nerve growth factor in inflammation. J Neurosci 1996;16:2716–23.
[139] Yaksh TL. Pharmacology and mechanisms of opioid analgesic activity. Acta Anaesthesiol Scand 1997;41:94–111.
[140] Yaksh TL, Elde RP. Factors governing release of methionine enkephalin-like immunoreactivity from mesencephalon and spinal cord of the cat in vivo. J Neurophysiol 1981;46:1056–75.
[141] Zadina JE, Hackler L, Ge LJ, Kastin AJ. A potent and selective endogenous agonist for the mu-opiate receptor. Nature 1997;386:499–502.
[142] Zagon IS, Verderame MF, McLaughlin PJ. The biology of the opioid growth factor receptor (OGFr). Brain Res Brain Res Rev 2002;38:351–76.
[143] Zorman G, Belcher G, Adams JE, Fields HL. Lumbar intrathecal naloxone blocks analgesia produced by microstimulation of the ventromedial medulla in the rat. Brain Res 1982;236:77–84.
[144] Zubieta JK, Bueller JA, Jackson LR, Scott DJ, Xu Y, Koeppe RA, Nichols TE, Stohler CS. Placebo effects mediated by endogenous opioid activity on mu-opioid receptors. J Neurosci 2005;25:7754–62.
[145] Zubieta JK, Smith YR, Bueller JA, Xu Y, Kilbourn MR, Jewett DM, Meyer CR, Koeppe RA, Stohler CS. Regional mu opioid receptor regulation of sensory and affective dimensions of pain. Science 2001;293:311–5.
[146] Zubieta JK, Yau WY, Scott DJ, Stohler CS. Belief or need? Accounting for individual variations in the neurochemistry of the placebo effect. Brain Behav Immun 2006;20:15–26.

Correspondence to: Christopher J. Evans, MPH, PhD, Department of Psychiatry and Biobehavioral Sciences, UCLA, Los Angeles, CA 90095, USA. Email: cevans@ucla.edu.

Pharmacology of the Cannabinoid System

6

Josée Guindon,[a] Pierre Beaulieu,[b] and Andrea G. Hohmann[a]

[a] *Neuroscience and Behavior Program, Psychology Department, University of Georgia, Athens, Georgia, USA;*
[b] *Departments of Anesthesiology and Pharmacology, University of Montreal, Montreal, Quebec, Canada*

History of Cannabis

The cannabis plant, which is also known as hemp or marijuana, was named after the Greek word for hemp, *kannabis.* It is most likely that cannabis was first cultivated in central Asia and that its use spread by trade and invasion [12]. Cannabis has been used for many different purposes for more than 12 thousand years; for example, hemp was cultivated for fiber to make clothes, ropes, and sails [12]. Cannabis is one of the oldest documented medicines in history. One of the earliest known references to the use of cannabis for medicinal purposes dates to its appearance in a Chinese pharmacopoeia in 2800 BCE. [12]. Archaeological evidence from Israel documents a therapeutic use for cannabis for alleviating pain during childbirth. Cannabis has been used throughout the centuries for the treatment of pain, asthma, dysentery, nausea, and vomiting and also to alleviate spasms and convulsions. In 1839, W.B. O'Shaughnessy, an Irish doctor working for the British army in India, described the virtue and efficacy of cannabis, facilitating the introduction of cannabis to England and Europe. In the early 20th century, the development of synthetic drugs reduced the use of cannabis in America and Europe. The 1960s ushered in a new era of experimentation with the use of marijuana for recreational purposes and for liberation of the spirit. Today, cannabis remains widely used, like other drugs including tobacco and alcohol [12]. The discovery by Gaoni and Mechoulam [40] of Δ^9-tetrahydrocannabinol (Δ^9-THC), the major

Pharmacology of Pain
edited by Pierre Beaulieu, David Lussier, Frank Porreca, and Anthony H. Dickenson
IASP Press, Seattle, © 2010

psychoactive ingredient in marijuana, ushered in a new age of research focused on understanding the mechanisms of action of the cannabinoids. The cloning of cannabinoid receptors [92,97] and the isolation of their endogenous ligands (endocannabinoids) [28,93,134] marked a transition in the cannabinoid field. Cannabinoids could no longer be thought of merely as drugs of abuse. These discoveries established the existence of an endocannabinoid signaling system in the nervous system, whose functions have only recently been explored.

The Cannabis Plant

Cannabis (a member of the botanical family *Cannabaceae*) is a highly adapted herbaceous annual that grows in temperate and tropical zones of the world. Many species of cannabis exist; the most well-known species are *Cannabis sativa* (native to Europe), *Cannabis indica* (native to India), and *Cannabis ruderalis* (native to Siberia and central Asia) [12]. Of all three species, *Cannabis sativa* is the most widespread and can grow in almost all climates. It is an open-branched plant that can grow up to 6 meters in height. Cannabis is a very versatile plant because it grows at altitudes up to 2400 meters (8000 feet), has a relatively short life cycle (3–5 months), germinates within 6 days, and grows up to 15 centimeters a day with very little water [12]. It is a dioecious plant; individual plants are either male (producing pollen) or female (producing seeds). Both male and female plants produce an amber-colored resin containing Δ^9-tetrahydrocannabinol, although female plants produce greater amounts.

Pharmacology of Cannabinoids

Cannabis has approximately 460 known chemical constituents; more than 60 of these have the structure of a cannabinoid. The best-characterized constituent is Δ^9-THC, the principal psychoactive component of cannabis. Other important constituents include cannabidiol (CBD) and cannabinol. The former was historically believed to lack psychoactive capabilities, whereas the latter is a mildly psychoactive chemical. The first major pharmacological discovery in the cannabinoid field was consequently the isolation, characterization, and partial synthesis of Δ^9-THC [40]. Following this major finding, research on the pharmacology of cannabinoids and its mechanisms of action burgeoned, due in part to interest in therapeutic properties of these compounds, including the treatment of different pain conditions (for review see [32,109]).

Cannabinoids produce their effects through the activation of two distinct G-protein-coupled receptors termed cannabinoid CB_1 [27,92] and CB_2 receptors [97]. These receptors have a protein structure defined by an array of seven membrane-spanning helices including intracellular loops and a C-terminal domain that can associate with G proteins. The CB_1 receptor is expressed, at high levels, in the central nervous system (CNS), where it exhibits a heterogeneous distribution [52]. It is most densely expressed in motor and limbic regions of the brain [52], but it is also found in the spinal cord, on sensory neurons in dorsal root ganglia (DRG), and in the periphery [1,59] (see [52,86] for reviews). The CB_2 receptor is found predominantly, although not exclusively, outside the CNS, where it is most densely expressed in peripheral tissues with immune functions (see [39,97]). Genes encoding these proteins have been identified [92,97,104]. These receptors have been cloned [92,97], and knockout mice lacking the CB_1 [84,151] or CB_2 receptor, or both receptors, have been generated [14,72]. Recent research also suggests the existence of novel non-CB_1 and non-CB_2 receptors (e.g., GPR55 and GPR3/GPR6/GPR12; see [83] for a review).

Pharmacology of the Cannabinoid CB_1 Receptor

A G-protein-coupled cannabinoid receptor was first characterized in rat brain [27], and was subsequently cloned both in rat [92] and human cells [42]. The human gene coding for CB_1 has been localized to the q14–q15 region of the chromosome 6 [55], whereas the mouse gene for CB_1 is localized proximally in chromosome 4 [104]. CB_1 is well conserved between species (e.g., humans, rats, and mice) [110]. Indeed, the human CB_1 receptor has a 97% sequence similarity with the mouse or rat CB_1 receptor for the whole protein [127].

Transduction Mechanisms for the CB_1 Receptor

Activation of cannabinoid CB_1 receptors inhibits adenylate cyclase activity in a stereoselective and dose-dependent manner by coupling to the α subunit of the G protein of the $G_{i/o}$ family (G_{i1-3} and G_{o1-2}) [92] (see [68] for a review). Signaling of cannabinoid receptors through G proteins results from interactions with the second, third, and fourth intracellular loops of the receptor (see [68] for a review). CB_1-receptor activation produces inhibitory coupling to voltage-dependent calcium channels of types L, N, and P/Q as well as to potassium channels of type D. CB_1-receptor activation also stimulates G-protein-regulated inwardly rectifying potassium (GIRK) channels, enhances the activation of voltage-sensitive A-type potassium channels, and activates mitogen-activated protein kinases (MAPK) through their associated G proteins to regulate nuclear transcription factors (see [68,69,110] for reviews) (Fig. 1). Furthermore, cannabinoids can also inhibit serotonin 5-HT_3 receptors via an allosteric modulatory site, modulate nitric oxide production, and mobilize arachidonic acid. Activation of CB_1 receptors can also modulate sodium channel conductance, induce expression of the immediate-early gene *Krox-24,* and activate the Na^+/H^+ exchanger (for reviews see [68,69,110]).

Localization of CB_1 Receptors

CB_1 receptors are expressed predominantly in the CNS and, to a lesser extent, in certain peripheral tissues [52]. They are localized in adrenal glands, adipose tissue, heart, liver, lungs, prostate, uterus, ovaries, testes, bone marrow, thymus, tonsils, and presynaptic nerve terminals (see [108,111] for reviews). Within the brain, CB_1 is found in the cerebral cortex, hippocampus (particularly in the dentate gyrus), amygdala, basal ganglia, substantia nigra pars reticulata, internal and external segment of the globus pallidus, and cerebellum

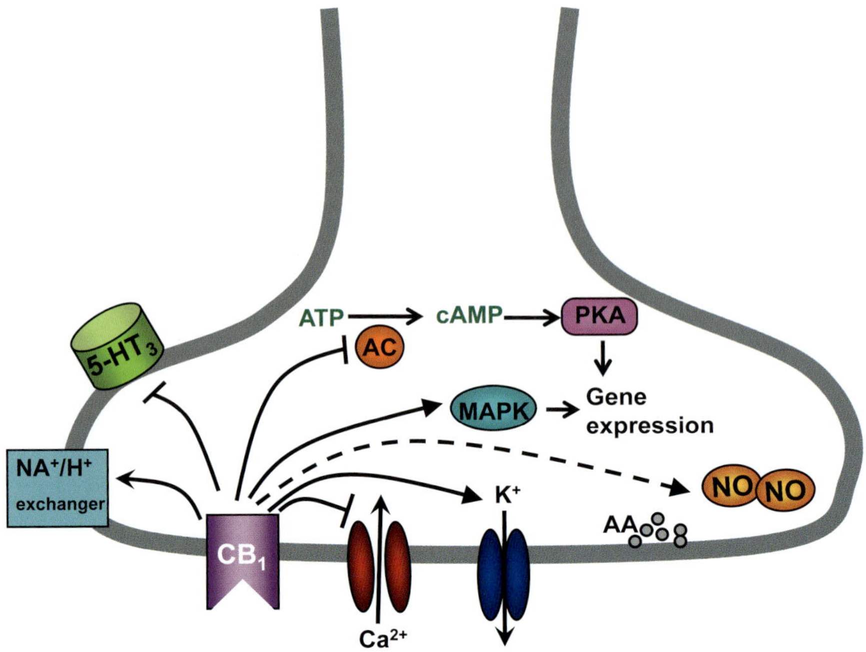

Fig. 1. Transduction mechanisms for the cannabinoid CB_1 receptors. Schematic representation of the main signalization pathways involving CB_1 receptors. Note that CB_1 receptors are found at the presynaptic level. Abbreviations: AA, arachidonic acid; AC, adenylate cyclase; cAMP, cyclic adenosine monophosphate; ATP, adenosine triphosphate; CB_1, cannabinoid receptor 1; 5-HT_3, 5-hydroxytryptamine 3; MAPK, mitogen-activated protein kinase; NO, nitric oxide; PKA, protein kinase A.

(molecular layer). This distribution provides an anatomical basis for the profound effects of cannabinoids on cognition and short-term memory (cerebral cortex and hippocampus), as well as on motor function (basal ganglia and cerebellum) (see [52,69,110] for reviews). Cannabinoid CB_1 receptors are among the most abundant G-protein-coupled receptors in the brain, with densities similar to γ-aminobutyric acid (GABA) and glutamate ion channels [69]. In contrast, CB_1 receptors are sparse in the brainstem [69], which accounts for the lack of toxicity associated with high doses of marijuana.

CB_1 receptors are found at supraspinal, spinal, and peripheral levels [1,58,59] (see [86] for a review). All these substrates contribute to the antinociceptive effects of cannabinoids (for a review, see [141]). CB_1 receptors are expressed presynaptically in GABAergic and glutamatergic neurons; activation of these receptors inhibits release of the primary neurotransmitter by decreasing calcium channel conductance and by increasing potassium channel conductance [111]. This distribution is consistent with functional evidence showing that CB_1 receptors serve as synaptic circuit breakers, regulating excitability throughout the nervous system.

Pharmacology of the Cannabinoid CB_2 Receptor

The CB_2 receptor was first described in the macrophage population of the spleen [97]. This G-protein-coupled receptor shares 44% identity with the amino acid sequence of the CB_1

receptor and 68% similarity when only the transmembrane region is considered [39]. The mouse CB_2 receptor shares 82% identity with the human CB_2 receptor. It differs from its human counterpart by 60 residues and is shorter at the carboxyl terminus by 13 residues [127].

Transduction Mechanisms for the CB_2 Receptor

Cannabinoid CB_2 receptors, like CB_1 receptors, are also members of the superfamily of G-protein-coupled receptors. CB_2-receptor activation inhibits the activity of adenylate cyclase through coupling to the α subunit of the G protein of the Gi/o family (see [68,110] for reviews). In comparison to CB_1 receptors, CB_2-receptor activation does not modulate calcium or potassium channel conductance (for a review, see [69]). However, CB_2-receptor activation stimulates MAPK activity and induces Krox-24 expression, presumably through activation of G-protein βγ subunits (see [68,69] for reviews).

Localization of CB_2 Receptors

CB_2 receptors are localized extensively in cells of the immune system. They are expressed in tissues involved in immune cell production and regulation such as the spleen, tonsils, and thymus (see [69] for a review). Immune cells bearing CB_2 receptors include mast cells, B cells, T4 and T8 cells, microglial cells, macrophages, natural killer cells, and to a lesser extent monocytes and polymorphonuclear neutrophils (see [69,108] for reviews). CB_2 receptors are found in immune tissues at levels 10–100 times greater than the CB_1 receptor [39]. Although previous reports suggested that CB_2 receptors were absent in the brain [97], they have recently been localized in the brain and spinal cord, on sensory neurons including DRG cells, and on microglia, although at lower levels than those observed in peripheral tissues [138] (see [74] for a review).

Signal transduction mechanisms associated with CB_1 and CB_2 receptors are summarized in Table I. Principal agonists and antagonists of the cannabinoid receptors are shown in Table II.

CB_1- and CB_2-Receptor Knockout Mice

The functional roles of cannabinoid receptors in different physiological processes involving the CNS and the cardiovascular, reproductive, endocrine, immune and gastrointestinal

Table I
Signal transduction mechanisms for cannabinoid CB_1 and CB_2 receptors

Mechanism	Receptor
$G_{i/o}$ protein activation	CB_1/CB_2 receptors
Inhibition of adenylate cyclase	CB_1/CB_2 receptors
Blockade of calcium channels type L, N, and P/Q	CB_1 receptors only
Activation of potassium channels type A and K_{ir}	CB_1 receptors only
Activation of mitogen-activated protein kinase	CB_1/CB_2 receptors

Table II
Principal agonists/antagonists for cannabinoid CB_1 and CB_2 receptors

Action	Agonist/Antagonist	CB_1	CB_2
Natural agonists	Δ^9-THC	++	++
	Cannabidiol* (no psychoactive properties)	0	0
	Cannabinol (psychoactive properties)	+	++
Synthetic agonists	Dronabinol (Marinol)	++	++
	Nabilone (Cesamet)	++	++
	THC-cannabidiol (1:1) (Sativex spray)	++	++
	Ajulemic acid (CT-3) (no psychoactive properties); binds to peroxisome proliferator-activated receptors	0	0
	Levonantradol	+	+
	HU-210	+++	+++
	WIN55,212-2	+++	+++
	CP55,940	+++	+++
	Methanandamide	++	+
	ACEA (arachidonyl-2'-chloroethylamide)	+++	+
	0-1812	+++	+
	JWH-051	+	++
	HU-308	+	+++
	AM1241	+	+++
	JWH-133	+	+++
	L-759633	+	+++
	GW405833 (L768242)	+	+++
	GW842166X	+	+++
	AM1714	+	+++
	JWH-015	+	+++
Antagonists/ inverse agonists	SR141716A	++	0
	LY-320135	++	0
	AM251	++	0
	AM281	++	0
	SR144528	0	++
	AM630	0	++

Symbols: 0 = no binding; + binding with low affinity; ++ binding with moderate affinity; +++ binding with high affinity.
* Cannabidiol has very low affinity at CB_1 and CB_2 receptors; it is a functional antagonist of cannabinoid agonists and a CB_2 inverse agonist.

systems have been elucidated, in part, through the generation of pharmacological tools such as subtype-selective agonists and antagonists and genetic tools such as knockout mice with disrupted genes for CB_1 [84,151] and/or CB_2 [14,72]. Mutant mice lacking CB_1 receptors are unresponsive to cannabinoid drugs, suggesting that CB_1 receptors mediate analgesia, hypothermia, hypolocomotion, and hypotension [84,151] as well as reinforcement [84]. In one study, CB_1-knockout mice still exhibited antinociceptive effects following administration of high doses of Δ^9-THC, although catalepsy, hypomobility, and hypothermia were absent [151]. Therefore, the majority, but not all, of the CNS effects attributed to the administration of Δ^9-THC are mediated by the CB_1 receptor.

CB_2-receptor knockout mice were initially characterized to clarify the role of CB_2 receptors in immune system regulation [14]. No differences in immune cell populations were revealed between CB_2-receptor knockout and wild-type mice. Δ^9-THC inhibited helper T-cell activation through macrophages found in wild-type, but not in CB_2-knockout mice, suggesting that these effects are mediated through the CB_2 receptor. In recent years, a novel role for CB_2 receptors in modulating persistent and neuropathic pain has been revealed through the use of CB_2-selective agonists and antagonists and CB_2 wild-type and knockout mice [70] (see [48] for review).

The generation of double knockout mice lacking both CB_1 and CB_2 receptors has been useful for evaluating the possible existence of other novel cannabinoid receptors [72]. Investigators have evaluated the persistence of cannabinoid agonist actions in mice lacking both CB_1 and CB_2 receptors. The ability of anandamide, an endocannabinoid, to produce mesenteric vasodilatation in double CB_1/CB_2 knockout mice suggests the existence of an unidentified endothelial receptor for anandamide [72]. Other targets of anandamide are described below.

Other Cannabinoid Receptors

As mentioned above, not all effects of cannabinoids are mediated by either CB_1 or CB_2 receptors (see [10,83] for reviews). The existence of cannabinoid receptors distinct from CB_1 or CB_2 receptors has been postulated. Recently, one receptor that has attracted particular interest is the orphan receptor GPR55 [123]. This G-protein-coupled receptor binds to $G\alpha_{13}$ and can mediate activation of the guanosine triphosphate-binding enzymes rhoA, cdc42, and rac1. GPR55 shows only low sequence similarity with either CB_1 (13.5%) or CB_2 (14.4%) receptors, and it lacks the functional fingerprint of a cannabinoid receptor. It is expressed in the CNS and peripheral tissues, including immune tissues such as the tonsils and spleen. It is also found in the adrenals and in parts of the gastrointestinal tract [123,131]. Although GPR55 mRNA is broadly distributed in brain tissue, it is found in much lower concentrations, in comparison to CB_1 receptors. GPR55 knockout mice were recently generated to investigate the functional role of this receptor in pain modulation [131]. GPR55 knockouts fail to develop mechanical hyperalgesia related to inflammatory or neuropathic pain [131]. Also of particular interest lately are the GPR3, GPR6, and GPR12 receptors, which are sphingosine-1-phosphate lipid receptors [80]. The relevance of these newly discovered receptors to the endocannabinoid system has not been established. Future investigations employing receptor-specific agonists and antagonists and reliable genetic tools (see [83] for a review on novel cannabinoid receptors) should facilitate the investigation of the role of these receptors in endocannabinoid signaling and their contribution to pain processing in states of health and disease.

The Endocannabinoid System

The endocannabinoid signaling system offers a large number of targets that exhibit therapeutic potential, and thus are of interest to the drug development sector (for review, see [32]). Endogenous cannabinoids, termed endocannabinoids, are the brain's own cannabis-like substances. Endocannabinoids are defined as endogenous lipid-signaling molecules that are generated in the cell membrane from phospholipid precursors. They possess cannabimimetic properties because they bind to and activate one or both major cannabinoid receptor subtypes [113]. Endocannabinoids are implicated in controlling different physiological and pathological conditions (e.g., regulation of food intake, immunomodulation, inflammation, analgesia, cancer, addictive behavior, and epilepsy) (for a review, see [32,105]). The best-studied endocannabinoids isolated to date are anandamide (arachidonoyl ethanolamine, AEA) and 2-arachidonoylglycerol (2-AG). Synthesis and metabolism of these endocannabinoids is controlled by distinct enzymatic pathways. Anandamide is hydrolyzed by the enzyme fatty-acid amide hydrolase (FAAH), whereas 2-arachidonoylglycerol (2-AG) is degraded, predominantly but not exclusively, by a distinct enzyme, monoacylglycerol lipase (MGL) (see [105] for a review).

Different Endocannabinoids

The discovery of AEA [28] was followed a few years later by the identification of 2-AG [93,134] (Fig. 2). Since then, several additional putative endocannabinoids have been isolated. These include noladin ether (2-AG ether), virodhamine, and N-arachidonoyl dopamine (NADA) (for reviews, see [13,29]). These putative endocannabinoids differ in their

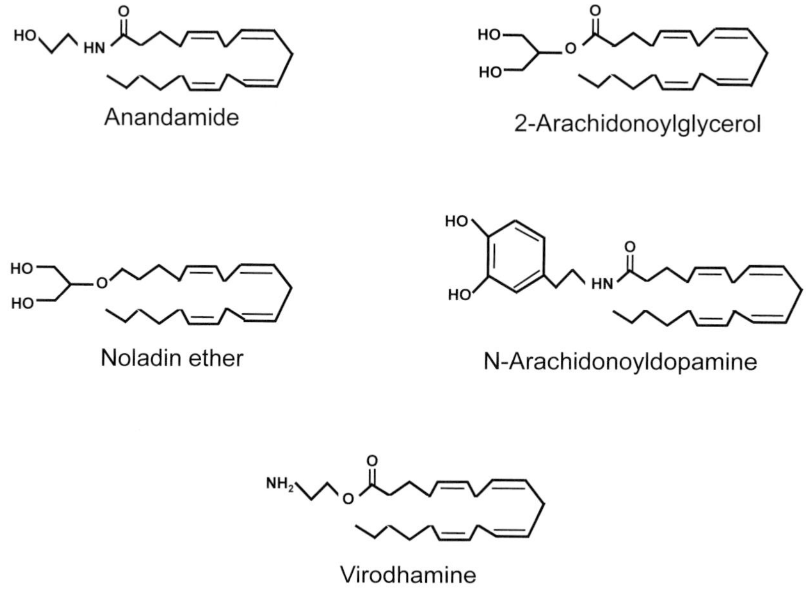

Fig. 2. Chemical structure of the main endogenous cannabinoids and endocannabinoids.

affinities for CB_1, CB_2, and transient receptor potential vanilloid 1 (TRPV1) receptors (Table III). The endocannabinoid-like properties of these endogenous ligands remain poorly characterized to date. Elucidation of the endogenous functions of these compounds in different physiological processes and their precise mechanisms of action requires further investigation [30,32]. Additional research is likely to identify other novel lipid mediators that possess cannabimimetic properties and serve as endogenous ligands for CB_1, CB_2, GPR55, or as-yet uncharacterized cannabinoid receptor subtypes.

Table III
Endocannabinoids and their selectivity for CB_1, CB_2, and TRPV1 receptors

Endocannabinoid	CB_1	CB_2	TRPV1
Anandamide	+++	+	+
2-arachidonoylglycerol	+++	++	0
Virodhamine (O-arachidonoyl-ethanolamine)	Agonist/partial antagonist	+	0
N-arachidonoyl-dopamine	++	0	+++
Noladin ether (2-arachidonoyl-glyceryl-ether)	+++	+	0

Symbols: 0 = no binding; + binding with low affinity; ++ binding with moderate affinity; +++ binding with high affinity.

Synthesis and Release of AEA and 2-AG

Endocannabinoids are produced upon demand by activity-dependent or receptor-stimulated cleavage of membrane lipid precursors. Endocannabinoids can be released from cells immediately after their production because they are highly lipophilic and are thus unlikely to be stored in vesicles (see [29,145] for reviews). Endocannabinoid signaling is regulated by synthesis, release, uptake, and degradation. Membrane depolarization, increases in intracellular calcium levels, and receptor stimulation can all activate enzymatic processes, leading to the cleavage of membrane phospholipid precursors and subsequent synthesis of endocannabinoids (for reviews see [29,30,145]). Different enzymes are implicated in the synthesis of AEA and 2-AG (Fig. 3). Anandamide biosynthesis was originally believed to occur from enzymatic cleavage of a phospholipid precursor, N-arachidonoyl-phosphatidylethanolamine (NAPE). NAPE is synthesized by the enzymatic transfer of arachidonic acid in the sn-1 position of a phosphatidylcholine to the amide group of a phosphatidylethanolamine under the supervision of the calcium-independent N-acyl-transferase (NAT) [75]. NAPE is then hydrolyzed to AEA by a specific phospholipase D (NAPE-PLD), which has recently been cloned and molecularly characterized [145]. However, NAPE-PLD knockout mice show no deficit in AEA production, a finding that calls into question the role of this enzyme in anandamide biosynthesis [85]. Indeed, conversion of synthetic NAPE to anandamide in mouse brain homogenate is processed through two additional parallel pathways: PLC/phosphatase and Abh4/phosphodiesterase [88]. Thus, multiple enzymatic pathways may be involved in the biosynthesis of anandamide, and NAPE-PLD is unlikely to exclusively control its biosynthesis [85].

2-Arachidonoylglycerol is synthesized in a two-step process. First, the 2-AG precursor diacylglycerol (DAG) is formed from enzymatic cleavage of membrane phospholipid precursors by the enzyme phospholipase C (PLC) (for review, see [18]). DAG is

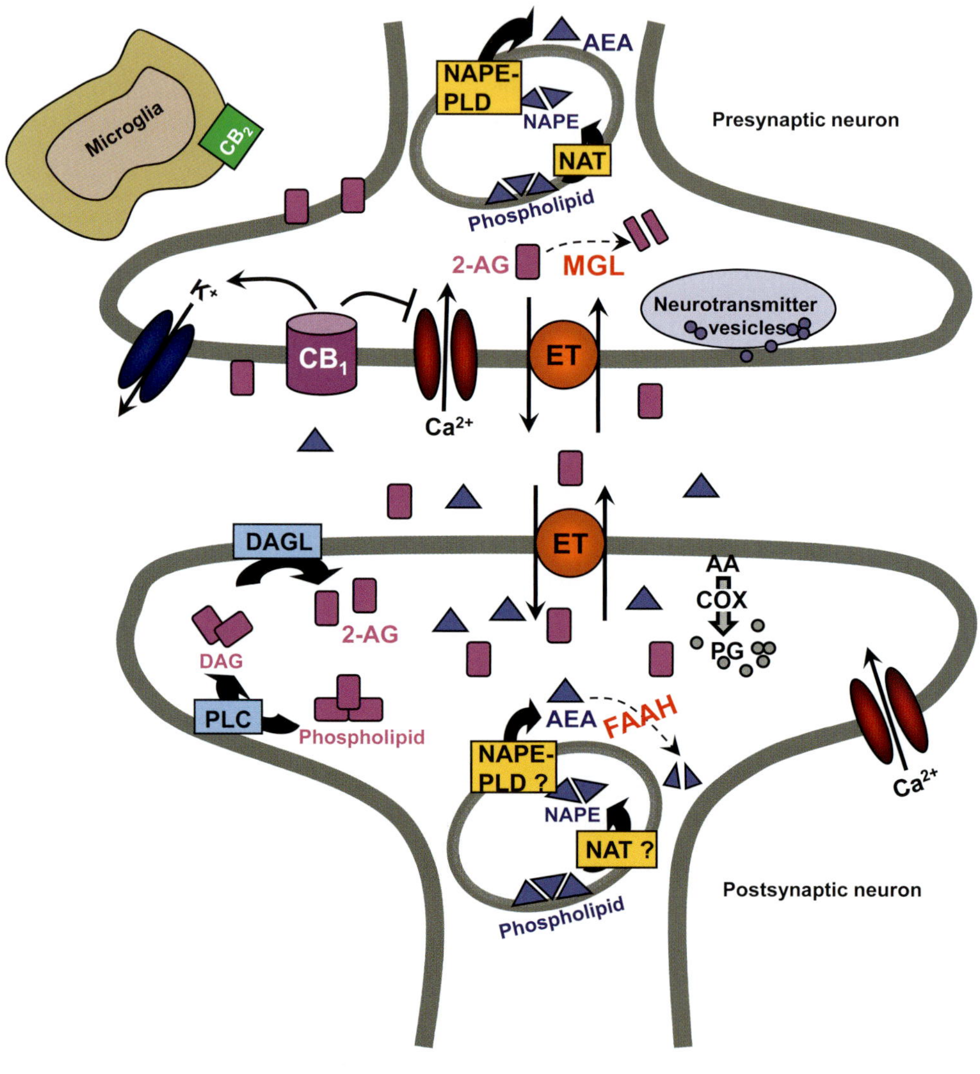

Fig. 3. Synthesis and inactivation of anandamide and 2-arachidonoylglycerol. The synthesis and metabolism of anandamide (involving NAT and NAPE-PLD) and 2-arachidonoylglycerol (involving PLC and DAGL) are controlled by distinct enzymatic pathways, as demonstrated in this figure. Anandamide is hydrolyzed by the enzyme FAAH in postsynaptic neurons, whereas 2-AG is degraded, predominantly, but not exclusively, by a distinct enzyme (MGL) in presynaptic neurons. Abbreviations: 2-AG, 2-arachidonoylglycerol; AA, arachidonic acid; AEA, anandamide; CB_1, cannabinoid receptor 1; CB_2, cannabinoid receptor 2; COX, cyclooxygenase; DAG, diacylglycerol; DAGL, diacylglycerol lipase; ET, endocannabinoid membrane transporter; FAAH, fatty acid amide hydrolase; MGL, monoacylglycerol lipase; NAPE, N-arachidonoyl-phosphatidylethanolamine; NAPE-PLD, N-arachidonoyl-phosphatidylethanolamine phospholipase D; NAT, N-acyltransferase; PG, prostaglandins; PLC, phospholipase C.

subsequently hydrolyzed by a diacylglycerol lipase (DAGL) selective for the sn-1 position to generate 2-AG [145]. Detailed reviews of these processes are available [29,30,105] (Fig. 3). Subsequent to their on-demand synthesis, endocannabinoids may activate cannabinoid receptors following their release into the extracellular space or their movement directly into the cell membrane [114]. Anandamide preferentially binds to CB_1 receptors in vitro, and it exhibits low affinity for TRPV1 receptors [31,107]. 2-arachidonoyl glycerol is known to activate both CB_1 and CB_2 receptors [93,134]. This compound is found in the brain in concentrations 170-fold higher than those of anandamide [132]. A role for endogenous 2-AG in pain modulation has only recently been described [62,103,137].

In addition to activating metabotropic CB_1 receptors, AEA can also activate ionotropic TRPV1 receptors as an endovanilloid. TRPV1 receptors are expressed in nociceptive sensory neurons and can detect and respond to noxious mechanical, thermal (i.e., heat), and chemical (i.e., capsaicin) stimuli [3,31]. Capsaicin and AEA share the same binding site, but AEA must be present at high concentrations to activate TRPV1 receptors. Activation of TRPV1 receptors increases intracellular levels of cations such as Ca^{2+} and depolarizes the cell; these effects can also liberate calcitonin gene-related peptide (CGRP) and substance P to produce vasodilatation [31]. At high concentrations, AEA can thus exert opposing effects through activation of cannabinoid and TRPV1 receptors, respectively. A functional relationship exists between TRPV1 and CB_1 receptors in the DRG [2], in the spinal cord and brain [21], and wherever these two receptors may be co-expressed in the same cell. Peripheral and central TRPV1 receptors therefore remain a viable therapeutic target.

Uptake of Endocannabinoids

Reuptake of endocannabinoids, and most notably AEA, in the synaptic space may be facilitated by a transporter that has yet to be molecularly cloned. Pharmacological inhibitors for endocannabinoid transport have nonetheless been developed (AM404, VDM11, and others) [29,105,107]. Anandamide may accumulate in neurons and other cells by facilitated diffusion rather than through a specific transport mechanism [54]. This process is saturable, is temperature-dependent, does not require ATP, and is driven by a transmembrane concentration gradient. The existence of a specific endocannabinoid transporter remains controversial, and new discoveries are necessary to establish beyond doubt the mechanism of endocannabinoid transport [43,54]. However, it is noteworthy that AEA uptake is selectively inhibited by a variety of pharmacological agents, consistent with the existence of a saturable component in the transport of anandamide [43,54] (see Fig. 3), and thus, uptake inhibitors represent useful research tools.

Degradation of AEA and 2-AG

Endocannabinoid signaling is limited by efficient degradation processes involving enzymatic hydrolysis mediated by specific intracellular enzymes. The enzymes that degrade endocannabinoids are quite well characterized and include fatty-acid amide hydrolase

(FAAH) and monoacylglycerol lipase (MGL) (see [29,30] for reviews). Inhibitors for FAAH (AM374, URB597, URB532, and others) or MGL (URB602, OMDM169, JZL184, and Compound 11) enzymes have been described (for review, see [105,126]), although selectivity of some agents may vary considerably. FAAH hydrolyzes AEA and related compounds [20,126], whereas MGL metabolizes 2-AG [33]. FAAH, a membrane-bound enzyme, hydrolyzes AEA in neurons and astrocytes into the breakdown products arachidonic acid and ethanolamine [20,32]. FAAH knockout mice exhibit a profound reduction in AEA hydrolysis and an increase in brain levels of endogenous AEA [19]. They display a phenotypic hypoalgesia, and exhibit antinociception, compared to their wild-type controls, in the hot-plate, tail immersion, and formalin tests [19]. The distribution of FAAH in organs of the rat has been described in detail; the activity of this enzyme is highest in the liver, followed by the small intestine, brain, and testes (see [26] for a review). Immunohistochemical studies have mapped the distribution of FAAH in the brain. FAAH is found in regions related to nociceptive transmission such as the termination zone of the spinothalamic tract in the ventral posterior lateral nucleus of the thalamus [35]. FAAH has also been found in Lissauer's tract, in neurons of the superficial dorsal horn of the spinal cord, and in DRG cells.

MGL, a serine hydrolase, hydrolyzes 2-AG into the breakdown products arachidonic acid and glycerol. MGL is located on presynaptic sites [29,33,62], whereas FAAH is found on postsynaptic sites [29,126]. Thus, FAAH may also regulate endocannabinoids near sites of synthesis, whereas MGL may terminate endocannabinoid actions following receptor activation. Northern blot, immunohistochemical, and in situ hybridization techniques have demonstrated that MGL is heterogeneously distributed in the rat brain, with the highest levels observed in regions expressing CB_1 receptors, such as the cortex, thalamus, hippocampus, and cerebellum [33]. MGL is localized exclusively to axon terminals, where it colocalizes with CB_1 [50]. Although the biosynthesis and metabolism of AEA and 2-AG have been simplified here to maintain the focus of this chapter, it is important to mention that, in addition to hydrolysis, alternative metabolic pathways exist [47,81]. Indeed, there is evidence for the metabolism of AEA and 2-AG by cyclooxygenase (COX), lipoxygenase, and cytochrome P450 enzymes, further adding to the complexity of endocannabinoid signaling mechanisms [47,81].

Endogenous Cannabinoids Act as Retrograde Synaptic Messengers

Given that endocannabinoids are produced on demand and can be released immediately from cells, they can regulate synaptic transmission, both excitatory and inhibitory. In the CNS, endocannabinoids act as neurotransmitters. Neurophysiological studies have provided insights into the physiological role of endocannabinoids acting as retrograde signaling molecules (for review, see [78]). Endocannabinoids, released from depolarized postsynaptic neurons, travel to presynaptic terminals, where they activate CB_1 receptors through a retrograde signaling mechanism [4,149] (see Fig. 3). The general effect is a decrease in the release of neurotransmitters such as GABA or glutamate. This retrograde signaling mechanism suggests an important modulatory role for endocannabinoids in controlling neuronal excitability and maintaining homeostasis [78].

Biological Actions of Cannabinoids and Endocannabinoids

Cannabinoids modulate responses in diverse physiological systems. An exhaustive description of all these effects is beyond the scope of this chapter (for reviews, see [30,69,109]). The principal actions of the cannabinoids are summarized in Table IV. Undesirable or toxic effects related to the consumption of either cannabis or cannabinoids have been described, which has made the use of centrally acting cannabinoid pharmacotherapies for pain controversial [144]. Cannabinoid signaling systems control the functions of diverse biological systems in physiological and pathological conditions (see Table IV). Therefore, pharmacotherapies engineered to modulate these systems show therapeutic potential for a broad array of disorders (see [105,109] for reviews). Strategies to exploit the analgesic potential of cannabinoid signaling systems while minimizing unwanted side effects have been described [5].

Table IV
Effects of cannabinoids on different physiological systems

System	Effects
Central nervous system	Euphoria—cannabinoid exhilaration Increased sensory perception Disruption of intellectual and psychomotor performance Temporospatial disorientation Impaired ideation/impaired memory Thermoregulation disorder Psychotic episodes Analgesia Antiemetic properties Antianxiety and antistress properties Appetite stimulant properties Neuroprotection Anticonvulsive properties
Cardiovascular system	Tachycardia Vasodilatation Decrease in blood pressure
Respiratory system	Bronchodilatation Cough suppression
Gastrointestinal system	Inhibition of intestinal transit Antiobesity/anorexic properties Anti-inflammatory effects in the colon
Reproductive system	Implantation Hormonal secretions
Locomotor system	Hypomotility/reduced movement Antispastic properties
Ocular system	Decrease in intraocular pressure
Other systems	Effects on immune functions Inhibition of tumor growth Tolerance phenomenon after prolonged use

Cannabinoids/Endocannabinoids and Pain

Cannabinoid receptors, endocannabinoids, and enzymes controlling their synthesis and degradation are localized in multiple levels of the neuraxis, from the periphery to the CNS [53] (for review, see [56]). The discovery of the endocannabinoid system, the availability of antagonists for cannabinoid receptors (CB_1 and CB_2), and the generation of transgenic mice lacking CB_1 and/or CB_2 and FAAH have spurred research in this growing field. Sites of action for endocannabinoids in suppressing pain were initially suggested by studies employing synthetic cannabinoids targeted at CB_1 and/or CB_2 receptors. These studies have recently been reviewed [48,56,117,141].

Supraspinal Analgesia

The antinociceptive [87] and electrophysiological [59] effects produced by the systemic administration of cannabinoids are attenuated following spinal transection. These studies implicate a role for supraspinal sites in contributing to cannabinoid analgesic action. Direct support for supraspinal sites of cannabinoid analgesic action was derived from studies injecting synthetic cannabinoid agonists intraventricularly and locally into various brain regions (for a review, see [141]). Structures targeted include the periaqueductal gray (PAG) [91], thalamus [90], rostral ventromedial medulla (RVM) [94], and amygdala [89], among others. These studies have permitted initial identification of brain regions responsible for the antinociceptive properties of cannabinoids. Activation of these sites by endocannabinoids may, therefore, produce antinociception under physiological conditions.

Neurophysiological studies by Walker's laboratory first documented that cannabinoids suppress nociceptive processing [90] (see [141] for a review). Cannabinoids, administered systemically, suppress the activity of nociceptive neurons in the spinal dorsal horn [60] and ventroposterior lateral nucleus of the thalamus, without altering the activity of purely non-nociceptive neurons. Importantly, these neurophysiological effects correlate highly with the antinociceptive effects of cannabinoids, and they cannot be attributed to the motor effects of the same compounds [90].

Walker's group first identified a role for endogenous AEA, released under physiological conditions, in pain modulation [142]. Electrical stimulation of the dorsolateral PAG produced antinociception in the tail-flick test and mobilized endogenous AEA, as measured by microdialysis. Importantly, this stimulation-produced analgesia was blocked by the CB_1 antagonist SR141716A, demonstrating mediation by CB_1. Intraplantar administration of formalin was also shown to increase levels of endogenous AEA in the dorsolateral PAG. Thus, noxious stimulation may produce endocannabinoid mobilization [142]. Exposure to an environmental stressor (brief continuous footshock) also produces endocannabinoid-mediated stress-induced analgesia that is associated with mobilization of endogenous 2-AG and anandamide [62]. Endocannabinoid mobilization was most pronounced in dorsal midbrain fragments containing the intact PAG [62]. Endocannabinoid-mediated stress-induced analgesia is blocked by CB_1, but not by CB_2, antagonists and is insensitive to blockade by opioid antagonists (naltrexone) and TRPV1 antagonists (capsazepine) [62,136]. Moreover, 2-AG mobilization in the PAG correlates highly with endocannabinoid-mediated stress antinociception [61]. These observations are also consistent with the ability of inhibitors of endocannabinoid uptake (e.g., VDM11) or FAAH (e.g. URB597, arachidonoyl-serotonin) and locally administered FAAH (e.g. URB597, arachidonoyl-serotonin) and MGL (URB602) inhibitors to enhance endocannabinoid-mediated stress antinociception through a CB_1-dependent mechanism [62,136,137]. These effects were all observed at doses that do not alter basal nociceptive thresholds. In the case of URB602, which is not appropriate for systemic use as a selective MGL inhibitor, biochemical studies confirmed that URB602, injected into the PAG, increased levels of 2-AG selectively without altering levels of AEA [62]. These studies collectively suggest a functional role for endogenous AEA and 2-AG in suppressing pain under physiological conditions.

Exogenous cannabinoids also modulate activity of ON and OFF cells in the rostral ventromedial medulla; here, inactivation of the RVM suppresses exogenous cannabinoid antinociception [94]. Pharmacological inactivation of the RVM also suppresses endocannabinoid-mediated analgesia in a rodent model of stress-induced analgesia [136]. Endocannabinoid-mediated stress-induced analgesia is also enhanced in a CB_1-dependent manner by intra-RVM administration of an FAAH inhibitor, administered at doses that do not alter the basal nociceptive threshold [137]. These studies support a role for endogenous AEA in the RVM in endocannabinoid-mediated analgesia, although a role for 2-AG has not been specifically assessed.

Endocannabinoid levels are altered in specific brain regions implicated in cannabinoid antinociceptive mechanisms following nerve injury. For example, injury of the sciatic nerve increases AEA and 2-AG levels in the PAG and RVM [112], structures implicated in both the descending modulation and descending facilitation of pain. Anandamide levels were also increased in the dorsal raphe following chronic constriction injury (CCI) [106,112].

Systemic administration of inhibitors of endocannabinoid uptake (VDM-11, OMDM-2, UCM-707, and LY2318912) increases AEA and/or 2-AG levels in brain [22]. Interestingly, FAAH inhibition by N-arachidonoyl-serotonin (AA-5-HT) was shown to increase brain levels of both AEA and 2-AG [22]. These studies suggest that inhibitors of endocannabinoid uptake and deactivation show therapeutic potential for increasing endocannabinoid levels, although selectivity for manipulations of AEA or 2-AG requires biochemical confirmation.

Spinal Analgesia

Intrathecal administration of cannabinoids produces antinociception [128], and suppresses nociceptive neuronal activity [63] (for review, see [141]). These studies initially documented the existence of spinal sites of cannabinoid antinociceptive actions. Indeed, behavioral [128], electrophysiological [63], and neurochemical [64] studies have demonstrated that cannabinoids act at the spinal level to modulate pain. Mixed cannabinoid agonists such as levonantradol, WIN55,212-2, and CP,55,940, at the spinal level, produce CB_1-mediated antinociceptive effects (see [141] for a detailed review). Moreover, cannabinoids suppress C-fiber-evoked responses of dorsal horn neurons recorded in normal, inflamed, and nerve-injured rats [36,99]. Furthermore, these data are consistent with the ability of cannabinoids to suppress Fos protein expression, a neurochemical marker of sustained neuronal activation, in different animal models of persistent pain through CB_1- and CB_2-specific mechanisms [64,98]. Cannabinoid receptors have been demonstrated on primary afferent neurons at pre- and postsynaptic sites in the spinal cord using receptor binding and quantitative autoradiography [57,103]. In the dorsal horn of the spinal cord, CB_1 receptors were initially found on terminals of spinal interneurons [37] and on astrocytes [125] using immunohistochemical methods. Cannabinoid receptors in the spinal cord reside on both presynaptic terminals [103] and postsynaptic sites (e.g., terminals of intrinsic spinal cord interneurons). The presence of CB_1 on both excitatory and inhibitory elements in the spinal cord makes the endocannabinoid system ideally situated to regulate neuronal excitability. Upregulation of cannabinoid receptors is also observed in the spinal cord following nerve injury [124], suggesting that both endocannabinoids and their receptors are regulated under conditions of injury.

A role for endocannabinoid release under physiological conditions in pain modulation is also supported at the spinal level; exposure to an acute environmental stressor increases accumulation of 2-AG, but not of anandamide, in the lumbar spinal cord [137]. 2-AG accumulation in the spinal cord correlates highly with the appearance of stress-induced antinociception [137]. In the spinal cord, the 2-AG-synthesizing enzyme DGL-α is found in postsynaptic elements that colocalize with metabotropic glutamate receptor 5 (mGluR5) [103], whose activation induces 2-AG biosynthesis in vitro. CB_1 receptors are localized presynaptically in DGL-α-expressing cells in the superficial dorsal horn, where they are found at excitatory synapses formed by C and Aδ fibers [103]. These observations confirm the molecular architecture of retrograde 2-AG signaling in the spinal cord. Moreover, intrathecal administration of both FAAH (URB597/AA5-HT) and MGL-preferring (URB602) inhibitors also enhance endocannabinoid-mediated stress-induced analgesia through a CB_1-dependent mechanism [137].

Anandamide and 2-AG are also increased in the spinal cord following induction of a neuropathic pain state produced by chronic constriction injury of the sciatic nerve [112]. The endocannabinoid system is similarly modulated in response to a spinal cord contusion in rats [41]. The early stages are marked by increases in AEA levels, upregulation of the putative synthetic enzyme NAPE-PLD, and downregulation of the degradative enzyme FAAH. The delayed stages are marked by increases in 2-AG, a marked upregulation of the 2-AG-synthesizing enzyme DAGL-α (i.e., in neurons, astrocytes and immune infiltrates), and a moderate increase in levels of the degradative enzyme MGL [41]. In this study, CB_1 receptors were expressed in neurons, oligodendrocytes, and astrocytes, whereas CB_2 receptors were strongly upregulated after the lesion and were expressed mainly in immune infiltrates and astrocytes [41]. The importance of the cannabinoid CB_2 receptor as a potential therapeutic target for treatment of pathological pain states with limited centrally mediated side effects has been demonstrated in behavioral, neurochemical, and electrophysiological studies (see [48] for a review). Indeed, the development and evaluation of CB_2-selective agonists such as HU308, AM1241, JWH-133, and GW405833 (L768242) have provided direct evidence to support the hypothesis that activation of CB_2 produces antinociceptive effects in persistent pain states (see [48] for a review on the subject). The complexity of the actions of CB_2 agonists on neuronal and non-neuronal cells and their signaling properties are only beginning to be explored. The available literature supports the efficacy of CB_2 agonists in suppressing persistent pain states following acute administration at multiple levels of the neuraxis, although the impact of long-term treatment on antinociceptive effects and immune functions remains unknown. More work is needed to identify clinical efficacy as well as limitations associated with therapeutic strategies targeting CB_2 receptors.

Peripheral Analgesia

Peripheral antinociceptive actions of cannabinoids have been demonstrated in numerous animal pain models (for review, see [48,56,117]). Harnessing these mechanisms shows considerable promise for separating the therapeutic effects of cannabinoids from unwanted CNS side effects. Cannabinoid receptors are synthesized in DRG cells, which are the source of primary afferent input to the spinal cord [1,2,58,59,121,129,140]. These afferent nerve fibers transmit information about sensory stimulation to the spinal cord, thereby enabling communication between the periphery and specific areas of the CNS that contribute to pain perception [38]. Following the induction of neuropathy (by spinal nerve ligation), cannabinoid receptors and their endogenous ligands (AEA and 2-AG) are increased in the DRG on the ipsilateral side of the injury [95]. Cannabinoid CB_1 [1,2,58,59] and CB_2 [121,140] receptors are detected in the DRG. DRG cells synthesize cannabinoid receptors and transport them to peripheral terminals of primary afferents [58,59]. Indeed, the specific deletion of CB_1 receptors in peripheral nociceptors reduces peripheral as well as systemic cannabinoid-induced analgesia [1]. Multiple approaches support the presence of cannabinoid receptors on primary afferent neurons [2,129]. CB_1 and CB_2 receptors are found in large myelinated and small unmyelinated human cutaneous nerve fibers [129]. Both cannabinoid receptor subtypes have also been found in different layers of the skin, and in some adnexal structures (sweat glands, sebaceous cells, and others), which may contribute to peripheral antinociceptive actions [45,70,129].

Endocannabinoid levels and FAAH activity have also been measured in rodent paw skin [16,49,66]. AEA is detected in paw tissue [16,49], and a decrease in FAAH activity is observed in the inflamed paw following carrageenan-induced inflammation [66]. In the formalin model, OMDM169, an inhibitor of 2-AG hydrolysis, increased levels of 2-AG, but not AEA, in the ipsilateral paw [11]. Intraplantar administration of exogenous AEA or the FAAH inhibitor URB597 also increased the local level of AEA in an animal model of bone cancer pain [79]. These studies suggest that the manipulation of peripheral endocannabinoids may be a promising strategy for the management of pain, either alone or as an adjuvant to existing analgesics (e.g., COX inhibitors).

Antinociceptive Effects of Cannabinoids in Different Pain Models

Early physiological support for the hypothesis that endocannabinoids suppress pain comes from studies evaluating hypersensitivity to pain (hyperalgesia) following pharmacological blockade of CB_1 receptors. Hyperalgesia has been observed in the hot-plate test following intrathecal administration of the CB_1 antagonist/inverse agonist SR141716A, and these effects are mimicked by CB_1 antisense knockdown at the spinal level [118,119]. Pharmacological blockade of CB_1 receptors with SR141716A has also been reported to produce hyperalgesia in the formalin test [16,133]. Moreover, the local administration of exogenous anandamide and/or 2-AG reduced pain induced by carrageenan [120], formalin injection [16,46], or nerve ligation [25,44,51]. However, one limitation of studies employing exogenous endocannabinoids is that they do not demonstrate whether the endogenous ligands play similar roles under physiological conditions.

Therefore, documentation of intrinsic effects of endocannabinoids released under physiological conditions is critical for understanding the functional roles of endocannabinoids in nociceptive processing. Studies employing stimulation-produced analgesia and stress-induced analgesia provide direct support for the hypothesis that endogenous AEA and 2-AG suppress pain through a CB_1-dependent mechanism. Stress-induced analgesia is CB_1-mediated; it is blocked by multiple CB_1 antagonists, involves the mobilization of endocannabinoids supraspinally (2-AG and AEA) [62] and spinally (2-AG alone) [137] and is enhanced by inhibitors of endocannabinoid deactivation (URB597, AA-5-HT, or URB602) or transport (VDM11). The failure of a CB_2 antagonist to block endocannabinoid-mediated stress-induced analgesia in these studies [62] may reflect the absence of a CB_2-mediated component in endocannabinoid-mediated stress analgesia or, alternately, the failure of the spinally mediated tail-flick test to detect a CB_2-mediated component of endocannabinoid analgesia. The existence of cross-tolerance and cross-sensitization between exogenous cannabinoid antinociception and endocannabinoid-mediated stress-induced analgesia suggests that these phenomena are linked by a common mechanism [135].

The development of drugs that inhibit the enzymatic degradation of endocannabinoids (i.e., through inhibition of FAAH or MGL) or their transport has improved our understanding of the functional roles of the endocannabinoid system in modulating pain under physiological conditions (for a review, see [73]). Effects of exogenous administration of cannabinoids (CB_1 agonists, CB_2 agonists, CB_1/CB_2 agonists), endocannabinoids (focusing on AEA and 2-AG), and the modulation of endocannabinoids (MGL, FAAH, or uptake inhibitors) in models of acute, inflammatory, and neuropathic pain are summarized in Table V. Behavioral and neurophysiological studies continue to reaffirm that cannabinoids produce antinociception in acute, inflammatory, and neuropathic pain models through CB_1- and/or CB_2-dependent mechanisms. Interested readers are referred to recent reviews [48,73,141].

Clinical Use of Cannabis and Cannabinoids in the Treatment of Pain

Cannabis has been used in medicine for millennia. O'Shaughnessy (a 19th-century Irish physician working in India) made the first scientific study of cannabis. Later, tincture of cannabis was available in some European countries and in the United States until the beginning of the 20th century. However, it was not until the discovery of the main psychoactive component of marijuana (THC) in 1964 [40] that interest in cannabis was rekindled. This research led 10 years later to the publication of the first clinical trials performed to investigate the role of cannabinoids in the treatment of pain. With the major pharmacological discoveries made in the 1990s (the cloning of the two cannabinoid receptors and discovery of the endocannabinoid system), a new interest in cannabinoids led to renewed clinical trials. There are to date 45 randomized clinical trials (and three follow-up studies) looking at the efficacy of various cannabinoids in the treatment of different pain conditions (for review, see [9,24,32,67,86,147]); however, it would be outside the scope of this chapter to review all these trials.

Acute Pain

Cannabinoids are least effective in alleviating acute pain. This conclusion is based upon studies conducted in the postoperative setting and in human volunteers. In some cases, administration of cannabinoids, especially in high doses, is associated with increased pain [8,82,115,143]. However, consider the following caveats before concluding that cannabinoids are not at all indicated in acute pain: (1) Some studies have demonstrated an analgesic effect in postoperative pain [65,71] and in human volunteers [116,122]. (2) In postoperative patients, a small number of patients have been studied, and the doses used may not have been adequate. For example, in one study [15], a higher dose of THC (10 mg) could have been tested because the THC dose employed (5 mg) is rarely effective in alleviating pain, according to the literature. (3) Potent and effective drugs such as opioids are often not necessarily very good analgesics in human volunteer studies when certain modalities of painful stimulus are used, for example heat pain [100]. (4) The combination of THC and CBD administered in an oromucosal spray in postoperative patients who cannot take oral medications after abdominal or major surgery may show therapeutic potential. A large multicenter study recruiting patients undergoing operations with a reproducible painful condition and using THC/CBD spray is needed before a conclusion can be drawn on the effect of cannabinoids in postoperative pain management.

Chronic Pain

Cannabinoids are, on the whole, effective for the treatment of chronic pain conditions [9]. A large number of recent studies using a substantial number of patients have shown that a THC/CBD combination (by oromucosal spray) is effective in alleviating pain in

Table V
Antinociceptive effects of modulators of cannabinoid signaling

Pain Model	Exogenous eCBs	CB_1 Agonists	CB_2 Agonists	CB_1/CB_2 Agonists	eCB Uptake Inhibitors	FAAH Inhibitors	MGL Inhibitors
Acute							
Tail-flick	AEA	ACEA	AM1241 GW405833 (L768242)	HU-210 CP55,940 WIN55,212-2	UCM707 VDM-11	AA-5-HT PMSF PTK URB597	URB602 JZL184 (in tail-immersion test)
Hotplate	AEA	NT	AM1241	HU-210 CP55,940 WIN55,212-2	AM404 OMDM-1 OMDM-2 UCM707 VDM-11	URB597 URB532	NT
Plantar	AEA	NT	AM1241 GW405833 (L768242) HU-308	CP55,940 WIN55,212-2	NT	Compound 17	NT
Inflammatory							
Formalin	AEA 2-AG	NT	AM1241 GW405833 (L768242) HU-308	CP55,940 HU-210 WIN55,212-2	AM404 LY2318912 LY2183240 OMDM132 UCM707	AA-5-HT Compound 17 Flurbiprofen Ibuprofen LY2183240 MAFP Propofol Rofecoxib OMDM106 OMDM119 OMDM122	OMDM169 URB602 JZL184 (also active in acetic acid-induced writhing test)

Carrageenan	AEA	ACEA	AM1241 GW405833 (L768242) JWH-133	CP55,940 HU-210 WIN55,212-2	NT	JNJ-1661010 URB597	Compound 21 URB602
Capsaicin	AEA	Methan-andamide	AM1241	CP55,940 HU-210 WIN55,212-2	NT	NT	NT
CFA	AEA	ACEA	A-796260 GW405833 (L768242) GW842166X	CP55,940 HU-210 WIN55,212-2	AM404	URB597	NT
Neuropathic							
CCI	NT	NT	A-796260 GW405833 (L768242)	Bay 59-3074 WIN55,212-2	AM404 VDM11	AA-5-HT OL-135 URB597	NT
PSNL	AEA 2-AG	NT	GW405833 (L768242)	CP55,940 HU-210 WIN55,212-2	AM404	Ibuprofen Rofecoxib URB597	URB602
SNL	NT	ACEA	AM1241 JWH-133 GW405833 (L768242)	HU-210 CP55,940 WIN55,212-2 Bay 59-3074	NT	URB597 Compound 17 Compound 34 JNJ-1661010	NT

Abbreviations: 2-AG, 2-arachidonoylglycerol; AA-5-HT, N-arachidonoyl serotonin; ACEA, arachidonyl-2′-chloroethylamide; AEA, anandamide; CB_1, cannabinoid receptor 1; CB_2, cannabinoid receptor 2; CCI, chronic constriction injury; CFA, complete Freund's adjuvant; eCBs, endocannabinoids; FAAH, fatty acid amide hydrolase; MAFP, methyl arachidonyl fluorophosphonate; MGL, monoacylglycerol lipase; NT, not tested; PMSF, phenylmethylsulfonyl fluoride; PSNL, partial sciatic nerve ligation; PTK, palmitoyl trifluoromethyl ketone; SNL, spinal nerve ligation.

neuropathic pain patients and especially in the subgroup of patients suffering from multiple sclerosis [9]. The use of cannabidiol and ajulemic acid was also associated with a positive outcome in pain treatment [9]. However, the outcome of two trials using dronabinol and nabilone was negative in patients with neuropathic pain [6a,38a]. It should be noted that these two trials are the only trials associated with a negative outcome in all published trials evaluating cannabinoids for chronic pain.

Smoked cannabis is also effective for the treatment of chronic pain, as reported in two very recent studies in HIV patients and in patients with neuropathic pain. The issue of whether smoked cannabis should be used in clinical practice has been recently discussed. Ware argues that until further trials of cannabis in conditions for which patients have already claimed benefit are completed, it is premature to claim that there is no future for herbal marijuana [146]. Another group does not see much of a future for it [77].

In other treatment outcome assessments of chronic pain, THC or its synthetic analogues were effective in relieving pain in patients with musculoskeletal disorders, fibromyalgia, spinal cord injury, or other chronic pain conditions [9,67,147].

Cancer Pain

Only four studies, performed more than 30 years ago, have evaluated the role of cannabinoids in relieving pain associated with cancer. Indeed, a preliminary trial of oral THC at 15 and 20 mg demonstrated an analgesic effect in patients experiencing cancer pain [102]. In a subsequent study, the administration of single oral doses of THC to patients with cancer pain demonstrated a mild analgesic effect. At doses of 10 mg, THC was well tolerated, whereas at 20 mg its administration was associated with unwanted side effects. However, the authors concluded that despite its sedative effect, THC at 10-mg doses has analgesic potential in these patients [101]. Another study on patients with cancer, using a nitrogen analogue of THC, showed that pain relief was superior to placebo and approximately equivalent to 50 mg of codeine phosphate [130]. Conversely, using a nitrogen analogue of THC in patients with chronic pain due to malignancies and compared with codeine and placebo, other authors found that benzopyranoperidine was not effective as an analgesic and even appeared to augment pain perception [76].

Side Effects

As with morphine, nonsteroidal anti-inflammatory drugs, and most other analgesics, cannabinoid use is associated with side effects. The studies outlined above suggest that there is therapeutic potential for cannabinoids in relieving pain in some conditions. However, significant hurdles exist in achieving clinically relevant outcomes with minimal side effects. Short-term side effects of cannabinoid therapy are largely expected and non-serious, but they remain the main drawbacks to patient compliance with therapy [9]. More specific information is required on the long-term side effects of cannabinoid therapy, including drug interactions, tolerance, cognitive impairment, and risks of addiction. However, it is important to emphasize that these issues are not unique to cannabinoids. Indeed, they point to the need for pain physicians to exercise diligence in following patients who are taking psychoactive medications [9,148].

A systematic review of safety studies of medical cannabinoids published over the past 40 years has recently been performed [144]. After exclusion of studies focusing on recreational cannabis use and studies that involved synthetic cannabinoids (e.g., nabilone, levonantradol), the authors included 31 randomized controlled trials and 8 observational studies in their review. The median cannabinoid exposure was 2 weeks. Most (96.6%) reported adverse effects that were not serious; dizziness (15.5%) was the most commonly reported event. Of the serious adverse events, the most common were relapse of multiple sclerosis (12.8%), vomiting (9.8%), and urinary tract infection (9.1%). It should be noted that 99% of the serious adverse events were reported in only two trials [139,150]. The authors advocate that high-quality trials with long-term exposure are required to further characterize safety issues related to the use of medical cannabinoids.

Conclusions on Cannabinoid Use in Patients for the Treatment of Pain

Preclinical evidence demonstrates the importance of cannabinoid receptors in controlling nociceptive transmission (see above). The publication, in the last 5 years, of several important clinical trials pointing to the potential role for cannabinoids in pain management, and ongoing work on the subject, make cannabinoids worthy of consideration for refractory pain conditions. However, it is crucial to fully inform patients of the side-effect profile associated with the use of cannabinoids, and to monitor them carefully.

The therapeutic potential of cannabis in pain medicine has recently been reviewed [67,86]. In acute pain studies using cannabis or cannabinoid agonists, many clinical trials have provided negative or equivocal results. The strongest evidence of their benefit is for the treatment of neuropathic pain, especially in multiple sclerosis patients. Guidelines for the use of cannabinoids in pain treatment have been published in Canada [17]. International guidelines for the treatment of neuropathic pain have included cannabinoids in their algorithm, not as a first-line treatment, but as a third or fourth option [7,34,96].

Clinicians working in pain management should be aware of the options becoming available from the cannabinoid class of medications. They should understand that THC or synthetic equivalents are different from smoked marijuana and from combined THC/CBD preparations. Furthermore, selective peripheral CB_1-receptor agonists and/or CB_2-receptor agonists deserve imminent clinical trials for nociceptive, inflammatory, and neuropathic pain [6] because their use will minimize central psychoactivity. Finally, the combination of opioids with cannabinoids in the treatment of pain is a potentially interesting option because cannabinoid synergism with opioid analgesics could reduce requirements for opioids [23]. Finally, the modulation of the endocannabinoid system, although not yet tested in clinical trials, is of great potential for future pain management, possibly in combination with other agents [24,32,113].

Acknowledgments

J. Guindon is supported by a Fonds de la Recherche en Santé du Québec (FRSQ) postdoctoral fellowship. P. Beaulieu is supported by a clinician-scientist grant from the FRSQ. A.G. Hohmann is supported by DA021644, DA022478, and DA022702.

References

[1] Agarwal N, Pacher P, Tegeder I, Amaya F, Constantin CE, Brenner GJ, Rubino T, Michalski CW, Marsicano G, Monory K, et al. Cannabinoids mediate analgesia largely via peripheral type 1 cannabinoid receptors in nociceptors. Nat Neurosci 2007;10:870–9.
[2] Ahluwalia J, Urban L, Capogna M, Bevan S, Nagy I. Cannabinoid 1 receptors are expressed in nociceptive primary sensory neurons. Neuroscience 2000;100:685–8.
[3] Akopian AN, Ruparel NB, Jeske NA, Patwardhan A, Hargreaves KM. Role of ionotropic cannabinoid receptors in peripheral antinociception and antihyperalgesia. Trends Pharmacol Sci 2009;30:79–84.
[4] Alger BE. Retrograde signaling in the regulation of synaptic transmission: focus on endocannabinoids. Prog Neurobiol 2002;68:247–86.
[5] Anand P, Whiteside G, Fowler CJ, Hohmann AG. Targeting CB_2 receptors and the endocannabinoid system for the treatment of pain. Brain Res Rev 2009;60:255–66.
[6] Anand U, Otto WR, Sanchez-Herrera D, Facer P, Yiangou Y, Korchev Y, Birch R, Benham C, Bountra C, Chessell IP, Anand P. Cannabinoid receptor CB2 localisation and agonist-mediated inhibition of capsaicin responses in human sensory neurons. Pain 2008;138:667–80.
[6a] Attal N, Brasseur L, Guirimand D, Clermond-Gnamien S, Atlami S, Bouhassira D. Are oral cannabinoids safe and effective in refractory neuropathic pain? Eur J Pain 2004;8:173–7.
[7] Attal N, Cruccu G, Haanpää M, Hansson P, Jensen TS, Nurmikko T, Sampaio C, Sindrup S, Wiffen P; EFNS Task Force. EFNS guidelines on pharmacological treatment of neuropathic pain. Eur J Neurol 2006;13:1153–69.
[8] Beaulieu P. Effects of nabilone, a synthetic cannabinoid, on postoperative pain. Can J Anesth 2006;53:769–75.
[9] Beaulieu P, Ware M. Reassessment of the role of cannabinoids in the management of pain and other symptoms. Curr Opin Anaesthesiol 2007;20:473–7.
[10] Begg M, Pacher P, Bátkai S, Osei-Hyiaman D, Offertáler L, Mo FM, Liu J, Kunos G. Evidence for novel cannabinoid receptors. Pharmacol Ther 2005;106:133–45.
[11] Bisogno T, Ortar G, Petrosino S, Morera E, Palazzo E, Nalli M, Maione S, Di Marzo V; Endocannabinoid Research Group. Development of a potent inhibitor of 2-arachidonoylglycerol hydrolysis with antinociceptive activity in vivo. Biochim Biophys Acta 2009;1791:53–60.
[12] Booth M. Cannabis: a history. New York: Picador (St. Martin's Press), 2003.
[13] Bradshaw HB, Walker JM. The expanding field of cannabimimetic and related lipid mediators. Br J Pharmacol 2005;144:459–65.
[14] Buckley NE, McCoy KL, Mezey E, Bonner T, Zimmer A, Felder CC, Glass M, Zimmer A. Immunomodulation by cannabinoids is absent in mice deficient for the cannabinoid CB2 receptor. Eur J Pharmacol 2000;396:141–9.
[15] Buggy DJ, Toogood L, Maric S, Sharpe P, Lambert DG, Rowbotham DJ. Lack of analgesic efficacy of oral delta-9-tetrahydrocannabinol in postoperative pain. Pain 2003;106:169–72.
[16] Calignano A, La Rana G, Giuffrida A, Piomelli D. Control of pain initiation by endogenous cannabinoids. Nature 1998;394:277–81.
[17] Clark AJ, Lynch ME, Ware M, Beaulieu P, McGilveray IJ, Gourlay D. Guidelines for the use of cannabinoids in chronic pain. Pain Res Manag 2005;10:44–6A.
[18] Cocco L, Faenza I, Fiume R, Maria Billi A, Gilmour RS, Manzoli FA. Phosphoinositide-specific phospholipase C (PI-PLC) beta1 and nuclear lipid-dependent signaling. Biochim Biophys Acta 2006;1761:509–21.
[19] Cravatt BF, Demarest K, Patricelli MP, Bracey MH, Giang DK, Martin BR, Lichtman AH. Supersensitivity to anandamide and enhanced endogenous cannabinoid signaling in mice lacking fatty acid amide hydrolase. Proc Natl Acad Sci USA 2001;98:9371–6.
[20] Cravatt BF, Giang DK, Mayfield SP, Boger DL, Lerner RA, Gilula NB. Molecular characterization of an enzyme that degrades neuromodulatory fatty-acid amides. Nature 1996;384:83–7.
[21] Cristino L, De Petrocellis L, Pryce G, Baker D, Guglielmotti V, Di Marzo V. Immunohistochemical localization of cannabinoid type 1 and vanilloid transient receptor potential vanilloid type 1 receptors in the mouse brain. Neuroscience 2006;139:1405–15.
[22] de Lago E, Petrosino S, Valenti M, Morera E, Ortega-Gutierrez S, Fernandez-Ruiz J, Di Marzo V. Effect of repeated systemic administration of selective inhibitors of endocannabinoid inactivation on rat brain endocannabinoid levels. Biochem Pharmacol 2005;70:446–52.
[23] Desroches J, Beaulieu P. Opioid and endocannabinoid interactions: roles in pain management. Current Drug Targets 2009; in press.
[24] Desroches J, Beaulieu P. The cannabinoid system and pain: a new therapeutic avenue? Rev Med Suisse 2008;4:1505–13.

[25] Desroches J, Guindon J, Lambert C, Beaulieu P. Modulation of the anti-nociceptive effects of 2-arachidonoyl glycerol by peripherally administered FAAH and MGL inhibitors in a neuropathic pain model. Br J Pharmacol 2008;155:913–24.
[26] Deutsch DG, Ueda N, Yamamoto S. The fatty acid amide hydrolase (FAAH). Prostaglandins Leukot Essent Fatty Acids 2002;66:201–10.
[27] Devane WA, Dysarz FA 3rd, Johnson MR, Melvin LS, Howlett AC. Determination and characterization of a cannabinoid receptor in rat brain. Mol Pharmacol 1988;34:605–13.
[28] Devane WA, Hanus L, Breuer A, Pertwee RG, Stevenson LA, Griffin G, Gibson D, Mandelbaum A, Etinger A, Mechoulam R. Isolation and structure of a brain constituent that binds to the cannabinoid receptor. Science 1992;258:1946–9.
[29] Di Marzo V. Endocannabinoids: synthesis and degradation. Rev Physiol Biochem Pharmacol 2006;160:1–24.
[30] Di Marzo. Targeting the endocannabinoid system: to enhance or reduce? Nat Rev Drug Discov 2008;7:438–55.
[31] Di Marzo V, Bisogno T, De Petrocellis L. Anandamide: some like it hot. Trends Pharmacol Sci 2001;22:346–9.
[32] Di Marzo V, De Petrocellis LD. Plant, synthetic, and endogenous cannabinoids in medicine. Annu Rev Med 2006;57:553–74.
[33] Dinh TP, Carpenter D, Leslie FM, Freund TF, Katona I, Sensi SL, Kathuria S, Piomelli D. Brain monoglyceride lipase participating in endocannabinoid inactivation. Proc Natl Acad Sci USA 2002;99:10819–24.
[34] Dworkin RH, O'Connor AB, Backonja M, Farrar JT, Finnerup NB, Jensen TS, Kalso EA, Loeser JD, Miaskowski C, Nurmikko TJ, et al. Pharmacologic management of neuropathic pain: evidence-based recommendations. Pain 2007;132:237–51.
[35] Egertova M, Cravatt BF, Elphick MR. Comparative analysis of fatty acid amide hydrolase and CB_1 cannabinoid receptor expression in the mouse brain: evidence of a widespread role for fatty acid amide hydrolase in regulation of endocannabinoid signaling. Neuroscience 2003;119:481–96.
[36] Elmes SJ, Jhaveri MD, Smart D, Kendall DA, Chapman V. Cannabinoid CB2 receptor activation inhibits mechanically evoked responses of wide dynamic range dorsal horn neurons in naïve rats and in rat models of inflammatory and neuropathic pain. Eur J Neurosci 2004;20:2311–20.
[37] Farquhar-Smith WP, Egertová M, Bradbury EJ, McMahon SB, Rice AS, Elphick MR. Cannabinoid CB_1 receptor expression in rat spinal cord. Mol Cell Neurosci 2000;15:510–21.
[38] Farquhar-Smith WP, Rice ASC. Peripheral mechanisms of inflammatory pain: towards the discovery of novel analgesics. In: Adams AP and Cashman JN, editors. Recent advances in anaesthesia and analgesia. London: Churchill Livingstone; 2000. p. 41–60.
[38a] Frank B, Serpell MG, Hughes J, Matthews JN, Kapur D. Comparison of analgesic effects and patient tolerability of nabilone and dihydrocodeine for chronic neuropathic pain: randomised, crossover, double blind study. BMJ 2008;336:199–201.
[39] Galiègue S, Mary S, Marchand J, Dussossoy D, Carrière D, Carayon P, Bouaboula M, Shire D, Le Fur G, Casellas P. Expression of central and peripheral cannabinoid receptors in human immune tissues and leukocyte subpopulations. Eur J Biochem 1995;232:54–61.
[40] Gaoni Y, Mechoulam R. Isolation, structure and partial synthesis of an active constituent of hashish. J Am Chem Soc 1964;86:1646–7.
[41] Garcia-Ovejero D, Arevalo-Martin A, Petrosino S, Docagne F, Hagen C, Bisogno T, Watanabe M, Guaza C, Di Marzo V, Molina-Holgado E. The endocannabinoid system is modulated in response to spinal cord injury in rats. Neurobiol Dis 2009;33:57–71.
[42] Gérard CM, Mollereau C, Vassart G, Parmentier M. Molecular cloning of a human cannabinoid receptor which is also expressed in testis. Biochem J 1991;279:129–34.
[43] Glaser ST, Kaczocha M, Deutsch DG. Anandamide transport: a critical review. Life Sci 2005;77:1584–604.
[44] Guindon J, Beaulieu P. Antihyperalgesic effects of local injections of anandamide, ibuprofen, rofecoxib and their combinations in a model of neuropathic pain. Neuropharmacology 2006;50:814–23.
[45] Guindon J, Beaulieu P. The role of the endogenous cannabinoid system in peripheral analgesia. Curr Mol Pharmacol 2009;2:134–9.
[46] Guindon J, De Léan A, Beaulieu P. Local interactions between anandamide, an endocannabinoid, and ibuprofen, a nonsteroidal anti-inflammatory drug, in acute and inflammatory pain. Pain 2006;121:85–93.
[47] Guindon J, Hohmann AG. A physiological role for endocannabinoid-derived products of cyclooxygenase-2-mediated oxidative metabolism. Br J Pharmacol 2008;153:1341–3.
[48] Guindon J, Hohmann AG. Cannabinoid CB2 receptors: a therapeutic target for the treatment of inflammatory and neuropathic pain. Br J Pharmacol 2008;153:319–34.
[49] Guindon J, LoVerme J, De Léan A, Piomelli D, Beaulieu P. Synergistic antinociceptive effects of anandamide, an endocannabinoid, and nonsteroidal anti-inflammatory drugs in peripheral tissue: a role for endogenous fatty-acid ethanolamides? Eur J Pharmacol 2006;550:68–77.
[50] Gulyas AI, Cravatt BF, Bracey MH, Dinh TP, Piomelli D, Boscia F, Freund TF. Segregation of two endocannabinoid-hydrolyzing enzymes into pre- and postsynaptic compartments in the rat hippocampus, cerebellum and amygdala. Eur J Neurosci 2004;20:441–58.
[51] Helyes Z, Németh J, Thán M, Bölcskei K, Pintér E, Szolcsányi J. Inhibitory effect of anandamide on resiniferatoxin-induced sensory neuropeptide release in vivo and neuropathic hyperalgesia in the rat. Life Sci 2003;73:2345–53.
[52] Herkenham M. Localization of cannabinoid receptors in brain and periphery. In: Pertwee RG, editor. Cannabinoid receptors. London: Academic Press; 1995. p. 145–66.
[53] Herkenham M, Lynn AB, Johnson MR, Melvin LS, de Costa BR, Rice KC. Characterization and localization of cannabinoid receptors in rat brain: a quantitative in vitro autoradiographic study. J Neurosci 1991;11:563–83.

[54] Hillard CJ, Jarrahian A. Cellular accumulation of anandamide: consensus and controversy. Br J Pharmacol 2003;140:802–8.
[55] Hoehe MR, Caenazzo L, Martinez MM, Hsieh WT, Modi WS, Gershon ES, Bonner TI. Genetic and physical mapping of the human cannabinoid receptor gene to chromosome 6q14-q15. New Biol 1991;3:880–5.
[56] Hohmann AG. Spinal and peripheral mechanisms of cannabinoid antinociception: behavioural, neurophysiological and neuroanatomical perspectives. Chem Phys Lipids 2002;121:173–90.
[57] Hohmann AG, Briley EM, Herkenham M. Pre- and postsynaptic distribution of cannabinoid and mu opioid receptors in rat spinal cord. Brain Res 1999;822:17–25.
[58] Hohmann AG, Herkenham M. Cannabinoid receptors undergo axonal flow in sensory nerves. Neuroscience 1999;92:1171–5.
[59] Hohmann AG, Herkenham M. Localization of central cannabinoid CB1 receptor messenger RNA in neuronal subpopulations of rat dorsal root ganglia: a double-label in situ hybridization study. Neuroscience 1999;90:923–31.
[60] Hohmann AG, Martin WJ, Tsou K, Walker JM. Inhibition of noxious stimulus-evoked activity of spinal cord dorsal horn neurons by the cannabinoid WIN 55,212-2. Life Sci 1995;56:2111–8.
[61] Hohmann AG, Suplita RL 2nd. Endocannabinoid mechanisms of pain modulation. AAPS J 2006;8:E693–708.
[62] Hohmann AG, Suplita RL, Bolton NM, Neely MH, Fegley D, Mangieri R, Krey JF, Walker JM, Holmes PV, Crystal JD, et al. An endocannabinoid mechanism for stress-induced analgesia. Nature 2005;435:1108–12.
[63] Hohmann AG, Tsou K, Walker JM. Cannabinoid modulation of wide dynamic range neurons in the lumbar dorsal horn of the rat by spinally administered WIN55,212-2.Neurosci Lett 1998;257:119–22.
[64] Hohmann AG, Tsou K, Walker JM. Cannabinoid suppression of noxious heat-evoked activity in wide dynamic range neurons in the lumbar dorsal horn of the rat. J Neurophysiol 1999;81:575–83.
[65] Holdcroft A, Maze M, Doré C, Tebbs S, Thompson S. A multicenter dose-escalation study of the analgesic and adverse effects of an oral cannabis extract (Cannador) for postoperative pain management. Anesthesiology 2006;104:1040–6.
[66] Holt S, Comelli F, Costa B, Fowler CJ. Inhibitors of fatty acid amide hydrolase reduce carrageenan-induced hind paw inflammation in pentobarbital-treated mice: comparison with indomethacin and possible involvement of cannabinoid receptors. Br J Pharmacol 2005;146:467–76.
[67] Hosking RD, Zacijek JP. Therapeutic potential of cannabis in pain medicine. Br J Anaesth 2008;101:58–68.
[68] Howlett AC. Cannabinoid receptor signaling. Handb Exp Pharmacol 2005;168:53–79.
[69] Howlett AC, Breivogel CS, Childers SR, Deadwyler SA, Hampson RE, Porrino LJ. Cannabinoid physiology and pharmacology: 30 years of progress. Neuropharmacology 2004;47:345–58.
[70] Ibrahim MM, Porreca F, Lai J, Albrecht PJ, Rice FL, Khodorova A, Davar G, Makriyannis A, Vanderah TW, Mata HP, Malan TP Jr. CB2 cannabinoid receptor activation produces antinociception by stimulating peripheral release of endogenous opioids. Proc Natl Acad Sci USA 2005;102:3093–8.
[71] Jain AK, Ryan JR, McMahon FG, Smith G. Evaluation of intramuscular levonantradol and placebo in acute postoperative pain. J Clin Pharmacol 1981;21:320S–6.
[72] Járai Z, Wagner JA, Varga K, Lake KD, Compton DR, Martin BR, Zimmer AM, Bonner TI, Buckley NE, Mezey E, et al. Cannabinoid-induced mesenteric vasodilation through an endothelial site distinct from CB1 or CB2 receptors. Proc Natl Acad Sci USA 1999;96:14136–41.
[73] Jhaveri MD, Richardson D, Chapman V. Endocannabinoid metabolism and uptake: novel targets for neuropathic and inflammatory pain. Br J Pharmacol 2007;152:624–32.
[74] Jhaveri MD, Sagar DR, Elmes SJ, Kendall DA, Chapman V. Cannabinoid CB2 receptor-mediated anti-nociception in models of acute and chronic pain. Mol Neurobiol 2007;36:26–35.
[75] Jin XH, Uyama T, Wang J, Okamoto Y, Tonai T, Ueda N. cDNA cloning and characterization of human and mouse Ca^{2+}-independent phosphatidylethanolamine N-acyltransferases. Biochim Biophys Acta 2009;1791:32–8.
[76] Jochimsen PR, Lawton RL, VerSteeg K, Noyes R Jr. Effect of benzopyranoperidine, a delta-9-THC congener, on pain. Clin Pharmacol Ther 1978;24:223–7.
[77] Kalant H. Smoked marijuana as medicine: not much future. Clin Pharmacol Ther 2008;83:517–9.
[78] Katona I, Freund TF. Endocannabinoid signaling as a synaptic circuit breaker in neurological disease. Nat Med 2008;14:923–30.
[79] Khasabova IA, Khasabov SG, Harding-Rose C, Coicou LG, Seybold BA, Lindberg AE, Steevens CD, Simone DA, Seybold VS. A decrease in anandamide signaling contributes to the maintenance of cutaneous mechanical hyperalgesia in a model of bone cancer pain. J Neurosci 2008;28:11141–52.
[80] Kostenis E. Novel clusters of receptors for sphingosine-1-phosphate, sphingosylphosphorylcholine, and (lyso)-phosphatidic acid: new receptors for "old" ligands. J Cell Biochem 2004;92:923–36.
[81] Kozak KR, Marnett LJ. Oxidative metabolism of endocannabinoids. Prostaglandins Leukot Essent Fatty Acids 2002;66:211–20.
[82] Kraft B, Frickey NA, Kaufmann RM, Reif M, Frey R, Gustorff B, Kress HG. Lack of analgesia by oral standardized cannabis extract on acute inflammatory pain and hyperalgesia in volunteers. Anesthesiology 2008;109:101–9.
[83] Kreitzer FR, Stella N. The therapeutic potential of novel cannabinoid receptors. Pharmacol Ther 2009;122:83–96.
[84] Ledent C, Valverde O, Cossu G, Petitet F, Aubert JF, Beslot F, Böhme GA, Imperato A, Pedrazzini T, Roques BP, et al. Unresponsiveness to cannabinoids and reduced addictive effects of opiates in CB1 receptor knockout mice. Science 1999;283:401–4.
[85] Leung D, Saghatelian A, Simon GM, Cravatt BF. Inactivation of N-acylphosphatidylethanolamine phospholipase D reveals multiple mechanisms for the biosynthesis of endocannabinoids. Biochemistry 2006;45:4720–6.
[86] Lever IJ, Rice AS. Cannabinoids and pain. Handb Exp Pharmacol 2007;177:265–306.
[87] Lichtman AH, Martin BR. Spinal and supraspinal components of cannabinoid-induced antinociception. J Pharmacol Exp Ther 1991;258:517–23.

[88] Liu J, Wang L, Harvey-White J, Huang BX, Kim HY, Luquet S, Palmiter RD, Krystal G, Rai R, Mahadevan A, et al. Multiple pathways involved in the biosynthesis of anandamide. Neuropharmacology 2008;54:1–7.
[89] Martin WJ, Coffin PO, Attias E, Balinsky M, Tsou K, Walker JM. Anatomical basis for cannabinoid-induced antinociception as revealed by intracerebral microinjections. Brain Res 1999;822:237–42.
[90] Martin WJ, Hohmann AG, Walker JM. Suppression of noxious stimulus-evoked activity in the ventral posterolateral nucleus of the thalamus by a cannabinoid agonist: correlation between electrophysiological and antinociceptive effects. J Neurosci 1996;16:6601–11.
[91] Martin WJ, Patrick SL, Coffin PO, Tsou K, Walker JM. An examination of the central sites of action of cannabinoid-induced antinociception in the rat. Life Sci 1995;56: 2103–9.
[92] Matsuda LA, Lolait SJ, Brownstein MJ, Young AC, Bonner TI. Structure of a cannabinoid receptor and functional expression of the cloned cDNA. Nature 1990;346:561–4.
[93] Mechoulam R, Ben-Shabat S, Hanus L, Ligumsky M, Kaminski NE, Schatz AR, Gopher A, Almog S, Martin BR, Compton DR, et al. Identification of an endogenous 2-monoglyceride, present in canine gut, that binds to cannabinoid receptors. Biochem Pharmacol 1995;50:83–90.
[94] Meng ID, Manning BH, Martin WJ, Fields HL. An analgesia circuit activated by cannabinoids. Nature 1998;395:381–3.
[95] Mitrirattanakul S, Ramakul N, Guerrero AV, Matsuka Y, Ono T, Iwase H, Mackie K, Faull KF, Spigelman I. Site-specific increases in peripheral cannabinoid receptors and their endogenous ligands in a model of neuropathic pain. Pain 2006;126:102–14.
[96] Moulin DE, Clark AJ, Gilron I, Ware MA, Watson CP, Sessle BJ, Coderre T, Morley-Forster PK, Stinson J, Boulanger A, et al.; Canadian Pain Society. Pharmacological management of chronic neuropathic pain: consensus statement and guidelines from the Canadian Pain Society. Pain Res Manag 2007;12:13–21.
[97] Munro S, Thomas KL, Abu-Shaar M. Molecular characterization of a peripheral receptor for cannabinoids. Nature 1993;365:61–5.
[98] Nackley AG, Makriyannis A, Hohmann AG. Selective activation of cannabinoid CB_2 receptors suppresses spinal fos protein expression and pain behavior in a rat model of inflammation. Neuroscience 2003;119:747–57.
[99] Nackley AG, Zvonok AM, Makriyannis A, Hohmann AG. Activation of cannabinoid CB2 receptors suppresses C-fiber responses and windup in spinal wide dynamic range neurons in the absence and presence of inflammation. J Neurophysiol 2004;92:3562–74.
[100] Naef M, Curatolo M, Petersen-Felix S, Arendt-Nielsen L, Zbinden A, Brenneisen R. The analgesic effect of oral delta-9-tetrahydrocannabinol (THC), morphine, and a THC-morphine combination in healthy subjects under experimental pain conditions. Pain 2003;105:79–88.
[101] Noyes R, Brunk SF, Avery DA, Canter AC. The analgesic properties of delta-9-tetrahydrocannabinol and codeine. Clin Pharmacol Ther 1975;18:84–9.
[102] Noyes R, Brunk SF, Baram DA, Canter A. Analgesic effect of delta-9-tetrahydrocannabinol. J Clin Pharmacol 1975;15:139–43.
[103] Nyilas R, Gregg LC, Mackie K, Watanabe M, Zimmer A, Hohmann AG, Katona I. Molecular architecture of endocannabinoid signalling at nociceptive synapses mediating analgesia. Eur J Neurosci 2009;29:1964–78.
[104] Onaivi ES, Chakrabarti A, Chaudhuri G. Cannabinoid receptors genes. Prog Neurobiol 1996;48:275–305.
[105] Pacher P, Batkai S, Kunos G. The endocannabinoid system as an emerging target of pharmacotherapy. Pharmacol Rev 2006;58:389–462.
[106] Palazzo E, de Novellis V, Petrosino S, Marabese I, Vita D, Giordano C, Di Marzo V, Mangoni GS, Rossi F, Maione S. Neuropathic pain and the endocannabinoid system in the dorsal raphe: pharmacological treatment and interactions with the serotonergic system. Eur J Neurosci 2006;24:2011–20.
[107] Palmer SL, Thakur GA, Makriyannis A. Cannabinergic ligands. Chem Phys Lipids 2002;121:3–19.
[108] Pertwee RG. Cannabinoid pharmacology: the first 66 years. Br J Pharmacol 2006;147:S163–71.
[109] Pertwee RG. Emerging strategies for exploiting cannabinoid receptor agonists as medicines. Br J Pharmacol 2009;156:397–411.
[110] Pertwee RG. Pharmacology of cannabinoid CB1 and CB2 receptors. Pharmacol Ther 1997;74:129–80.
[111] Pertwee RG, Ross RA. Cannabinoid receptors and their ligands. Prostaglandins Leukot Essent Fatty Acids 2002;66:101–21.
[112] Petrosino S, Palazzo E, de Novellis V, Bisogno T, Rossi F, Maione S, Di Marzo V. Changes in spinal and supraspinal endocannabinoid levels in neuropathic rats. Neuropharmacology 2007;52:415–22.
[113] Piomelli D. The endocannabinoid system: a drug discovery perspective. Curr Opin Invest Drugs 2005;6:672–9.
[114] Piomelli D. The molecular logic of endocannabinoid signalling. Nat Rev Neurosci 2003;4:873–84.
[115] Raft D, Gregg J, Ghia J, Harris L. Effects of intravenous tetrahydrocannabinol on experimental and surgical pain. Psychological correlates of the analgesic response. Clin Pharmacol Ther 1977;21:26–33.
[116] Redmond WJ, Goffaux P, Potvin S, Marchand S. Analgesic and antihyperalgesic effects of nabilone on experimental pain. Curr Med Res Opin 2008;24:1017–24.
[117] Rice AS, Farquhar-Smith WP, Nagy I. Endocannabinoids and pain: spinal and peripheral analgesia in inflammation and neuropathy. Prostaglandins Leukot Essent Fatty Acids 2002;66:243–56.
[118] Richardson JD, Aanonsen L, Hargreaves KM. Hypoactivity of the spinal cannabinoid system results in NMDA-dependent hyperalgesia. J Neurosci 1998;18:451–7.
[119] Richardson JD, Aanonsen L, Hargreaves KM. SR 141716A, a cannabinoid receptor antagonist, produces hyperalgesia in untreated mice. Eur J Pharmacol 1997;319:R3–4.
[120] Richardson JD, Kilo S, Hargreaves KM. Cannabinoids reduce hyperalgesia and inflammation via interaction with peripheral CB1 receptors. Pain 1998;75:111–9.

[121] Ross RA, Coutts AA, McFarlane SM, Anavi-Goffer S, Irving AJ, Pertwee RG, MacEwan DJ, Scott RH. Actions of cannabinoid receptor ligands on rat cultured sensory neurones: implications for antinociception. Neuropharmacology 2001;40:221–32.
[122] Rukwied R, Watkinson A, McGlone F, Dvorak M. Cannabinoid agonists attenuate capsaicin-induced responses in human skin. Pain 2003;102:283–8.
[123] Ryberg E, Larsson N, Sjögren S, Hjorth S, Hermansson NO, Leonova J, Elebring T, Nilsson K, Drmota T, Greasley PJ. The orphan receptor GPR55 is a novel cannabinoid receptor. Br J Pharmacol 2007;152:1092–101.
[124] Sagar DR, Kelly S, Millns PJ, O'Shaughnessey CT, Kendall DA, Chapman V. Inhibitory effects of CB1 and CB2 receptor agonists on responses of DRG neurons and dorsal horn neurons in neuropathic rats. Eur J Neurosci 2005;22:371–9.
[125] Salio C, Doly S, Fischer J, Franzoni MF, Conrath M. Neuronal and astrocytic localization of the cannabinoid receptor-1 in the dorsal horn of the rat spinal cord. Neurosci Lett 2002;329:13–6.
[126] Seierstad M, Breitenbucher JG. Discovery and development of fatty acid amide hydrolase (FAAH) inhibitors. J Med Chem 2008;51:7327–43.
[127] Shire D, Calandra B, Rinaldi-Carmona M, Oustric D, Pessègue B, Bonnin-Cabanne O, Le Fur G, Caput D, Ferrara P. Molecular cloning, expression and function of murine CB2 peripheral cannabinoid receptor. Biochim Biophys Acta 1996;1307:132–6.
[128] Smith PB, Martin BR. Spinal mechanisms of delta 9-tetrahydrocannabinol-induced analgesia. Brain Res 1992;578:8–12.
[129] Ständer S, Schmelz M, Metze D, Luger T, Rukwied R. Distribution of cannabinoid receptor 1 (CB1) and 2 (CB2) on sensory nerve fibers and adnexal structures in human skin. J Dermatol Sci 2005;38:177–88.
[130] Staquet M, Gantt C, Machin D. Effect of a nitrogen analog of tetrahydrocannabinol on cancer pain. Clin Pharmacol Ther 1978;23:397–401.
[131] Staton PC, Hatcher JP, Walker DJ, Morrison AD, Shapland EM, Hughes JP, Chong E, Mander PK, Green PJ, Billinton A, et al. The putative cannabinoid receptor GPR55 plays a role in mechanical hyperalgesia associated with inflammatory and neuropathic pain. Pain 2008;139:225–36.
[132] Stella N, Schweitzer P, Piomelli D. A second endogenous cannabinoid that modulates long-term potentiation. Nature 1997;388:773–8.
[133] Strangman NM, Patrick SL, Hohmann AG, Tsou K, Walker JM. Evidence for a role of endogenous cannabinoids in the modulation of acute and tonic pain sensitivity. Brain Res 1998;813:323–8.
[134] Sugiura T, Kondo S, Sukagawa A, Nakane S, Shinoda A, Itoh K, Yamashita A, Waku K. 2-Arachidonoylglycerol: a possible endogenous cannabinoid receptor ligand in brain. Biochem Biophys Res Commun 1995;215:89–97.
[135] Suplita RL 2nd, Eisenstein SA, Neely MH, Moise AM, Hohmann AG. Cross-sensitization and cross-tolerance between exogenous cannabinoid antinociception and endocannabinoid-mediated stress-induced analgesia. Neuropharmacology 2008;54:161–71.
[136] Suplita RL 2nd, Farthing JN, Gutierrez T, Hohmann AG. Inhibition of fatty-acid amide hydrolase enhances cannabinoid stress-induced analgesia: sites of action in the dorsolateral periaqueductal gray and rostral ventromedial medulla. Neuropharmacology 2005;49:1201–9.
[137] Suplita RL 2nd, Gutierrez T, Fegley D, Piomelli D, Hohmann AG. Endocannabinoids at the spinal level regulate, but do not mediate, nonopioid stress-induced analgesia. Neuropharmacology 2006;50:372–9.
[138] Van Sickle MD, Duncan M, Kingsley PJ, Mouihate A, Urbani P, Mackie K, Stella N, Makriyannis A, Piomelli D, Davison JS, et al. Identification and functional characterization of brainstem cannabinoid CB2 receptors. Science 2005;310:329–32.
[139] Wade DT, Makela PM, House H, Bateman C, Robson P. Long-term use of a cannabis-based medicine in the treatment of spasticity and other symptoms in multiple sclerosis. Mult Scler 2006;12:639–45.
[140] Walczak JS, Pichette V, Leblond F, Desbiens K, Beaulieu P. Behavioral, pharmacological and molecular characterization of the saphenous nerve partial ligation: a new model of neuropathic pain. Neuroscience 2005;132:1093–102.
[141] Walker JM, Hohmann AG. Cannabinoid mechanisms of pain suppression. Handb Exp Pharmacol 2005;168:509–54.
[142] Walker JM, Huang SM, Strangman NM, Tsou K, Sañudo-Peña MC. Pain modulation by release of the endogenous cannabinoid anandamide. Proc Natl Acad Sci USA 1999;96:12198–203.
[143] Wallace M, Schulteis G, Atkinson JH, Wolfson T, Lazzaretto D, Bentley H, Gouaux B, Abramson I. Dose-dependent effects of smoked cannabis on capsaicin-induced pain and hyperalgesia in healthy volunteers. Anesthesiology 2007;107:785–96.
[144] Wang T, Collet J-P, Shapiro S, Ware MA. Adverse effects of medical cannabinoids: a systematic review. CMAJ 2008;178:1669–78.
[145] Wang J, Ueda N. Biology of endocannabinoid synthesis system. Prostaglandins Other Lipid Mediat 2008;Epub Dec 14.
[146] Ware MA. Marijuana as medicine: does it have a future? Clin Pharmacol Ther 2008;83:515–7.
[147] Ware M, Beaulieu P. Cannabinoids for the treatment of pain: an update on recent clinical trials. Pain Res Manage 2005;10:27A–30.
[148] Ware MA, Tawfik VL. Safety issues concerning the medical use of cannabis and cannabinoids. Pain Res Manag 2005;10:31–7A.
[149] Wilson RI, Nicoll RA. Endocannabinoid signaling in the brain. Science 2002;296:678–82.
[150] Zajicek J, Fox P, Sanders H, Wright D, Vickery J, Nunn A, Thompson A; UK MS Research Group. Cannabinoids for treatment of spasticity and other symptoms related to multiple sclerosis (CAMS study): multicentre randomised placebo-controlled trial. Lancet 2003;362:1517–26.

Correspondence to: Andrea G. Hohmann, PhD, Neuroscience and Behavior Program, Psychology Department, University of Georgia, Athens, GA 30602-3013, USA. Email: ahohmann@uga.edu.

7

Sodium Channels in Pain Pharmacology

Theodore R. Cummins[a] and Stephen G. Waxman[b,c]

[a]Department of Pharmacology & Toxicology, Stark Neurosciences Research Institute, Indiana University School of Medicine, Indianapolis, Indiana, USA; [b]Department of Neurology and Center for Neuroscience and Regeneration Research, Yale University School of Medicine, New Haven, Connecticut, USA; [c]Rehabilitation Research Center, VA Connecticut Healthcare System, West Haven, Connecticut, USA

Dorsal root ganglion (DRG) and trigeminal neurons are the first elements in the chain of neurons making up the somatosensory system, which includes the nociceptive pathways. These neurons encode and transmit information from the periphery to the spinal cord in the form of action potentials, transient all-or-none alterations in the electrical potential (action potentials) across the plasma membrane of neurons that result from highly regulated changes in specific ionic conductances. The rapid depolarizing upstroke of the action potential is produced by voltage-gated sodium channels; in addition, some sodium channels (termed "threshold channels" by some investigators) work in the voltage range below the action potential threshold, amplifying small depolarizations and thereby increasing cell excitability. Under normal circumstances, DRG and trigeminal neurons involved in nociception are relatively quiescent unless they are stimulated; however, following peripheral inflammation and some nerve injuries, primary sensory neurons can become hyperexcitable, leading to unprovoked spontaneous action potential activity or pathological bursting, which can contribute to chronic pain [85,108]. Evidence indicates that multiple classes of peripheral sensory neurons, both nociceptors and sensory neurons that are not normally involved in nociception, can contribute to neuropathic pain in various situations. Alterations in the properties of voltage-gated sodium channels have been implicated as important contributors to both inflammatory and neuropathic pain. Although voltage-gated sodium channels have long been considered important targets of pain therapeutics, recent

Pharmacology of Pain
edited by Pierre Beaulieu, David Lussier, Frank Porreca, and Anthony H. Dickenson
IASP Press, Seattle, © 2010

advances indicate that the targeting of specific voltage-gated sodium channel isoforms that are preferentially expressed in peripheral sensory neurons may provide a powerful new approach to the more effective treatment of pain. In this chapter we review the understanding of sodium channel expression in peripheral sensory neurons, the roles that different voltage-gated sodium channel isoforms play in normal and abnormal pain sensations, and the pharmacology of voltage-gated sodium channels.

Multiple Sodium Channels in Dorsal Root Ganglion Neurons

Voltage-gated sodium channels are transmembrane proteins that form a conductance pathway across the cytoplasmic membranes of cells that is selective for sodium ions and is controlled or gated by changes in the transmembrane voltage. The first two sodium channel isoforms identified in mammals ($Na_V1.1$ and $Na_V1.2$) were cloned from rat brain [84] and are comprised of ~2000 amino acids. Noda and colleagues proposed that these channels contain 24 transmembrane segments (Fig. 1A), arranged in four homologous internal repeats (often referred to as domains I–IV). They further proposed that the fourth (S4) segments of the different domains, which contain 4–8 evenly spaced positively charged amino acid residues, are important components of the sodium channel voltage sensors. Over the next 20 years, numerous studies investigated the molecular determinants of ion channel gating. Many studies have confirmed that the acidic charges in the S4 segments are indeed important determinants of voltage-dependent gating [97]. Based on homology with voltage-dependent potassium channels and the crystal structure of the $K_V1.2$ potassium channel [75], it is likely that the voltage sensor units of sodium channels are formed by a complex of segments 1–4 of each domain. While the S4 segments of domains I, II, and III are especially important in activation, the S4 segment of domain IV is crucial for inactivation [27,28]. The core of sodium channels is believed to be formed by the S5 and S6 segments, with the loops between the S5 and S6 segments lining the outer portion of the pore and the second half of the S6 segments lining the inner, or cytoplasmic, portion of the pore. It has been proposed, mainly based on the structural studies of voltage-gated potassium channels, that the S4–S5 linkers of each domain couple the voltage sensor units to the S6 segments, providing mechanical force that works to open or close the inner portion of the pore, controlling channel activation. Other studies have determined that specific residues in the cytoplasmic linker between domains III and IV are critical determinants of sodium channel inactivation. These residues, often referred to as the inactivation particle or the IFM (isoleucine, phenylalanine, methionine) motif, may act as a "hinged lid" that binds to the inner aspect of the pore and blocks ionic conductance following depolarization. A total of nine distinct sodium channel genes have been cloned from mammals [60]. Although homology between the different isoforms ($Na_V1.1$– $Na_V1.9$) ranges from ~87% to ~45% (Fig. 1B), all nine of the known mammalian sodium channel genes have the same basic overall structure described above.

In many excitable cells, sodium currents appear rather homogeneous, with rapid activation and inactivation kinetics that can often be described by simple exponential functions. This observation was consistent with the proposal that sodium channels had but one primary function—to give rise to the rapid upstroke of the regenerative action potential [66]. Indeed, in the first edition of his authoritative book on ion channels, Bertil Hille wrote that with sodium channels "one is impressed more with the similarity of function than with the differences" because "their activation and inactivation time constants would not differ by more than twofold" and "the pharmacology of all [sodium] channels shows similarities." Sodium channels in central nervous system (CNS) neurons, in skeletal muscle, and even in squid giant axons generate currents with similar kinetics that are all sensitive to nanomolar concentrations of the puffer fish toxin tetrodotoxin (TTX). However, it was demonstrated in the late 1970s that dorsal root ganglion (DRG) neurons could express TTX-resistant as well as TTX-sensitive sodium currents [77]. Kostyuk et al. subsequently showed that the TTX-resistant sodium currents in DRG neurons exhibited kinetics of activation and inactivation that were about 10 times slower than those of the

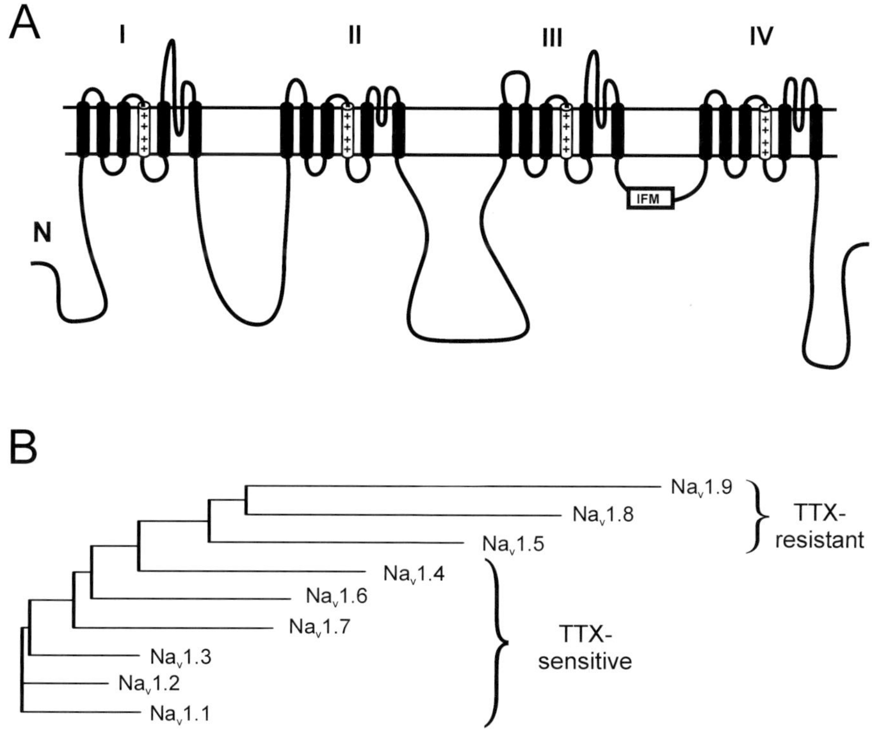

Fig. 1. (A) Schematic diagram of the secondary structure of voltage-gated sodium channels. The fourth transmembrane segments (shown in white) of each of the four homologous domains contain several positively charged residues that contribute to voltage sensitivity. The isoleucine, phenylalanine, and methionine (IFM) motif between domains II and IV is crucial to fast inactivation of the channels. (B) Phylogenetic tree of the voltage-gated sodium channels. The tree was constructed by comparing the amino acid sequences of the nine human voltage-gated sodium channel isoforms. Na$_V$1.1 and Na$_V$1.2 show the highest homology (87% identical). The three tetrodotoxin (TTX)-resistant channels show less homology than the TTX-sensitive channels. Na$_V$1.9 has the lowest homology, with only ~45% identity to the other voltage-gated sodium channels.

TTX-sensitive currents in DRG neurons [72]. These data clearly suggested that sodium channels might be more diverse in DRG neurons than in other tissues. We now know that DRG sensory neurons can express a complex array of sodium currents, with multiple TTX-resistant and TTX-sensitive components generated by distinct channels encoded by up to seven different sodium channel genes.

Contribution of Sodium Channels to Pain Mechanisms

Over the last two decades a good deal has been learned about the expression patterns of the different mammalian sodium channel isoforms. Study of the mRNAs encoding the various channels, by reverse transcription polymerase chain reaction (RT-PCR) or in situ hybridization, provides precise information about which sodium channel genes are transcriptionally active in different tissues [15]. Isoform-specific antibodies can help determine which channels are expressed at the protein level in different tissues, cell populations, and regions of individual cells. There is solid evidence that DRG neurons can express $Na_V1.1$, $Na_V1.3$, $Na_V1.5$, $Na_V1.6$, $Na_V1.7$, $Na_V1.8$, and $Na_V1.9$. The only two isoforms that are not found to be expressed to any significant extent in the DRG are $Na_V1.4$ (which is predominantly expressed in skeletal muscle) and $Na_V1.2$ (which is predominantly expressed in neurons of the CNS). Although $Na_V1.5$ message and current can be identified in embryonic and neonatal DRG [90], $Na_V1.5$ is not likely to be an important contributor to sensory neuron excitability. The currents generated by $Na_V1.5$ are very small compared to those produced by other isoforms, and in adult DRG neurons $Na_V1.5$ message and current are difficult to detect. Furthermore, $Na_V1.5$, which exhibits an intermediate sensitivity to TTX, is the predominant sodium channel in cardiac muscle, and therefore it is generally not considered to be a valid target for analgesics.

In the uninjured nervous system, levels of $Na_V1.3$ message and current are also higher in embryonic and neonatal DRG neurons than in adult neurons. Interestingly, as discussed below, $Na_V1.3$ mRNA and protein levels significantly increase in adult DRG neurons following nerve injury and also with chronic inflammation, suggesting that this channel isoform might be important in pain [16,105]. $Na_V1.1$ and $Na_V1.6$ are highly expressed in peripheral sensory neurons. These isoforms are expressed at the highest levels in large-diameter fibers and their cells of origin (which tend not to be nociceptive), although $Na_V1.6$ protein immunoreactivity has been observed in small-diameter unmyelinated fibers and their cells of origin (which tend to be nociceptive) [15,18]. As $Na_V1.1$.and $Na_V1.6$ are also expressed at high levels in CNS neurons, it is not clear if they are the best targets for analgesics.

The remaining three isoforms ($Na_V1.7$, $Na_V1.8$, and $Na_V1.9$) are predominantly expressed in the peripheral nervous system (PNS). $Na_V1.7$ is found in both sensory neurons and sympathetic neurons [102]. $Na_V1.8$ may be exclusively expressed in sensory neurons [4], although some disease states, such as multiple sclerosis, can induce aberrant expression of $Na_V1.8$ in CNS neurons [14]. $Na_V1.9$ is expressed in sensory neurons and in the enteric nervous system [38]. In the DRG, $Na_V1.7$, $Na_V1.8$, and $Na_V1.9$ are preferentially expressed in small-diameter neurons that exhibit nociceptive properties [43,44,53]. Because of their preferential expression in sensory neurons, $Na_V1.7$, $Na_V1.8$, and $Na_V1.9$ could be important targets for analgesics.

The functional properties of the various voltage-gated sodium channels that are expressed in sensory neurons are quite diverse and have been studied in DRG and trigeminal neurons as well as in heterologous expression systems (Table I). The TTX-sensitive currents in sensory neurons have similar voltage dependence of activation and inactivation to the TTX-sensitive currents in CNS neurons. However, the TTX-sensitive currents in small-diameter DRG neurons are known to exhibit relatively slow kinetics for recovery from inactivation (often referred to as repriming) compared to the kinetics of the TTX-resistant current in DRG neurons and TTX-sensitive currents in cortical neurons [48]. Subsequent studies found that although the TTX-sensitive currents in small-diameter neurons recovered from inactivation slowly, those in large-diameter sensory neurons recovered from inactivation about seven times faster [64]. It is highly likely that differential expression of TTX-sensitive sodium channel isoforms is a major contributor to the difference in recovery from inactivation kinetics. $Na_V1.7$ channels exhibit very slow recovery from inactivation kinetics, similar to the TTX-sensitive currents in small-diameter neurons, whereas $Na_V1.6$ channels exhibit very rapid recovery from inactivation kinetics, similar to the TTX-sensitive currents in large-diameter neurons [36,64].

Interestingly, ~40% of medium- and large-diameter neurons can also generate specialized TTX-sensitive sodium currents called resurgent currents [35]. Resurgent currents

Table I
Properties of voltage-gated sodium channels

Isoform	Primary Tissue(s)	TTX Sensitivity	Kinetics	Unique Properties in DRG Neurons
$Na_V1.1$	CNS and PNS	Sensitive	Fast	
$Na_V1.2$	CNS	Sensitive	Fast	
$Na_V1.3$	Immature CNS and PNS	Sensitive	Fast	Rapid repriming and large-ramp currents
$Na_V1.4$	Skeletal muscle	Sensitive	Fast	
$Na_V1.5$	Cardiac muscle	Resistant	Fast	Hyperpolarized voltage dependence
$Na_V1.6$	CNS and PNS	Sensitive	Fast	Rapid repriming and resurgent currents
$Na_V1.7$	PNS	Sensitive	Fast	Slow closed-state inactivation, large-ramp currents
$Na_V1.8$	PNS	Very resistant	Slow	Depolarized voltage dependence
$Na_V1.9$	PNS	Very resistant	Ultra-slow	Persistent currents at hyperpolarized voltages

Abbreviations: CNS = central nervous system; PNS = peripheral nervous system; TTX = tetrodotoxin; DRG = dorsal root ganglion.

are unusual inward currents that arise during moderate hyperpolarizations following depolarizations that seem to produce complete sodium channel inactivation; they were first identified in cerebellar Purkinje neurons and can contribute to spontaneous and burst firing [69]. Cummins et al. demonstrated that Na_V1.6 is necessary and sufficient to produce resurgent currents in DRG neurons [35]. It is not known whether resurgent sodium currents contribute to pain sensations.

Na_V1.8 and Na_V1.9 generate sodium currents that are ~5,000-fold less sensitive to TTX than TTX-sensitive channels in DRG neurons [4,34,74,98]. Na_V1.8 underlies the classic TTX-resistant sodium current in DRG neurons characterized by Kostyuk et al. [72]. The voltage-dependencies of activation and inactivation of Na_V1.8 currents are much more depolarized than those of TTX-sensitive currents [4]. While the time constants for inactivation of Na_V1.8 currents are about 10-fold slower than those of TTX-sensitive channels, the kinetics for recovery from inactivation are faster than those of Na_V1.6. There is convincing evidence that TTX-resistant sodium channels (most likely Na_V1.8) can participate in the conduction of action potentials within nociceptive sensory neurons and their axons [21] and that Na_V1.8 is an important contributor to the inward membrane current that flows during the rising phase of the action potential in many small-diameter sensory neurons [89]. By contrast, it is unlikely that Na_V1.9 contributes to the upstroke of the action potential (Fig. 2). Na_V1.9 produces sodium currents that activate at potentials that are more negative than those that activate either Na_V1.8 currents or TTX-sensitive currents in DRG neurons [34,38]. At voltages near neuronal resting membrane potentials (~65 mV), Na_V1.9 generates currents that persist for several seconds. At –40 mV, the time constant for inactivation of Na_V1.9 currents is ~ 4-fold slower than that of Na_V1.8 currents and ~ 24-fold slower than that of Na_V1.7 currents [34]. These observations and computer simulation of DRG neuron excitability indicate that the persistent currents generated by Na_V1.9 probably modulate resting membrane potential and amplify subthreshold depolarizing stimuli [34,38,65]. TTX-sensitive persistent sodium currents have also been observed in both small-diameter [71] and large-diameter [8] DRG neurons, although the precise isoforms that contribute to these TTX-sensitive persistent sodium currents have not been determined.

Experimental models of pain, including chronic inflammation and nerve injury models, have provided important insight into how sensory neuron voltage-gated sodium channels might contribute to pain. While under normal conditions sensory neurons are typically quiescent [42], peripheral sensory neurons can become hyperexcitable after nerve injury [108] or in response to inflammation [42]. This hyperexcitability is likely to contribute to enhanced pain sensations, and given that voltage-gated sodium channels are a crucial component of neuronal excitability, there is good reason to believe that changes in voltage-gated sodium channel expression and function could be important contributors to the neuronal hyperexcitability associated with inflammatory and neuropathic pain. Chronic peripheral inflammation upregulates mRNA and protein levels for Na_V1.3, Na_V1.7, and Na_V1.8 in DRG neurons and increases current amplitudes for both TTX-resistant and TTX-sensitive sodium currents in DRG neurons [16,101], in part because of the effects of inflammatory mediators such as nerve growth factor (NGF) [55]. NGF and other inflammatory mediators can also have acute effects on sodium currents in DRG neurons. Prostaglandin E_2 (PGE_2) and ATP can increase the TTX-resistant persistent current in DRG neurons [7,93]. PGE_2 and serotonin also produce an increase in $Na_V1.8$ current amplitude and, in addition, a hyperpolarizing shift in activation [23,57]. All of these changes are likely to increase sensory neuron excitability. Indeed, decreasing $Na_V1.8$ mRNA levels using antisense oligodeoxynucleotides is effective at reducing pain behaviors associated with peripheral inflammation in rats [70]. Moreover, knockdown of $Na_V1.7$ in the DRG of adult mice, via hindpaw application of viruses containing short hairpin RNA (shRNA) that reduce expression of $Na_V1.7$ through RNA interference, reduces inflammatory pain-related behaviors [107].

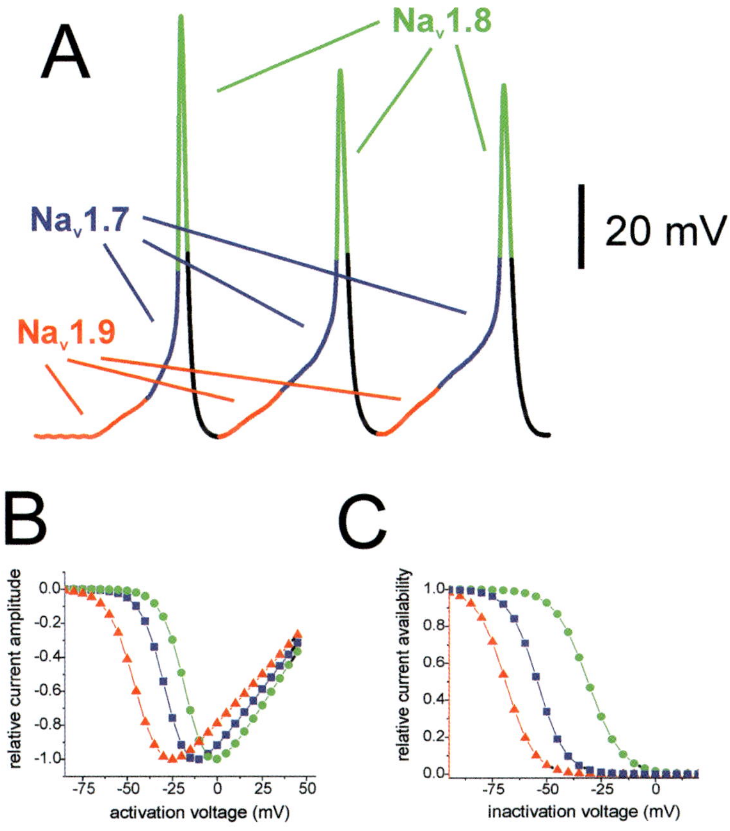

Fig. 2. Voltage-gated sodium channels differ in their contribution to action potential generation and in their voltage-dependent properties. (A) $Na_V1.8$ channels are largely responsible for the overshooting action potential. $Na_V1.7$ channels are a crucial determinant of subthreshold activity and of the initial upstroke of the action potential. $Na_V1.9$ channels are likely to contribute to subthreshold activity and to modulate the resting membrane potential, especially under sensitizing conditions such as those associated with peripheral inflammation. (B) While $Na_V1.9$ currents (red triangles) exhibit a hyperpolarized voltage dependence of activation compared to $Na_V1.7$ currents (blue squares), $Na_V1.8$ currents (green circles) have a comparatively depolarized voltage dependence of activation. (C) Similarly, the voltage dependence of steady-state inactivation is more negative for $Na_V1.9$ channels (red triangles) than for $Na_V1.7$ channels (blue squares), while that of $Na_V1.8$ channels (green circles) is much more depolarized.

Transection of the sciatic nerve can also induce dramatic changes in the sodium channels and currents of DRG neurons. Early studies [105] demonstrated a significant upregulation of expression of the previously silent $Na_V1.3$ sodium channel gene in DRG neurons following axonal transection within the sciatic nerve. Interestingly, abnormal accumulations of $Na_V1.3$ protein can be detected close to the tips of injured axons within the experimental neuromas [13], a site where aberrant hyperexcitability has been demonstrated. In human painful neuromas, accumulations of $Na_V1.3$, $Na_V1.7$, $Na_V1.8$, and mitogen-activated protein kinases, which can upregulate the currents generated by these channels, have all been found at the blindly ending axon tips near the site of injury [17]. The properties of the TTX-sensitive sodium currents are also altered in DRG neurons following axotomy, with the emergence of a current that reprimes about four times more rapidly than the TTX-sensitive current in uninjured neurons [37]. It has been proposed that the expression of $Na_V1.3$ underlies the emergence of the rapidly repriming sodium current [37], and this suggestion is supported by a study showing that $Na_V1.3$ displays rapid repriming when expressed in a mammalian expression system (HEK 293 cells) [33]. Conversely, transection of the sciatic nerve induces a pronounced downregulation of $Na_V1.8$ and $Na_V1.9$ gene expression in DRG neurons, which can persist for months following axotomy [39]. Patch-clamp studies have identified a significant attenuation of TTX-resistant sodium currents, including persistent currents, in DRG neurons following axonal transection within the sciatic nerve, consistent with the long-lasting changes in sodium channel gene expression that have been described in these cells [37]. Based on these observations, one might predict that $Na_V1.8$ and $Na_V1.9$ might be unlikely to contribute to neuropathic pain associated with peripheral nerve injury. However, specific knockdown of $Na_V1.8$ in rats by specific antisense oligodeoxynucleotides or small interfering RNAs is reported to be antiallodynic and antihyperalgesic in response to nerve injuries used to mimic neuropathic pain conditions [45,73]. This knockdown, which is rapidly reversible, indicates that $Na_V1.8$ can play an important role in the onset of neuropathic pain. An intriguing explanation for this paradox, proposed by Gold et al. [58], is that alterations in the activity, or redistribution, of $Na_V1.8$ channels in the remaining ***uninjured*** neurons are important determinants of the hyperexcitability and hyperalgesia associated with injuries that cause neuropathic pain.

Lessons from Transgenic Models

Transgenic knockout animals have been used to investigate the roles of different voltage-gated sodium channel isoforms in pain. $Na_V1.8$-null transgenic mice have deficits in acute mechanical sensation, noxious cold sensation, NGF-induced hyperalgesia, inflammatory pain [5], and visceral pain [1]. $Na_V1.9$-null transgenic mice show reduced hypersensitivity to inflammatory hyperalgesia induced by formalin, carrageenan, complete Freund's adjuvant (CFA), and PGE_2 [87] and a reduced sensitivity to specific inflammatory mediators such as bradykinin, serotonin, and ATP, while responding normally to NGF [6].

$Na_V1.7$-null mice die soon after birth if $Na_V1.7$ is knocked out globally. However, if $Na_V1.7$ is selectively knocked out in neurons that transcribe $Na_V1.8$ (using mice that express Cre recombinase from the $Na_V1.8$ locus), major deficits are observed in inflammatory pain behaviors [82]. These data suggest that $Na_V1.7$, $Na_V1.8$, and $Na_V1.9$ are all valid targets for new drugs to treat inflammatory pain. Interestingly, $Na_V1.3$-null mice did not show obvious deficits in either inflammatory pain or in neuropathic pain behaviors, a result that was interpreted as suggesting that $Na_V1.3$ is neither necessary nor sufficient to produce inflammatory or neuropathic pain [80]. In addition, $Na_V1.3$-null, $Na_V1.7$-null (nociceptor-selective), $Na_V1.8$-null, and $Na_V1.9$-null mice all fail to exhibit deficits in neuropathic pain behaviors [1,6,80,82]. Mice that lack *both* $Na_V1.7$ and $Na_V1.8$ expression in their DRG neurons also appear to normally develop neuropathic pain behaviors (Fig. 3) [81]. These data are somewhat perplexing given that $Na_V1.8$ antisense oligodeoxynucleotides or small interfering RNAs appear effective against neuropathic pain [45,73], but they may indicate that $Na_V1.1$ and/or $Na_V1.6$ are potentially important in neuronal activity that underlies neuropathic pain.

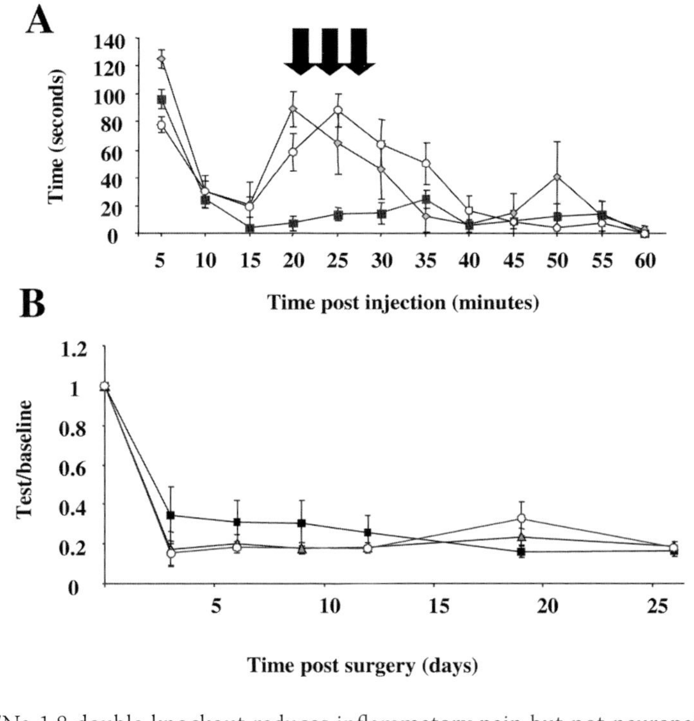

Fig. 3. The $Na_V1.7/Na_V1.8$ double knockout reduces inflammatory pain but not neuropathic pain behaviors. (A) Following formalin injection, the second phase (arrows) of the inflammatory pain response in greatly reduced in the $Na_V1.7/Na_V1.8$ double knockout mice (black squares) compared to wild-type (WT) mice (open circles) and $Na_V1.8$ knockout mice (gray diamonds). (B) Ligation of spinal nerve L5 causes pronounced neuropathic pain behavior (mechanical allodynia) in WT mice (open circles), $Na_V1.7$ knockout mice (gray triangles), and $Na_V1.7/Na_V1.8$ double knockout mice (black squares). Modified with permission from Biomed Central [81].

Human Hereditary Pain Syndromes

Studies of humans with inherited pain syndromes provide compelling evidence that changes in $Na_V1.7$ channel and current properties are sufficient to cause neuropathic pain. As a result of its voltage dependence and slow inactivation from the closed state, $Na_V1.7$ can produce a depolarization in response to small, subtle depolarizations near resting potential [36], poising it to set the gain on nociceptors [104]. Single point mutations in $Na_V1.7$ have been identified as underlying two distinct autosomal dominant chronic pain syndromes in humans: inherited erythromelalgia (IE) and paroxysmal extreme pain disorder (PEPD) [40]. At least 11 distinct point mutations in *SCN9A*, the gene that encodes $Na_V1.7$, have been identified in patients with IE, who experience severe burning sensations, primarily in their hands and feet. All of the IE mutations cause significant hyperpolarizing shifts in the voltage dependence of activation, and most of them also produce larger currents in response to slow ramp depolarizations. These functional alterations are likely to contribute to enhanced excitability. Indeed, DRG neurons transfected with recombinant $Na_V1.7$-containing IE mutations exhibit lower thresholds for firing action potentials, and they fire at higher-than-normal frequencies [40,92], showing that IE mutations can increase the excitability of sensory neurons. Interestingly, the hyperexcitability produced by the IE mutations appears to be dependent on the coexpression of $Na_V1.8$ channels in the neurons [92]. The majority of the IE mutations are located at or near parts of the channel that are associated with activation gating.

Eight $Na_V1.7$ missense mutations, distinct from the IE mutations, have been identified in families with PEPD [54]. Patients with these mutations typically experience severe burning sensations in rectal, ocular, and submandibular regions. The PEPD mutations are predominantly located in regions of the sodium channel associated with inactivation gating, and the PEPD mutations mainly cause depolarizing shifts in voltage dependence of steady-state inactivation and slow the rate of fast inactivation, leading to enhanced persistent currents [54]. Thus, while IE mutations predominantly enhance activation, PEPD mutations impair inactivation. Interestingly, a mutation that alters both activation and inactivation of $Na_V1.7$ causes a mixed IE/PEPD clinical phenotype (Fig. 4) [52]. These studies demonstrate that alterations in $Na_V1.7$ currents are sufficient to cause severe chronic pain in humans and that alterations of different properties of $Na_V1.7$ determine the clinical manifestations of the pain associated with the mutations. Interestingly, while PEPD patients often respond well to treatment with carbamazepine, IE patients reportedly do not [54].

Recent studies of individuals and families with complete insensitivity to pain or congenital insensitivity to pain (CIP) provide very strong confirmation that $Na_V1.7$ plays a crucial role in human ability to perceive pain [3,30,59]. Distinct homozygous or heterozygous nonsense mutations were identified in each of the individuals with CIP, and these truncating mutations were either shown to, or are predicted to, result in a complete loss of functional $Na_V1.7$ currents. Although some individuals with CIP have deficits in olfaction or exhibit an awkward gait, the study subjects otherwise appeared normal based on neurological examinations [3,30,59]. Autonomic function, evaluated by testing sweating, tear formation, blood pressure regulation, and temperature regulation, is reported to be normal in patients with CIP [59]. This lack of effect on autonomic functions is surprising, as $Na_V1.7$ is expressed in sympathetic neurons as well as in small-diameter sensory neurons. One possibility is that the lack of functional $Na_V1.7$ channels throughout development may have induced compensatory changes in the sympathetic nervous system, and therefore, it cannot necessarily be concluded from these patients that $Na_V1.7$ does not make important contributions to sympathetic neuron excitability in humans. It is also possible that some patients with CIP might develop autonomic abnormalities later in life. It should also be noted that is not yet clear if individuals who lack $Na_V1.7$ have a complete inability to develop neuropathic pain. For example, it remains to be determined if patients with CIP could develop specific neuropathic pain disorders such as painful diabetic neuropathy or traumatic nerve injury. Thus, although $Na_V1.7$ appears to play a crucial role in pain sensations, drugs that specifically target $Na_V1.7$ may not target all types of neuropathic pain and will need to be carefully evaluated for sympathetic effects.

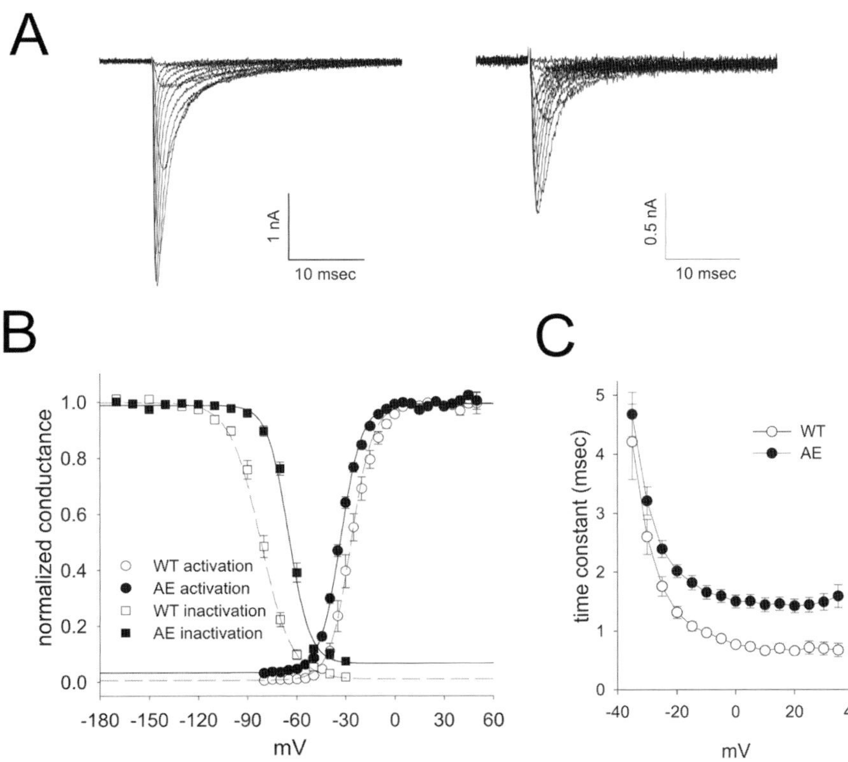

Fig. 4. Inherited mutations in $Na_V1.7$ that cause chronic burning pain syndromes alter functional properties of $Na_V1.7$ sodium currents. (A) Representative currents from wild-type (WT) $Na_V1.7$ and A1623E mutant (AE) $Na_V1.7$ channels. The A1623E mutation causes a mixed erythromelalgia/paroxysmal extreme pain disorder (PEPD) phenotype in patients. (B) The A1623E mutation shifts the voltage dependence of $Na_V1.7$ inactivation in the depolarizing direction, similar to other PEPD mutations, and the voltage dependence of activation in the hyperpolarizing direction, similar to other erythromelalgia mutations. (C) The A1623E mutation also increases the time constants for fast inactivation, which is consistent with other PEPD mutations. Modified with permission from [52].

Pharmacology of Sodium Channels

Voltage-gated sodium channels are clearly promising targets for pain therapeutics. Indeed, the primary mechanism of action for several drugs that are currently used to treat pain, such as lidocaine and carbamazepine, is thought to involve inhibition of voltage-gated sodium channels. However, although these drugs show a degree of clinical efficacy, they tend to have broad-spectrum sodium channel activity and therefore are often associated with adverse effects and narrow therapeutic windows. Although many of the currently available drugs that target sodium channels seem to act by the same general mechanism, sodium channels are sensitive to modulation by a wide variety of pharmacological agents that interact with them in different ways [24,25]. It is possible that some of these alternative mechanisms might be used to help develop better sodium channel modulators. In this section we discuss the pharmacology of voltage-gated sodium channels and highlight areas that show promise for the development of more effective and selective analgesics.

Drugs such as lidocaine and carbamazepine, which are widely used for treating pain and other disorders of excitability, produce both tonic and phasic (or use-dependent) block of sodium currents. The tonic block is generally a lower affinity block that results from interaction of the compound with resting channels that are closed but available for activation. The phasic block involves higher affinity interactions with open or inactivated channels, which can induce shifts in the voltage dependence of steady-state inactivation. This type of state-dependent modulation is typical for most of the local anesthetics, anticonvulsants, and antiarrhythmics that interact with voltage-gated sodium channels. Although these drugs show some clinical efficacy, they do not always show high specificity for sodium channels over other types of ion channels, and in general there are only subtle differences in their effects on the different sodium channel isoforms. The specificity of action of these state-dependent modulators arises from their propensity to target channels that are repetitively activated, such as those in neurons that are firing repetitive action potentials, or that are chronically depolarized, which can occur following injury or inflammation. The analgesic activity of these drugs is generally fully reversible.

Lidocaine is the most widely used of the state-dependent modulators for treating pain. Lidocaine is effective at inhibiting sensory neuronal sodium channels [19], evoked and spontaneous peripheral nerve activity in experimental systems [26], and pain in animal models [99]. Lidocaine and other local anesthetics can be applied topically to provide localized, superficial anesthesia. Local anesthetics that are readily absorbed have the potential to produce systemic toxicity. Benzocaine, which is poorly soluble in water, is used in many non-prescription preparations because it is not generally toxic. A mixture of lidocaine and prilocaine (EMLA: eutectic mixture of local anesthetics) has been developed that has a relatively low melting point, readily penetrates intact skin, and therefore can produce analgesia at a depth of up to 5 mm. Another preparation for topical application of local anesthetics is the lidocaine patch (5% lidocaine), which is considered one of the most effective treatments for postherpetic neuropathic pain [78] and can also be effective at treating painful diabetic neuropathy [9] and painful idiopathic distal polyneuropathy [63]. The lidocaine patch allows for prolonged transdermal delivery of lidocaine and produces a low steady-state plasma concentration of lidocaine that is well tolerated [56]. Systemic lidocaine can also be delivered by intravenous injection, although this approach has had mixed results in providing substantial pain relief [76].

Interestingly, although lidocaine can inhibit cardiac sodium channels [10], clinically significant cardiotoxicity is generally not a problem except at very high dosages. Lidocaine dissociates relatively rapidly from hyperpolarized sodium channels, and therefore cardiac sodium channels are probably able to recover from lidocaine block during the prolonged interval between cardiac action potentials. However, side effects such as lightheadedness, drowsiness, and confusion can result from altered function of neurons other than DRG neurons and can be a problem with systemic lidocaine. Mexiletine, an orally active analogue of lidocaine that is used for treating ventricular arrhythmias, has shown some efficacy in animal studies on the treatment of pain [49]; however, although mexiletine can reduce pain associated with diabetic neuropathy, it is not considered effective compared to other treatment options [2].

Anticonvulsants, such as phenytoin and carbamazepine, are state-dependent blockers of voltage-gated sodium channels and can be effective at blocking migraine and neuropathic pain [46]. Interestingly, carbamazepine is often effective at treating inherited paroxysmal extreme pain disorder [54], but it is generally not effective at treating inherited erythromelalgia pain. This difference is perplexing, as both of these inherited painful disorders result from gain-of-function single point mutations in $Na_V1.7$. Carbamazepine is also not considered very effective for treating painful diabetic neuropathy [2]. Oxcarbazepine, a newer analogue of carbamazepine with reduced liver metabolism that is also likely to interact with sodium channels, has shown potential for treating allodynia and hyperalgesia in animal models of neuropathic pain [79]. Clinical studies suggest that oxcarbazepine may be effective at treating several types of pain, including pain associated with multiple sclerosis and trigeminal neuralgia. However, the analgesic efficacy of oxcarbazepine in painful diabetic neuropathy is less clear [79]. Lamotrigine, another anticonvulsant whose activity is due, at least in part, to inhibition of voltage-gated sodium channels, is also reported to be effective at treating several different neuropathic pain states [46], including HIV-associated neuropathy, trigeminal neuralgia, and diabetic neuropathy. However, in a large placebo-controlled study on pain associated with diabetic neuropathy, lamotrigine was reported to be inconsistently effective at reducing pain [103].

Lacosamide, a novel functionalized amino acid [11] that was approved by the U.S. Food and Drug Administration (FDA) in 2008 for adjunctive treatment of partial-onset seizures has also shown promise as an analgesic. In acute, inflammatory and neuropathic animal pain models lacosamide effectively reduced pain-associated behaviors with minimal adverse effects [11]. Lacosamide has also been reported to have some success in clinical trials for diabetic neuropathic pain [95]. Interestingly, lacosamide weakly displaces batrachotoxin binding from voltage-gated sodium channels [50] and reduces action potential firing during prolonged depolarizations, indicating that the mechanism of action of this agent involves attenuation of sodium currents in neurons [50]. However, lacosamide does not display use-dependent inhibition or alter fast inactivation of the sodium currents, but rather seems to selectively enhance slow inactivation of sodium channels, a mechanistically distinct form of inactivation [51]. Lacosamide potently inhibits $Na_V1.3$, $Na_V1.7$, and $Na_V1.8$-type sodium currents and, compared to carbamazepine and lidocaine, exhibits a much greater ability to discriminate between resting and inactivated voltage-gated sodium channels [96]. These data suggest that lacosamide is likely to be selective at inhibiting the activity of neurons with depolarized membrane potentials compared to neurons with normal resting membrane potentials and further raise the possibility that drugs specifically targeting slow inactivation of voltage-gated sodium channels might target sodium channels in neurons with abnormal resting potentials and pathological electrical activity.

Tricyclic antidepressants have been successfully used for several decades to treat pain and are considered by some clinicians as a first-line treatment for some types of neuropathic pain. Amitriptyline is the most commonly used antidepressant for neuropathic pain. A study comparing the analgesic effects of nine tricyclic antidepressants and three local anesthetics administered intrathecally in rats determined that although all of the compounds had analgesic activity, amitriptyline was the most potent and provided the longest duration of spinal anesthesia [29]. Amitriptyline inhibits voltage-dependent sodium channels at concentrations that are effective for treating neuropathic pain, shows higher affinity for inactivated sodium channels, and exhibits use-dependent binding of sodium channels [41]. Although tricyclic antidepressants have been shown to interact with several different molecular targets, it is hypothesized that sodium channel blockade is important for the tricyclic antidepressants that are effective against neuropathic pain.

The Local Anesthetic Binding Site

Many of the local anesthetics, anticonvulsants, and tricyclic compounds that inhibit voltage-gated sodium channels interact with a common binding site [88]. This site, often referred to as the local anesthetic binding site, is formed by residues in the portion of the pore of the channel that is formed by the S6 segments (Fig. 5A,C) [83,88]. In general, it is believed that these compounds bind with higher affinity to activated (or partially activated) channels and stabilize the binding of the inactivation particle to the inner mouth of the channel pore. Although local anesthetics, anticonvulsants, and tricyclic compounds that inhibit voltage-gated sodium channels show some efficacy in treating neuropathic pain, they typically have narrow therapeutic windows that limit their ability to provide adequate pain relief. The S6 segments of the voltage-gated sodium channels are highly conserved, which probably contributes to the lack of specificity for state-dependent modulators that interact with the local anesthetic binding site. However, the sequence of $Na_V1.8$ differs at several residues implicated in the local anesthetic binding site, and $Na_V1.8$ currents exhibit notable differences in the pharmacodynamics of inhibition by local anesthetics, anticonvulsants, and tricyclic compounds [22].

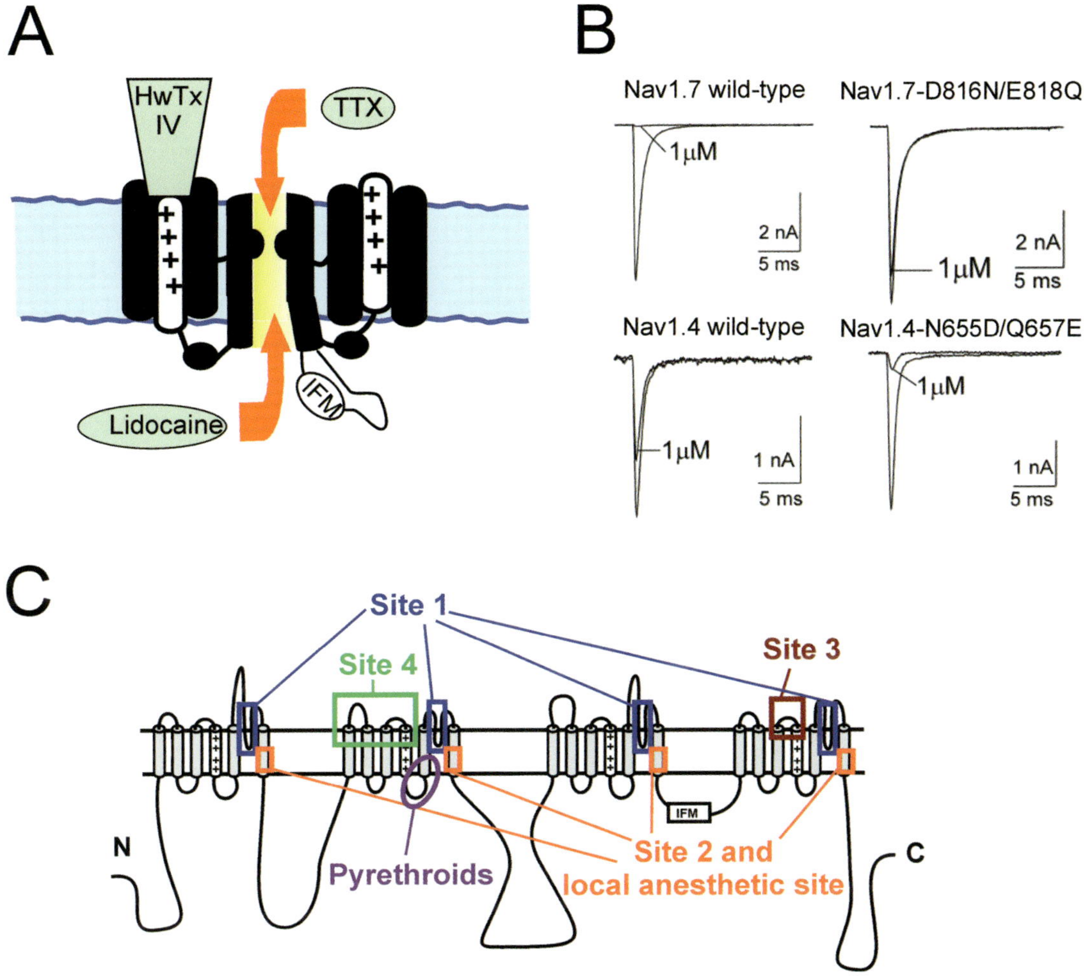

Fig. 5. Sodium channels are inhibited by a variety of different compounds. (A) Illustration of the sites of interaction of several compounds that inhibit voltage-gated sodium channels. Lidocaine and other modulators bind in the inner aspect of the pore. Tetrodotoxin (TTX) binds in the outer aspect of the pore. Tarantula toxins such as huwentoxin-IV (HwTX-IV) bind to the cytoplasmic end of the S4 segment of domain II. (B) Huwentoxin-IV inhibits $Na_V1.7$ channels with high affinity, but it has a greatly reduced effect on $Na_V1.4$ channels. Exchanging two specific amino acid residues at the cytoplasmic end of S4 of domain II renders $Na_V1.7$ insensitive to HwTX-IV and $Na_V1.4$ highly sensitive to HwTX-IV. Modified with permission from [106]. (C) Schematic diagram of the secondary structure of voltage-gated sodium channels showing the regions of the channel that have been identified as neurotoxin binding sites 1–4. A region of the sodium channel that has been identified as critical for the action of pyrethroids is also indicated. Note that the local anesthetic binding site overlaps with neurotoxin binding site 2.

Newer Pharmacological Approaches

Several different approaches are being pursued to develop sodium channel inhibitors that are more effective at treating pain. It has been proposed that broad spectrum sodium channel blockers with enhanced potency would be less likely to alter the activity of other channels or proteins, thus reducing side effects and providing better pain relief at lower dosages. Potent broad-spectrum sodium channel inhibitors should inhibit PNS as well as CNS sodium channels and therefore might target pain activity at multiple levels. The compound PPPA (2-[4-(4-chloro-2-fluorophenoxy)phenyl]-pyrimidine-4-carboxamide) is a novel use-dependent blocker that exhibits 1,000-fold greater potency for sodium channels compared to carbamazepine and lamotrigine [67]. PPPA effectively reduced pain behaviors in animal models of inflammatory and neuropathic pain at doses that had negligible effects on motor performance.

An alternative approach to reducing CNS side effects is to identify sodium channel blockers that do not penetrate the blood-brain barrier. Cyclopentane dicarboxamide (CDA54), an example compound [20], exhibits 33-fold lower concentrations in the brain than in plasma when given orally to rats, preferentially inhibits inactivated sodium channels, and was effective in two different animal neuropathic pain models. Importantly, although CDA54 blocks $Na_V1.2$, $Na_V1.5$, $Na_V1.7$, and $Na_V1.8$ channels at roughly the same range of concentrations in vitro, CDA54 showed significantly lower CNS side effects and cardiotoxicity than mexiletine [20].

A novel strategy for specifically targeting sodium channels in nociceptive neurons was recently proposed [12], whereby the application of a membrane-impermeant lidocaine derivative (QX-314) is combined with capsaicin application. Capsaicin is a selective agonist for the TRPV1 (transient receptor potential vanilloid 1) channel, a molecular sensor for noxious heat that is predominantly expressed on nociceptive sensory neurons. The pore of TRPV1 is large enough to allow small charged molecules such as QX-314 to pass through it, thus allowing extracellularly applied QX-314 to enter nociceptive neurons, gain access to the local anesthetic binding site, and inhibit nociceptor excitability. Because QX-314 does not cross the blood-brain barrier and non-nociceptive neurons do not seem to express TRPV1 channels, the QX-314 does not alter the activity of other neurons. In rats, capsaicin injected with QX-314 into the hindpaw, or near the sciatic nerve, was able to significantly decrease pain sensitivity without apparent motor or tactile deficits.

Another way to target peripheral sensory neuron activity is to identify sodium channel inhibitors that selectively target the sodium channels that contribute to the pain-related activity in peripheral neurons. TTX, which can block voltage-gated sodium currents with a high degree of selectivity over other types of ionic currents, is a classic example of a simple pore blocker that shows some isoform selectivity. TTX blocks six of the nine sodium channel isoforms at nanomolar concentrations ($Na_V1.1$–$Na_V1.4$, $Na_V1.6$, and $Na_V1.7$), but it has greatly reduced activity at the remaining three ($Na_V1.5$, $Na_V1.8$, and $Na_V1.9$). We have extensive knowledge of how TTX, and similar toxins such as saxitoxin

(STX), bind within the channel pore and block the conductance pathway. The residues that are involved in the binding of these toxins have been extensively investigated, and the binding site has been designated as toxin binding site 1. TTX and STX bind within the outer portion of the channel pore (Fig. 5A,C) that is formed by the pore loops between the S5 and S6 segments [25]. Although several different residues are involved in the binding of these toxins, most of these residues are fully conserved among the nine channel isoforms. A single residue in the pore loop of domain I dictates the resistance of $Na_V1.5$, $Na_V1.8$, and $Na_V1.9$ channels to TTX and STX [62,74,98]. This residue is a phenylalanine or tyrosine in TTX-sensitive channels, a cysteine in $Na_V1.5$ and serine in $Na_V1.8$ and $Na_V1.9$. TTX can inhibit ectopic activity in animal models of neuropathic pain [86] and has been used in limited clinical trials for treating pain, such as severe cancer pain [61]. Neosaxitoxin, an analogue of STX, has also been investigated as an analgesic in humans. However, these small, water-soluble guanidine toxins target the most prevalent CNS neuronal sodium channels, raising concern about systemic toxicity. The cardiac channel, $Na_V1.5$, is ~50-fold less sensitive and the peripheral neuronal channels $Na_V1.8$ and $Na_V1.9$ are ~5,000-fold less sensitive to STX and TTX [4,62,74]. Interestingly, a TTX analogue that shows pronounced selectivity for $Na_V1.6$ has recently been reported [91], suggesting that it may be feasible to develop other isoform-selective small-molecule pore blockers that target toxin site 1. A TTX analog that selectively targets site 1 in $Na_V1.8$ and $Na_V1.9$ channels could present interesting possibilities.

Another group of molecules that selectively target sodium channels and bind at site 1 are the μ-conotoxins (e.g. GIIIA), which are large peptide toxins of ~22 amino acids isolated from the venom of marine cone snails [31]. GIIIA potently inhibits rat $Na_V1.4$ channels but has ~20-fold lower affinity for neuronal TTX-sensitive channels. Although μ-conotoxins also bind at site 1, the isoform specificity is due to specific amino-acid residues at the outer edge of the channel pore [32]. There is significant diversity in these residues among the different isoforms, suggesting that large peptide toxins that target site 1 may have more potential as isoform-specific blockers than small molecules such as TTX that interact with fewer residues within the pore. MrVIb, another peptide toxin isolated from marine cone snails, has substantial analgesic activity in animal models of pain and exhibits ~10-fold higher affinity for $Na_V1.8$ block compared to $Na_V1.5$ and $Na_V1.7$ [47]. Although this difference is small, it is hoped that analogues of MrVIb that are more selective for $Na_V1.8$, if they can be developed, might effectively decrease chronic pain with better therapeutic indices than the nonselective sodium channel inhibitors currently available.

A very intriguing small-molecule blocker of $Na_V1.8$, A-803467, was discovered in an extensive screen for blockers of $Na_V1.8$ [68]. The discovery of A-803467 provides proof-of-principle that demonstrates that small-molecule inhibitors of $Na_V1.8$ are feasible and have the potential to be useful as analgesics. A-803467 blocks recombinant $Na_V1.8$ channels with ~100-fold higher selectivity over recombinant $Na_V1.2$, $Na_V1.3$, $Na_V1.5$, and $Na_V1.7$ channels and therefore is the first small molecule to be reported that has selectivity for $Na_V1.8$ over cardiac and TTX-sensitive neuronal channels (it is not clear if A-803467 has activity against $Na_V1.9$ currents). A-803467 blocks spontaneous and evoked action potentials in sensory neurons and exhibits analgesic activity in several inflammatory and neuropathic models of pain at free plasma concentrations of ~200–300 nM. However, A-803467 was not very effective in skin incision models of postoperative pain, in a chemotherapy-induced pain model, or in a visceral pain model, raising the possibility that $Na_V1.8$ activity is not critical in all types of pain. Importantly, A-803467 did not adversely affect spontaneous exploratory behavior or motor coordination of rats, supporting the proposal that this drug is selective in vivo for $Na_V1.8$ channels [68]. Like many drugs with analgesic activity that target sodium channels, A-803467 showed higher affinity for inactivated $Na_V1.8$ channels than for resting $Na_V1.8$ channels. This finding suggests that it might not be a pore blocker. However A-803467 did not show significant use-dependent block, possibly suggesting that A-803467 might not bind to the local anesthetic binding site of $Na_V1.8$.

Multiple Toxin Binding Sites and Their Pharmacological Implications

Several other toxin binding sites have been identified on sodium channels in addition to site 1 [25]. Many of the toxins that bind at these other sites are considered as gating modifiers because the toxins do not simply block the flow of ions through the channel pore but rather alter the gating conformations associated with channel activity. It is important to note that many of these gating modifier toxins (e.g., batrachotoxin) do not inhibit but actually promote channel activity by enhancing activation gating or impairing inactivation gating. These biological toxins are unlikely to be good candidates for reducing the neuronal activity associated with pain but rather are likely to be proalgesic. However, understanding how and where different toxins interact with voltage-gated sodium channels can help identify strategies and compounds for inhibiting sodium channel activity. For example, veratridine and batrachotoxin, which promote sodium channel activity, bind to residues in the S6 segments that overlap the local anesthetic binding site [83]. These toxins, which are classified as site 2 toxins, have been used in high-throughput screening assays to help identify compounds that inhibit active channels. Pyrethroids, synthetic compounds that selectively target insect sodium channels, have similar actions to veratridine. However, these compounds appear to interact with distinct amino acid residues in the S4–S5 linker of domain 2 (Fig. 5C).

Scorpion α-toxins and sea anemone toxins bind to neurotoxin receptor site 3 at the extracellular S3–S4 linker on domain IV (Fig. 5C). These toxins slow inactivation kinetics by trapping the domain IV voltage sensor in the closed position, and it has been proposed that compounds that trap the domain IV voltage sensor in the open position should be able to enhance sodium channel inactivation [25].

Scorpion β-toxins, which enhance activation, do so by binding to neurotoxin receptor site 4 (Fig. 5C) at the extracellular S3–S4 linker on domain II and trapping the

IIS4 voltage sensor in the outward, activated configuration [25]. Conversely, three spider toxins (huwentoxin-I, huwentoxin-IV, and ProTx-II) have been identified that block channel activation, and thus channel activity, by binding at or near to neurotoxin receptor site 4, trapping the voltage sensor of domain II in the inward, closed configuration (Fig. 5A) [100,106]. These spider toxins also exhibit interesting isoform specificities. The tarantula toxins huwentoxin-I and huwentoxin-IV have virtually no effect on muscle sodium channels ($Na_V1.4$ and $Na_V1.5$) or on the TTX-resistant current in DRG neurons, but they are potent inhibitors of neuronal TTX-sensitive channels. Of the neuronal TTX-sensitive channels that were tested ($Na_V1.2$, $Na_V1.3$, and $Na_V1.7$), huwentoxin-IV showed the highest affinity for $Na_V1.7$ (IC50 ~ 8nM). Xiao et al. showed that exchanging just two amino-acid residues between the IIS3–S4 linker of $Na_V1.4$ and $Na_V1.7$ results in a near-complete switch in the sensitivity of these channels to the huwentoxins (Fig. 5B) [106]. ProTx-II, which also binds at or near site 4, is ~50 to 500-fold more selective for $Na_V1.7$ channels over other voltage-gated sodium channels [94]. Although these spider toxins are voltage-gating modifiers that block channel activity by locking the voltage-sensor of domain II in the closed configuration, functionally they can behave as simple channel blockers [106]. Overall, this research indicates that the voltage sensors are viable targets for the development of sodium channel inhibitors and analgesics.

There is considerable variability among the different isoforms in the amino acid sequences of the external faces of the voltage sensor units. Large peptide toxins are likely to interact with numerous residues on voltage-gated sodium channels, which increases the potential for isoform specificity. As many of these peptidic toxins are charged, they are also unlikely to cross the blood-brain barrier, which could be an advantage for their use as peripheral analgesics. However, although ProTx-II may have a better selectivity profile than the huwentoxins and is able to block peripheral C-fiber nerve conduction when applied to desheathed cutaneous nerves, it failed to block nerve conduction when applied to intact nerves and did not demonstrate analgesic activity in animal models of acute and inflammatory pain [94], reflecting the pharmacokinetic problems that can be associated with large peptide compounds.

Overview and Prospects

Sodium channels contribute in multiple ways to sensory neuron hyperexcitability and pain sensations. Inflammation and nerve injury can significantly alter sodium channel expression and sodium currents in DRG neurons. $Na_V1.7$, $Na_V1.8$, and $Na_V1.9$ are preferentially expressed in nociceptors, are likely to play important roles in nociception, and are currently being investigated as potential therapeutic targets for pain. Studies of human inherited disorders of pain show that loss-of-function mutations in $Na_V1.7$ can result in an apparent complete insensitivity to pain, and gain-of-function mutations in $Na_V1.7$ can cause severe chronic pain. Unfortunately, the drugs targeting sodium channels that are currently available for clinical use are not highly isoform-specific and are often associated with unwanted cardiac and CNS side effects. Importantly, high-throughput screening has begun to identify compounds with a degree of subtype selectivity, and at least seven distinct binding sites have been identified on sodium channel α-subunits, with several of these sites exhibiting substantial isoform-specific differences. As a result of major advances in our understanding of the cellular, molecular, and pharmacological properties of voltage-gated sodium channels, it now appears feasible to develop drugs that will specifically target peripheral neuronal sodium channels, an advance that may bring us closer to more effective pharmacotherapy for pain.

References

[1] Abrahamsen B, Zhao J, Asante CO, Cendan CM, Marsh S, Martinez-Barbera JP, Nassar MA, Dickenson AH, Wood JN. The cell and molecular basis of mechanical, cold, and inflammatory pain. Science 2008;321:702–5.

[2] Adriaensen H, Plaghki L, Mathieu C, Joffroy A, Vissers K. Critical review of oral drug treatments for diabetic neuropathic pain: clinical outcomes based on efficacy and safety data from placebo-controlled and direct comparative studies. Diabetes Metab Res Rev 2005;21:231–40.

[3] Ahmad S, Dahllund L, Eriksson AB, Hellgren D, Karlsson U, Lund PE, Meijer IA, Meury L, Mills T, Moody A, Morinville A, Morten J, O'Donnell D, Raynoschek C, Salter H, Rouleau GA, Krupp JJ. A stop codon mutation in SCN9A causes lack of pain sensation. Hum Mol Genet 2007;16:2114–21.

[4] Akopian AN, Sivilotti L, Wood JN. A tetrodotoxin-resistant voltage-gated sodium channel expressed by sensory neurons. Nature 1996;379:257–62.

[5] Akopian AN, Souslova V, England S, Okuse K, Ogata N, Ure J, Smith A, Kerr BJ, McMahon SB, Boyce S, Hill R, Stanfa LC, Dickenson AH, Wood JN. The tetrodotoxin-resistant sodium channel SNS has a specialized function in pain pathways. Nat Neurosci 1999;2:541–8.

[6] Amaya F, Wang H, Costigan M, Allchorne AJ, Hatcher JP, Egerton J, Stean T, Morisset V, Grose D, Gunthorpe MJ, et al. The voltage-gated sodium channel $Na_V1.9$ is an effector of peripheral inflammatory pain hypersensitivity. J Neurosci 2006;26:12852–60.

[7] Baker MD. Protein kinase C mediates up-regulation of tetrodotoxin-resistant, persistent Na^+ current in rat and mouse sensory neurones. J Physiol 2005;567:851–67.

[8] Baker MD, Bostock H. Low-threshold, persistent sodium current in rat large dorsal root ganglion neurons in culture. J Neurophysiol 1997;77:1503–13.

[9] Barbano RL, Herrmann DN, Hart-Gouleau S, Pennella-Vaughan J, Lodewick PA, Dworkin RH. Effectiveness, tolerability, and impact on quality of life of the 5% lidocaine patch in diabetic polyneuropathy. Arch Neurol 2004;61:914–8.

[10] Bean BP, Cohen CJ, Tsien RW. Lidocaine block of cardiac sodium channels. J Gen Physiol 1983;81:613–42.

[11] Beyreuther BK, Freitag J, Heers C, Krebsfanger N, Scharfenecker U, Stohr T. Lacosamide: a review of preclinical properties. CNS Drug Rev 2007;13:21–42.

[12] Binshtok AM, Bean BP, Woolf CJ. Inhibition of nociceptors by TRPV1-mediated entry of impermeant sodium channel blockers. Nature 2007;449:607–10.

[13] Black JA, Cummins TR, Plumpton C, Chen YH, Hormuzdiar W, Clare JJ, Waxman SG. Upregulation of a silent sodium channel after peripheral, but not central, nerve injury in DRG neurons. J Neurophysiol 1999;82:2776–85.

[14] Black JA, Dib-Hajj S, Baker D, Newcombe J, Cuzner ML, Waxman SG. Sensory neuron-specific sodium channel SNS is abnormally expressed in the brains of mice with experimental allergic encephalomyelitis and humans with multiple sclerosis. Proc Natl Acad Sci USA 2000;97:11598–602.

[15] Black JA, Dib-Hajj S, McNabola K, Jeste S, Rizzo MA, Kocsis JD, Waxman SG. Spinal sensory neurons express multiple sodium channel alpha-subunit mRNAs. Brain Res Mol Brain Res 1996;43:117–31.

[16] Black JA, Liu S, Tanaka M, Cummins TR, Waxman SG. Changes in the expression of tetrodotoxin-sensitive sodium channels within dorsal root ganglia neurons in inflammatory pain. Pain 2004;108:237–47.

[17] Black JA, Nikolajsen L, Kroner K, Jensen TS, Waxman SG. Multiple sodium channel isoforms and mitogen-activated protein kinases are present in painful human neuromas. Ann Neurol 2008;64:644–53.

[18] Black JA, Renganathan M, Waxman SG. Sodium channel $Na_V1.6$ is expressed along nonmyelinated axons and it contributes to conduction. Brain Res Mol Brain Res 2002;105:19–28.

[19] Brau ME, Dreimann M, Olschewski A, Vogel W, Hempelmann G. Effect of drugs used for neuropathic pain management on tetrodotoxin-resistant Na^+ currents in rat sensory neurons. Anesthesiology 2001;94:137–44.

[20] Brochu RM, Dick IE, Tarpley JW, McGowan E, Gunner D, Herrington J, Shao PP, Ok D, Li C, Parsons WH, et al. Block of peripheral nerve sodium channels selectively inhibits features of neuropathic pain in rats. Mol Pharmacol 2006;69:823–32.

[21] Brock JA, McLachlan EM, Belmonte C. Tetrodotoxin-resistant impulses in single nociceptor nerve terminals in guinea-pig cornea. J Physiol 1998;512:211–17.

[22] Cardenas CA, Cardenas CG, de Armendi AJ, Scroggs RS. Carbamazepine interacts with a slow inactivation state of $Na_V1.8$-like sodium channels. Neurosci Lett 2006;408:129–34.
[23] Cardenas LM, Cardenas CG, Scroggs RS. 5HT increases excitability of nociceptor-like rat dorsal root ganglion neurons via cAMP-coupled TTX-resistant Na^+ channels. J Neurophysiol 2001;86:241–8.
[24] Catterall WA. Molecular properties of brain sodium channels: an important target for anticonvulsant drugs. Adv Neurol 1999;79:441–56.
[25] Cestele S, Catterall WA. Molecular mechanisms of neurotoxin action on voltage-gated sodium channels. Biochimie 2000;82:883–92.
[26] Chabal C, Russell LC, Burchiel KJ. The effect of intravenous lidocaine, tocainide, and mexiletine on spontaneously active fibers originating in rat sciatic neuromas. Pain 1989;38:333–8.
[27] Chahine M, George AL Jr, Zhou M, Ji S, Sun W, Barchi RL, Horn R. Sodium channel mutations in paramyotonia congenita uncouple inactivation from activation. Neuron 1994;12:281–94.
[28] Chanda B, Bezanilla F. Tracking voltage-dependent conformational changes in skeletal muscle sodium channel during activation. J Gen Physiol 2002;120:629–45.
[29] Chen YW, Huang KL, Liu SY, Tzeng JI, Chu KS, Lin MT, Wang JJ. Intrathecal tri-cyclic antidepressants produce spinal anesthesia. Pain 2004;112:106–12.
[30] Cox JJ, Reimann F, Nicholas AK, Thornton G, Roberts E, Springell K, Karbani G, Jafri H, Mannan J, Raashid Y, et al. An *SCN9A* channelopathy causes congenital inability to experience pain. Nature 2006;444:894–8.
[31] Cruz LJ, Gray WR, Olivera BM, Zeikus RD, Kerr L, Yoshikami D, Moczydlowski E. *Conus geographus* toxins that discriminate between neuronal and muscle sodium channels. J Biol Chem 1985;260:9280–8.
[32] Cummins TR, Aglieco F, Dib-Hajj SD. Critical molecular determinants of voltage-gated sodium channel sensitivity to mu-conotoxins GIIIA/B. Mol Pharmacol 2002;61:1192–201.
[33] Cummins TR, Aglieco F, Renganathan M, Herzog RI, Dib-Hajj SD, Waxman SG. $Na_V1.3$ sodium channels: rapid repriming and slow closed-state inactivation display quantitative differences after expression in a mammalian cell line and in spinal sensory neurons. J Neurosci 2001;21:5952–61.
[34] Cummins TR, Dib-Hajj SD, Black JA, Akopian AN, Wood JN, Waxman SG. A novel persistent tetrodotoxin-resistant sodium current in SNS-null and wild-type small primary sensory neurons. J Neurosci 1999;19:RC43.
[35] Cummins TR, Dib-Hajj SD, Herzog RI, Waxman SG. $Na_V1.6$ channels generate resurgent sodium currents in spinal sensory neurons. FEBS Lett 2005;579:2166–70.
[36] Cummins TR, Howe JR, Waxman SG. Slow closed-state inactivation: a novel mechanism underlying ramp currents in cells expressing the hNE/PN1 sodium channel. J Neurosci 1998;18:9607–19.
[37] Cummins TR, Waxman SG. Downregulation of tetrodotoxin-resistant sodium currents and upregulation of a rapidly repriming tetrodotoxin-sensitive sodium current in small spinal sensory neurons after nerve injury. J Neurosci 1997;17:3503–14.
[38] Dib-Hajj S, Black JA, Cummins TR, Waxman SG. NaN/$Na_V1.9$: a sodium channel with unique properties. Trends Neurosci 2002;25:253–9.
[39] Dib-Hajj S, Black JA, Felts P, Waxman SG. Down-regulation of transcripts for Na channel alpha-SNS in spinal sensory neurons following axotomy. Proc Natl Acad Sci USA 1996;93:14950–4.
[40] Dib-Hajj SD, Cummins TR, Black JA, Waxman SG. From genes to pain: $Na_V1.7$ and human pain disorders. Trends Neurosci 2007;30:555–63.
[41] Dick IE, Brochu RM, Purohit Y, Kaczorowski GJ, Martin WJ, Priest BT. Sodium channel blockade may contribute to the analgesic efficacy of antidepressants. J Pain 2007;8:315–24.
[42] Djouhri L, Dawbarn D, Robertson A, Newton R, Lawson SN. Time course and nerve growth factor dependence of inflammation-induced alterations in electrophysiological membrane properties in nociceptive primary afferent neurons. J Neurosci 2001;21:8722–33.
[43] Djouhri L, Fang X, Okuse K, Wood JN, Berry CM, Lawson SN. The TTX-resistant sodium channel $Na_V1.8$ (SNS/PN3): expression and correlation with membrane properties in rat nociceptive primary afferent neurons. J Physiol 2003;550:739–52.
[44] Djouhri L, Newton R, Levinson SR, Berry CM, Carruthers B, Lawson SN. Sensory and electrophysiological properties of guinea-pig sensory neurones expressing $Na_V1.7$ (PN1) Na^+ channel alpha subunit protein. J Physiol 2003;546:565–76.
[45] Dong XW, Goregoaker S, Engler H, Zhou X, Mark L, Crona J, Terry R, Hunter J, Priestley T. Small interfering RNA-mediated selective knockdown of $Na_V1.8$ tetrodotoxin-resistant sodium channel reverses mechanical allodynia in neuropathic rats. Neuroscience 2007;146:812–21.
[46] Eisenberg E, River Y, Shifrin A, Krivoy N. Antiepileptic drugs in the treatment of neuropathic pain. Drugs 2007;67:1265–89.
[47] Ekberg J, Jayamanne A, Vaughan CW, Aslan S, Thomas L, Mould J, Drinkwater R, Baker MD, Abrahamsen B, Wood JN, et al. MuO-conotoxin MrVIB selectively blocks $Na_V1.8$ sensory neuron specific sodium channels and chronic pain behavior without motor deficits. Proc Natl Acad Sci USA 2006;103:17030–5.
[48] Elliott AA, Elliott JR. Characterization of TTX-sensitive and TTX-resistant sodium currents in small cells from adult rat dorsal root ganglia. J Physiol 1993;463:39–56.
[49] Erichsen HK, Hao JX, Xu XJ, Blackburn-Munro G. A comparison of the antinociceptive effects of voltage-activated Na^+ channel blockers in two rat models of neuropathic pain. Eur J Pharmacol 2003;458:275–82.
[50] Errington AC, Coyne L, Stohr T, Selve N, Lees G. Seeking a mechanism of action for the novel anticonvulsant lacosamide. Neuropharmacology 2006;50:1016–29.
[51] Errington AC, Stohr T, Heers C, Lees G. The investigational anticonvulsant lacosamide selectively enhances slow inactivation of voltage-gated sodium channels. Mol Pharmacol 2008;73:157–69.

[52] Estacion M, Dib-Hajj SD, Benke PJ, Te Morsche RH, Eastman EM, Macala LJ, Drenth JP, Waxman SG. $Na_V1.7$ gain-of-function mutations as a continuum: A1632E displays physiological changes associated with erythromelalgia and paroxysmal extreme pain disorder mutations and produces symptoms of both disorders. J Neurosci 2008;28:11079–88.
[53] Fang X, Djouhri L, Black JA, Dib-Hajj SD, Waxman SG, Lawson SN. The presence and role of the tetrodotoxin-resistant sodium channel $Na_V1.9$ (NaN) in nociceptive primary afferent neurons. J Neurosci 2002;22:7425–33.
[54] Fertleman CR, Baker MD, Parker KA, Moffatt S, Elmslie FV, Abrahamsen B, Ostman J, Klugbauer N, Wood JN, Gardiner RM, Rees M. *SCN9A* mutations in paroxysmal extreme pain disorder: allelic variants underlie distinct channel defects and phenotypes. Neuron 2006;52:767–74.
[55] Fjell J, Cummins TR, Fried K, Black JA, Waxman SG. In vivo NGF deprivation reduces SNS expression and TTX-R sodium currents in IB4-negative DRG neurons. J Neurophysiol 1999;81:803–10.
[56] Gammaitoni AR, Alvarez NA, Galer BS. Safety and tolerability of the lidocaine patch 5%, a targeted peripheral analgesic: a review of the literature. J Clin Pharmacol 2003;43:111–7.
[57] Gold MS, Reichling DB, Shuster MJ, Levine JD. Hyperalgesic agents increase a tetrodotoxin-resistant Na^+ current in nociceptors. Proc Natl Acad Sci USA 1996;93:1108–12.
[58] Gold MS, Weinreich D, Kim CS, Wang R, Treanor J, Porreca F, Lai J. Redistribution of $Na_V1.8$ in uninjured axons enables neuropathic pain. J Neurosci 2003;23:158–66.
[59] Goldberg YP, MacFarlane J, MacDonald ML, Thompson J, Dube MP, Mattice M, Fraser R, Young C, Hossain S, Pape T, et al. Loss-of-function mutations in the $Na_V1.7$ gene underlie congenital indifference to pain in multiple human populations. Clin Genet 2007;71:311–9.
[60] Goldin AL, Barchi RL, Caldwell JH, Hofmann F, Howe JR, Hunter JC, Kallen RG, Mandel G, Meisler MH, Netter YB, et al. Nomenclature of voltage-gated sodium channels. Neuron 2000;28:365–8.
[61] Hagen NA, du Souich P, Lapointe B, Ong-Lam M, Dubuc B, Walde D, Love R, Ngoc AH. Tetrodotoxin for moderate to severe cancer pain: a randomized, double blind, parallel design multicenter study. J Pain Symptom Manage 2008;35:420–9.
[62] Heinemann SH, Terlau H, Imoto K. Molecular basis for pharmacological differences between brain and cardiac sodium channels. Pflugers Arch 1992;422:90–2.
[63] Herrmann DN, Barbano RL, Hart-Gouleau S, Pennella-Vaughan J, Dworkin RH. An open-label study of the lidocaine patch 5% in painful idiopathic sensory polyneuropathy. Pain Med 2005;6:379–84.
[64] Herzog RI, Cummins TR, Ghassemi F, Dib-Hajj SD, Waxman SG. Distinct repriming and closed-state inactivation kinetics of $Na_V1.6$ and $Na_V1.7$ sodium channels in mouse spinal sensory neurons. J Physiol 2003;551:741–50.
[65] Herzog RI, Cummins TR, Waxman SG. Persistent TTX-resistant Na^+ current affects resting potential and response to depolarization in simulated spinal sensory neurons. J Neurophysiol 2001;86:1351–64.
[66] Hille B. Ion channels of excitable membranes. Sunderland, MA: Sinauer; 1984.
[67] Ilyin VI, Pomonis JD, Whiteside GT, Harrison JE, Pearson MS, Mark L, Turchin PI, Gottshall S, Carter RB, Nguyen P, et al. Pharmacology of 2-[4-(4-chloro-2-fluorophenoxy)phenyl]-pyrimidine-4-carboxamide: a potent, broad-spectrum state-dependent sodium channel blocker for treating pain states. J Pharmacol Exp Ther 2006;318:1083–93.
[68] Jarvis MF, Honore P, Shieh CC, Chapman M, Joshi S, Zhang XF, Kort M, Carroll W, Marron B, Atkinson R, et al. A-803467, a potent and selective $Na_V1.8$ sodium channel blocker, attenuates neuropathic and inflammatory pain in the rat. Proc Natl Acad Sci USA 2007;104:8520–5.
[69] Khaliq ZM, Gouwens NW, Raman IM. The contribution of resurgent sodium current to high-frequency firing in Purkinje neurons: an experimental and modeling study. J Neurosci 2003;23:4899–912.
[70] Khasar SG, Gold MS, Levine JD. A tetrodotoxin-resistant sodium current mediates inflammatory pain in the rat. Neurosci Lett 1998;256:17–20.
[71] Kiernan MC, Baker MD, Bostock H. Characteristics of late Na^+ current in adult rat small sensory neurons. Neuroscience 2003;119:653–60.
[72] Kostyuk PG, Veselovsky NS, Tsyndrenko AY. Ionic currents in the somatic membrane of rat dorsal root ganglion neurons-I. Sodium currents. Neuroscience 1981;6:2423–30.
[73] Lai J, Gold MS, Kim CS, Bian D, Ossipov MH, Hunter JC, Porreca F. Inhibition of neuropathic pain by decreased expression of the tetrodotoxin-resistant sodium channel, $Na_V1.8$. Pain 2002;95:143–52.
[74] Leffler A, Herzog RI, Dib-Hajj SD, Waxman SG, Cummins TR. Pharmacological properties of neuronal TTX-resistant sodium channels and the role of a critical serine pore residue. Pflugers Arch 2005;451:454–63.
[75] Long SB, Campbell EB, Mackinnon R. Crystal structure of a mammalian voltage-dependent Shaker family K^+ channel. Science 2005;309:897–903.
[76] Mao J, Chen LL. Systemic lidocaine for neuropathic pain relief. Pain 2000;87:7–17.
[77] Matsuda Y, Yoshida S, Yonezawa T. Tetrodotoxin sensitivity and Ca component of action potentials of mouse dorsal root ganglion cells cultured in vitro. Brain Res 1978;154:69–82.
[78] Meier T, Wasner G, Faust M, Kuntzer T, Ochsner F, Hueppe M, Bogousslavsky J, Baron R. Efficacy of lidocaine patch 5% in the treatment of focal peripheral neuropathic pain syndromes: a randomized, double-blind, placebo-controlled study. Pain 2003;106:151–8.
[79] Nasreddine W, Beydoun A. Oxcarbazepine in neuropathic pain. Expert Opin Investig Drugs 2007;16:1615–25.
[80] Nassar MA, Baker MD, Levato A, Ingram R, Mallucci G, McMahon SB, Wood JN. Nerve injury induces robust allodynia and ectopic discharges in $Na_V1.3$ null mutant mice. Mol Pain 2006;2:33.
[81] Nassar MA, Levato A, Stirling LC, Wood JN. Neuropathic pain develops normally in mice lacking both $Na_V1.7$ and $Na_V1.8$. Mol Pain 2005;1:24.
[82] Nassar MA, Stirling LC, Forlani G, Baker MD, Matthews EA, Dickenson AH, Wood JN. Nociceptor-specific gene deletion reveals a major role for $Na_V1.7$ (PN1) in acute and inflammatory pain. Proc Natl Acad Sci USA 2004;101:12706–11.

[83] Nau C, Wang GK. Interactions of local anesthetics with voltage-gated Na^+ channels. J Membr Biol 2004;201:1–8.
[84] Noda M, Ikeda T, Kayano T, Suzuki H, Takeshima H, Kurasaki M, Takahashi H, Numa S. Existence of distinct sodium channel messenger RNAs in rat brain. Nature 1986;320:188–92.
[85] Nordin M, Nystrom B, Wallin U, Hagbarth KE. Ectopic sensory discharges and paresthesiae in patients with disorders of peripheral nerves, dorsal roots and dorsal columns. Pain 1984;20:231–45.
[86] Omana-Zapata I, Khabbaz MA, Hunter JC, Clarke DE, Bley KR. Tetrodotoxin inhibits neuropathic ectopic activity in neuromas, dorsal root ganglia and dorsal horn neurons. Pain 1997;72:41–9.
[87] Priest BT, Murphy BA, Lindia JA, Diaz C, Abbadie C, Ritter AM, Liberator P, Iyer LM, Kash SF, Kohler MG, et al. Contribution of the tetrodotoxin-resistant voltage-gated sodium channel $Na_V1.9$ to sensory transmission and nociceptive behavior. Proc Natl Acad Sci USA 2005;102:9382–7.
[88] Ragsdale DS, McPhee JC, Scheuer T, Catterall WA. Common molecular determinants of local anesthetic, antiarrhythmic, and anticonvulsant block of voltage-gated Na^+ channels. Proc Natl Acad Sci USA 1996;93:9270–5.
[89] Renganathan M, Cummins TR, Waxman SG. Contribution of $Na_V1.8$ sodium channels to action potential electrogenesis in DRG neurons. J Neurophysiol 2001;86:629–40.
[90] Renganathan M, Dib-Hajj S, Waxman SG. $Na_V1.5$ underlies the 'third TTX-R sodium current' in rat small DRG neurons. Brain Res Mol Brain Res 2002;106:70–82.
[91] Rosker C, Lohberger B, Hofer D, Steinecker B, Quasthoff S, Schreibmayer W. The TTX metabolite 4,9-anhydro-TTX is a highly specific blocker of the Na(v1.6) voltage-dependent sodium channel. Am J Physiol Cell Physiol 2007;293:C783–9.
[92] Rush AM, Dib-Hajj SD, Liu S, Cummins TR, Black JA, Waxman SG. A single sodium channel mutation produces hyper- or hypoexcitability in different types of neurons. Proc Natl Acad Sci USA 2006;103:8245–50.
[93] Rush AM, Waxman SG. PGE2 increases the tetrodotoxin-resistant $Na_V1.9$ sodium current in mouse DRG neurons via G-proteins. Brain Res 2004;1023:264–71.
[94] Schmalhofer WA, Calhoun J, Burrows R, Bailey T, Kohler MG, Weinglass AB, Kaczorowski GJ, Garcia ML, Koltzenburg M, Priest BT. ProTx-II, a selective inhibitor of $Na_V1.7$ sodium channels, blocks action potential propagation in nociceptors. Mol Pharmacol 2008;74:1476–84.
[95] Shaibani A, Biton V, Rauck R, Koch B, Simpson J. Long-term oral lacosamide in painful diabetic neuropathy: a two-year open-label extension trial. Eur J Pain 2009;13:458–63.
[96] Sheets PL, Heers C, Stoehr T, Cummins TR. Differential block of sensory neuronal voltage-gated sodium channels by lacosamide [(2R)-2-(acetylamino)-N-benzyl-3-methoxypropanamide], lidocaine, and carbamazepine. J Pharmacol Exp Ther 2008;326:89–99.
[97] Sigworth FJ. Voltage gating of ion channels. Q Rev Biophys 1994;27:1–40.
[98] Sivilotti L, Okuse K, Akopian AN, Moss S, Wood JN. A single serine residue confers tetrodotoxin insensitivity on the rat sensory-neuron-specific sodium channel SNS. FEBS Lett 1997;409:49–52.
[99] Smith LJ, Shih A, Miletic G, Miletic V. Continual systemic infusion of lidocaine provides analgesia in an animal model of neuropathic pain. Pain 2002;97:267–73.
[100] Sokolov S, Kraus RL, Scheuer T, Catterall WA. Inhibition of sodium channel gating by trapping the domain II voltage sensor with protoxin II. Mol Pharmacol 2008;73:1020–8.
[101] Tanaka M, Cummins TR, Ishikawa K, Dib-Hajj SD, Black JA, Waxman SG. SNS Na^+ channel expression increases in dorsal root ganglion neurons in the carrageenan inflammatory pain model. Neuroreport 1998;9:967–72.
[102] Toledo-Aral JJ, Moss BL, He ZJ, Koszowski AG, Whisenand T, Levinson SR, Wolf JJ, Silos-Santiago I, Halegoua S, Mandel G. Identification of PN1, a predominant voltage-dependent sodium channel expressed principally in peripheral neurons. Proc Natl Acad Sci USA 1997;94:1527–32.
[103] Vinik AI, Tuchman M, Safirstein B, Corder C, Kirby L, Wilks K, Quessy S, Blum D, Grainger J, White J, Silver M. Lamotrigine for treatment of pain associated with diabetic neuropathy: results of two randomized, double-blind, placebo-controlled studies. Pain 2007;128:169–79.
[104] Waxman SG. Neurobiology: a channel sets the gain on pain. Nature 2006;444:831–2.
[105] Waxman SG, Kocsis JD, Black JA. Type III sodium channel mRNA is expressed in embryonic but not adult spinal sensory neurons, and is reexpressed following axotomy. J Neurophysiol 1994;72:466–70.
[106] Xiao Y, Bingham JP, Zhu W, Moczydlowski E, Liang S, Cummins TR. Tarantula huwentoxin-IV inhibits neuronal sodium channels by binding to receptor site 4 and trapping the domain II voltage sensor in the closed configuration. J Biol Chem 2008;283:27300–13.
[107] Yeomans DC, Levinson SR, Peters MC, Koszowski AG, Tzabazis AZ, Gilly WF, Wilson SP. Decrease in inflammatory hyperalgesia by herpes vector-mediated knockdown of $Na_V1.7$ sodium channels in primary afferents. Hum Gene Ther 2005;16:271–7.
[108] Zhang JM, Donnelly DF, Song XJ, Lamotte RH. Axotomy increases the excitability of dorsal root ganglion cells with unmyelinated axons. J Neurophysiol 1997;78:2790–4.

Correspondence to: Stephen G. Waxman, MD, PhD, Department of Neurology, LCI 707, Yale University School of Medicine, 333 Cedar Street, New Haven, CT 06510, USA. Email: stephen.waxman@yale.edu.

Potassium and Calcium Channels in Pain Pharmacology

Sérgio H. Ferreira, Wiliam A. Prado, and Luiz F. Ferrari

Department of Pharmacology, Faculty of Medicine of Ribeirão Preto, University of São Paulo, Ribeirão Preto, Brazil

Pain can be described as "an unpleasant and emotional perception of a nociceptive sensation." This simple pragmatic concept implies that a pharmacologist has few basic neuronal general targets for therapeutic control of pain. The nociceptive stimulus that directly activates the nociceptive system may originate from within or outside the body, within or outside the central nervous system (CNS). The process of natural selection during evolution involved the development of several physiological and pathological mechanisms that contributed to animal survival. An animal's ability to feel immediate pain upon an environmental threat and to rapidly defend itself from attack by predators was certainly a major contribution to natural selection.

To abolish the perception of immediate pain, central anesthetics are the drugs of choice for surgical and trauma-related pain. The nociceptive sensation of immediate pain can also be blocked at the moment of transduction of a peripheral stimulus by a local anesthetic. Unpleasantness and emotional responses to pain may be controlled by centrally acting drugs such as opioids and tranquilizers. On the other hand, analgesia for inflammatory pain is based on drugs that (1) prevent the development of the sensitization of nociceptors, (2) directly block ongoing sensitization, or (3) interfere with the release of mediators responsible for transmission in the nociceptive system (glutamate, substance P, etc.).

Inflammatory pain involves the sensitization and activation of a special class of primary sensory neurons that normally are quiescent (the sleeping or silent nociceptors)

Pharmacology of Pain
edited by Pierre Beaulieu, David Lussier, Frank Porreca, and Anthony H. Dickenson
IASP Press, Seattle, © 2010

[64,95]. Depending on the inflammatory scenario, we may end up with a soup of inflammatory mediators, but frequently, the prostaglandins are the major sensitizing mediator, as described by several studies showing the analgesic effectiveness of cyclooxygenase (COX) inhibitors (see Chapter 3 by Vergne-Salle and Beneytout). During inflammation, however, the generation of prostaglandins is also prevented by inhibition of the release of proinflammatory cytokines (tumor necrosis factor-α, interleukin-6, and interleukin-1) by corticosteroids or specific antagonists, which explains the analgesic effect of these substances [25].

The nociceptor has a peripheral axon that conducts action potentials from its terminal to the cell body (localized in the dorsal root ganglion [63]) that controls the identity and integrity of the neuron, and to a central axon with a terminal that forms the presynaptic element of the first synapse in the sensory pathway in the CNS [115] (see Chapter 1 by Marchand). The cell bodies are informed about the status of their peripheral terminals whenever a noxious stimulus occurs. Retrograde signals in nociceptor neurons increase the transcription of several intracellular proteins, including neuropeptides, brain-derived neurotrophic factor (BDNF), and sodium channels, as well as the translation of transient receptor potential (TRP) channels to augment both central transmission and peripheral sensitization [47,58]. Furthermore, inflammation induced via nerve growth factor (NGF) release increases the expression of μ-opioid receptors, resulting in enhanced sensitivity to opioids [84]. In this context, it should be pointed out that morphine has little or no effect in normal rat paws, but it has a peripheral antinociceptive effect when the paws are sensitized by prostaglandins or inflammation [30]. The physiological response to noxious stimulation initiates in the peripheral terminal, but ectopic nonphysiological firings that produce noxious inputs in the absence of stimuli may originate from the axon or cell body [24], or even from neighboring intact fibers [19]. Peripheral nerve injury changes the expression of neurotransmitters, neuromodulators, their respective receptors, transcription factors, and other molecules implicated in cell signaling [44].

Prostaglandin E_2 (PGE_2) sensitizes C fibers via the activation of adenyl cyclase, protein kinase A (PKA), and protein kinase C (PKC) [1,15,29] to modulate the voltage-sensitive, tetrodotoxin-resistant (TTX-r) sodium channels [22,35] and potassium channels [48,68], thereby facilitating the induction of action potentials and their neuronal conduction. We have also proposed that, during hypernociception, there is a phenomenon described as *retrograde sensitization* [27,28], in which the glutamate released by the peripheral nerve acts in the presynaptic terminal, allowing calcium (Ca^{2+}) influx, which may help to integrate all regions of the neuron [75]. Moreover, abnormal or disproportional severe sensitization of the nociceptors may occur during or after tissue injury, especially when there is damage to a peripheral nerve. In this case, myelinated nociceptive fibers also will be affected and begin to respond abnormally to stimulation. This neuropathic sensitization is related to permanent spinal sensitization and is not amenable to classic anti-inflammatory analgesics. However, drugs that directly influence ion flux through membrane channels, in addition to tricyclic antidepressants and anticonvulsants, have been reported to be effective in the control of neuropathic pain symptoms.

Ionic conductance through the neuronal membrane is the main mechanism by which electrical information is conducted along the axons. Thus, the information produced by a noxious stimulus may reach the upper regions of the nervous system and be perceived as pain. In this sense, knowing how to control this flow of information may lead to the development of effective analgesic and anesthetic drugs.

Potassium Channels in Pain and Analgesia

The last decades of the 20th century were very prolific in terms of elucidating the mechanism of pain transduction. For example, researchers demonstrated that a diverse group of ligand- and voltage-gated ion channels transduce innocuous and noxious stimuli into depolarizations that are conducted along the axons and finally converted into neurotransmitter release. Indeed, these ion channels may be considered attractive targets for therapeutic intervention in peripheral pain. In this sense, the observation that agonists of G-protein-coupled receptors (opioid receptors, for instance) open specific potassium (K^+) channels in neurons [69] and induce antinociception led to the hypothesis that the opening of this type of ion channel was involved in the antinociceptive effect of opioid drugs. Later, this hypothesis was confirmed in both the central and peripheral nervous system by the inhibition of opioid-induced analgesia by specific K^+ channel blockers, which also helped to determine the mechanism of action of such drugs.

Potassium channels are found in every cell and have an essential role in the membrane resting potential. The closing of these channels facilitates membrane depolarization, while their opening (activation) takes the membrane potential to electronegative values. Modulators of K^+ channels change their properties, leading to alterations in the membrane charge, or induce intracellular processes as a direct consequence of the membrane potential change. The study of the structure of different K^+ channels has shown that most of the blockers of these channels act at sites located inside the pore (mainly the voltage-activated K^+ channels).

More recently, new strategies were used to evaluate the role of these channels in the sensory process and to identify the subtypes involved in pain signaling. The antinociceptive effect of drugs was tested in animals treated with antisense oligodeoxynucleotides to knock down the expression of particular K^+-channel subtypes [33] or in animals genetically modified to knock out the expression of specific K^+ channels [13]. These studies indicated that new antinociceptive drugs could be developed, focusing on the direct interaction with K^+ channels as the mechanism of action. Moreover, the evaluation of these drugs in models of acute and chronic pain was essential for this research.

The demonstration that the opening of K^+ channels plays a role in the antinociceptive effect induced by various analgesic drugs (nonsteroidal anti-inflammatory and opioid drugs) has helped to increase our knowledge of the mechanisms of neuronal sensitization. There are many types of K^+ channels that differ in structure, functional characteristics, and pharmacological sensitivity, and the identification of the differential importance of each subtype for pain processing may be enlightening.

The activation of K^+ channels present in neurons reestablishes the resting potential after depolarization. Their opening allows the outflow of K^+ and the decrease of membrane electrical potential to an electronegative condition, i.e., the resting potential. In other words, these channels play a key role in the control of neuronal activity and signal propagation throughout the nerve [56,92]. Changes in membrane voltage or in intracellular levels of other ions and proteins [56,92] regulate the opening and closing of K^+ channels, such that agents that interfere with these factors may also be considered in pharmacological intervention. Given that the different subtypes of K^+ channels may act differentially in the electrical signaling of the cells, studies are very numerous and sometimes contradictory. In order to unify and update the different classifications published previously, the International Union of Pharmacology (IUPHAR) proposed a standardized K^+ channel nomenclature based on the structural and phylogenetic relationships of the proteins that constitute the channels [39,92].

Voltage-Gated Potassium Channels

The K^+ channels that are activated by changes in the cell membrane potential are known as voltage-gated K^+ or K_V channels. There are many subtypes of these channels, comprising 12 different families, designated K_V1 to K_V12. Many of these families consist of more than one channel (for example, the K_V1 family has eight different channels: $K_V1.1$ to $K_V1.8$). All members of this group share the same structural characteristics and are tetramers of α subunits (proteins with six transmembrane domains and N- and C-terminal regions located intracellularly). The pore is formed by the fifth and sixth transmembrane domains and the region between them, and the fourth transmembrane domain contains part of the voltage sensor that permits the opening of the channel when the cell is depolarized [39,56,92]. There are also β subunits, which, when present, alter some properties of the channel. Fig. 1 shows the basic structure of the K_V channels.

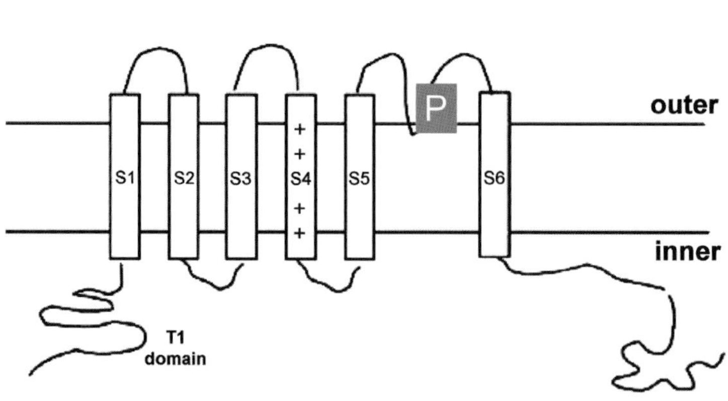

Fig. 1. Structure of voltage-gated potassium channels: topology cartoon for one K_V subunit. S1–S6: transmembrane segments; pore-forming "P"; S4: the voltage-sensor helix. The N-terminal T1-domain and the C-terminal tail are shown (after Pischalnikova and Sokolova [81]).

The majority of the K_V1 channels present in myelinated nerve fibers comprises $K_V1.1$, $K_V1.2$, and $K_V\beta2.1$ subunits [89,110]. Distinct populations of DRG neurons express a variety of K_V currents, and pharmacological blockade of these currents affects neuronal excitability [36]. Moreover, nerve injury is believed to result in a reduction in K_V currents (downregulation of K_V channels), leading to hyperexcitability and hyperalgesia [88], as observed in experimental models of neuropathic pain [88]. It is also known that hyperalgesic (inflammatory) agents, while increasing tetrodotoxin-resistant (TTX-r) sodium (Na^+) currents in nociceptors, reduce K_V currents, which contributes to increased sensitivity to mechanical stimuli (see Chapter 7 by Cummins and Waxman). Given that axotomy results in upregulation of $Na_V1.3$ and downregulation of $Na_V1.8$ and $Na_V1.9$ [70,113], along with downregulation of K_V channels, it is reasonable to conclude that the interaction between Na_V and K_V currents contributes to the resting membrane electrical potential [70,113]. However, there are also demonstrations of downregulation of K^+ channels in neuropathic pain models, which may contribute to the hyperexcitable state [88].

Many synthetic drugs are able to block K_V channels. For example, 4-aminopyridine (4-AP) and tetraethylammonium (TEA) have frequently been used in studies of ionic mechanisms of nociception. However, these drugs are not selective for a particular type of K_V channel (and can even block some calcium channels at high concentrations) [50], and therefore, more specific K_V subtype blockers are needed. Interestingly, many toxins from scorpions and spiders are K_V blockers and are apparently more specific [50].

The hyperalgesic effect of inflammatory mediators such as prostaglandin also depends, to a certain extent, on changes in K_V channels. The enhanced sensitivity of sensory neurons induced by PGE_2 results, at least in part, from the suppression of delayed-rectifying K^+ channel currents, more specifically $K_V1.1$ [48]. Interestingly, knockout mice that lack $K_V1.1$ channels apparently are naturally hyperalgesic, and these data are in line with a study by Boland and Jackson [9] that showed inhibition of $K_V1.1$ function by PKC, one of the second intracellular messengers activated by PGE_2. On the other hand, the observed absence of antinociception induced by morphine in mutant mice lacking $K_V1.1$ channels suggests a role of this subtype in the effect of this drug [13], although it is believed that opioids act more intensely via other types of K^+ channels (e.g., K_{ATP}, discussed below) [13].

Alternatively, voltage-activated K^+ channels can show a rapid inactivation when depolarization is sustained. These channels, in which activation produces transient outward currents, are called K^+_A channels (the current produced is called an A-current). According to Rasband et al. [88], small-diameter DRG neurons predominantly express A-type K^+ currents whose properties correspond to those expected for channels formed by $K_V1.4$ subunits. Three other transient K_V currents have been identified in small-diameter neurons [36]. Chronic inflammation increases the excitability of C fibers through the suppression of A-type K_V channels, which, together with channels formed by $K_V1.4$ subunits, are considered a major determinant of C-fiber excitability [88]. Moreover, homotetrameric $K_V1.4$ channels may contribute directly to regulating conduction in C fibers, which should be of special importance when considering pharmacological treatment of pain. In this sense, an alternative to reducing nociceptor excitability through the blockade of action potential depolarization, as achieved by the use of Na^+ antagonists, should lie in enhancing or prolonging the activity of $K_V1.4$. Neuronal homotetrameric $K_V1.4$ channels are thought to be unusual, because these channels exist primarily as heteromultimeric complexes in most other neurons [23,89], and thus an agonist specific for homotetrameric $K_V1.4$ channels would be expected to exhibit selectivity for small-diameter sensory neurons.

Calcium-Activated Potassium Channels

Calcium-activated K^+ channels were first described in neurons and are not as numerous as the K_V channels. They are classified into three families, according to their conductance properties, as large-conductance (BK), intermediate-conductance (IK), and small-conductance (SK) Ca^{2+}-activated K^+ channels [108]. A common characteristic of all Ca^{2+}-activated K^+ channels is that they are activated when the cytoplasmic concentration of Ca^{2+} is increased, although the BK channels are also voltage-sensitive [108]. Moreover, there are differences in the pharmacological modulation of the subtypes of these channels. The main pharmacological feature of BK channels is their sensitivity to charybdotoxin, a scorpion toxin (see Fig. 2 and Table I). This toxin also blocks other types of K^+ channels, such as IK and some K_V channels [12]. Besides charybdotoxin, iberiotoxin also inhibits BK currents, but in a more specific manner. Both charybdotoxin and iberiotoxin have been used to determine the role of BK channels in the antinociception induced by various drugs. Intracerebroventricular

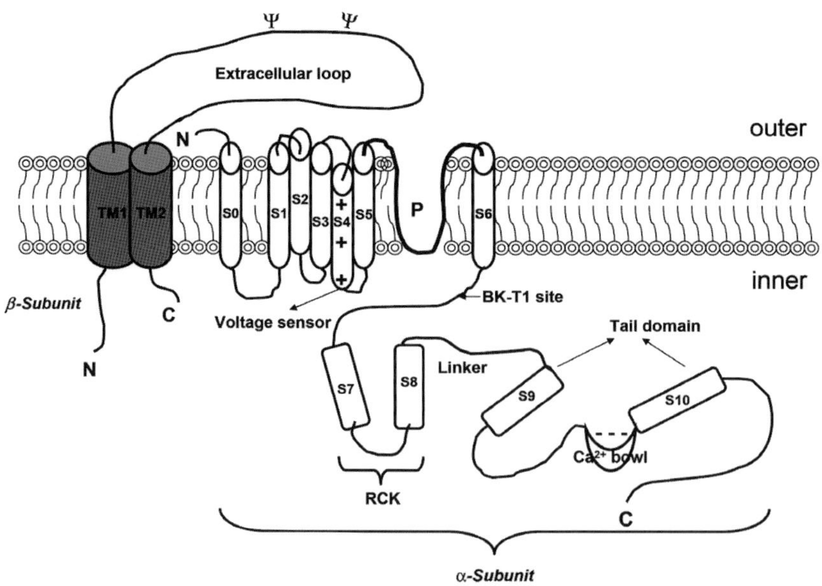

Fig. 2. Schematic representation of the structure of the α and β subunits of the BK (large-conductance Ca^{2+}-activated K^+) channel. The scheme shows the N-terminus, the S0–S6 domains, the pore region, the S7–S10 domains, the calcium bowl, and the long C-terminus of the α subunit and the TM1 and TM2 domains of the β subunit (after Ghatta et al. [34]).

(i.c.v.) injection of charybdotoxin prevents the antinociception mediated by tricyclic antidepressants [96]. On the other hand, endothelin-1 seems to increase the activity of BK channels at low concentrations (1 nM), while at high doses, it acts as a blocker.

Table I
Some agonists and antagonists of large-conductance Ca^{2+}-activated K^+ (BK) channels

	BK Channel Modulatory Molecules
Blockers	*Peptide blockers:* iberiotoxin, charybdotoxin, slotoxin *Nonpeptide blockers:* paxilline, penitrem, tetrandrine *Nonspecific blockers:* tetraethylammonium, tetrabutylammonium, clotrimazole, ruthenium red
Openers	NS004, NS619, NS8, and NS1608 Estradiol, dihydrosoyasaponin-I, maxikdiol, pimaric acid Flufenamic acid, mefenamic acid, niflumic acid

Source: Ghatta et al. [34].

Inwardly Rectifying Potassium Channels

Inwardly rectifying K^+ (K_{ir}) channels work exactly as their name states, rectifying the direction of the ion flux. In other words, the influx current becomes more intense than the efflux current. These channels used to be called "anomalous," because their properties contrast with the "normal" delayed-rectifying K^+ channels (the K_V channels). The function of the inward and outward currents is to keep the membrane potential within certain limits, thus preventing abrupt changes in the membrane charge.

The K_{ir} channels are numerous and comprise seven different families ($K_{ir}1$–$K_{ir}7$) [67]. Two of these families are particularly important for nociception: the G-protein-regulated inwardly rectifying K^+ channels (GIRK or $K_{ir}3$) and the adenosine triphosphate (ATP)-sensitive K^+ channels (K_{ATP} or $K_{ir}6$) (Fig. 3). The GIRK channels contain cytoplasmic structures that permit interaction with the G-βγ subunits of G proteins [92]. Also, this type of channel is blocked by tertiapin, a drug used in some experiments involving GIRK channels and nociception [59]

The K_{ATP} channels are found in muscles and neurons, as well as in β-pancreatic cells, where they regulate insulin release. They are composed of two subunits, the $K_{ir}6$ channel and the sulfonylurea receptor (SUR) subunit. Several subtypes of $K_{ir}6$ ($K_{ir}6.1$ and $K_{ir}6.2$) and SUR (SUR1, SUR2A, and SUR2B) have been identified. This diversity permits many combinations of subunits to constitute the functional K_{ATP} channels, which are tetramers of $K_{ir}6$-SUR complexes. The SUR subunit permits blockade of the K_{ATP} channels by sulfonylureas and their opening by several K_{ATP} openers, such as cromakalim, pinacidil, minoxidil, nicorandil, and diazoxide, and regulation of K_{ATP} channel activity by G proteins.

In fact, the K_{ATP} channels have been intensely studied because of the many lines of evidence pointing to their role in morphine-induced antinociception. The i.c.v. injection of specific K_{ATP} blockers, such as glibenclamide or tolbutamide, has been shown to

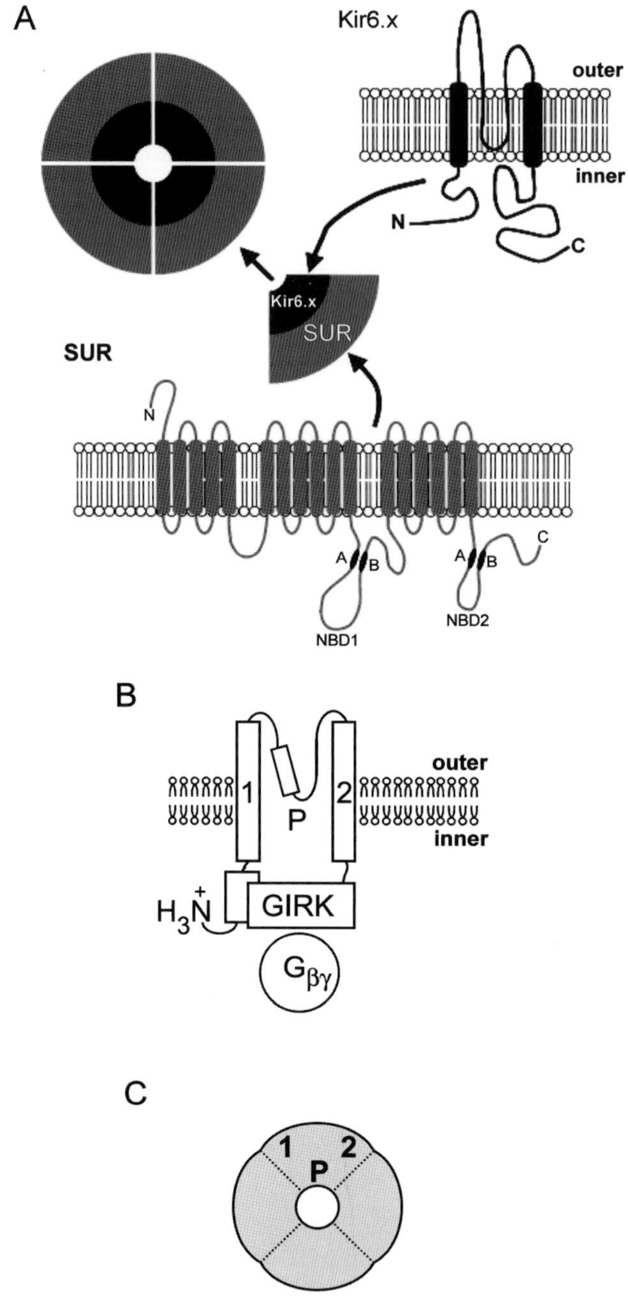

Fig. 3. Diagrammatic representation of the structure of (A) adenosine triphosphate (ATP)-sensitive and (B and C) G-protein-regulated inwardly rectifying (GIRK) potassium channels. (A) K_{ATP} channels are composed of two subunits: the sulfonylurea receptor (SUR) and the inwardly rectifying K^+ channel ($K_{ir}6.x$) in an octameric complex. The central four $K_{ir}6.x$ subunits form the pore through which K^+ ions move; the SURs are regulatory. Different forms of the subunits give different affinities for K^+ channel regulators (after Davies et al. [16]). (B) GIRK channels structure comprises only two transmembrane domains and a P-loop. The N and C termini are intracellular and contain domains that interact with the Gβγ subunits of G proteins, which regulate channel opening. (C) Schematic quaternary structure of the GIRK channels: the channel is a tetramer of α subunits (after Ocaña et al. [72]).

antagonize morphine-induced antinociception [71,73,90]. Moreover, according to many authors, opioid drugs, by activating metabotropic receptors, produce an inhibitory effect on cellular excitability, in part by activating $G_{i/o}$-protein-coupled K^+ channels, thereby hyperpolarizing the membrane potential.

When it was discovered that the endothelial relaxing factor was nitric oxide (NO), acting via the stimulation of guanylate cyclase, it had already been established that cyclic guanosine monophosphate (cGMP) could abolish ongoing hypernociception [29]. The effect of opioid drugs was shown to be inhibited by nonselective inhibitors of the enzyme NO synthase (L-NMMA), guanylate cyclase inhibitors, protein kinase G (PKG) inhibitors, and K^+_{ATP} channel blockers as well [21,26,94]. Furthermore, direct blockade of ongoing mechanical hyperalgesia has been observed after the administration of substances that stimulate neuronal soluble guanylate cyclase—NO donors (SNAP and sodium nitroprusside), or K^+_{ATP} channel openers (e.g., diazoxide). Thus, it was concluded that morphine analgesia was due to the stimulation of the arginine/NO/cGMP pathway.

These types of peripheral analgesics seem to act by restoring the activation threshold of nociceptors via an increase in K^+ permeability. In support of this idea, it was also demonstrated, by using patch-clamp electrophysiological recordings, that the activation of K^+_{ATP} channels reversed the sensitization produced by PGE_2 in DRG neurons [11]. Other anti-inflammatory analgesics and peripheral-acting agents have been described as acting by the same route, such as dipyrone, ketorolac, diclofenac, the κ-opioid agonist bremazocine, and agents such as sildenafil and *Crotalus durissus terrificus* venom [6,21,37,45,55,80,107].

KCNQ Potassium Channels

One family of K^+ channels that are known to regulate excitability in a variety of central and peripheral neurons are the M channels (K_M or K_V7) [61]. Also known as KCNQ channels, this family of K^+ channels stirred considerable interest because of certain peculiarities observed. For example, most of the KCNQ genes expressed have a clear physiological correlate, and it is the first K^+ channel family in which mutations have been directly linked to human diseases. Some pharmacological agents show selectivity for these currents and may represent novel clinically useful drugs.

The current produced by activation of KCNQ channels is called an M-current because it is blocked by muscarinic agonists [111]. Their activation in the subthreshold voltage range critically determines cellular excitability and responsiveness to synaptic inputs.

All KCNQ channels are voltage gated. Depolarization increases the probability of their opening, although other elements modulate the channels' response to voltage. For example, KCNQ1 current has been shown to be enhanced when intracellular cAMP levels are raised with forskolin [116]. In general, the expression of these channels induces outwardly rectifying voltage-dependent K^+ currents.

Heteromeric K^+ channels known as KCNQ2 and KCNQ3 seem to be exclusively expressed in the nervous system, with a high abundance in the cortical and hippocampal regions, as well as in the sympathetic ganglia and DRG. Their presence in sensory neurons has also been observed, indicating their importance in pain therapy. For instance, the anticonvulsant drug retigabine, which enhances the activity of these channels [17,41] can alleviate some forms of chronic pain [8]. In animal models, retigabine enhanced the activity of K_M and its respective subunits in the DRG of rats. In addition, this drug reduced electrophysiological and behavioral manifestations of enhanced nociceptive activity in experimental models of persistent, but not acute, pain. These findings suggest that this type of channel regulates the activity of nociceptive sensory neurons [57,76,93].

In pharmacological terms, a number of K^+ channel blockers have been tested on the KCNQ family. However, the drugs most often used to study these channels are retigabine and flupirtine (openers) and linopiridine and its analogues (blockers). Although retigabine is a derivative of the analgesic flupirtine, the pharmacological profiles of the two agents are different. Moreover, retigabine has antihyperalgesic properties: it inhibits the second phase of the formalin test, besides exerting a strong antiallodynic effect in models of neuropathy (chronic sciatic nerve constriction) [20].

Two-Pore-Domain Potassium Channels

A large number of this type of K^+ channels (K_{2P}) are described in the literature. The channels included in this family have some peculiarities that influence their properties in a unique manner. The alpha subunit that constitutes the K_{2P} contains two-pore-forming motifs linked in tandem, and that is why they are designated as such (Fig. 4B). Although many authors have studied the involvement of tandem-pore or two-pore domain K^+ channels in physiological processes, the pharmacological characteristics of these channels are not well known. In fact, their importance in physiological mechanisms is still emerging [77]. Moreover, the few existing studies that have shown their role in nociception have focused mainly on their role in the CNS.

These channels appear to be an ancient class of ion channels and have a wide distribution. Many authors have suggested a role for K_{2P} channels in the physiological actions of local anesthetics, in such a way that the local anesthetic inhibition of K_{2P} channels would block repolarization currents, delaying recovery of membrane potential after a depolarization and contributing to action potential prolongation. Recently, the complete family of K_{2P} channels has been identified in the human genome. This breakthrough may lead to a better understanding of how physiological actions of these channels can be modified by local anesthetic drugs to produce altered perception of painful stimuli.

It has also been demonstrated that K_{2P} channels are involved in the control of the resting membrane potential and the firing pattern of excitable cells. Hence, the two-pore-domain K^+ channels have emerged as possible substrates for the action of anesthetics such as halothane and isoflurane [78]. In this context, the subtypes TASK-1 and TASK-3 are of particular interest, because they contribute to resting K^+ currents in neurons that are potentially involved in the clinical effects of these drugs [99,112].

Other K_{2P} channels such as TREK-1 and TREK-2 participate in the CNS actions of general anesthetics. Possible roles for these channels in such actions have been investigated, and a number of K_{2P} channels that are not prominently expressed in the CNS are affected by clinically relevant doses of general anesthetics [77], thus contributing to some of their well-known peripheral effects. In addition, some of these channels are sensitive to the actions of local anesthetics and may participate in the clinical effects of these drugs [77].

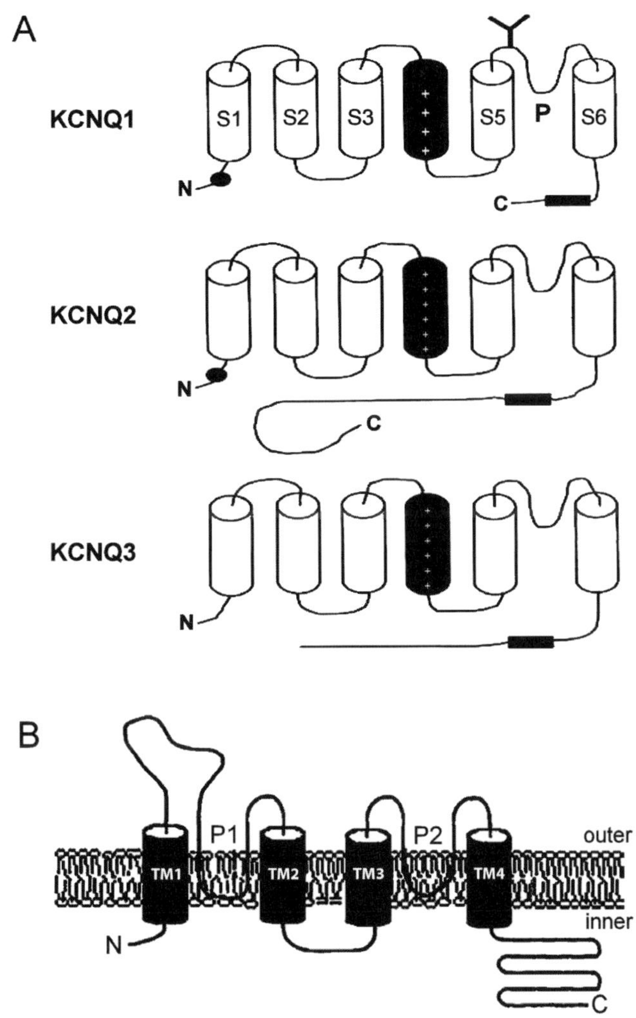

Fig. 4. (A) Structural characteristics of KCNQ K^+ channel 1, 2, and 3 subtypes. The six transmembrane domains (S1–S6) and the P-loop (P) indicated on KCNQ1 apply to the others. Glycosylation (Y), protein kinase A (PKA) phosphorylation (●), and A-domains (■) are also indicated. The length of the COOH terminus (C) is representative of the relative size of the different subunits. The numbers of charged residues (+) in the S4 domain are indicated (after Robbins [91]). (B) Predicted transmembrane topology of a mammalian K2P channel subunit. Transmembrane domains (TM1–TM4), pore regions (P1, P2), and the amino (N) and carboxyl (C) termini are shown (after Kindler and Yost [52]).

Role of Potassium Channels in Opioid Antinociception

Many studies performed with electrophysiological methods have demonstrated that agonists of μ- and δ-opioid receptors open K_{ir} channels in neurons through the activation of $G_{i/o}$ proteins [69]. According to several authors, these G proteins are able to open two different types of K_{ir} channels: K_{ATP}, the first one to be proposed to play a role in μ-opioid-induced antinociception [73,90], and GIRK, demonstrated to be important for the expression of the spinal antinociceptive effect of morphine [60]. Thus, these two types of K^+ channels have been involved in many studies on opioid-induced antinociception, where activation leads to cell membrane hyperpolarization [59]. In addition, morphine activates presynaptic opioid G-protein-coupled μ-opioid receptors or inhibits calcium currents, mainly those of N-type channels [98], thereby reducing neurotransmitter release (see Chapter 5 by Marvizon et al.).

A great number of studies have suggested that the opening of K_{ATP} channels plays an important role in the antinociception induced by morphine at the supraspinal, spinal, and peripheral (primary afferent nerve endings) levels. The opening of these channels by morphine could be due to its capacity to activate $G_{i/o}$ proteins, since both G_α and $G_{\beta\gamma}$ subunits of these proteins are able to activate K_{ATP} channels. Moreover, their activation was also demonstrated to be involved in the antinociception induced by δ-opioid agonists, although additional studies are needed to define the involvement of other K^+ channels in δ-opioid-receptor-mediated antinociception and to uncover the possible differences between the K^+ channels involved in the analgesic effect of agonists selective for the δ-opioid receptor subtype. On the other hand, some authors state that the opening of K_{ATP} channels does not play a role in the antinociceptive effect of agonists of κ-opioid receptors [66,79].

Role of Potassium Channels in Antinociception Induced by Other Drugs

For a long time, K_{ATP} channels were generally believed to be the main K^+ channel involved in antinociception. Demonstrations of their involvement in the effect of several drugs led to further investigations of the role of other subtypes in analgesia/antinociception. It was also observed that the activation of GIRK, K_V, or Ca^{2+}-activated K^+ channels was important for changes in nociceptive threshold. Peripherally mediated antinociception in rats induced by intraplantar administration of diclofenac or ketorolac was found to be antagonized by intraplantar injection of sulfonylureas, such as glibenclamide and tolbutamide [53,74]. However, using the inflammatory model of hyperalgesia induced by PGE_2, investigators obtained similar results with dipyrone and diclofenac [3,4]. In addition, peripheral administration of K_{ATP} openers such as pinacidil and diazoxide also produced antinociception that was blocked by sulfonylureas [4]. Taken together, these results suggest that the opening of K_{ATP} channels in peripheral neurons is important for the antinociceptive effect of several nonsteroidal anti-inflammatory drugs (NSAIDs). However, the role of other subtypes of K^+ channels needs to be investigated.

Blockers of K_V channels (4-AP, TEA) and of Ca^{2+}-activated K^+ channels (charybdotoxin, a BK blocker, and apamin, an SK blocker), when peripherally administered, were found to have an apparent effect on some NSAID-induced antinociception, although they were not able to alter the antinociception induced by dipyrone and indomethacin [3,74]. For instance, charybdotoxin antagonized the effect of diclofenac in the formalin test [74], but showed no effect in diclofenac-induced antinociception in PGE_2-induced inflammatory hypernociception [4].

Analgesics that owe their effects to activation of the NO pathway, which increases intracellular levels of cGMP, have also been demonstrated to induce the opening of K^+ channels [101]. The inhibition of antinociception induced by NO donors (such as sodium nitroprusside) or dibutyryl-cGMP (an analogue of cGMP) by sulfonylureas (glibenclamide or tolbutamide), and the potentiation of analgesia by K_{ATP} channel openers (such as diazoxide), have been found to be associated with this specific type of K^+ channel [5,101,102]. Together with data showing no changes in the antinociception induced by such drugs administered in combination with 4-AP or TEA (K_V blockers), or with charybdotoxin or apamin (Ca^{2+}-activated K^+ channel blockers), these findings confirm the important role of K_{ATP} in the antinociceptive effect induced by analgesics that act via the NO pathway. Moreover, the findings offer a mechanistic explanation for the differential involvement of K_{ATP} channels in the analgesia produced by some NSAIDs. This list includes dipyrone and diclofenac, and even cyclooxygenase-2 (COX-2)-specific inhibitors such as rofecoxib [3,18,53,74].

Similarly, some other types of drugs have been demonstrated to act via the activation of K^+ channels. Several tricyclic antidepressants and antihistamines specific for the H1 subtype of histamine receptor activate G-protein-coupled receptors, an effect related to their action on nociception [32,33]. Since the activation of many G-protein-coupled receptors produces antinociception through the opening of K^+ channels, it has been proposed that the analgesic effect of these drugs occurs via this mechanism. Peripheral administration (s.c.) of the tricyclic antidepressants amitriptyline or clomipramine was shown to induce antinociception in the hotplate test, which was antagonized by i.c.v. TEA and apamin, indicating an effect dependent on central K_V or SK channels [33].

Pyrilamine, diphenhydramine and promethazine, all H1-specific antagonists, were also demonstrated to show an effect dependent on K^+ channels, because they were sensitive to K^+ channel blockers, similar to the tricyclic antidepressants [32]. Moreover, as occurred with the latter drugs, their effect was potentiated by K^+ channel openers.

The antinociceptive effect of antiepileptic drugs has also been evaluated in terms of their actions on K^+ channels. The antiallodynic effect of intrathecal (i.t.) gabapentin, observed in a model of neuropathic pain induced by spinal nerve ligation, was antagonized by i.t. glibenclamide, apamin, or charybdotoxin [65]. These results suggest that gabapentin could act as an analgesic by opening K_{ATP}, SK, and BK channels.

Calcium Channels in Pain and Analgesia

Calcium ions (Ca^{2+}) play a pivotal role in mechanisms that control pain and antinociception [83]. The start and transmission of nociceptive impulses as well as the perception of pain are all influenced by changes in the intracellular concentration of Ca^{2+} [40], which also may occur in some painful pathological states [42]. The concentration of Ca^{2+} is normally much higher in the extracellular (1.5 mM) than in the intracellular (0.1 nM) medium. This steep gradient is due to the selective ion permeability of the cell membrane and to metabolic pumps that act to restore the original gradient whenever changes occur in the cytoplasmic Ca^{2+} concentration. A transient increase in cytoplasmic free Ca^{2+} concentration works as an intracellular signaling to trigger or regulate intracellular events such as muscle contraction, secretion of hormones, neurotransmitter release, cell differentiation, and gene expression.

Alternatively, cytoplasmic Ca^{2+} is taken up by Ca^{2+}-binding proteins or is sequestered by mitochondria or by the sarcoplasmic/endoplasmic reticulum via Ca^{2+}-ATPase or the plasma membrane Ca^{2+}-ATPase pump [109]. The influx of Ca^{2+} from the extracellular fluid involves voltage-operated Ca^{2+} channels (VOCCs), which are activated directly by depolarization of the cell membrane. Calcium ions can also enter cells through a ligand-operated ion channel (or second messenger-operated channel), usually a nonspecific cation channel that is able to produce a Ca^{2+}-mediated current. One subset of ligand-operated channels is represented by the receptor-operated channels, in which the ion channel and the receptor are one and the same molecular entity [46]. Calcium ions that enter the cytoplasm are extruded from the cell by Na^+/Ca^{2+} exchangers. Alternatively, cytoplasmic Ca^{2+} is taken up by Ca^{2+}-binding proteins or is sequestered by mitochondria or by the sarcoplasmic/endoplasmic reticulum via the intracellular sarcoplasmic/endoplasmic reticulum Ca^{2+}-ATPase or the plasma membrane Ca^{2+}-ATPase pump [109]. Free Ca^{2+} present in the sarcoplasmic/endoplasmic reticulum stores is released back to the cytoplasm via Ca^{2+} channels formed by inositol 1,4,5-trisphosphate (IP_3) receptors and ryanodine receptors, which are activated by IP_3 and cyclic adenosine diphosphate-ribose, respectively. The influx of Ca^{2+} inducing a further release of Ca^{2+} from internal stores via ryanodine receptors is a mechanism known as Ca^{2+}-induced Ca^{2+} release. A receptor-operated channel coupled to phospholipase C generates IP_3, which in turn mediates the discharge of Ca^{2+} from intracellular stores [85]. A decrease of Ca^{2+} in the sarcoplasmic/endoplasmic reticulum activates a subset of plasma membrane Ca^{2+} channels known as store-operated Ca^{2+} channels [86]. The retrograde process by which plasma membrane Ca^{2+} channels are signaled by the endoplasmic reticulum has been called "capacitative calcium entry," or "store-operated calcium entry" [85]. The capacitative Ca^{2+} entry provides prolonged and sustained elevation of intracellular Ca^{2+} concentration in order to maintain the constant amplitude of each spike in intracellular Ca^{2+} concentration [86].

Transient Receptor Potential Family

The transient receptor potential (TRP) family includes specific "pain receptors" necessary for the peripheral reception of nociceptive stimuli [14] (see Chapter 15 by Chung et al.). These receptors/channels are located on the cell membrane of nociceptive neurons as well as in membranes of intracellular Ca^{2+} stores such as the endoplasmic reticulum. An increase in intracellular Ca^{2+} activates protein kinase C and calcium/calmodulin-dependent protein kinase II. Bradykinin excites sensory neurons, activating the capsaicin receptor (TRPV1) via phospholipase A_2 and the lipoxygenase cascade in sensory neurons [54]. Bradykinin also activates protein kinase C, resulting in the phosphorylation of TRPV1 and sensitization [49]. Sensitization occurs in damaged and surrounding intact axons and in the cell body, during the course of a neuropathy [82]. TRPA1 channels have been demonstrated in many cell types, including sensory neurons that detect noxious cold temperatures, resulting in the perception of a "burning" pain [7]. Most TRP channels are nonselective cation channels with variable permeability to Ca^{2+}. They serve as sensors for various stimuli, including noxious ones [54].

Voltage-Operated Calcium Channels

The voltage-operated Ca^{2+} channels (VOCCs) are complex proteins composed of a single α_1 subunit, together with several other $\alpha_2\delta$, β, and γ auxiliary subunits that modulate the expression of the α_1 subunit, which is organized in four repeat domains, known as domains I–IV, each with a six-transmembrane helical structure [38] (Fig. 5).

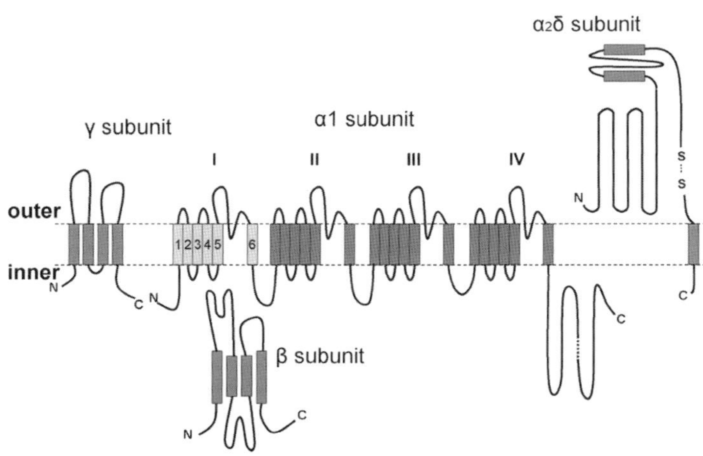

Fig. 5. Schematic representation of the subunit structure of voltage-operated calcium channels. The pore-forming α_1 subunit has I–IV domains of six transmembrane segments each. Segment 4 is responsible for voltage dependence; segments 5 and 6 represent the pore region. Modified from Gribkoff [38].

At least five VOCCs have been described, differing in their gating kinetics, mode of inactivation, regulation by Ca^{2+}, and sensitivity to toxins [10]. The VOCCs are classified according to their voltages of activation as low-threshold T-type or high-threshold L, N, P/Q, and R channels. The VOCCs are also classified in subfamilies on the basis of their structural similarity of the pore-forming α_1 subunit and pharmacological characteristics: $Ca_V1.1–1.4$ (L-type), $Ca_V2.1–2.3$ (P/Q, N and R-type), and $Ca_V3.1–3.3$ (T-type). Associated with this major subunit are $\alpha_2\delta$-1–4, β-1–4, and γ-1–8 subunits. Ten different α_1 subunits have been discovered and are classified as L (α_{1S}, α_{1C}, α_{1D}, and α_{1F}), P/Q (α_{1A}), N (α_{1B}), R (α_{1E}), and T (α_{1G}, α_{1H}, and α_{1I}) types. Neurons often express all types of VOCC, but the presynaptic Ca^{2+} influx compulsory for exocytosis is associated mainly with the P/Q- and N-types (Table II).

Table II
Subtype classification of voltage-operated calcium channels

Channel	Current	Localization	Functions
Cav1.1	L	Skeletal muscle; transverse tubules	Excitation-contraction coupling
Cav1.2	L	Cardiac and smooth muscle myocytes; endocrine cells; neuronal cell bodies and proximal dendrites	Excitation-contraction coupling; hormone release; regulation of transcription; synaptic integration
Cav1.3	L	Neuronal cell bodies and dendrites; endocrine cells; cardiac atrial myocytes and pacemaker cells; cochlear hair cells	Hormone release; cardiac pacemaking; hearing; neuro-transmitter release from sensory cells
Cav1.4	L	Retinal cells; spinal cord; adrenals; mast cells	Neurotransmitter release from photoreceptors
Cav2.1	P/Q	Nerve terminals and dendrites; neuroendocrine cells	Neurotransmitter release; hormone release
Cav2.2	N	Nerve terminals and dendrites; neuroendocrine cells	Neurotransmitter release; hormone release
Cav2.3	R	Neuronal cell bodies and dendrites	Repetitive firing; dendritic calcium transients
Cav3.1	T	Neuronal cell bodies and dendrites; cardiac and smooth muscle myocytes	Pacemaking; repetitive firing
Cav3.2	T	Neuronal cell bodies and dendrites; cardiac and smooth muscle myocytes	Pacemaking; repetitive firing
Cav3.3	T	Neuronal cell bodies and dendrites	Pacemaking; repetitive firing

In sensory neurons, nociceptive neurotransmitters such as substance P and calcitonin gene-related peptide are released upon activation of L-, N-, and P/Q-type Ca^{2+} channels [54]. Cell bodies of sensory neurons in the DRG express L- and N-type (all neurons), P/Q-type (few neurons), and T-type (primarily in nociceptive neurons) channels [104].

Each VOCC is subject to modulation and may be changed by the biochemical environment in which the channel is immersed, or in response to injury and disease [114]. Mutations in proteins of the membrane channels responsible for the influx of Ca^{2+} ions have allowed researchers to determine which channels are linked to human disease. Sciatic nerve ligature increases the protein and mRNA levels of $\alpha_2\delta$-1 subunit in the spinal cord and DRG, respectively, providing evidence for a peripheral injury-induced upregulation of the $\alpha_2\delta$ subunit in primary afferent terminals. Also, a reduction in the Ca^{2+} signal in axotomized neurons may be due to a certain extent to the loss of Ca^{2+} influx through voltage-gated Ca^{2+} channels. These changes in the critical Ca^{2+} signal may mediate various injury-related abnormalities in Ca^{2+}-dependent neuronal functions. The L-type and T-type currents are both reduced in nociceptive sensory neurons after chronic constriction injury of the sciatic nerve [43,62]. In contrast, the N-type calcium channel is upregulated in injured DRG. A marked upregulation of the $\alpha_2\delta$-1 subunit in rat DRG and in spinal dorsal horn has been demonstrated in some models of neuropathy but not in others, thus suggesting an injury type-specific regulation of the subunit.

The participation of L-type Ca^{2+} channels in nociception depends on the drug, dosage, and route of administration. Nifedipine inhibits the release of substance P induced in inflammatory processes [87], and verapamil reduces mechanical and thermal pain. After a nerve dissection, gene expression of α_{1C}, α_{1D}, α_{1H}, and α_{1I} in the correspondent dorsal ganglia is downregulated after about 7 days [51]. Antagonists of L-type channels also produce analgesia in models of noxious thermal and mechanical stimuli, but they are frequently very weak in models of phasic pain or when used for the management of postoperative pain [83].

The N-type channels have generated increased interest with regard to nociception and are now generally considered to be the major VOCC in nociceptors. The N-type calcium channels are expressed in neuronal tissue, and their expression is particularly high in the superficial layer of the dorsal horn. Blockers of N-type channels stop the release of neuropeptides such as substance P [100]. Lastly, knockout mice that lack the gene that encodes the N-type Ca^{2+} channel are less sensitive to neuropathic and inflammatory pain, compared to wild-type mice, despite being otherwise normal [94]. Pain states are characterized by high discharge frequencies in neurons of nociceptive pathways, including those in the DRG, where N-type channels are typically activated by high-frequency depolarization. In addition, the intrathecal administration of specific N-type calcium channel blockers such as ω-conotoxin MVIIA or ω-conotoxin GVIA (isolated from the venom of the cone snails *Conus magus* and *C. geographus*, respectively) reduces inflammation-induced hyperalgesia and neuropathic pain and reduces the spontaneous ectopic firing in the DRG 7–14 days after the experimental neuronal damage [2]. These findings suggest that the N-type Ca^{2+} channel mediates nociception in the spinal cord. The peptide ω-conotoxin MVIIA is also known as ziconotide. Used intrathecally, this drug induces antinociception and reduces tactile allodynia, and it was recently approved by the U.S. FDA for managing neuropathic pain [114]. Ziconotide is also effective for the management of cancer pain, but its side effects require intrathecal delivery, which limits its usefulness [114].

The blockade of P/Q-type channels with intrathecal ω-agatoxin IVA does not change the mechanical allodynia in an animal neuropathic pain model. On the other hand, the P/Q- type channels have been implicated in the physiopathology of familiar hemiplegic migraine [114].

The literature has provided evidence for the involvement of T-type channels in nociception. The intravenous injection of mibefradil, a partial blocker of T-type channels, has been shown to induce analgesia [106], whereas α_{1G}-deficient mice displayed hyperalgesic responses in the writhing test [51]. Mibefradil was also demonstrated to prevent the hyperalgesia induced by the intraplantar injection of reducing agents such a dithiothreitol or L-cysteine [105]. The intraperitoneal administration of ethosuximide, a T-type channel blocker, abolished the hyperalgesia and the mechanical and thermal allodynia induced in rats by paclitaxel [31], an antineoplastic agent that promotes peripheral neuropathy in rats [97].

T-type channels regulate cellular excitability and rhythmic activity. Originally, they were found in small sensory neurons, in small and medium-sized DRG neurons, and in neurons of the spinal dorsal horn lamina I. Spinal motor neurons do not express T-type channels, and thus the blockade of these channels may suppress nociception without alteration of other modalities of sensory transmission or motor function [103]. Intrathecal injection of antisense oligonucleotides for the T-type channel may result in analgesic or hyperalgesic effects [115]. The T-type channels that are pronociceptive are likely to be either $Ca_V3.2$ or $Ca_V3.3$ subtypes. Thus, the challenge for drug development is to design T-type Ca_V2C-channel blockers with selective $Ca_V3.2$-channel-blocking activity.

Gabapentin and pregabalin are effective in neuropathic pain management [16]. Intrathecal gabapentin abolishes the sciatic nerve ligature-induced decrease in the latency of paw withdrawal against thermal or tactile stimulation in mice. Gabapentin reduces Ca^{2+} currents in DRG neurons and synaptosomes, and it inhibits the release of excitatory amino acids in neocortical slices. These agents are not Ca^{2+} channel blockers, but they may reduce transmitter release following binding to the accessory $\alpha_2\delta$-1 subunit [31]. The $\alpha_2\delta$-1 subunit is upregulated in nociceptor terminals after peripheral axonal injury, and evidence suggests a common role of T-type Ca^{2+} channels and $\alpha_2\delta$-1 subunits in the perception of neuropathic pain. Gabapentin suppresses KCl-induced extracellular Ca^{2+} influx, but not IP_3-induced intracellular Ca^{2+} release in cultured spinal neurons [63]. The most prominent effect of gabapentin involves the inhibition of N-type Ca^{2+} currents in DRG neurons, which accounts for the clinical efficacy of this drug against neuropathic pain.

Conclusions

What we have learned in the last few years is that in various pain scenarios, the final actors are always the ion channels. They contribute to our present understanding of the perception of nociceptive sensations. It has not escaped our attention that the stimulus that induces nociceptive perceptions can originate in the CNS, i.e., it can be psychogenic in nature. Possibly the difficulties that arise in the treatment of some patients with chronic pain may be due to a considerable contribution of this type of stimulus, as indicated by the positive effect of some antidepressants. At present, the key mechanism of useful analgesics is their action on the disrupted function of ion channels (K^+, Ca^{2+}, or Na^+). In this way, these drugs help to restore the normal physiological functioning of the cells (by restoring their threshold) or the neuronal system involved (by normalizing the release of neuronal mediators).

Acknowledgments

We thank Mrs. Vanessa Rinhel Del Bem Mariotto for expert assistance with the manuscript.

References

[1] Aantaa R, Marjamaki A, Scheinin M. Molecular pharmacology of alpha 2-adrenoceptor subtypes. Ann Med 1995;27:439–49.
[2] Altier C, Zamponi GW. Targeting Ca^{2+} channels to treat pain: T-type versus N-type. Trends Pharmacol Sci 2004;25:465–70.
[3] Alves D, Duarte I. Involvement of ATP-sensitive K^+ channels in the peripheral antinociceptive effect induced by dipyrone. Eur J Pharmacol 2002;444:47–52.
[4] Alves DP, Soares AC, Francischi JN, Castro MS, Perez AC, Duarte ID. Additive antinociceptive effect of the combination of diazoxide, an activator of ATP-sensitive K^+ channels, and sodium nitroprusside and dibutyryl-cGMP. Eur J Pharmacol 2004;489:59–65.
[5] Alves DP, Tatsuo MA, Leite R, Duarte ID. Diclofenac-induced peripheral antinociception is associated with ATP-sensitive K^+ channel activation. Life Sci 2004;74:2577–91.
[6] Amarante LH, Duarte ID. The kappa-opioid agonist (+/-)-bremazocine elicits peripheral antinociception by activation of the L-arginine/nitric oxide/cyclic GMP pathway. Eur J Pharmacol 2002;454:19–23.
[7] Bandell M, Story GM, Hwang SW, Viswanath V, Eid SR, Petrus MJ, Earley TJ, Patapoutian A. Noxious cold ion channel TRPA1 is activated by pungent compounds and bradykinin. Neuron 2004;41:849–57.
[8] Blackburn-Munro G, Jensen BS. The anticonvulsant retigabine attenuates nociceptive behaviours in rat models of persistent and neuropathic pain. Eur J Pharmacol 2003;460:109–16.
[9] Boland LM, Jackson KA. Protein kinase C inhibits Kv1.1 potassium channel function. Am J Physiol 1999;277:C100–10.
[10] Catterall WA, Perez-Reyes E, Snutch TP, Striessnig J. International Union of Pharmacology. XLVIII. Nomenclature and structure-function relationships of voltage-gated calcium channels. Pharmacol Rev 2005;57:411–25.
[11] Chi XX, Jiang X, Nicol GD. ATP-sensitive potassium currents reduce the PGE2-mediated enhancement of excitability in adult rat sensory neurons. Brain Res 2007;1145:28–40.
[12] Christie MJ, Adelman JP, Douglass J, North RA. Expression of a cloned rat brain potassium channel in *Xenopus* oocytes. Science 1989;244:221–4.
[13] Clark JD, Tempel BL. Hyperalgesia in mice lacking the Kv1.1 potassium channel gene. Neurosci Lett 1998;251:121–4.
[14] Cortright DN, Krause JE, Broom DC. TRP channels and pain. Biochim Biophys Acta 2007;1772:978–88.
[15] Cunha FQ, Teixeira MM, Ferreira SH. Pharmacological modulation of secondary mediator systems—cyclic AMP and cyclic GMP—on inflammatory hyperalgesia. Br J Pharmacol 1999;127:671–8.
[16] Davies A, Hendrich J, Van Minh AT, Wratten J, Douglas L, Dolphin AC. Functional biology of the alpha$_2$delta subunits of voltage-gated calcium channels. Trends Pharmacol Sci 2007;28:220–8.
[17] De SG, Di Paola ED, Conte G, Pasculli MP, De SA. Influence of retigabine on the anticonvulsant activity of some antiepileptic drugs against audiogenic seizures in DBA/2 mice. Naunyn Schmiedebergs Arch Pharmacol 2001;363:330–6.
[18] Deciga-Campos M, Lopez-Munoz FJ. Participation of the L-arginine-nitric oxide-cyclic GMP-ATP-sensitive K^+ channel cascade in the antinociceptive effect of rofecoxib. Eur J Pharmacol 2004;484:193–9.
[19] Djouhri L, Koutsikou S, Fang X, McMullan S, Lawson SN. Spontaneous pain, both neuropathic and inflammatory, is related to frequency of spontaneous firing in intact C-fiber nociceptors. J Neurosci 2006;26:1281–92.
[20] Dost R, Rostock A, Rundfeldt C. The anti-hyperalgesic activity of retigabine is mediated by KCNQ potassium channel activation. Naunyn Schmiedebergs Arch Pharmacol 2004;369:382–90.
[21] Duarte ID, dos S, I, Lorenzetti BB, Ferreira SH. Analgesia by direct antagonism of nociceptor sensitization involves the arginine-nitric oxide-cGMP pathway. Eur J Pharmacol 1992;217:225–7.
[22] England S, Bevan S, Docherty RJ. PGE2 modulates the tetrodotoxin-resistant sodium current in neonatal rat dorsal root ganglion neurones via the cyclic AMP-protein kinase A cascade. J Physiol 1996;495(Pt 2):429–40.
[23] Felix JP, Bugianesi RM, Schmalhofer WA, Borris R, Goetz MA, Hensens OD, Bao JM, Kayser F, Parsons WH, Rupprecht K, Garcia ML, Kaczorowski GJ, Slaughter RS. Identification and biochemical characterization of a novel nortriterpene inhibitor of the human lymphocyte voltage-gated potassium channel, Kv1.3. Biochemistry 1999;38:4922–30.
[24] Ferreira SH. Local analgesic effect of morphine on the hyperalgesia induced by cAMP, Ca^{2+}, isoprenaline, and PGE_2. Adv Prostaglandin Thromboxane Res 1980;8:1207–15.
[25] Ferreira SH, Cunha FQ, Lorenzetti BB, Michelin MA, Perretti M, Flower RJ, Poole S. Role of lipocortin-1 in the antihyperalgesic actions of dexamethasone. Br J Pharmacol 1997;121:883–8.
[26] Ferreira SH, Duarte ID, Lorenzetti BB. The molecular mechanism of action of peripheral morphine analgesia: stimulation of the cGMP system via nitric oxide release. Eur J Pharmacol 1991;201:121–2.
[27] Ferreira SH, Lorenzetti BB. Glutamate spinal retrograde sensitization of primary sensory neurons associated with nociception. Neuropharmacology 1994;33:1479–85.
[28] Ferreira SH, Lorenzetti BB. Intrathecal administration of prostaglandin E2 causes sensitization of the primary afferent neuron via the spinal release of glutamate. Inflamm Res 1996;45:499–502.

[29] Ferreira SH, Nakamura M. I - Prostaglandin hyperalgesia, a cAMP/Ca^{2+} dependent process. Prostaglandins 1979;18:179–90.
[30] Ferreira SH, Nakamura M. II - Prostaglandin hyperalgesia: the peripheral analgesic activity of morphine, enkephalins and opioid antagonists. Prostaglandins 1979;18:191–200.
[31] Flatters SJ, Bennett GJ. Ethosuximide reverses paclitaxel- and vincristine-induced painful peripheral neuropathy. Pain 2004;109:150–61.
[32] Galeotti N, Ghelardini C, Bartolini A. The role of potassium channels in antihistamine analgesia. Neuropharmacology 1999;38:1893–1901.
[33] Galeotti N, Ghelardini C, Bartolini A. Involvement of potassium channels in amitriptyline and clomipramine analgesia. Neuropharmacology 2001;40:75–84.
[34] Ghatta S, Nimmagadda D, Xu X, O'Rourke ST. Large-conductance, calcium-activated potassium channels: structural and functional implications. Pharmacol Ther 2006;110:103–16.
[35] Gold MS, Levine JD, Correa AM. Modulation of TTX-R INa by PKC and PKA and their role in PGE_2-induced sensitization of rat sensory neurons in vitro. J Neurosci 1998;18:10345–55.
[36] Gold MS, Shuster MJ, Levine JD. Characterization of six voltage-gated K^+ currents in adult rat sensory neurons. J Neurophysiol 1996;75:2629–46.
[37] Granados-Soto V, Flores-Murrieta FJ, Castaneda-Hernandez G, Lopez-Munoz FJ. Evidence for the involvement of nitric oxide in the antinociceptive effect of ketorolac. Eur J Pharmacol 1995;277:281–4.
[38] Gribkoff VK. The role of voltage-gated calcium channels in pain and nociception. Semin Cell Dev Biol 2006;17:555–64.
[39] Gutman GA, Chandy KG, Adelman JP, Aiyar J, Bayliss DA, Clapham DE, Covarriubias M, Desir GV, Furuichi K, Ganetzky B, et al. International Union of Pharmacology. XLI. Compendium of voltage-gated ion channels: potassium channels. Pharmacol Rev 2003;55:583–6.
[40] Hagenacker T, Ledwig D, Busselberg D. Feedback mechanisms in the regulation of intracellular calcium ([Ca^{2+}]i) in the peripheral nociceptive system: role of TRPV-1 and pain related receptors. Cell Calcium 2008;43:215–27.
[41] Hetka R, Rundfeldt C, Heinemann U, Schmitz D. Retigabine strongly reduces repetitive firing in rat entorhinal cortex. Eur J Pharmacol 1999;386:165–71.
[42] Hilaire C, Inquimbert P, Al-Jumaily M, Greuet D, Valmier J, Scamps F. Calcium dependence of axotomized sensory neurons excitability. Neurosci Lett 2005;380:330–34.
[43] Hogan QH, McCallum JB, Sarantopoulos C, Aason M, Mynlieff M, Kwok WM, Bosnjak ZJ. Painful neuropathy decreases membrane calcium current in mammalian primary afferent neurons. Pain 2000;86:43–53.
[44] Hokfelt T, Zhang X, Wiesenfeld-Hallin Z. Messenger plasticity in primary sensory neurons following axotomy and its functional implications. Trends Neurosci 1994;17:22–30.
[45] Jain NK, Patil CS, Singh A, Kulkarni SK. Sildenafil-induced peripheral analgesia and activation of the nitric oxide-cyclic GMP pathway. Brain Res 2001;909:170–8.
[46] Janssen LJ, Kwan CY. ROCs and SOCs: what's in a name? Cell Calcium 2007;41:245–7.
[47] Ji RR, Samad TA, Jin SX, Schmoll R, Woolf CJ. p38 MAPK activation by NGF in primary sensory neurons after inflammation increases TRPV1 levels and maintains heat hyperalgesia. Neuron 2002;36:57–68.
[48] Jiang X, Zhang YH, Clark JD, Tempel BL, Nicol GD. Prostaglandin E2 inhibits the potassium current in sensory neurons from hyperalgesic Kv1.1 knockout mice. Neuroscience 2003;119:65–72.
[49] Julius D, Basbaum AI. Molecular mechanisms of nociception. Nature 2001;413:203–10.
[50] Kaczorowski GJ, Garcia ML. Pharmacology of voltage-gated and calcium-activated potassium channels. Curr Opin Chem Biol 1999;3:448–58.
[51] Kim DS, Yoon CH, Lee SJ, Park SY, Yoo HJ, Cho HJ. Changes in voltage-gated calcium channel alpha(1) gene expression in rat dorsal root ganglia following peripheral nerve injury. Brain Res Mol Brain Res 2001;96:151–6.
[52] Kindler CH, Yost CS. Two-pore domain potassium channels: new sites of local anesthetic action and toxicity. Reg Anesth Pain Med 2005;30:260–74.
[53] Lazaro-Ibanez GG, Torres-Lopez JE, Granados-Soto V. Participation of the nitric oxide-cyclic GMP-ATP-sensitive K^+ channel pathway in the antinociceptive action of ketorolac. Eur J Pharmacol 2001;426:39–44.
[54] Lee Y, Lee CH, Oh U. Painful channels in sensory neurons. Mol Cells 2005;20:315–24.
[55] Lorenzetti BB, Ferreira SH. Activation of the arginine-nitric oxide pathway in primary sensory neurons contributes to dipyrone-induced spinal and peripheral analgesia. Inflamm Res 1996;45:308–11.
[56] MacKinnon R. Potassium channels. FEBS Lett 2003;555:62–5.
[57] Main MJ, Cryan JE, Dupere JR, Cox B, Clare JJ, Burbidge SA. Modulation of KCNQ2/3 potassium channels by the novel anticonvulsant retigabine. Mol Pharmacol 2000;58:253–62.
[58] Mannion RJ, Costigan M, Decosterd I, Amaya F, Ma QP, Holstege JC, Ji RR, Acheson A, Lindsay RM, Wilkinson GA, Woolf CJ. Neurotrophins: peripherally and centrally acting modulators of tactile stimulus-induced inflammatory pain hypersensitivity. Proc Natl Acad Sci USA 1999;96:9385–90.
[59] Marker CL, Lujan R, Loh HH, Wickman K. Spinal G-protein-gated potassium channels contribute in a dose-dependent manner to the analgesic effect of mu- and delta- but not kappa-opioids. J Neurosci 2005;25:3551–9.
[60] Marker CL, Stoffel M, Wickman K. Spinal G-protein-gated K^+ channels formed by GIRK1 and GIRK2 subunits modulate thermal nociception and contribute to morphine analgesia. J Neurosci 2004;24:2806–12.
[61] Marrion NV. Control of M-current. Annu Rev Physiol 1997;59:483–504.
[62] McCallum JB, Kwok WM, Mynlieff M, Bosnjak ZJ, Hogan QH. Loss of T-type calcium current in sensory neurons of rats with neuropathic pain. Anesthesiology 2003;98:209–16.
[63] McClelland D, Evans RM, Barkworth L, Martin DJ, Scott RH. A study comparing the actions of gabapentin and pregabalin on the electrophysiological properties of cultured DRG neurones from neonatal rats. BMC Pharmacol 2004;4:14.

[64] McMahon S, Koltzenburg M. The changing role of primary afferent neurones in pain. Pain 1990;43:269–72.
[65] Mixcoatl-Zecuatl T, Medina-Santillan R, Reyes-Garcia G, Vidal-Cantu GC, Granados-Soto V. Effect of K^+ channel modulators on the antiallodynic effect of gabapentin. Eur J Pharmacol 2004;484:201–8.
[66] Narita M, Suzuki T, Misawa M, Nagase H. Role of central ATP-sensitive potassium channels in the hyperthermic effect of morphine in mice. Psychopharmacology (Berl) 1992;109:239–40.
[67] Nichols CG, Lopatin AN. Inward rectifier potassium channels. Annu Rev Physiol 1997;59:171–91.
[68] Nicol GD, Vasko MR, Evans AR. Prostaglandins suppress an outward potassium current in embryonic rat sensory neurons. J Neurophysiol 1997;77:167–76.
[69] North RA. Twelfth Gaddum memorial lecture. Drug receptors and the inhibition of nerve cells. Br J Pharmacol 1989;98:13–28.
[70] Novakovic SD, Tzoumaka E, McGivern JG, Haraguchi M, Sangameswaran L, Gogas KR, Eglen RM, Hunter JC. Distribution of the tetrodotoxin-resistant sodium channel PN3 in rat sensory neurons in normal and neuropathic conditions. J Neurosci 1998;18:2174–87.
[71] Ocana M, Baeyens JM. Differential effects of K^+ channel blockers on antinociception induced by alpha 2-adrenoceptor, $GABA_B$ and kappa-opioid receptor agonists. Br J Pharmacol 1993;110:1049–54.
[72] Ocana M, Cendan CM, Cobos EJ, Entrena JM, Baeyens JM. Potassium channels and pain: present realities and future opportunities. Eur J Pharmacol 2004;500:203–19.
[73] Ocana M, Del PE, Barrios M, Robles LI, Baeyens JM. An ATP-dependent potassium channel blocker antagonizes morphine analgesia. Eur J Pharmacol 1990;186:377–8.
[74] Ortiz MI, Granados-Soto V, Castaneda-Hernandez G. The NO-cGMP-K^+ channel pathway participates in the antinociceptive effect of diclofenac, but not of indomethacin. Pharmacol Biochem Behav 2003;76:187–95.
[75] Parada CA, Vivancos GG, Tambeli CH, Cunha FQ, Ferreira SH. Activation of presynaptic NMDA receptors coupled to Na_V1.8-resistant sodium channel C-fibers causes retrograde mechanical nociceptor sensitization. Proc Natl Acad Sci USA 2003;100:2923–8.
[76] Passmore GM, Selyanko AA, Mistry M, Al-Qatari M, Marsh SJ, Matthews EA, Dickenson AH, Brown TA, Burbidge SA, Main M, Brown DA. KCNQ/M currents in sensory neurons: significance for pain therapy. J Neurosci 2003;23:7227–36.
[77] Patel AJ, Honore E. Anesthetic-sensitive 2P domain K^+ channels. Anesthesiology 2001;95:1013–21.
[78] Patel AJ, Honore E, Lesage F, Fink M, Romey G, Lazdunski M. Inhalational anesthetics activate two-pore-domain background K^+ channels. Nat Neurosci 1999;2:422–6.
[79] Picolo G, Cassola AC, Cury Y. Activation of peripheral ATP-sensitive K^+ channels mediates the antinociceptive effect of *Crotalus durissus terrificus* snake venom. Eur J Pharmacol 2003;469:57–64.
[80] Picolo G, Giorgi R, Cury Y. Delta-opioid receptors and nitric oxide mediate the analgesic effect of *Crotalus durissus terrificus* snake venom. Eur J Pharmacol 2000;391:55–62.
[81] Pischalnikova AV, Sokolova OS. The domain and conformational organization in potassium voltage-gated ion channels. J Neuroimmune Pharmacol 2009;4:71–82.
[82] Porreca F, Lai J, Bian D, Wegert S, Ossipov MH, Eglen RM, Kassotakis L, Novakovic S, Rabert DK, Sangameswaran L, Hunter JC. A comparison of the potential role of the tetrodotoxin-insensitive sodium channels, PN3/SNS and NaN/SNS2, in rat models of chronic pain. Proc Natl Acad Sci USA 1999;96:7640–4.
[83] Prado WA. Involvement of calcium in pain and antinociception. Braz J Med Biol Res 2001;34:449–61.
[84] Puehler W, Zollner C, Brack A, Shaqura MA, Krause H, Schafer M, Stein C. Rapid upregulation of mu opioid receptor mRNA in dorsal root ganglia in response to peripheral inflammation depends on neuronal conduction. Neuroscience 2004;129:473–9.
[85] Putney JW Jr. Pharmacology of capacitative calcium entry. Mol Interv 2001;1:84–94.
[86] Putney JW, Bird GS. Cytoplasmic calcium oscillations and store-operated calcium influx. J Physiol 2008;586:3055–9.
[87] Rane SG, Holz GG, Dunlap K. Dihydropyridine inhibition of neuronal calcium current and substance P release. Pflugers Arch 1987;409:361–6.
[88] Rasband MN, Park EW, Vanderah TW, Lai J, Porreca F, Trimmer JS. Distinct potassium channels on pain-sensing neurons. Proc Natl Acad Sci USA 2001;98:13373–8.
[89] Rhodes KJ, Strassle BW, Monaghan MM, Bekele-Arcuri Z, Matos MF, Trimmer JS. Association and colocalization of the Kvbeta1 and Kvbeta2 beta-subunits with Kv1 alpha-subunits in mammalian brain K^+ channel complexes. J Neurosci 1997;17:8246–58.
[90] Roane DS, Boyd NE. Reduction of food intake and morphine analgesia by central glybenclamide. Pharmacol Biochem Behav 1993;46:205–7.
[91] Robbins J. KCNQ potassium channels: physiology, pathophysiology, and pharmacology. Pharmacol Ther 2001;90:1–19.
[92] Roosild TP, Le KT, Choe S. Cytoplasmic gatekeepers of K^+-channel flux: a structural perspective. Trends Biochem Sci 2004;29:39–45.
[93] Rundfeldt C, Netzer R. The novel anticonvulsant retigabine activates M-currents in Chinese hamster ovary-cells tranfected with human KCNQ2/3 subunits. Neurosci Lett 2000;282:73–6.
[94] Saegusa H, Kurihara T, Zong S, Kazuno A, Matsuda Y, Nonaka T, Han W, Toriyama H, Tanabe T. Suppression of inflammatory and neuropathic pain symptoms in mice lacking the N-type Ca^{2+} channel. EMBO J 2001;20:2349–56.
[95] Schaible HG, Schmidt RF. Time course of mechanosensitivity changes in articular afferents during a developing experimental arthritis. J Neurophysiol 1988;60:2180–95.
[96] Schroder W. Potassium Channels. In: Buschmann H, Bahrenberg G, editors. Analgesics: from chemistry and pharmacology to clinical application. Berlin: Wiley-VCH, 2002. p. 333–52.
[97] Scripture CD, Figg WD, Sparreboom A. Peripheral neuropathy induced by paclitaxel: recent insights and future perspectives. Curr Neuropharmacol 2006;4:165–72.

[98] Seward E, Hammond C, Henderson G. Mu-opioid-receptor-mediated inhibition of the N-type calcium-channel current. Proc Biol Sci 1991;244:129–35.
[99] Sirois JE, Lei Q, Talley EM, Lynch C, III, Bayliss DA. The TASK-1 two-pore domain K^+ channel is a molecular substrate for neuronal effects of inhalation anesthetics. J Neurosci 2000;20:6347–54.
[100] Smith MT, Cabot PJ, Ross FB, Robertson AD, Lewis RJ. The novel N-type calcium channel blocker, AM336, produces potent dose-dependent antinociception after intrathecal dosing in rats and inhibits substance P release in rat spinal cord slices. Pain 2002;96:119–27.
[101] Soares AC, Duarte ID. Dibutyryl-cyclic GMP induces peripheral antinociception via activation of ATP-sensitive K^+ channels in the rat PGE2-induced hyperalgesic paw. Br J Pharmacol 2001;134:127–31.
[102] Soares AC, Leite R, Tatsuo MA, Duarte ID. Activation of ATP-sensitive K^+ channels: mechanism of peripheral antinociceptive action of the nitric oxide donor, sodium nitroprusside. Eur J Pharmacol 2000;400:67–71.
[103] Todorovic SM, Jevtovic-Todorovic V. The role of T-type calcium channels in peripheral and central pain processing. CNS Neurol Disord Drug Targets 2006;5:639–53.
[104] Todorovic SM, Jevtovic-Todorovic V, Meyenburg A, Mennerick S, Perez-Reyes E, Romano C, Olney JW, Zorumski CF. Redox modulation of T-type calcium channels in rat peripheral nociceptors. Neuron 2001;31:75–85.
[105] Todorovic SM, Lingle CJ. Pharmacological properties of T-type Ca^{2+} current in adult rat sensory neurons: effects of anticonvulsant and anesthetic agents. J Neurophysiol 1998;79:240–52.
[106] Todorovic SM, Meyenburg A, Jevtovic-Todorovic V. Mechanical and thermal antinociception in rats following systemic administration of mibefradil, a T-type calcium channel blocker. Brain Res 2002;951:336–40.
[107] Tonussi CR, Ferreira SH. Mechanism of diclofenac analgesia: direct blockade of inflammatory sensitization. Eur J Pharmacol 1994;251:173–9.
[108] Vergara C, Latorre R, Marrion NV, Adelman JP. Calcium-activated potassium channels. Curr Opin Neurobiol 1998;8:321–9.
[109] Verkhratsky A. Endoplasmic reticulum calcium signaling in nerve cells. Biol Res 2004;37:693–9.
[110] Wang H, Kunkel DD, Martin TM, Schwartzkroin PA, Tempel BL. Heteromultimeric K^+ channels in terminal and juxtaparanodal regions of neurons. Nature 1993;365:75–9.
[111] Wang W, Xia J, Kass RS. MinK-KvLQT1 fusion proteins, evidence for multiple stoichiometries of the assembled IsK channel. J Biol Chem 1998;273:34069–74.
[112] Washburn CP, Sirois JE, Talley EM, Guyenet PG, Bayliss DA. Serotonergic raphe neurons express TASK channel transcripts and a TASK-like pH- and halothane-sensitive K^+ conductance. J Neurosci 2002;22:1256–65.
[113] Waxman SG, Dib-Hajj S, Cummins TR, Black JA. Sodium channels and pain. Proc Natl Acad Sci USA 1999;96:7635–9.
[114] Weiss N, De WM. [Voltage-dependent calcium channels at the heart of pain perception]. Med Sci (Paris) 2006;22:396–404.
[115] Wen XJ, Li ZJ, Chen ZX, Fang ZY, Yang CX, Li H, Zeng YM. Intrathecal administration of Cav3.2 and Cav3.3 antisense oligonucleotide reverses tactile allodynia and thermal hyperalgesia in rats following chronic compression of dorsal root of ganglion. Acta Pharmacol Sin 2006;27:1547–52.
[116] Yang WP, Levesque PC, Little WA, Conder ML, Shalaby FY, Blanar MA. KvLQT1, a voltage-gated potassium channel responsible for human cardiac arrhythmias. Proc Natl Acad Sci USA 1997;94:4017–21.

Correspondence to: Prof. Sérgio Henrique Ferreira, University of São Paulo, Faculty of Medicine of Ribeirão Preto, Department of Pharmacology, Av. Dos Bandeirantes, 3900 Campus USP, CEP 14049-900, Ribeirão Preto, SP, Brazil. Tel: +55 16 3602-3222; fax: +55 16 3623-2792; email: shferrei@fmrp.usp.br.

9

Toward Deciphering the Respective Roles of Multiple 5-HT Receptors in the Complex Serotonin-Mediated Control of Pain

Valérie Kayser, Sylvie Bourgoin, Florent Viguier, Benoît Michot, and Michel Hamon

Faculty of Medicine, Pierre et Marie Curie-Paris University, INSERM/CPN U894, Paris, France

Serotonin (5-hydroxytryptamine, 5-HT) is a monoamine neurotransmitter that is widely distributed in the central nervous system (CNS) and the periphery in mammals. The serotoninergic neurons that release 5-HT in the spinal cord have cell bodies within the caudal brainstem raphe nuclei. The major contributors are the nucleus raphe magnus (NRM), which projects mainly to the dorsal horn via the dorsolateral funiculus, and the nuclei raphe pallidus and raphe obscurus, which project mainly to the ventral horn and the intermediolateral cell column through the ventrolateral funiculus [92]. Extensive studies in rodents suggest that 5-HT in the periphery and at the spinal level modulates nociceptive responses. However, the involvement of 5-HT in pain processing is complex because this transmitter can inhibit or facilitate nociceptive transmission, depending on the nature of nociceptive stimuli applied, its site of action, and the receptor subtype it acts on [11,41,65]. In the periphery, 5-HT acting in combination with other inflammatory mediators may excite and sensitize primary afferent nerve fibers, thus contributing to peripheral sensitization and hyperalgesia following both inflammation and nerve injury [85]. At the spinal level, 5-HT has long been implicated in the processing and modulation of pain, with both pronociceptive and antinociceptive actions through bulbospinal descending projections [41,65]. In the brain, antinociceptive effects of 5-HT as part of an ascending component involving thalamic nuclei have been described [42,94]. Recently, Qu et al. [78] reported that microinjection of 5-HT directly into the ventrolateral orbital cortex also exerts clear

Pharmacology of Pain
edited by Pierre Beaulieu, David Lussier, Frank Porreca, and Anthony H. Dickenson
IASP Press, Seattle, © 2010

antinociceptive effects, probably through the activation of the cortico-periaqueductal gray (PAG) descending pathway. Such complex pro- and antinociceptive effects could be related to the existence of multiple 5-HT receptors expressed both at the periphery and in the CNS [41]. Recent studies have found that mice that lack central 5-HT neurons [100] or that do not express various types of 5-HT receptors or the transporter mediating 5-HT reuptake [52] have altered mechanical, thermal, and inflammatory-induced nociception compared with their control littermates. These findings stress the *physiological* nature of the complex role of the 5-HT system in pain control.

Much effort has been directed toward understanding the role of individual classes of 5-HT receptors in nociception [48,65]. At present, seven classes of these receptors (5-HT_1 to 5-HT_7) have been identified that comprise a total of at least 15 subtypes (Table I). Except for the 5-HT_3 receptor, which is a 5-HT-gated cation channel, all 5-HT receptors belong to the seven-transmembrane-domain G-protein-coupled receptor superfamily, and they act through modulation of cyclic adenosine monophosphate (cAMP) production, phospholipid metabolism, and/or cation channel conductance. Most of these receptors are expressed in the spinal cord, especially within the superficial layers of the dorsal horn, which receive nociceptive signals generated from peripheral nociceptors [41,65]. The receptors are located on the terminals of afferent fibers to control neurotransmitter release, on the soma and dendrites of intrinsic spinal interneurons and of spinal neurons projecting to supraspinal structures, and on the terminals of descending fibers, where they act as autoreceptors (on serotoninergic projections) or heteroreceptors (on nonserotoninergic projections). In addition, some of these receptor types can also be expressed by astroglial cells. Among them, 5-HT_{1A}, 5-$HT_{1B,}$ 5-HT_{1D}, 5-HT_{2A}, 5-HT_{2C}, and 5-HT_3 receptors have received much attention. In addition, evidence indicates that 5-HT_4 and 5-HT_7 receptors may play a role in nociceptive processing, but relevant data are still relatively scarce, mainly because ligands acting selectively at these receptor types have only recently become available.

This chapter focuses on 5-HT_{1A}, 5-$HT_{1B/1D}$, 5-HT_{2A}, 5-HT_{2C}, 5-HT_3, 5-HT_4, 5-HT_6, and 5-HT_7 receptors (Table I), which may be considered as potential targets for pain therapy, with special interest with regard to neuropathic pain.

5-HT_{1A} Receptors in Pain Processing and Control

The 5-HT_{1A} receptor is an inhibitory G-protein-coupled receptor, which is located on the soma and dendrites of various neuron types, including 5-HT neurons, where it acts as an autoreceptor. Somatodendritic 5-HT_{1A} autoreceptor activation leads to decreased 5-HT release into the synaptic cleft, whereas activation of postsynaptic 5-HT_{1A} heteroreceptors causes inhibition/hyperpolarization of target neurons of serotoninergic projections [54]. More specifically, with respect to the bulbospinal serotoninergic system, 5-HT_{1A} autoreceptors are located on the soma and dendrites of 5-HT neurons in the nucleus raphe magnus (and other bulbar raphe nuclei; see [13]), and postsynaptic 5-HT_{1A} heteroreceptors are

Table I
Main pharmacological characteristics, signaling mechanisms, and expression levels of the various types of 5-HT receptors in the dorsal horn of the spinal cord and dorsal root ganglia (in rodents)

Receptor Type	Agonists	Antagonists	G Protein	Transduction Mechanism	Spinal Cord Dorsal Horn (Protein)	DRG (mRNA)
5-HT$_{1A}$	8-OH-DPAT, alnespirone, F-13640	WAY-100635, NAD 299	G$_{i/o}$	cAMP ↘	+++	—
5-HT$_{1B}$	CP 93129, triptans	GR 555622, SB 242289, F-11648	G$_{i/o}$	cAMP ↘	++	+
5-HT$_{1D}$	GR 46611, L 694,247, triptans	GR 127935	G$_{i/o}$	cAMP ↘	+	++
5-HT$_{1E}$	—	—	G$_{i/o}$	cAMP ↘	+	—
5-HT$_{1F}$	LY 334370, sumatriptan	—	G$_{i/o}$	cAMP ↘	+	+
5-HT$_{2A}$	α-Me-5-HT, DOI	MDL-100,907, MDL-11,939, ketanserin	G$_{q/11}$	PLC ↗ PLA$_2$ ↗	(+)	+
5-HT$_{2B}$	α-Me-5-HT, BW 723686	SB 206553, SB 266097	G$_{q/11}$	PLC ↗	+	—?
5-HT$_{2C}$	α-Me-5-HT, MK-212, mCPP, TFMPP	RS-102221, SB 206553, SB 221284	G$_{q/11}$	PLC ↗	+	+
5-HT$_4$	BIMU-1, BIMU-8, BZTZ, RS 67333, RS 67506, tegaserod	GR 113808, LY 297582, SDZ-205,557	G$_s$	cAMP ↗	+	+
5-HT$_{5A}$	—	—	G$_i$	cAMP ↘	+	+
5-HT$_{5B}$	—	—	?	?	+	+
5-HT$_6$	—	SB-271046	G$_s$	cAMP ↗	+	—
5-HT$_7$	AS-19, E-55888, MSD-5a	SB-258719, SB-269970	G$_s$	cAMP ↗	+	+
5-HT$_3$	m-Cl-phenyl-biguanide, SR 57277 A	Ondansetron, granisetron, tropisetron	None	Na^+, K^+, Ca^{2+} channels	++	++

Abbreviations and symbols: ↗ = activation; ↘ = inhibition; +, ++, +++ = graded levels of expression; — = no expression; ? = unknown; 5-HT = 5-hydroxytryptamine; cAMP = cyclic adenosine monophosphate; DRG = dorsal root ganglia; PLC = phospholipase C; PLA$_2$ = phospholipase A$_2$.

expressed by both interneurons and spinothalamic neurons within the dorsal horn [11,41]. Interestingly, no 5-HT$_{1A}$ receptor mRNA could be detected in dorsal root (or trigeminal) ganglia, indicating that primary afferent fibers are not endowed with 5-HT$_{1A}$ receptors and thus cannot be directly modulated by 5-HT$_{1A}$-receptor ligands [76]. Therefore, in the early 1980s, researchers began to realize that 5-HT$_{1A}$ receptors may contribute to medullospinal regulation of pain. Numerous data have supported this influence. In particular, Wei and Pertovaara [91] reported that administration of WAY-100635, a potent and selective 5-HT$_{1A}$-receptor antagonist, into the rostroventromedial medulla attenuated neuropathic hypersensitivity. These findings suggest that endogenous release of 5-HT, through the activation of medullary 5-HT_{1A} receptors, tonically suppresses descending pain inhibition mechanisms, thereby promoting neuropathic hypersensitivity. Accordingly, other studies have shown that the blockade of 5-HT_{1A}-autoreceptor-mediated inhibitory control of 5-HT release promotes the analgesic effects of antidepressants by facilitating descending pathways involved in pain modulation. In particular, in two models of neurogenic sustained pain (experimentally induced mononeuropathic and diabetic states in rats), the selective 5-HT_{1A}-receptor antagonist WAY-100635 was found to reduce the delay of onset and increase the maximal antinociceptive effects of the tricyclic antidepressant, clomipramine, a preferential 5-HT reuptake inhibitor [6], probably through the blockade of a negative feedback mechanism involving somatodendritic 5-HT_{1A} autoreceptors. Also in mononeuropathic rats, blockade of supraspinal 5-HT_{1A} receptors by repeated intracerebroventricular administration of WAY-100635 increased the inhibitory effect of the antidepressant venlafaxine, a mixed monoamine reuptake inhibitor with preferential action on 5-HT reuptake, on spinal wind-up activity [14,61]. Relevant data have also been obtained with tramadol, an atypical centrally acting analgesic agent with relatively weak opioid receptor affinity, as well as 5-HT (and norepinephrine) reuptake inhibitory properties that account for some antidepressant efficacy [64]. For example, Rojas-Corrales et al. [79] reported that systemic administration of WAY-100635 enhanced the antinociceptive effect of tramadol in the hot-plate test in mice, as would be expected from a negative influence of somatodendritic 5-HT_{1A} receptors on the analgesic action of this atypical antidepressant.

At the spinal level, however, 5-HT_{1A}-receptor agonists are regularly reported to reduce pain-related behavioral and electrophysiological responses in healthy, inflamed, and neuropathic animals [48]. Systemic administration of 5-HT_{1A}-receptor agonists can also produce antinociception in a number of pain models [41], and recent studies in validated animal models emphasize that high-efficacy 5-HT_{1A}-receptor stimulation might be a new approach to alleviate a variety of pain states [23]. Indeed, in the formalin model of pain in rats, acute, systemic administration of a high-efficacy 5-HT_{1A}-receptor agonist, F-13640, was especially potent in abolishing nociceptive behavior at the early and late phases after formalin injection [9]. In a model of intra- and postoperative pain caused by surgery in rats, pretreatment with F-13640 lowered the requirement of intraoperative isoflurane anesthesia, and F-13640 administered after surgery produced a long-lasting and powerful suppression of postoperative pain behaviors [53]. Furthermore, in arthritic rats, continuous systemic infusion of F-13640 from an osmotic minipump induced a dose-dependent analgesia that could equal that obtained with 5 mg/day of morphine [21]. Altogether, the data suggest that high-efficacy 5-HT_{1A}-receptor activation can alleviate chronic nociceptive pain with an efficacy that is rivaled only by morphine-like opioids.

In rats that presented lowered paw-withdrawal thresholds to von Frey filament stimulation after chronic constriction injury (CCI) to the sciatic nerve, a 2-week systemic infusion of F-13640 significantly reduced these allodynia-like responses [21]. We investigated whether normalization of paw withdrawal and vocalization thresholds to paw pressure (the Randall-Selitto test) could also be achieved in this model after acute administration of F-13640, further demonstrating the marked efficacy of 5-HT_{1A}-receptor activation to reduce sciatic nerve ligature-evoked hyperalgesia (Fig. 1). Moreover, in rats suffering from ischemic injury to the spinal cord and developing allodynic responses to cutaneous stimulations such as von Frey filament application, a gentle brush, or a cold spray, F-13640 robustly inhibited such manifestations of neuropathic pain [21]. Finally, in rats with CCI to the infraorbital nerve, a model of trigeminal neuropathic pain, acute administration of F-13640 counteracted allodynic responses to von Frey filament stimulation, and this effect not only persisted but even became more pronounced during a 2-week infusion of the 5-HT_{1A}-receptor agonist from an implanted osmotic minipump [25]. These results suggest that, at least in the rat, the 5-HT_{1A} receptors that mediate the antinociceptive action of high-efficacy agonists do not become desensitized but may even develop supersensitive downstream signaling mechanisms under chronic treatment conditions.

Conversely, other data show that spinal administration of 5-HT_{1A}-receptor agonists may promote nociception under different experimental conditions [3,48,56]. Interestingly, the direction of the pain-modulatory effect induced by 5-HT_{1A}-receptor activation appeared to vary from facilitation to inhibition within the same study, depending on a

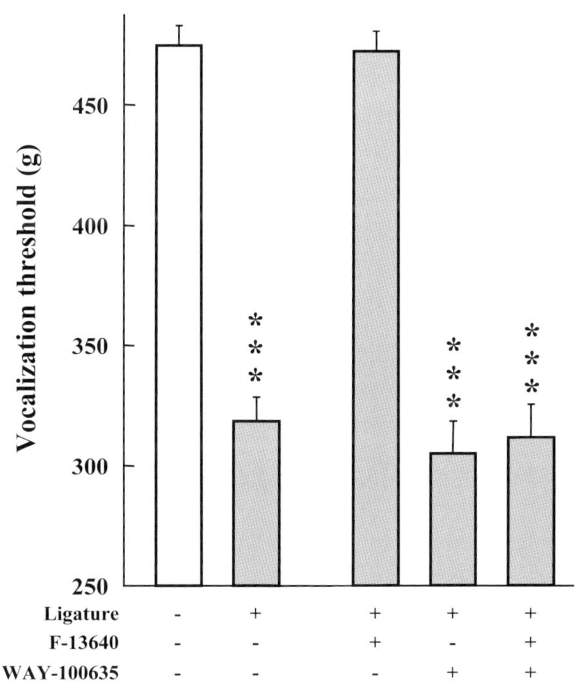

Fig. 1. Antihyperalgesic effects of 5-HT_{1A}-receptor activation. Mean vocalization thresholds (expressed in grams) were measured using the Randall and Selitto paw pressure test in rats that had undergone unilateral constriction injury to the sciatic nerve 2 weeks previously and had subsequently received acute treatment with the 5-HT_{1A}-receptor agonist F-13640 (0.2 mg/kg i.p.), the 5-HT_{1A}-receptor antagonist WAY-100635 (2 mg/kg s.c.), or a combination of both drugs (10 minutes prior to the test). Each bar is the mean ± SEM of six independent determinations. Hyperalgesia observed 2 weeks after sciatic nerve ligature was reversed by 5-HT_{1A}-receptor activation with F-13640. ***$P < 0.001$ as compared with threshold values in control "sham" rats (empty bar), Student's *t* test.

number of experimental factors such as modalities of test stimulation, dose of receptor agonist, duration of treatment, and pathophysiological condition [14,21]. A mechanism that may be involved in such variability in the effects of 5-HT$_{1A}$-receptor activation is the well-established regional difference in functional adaptation of 5-HT$_{1A}$ receptors upon long-term stimulation by agonists. Thus, chronic treatment with direct or indirect (i.e., 5-HT reuptake inhibitors) agonists produces a marked desensitization of 5-HT$_{1A}$ autoreceptors on 5-HT neurons in raphe nuclei, without altering the functional characteristics of postsynaptic 5-HT$_{1A}$ receptors in most, if not all, projection areas of these neurons [54], such as the dorsal horn of the spinal cord [41]. As a result, the 5-HT$_{1A}$-autoreceptor-mediated inhibitory feedback control of 5-HT neurotransmission vanishes, which allows maximal 5-HT$_{1A}$ signaling at postsynaptic receptors [54]. In consistency with these findings, recent observations from our laboratory using a large range of systemic doses of the 5-HT$_{1A}$-receptor agonists 8-OH-DPAT and F-13640 in mice lacking the 5-HT$_{1A}$ receptor or that do not express the 5-HT transporter (5-HTT) indicated that 5-HT$_{1A}$-receptor activation exerts bidirectional effects, depending on the respective contribution of auto- versus hetero- (postsynaptic) receptors. Indeed, the pronociceptive effects of 5-HT$_{1A}$-receptor agonists appeared to be predominantly mediated by presynaptic 5-HT$_{1A}$ autoreceptors, whereas their antinociceptive effects most probably resulted from the stimulation of postsynaptic 5-HT$_{1A}$ heteroreceptors [22]. In line with this interpretation, 5-HT$_{1A}$-receptor agonists only exerted antinociceptive effects in the formalin test applied to 5-HTT$^{-/-}$ knockout mice, in which 5-HT$_{1A}$ autoreceptors are deeply desensitized [31], whereas dose-dependent, pronociceptive effects (at low doses) and then antinociceptive effects (at high doses) were noted in wild-type mice. A strong inhibitory action of 5-HT$_{1A}$-receptor activation on NMDA-receptor-mediated ionic and synaptic currents has recently been characterized in the rat prefrontal cortex [97], and it remains to be investigated whether such a mechanism underlies the antinociceptive effects of 5-HT$_{1A}$-receptor agonists acting at postsynaptic sites within the dorsal horn of the spinal cord, especially in neuropathic pain conditions, when glutamatergic neurotransmission is tonically activated.

5-HT$_{1B/1D}$ Receptors in Pain Processing and Control

Although 5-HT$_{1B}$ and 5-HT$_{1D}$ receptors are encoded by different genes, they are highly homologous regarding their amino acid sequences, downstream signaling mechanisms, regional and subcellular localizations, and pharmacological properties, which explains why their respective contributions to the effects of agonists are often difficult to assess. It must be emphasized, however, that the density of 5-HT$_{1B}$ receptors is much higher than that of 5-HT$_{1D}$ receptors in the CNS [11]. Both 5-HT$_{1B}$ and 5-HT$_{1D}$ receptors are expressed within the superficial laminae of the dorsal horn of the spinal cord, where nociceptive messages are relayed from primary afferent fibers to ascending spinal neurons [41]. Decreased responses to nociceptive stimulation have generally been reported after intrathecal or topical administration of 5-HT$_{1B/1D}$-receptor agonists [3,48,56]. This antinociceptive effect of

5-HT$_{1B}$ receptor stimulation seems to occur under physiological conditions because it has been demonstrated in the absence of any drug treatment aimed at affecting 5-HT neurotransmission. Indeed, in 5-HT$_{1B}^{-/-}$ knockout mice, nociceptive responses to noxious heat and to intraplantar injection of formalin (during the early and late phases) were exacerbated in comparison with paired wild-type animals [52]. Pharmacological blockade of 5-HT$_{1B}$ receptors by the selective antagonist F-11648 enhanced these responses in wild-type, but not knock-out, mice, thereby supporting the idea that 5-HT$_{1B}$ receptors mediate a 5-HT inhibitory control of noxious heat- and formalin-evoked nociceptive messages in mice [52].

5-HT$_{1B}$ receptors are notably located on axon terminals of primary afferent fibers, and 5-HT acting at these receptors exerts an inhibitory influence on neurotransmitter release from primary afferent terminals [7,41]. Accordingly, it can be proposed that, under physiological conditions, activation of descending 5-HT bulbospinal pathways enhances spinal 5-HT release, which, in turn, activates terminal 5-HT$_{1B}$ receptors to reduce evoked release of nociceptive neurotransmitters—glutamate, substance P, and calcitonin-gene-related peptide (CGRP)—within the dorsal horn of the spinal cord.

Triptans are potent agonists that act at 5-HT$_{1B}$, 5-HT$_{1D}$, and 5-HT$_{1F}$ receptors, and their utility in the treatment of migraine pain is well established. At the periphery, triptans prevent or block neurogenic inflammation, at least in part, by inhibiting the release of substance P and CGRP from peptidergic afferents [19]. There is also evidence for a central action of triptans [49], including presynaptic inhibition of neurotransmitter release from the central terminals of primary afferents in the trigeminal nucleus caudalis [47,55], post-synaptic inhibition of the responses of trigeminal caudalis neurons to glutamate or to an *N*-methyl D-aspartate (NMDA) receptor agonist [38], and activation of 5-HT$_{1B}$/$_{1D}$ receptors expressed by pain-modulatory neurons in the periaqueductal gray [10]. The specificity of triptans against migraine and cluster headache and their lack of effect in other pain disorders raise puzzling questions concerning their mechanisms of action [1].

In convergence with the idea that triptans may act selectively on pain associated with the trigeminal region, we found that systemic administration of sumatriptan, zolmitriptan, and naratriptan, at a clinically relevant dose (100 μg/kg s.c.), led to a significant reduction of nociceptive behaviors in rats following CCI to the infraorbital nerve (a validated model of trigeminal neuropathic pain), but was inactive in rats showing signs of extracephalic neuropathic pain caused by unilateral CCI to the sciatic nerve [51]. Given that 5-HT$_{1B}$ and 5-HT$_{1D}$ receptors are both expressed by trigeminal and dorsal root ganglion (DRG) neurons in the rat [77], the lack of effect of triptans on neuropathic pain caused by sciatic nerve injury strongly suggests that the functional state of these receptors—or their intracellular signaling pathways—could be different in the cephalic versus extracephalic territory following peripheral nerve injury. Recent data have reported variations in G proteins interacting with the same receptor, depending either on the cell type expressing the receptor [60] or on the degree of activation of the receptor [87]. Direct investigations of the G-protein coupling of 5-HT$_{1B/1D}$ receptors in rats that underwent a unilateral CCI to the infraorbital nerve versus the sciatic nerve should be especially informative in this regard.

Very recently, Nikai et al. [70] reported that sumatriptan can significantly reduce inflammatory pain in noncranial regions of the body, when given intrathecally in mice. Importantly, systemic administration of sumatriptan had no effect, even at doses 200-fold higher than the effective intrathecal dose. Accordingly, the capacity of 5-$HT_{1B}/_{1D}$-receptor agonists to cross the blood-brain barrier must also be considered in their effectiveness or failure in reducing nociceptive responses in validated models. Whether or not systemically administered triptans reach more easily central structures involved in cephalic compared to extracephalic (spinally mediated) pain is also a relevant question to be addressed regarding the potential development of these drugs for the alleviation of severe peripheral inflammatory pain.

5-HT_{2A} Receptors in Pain Processing and Control

The 5-HT_{2A} receptor is a G-protein-coupled receptor that is functionally coupled to phospholipase C and phospholipase A_2, leading to the production of inositol phosphates, diacylglycerol, and arachidonic acid as second messengers and the facilitation of nociceptive spinal transmission upon its activation by selective agonists. 5-HT_{2A}-receptor activation also inhibits K^+ channel conductance, thereby causing neuronal excitation. 5-HT_{2A} receptors are notably expressed by primary afferent fibers that convey nociceptive messages from the periphery to the CNS [41]. Through these receptors, 5-HT, acting in combination with other inflammatory mediators, has been reported to ectopically excite and sensitize acutely axotomized afferent nerve fibers [63]. In line with the idea that peripheral 5-HT_{2A} receptors may mediate pronociceptive effects of 5-HT, intraplantar administration of 5-HT_{2A}-receptor antagonists has been shown to exert antinociceptive effects in rodent models of inflammatory pain. These considerations led us to use mutant mice that do not express 5-HT_{2A} receptors as an indirect approach to further assess the role of these receptors in the *physiological* control of nociceptive responses to a wide range of noxious mechanical and thermal stimuli and to intraplantar injection of formalin [52]. Our results showed that 5-$HT_{2A}^{-/-}$ mutants exhibited markedly decreased responses to formalin-induced prolonged noxious stimulation, indicating that these receptors may play a role in the development of inflammation-associated hyperalgesia. In contrast, no changes in mechano- or thermonociceptive responses were seen in the mutants. As expected, acute blockade of 5-HT_{2A} receptors by the selective antagonist MDL-100,907 in wild-type mice replicated the findings in knockout mice.

Convergent data in the literature show that 5-HT_{2A}-receptor antagonists specifically reduce hyperalgesia without affecting normal nociceptive reactions, probably by inhibiting sensitization of primary sensory neurons associated with inflammatory [71] and neuropathic [72] pain. Indeed, 5-HT is released from platelets and mast cells in injured/inflamed tissues, and it is one of the substances involved in the late-phase response in the formalin test [84]. By stimulating 5-HT$_{2A}$ receptors, 5-HT activates C-fiber afferents and increases the excitability of small-diameter neurons in the DRG, thereby promoting CGRP release [90]. These characteristics may underlie the key role of 5-HT$_{2A}$ receptors in pain associated with inflammation. Indeed, numerous data support the idea that 5-HT$_{2A}$ receptors are responsible for 5-HT-induced hyperalgesia at the peripheral level in inflammatory states [83,90]. Furthermore, inflammation strongly upregulates 5-HT$_{2A}$-receptor expression in the DRG [56], and this change may participate in some of the mechanisms that exacerbate inflammatory pain. Very recently, however, Yu et al. [96] reported an extraordinary potency of the 5-HT$_{2A}$-receptor agonist DOI (in the range of 10^{-12} to 10^{-9} M), in suppressing TNF-α-induced inflammatory processes in primary aortic smooth muscle cells. This finding suggests that 5-HT$_{2A}$ receptors can mediate variable effects of 5-HT on inflammation, depending on the cell type and cytokine involved, possibly explaining why 5-HT$_{2A}$ receptor ligands have low therapeutic potential for alleviating inflammatory pain. In contrast, neuropathic pain might be more consistently alleviated by 5-HT$_{2A}$-receptor blockade. Indeed a peripherally acting 5-HT$_{2A}$-receptor antagonist, sarpogrelate, used in Japan as an antiplatelet agent to treat patients with arteriosclerosis, significantly attenuated allodynia in neuropathic rats [43].

On the whole, 5-HT$_{2A}$ receptors at the central level also participate in the control of nociception and pain [41]. In particular, the implication of 5-HT$_{2A}$ receptors in neuropathic pain could be recently demonstrated in a model of peripheral neuropathy induced by 2',3'-dideoxycytidine, a nucleoside analogue with reverse transcriptase inhibitory properties used in HIV/AIDS therapy [89]. Four days after systemic 2',3'-dideoxycytidine administration, rats developed thermal allodynia as well as mechanical hyperalgesia and allodynia, which could be dose-dependently reversed by epidural injection of MDL-11,939, a selective 5-HT$_{2A}$-receptor antagonist, thereby suggesting that the intensity of neuropathic pain depended on the expression of 5-HT$_{2A}$ receptors. In line with this inference, 5-HT$_{2A}$-receptor knockout mice did not develop 2',3'-dideoxycytidine-induced neuropathic pain, whereas their control littermates displayed allodynia and hyperalgesia comparable to those observed in rats [89]. Interestingly, similar findings were recently described in neuropathic pain evoked by systemic treatment with vincristine [88]. Furthermore, an upregulation of 5-HT$_{2A}$ receptors within the dorsal horn of the spinal cord was evidenced in rats rendered neuropathic by either 2',3'-dideoxycytidine or vincristine [88,89].

In addition to primary sensory neurons and spinal neurons [27,89], several other neuronal populations express 5-HT$_{2A}$ receptors, notably in brain structures involved in the control and transmission of nociceptive messages, including the reticular formation, the nucleus raphe magnus, the central gray, the thalamus, the cerebral cortex, and limbic structures [24]. In line with the idea that these supraspinal receptors may also participate in pain signal processing, a significant upregulation of 5-HT$_{2A}$ receptor mRNA has been reported to occur not only in the dorsal spinal cord, but also in the nucleus raphe magnus, the ventrolateral gray, and the dorsal raphe nucleus [99] 3 hours after peripheral carrageenan-induced inflammation in rats.

Therefore, 5-HT_{2A}-receptor blockade might help to alleviate various kinds of pain, both at the periphery and in the CNS, and the therapeutic potential of selective 5-HT_{2A}-receptor antagonists deserves further research.

5-HT_{2C} Receptors in Pain Processing and Control

The 5-HT_{2C} receptor is a G-protein-coupled receptor. Its stimulation activates phospholipase C, thereby increasing intracellular Ca^{2+} levels and mediating an excitatory influence of 5-HT [41]. 5-HT_{2C} receptors are present in the dorsal horn of the spinal cord, mainly in the deeper laminae [35], and their stimulation by specific agonists has been reported to mediate antinociception, through γ-aminobutyric acid (GABA)-dependent mechanisms [15,46]. Indeed, clear evidence indicates that the great majority of 5-HT_{2C} receptors are expressed by GABAergic interneurons, thereby converting the expected excitatory action of 5-HT_{2C}-receptor stimulation into an inhibitory influence throughout the CNS [11].

Mediation by 5-HT_{2C} receptors of the antinociceptive effect of spinally administered 5-HT has been clearly demonstrated in a mechanical pain test in rats [8]. Through these receptors, intrathecal 5-HT also attenuated the flinching responses in phase 1 and phase 2 of the formalin test in the rat, an effect that could be mimicked by a direct 5-HT_{2C}-receptor agonist, MK-212 [48]. In line with the idea that spinal 5-HT_{2C} receptors may mediate antinociception in sustained pain models, intrathecal administration of the mixed 5-$HT_{2A/2C}$-receptor agonist, α-methyl-5-HT, was shown to exert antinociceptive effects in rats with behavioral signs of neuropathic pain caused by CCI to the sciatic nerve [82]. Furthermore, clear-cut evidence indicates that 5-$HT_{2A/2C}$-receptor activation plays an essential role in the antinociceptive action of the selective serotonin reuptake inhibitors fluoxetine and fluvoxamine in mice with streptozotocin-induced diabetic neuropathy [5,45]. That 5-HT_{2C}, rather than 5-HT_{2A}, receptors, mediated such antinociceptive actions is strongly suggested by the findings of Obata et al. [74] showing that the intrathecal administration of 5-HT_{2C}-receptor agonists—MK-212, mCPP, and TFMPP—produced antiallodynic effects in rats with tight ligation of the L5 and L6 spinal nerves. Indeed, as expected, intrathecal pretreatment with the selective 5-HT_{2C}-receptor antagonist, RS-102221, markedly attenuated the effects of these agonists.

Possible involvement of spinal noradrenergic mechanisms in the antiallodynic effects of intrathecally administered 5-HT_{2C}-receptor agonists in rats with peripheral nerve injury is supported by the observation that yohimbine, an α_2-adrenoceptor antagonist, reversed these effects. Furthermore, intrathecal pretreatment with 6-hydroxydopamine, which causes the degeneration of bulbospinal catecholaminergic projections, also inhibited the antiallodynic effects of MK-212 [75].

Very recently, investigations in various animal models of central or peripheral neuropathic pain (contusive spinal cord injury or CCI to the infra-orbital nerve) have shown that modulation of 5-HT_{2C}-receptor mRNA editing could be an adaptive response accompanying the sensitization of nociceptive signaling mechanisms [67,68]. Because

5-HT$_{2C}$-receptor mRNA editing produces 5-HT$_{2C}$ receptor isoforms less efficiently coupled to downstream intracellular signaling mechanisms, such adaptive changes, by reducing antinociceptive responses to 5-HT$_{2C}$-receptor activation, might also contribute to the development and maintenance of neuropathic pain.

5-HT$_3$ Receptors in Pain Processing and Control

5-HT$_3$ receptors are 5-HT-receptor-gated cation channels, activation of which increases the plasma membrane conductance for Na^+, K^+, and Ca^{2+} ions [11]. At the periphery, 5-HT$_3$ receptors are located notably on the terminals of nociceptors, where they mediate an excitatory influence of 5-HT. 5-HT$_3$ receptors are also abundant in the superficial layers of the dorsal horn of the spinal cord, where they are expressed by both the central terminals of primary afferent fibers and interneurons (especially those of GABAergic phenotype). However, to date, their possible function in pain control mechanisms has not been satisfactorily clarified, and studies have yielded partly contradictory results [32].

In line with the idea that peripheral 5-HT$_3$ receptors may mediate pronociceptive effects of 5-HT, intraplantar administration of ondansetron, a 5-HT$_3$-receptor antagonist, showed antinociceptive effects in the model of formalin-induced inflammatory pain in mice [98]. Similarly, in 5-HT$_{3A}$ knockout mice, nociceptive responses to mechanical and thermal stimuli are similar to those in wild-type mice, but those for the second phase in the formalin test are markedly reduced [52]. In the CNS, the situation is more confusing because activation of spinal 5-HT$_3$ receptors has been reported to produce pronociceptive as well as antinociceptive actions [65].

An initial series of data supports the idea that spinal 5-HT$_3$ receptors mediate, at least in part, the antinociceptive effect of intrathecally administered 5-HT [8,37,48,56]. In convergence with this idea, Yokogawa et al. [95] reported that in the formalin model of pain in rats, the 5-HT$_3$-receptor antagonist ondansetron significantly antagonizes the 5-HT (and norepinephrine)-mediated antinociception induced by the tricyclic antidepressant imipramine. In line with the evidence discussed above regarding the antinociceptive effects of 5-HT$_{2C}$-receptor agonists administered directly at the spinal level, evidence has been provided that spinal 5-HT$_3$-receptor activation exerts an antinociceptive influence through a local release of GABA, ending with the stimulation of inhibitory GABA$_A$ receptors [2]. In contrast, other data show that spinally administered 5-HT$_3$-receptor agonists may facilitate nociceptive responses [4,39], strongly suggesting that spinal 5-HT$_3$ receptors participate in a descending 5-HT facilitatory influence on nociceptive transmission. In line with this inference, spinally administered ondansetron has been reported to reduce responses to mechanical and thermal stimuli in a rat model of cancer-induced bone pain [29].

The 5-HT$_3$ receptors that mediate the pronociceptive effects of 5-HT are probably those located on nerve terminals of small-diameter afferent fibers [98]. Indeed, by blocking these receptors, which mediate an excitatory action of 5-HT, 5-HT$_3$-receptor antagonists inhibit the release of substance P, neurokinin A, and CGRP from primary afferent terminals within the dorsal horn of the spinal cord [81]. The existence of descending 5-HT_3-receptor-mediated facilitation of pain-signaling mechanisms has been further confirmed by data showing that the efficacy of ondansetron to suppress spinal responses to von Frey filament stimulation was significantly enhanced after spinal nerve ligation, as expected from an increase in descending 5-HT facilitatory drive to the spinal cord [86]. Furthermore, depletion of spinal 5-HT caused by intrathecal administration of 5,7-dihydroxytryptamine was found to attenuate signs of behavioral hypersensitivity after nerve ligation. This 5-HT facilitatory drive, mediated through spinal 5-HT_3 receptors, is thought to involve a spinal-brainstem-spinal loop originating from superficial dorsal horn neurokinin-1-expressing neurons, with projections to the parabrachial complex and rostroventral medial medulla, from which descending excitatory pathways project onto deep dorsal horn neurons [86].

In animal models, painful colonic distension enhances c-fos expression in diverse brain nuclei, including the rostral ventrolateral medulla and the nucleus tractus solitarii, and pretreatment with granisetron can significantly reduce this response [66]. This finding supports the idea that 5-HT_3 receptors play a key role in the activation of the pain facilitatory spinal-brainstem-spinal loop. Similar mechanisms probably occur in humans, because ondansetron, currently used as an antiemetic, exhibits some analgesic properties in patients with chronic neuropathic pain [58]. Furthermore, beneficial effects of 5-HT_3-receptor antagonists have also been reported in fibromyalgia [33] and irritable bowel syndrome, especially in women [59].

5-HT_4 Receptors in Pain Processing and Control

The 5-HT_4 receptor is a G-protein-coupled receptor that exerts its actions through an increase in adenylyl cyclase activity and subsequent protein kinase A activation [41]. 5-HT_4 receptors are expressed in the spinal cord, with a marked enrichment within the superficial layers of the dorsal horn (layers 1 and 2), where they mostly correspond to presynaptic receptors located on the terminals of capsaicin-sensitive primary afferent sensory fibers that convey nociceptive messages from the periphery [20]. This location suggests that 5-HT_4 receptors are possibly involved in a 5-HT-mediated control of pain-signaling mechanisms. However, to date, relatively few studies have addressed this question. Two 5-HT_4-receptor agonists, BIMU-1 and BIMU-8, have been shown to exert potent antinociceptive activity through a central cholinergic mechanism [36]. However, 5-HT_4-receptor blockade by GR113808 had no significant effect on antinociception evoked by intrathecal administration of 5-HT in a mechanical pain test, which seems to exclude a mediation by 5-HT_4 receptors of the antinociceptive effect of 5-HT at the spinal level [8]. In contrast, other tests allowed the opposite conclusion, because antinociception produced by intrathecal administration of 5-HT in the rat formalin test could be blocked by SDZ-205,557, another potent 5-HT_4-receptor antagonist, and was mimicked by the 5-HT_4-receptor agonist BZTZ, also administered via the intrathecal route [48].

Electrophysiological recordings of wide-dynamic-range (WDR) neurons, which can be excited by both noxious and innocuous stimuli of different modalities, were used to systematically evaluate the roles of 5-HT_4 receptors in spinal nociceptive modulation [56]. It was found that the spinally applied 5-HT_4-receptor antagonist GR113808 reduced the inhibitory effects of 5-HT on C-fiber responses. Coincidentally, the 5-HT_4-receptor agonist BZTZ mimicked the inhibitory influence of 5-HT on these responses. These results support the concept that 5-HT_4 receptors mediate 5-HT-induced inhibition of C-fiber responses, in sharp contrast with an expected direct excitatory effect through 5-HT_4 receptors expressed by primary sensory C fibers [20]. As already discussed above with regard to 5-HT_{2C} and 5-HT_3 receptors, it is possible that the observed 5-HT_4-receptor-mediated inhibition by 5-HT relied on excitation of inhibitory interneurons influencing the WDR neurons recorded in laminae IV–VI of the dorsal spinal cord. In fact, 5-HT_4-receptor activation does increase GABA release in the CNS [12]. GABA-mediated inhibitory mechanisms are therefore probably responsible for the ability of tegaserod, a 5-HT_4-receptor agonist, to decrease nociceptive responses to rectal distension and significantly improve abdominal pain in humans [40]. Conversely, 5-HT_4-receptor activation at the periphery seems to increase visceral pain [30], which might counteract the antinociceptive effects of spinal 5-HT_4-receptor activation.

Because of such dual, mutually antagonizing effects, the potential for clinical use of 5-HT_4-receptor ligands to alleviate pain requires further investigation.

5-HT_6 Receptors in Pain Processing and Control

The 5-HT_6 receptor is a G-protein-coupled receptor that is positively coupled to adenylyl cyclase; it is expressed almost exclusively in the CNS [17,93]. Given the extensive expression of the 5-HT_6 receptor in the basal ganglia, the limbic system, and the cerebral cortex, much attention has focused on its potential role in psychotic disorders, in affective disorders, and in cognitive function. The distribution of the 5-HT_6 receptor and/or its mRNA in regions such as the amygdala, thalamus, and periaqueductal gray and in the dorsal horn of the spinal cord is also consistent with a potential role in nociceptive control mechanisms. However, to date, few studies have investigated the possible implication of 5-HT_6 receptors in nociception. Bourson et al. [16] reported that repeated intracerebroventricular administration of an antisense oligonucleotide sequence, designed to block 5-HT_6-receptor expression, had no effect on paw-lick latency in the hot-plate test in rats. More recently, acute systemic administration of the 5-HT_6-receptor antagonist SB-271046 was found to reduce formalin-evoked nociceptive behavior in rats [34]. Such findings should prompt the design of further studies aimed at investigating the analgesic potential, together with the sites and mechanism of action, of selective 5-HT_6-receptor antagonists in models of acute and chronic pain. Indeed, such studies were impossible because of a lack of agonists and antagonists acting selectively at 5-HT_6 receptors, but fortunately, the situation has changed with the recent development of appropriate ligands (mainly because of the potential usefulness of 5-HT$_6$-receptor antagonists in counteracting cognitive deficits).

5-HT$_7$ Receptors in Pain Processing and Control

One of the most recently identified 5-HT-receptor subtypes that may play a role in nociceptive signal processing is the 5-HT$_7$ receptor. This receptor is positively coupled to adenylyl cyclase, and its activation causes neuronal excitation [44]. The pharmacological properties of 5-HT$_7$ receptors resemble to some extent those of 5-HT$_{1A}$ receptors [57], suggesting that certain actions initially attributed to 5-HT$_{1A}$ agonists could indeed be mediated, at least in part, by 5-HT$_7$ receptors.

Several lines of evidence suggest that 5-HT$_7$ receptors could be involved in pain control at the peripheral, spinal, and/or supraspinal level. First, anatomical studies demonstrated the expression of 5-HT$_7$ receptors at critical synaptic relays along nociceptive neuronal pathways. In particular, Pierce et al. [76] detected the presence of 5-HT$_7$-receptor mRNA in rat and human DRG, and Doly et al. [28] described the immunocytochemical localization of 5-HT$_7$ receptors at the lumbar level in small and medium-sized DRG cells as well as in the superficial laminae of the dorsal horn. As illustrated in Fig. 2, a dense immunocytochemical labeling of 5-HT$_7$ receptors is observed not only in the latter areas but also in superficial layers of the caudal trigeminal nucleus (Sp5c). Electron microscopic examination of the dorsal horn revealed both a presynaptic localization (in axon terminals from primary afferents and spinal interneurons) and a postsynaptic localization (mainly in cell bodies and synaptic differentiations of dendrites belonging to local interneurons). At the supraspinal level, the distribution of 5-HT$_7$ receptors in cortical areas, thalamic nuclei, and several nuclei in the midbrain, pons, and medulla [69] is also compatible with a role in the control of pain.

The definitive demonstration of the implication of 5-HT$_7$ receptors in nociception could be made only recently thanks to the development of selective agonists and antagonists in the last few years. Using SB-269970 as a selective 5-HT$_7$-receptor antagonist (administered via the intrathecal route), researchers established that the pharmacological blockade of spinal 5-HT$_7$ receptors prevented the antinociceptive effect of systemic morphine in the tail-flick test [26]. This effect was not seen with 5-HT$_{1A}$- or 5-HT$_2$-receptor antagonists (also injected intrathecally), supporting that activation of spinal 5-HT$_7$ receptors underlies, at least in part, the action of morphine in this nociceptive test. It is unlikely that activation of 5-HT$_7$ receptors could directly inhibit primary afferents or nociceptive dorsal horn neurons because 5-HT$_7$-receptor stimulation is excitatory [44]. One plausible explanation could be that the 5-HT$_7$ receptors involved are those localized on spinal inhibitory enkephalinergic or GABAergic interneurons. 5-HT$_7$-receptor activation would then evoke the release of enkephalins and/or GABA, which, in turn, could inhibit nociceptive transmission at either pre- or postsynaptic sites. In consistency with this hypothesis, Kawamata et al. [50] demonstrated that the GABAergic system contributes to spinal 5-HT-mediated antinociception. Furthermore, evidence has also been reported that the opioidergic system is involved in the antinociceptive effect of selective 5-HT reuptake inhibitors [73].

However, the most convincing data were obtained by using high-affinity and selective agonists to directly activate 5-HT_7 receptors. Thus, in a recent study, Brenchat et al. [18] provided the first demonstration that subcutaneous administration of AS-19, MSD-5a, and E-55888, all 5-HT_7-receptor agonists, exerted a clear-cut dose-dependent inhibition of mechanical allodynia induced by intraplantar injection of capsaicin in mice. Indeed, all three agonists suppressed this behavioral manifestation of pain and restored the nociceptive response of capsaicin-sensitized mice to values similar to those found in control mice. The order of efficacy was E-55888 > AS-19 > MSD-5a, in line with their respective in vitro efficacy as 5-HT_7-receptor agonists to enhance cAMP production in 5-HT_7-receptor-expressing cell lines. Furthermore, as expected, the antiallodynic effects

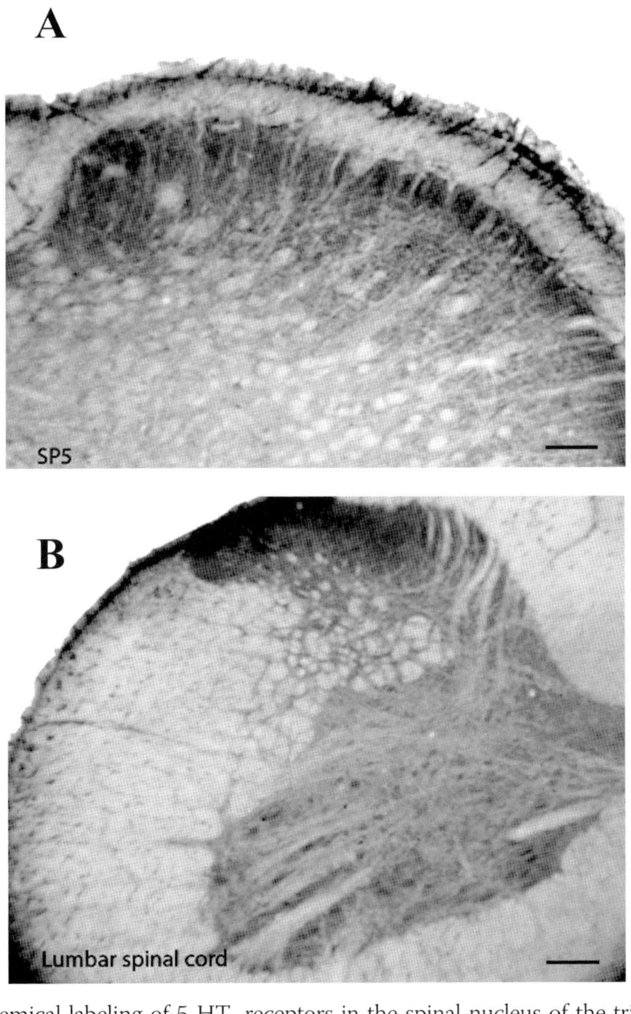

Fig. 2. Immunohistochemical labeling of 5-HT_7 receptors in the spinal nucleus of the trigeminal nerve (Sp5; A) and in the lumbar spinal cord (B) in the rat. At both levels, 5-HT_7-receptor immunoperoxidase labeling is confined within the superficial layers, which receive nociceptive signals generated at the periphery. Scale bars: 200 μm.

of agonists were prevented by the systemic administration of two different 5-HT$_7$-receptor antagonists (SB-258719 and SB-269970). In agreement with the antiallodynic effect exerted by agonists, a dose-dependent proallodynic effect was observed when the 5-HT$_7$-receptor antagonist SB-258719 was given to mice that had been injected with a low, subactive dose of capsaicin, but not in mice given an intraplantar injection of vehicle, thus suggesting that endogenous activation of the receptor takes place only in the presence of a sensitizing stimulus.

In rats with unilateral constriction injury to the sciatic nerve, we investigated whether and how 5-HT$_7$ receptors participate in the modulation of neuropathic pain. Blockade of 5-HT$_7$ receptors (by SB-269970) caused a transient and limited increase in vocalization threshold (but not in paw-withdrawal threshold) to paw pressure using the Randall and Selitto test. In contrast, 5-HT$_7$-receptor activation by MSD-5a, E-55888, or AS-19 markedly increased paw withdrawal and vocalization thresholds to hindpaw pressure and increased struggle latency to hindpaw immersion into a noxious (46°C) hot water bath. Blockade of 5-HT$_7$ receptors by SB-269970 prevented the effects of all three agonists (Fig. 3 and unpublished observations). Because 5-HT$_7$-receptor stimulation is excitatory,

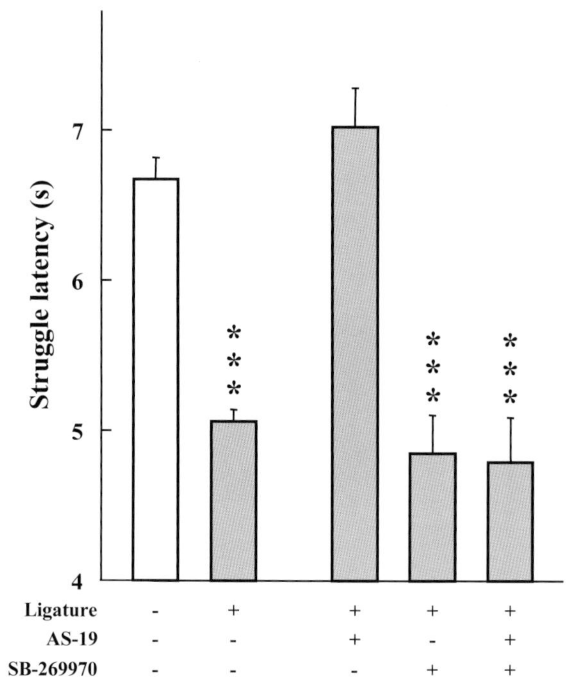

Fig. 3. Antihyperalgesic effects of 5-HT$_7$-receptor activation. Mean struggle latencies (expressed in seconds) after immersion of the nerve-injured hindpaw into a hot (46°C) water bath in rats that had undergone unilateral constriction injury to the sciatic nerve 2 weeks previously and had subsequently received acute treatment with the 5-HT$_7$-receptor agonist AS-19 (10 mg/kg s.c.), the 5-HT$_7$-receptor antagonist SB-269970 (3 mg/kg i.p.), or a combination of both drugs (10 minutes prior to the test). Each bar is the mean ± SEM of six independent determinations. Hyperalgesia observed 2 weeks after sciatic nerve ligature was reversed by 5-HT$_7$-receptor activation with AS-19. ***$P < 0.001$ as compared with values in control "sham" rats (empty bar), Student's *t* test.

we hypothesized that the antihyperalgesic effects of all three agonists were mediated by activation of inhibitory interneurons rather than through presynaptic 5-HT$_7$ receptors on primary afferent fibers. Accordingly, rats were given E-55888 plus either naloxone or bicuculline to block any 5-HT$_7$-receptor-mediated activation of opioidergic or GABAergic neurotransmission, respectively. Blockade of spinal GABA$_A$ receptors by intrathecal administration of bicuculline was found to significantly counteract the antihyperalgesic effects of E-55888. In contrast, blockade of spinal opioid receptors by naloxone was only marginally effective. These data therefore support the idea that 5-HT$_7$-receptor stimulation induced antihyperalgesic effects mainly through the release of GABA at the spinal level in neuropathic rats. Accordingly, effective 5-HT$_7$ receptors are very probably those expressed by GABAergic interneurons within the dorsal horn.

In contrast to the studies mentioned above, which strongly suggest that 5-HT$_7$-receptor activation exerts antinociceptive effects, two reports have described a pronociceptive modulation by 5-HT acting at 5-HT$_7$ receptors. First, Rocha-Gonzalez et al. [80] noted that local injection (into the hindpaw) or intrathecal administration of 5-HT or of 5-carboxamidotryptamine, a nonselective 5-HT$_7$-receptor agonist, enhanced nociceptive responses to intraplantar injections of formalin. This effect could be prevented by the 5-HT$_7$-receptor antagonist SB-269970. The second study described an activation of primary sensory nociceptive pathways accompanied by an increase of c-fos expression in the dorsal horn when 8-OH-DPAT, acting via the stimulation of 5-HT$_7$ receptors, was administered intra-articularly in rats [62]. Therefore, an important question to be addressed is whether activation of 5-HT$_7$ receptors can elicit a spectrum of pro- and antinociceptive actions depending on the location of the receptors and/or the quality and modality of the stimulus. So far, the available data point to a central antinociceptive action, whereas activation of peripheral receptors seems to exert a pronociceptive effect. If a balance between pro- and antinociceptive actions really exists, at least in conditions involving central sensitization (capsaicin or neuropathy models), the overall effect of systemically administered 5-HT$_7$-receptor agonists is clearly analgesic, which points to the potential therapeutic interest of such ligands for alleviating neuropathic pain.

Conclusion

Since the discovery, in the 1970s, that direct electrical stimulation of the nucleus raphe magnus produces a strong analgesic effect through the activation of descending bulbospinal serotoninergic projections, a considerable number of investigations have been devoted to identifying which types among the 15 different classes of 5-HT receptors are responsible for this effect. Relevant studies in various animal models showed that at least seven different receptor types—5-HT$_{1A}$, 5-HT$_{1B}$, 5-HT$_{2A}$, 5-HT$_{2C}$, 5-HT$_3$, 5-HT$_4$, and 5-HT$_7$—are potentially involved in 5-HT-mediated modulatory mechanisms of nociception and chronic pain. As detailed in the sections above, either direct actions or indirect mechanisms (i.e., through inhibitory interneurons) underlie the antinociceptive effects of 5-HT mediated by these receptors (Fig. 4).

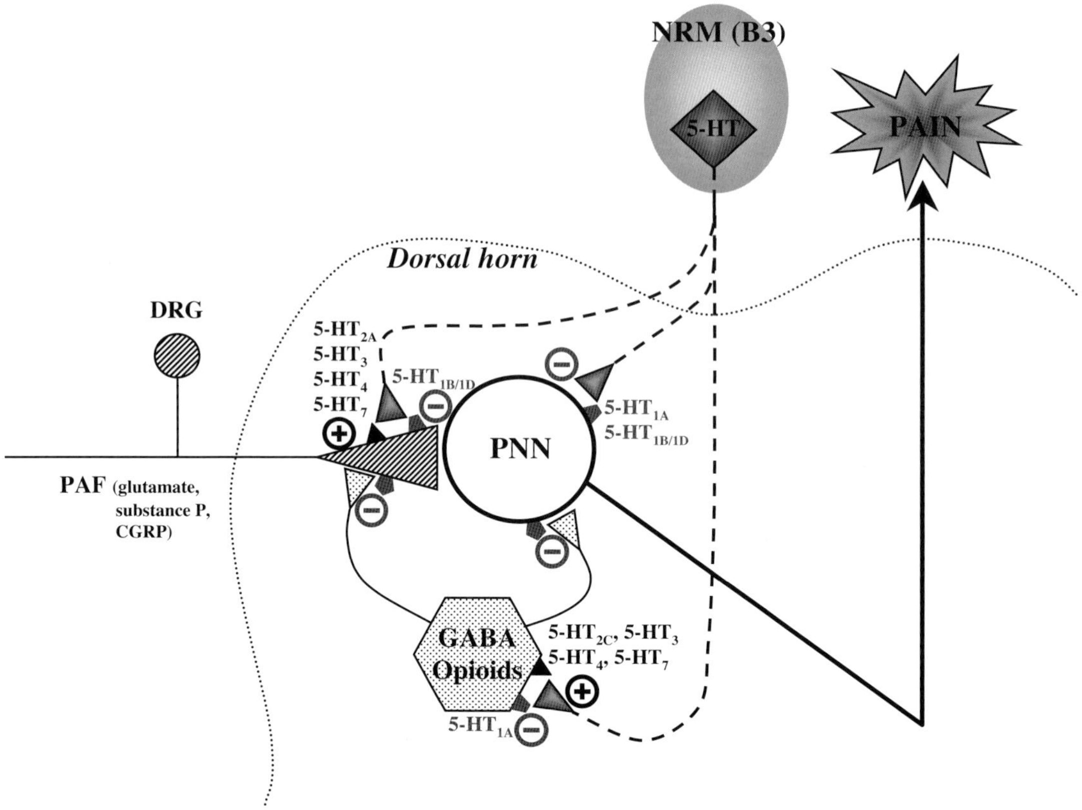

Fig. 4. Schematic representation of direct and indirect mechanisms underlying 5-HT-induced antinociceptive effects at the spinal level in rodents. Through the stimulation of 5-HT$_{1A}$ and 5-HT$_{1B/1D}$ receptors, 5-HT directly inhibits (pre- and/or postsynaptic) nociceptive signaling in superficial laminae of the dorsal horn. On the other hand, thanks to the expression of excitatory receptors (5-HT$_{2C}$, 5-HT$_3$, 5-HT$_4$, and 5-HT$_7$) on GABAergic (and opioidergic) inhibitory interneurons, 5-HT exerts an indirect, GABA- and/or opioid-mediated inhibition of nociceptive signaling mechanisms. Both direct and indirect mechanisms contribute to the antinociceptive effects of intrathecally administered 5-HT in rodents. CGRP: calcitonin-gene-related peptide; DRG: dorsal root ganglion; GABA: γ-aminobutyric acid; NRM: nucleus raphe magnus; PAF: primary afferent (nociceptive) fibers; PNN: postsynaptic nociceptive neuron.

However, depending on their peripheral versus central distribution, on the cell phenotypes expressing the receptors, on their subcellular location (somatodendritic versus axonal; postsynaptic versus presynaptic), they can in fact mediate not only antinociceptive but also pronociceptive effects of 5-HT. Such complex functional implications explain why, after more than 30 years of extensive research, numerous important questions regarding the exact role of 5-HT in pain control are still unsolved. Nevertheless, major achievements have been made with the development of triptans, which act as 5-HT$_{1B/1D}$-receptor agonists, for alleviating migraine pain, and most recent studies with 5-HT$_{1A}$- and 5-HT$_7$-receptor agonists seem to open very promising perspectives for the therapeutic treatment of pain with these ligands, either alone or most probably in combination with other drugs.

Acknowledgments

The team activity is supported by grants from INSERM, Université Pierre et Marie Curie (Paris 6) and Institut UPSA de la Douleur.

References

[1] Ahn AH, Basbaum AI. Tissue injury regulates serotonin 1D receptor expression: implications for the control of migraine and inflammatory pain. J Neurosci 2006;26:8332–8.
[2] Alhaider AA, Lei SZ, Wilcox GL. Spinal 5-HT3-mediated anti-nociception-possible release of GABA. J Neurosci 1991;11:1881–8.
[3] Alhaider AA, Wilcox GL. Differential roles of 5-hydroxytryptamine1A and 5-hydroxytryptamine1B receptor subtypes in modulating spinal nociceptive transmission in mice. J Pharmacol Exp Ther 1993;265:378–85.
[4] Ali Z, Wu G, Kozlov A, Barasi S The role of 5HT3 in nociceptive processing in the rat spinal cord: results from behavioral and electrophysiological studies. Neurosci Lett 1996;208:203–7.
[5] Anjaneyulu M, Chopra K. Fluoxetine attenuates thermal hyperalgesia through 5-HT1/2 receptors in streptozotocin-induced diabetic mice. Eur J Pharmacol 2004;497:285–92.
[6] Ardid D, Alloui A, Brousse G, Jourdan D, Picard P, Dubray C, Eschalier A. Potentiation of the antinociceptive effect of clomipramine by a 5-HT_{1A} antagonist in neuropathic pain in rats. Br J Pharmacol 2001;132:1118–26.
[7] Arvieu L, Mauborgne A, Bourgoin S, Oliver C, Feltz P, Hamon M, Cesselin F. Sumatriptan inhibits the release of CGRP and substance P from the rat spinal cord. Neuroreport 1996;7:1973–6.
[8] Bardin L, Lavarenne J, Eschalier A. Serotonin receptor subtypes involved in the spinal antinociceptive effect of 5-HT in rats. Pain 2000;86:11–8.
[9] Bardin L, Tarayre JP, Malfetes N, Koek W, Colpaert FC. Profound, non-opioid analgesia produced by the high-efficacy 5-HT_{1A} agonist F 13640 in the formalin model of tonic nociceptive pain. Pharmacology 2003;67:182–94.
[10] Bartsch T, Knight YE, Goadsby PJ. Activation of 5-$HT_{1B/1D}$ receptor in the periaqueductal gray inhibits nociception. Ann Neurol 2004;56:371–81.
[11] Barnes NM, Sharp T, A review of central 5-HT receptors and their function. Neuropharmacology 1999;38:1083–152.
[12] Bianchi C, Rodi D, Marino S, Beani L, Siniscalchi A. Dual effects of 5-HT4 receptor activation on GABA release from guinea pig hippocampal slices. Neuroreport 2002;13:2177–80.
[13] Bonnavion P, Bernard JF, Hamon M, Adrien J, Fabre V. Heterogeneous distribution of the 5-HT1A receptor mRNA in chemically identified neurons of the mouse rostral brainstem. J Sleep Res 2008;17:Suppl 1.
[14] Bonnefont J, Chapuy E, Clottes E, Alloui A, Eschalier A. Spinal 5-HT1A receptors differentially influence nociceptive processing according to the nature of the noxious stimulus in rats: effect of WAY-100635 on the antinociceptive activities of paracetamol, venlafaxine and 5-HT. Pain 2005;114:482–90.
[15] Boothman L, Raley J, Denk F, Hirani E, Sharp T. In vivo evidence that 5-HT_{2C} receptors inhibit 5-HT neuronal activity via a GABAergic mechanism. Br J Pharmacol 2006;149:861–9.
[16] Bourson A, Borroni E, Austin RH, Monsma FJ, Sleight AJ. Determination of the role of the 5-HT6 receptor in the rat brain: a study using antisense oligonucleotides. J Pharmacol Exp Ther 1995;274:173–80.
[17] Branchek TA, Blackburn TP. 5-HT6 receptors as emerging targets for drug discovery. Annu Rev Pharmacol Toxicol 2000;40:319–34.
[18] Brenchat A, Romero L, Torrens A, García M, Pujol M, Burgueño J, Hamon M, Baeyens JM, Buschmann H, Zamanillo D, Vela JM. 5-HT7 receptor activation inhibits mechanical allodynia secondary to capsaicin sensitization in mice. Pain 2009;141:239–47.
[19] Buzzi MG, Carter WB, Shimizu T, Heath H 3rd, Moskowitz MA. Dihydroergotamine and sumatriptan attenuate levels of CGRP in plasma in rat superior sagittal sinus during electrical stimulation of the trigeminal ganglion. Neuropharmacology 1991;30:1193–200.
[20] Cardenas CG, Del Mar LP, Cooper BY, Scroggs RS. 5HT4 receptors couple positively to tetrodotoxin-insensitive sodium channels in a subpopulation of capsaicin-sensitive rat sensory neurons. J Neurosci 1997;17:7181–9.
[21] Colpaert FC, Tarayre JP, Koek W, Pauwels PJ, Bardin L, Xu XJ, Wiesenfeld-Hallin Z, Cosi C, Carilla-Durand E, Assié MB, et al. Large-amplitude 5-HT1A receptor activation: a new mechanism of profound, central analgesia. Neuropharmacology 2002;43:945–58.
[22] Colpaert FC, Hamon H, Wiesenfeld-Hallin Z. 5-HT1A receptors in chronic pain processing and control. In: Flor H, Kalso E, Dostrovsky JO, editors. Proceedings of the 11th World Congress on Pain. Seattle: IASP Press; 2006. p. 147–54.
[23] Colpaert FC. 5-HT_{1A} receptor activation: new molecular and neuroadaptive mechanisms of pain relief. Curr Opin Investig Drugs 2006;7:40–7.
[24] Cornea-Hebert V, Riad M, Wu C, Singh SK Descarries L. Cellular and subcellular distribution of the serotonin 5-HT2A receptor in the central nervous system of adult rat. J Comp Neurol 1999;409:187–209.
[25] Deseure K, Koek W, Colpaert FC, Adriaensen H. The 5-HT_{1A} receptor agonist F 13640 attenuates mechanical allodynia in a rat model of trigeminal neuropathic pain. Eur J Pharmacol 2002;456:51–7.
[26] Dogrul A, Seyrek M. Systemic morphine produce antinociception mediated by spinal 5-HT7, but not 5-HT1A and 5-HT2 receptors in the spinal cord. Br J Pharmacol 2006;149:498–505.

[27] Doly S, Madeira A, Fischer J, Brisorgueil MJ, Daval G, Bernard R, Vergé D, Conrath M. The 5-HT2A receptor is widely distributed in the rat spinal cord and mainly localized at the plasma membrane of postsynaptic neurons. J Comp Neurol 2004;472:496–511.

[28] Doly S, Fischer J, Brisorgueil MJ, Vergé D, Conrath M. Pre- and postsynaptic localization of the 5-HT7 receptor in rat dorsal spinal cord: immunocytochemical evidence. J Comp Neurol 2005;490:256–69.

[29] Donovan-Rodriguez T, Urch CE, Dickenson AH. Evidence of a role for descending serotonergic facilitation in a rat model of cancer-induced bone pain. Neurosci Lett 2006;393:237–42.

[30] Espejo, EF, Gil, E. Antagonism of peripheral 5-HT4 receptors reduces visceral and cutaneous pain in mice, and induces visceral analgesia after simultaneous inactivation of 5HT3 receptors. Brain Res 1998;788:20–4.

[31] Fabre V, Beaufour C, Evrard A, Rioux A, Hanoun N, Lesch KP, Murphy DL, Lanfumey L, Hamon M, Martres MP. Altered expression and functions of serotonin 5-HT1A and 5-HT1B receptors in knock-out mice lacking the 5-HT transporter. Eur J Neurosci 2000;12:2299–310.

[32] Faerber L, Drechsler S, Ladenburger S, Gschaidmeier H, Fischer W. The neuronal 5-HT3 receptor network after 20 years of research–¬|¬Evolving concepts in management of pain and inflammation. Eur J Pharmacol 2007;560:1–8.

[33] Färber L, Stratz TH, Brückle W, Späth M, Pongratz D, Lautenschläger J, Kötter I, Zöller B, Peter HH, Neeck G, et al. German Fibromyalgia Study Group. Short-term treatment of primary fibromyalgia with the 5-HT3 receptor antagonist tropisetron. Results of a randomized, double-blind, placebo-controlled multicenter trial in 418 patients, Int J Clin Pharmacol Res 2001;21:1–13.

[34] Finn DP, Fone KC, Beckett SR, Baxter JA, Ansell L, Marsden CA, Chapman V. The effects of pharmacological blockade of the 5-HT_6 receptor on formalin-evoked nociceptive behaviour, locomotor activity and hypothalamo-pituitary-adrenal axis activity in rats. Eur J Pharmacol 2007;569:59–63.

[35] Fonseca MI, Ni YG, Dunning DD, Miledi R. Distribution of serotonin 2A, 2C and 3 receptor mRNA in spinal cord and medulla oblongata. Mol Brain Res 2001;89:11–9.

[36] Ghelardini C, Galeotti N, Casamenti F, Malmberg-Aiello P, Pepeu G, Gualtieri F, Bartolini A. Central cholinergic antinociception induced by 5HT4 agonists: BIMU 1 and BIMU 8. Life Sci 1996;58:2297–309.

[37] Glaum SR, Proudfit HK, Anderson EG. 5-HT3 receptors modulate spinal nociceptive reflexes. Brain Res 1990;510:12–6.

[38] Goadsby PJ, Akerman S, Storer RJ. Evidence for postjunctional serotonin (5-HT1) receptors in the trigeminocervical complex. Ann Neurol 2001;50:804–7.

[39] Green GM, Scarth J, Dickenson A. An excitatory role for 5-HT in spinal inflammatory nociceptive transmission: state-dependent actions via dorsal horn 5-HT3 receptors in the anesthetized rat. Pain 2000;89:81–8.

[40] Hammerle CW, Surawicz CM. Updates on treatment of irritable bowel syndrome. World J Gastroenterol 2008;14:2639–49.

[41] Hamon M, Bourgoin S. Serotonin and its receptors in pain control. In: Sawynok J, Cowan A. editors. Novel aspects of pain management: opioids and beyonds. New York: John Wiley and Sons; 1999. p. 203–28.

[42] Harte SE, Kender RG, Borszcz GS. Activation of 5-HT1A and 5-HT7 receptors in the parafascicular nucleus suppresses the affective reaction of rats to noxious stimulation. Pain 2005;113:405–15.

[43] Hashizume H, Kawakami M, Yoshida M, Okada M, Enyo Y, Inomata Y. Sarpogrelate hydrochloride, a 5-HT2A receptor antagonist, attenuates neurogenic pain induced by nucleus pulposus in rats. Spine 2007;32:315–20.

[44] Hedlund PB, Sutcliffe JG. Functional, molecular and pharmacological advances in 5-HT7 receptor research. Trends Pharmacol Sci 2004;25:481–6.

[45] Honda M, Uchida K, Tanabe M, Ono H. Fluvoxamine, a selective serotonin reuptake inhibitor, exerts its antiallodynic effects on neuropathic pain in mice via 5-HT2A/2C receptors. Neuropharmacology 2006;5:866–72.

[46] Invernizzi RW, Pierucci M, Calcagno E, Di Giovanni G, Di Matteo V, Benigno A, Esposito E. Selective activation of 5-HT_{2C} receptors stimulates GABA-ergic function in the rat substantia nigra pars reticulata: a combined in vivo electrophysiological and neurochemical study. Neuroscience 2007;144:15231–535.

[47] Jennings EA, Ryan RM, Christie MJ. Effects of sumatriptan on rat medullary dorsal horn neurons. Pain 2004;111:30–37.

[48] Jeong CY, Choi JI, Yoon MH. Roles of serotonin receptor subtypes for the antinociception of 5-HT in the spinal cord of rats. Eur J Pharmacol 2004;502:205–11.

[49] Kaube H, Hoskin KL, Goadsby PJ. Inhibition by sumatriptan of central trigeminal neurones only after blood-brain barrier disruption. Br J Pharmacol 1993;109:788–92.

[50] Kawamata T, Omote K, Toriyabe M, Kawamata M, Namiki A. Intracerebroventricular morphine produces antinociception by evoking gamma-aminobutyric acid release through activation of 5-hydroxytryptamine 3 receptors in the spinal cord. Anesthesiology 2002;96:1175–82.

[51] Kayser V, Aubel B, Hamon M, Bourgoin S. The antimigraine 5-HT1B/1D receptor agonists, sumatriptan, zolmitriptan and dihydroergotamine, attenuate pain-related behaviour in a rat model of trigeminal neuropathic pain. Br J Pharmacol 2002;137:1287–97.

[52] Kayser V, Elfassi IE, Aubel B, Melfort M, Julius D, Gingrich JA, Hamon M, Bourgoin S. Mechanical, thermal and formalin-induced nociception is differentially altered in 5-HT1A-/-, 5-HT1B-/-, 5-HT2A-/-, 5-HT3A-/- and 5-HTT-/- knock-out male mice. Pain 2007;130:235–48.

[53] Kiss I, Degryse AD, Bardin L, Gomez de Segura IA, Colpaert FC. The novel analgesic, F 13640, produces intra- and postoperative analgesia in a rat model of surgical pain. Eur J Pharmacol 2005;523:29–39.

[54] Lanfumey L, Hamon M. 5-HT1 receptors. Curr Drug Targets CNS Neurol Disord 2004;3:1–10.

[55] Levy D, Jakubowski M, Burstein R. Disruption of communication between peripheral and central trigeminovascular neurons mediates the antimigraine action of 5-HT 1B/1D receptor agonists. Proc Natl Acad Sci USA 2004;101:4274–9.

[56] Liu FY, Xing GG, Qu XX, Xu IS, Han JS, Wan Y. Roles of 5-hydroxytryptamine (5-HT) receptor subtypes in the inhibitory effects of 5-HT on C-fiber responses of spinal wide dynamic range neurons in rats. J Pharmacol Exp Ther 2007;321:1046–53.
[57] Lovenberg TW, Baron BM, de Lecea L, Miller JD, Prosser RA, Rea MA, Foye PE, Racke M, Slone AL, Siegel BW, et al. A novel adenylyl cyclase-activating serotonin receptor (5-HT7) implicated in the regulation of mammalian circadian rhythms. Neuron 1993;11:449–58.
[58] McCleane GJ, Suzuki R, Dickenson AH. Does a single intravenous injection of the 5HT3 receptor antagonist ondansetron have an analgesic effect in neuropathic pain? A double-blinded, placebo-controlled cross-over study. Anesth Analg 2003;97:1474–8.
[59] Mangel AW, Northcutt AR. Review article: the safety and efficacy of alosetron, a 5-HT3 receptor antagonist, in female irritable bowel syndrome patients. Aliment Pharmacol Ther 1999;13:77–82.
[60] Mannoury la Cour C, El Mestikawy S, Hanoun N, Hamon M, Lanfumey L. Regional differences in the coupling of 5-hydroxytryptamine-1A receptors to G proteins in the rat brain. Mol Pharmacol 2006;70:1013–21.
[61] Marchand F, Pelissier T, Eschalier A, Ardid D, Alloui A, Soto-Moyano R, Mondaca M, Laurido C, Constandil L, Hernández A. Blockade of supraspinal 5-HT1A receptors potentiates the inhibitory effect of venlafaxine on wind-up activity in mononeuropathic rats. Brain Res 2004;1008:288–92.
[62] Meuser T, Pietruck C, Gabriel A, Xie GX, Lim KJ, Pierce Palmer P. 5-HT7 receptors are involved in mediating 5-HT-induced activation of rat primary afferent neurons. Life Sci 2002;71:2279–89.
[63] Michaelis M, Vogel C, Blenk KH, Arnason A, Jänig W. Inflammatory mediators sensitize acutely axotomized nerve fibers to mechanical stimulation in rats. J Neurosci 1998;18:7581–7.
[64] Micó JA, Ardid D, Berrocoso E, Eschalier A. Antidepressants and pain. Trends Pharmacol Sci 2006;27:348–54.
[65] Millan MJ. Descending control of pain. Prog Neurobiol 2002;66:355–474.
[66] Monnikes H, Rüter J, Konig M, Grote C, Kobelt P, Klapp BF, Arnold R, Wiedenmann B, Tebbe JJ. Differential induction of c-fos expression in brain nuclei by noxious and non-noxious colonic distension: role of afferent C-fibers and 5-HT3 receptors. Brain Res 2003;966:253–64.
[67] Nakae A, Nakai K, Tanaka T, Takashina M, Hagihira S, Shibata M, Ueda K, Mashimo T. Serotonin2C receptor mRNA editing in neuropathic pain model. Neurosci Res 2008;60:228–31.
[68] Nakae A, Nakai K, Tanaka T, Hagihira S, Shibata M, Ueda K, Masimo T. The role of RNA editing of the serotonin 2C receptor in a rat model of oro-facial neuropathic pain. Eur J Neurosci 2008;27:2373–9.
[69] Neumaier JF, Sexton TJ, Yracheta J, Diaz AM, Brownfield M. Localization of 5-HT7 receptors in rat brain by immunocytochemistry, in situ hybridization, and agonist stimulated cFos expression. J Chem Neuroanat 2001;21:63–73.
[70] Nikai T, Basbaum AI, Ahn AH. Profound reduction of somatic and visceral pain in mice by intrathecal administration of the anti-migraine drug, sumatriptan. Pain 2008;139:533–40.
[71] Nishiyama T. Effects of a 5-HT2A receptor antagonist, sarpogrelate, on thermal or inflammatory pain. Eur J Pharmacol 2005;516:18–22.
[72] Nitanda A, Yasunami N, Tokumo K, Fujii H, Hirai T, Nishio H. Contribution of the peripheral 5-HT2A receptor to mechanical hyperalgesia in a rat model of neuropathic pain. Neurochem Int 2005;47:394–400.
[73] Nozaki C, Kamei J. Possible involvement of opioidergic systems in the antinociceptive effect of the selective serotonin reuptake inhibitors in sciatic nerve injured mice. Eur J Pharmacol 2006;552:99–104.
[74] Obata H, Saito S, Sakurazawa S, Sasaki M, Usui T, Goto F. Antiallodynic effects of intrathecally administered 5-HT_{2C} receptor agonists in rats with nerve injury. Pain 2004;108:163–9.
[75] Obata H, Ito N, Sasaki M, Saito S, Goto F. Possible involvement of spinal noradrenergic mechanisms in the antiallodynic effect of intrathecally administered 5-HT2C receptor agonists in the rats with peripheral nerve injury. Eur J Pharmacol 2007;567:89–94.
[76] Pierce PA, Xie GX, Meuser T, Peroutka SJ. 5-Hydroxytryptamine receptor subtype messenger RNAs in human dorsal root ganglia: a polymerase chain reaction study. Neuroscience 1997;81:813–9.
[77] Potrebic S, Ahn AH, Skinner K, Fields HL, Basbaum AI. Peptidergic nociceptors of both trigeminal and dorsal root ganglia express serotonin 1D receptors: implications for the selective antimigraine action of triptans. J Neurosci 2003;23:10988–97.
[78] Qu CL, Huo FQ, Huang FS, Li YQ, Tang JS, Jia H. The role of 5-HT receptor subtypes in the ventrolateral orbital cortex of 5-HT-induced antinociception in the rat. Neuroscience 2008;152:487–94.
[79] Rojas-Corrales MO, Berrocoso E, Micó JA. Role of 5-HT1A and 5-HT1B receptors in the antinociceptive effect of tramadol. Eur J Pharmacol 2005;511:21–6.
[80] Rocha-González HI, Meneses A, Carlton SM, Granados-Soto V. Pronociceptive role of peripheral and spinal 5-HT7 receptors in the formalin test. Pain 2005;117:182–92.
[81] Saria A, Javorsky F, Humpel C, Gamse R, 5-HT3-receptor antagonists inhibit sensory neuropeptide release from the rat spinal cord. NeuroReport 1990;1:104–6.
[82] Sasaki M, Obata H, Saito S, Goto F. Antinociception with intrathecal alpha-methyl-5-hydroxytryptamine, a 5-hydroxytryptamine 2A/2C receptor agonist, in two rat models of sustained pain. Anesth Analg 2003;96:1072–8.
[83] Sasaki M, Obata H, Kawahara K, Saito S, Goto F. Peripheral 5-HT2A receptor antagonism attenuates primary thermal hyperalgesia and secondary mechanical allodynia after thermal injury in rats. Pain 2006;122:130–6.
[84] Shibata M, T. Ohkubo T, Takahashi H, Inoki R Modified formalin test: characteristic biphasic pain response. Pain 1989;38:347–52.
[85] Sommer C. Serotonin in pain and analgesia: actions in the periphery. Mol Neurobiol 2004;30:117–25.
[86] Suzuki R, Rygh LJ, Dickenson AH. Bad news from the brain: descending 5-HT pathways that control spinal pain processing. Trends Pharmacol Sci 2004;25:613–7.

[87] Tateyama M, Kubo Y. Dual signaling is differentially activated by different active states of the metabotropic glutamate receptor1alpha Proc Natl Acad Sci USA 2006;103:1124–8.
[88] Thibault K, van Steenwinckel J, Brisorgueil MJ, Fischer J, Hamon M, Calvino B, Conrath M. Serotonin 5-HT2A receptor involvement and Fos expression at the spinal level in vincristine-induced neuropathy in the rat. Pain 2008;140:305–22.
[89] Van Steenwinckel J, Brisorgueil MJ, Fischer J, Vergé D, Gingrich JA, Bourgoin S, Hamon M, Bernard R, Conrath M. Role of spinal serotonin 5-HT2A receptor in 2',3'-dideoxycytidine-induced neuropathic pain in the rat and the mouse. Pain 2008;137:66–80.
[90] Wei H, Chen Y, Hong Y. The contribution of peripheral 5-hydroxytryptamine2A receptor to carrageenan-evoked hyperalgesia, inflammation and spinal Fos protein expression in the rat. Neuroscience 2005;132:1073–82.
[91] Wei H, Pertovaara A. 5-HT_{1A} receptors in endogenous regulation of neuropathic hypersensitivity in the rat. Eur J Pharmacol 2006;535:157–65.
[92] Willis WD, Coggeshall RE. Sensory mechanisms of the spinal cord. New York: Kluwer Academic/Plenum; 2004.
[93] Woolley ML, Marsden CA, Fone KC. 5-HT6 receptors. Curr Drug Targets CNS Neurol Disord 2004;3:59–79.
[94] Xiao DQ, Zhu JX, Tang JS, Jia H. GABAergic modulation mediates antinociception produced by serotonin applied into thalamic nucleus submedius of the rat. Brain Res 2005;1057:161–7.
[95] Yokogawa F, Kiuchi Y, Ishikawa Y, Otsuka N, Masuda Y, Oguchi K, Hosoyamada A. An investigation of monoamine receptors involved in antinociceptive effects of antidepressants. Anesth Analg 2002;95:163–8.
[96] Yu B, Becnel J, Zerfaoui M, Rohatgi R, Boulares AH, Nichols CD. Serotonin 5-hydroxytryptamine(2A) receptor activation suppresses tumor necrosis factor-alpha-induced inflammation with extraordinary potency. J Pharmacol Exp Ther 2008;327:316–32.
[97] Yuen EY, Jiang Q, Chen P, Gu Z, Feng J, Yan Z. Serotonin 5-HT1A receptors regulate NMDA receptor channels through a microtubule-dependent mechanism. J Neurosci 2005;25:5488–501.
[98] Zeitz KP, Guy N, Malmberg AB, Dirajlal S, Martin WJ, Sun L, Bonhaus DW, Stucky CL, Julius D, Basbaum AI. The 5-HT3 subtype of serotonin receptor contributes to nociceptive processing via a novel subset of myelinated and unmyelinated nociceptors. J Neurosci 2002;22:1010–9.
[99] Zhang YQ, Gao X, Ji GC, Wu GC. Expression of 5-HT2A receptor mRNA in rat spinal dorsal horn and some nuclei of brainstem after peripheral inflammation. Brain Res 2001;900:146–51.
[100] Zhao ZQ, Chiechio S, Sun YG, Zhang KH, Zhao CS, Scott M, Johnson RL, Deneris ES, Renner KJ, Gereau RW, et al. Mice lacking central serotonergic neurons show enhanced inflammatory pain and an impaired analgesic response to antidepressant drugs. J Neurosci 2007;27:6045–53.

Correspondence to: Valérie Kayser, PhD, Faculté de médecine, Université Pierre et Marie Curie-Paris, site Pitié-Salpêtrière, INSERM/CPN U894, 91, Boulevard de l'Hôpital, 75013 Paris, France. Email: valerie.kayser@upmc.fr.

10

Glutamate and GABA Receptors in Pain Transmission

Ke Ren and Ronald Dubner

Department of Neural and Pain Sciences, Dental School; and Program in Neuroscience, University of Maryland, Baltimore, Maryland, USA

Glutamate and γ-aminobutyric acid (GABA) are metabolically related and represent the two most abundant amino acid neurotransmitters in the mammalian central nervous system (CNS), although they produce opposite effects. Glutamate mainly produces synaptic excitation and GABA predominantly induces inhibition. Glutamate and GABA both act on their respective ionotropic and metabotropic receptors and contribute to pain transmission at multiple levels of the CNS. More importantly, alterations in glutamatergic and GABAergic synaptic activity play critical roles in the development of pain hypersensitivity. Recent advances have corroborated and elaborated multiple modulatory sites on glutamate and GABA receptors and key mediators in their signal transduction, which are attractive targets for developing specific drugs for pain control. This chapter will briefly discuss the roles of glutamatergic and GABAergic synapses in spinal nociceptive transmission and mechanisms of persistent pain. Interested readers may consult extensive reviews for further information [121,200].

Glutamate Receptors in Pain Transmission

Since a series of observations a half-century ago by Curtis et al. [31] that L-glutamate produces powerful excitation of spinal neurons, it has been well established that glutamate is a prototypic amino acid transmitter at CNS excitatory synapses (for review, see [108]). Via

Pharmacology of Pain
edited by Pierre Beaulieu, David Lussier, Frank Porreca, and Anthony H. Dickenson
IASP Press, Seattle, © 2010

the ionotropic and metabotropic receptor families, glutamate-mediated synaptic activity contributes to enhanced excitability of dorsal horn neurons and behavioral hyperalgesia after injury.

Ionotropic Glutamate Receptors

The ionotropic glutamate receptors (iGluRs) consist of three major subtypes that are activated preferably by *N*-methyl-D-aspartate (NMDA), α-amino-3-hydroxy-5-methyl-4-isoxazolepropionic acid (AMPA), and 2-carboxy-3-carboxymethyl-4-isopropenylpyrrolidine (kainate) and are named after these agonists, respectively. All iGluRs are composed of multiple subunits (Table I) [28], which are likely to be tetramers, assembled as dimers of dimers [90]. Each iGluR subunit has four hydrophobic membrane domains (M1–M4),

Table I
Ionotropic glutamate receptor family subunits

iGluR Subtypes	Nomenclatures		
	Current*	NC-IUPHAR†	Others‡
NMDAR	NR1	GluN1	GluRζ1
	NR2A	GluN2A	GluRε1
	NR2B	GluN2B	GluRε2
	NR2C	GluN2C	GluRε3
	NR2D	GluN2D	GluRε4
	NR3A	GluN3A	
	NR3B	GluN3B	
AMPAR	GluR1	GluA1	GluRA
	GluR2	GluA2	GluRB
	GluR3	GluA3	GluRC
	GluR4	GluA4	GluRD
KAR	GluR5	GluK1	EAA3
	GluR6	GluK2	EAA4
	GluR7	GluK3	EAA5
	KA1	GluK4	EAA1
	KA2	GluK5	EAA2
Orphan	GluRδ1	GluD1	
	GluRδ2	GluD2	

Abbreviations: AMPAR = α-amino-3-hydroxy-5-methyl-4-isoxazolepropionic acid (AMPA) receptor; iGluR = ionotropic glutamate receptor; KAR = kainate receptor; NMDAR = *N*-methyl-D-aspartate (NMDA) receptor.

* Currently and commonly used nomenclatures for the iGluR family subunits.

† Updated nomenclature proposed by The International Union of Pharmacology Committee on Receptor Nomenclature and Drug Classification (NC-IUPHAR) (www.iuphar-db.org) [28]. Note that the letter "R" for receptor is removed to indicate the fact that these proteins are receptor subunits and should not be labeled as receptors.

‡ Other names used for iGluR family subunits. Greek letters in NMDAR subunits are used only for mice.

in which M1 and M3–4 are transmembrane-spanning domains and M2 makes a hairpin turn within the membrane and contributes to the ion pore (Fig. 1). The agonist-binding domain has been crystallized and is organized in a pocket between the pre-M1 region (S1 domain) and an extracellular loop between M3 and M4 (S2 domain) (Fig. 1) [90]. Based on amino acid sequence homology, GluRδ1 and δ2 subunits also belong to the iGluR family [115]. However, they are currently classified as orphan iGluRs because it is unclear whether they form functional channels, and their ligands are unknown. Whether GluRδ receptors contribute to pain transmission and thus constitute a therapeutic target has not been explored.

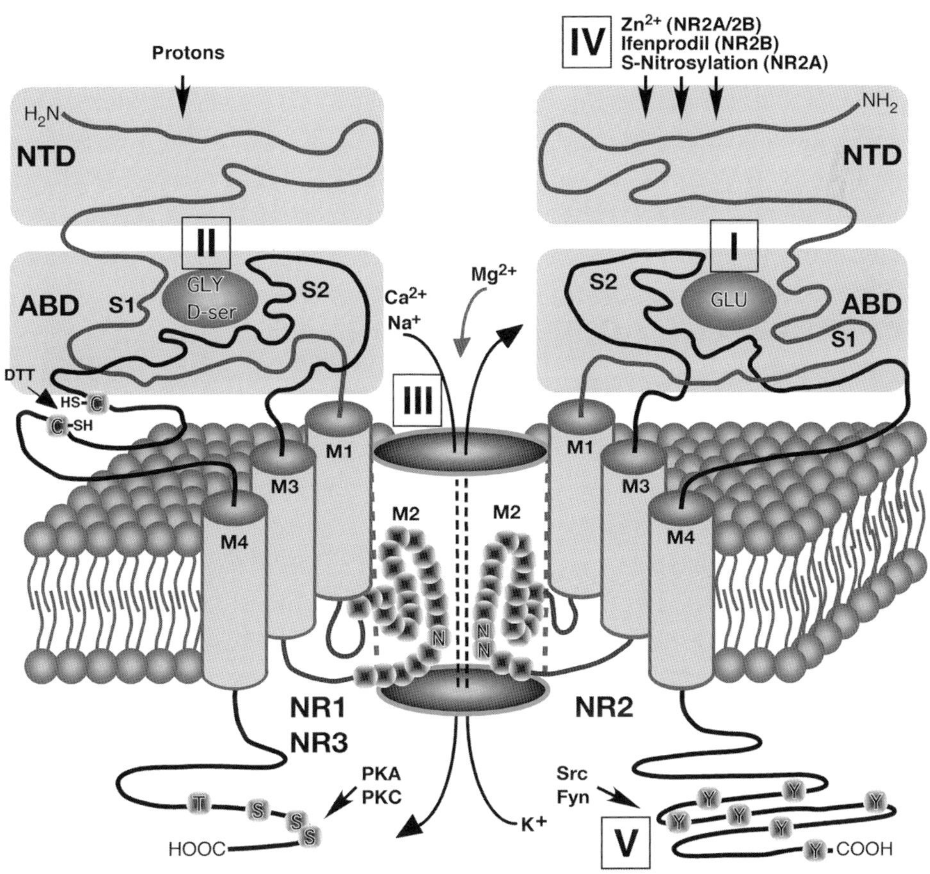

Fig. 1. The molecular and functional model of the *N*-methyl D-aspartate receptor (NMDAR)–ion channel complex. One NR1 (or NR3)/NR2 heterodimer is shown. Note that the extracellular region of each subunit consists of an N-terminal domain (NTD) and an agonist-binding domain (ABD) (gray-shaded rectangles). All ionotropic glutamate receptors (iGluRs) share the same membrane topology and have a similar agonist-binding domain structure that includes the S1 and S2 regions. Note that the asparagine (N) sites in the M2 segment of the NR1 and NR2 subunits govern both Ca^{2+} permeability and Mg^{2+} block in the NMDAR channel. The NMDAR can be modulated at multiple sites: (I) NR2 agonist recognition sites, (II) NR1/NR3 co-agonist sites, (III) ion channels, (IV) modulatory sites (note subunit specificity), and (V) C-terminal phosphorylation sites. See text for details.

NMDA Receptors

The NMDA glutamate receptor (NMDAR) is a receptor-ion channel complex (Fig. 1), characterized by a voltage-dependent block by Mg^{2+}, significant Ca^{2+} inflow upon activation, and slow kinetics [90,137]. Seven subunits contribute to the formation of the NMDAR: NR1 (GluN1 or GluRζ1), NR2A–D (GluN2A–D or GluRε1–4), and NR3A/B (GluN3A/B) (Table I). Alternative splicing of the NR1 gene further generates eight variants of the NR1 subunit. The native NMDAR channel consists of two NR1 and two NR2 subunits. Alternatively, an NR3 subunit may replace an NR1, resulting in ternary NR1/NR2/NR3 tetrameric NMDARs [22]. However, insertion of the NR3 subunit is associated with a reduced Ca^{2+} permeability of the NMDAR [22]. Glial NMDARs are weakly sensitive to magnesium block [98], which may indicate a predominant expression of the NR3 subunit. The large extracellular loop of the NMDAR subunits consists of a tandem of two regions, the N-terminal domain and the agonist-binding domain (Fig. 1). The site for allosteric inhibitors such as Zn^{2+} and ifenprodil is located in the N-terminal domain of the NR2A/B subunits. Glutamate binds to the agonist-binding domain of NR2, and the co-agonist glycine or D-serine binds to the NR1 or NR3 agonist-binding domain.

All NMDAR subunits are distributed in the spinal cord, and they may assemble into functionally different NMDARs that exhibit different sensitivity to glutamate [85,184,212]. While postsynaptic NMDARs facilitate pain transmission, interestingly, presynaptic NMDARs may also facilitate pain transmission by enhancing substance P release from primary afferent terminals [107]. Differential distribution of the NR2 subunits in synaptic versus extrasynaptic sites in the spinal dorsal horn has been reported, with NR2B located preferentially in extrasynaptic and NR2A in synaptic sites [125]. However, the role of extrasynaptic NMDARs in nociception is unclear.

The NMDAR plays an important role in processing nociceptive input to the spinal dorsal horn and is involved in dorsal horn hyperexcitability after injury [32,36,60,121,131,202]. An important observation is that wind-up of dorsal horn nociceptive neurons is selectively reduced by NMDAR antagonists [32,93]. Wind-up of dorsal horn neurons may trigger central hyperexcitability and result in prolonged nociceptive states. This phenomenon has been used to explain pain summation with repetitive stimulation. Further studies have shown that NMDARs are involved in increased excitability of dorsal horn neurons, a form of activity-dependent plasticity that is often referred to as central sensitization [202,203], and that they share some similar physiological properties with long-term potentiation (LTP) [35]. The alteration of receptive fields is a reflection of the activity-dependent plasticity of dorsal horn neurons. The expanded receptive fields of dorsal horn nociceptive neurons following inflammation induced by complete Freund's adjuvant (CFA) are also sensitive to the NMDAR antagonist [36]. The properties of NMDAR channels are altered by inflammation. Rat dorsal horn neurons that receive inputs from the inflamed hind paw exhibit a reduced Mg^{2+} block and enhanced NMDA responses [59]. Conditional deletion of the NR1 subunit in the spinal cord [26,172] and intrathecal injection of small interfering RNAs (siRNAs) targeting the NR2B subunit [179] reduced the formalin- and CFA-induced nocifensive behavior.

The increased NMDAR function involves post-translational modulation. Multiple sites at the C-termini of the NR1/NR2 subunits can be phosphorylated by protein kinase A (PKA), protein kinase C (PKC), or protein tyrosine kinases [3,13,183] (Fig. 1). A time-dependent and lasting NR1 phosphorylation at serine (ser) 896/897 after noxious stimulation has been observed [13,19,49,60,220]. The NMDAR gating is closely regulated by tyrosine kinase Src [3]. Seven specific tyrosine residues on the C-terminus of the NR2B subunit are phosphorylated by Fyn, an Src family tyrosine kinase, in vitro [130]. Src also regulates injury-activated ERK (extracellular signal-regulated kinase) [86]. Levels of NR2B tyrosine phosphorylation in the ipsilateral spinal dorsal horn are selectively increased after inflammation [62,142]. The wind-up of dorsal horn neurons appears to involve NR2 tyrosine phosphorylation and phosphatidylinositol 3-kinase signaling [142]. Abe et al. [1] show that Fyn kinase-mediated NR2B tyrosine phosphorylation at tyr1472 is essential for the maintenance of neuropathic pain. The phosphorylation of the NMDAR is regulated by protein phosphatases. Capsaicin injection also upregulates serine/threonine protein phosphatase 2A [217], which should facilitate dephosphorylation of the NMDAR. Application of phosphatase inhibitors enhances capsaicin-induced NMDAR phosphorylation and behavioral sensitization [216,217].

A key phenomenon with regard to NMDAR phosphorylation is that the changes in phosphorylation depend on primary afferent drive and occur within a few minutes after peripheral insult [61,62]. Importantly, thermal hyperalgesia and mechanical allodynia can also be detected within minutes after inflammation [62,78]. These correlated behavioral and biochemical findings indicate that NMDAR phosphorylation plays a key role in the *initiation* of pain hypersensitivity. Phosphorylation of the NR1/NR2 subunit wanes around 7 days, and no significant increase in phosphorylation is found at 14 days after inflammation [60–62]. The attenuation of CFA-induced hyperalgesia in mice with conditional knockout of the dorsal horn NR1 subunit occurred at 24 hours, but not at 48 hours, post-CFA [26]. However, CFA-induced hyperalgesia does not fully resolve until 2 weeks after inflammation [36]. Thus, the NMDAR phosphorylation may play less of a role, and other factors such as cyclooxygenase-2 expression and glial activation may participate in maintaining the late persistent phase of hyperalgesia [26].

The NMDAR forms multiprotein complexes with postsynaptic density (PSD) proteins including receptors, adaptor proteins, and protein kinases. The interactions between PSD proteins and kinases regulate synaptic trafficking and function of the receptor. For example, the N-terminal region of PSD-95 interacts with Src to suppress Src-mediated NMDAR phosphorylation [84] (Fig. 2). The functional integrity of the PSD is necessary for the expression of persistent pain behaviors. Mice with a mutated PSD-95 gene do not develop NMDAR-dependent hyperalgesia after neuropathy [52]. Inhibiting the expression of PSD-95 in spinal neurons significantly attenuates nocifensive facilitation by NMDA [181]. Targeted disruption of the PSD-93 gene attenuates NMDAR-dependent

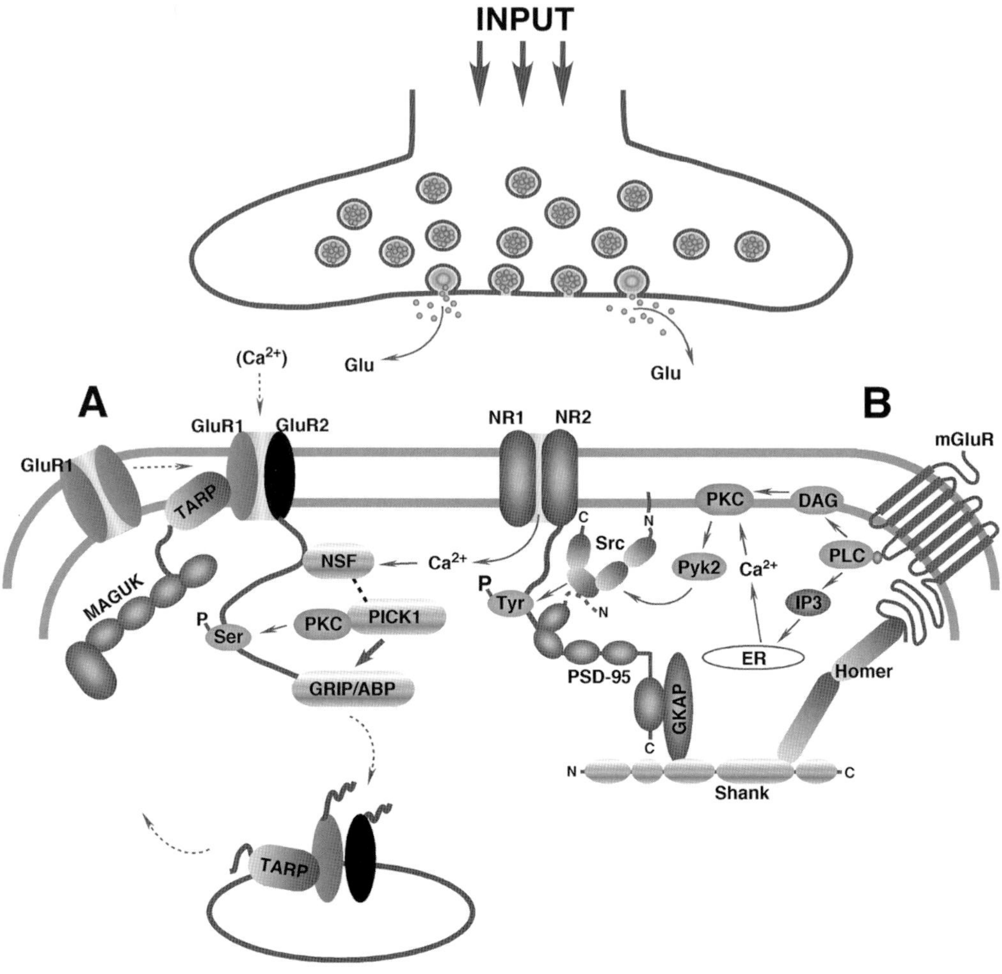

Fig. 2. Model of postsynaptic interactions between metabotropic glutamate receptors (mGluRs), NMDA glutamate receptors (NMDARs), and AMPA glutamate receptors (AMPARs). A glutamatergic presynaptic terminal bouton is shown on top. (A) Protein-protein interactions involved in AMPAR trafficking. (1) Transmembrane AMPAR regulatory proteins (TARPs), a family of auxiliary subunits of the AMPAR, bind to an AMPAR subunit and interact with synaptic scaffolding proteins of the membrane-associated guanylate kinase (MAGUK) family. This interaction leads to synaptic targeting/insertion of AMPARs and prevents their diffusion from the synapse. (2) Synaptic AMPARs are stabilized by interacting with glutamate receptor-interacting protein (GRIP) and AMPA-receptor binding protein (ABP) at the C-terminal PDZ binding sites. N-ethylmaleimide-sensitive factor (NSF) binds to GluR2 at a more proximal site on C-terminal and interacts with PICK1 (protein interacting with C kinase). The NSF-PICK1 interaction prevents PICK1 from unbinding GRIP/ABP by competition. (3) Two forces may drive unbinding of GRIP/ABP: protein kinase C (PKC)-triggered phosphorylation of Ser880 in the GluR2 and Ca^{2+} ions entering through NMDAR channels or another source (not shown). Ca^{2+} can bind to NSF and disrupt the NSF-GluR2 interaction, which allows PICK1 to replace ABP/GRIP at the GluR2 C-terminus. Association of PICKI with GluR2 leads to internalization of GluR2-containing AMPARs and insertion of Ca^{2+}-permeable AMPARs (GluR1 dimer, horizontal dashed arrow) to the synaptic site via lateral diffusion. The PICK1-mediated trafficking is crucial in determining the presence or absence of the GluR2 subunit in the AMPAR assembly and thus Ca^{2+} permeability. Influx of Ca^{2+} through AMPARs (vertical dashed arrow) contributes to central sensitization and hyperalgesia. Internalized GluR2-containing AMPARs can be recycled to the membrane (curved dashed arrows). (B) mGluR-NMDAR interaction. The NMDAR and group I mGluRs-Homer complex are associated via binding of postsynaptic density-95 protein (PSD-95), guanylate kinase-associated protein (GKAP), and Shank. Src, a protein tyrosine (Tyr) kinase, is associated with NMDAR via interaction with →

persistent pain after injury [182]. Brenner et al. [13] show that NR1 ser896 phosphorylation occurs in the endoplasmic reticulum, suggesting a role in trafficking of the NR1 subunit to the cell membrane. However, the role of NMDAR trafficking in persistent pain is not well understood.

Theoretically, drugs can target the following sites to affect the activity of the NMDAR, thus achieving a variety of therapeutic goals, including control of chronic pain (Fig. 1) [24,34,131,137].

I. Agonist recognition site: Compete for the recognition site of L-glutamate on the NR2 subunit. Antagonists include (±)-2-amino-5-phosphonopentanoic acid (AP-5) and (±)-3-(2-carboxypiperazin-4-yl)-propyl-1-phosphonic acid (CPP).

II. Co-agonist site: Modulate the binding of the co-agonist glycine or D-serine to the NR1 subunit. Antagonists include HA-966, 7-chlorokynurenic acid, and GVI196771. However, partial agonists, such as (+)-HA 966 or GLYX-13, at the glycine site are antinociceptive against the formalin response and neuropathic pain [122,201].

III. The ion channel: Act at the intra-ion channel sites to inhibit NMDAR channels. These agents include Mg^{2+}, dextromethorphan, dizocilpine maleate (MK-801), ketamine, and memantine.

IV. Modulatory sites: Zinc inhibits NMDAR function through both voltage-dependent and voltage-independent mechanisms [136,189]. Protons inhibit NMDAR function through interactions with the NR1 subunit [190]. Polyamines increase the binding of [^{3}H] MK-801 [152], suggesting that they could facilitate activation of the NMDAR by glutamate. Polyamines may also suppress the NMDAR function under certain conditions. The N1 insert (including Lys211) from exon 5 of the NR1 gene is involved in regulating pH sensitivity and the effects of zinc and polyamines on NMDAR [208]. Dithiothreitol, a sulfhydryl (SH) group reducing agent, enhances NMDAR responses via two cysteine residues (C744 and C798) of the NR1 subunit [158] (Fig. 1). Nitric oxide interacts with Cys399 on the NR2A subunit to induce S-nitrosylation and lead to desensitization of the NMDAR [24].

V. Protein phosphorylation sites: These sites include components of the signal transduction pathways such as protein kinases and phosphatases, cofactors, and scaffold proteins in the PSD.

VI. RNA transcription (not shown in Fig. 1): Pending efficient delivery, RNA interference can produce subtype-specific and localized silencing of NMDAR function [51,179].

PSD-95. After primary afferent activation, Tyr residues in the C-terminus of the NR2B subunits are phosphorylated through proline-rich tyrosine kinase 2 (Pyk2)-Src pathways. The N-terminal region of PSD-95 interacts with Src to produce negative regulation of Src-mediated phosphorylation. The upstream events leading to Src-Tyr signaling most likely involve activation of group I mGluRs, an increase in intracellular Ca^{2+} through inositol triphosphate (IP_3)-endoplastic reticulum (ER) pathways, and PKC activation through the diacylglycerol (DAG) pathway. Tyrosine phosphorylation of the NMDAR will potentiate NMDAR channel gating and trigger a cascade leading to increased gene transcription of the target genes. These events contribute to amplification of synaptic input, central sensitization, and the development of hyperalgesia.

AMPA Receptors

AMPARs are assembled from four subunits named GluR1–4 (alternatively known as GluA1–4; see Table I) [28]. Each subunit of the AMPAR exists in two isoforms, so called "flip" and "flop," due to alternative splicing of a 115-base pair region within the ligand binding (S2) domain [101]. The flip-flop splice forms affect kinetic and gating properties of the AMPAR channel, with the flop form mediating the fast desensitizing component and the flip form governing the steady-state current component. The eight AMPAR mRNA species are differentially distributed in the spinal cord with GluR1 (mainly the flop form) and GluR2 (mainly the flip form) subunits predominantly found in the dorsal horn and GluR3/4 subunits primarily located in ventral horn [185]. However, all AMPAR subunits have been found in the superficial laminae of the spinal cord [146,178]. AMPARs are present at dorsal horn synapses receiving unmyelinated fibers [147] and are involved in fast monosynaptic activation of spinal neurons and the basal level of pain processing [121].

AMPARs are involved in injury-induced synaptic plasticity and hyperalgesia. The AMPAR subunit mRNAs and proteins are upregulated after inflammation and nerve injury with a time course correlating with the early development of behavioral hyperalgesia and allodynia, and the upregulation is somatotopically relevant [68,219]. Downregulation of AMPAR subunits has also been observed [45,219]. Increased GluR1 phosphorylation at ser831/845 has been found within minutes after administration of capsaicin or inflammation [43,63]. Also shown in a sciatic nerve transection model, the AMPAR GluR2/3 subunit is selectively increased on the side ipsilateral to the injury, and the increase is restricted to the synapses of primary afferent terminals [148]. Coactivation of AMPAR and metabotropic glutamate receptors (mGluRs) produces mechanical hyperalgesia in rats [118]. Selective AMPAR/kainate receptor (KAR) antagonists reduce responses of dorsal horn neurons to noxious somatic and visceral stimulation [21,79] and produce analgesia in rats in a variety of preclinical models [66,80,134,167]. LY293558, a GluR5 antagonist, is efficacious and well tolerated in acute migraine patients [34,160]. The dorsal horn hyperexcitability associated with the incisional pain model can be selectively blocked by the AMPAR/KAR antagonist NBQX, but not by the NMDAR antagonist MK-801 [213].

The stoichiometry of the AMPAR is variable and dependent on functional necessity of the synapse. Apparently, alterations in composition of flip/flop isoforms may lead to altered synaptic efficacy and fast synaptic transmission, thus affecting pain transmission. However, any conclusions about the specific contribution of the GluR flip/flop splice variants to nociceptive transmission and persistent pain are currently only speculative [219]. The presence of the GluR2 subunit determines the permeability of the AMPAR channel for calcium ions. Due to Q/R (glutamine/arginine) RNA editing in the M2 pore loop domain, most adult GluR2 mRNAs encode arginine at this site, which denies Ca^{2+} permeability. Homomeric AMPAR complexes consisting of GluR1/3, or GluR4, proteins are permeable to Ca^{2+}, while homomeric GluR2 complexes or the heteromeric assembly of GluR2 with any of the other AMPAR subunits are not permeable to Ca^{2+} [90].

Both Ca^{2+}-permeable and Ca^{2+}-impermeable AMPAR assemblies are present in the superficial dorsal horn, and their distribution corresponds to the immunostaining of GluR1 and GluR2 receptors, respectively [38,147,178]. In lamina I of the dorsal horn, a population of neurons expressing Ca^{2+}-permeable AMPARs colocalize with the neurokinin-1 receptor (NK1R) [38,186]. A large population of lamina III/IV NK1R-bearing neurons also have postsynaptic Ca^{2+}-permeable AMPARs [186]. Apparently, both Ca^{2+}-permeable and Ca^{2+}-impermeable AMPARs receive primary synaptic drive. Synaptic localization of Ca^{2+}-permeable AMPARs in the spinal dorsal horn suggests that these receptors are capable of mediating noxious input from thin primary afferents as well as low-threshold sensory input.

Ca^{2+}-permeable AMPARs contribute to synaptic plasticity in dorsal horn circuitry. In mice deficient in the GluR2 subunit, there is an increase in rectification of excitatory postsynaptic current (EPSC), suggesting an increased expression of Ca^{2+}-permeable AMPARs [210]. As a result, LTP evoked by high-frequency stimulation of Aδ/C fibers is enhanced and long-term depression (LTD) is reduced in the spinal dorsal horn of the GluR2 mutants. In mice lacking GluR1 or GluR2 subunits, researchers have found the number of Ca^{2+}-permeable AMPARs and the density of AMPA channel currents to be decreased or increased, respectively [69]. Inflammatory hyperalgesia is enhanced in GluR2-deficient mice but reduced in GluR1-deficient mice [69]. In CFA-induced inflammation, there appears to be an increased contribution of Ca^{2+}-permeable AMPARs to nociceptive synaptic transmission in the dorsal horn, as seen by a significant shortening of the quantal AMPA current decay, a greater inward rectification of the AMPAR-mediated evoked EPSC amplitude and an increased sensitivity to the Ca^{2+}-permeable AMPAR channel blocker [196].

Thus, Ca^{2+}-permeable AMPAR channels appear to be a pharmacological target for analgesics. Several polyamine derivatives and toxins can be used to block Ca^{2+}-permeable AMPAR, including philanthotoxin, joro spider toxin (JSTx), argiotoxin, and 1-naphthylacetyl spermine. Pretreatment with JSTx in the rat spinal cord prevented the development of allodynia after a mild burn [170]. The antagonists of Ca^{2+}-permeable AMPARs are antinociceptive against thermal injury-induced mechanical allodynia and carrageenan-induced hyperalgesia/allodynia, but without an effect on the formalin model and allodynia after spinal nerve ligation [171]. Ca^{2+}-permeable AMPARs may also exist in spinal inhibitory interneurons [173]. Low doses of JSTx produce facilitation of C-fiber responses of dorsal horn neurons, suggesting a role of Ca^{2+}-permeable AMPARs in spinal inhibitory synaptic activity [175]. Synaptic AMPARs are dynamically regulated, including the trafficking to and from the synapse and modulation of subunit composition. Membrane trafficking of AMPARs is critical for adjusting synaptic strength to meet functional requirements in different types of synaptic plasticity. The different sensitivity or modulatory effect of JSTx on different pain models and dorsal horn neurons may be explained by varying numbers of synaptic GluR1/GluR2 subunits under different conditions.

Interactions among proteins are involved in AMPAR trafficking, including endocytosis and reinsertion/diffusion of the receptor to the synapse [67] (Fig. 2). The insertion of AMPARs to the synapse requires transmembrane AMPAR regulatory proteins (TARPs), a family of auxiliary subunits of the AMPAR. Stargazin (also called γ2), a member of the TARP family, binds to AMPAR subunits and interacts with membrane-associated guanylate kinases (MAGUKs), a family of synaptic scaffolding proteins including PSD-95, PSD-93, SAP-97 and SAP-102 [133]. This interaction leads to synaptic targeting/insertion of AMPARs and prevents their diffusion from the synapse [133].

One model of regulated removal of GluR2 from the synapse involves GRIP (or GRIP1, glutamate receptor-interacting protein), ABP (AMPAR-binding protein, or GRIP2) and PICK1 (protein interacting with C kinase) [67] (Fig. 2). The synaptic presence of AMPARs is favored by interactions with ABP/GRIP at their C-terminal PDZ binding sites. (PDZ is an initialism based on the first letters of the three first proteins that were determined to share this domain, including PSD-95.). NSF (N-ethylmaleimide-sensitive factor), a non-PDZ domain protein involved in membrane fusion, binds to GluR2 at a more proximal site on its C-terminal to favor interaction with PICK1. The NSF-PICK1 interaction interrupts PICK1-GluR2 contact and prevents GRIP/ABP unbinding by competition from PICK1. Upon the arrival of calcium signals and phosphorylation of Ser880 in the GluR2, NSF-GluR2 interaction is disrupted, allowing PICK1 to replace ABP/GRIP at the GluR2 C-terminus. Association of PICK1 with GluR2 leads to removal of GluR2-containing AMPARs from the synapse [67]. The PICK1-mediated trafficking is crucial in determining the presence or absence of the GluR2 subunit in the AMPAR assembly and thus Ca^{2+} permeability.

Only a few studies have addressed the role of AMPAR trafficking in pain transmission. An increase in GluR1 at the plasma membrane in the spinal cord has been observed following intracolonic capsaicin-induced referred hyperalgesia [48] and administration of formalin [142]. Serotonin unmasks dorsal horn silent glutamatergic synapses in neonatal rats [104]. When a synthetic peptide is used to disrupt binding of GluR2 to GRIP/ABP, serotonin-induced facilitation of dorsal horn neurons is blocked, although there is no effect on basal synaptic responses [103]. However, use of the same strategy to block GluR2–PICK1 interaction did not produce an effect on serotonin-induced facilitation. These results are consistent with a role of GRIP/ABP in maintaining synaptic AMPARs, which is the opposite to that of the GluR2–PICK1 interaction, leading to AMPAR removal from the synapse. Intrathecal administration of cell-permeable peptides to block GluR2–NSF and GluR2/3–GRIP/PICK1 interactions produces antihyperalgesia in a rat neuropathic pain model [53]. Antisense knockdown of stargazin in the spinal cord dose-dependently inhibited the second-phase response to formalin [180]. It is also likely that the effect of PSD-95 inhibition or mutation on pain behavior is related to an effect on synaptic AMPAR targeting through stargazin [52,181]. These findings indicate that protein interactions related to AMPAR trafficking help to maintain synaptic strength and efficacy in pain-processing circuitry and are particularly important in response to prolonged nociception.

Interaction of NMDA and AMPA Receptors in Pain Transmission

Both NMDAR and AMPAR subunits are present in spinothalamic tract cells [208,220]. Most glutamatergic synapses in the superficial dorsal horn are mixed, containing both NMDARs and AMPARs [7]. The interactions between these receptors are required to support regular synaptic activity and further modulate synaptic strength. A typical example is the existence of so-called silent synapses in neonatal animals, where NMDARs are essentially nonfunctional at the resting membrane potential due to a lack of the functional AMPARs in the synapse [74,104]. AMPA-mediated EPSCs appear upon LTP induction, involving trafficking of AMPAR to the membrane, which leads to conversion of the silent synapses to functional ones.

Synaptic responses evoked by primary afferent fibers are mediated differentially by all iGluR subtypes in the dorsal horn [121]. In the deep dorsal horn, dorsal root stimulation-induced EPSC contains initial fast AMPAR and late slow NMDAR components [55]. Seagrove et al. [165] showed that lamina I nociceptive neurons do not exhibit wind-up phenomena and are insensitive to NMDAR antagonists, and they are sensitive to NBQX. This quality is in contrast to deep dorsal horn neurons that show NMDAR-sensitive wind-up [32]. Interestingly, a transient noxious stimulus evokes glutamate and aspartate release from the superficial dorsal horn, and inflammation induces release of these molecules from both the superficial and deep dorsal horn [33]. These results suggest differential roles of NMDAR and AMPAR/KAR in the superficial and deep spinal dorsal horn in the processing of transient and persistent noxious information.

Interactions between NMDAR and AMPAR are implicated during normal nociception and central sensitization and hyperalgesia. A combination of the NMDAR and AMPAR antagonists AP-5 and YM872 acts synergistically to suppress the nociceptive tail-flick reflex and both phases of the formalin response [134]. Ca^{2+}-permeable AMPARs contribute to injury-dependent synaptic plasticity in dorsal horn circuitry and hyperalgesia [69,170,171,196,210]. Interestingly, most excitatory neurons in the superficial dorsal horn are associated with GluR2 subunits [88]. An increased NMDAR activity with Ca^{2+} influx may contribute to increased synaptic Ca^{2+}-permeable AMPARs through PICK1-mediated removal of GluR2 from the synapse (Fig. 2). Increased Ca^{2+} influx through AMPARs may desensitize neighboring NMDARs [95], and Ca^{2+}-permeable AMPARs would then become the major source of synaptic Ca^{2+}. Thus, the outcome of the interaction may be either facilitatory or inhibitory. In response to injury, neuronal excitation is predominant, such that the net effect is increased pain sensitivity.

Kainate Receptors

The native kainate receptor is formed by a heteromeric combination of five subunits, GluK1–5, comprising KA1,2 (high-affinity subunits) and GluR5,6,7 (low-affinity subunits) (Table I) [28]. Homomeric KA1 or KA2 subunit clones do not appear to form functional channels, but they may contribute to KAR channel activity when they form heteromeric receptors with GluR5–7 subunits. Alternative splicing of GluR5–7 mRNAs, mainly in the C-terminal region, generates further molecular diversity of KARs. Alterations in the C-terminal domains of the KAR subunits due to alternative splicing have a major impact on intracellular trafficking of KARs [143].

Kainate receptor subunits are expressed in the spinal dorsal horn and dorsal root ganglion (DRG) cells [64,112,184,204]. All KAR mRNA species have been found in the trigeminal ganglion [157], indicating a possible presynaptic or peripheral site of action, or both. GluR5 is the major low-affinity KAR subunit at the presynaptic site of primary nociceptive afferents [112], and it seems to play a role in inhibition of C-fiber-related input [209]. ATPA, a selective GluR5 agonist, increases GABAergic or glycinergic spontaneous inhibitory postsynaptic currents (sIPSCs) in substantia gelatinosa neurons and inhibits NMDAR and AMPAR-mediated EPSCs evoked by dorsal root stimulation, probably via a presynaptic site [87,205]. High-intensity stimulation of primary afferents, but not activation of low-threshold afferents, induces KAR-mediated synaptic current in dorsal horn neurons [204], suggesting a selective role in relaying nociceptive input. Bidirectional modulation of excitatory synaptic transmission in the superficial dorsal horn by KARs has been reported [209]. Evidence suggests that KARs are involved in both pre- and postsynaptic modulation of spinal sensory transmission [72,87,204].

Kainate receptors are involved in persistent pain states [204]. Systemic administration of kainate produces zinc-dependent hyperalgesia [99]. Selective KAR antagonists attenuate nocifensive responses to formalin and behavioral hyperalgesia [64,81]. Gene knockout studies indicate that GluR5 is critical in inflammatory pain [92]. Among the five KAR subunits, only GluR5 and GluR6 mRNAs were significantly regulated in the spinal cord by inflammation [64], supporting the view that GluR5/6 are "modulatory" subunits that are responsible for adjustment of KAR function in response to dramatic increases in synaptic input. This view is consistent with in vitro studies showing that GluR5/6 subunits are major contributors to kainate-gated current [143]. Selective upregulation of the GluR5/6 subunits may result in an altered composition of the KARs and changes in channel kinetics with increased functional activity. The role of KARs in spinal dorsal horn nociceptive processing appears to be enhanced after inflammation [150,174], which may explain why GluR5-receptor antagonists are less effective in reducing spinal nociceptive transmission in uninjured animals [174].

Similar to the GluR2 subunit of the AMPAR, an RNA Q/R editing occurs in the M2 of GluR5/6, and calcium permeability is reduced after Q/R editing [101]. Unlike the GluR2 receptors, Q/R editing is incomplete for GluR6 receptors in adults. Only about 50% of GluR6 mRNAs are edited in the adult rat spinal cord [9]. Analysis of the PCR product cDNA sequence and the *BbvI* endonuclease digestion assay revealed that the inflammation-upregulated GluR6 mRNAs were predominantly the unedited form (Q); the edited form (R) of GluR6 mRNA did not show a significant change after inflammation [64]. Although the molecular mechanisms of GluR editing have been studied in great detail, the physiological or pathophysiological significance of this process is less well understood. Studies have suggested a role of GluR6 Q/R editing in synaptic plasticity. Mice deficient in GluR6 Q/R editing, which have increased GluR6(Q), are more vulnerable to kainate-induced seizures [9,197]. The Q/R editing site of the GluR6 receptor may be a point of regulation after environmental challenge. An increase in GluR6(Q) will result in greater calcium flow into spinal neurons through the KAR and increased channel conductance, leading to neuronal hyperexcitability.

Metabotropic Glutamate Receptors

Metabotropic glutamate receptors were identified after the finding that glutamate-induced phosphoinositide hydrolysis was independent of iGluRs. The term "metabotropic" is used to describe these G-protein-coupled GluRs, which now have eight members, $mGluR_{1-8}$ ($mGlu_{1-8}$), numbered by the order in which they were cloned (Table II). Alternative splicing in the C-terminal region of $mGluR_{1,4,5}$ subtypes further results in a number of isoforms [90]. Based on sequence homology, second messenger coupling, and pharmacological profiles, mGluRs are divided into group I ($mGluR_{1,5}$) subunits that are coupled to G_q and primarily stimulate phospholipase C (PLC) and phosphoinositide hydrolysis, and group II ($mGluR_{2,3}$) and III ($mGluR_{4,6-8}$) subunits that are coupled to G_i/G_o proteins and inhibit adenylyl cyclase and cyclic adenosine monophosphate formation. Functional mGluRs are assembled as homodimers, present at both pre- and postsynaptic sites and mainly involved in modulating synaptic activity by interacting with other receptors [90]. In general, group I mGluRs are pronociceptive and groups II/III mGluRs are antinociceptive.

Table II
Metabotropic glutamate receptors

Group	Subunits*	G-Protein Coupling	Signal Transduction
I	$mGluR_1/mGlu_1$	G_q	Phospholipase C
	$mGluR_5/mGlu_5$	G_q	activation
II	$mGluR_2/mGlu_2$	G_i/G_o	Adenylate cyclase
	$mGluR_3/mGlu_3$	G_i/G_o	inhibition
III	$mGluR_4/mGlu_4$	G_i/G_o	Adenylate cyclase
	$mGluR_6/mGlu_6$	G_i/G_o	inhibition
	$mGluR_7/mGlu_7$	G_i/G_o	
	$mGluR_8/mGlu_8$	G_i/G_o	

* The NC-IUPHAR nomenclature avoids "R" when referring to a single subunit.

Group I mGluRs are distributed in the superficial spinal dorsal horn of the rat [10] and are localized on peripheral unmyelinated nerve terminals [11]. Studies have indicated a role of group I mGluRs in central sensitization and hyperalgesia [e.g., 2,61,83,132,164,192]. The selective group I mGluR agonist DHPG enhances Ca^{2+} signaling in superficial dorsal horn neurons, mediated by the release of Ca^{2+} from inositol triphosphate (IP_3)-sensitive intracellular stores and by an influx through L-type voltage-dependent Ca^{2+}-channels [71].

The induction of LTP of C-fiber-evoked field potentials involves group I mGluRs but not group II/III mGluRs [6]. The group I mGluR antagonist AIDA, the PLC inhibitor U-73122, and the IP_3R blocker 2-APB converted LTP of substantia gelatinosa neurons to LTD without affecting acute synaptic transmission [83], suggesting a role of postsynaptic group I mGluR/PLC/IP_3-gated Ca^{2+} stores in central sensitization. Group I mGluRs may also be involved in synaptic inhibition in the spinal cord, as shown by DHPG-induced LTD [70]. The signaling pathways involved in DHPG-induced LTD in superficial dorsal horn neurons are independent of PKC activity but require L-type voltage-dependent Ca^{2+}-channels and IP_3.

Consistent with a role in nociception, activation of group I mGluRs produces nocifensive behaviors in rats [110], and antisense treatment against $mGluR_1$ mRNA significantly inhibits nocifensive tail-flick reflex and reduces responses of dorsal horn neurons [211]. Pretreatment with $mGluR_1$ or $mGluR_5$ antagonists significantly delayed the development of mechanical hyperalgesia after inflammation [61]. DHPG further enhances nocifensive behavior in rat models of neuropathic and inflammatory pain through activation of the ERK pathway [2,164]. In a spinal cord injury model, $mGluR_1$ and $mGluR_5$ seem to contribute differentially to mechanical allodynia and thermal hyperalgesia, respectively [123]. Intradermal injection of group I mGluR antagonists CPCCOEt (mGluR1) and MPEP ($mGluR_5$) suppressed the second, but not the first, phase of the formalin response [11], suggesting that $mGluR_1$ and $mGluR_5$ are selectively involved in peripheral nociceptive sensitization associated with tissue injury.

In contrast to group I mGluRs, activation of group II and III mGluRs produces antinociception [58,82]. In rats, injection of interleukin-1β into the vibrissa pad produced mechanical allodynia in the orofacial area, which was attenuated by intracisternal administration of APDC, a group II mGluR agonist, and L-AP4, a group III mGluR agonist [82]. APDC and L-AP4 also attenuated scratching behavior induced by injection of formalin into the temporomandibular joint [102]. Intrathecal L-AP4 attenuated allodynia and responses of dorsal horn neurons in nerve-injured rats but had no antinociceptive effect in normal rats [25]. Elevation of extracellular N-acetylaspartylglutamate (NAAG), a functional agonist of group II mGluRs, by inhibition of NAAG peptidase, produces antinociception in neuropathic and inflammatory pain models [206]. The contrasting actions of group I versus II/III mGluRs are also seen at supraspinal sites, but with opposite polarity. In the midbrain periaqueductal gray, group I mGluRs enhance descending inhibition, but groups II/III mGluRs reduce descending modulation [113].

One should be cautious in interpreting findings related to the use of different classes of mGluR antagonists. Recent studies suggest that MPEP, extensively used as a selective mGluR5 antagonist, has other actions including inhibition of NMDARs and that MTEP has been shown to be a more selective $mGluR_5$ antagonist [100]. Nevertheless, there has been great interest in developing specific mGluR antagonists as therapeutic agents [34,192]. Recent effort in developing allosteric modulators of mGluRs may bring new tools and promise to the mGluR field [89]. For example, negative allosteric modulators of group I mGluRs and positive allosteric modulators of group II mGluRs are potential analgesics.

Signaling Coupling of mGluR to NMDAR

In CNS neurons, NMDA receptors are physically linked to mGluRs in the postsynaptic membrane. The group I mGluRs bind Homer (a family of dendritic proteins), and the latter binds Shank, a family of postsynaptic proteins [191]. Shank proteins are also linked to PSD-95 via binding with guanylate kinase-associated protein [129]. PSD-95 protein is known to interact with NR2A/B subunits of the NMDAR in spinal neurons [181]. In the spinal dorsal horn, the mGluR-Homer-Shank complex and NMDARs appear to be biochemically linked through PSD-95 (Fig. 2) [61].

The interaction between the mGluRs and NMDARs has received increased attention as a mechanism of modulation of neuronal plasticity [61,121]. Group I mGluRs have been implicated in a variety of pain conditions. The mGluR agonist-evoked response is enhanced in the spinal cord in hyperalgesic but not in naive animals, and this effect is reversed by an NMDAR antagonist [12]. Intrathecal administration of the $mGluR_{1,5}$ agonist (S)-3,5-DHPG in mice produced hyperalgesia that was attenuated by NMDAR antagonists. The DHPG-produced hyperalgesia was also suppressed by silencing the NR2B subunit by a specific short-hairpin RNA [47]. DHPG further enhances nocifensive behaviors after tissue and nerve injury, consistent with a positive modulatory role of group I mGluRs in central sensitization [2,164].

One important signaling pathway for inflammation-induced NR2B tyrosine phosphorylation involves the interaction or coupling between group I mGluRs and NMDARs [61]. The group I mGluR antagonists block inflammation-induced NR2B phosphorylation. In a dorsal horn slice preparation, the group I mGluR agonists (DHPG), but not agonists of group II (APDC) and III (L-AP4), induce NR2B tyrosine phosphorylation similar to that seen in vivo after inflammation [61]. These results demonstrate a role for the linking or coupling of group I mGluR and NMDARs in the development of spinal plasticity. The signal transduction pathways coupling mGluR and NR2B tyrosine phosphorylation involve PLC activation, IP_3-mediated intracellular calcium release, and activation of PKC and Src family protein tyrosine kinases. These biochemical events are correlated with the development of inflammatory hyperalgesia and may underlie the mechanisms of spinal sensitization. An important implication is that a functional consequence of group I mGluR activation after inflammation is to prime NMDARs for further enhanced hyperexcitability [61]. This mechanism may be a critical initiator for central nociceptive sensitization.

GABA Receptors in Pain Transmission

Iontophoretic application of GABA inhibits responses of dorsal horn neurons to primary afferent input, an effect first reported by Curtis et al. [31] at the same time that glutamate-induced excitation of spinal neurons was demonstrated. GABA has an established role as a major inhibitory transmitter in the dorsal horn pain-processing circuitry. Recent findings have further suggested several interesting possibilities regarding the contribution of spinal GABAergic mechanisms to hyperalgesia [20,29,149].

GABA acts at ionotropic $GABA_A/GABA_C$ and metabotropic $GABA_B$ receptors that in general mediate slow and prolonged inhibition, respectively. In the monkey and cat spinal cord, Aδ high-threshold mechanoreceptor primary afferent terminals receive GABAergic synaptic contact, and GABAergic axons also synapse on dendrites postsynaptic to the Aδ primary afferents, indicating that GABAergic control of nociceptive input involves both presynaptic and postsynaptic mechanisms [4]. The contribution of the GABA system to nociceptive processing and mechanisms of persistent pain after tissue and nerve injury prompts the targeting of GABAergic synapses for pain control [32,41].

Ionotropic GABA Receptors

The ionotropic GABA receptors (GABARs) gate the Cl^- ionophore and possess multiple modulatory sites (Fig. 3). The $GABA_A$Rs are assembled as heteropentamers from 18 homologous subunits [76] (Table III). The $GABA_C$Rs are composed of ρ1–3 subunits [23] (Table III). The ionotropic GABAR subunits share the same membrane topology with four transmembrane domains and extracellular amino- and carboxyl-terminals. Understanding the molecular composition of the GABARs, particularly the $GABA_A$ subtype, has helped researchers design genetic manipulations in the development of subtype-specific GABAergic analgesic agents with reduced side effects [91].

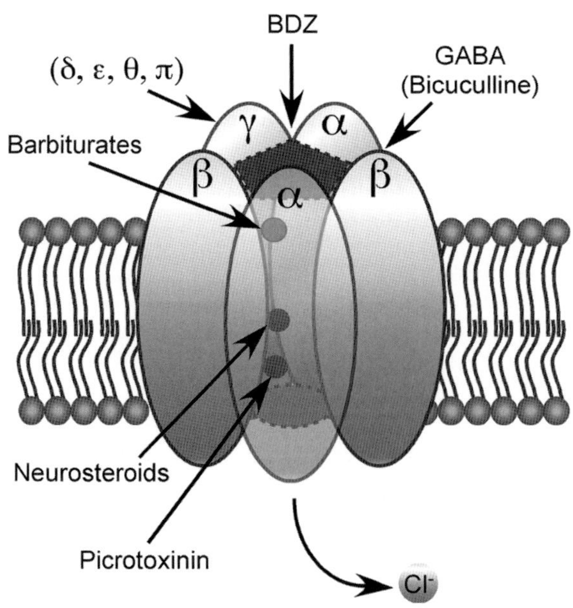

Fig. 3. Gamma-aminobutyric acid A ($GABA_A$) receptor model. Most neuronal surface $GABA_A$Rs are assembled by two α, two β, and one γ subunit. The γ subunit may be replaced by an ε, θ, or π subunit. The GABA and the competitive antagonist bicuculline site is presumably located at the α–β interface and the benzodiazepine (BDZ) site at the α–γ interface. The barbiturates and neurosteroids modulatory sites, and the non-competitive antagonist picrotoxin site are illustrated. Opening of the $GABA_A$R channel allows inflow of Cl^- when its reversal potential is more negative than resting membrane potential.

Table III
Ionotropic GABA receptors

Subtype	Subunits	Differential Pharmacological Sensitivity: CACA, (+)-CAMP	Bicuculline	TPMPA	Benzodiazepines, Barbiturates, Neurosteroids
$GABA_A$	α1–6, β1–3, γ1–3, δ, ε1–3, θ, π	No	Yes	No	Yes
$GABA_C$	ρ1-3	Yes	No	Yes	No

Abbreviations: CACA = *cis*-4-amino-crotonic acid; (+)-CAMP = (+)-*cis*-2-aminomethylcyclopropane carboxylic acid; GABA = γ-aminobutyric acid; TPMPA = (1,2,5,6-tetrahydropyridine-4-yl) methylphosphinic acid.

$GABA_A$ Receptors

The most common $GABA_A$Rs consist of α_1, β_2, and γ_2 subunits (Fig. 3). GABA binds to the α–β interface, and benzodiazepines probably interact with the α–γ interface. $GABA_A$Rs are sensitive to bicuculline and have distinct modulatory binding sites including barbiturates and neurosteroids. In general, synaptic $GABA_A$Rs are sensitive to benzodiazepines and mediate phasic inhibition and extrasynaptic $GABA_A$Rs are insensitive to benzodiazepines and mediate tonic synaptic inhibition [see 76]. In the spinal cord, the benzodiazepine diazepam produces analgesia via α_2- and α_3-containing, but not α_1-containing, $GABA_A$Rs [91].

Together with strychnine-sensitive glycine receptors (GlyR), $GABA_A$R mediates inhibition of pain transmission in the spinal dorsal horn [121]. Responses of lamina I neurons to Aδ-fiber input is controlled by $GABA_A$Rs [4,165]. Interestingly, there was an increase in $GABA_A$R-mediated sIPSCs in laminae I, III, and IV after capsaicin stimulation, which was blocked by an NK1R antagonist. This finding suggests that substance P released from primary afferents containing vanilloid receptors (TRPV1) also excites "inhibitory" neurons [4]. It is consistent with the view that NK1Rs are involved in the maintenance of the inhibitory tone of substantia gelatinosa interneurons [193]. Evidence indicates that $GABA_A$Rs colocalize with NK1Rs in spinal dorsal horn neurons and can be removed after treatment with substance P-saporin (SP-SAP) conjugate [151]. Interestingly, although bicuculline-induced facilitation is lost after SP-SAP treatment, nocifensive behaviors are attenuated, suggesting that the net contribution of these NK1-$GABA_A$R-bearing neurons to pain transmission circuitry is facilitation. Additionally, descending input also activates spinal $GABA_A$Rs [106].

In animals exhibiting hyperalgesia after chronic constriction injury of the sciatic nerve, spinal application of the $GABA_A$R agonist muscimol before high-frequency (50 Hz) tetanus stimulation produced a long-lasting depression of spinal dorsal horn field potentials [119]. The intrathecal $GABA_A$R agonist isoguvacine reversed tactile allodynia and thermal hyperalgesia after spinal nerve ligation [114]. The antiepileptic agents carbamazepine and oxcarbazepine suppressed inflammatory hyperalgesia, an effect that was reversed by bicuculline, suggesting the involvement of $GABA_A$Rs [176]. However, the

$GABA_AR$ agonist gaboxadol does not affect aversive behavior after nerve injury, as assessed with the place escape/avoidance paradigm [140].

Allosteric modulation of the $GABA_AR$ affects potency of $GABA_A$-mediated inhibition. Benzodiazepines, barbiturates, and neurosteroids interact with their respective specific sites to potentiate $GABA_AR$-mediated synaptic inhibition. In juvenile rats (15–21 days old), 5',3'-reduced neurosteroids such as endogenous 5'-pregnan-3'-ol-20-one (allopregnanolone) prolong $GABA_AR$-mediated miniature IPSCs of lamina II neurons, most likely via extrasynaptic $GABA_ARs$ [124]. Although the positive modulatory effect of neurosteroids on GABAergic transmission wanes and is gradually lost during postnatal life, reduced neurosteroids can be produced locally in superficial dorsal horn, and their effect on GABAergic synapses may be rekindled [161]. After carrageenan-induced inflammation, there is an increase in $GABA_AR$-mediated synaptic inhibition, associated with upregulation of 5'-reduced neurosteroids in the spinal cord. Curiously, the use of 5'-reductase inhibitor finasteride revealed that thermal hyperalgesia, but not mechanical allodynia, was correlated with upregulation of 5'-reduced neurosteroids [145].

$GABA_C$ Receptors

A distinct pharmacological profile differentiates $GABA_CRs$ from $GABA_ARs$ [23] (Table III). $GABA_CRs$ are selectively activated by *cis*-4-amino-crotonic acid (CACA) and (+)-*cis*-2-aminomethylcyclopropane carboxylic acid [(+)-CAMP] and are blocked by TPMPA [(1,2,5,6-tetrahydropyridine-4-yl) methylphosphinic acid], and they are insensitive to bicuculline, benzodiazepine, barbiturates, and neurosteroids (Table III). Unlike the $GABA_BRs$, the $GABA_CRs$ are not activated by baclofen. The $GABA_AR$ channel blocker picrotoxin also blocks $GABA_CRs$ composed of homomeric ρ1 subunits.

Initial studies primarily located $GABA_CRs$ in the vertebrate retina. Some studies show that there may also be functional $GABA_CRs$ in the spinal dorsal horn [138,156]. In the spinal cord, $GABA_CRs$ colocalize with $GABA_AR$ and GlyRs in approximately 25% of synapses [46]. Recordings from neurons in the substantia gelatinosa of the dorsal horn have shown that Cl^- channel-mediated responses to GABA include a component that is insensitive to bicuculline and is not modulated by benzodiazepines (glunitrazepam) or barbiturates (thiopental) [138]. These neurons receive nociceptive input and may use $GABA_CRs$ for regulation of pain transmission in the spinal cord. CACA injected into the hindpaw produced dose-dependent analgesia that was blocked by TPMPA and picrotoxin [153], suggesting the presence of peripheral $GABA_CRs$ in primary afferents that are involved in pain transmission.

Metabotropic GABA Receptors

Despite functional and pharmacological diversities, $GABA_BR$ is the only type of metabotropic GABAR that has been identified, which is in sharp contrast with the multiplicity of mGluR subtypes. $GABA_BRs$ exist as heterodimer assembled with B1 and B2 subunits.

Although two isoforms of the B1 subunits B1a and B1b have been identified, their differential involvement in specific neuronal functions is elusive. All $GABA_BR$ subunits including the B1 isoforms are present in the spinal dorsal horn [40,116]. However, only the two B1 isoforms are detected in the DRG, suggesting the presence of atypical $GABA_B$ homodimers there [54]. $GABA_BRs$ are coupled to $G_{\alpha i/o}$ subunits to produce inhibition of adenylyl cyclase and are involved in slow inhibitory regulation via pre- and postsynaptic mechanisms. Presynaptic $GABA_BRs$ inhibit voltage-dependent Ca^{2+}-channels to reduce transmitter release, and postsynaptic $GABA_BRs$ activate Kir3-type K^+ channels to hyperpolarize the postsynaptic membrane.

$GABA_BRs$ mediate inhibitory regulation of spinal pain transmission and have been a target of analgesic drug development [see 55,135]. Spinal administration of the $GABA_BR$ agonist baclofen, but not the $GABA_AR$ agonists muscimol or isoguvacine, in the rat significantly reduced NK-1R internalization of lamina I neurons in response to noxious stimulation, suggesting reduced presynaptic substance P release by baclofen [155]. Both excitatory glutamatergic and inhibitory GABAergic terminals in the substantia gelatinosa possess the $GABA_BR$. Baclofen dose-dependently reduced the frequency of both miniature excitatory (glutamatergic) and inhibitory (GABAergic) postsynaptic currents with similar potency in substantia gelatinosa neurons [75], suggesting that the net effect of $GABA_BR$ activation would also depend on its action on postsynaptic neurons [17]. The $GABA_BR$ agonists CGP35024 and L-baclofen inhibited capsaicin-evoked ventral root potentials and the "wind-up" response to repetitive stimulation, and reversed neuropathic mechanical hyperalgesia following single subcutaneous or intrathecal administration, but did not affect inflammatory mechanical hyperalgesia [139].

Baclofen has also been shown to reverse thermal hyperalgesia after spinal nerve ligation [114]. However, baclofen apparently impairs locomotor function at the antihyperalgesic dose. The novel $GABA_BR$ agonist CGP35024 appears to have an improved therapeutic window. In rats, CGP35024 is seven times more potent against neuropathic pain than in the rotarod test for motor coordination, while baclofen is approximately equipotent in the analgesic and motor function tests [139]. It is worth noting that at supraspinal levels of the brain, selectively activating $GABA_BR$-bearing rostral agranular insular cortex neurons produces hyperalgesia through projections to the amygdala [77]. Brainstem descending pathways produce antinociception via spinal $GABA_BRs$ [117].

GABAergic Mechanisms of Pain Hypersensitivity

As an important component consistent with the gate control theory of pain transmission, GABAergic synaptic activity in the spinal cord provides major inhibitory control over the passage of nociceptive information to supraspinal sites. Perturbations or alterations of GABAergic synapses and related function under different conditions have been attractive mechanisms for explaining hyperalgesia. Several hypotheses have emerged to attribute roles of the spinal GABAergic system to the development of persistent pain. In essence, most hypotheses emphasize disinhibition of GABAergic inhibition, whether by reduced/blocked GABAergic synaptic activity, by increased primary afferent depolarization (PAD), or by a change in the valence/polarity of GABAergic modulation.

Reduced/Blocked GABAergic Synaptic Activity

Blocking spinal $GABA_A$Rs by bicuculline or using strychnine to block GlyRs (1) produces changes in the high-threshold nociceptive flexion withdrawal reflex similar to those induced by C-fiber input and touch-evoked allodynia [166]; (2) produces an AMPAR-dependent spread of excitation from the deep to superficial dorsal horn in neuropathic rats [162]; and (3) reveals a novel Aβ-mediated and NMDAR-dependent input to lamina I NK1R-containing neurons [188]. Partial nerve injury but not complete nerve transection reduces $GABA_A$R-mediated IPSCs in lamina II neurons recorded from rat spinal cord slices, and this reduction is associated with neuronal apoptosis and reduced presynaptic GABA release [126]. These events may lead to loss of GABAergic inhibition in the superficial dorsal horn. On the other hand, targeting specific spinal $GABA_A$R subtypes can restore synaptic inhibition and reverse pain hypersensitivity [214]. For example, potent antihyperalgesia is produced when L-838,417, the nonsedative (due to α_1-sparing) benzodiazepine ligand, is used to selectively target $GABA_A$Rs containing the α_2 and α_3 subunits [91].

There is a loss of GABA immunoreactivity [73], along with reduced levels of the GABA-synthesizing enzyme glutamic acid decarboxylase (GAD) [37,65,126] and the GABA transporter GAT-1 [119], in the spinal dorsal horn after spinal cord or nerve injury. These results suggest a depletion of GABA from its terminals and reduced GABAergic inhibition in spinal circuitry in the development of neuropathic pain. However, there have been reports of increased GABA and GAD immunoreactivity in the spinal dorsal horn after inflammation, which was interpreted as a compensatory response in the face of enhanced excitatory input from the inflamed tissue [18,128]. Consistent with this suggestion, the increased GABA and GAD immunoreactivity was observed 3–7 days after injection of complete Freund's adjuvant when the hyperalgesia wanes. Thus, an increase in GABA at the later time of inflammation may contribute to the recovery of pain sensitivity toward the normal level. However, an increased GABA level seems to be consistent with the proposed exaggerated PAD that may contribute to the appearance of mechanical allodynia after tissue injury [20].

Altered $GABA_B$R gene expression after partial sciatic nerve ligation and sciatic nerve transection has been reported [116,207]. However, a careful time-course analysis indicates that both $GABA_B$R subunit isoforms in the rat spinal dorsal horn are unaffected by L5 spinal nerve ligation, despite the presence of mechanical allodynia and spontaneous pain behavior [40]. These results suggest a discrepancy in $GABA_B$R gene transcription and translation and may indicate that a loss of $GABA_B$R-mediated inhibition is unlikely to mediate the development or maintenance of allodynia or spontaneous pain behaviors after spinal nerve injury. In consistency with this possibility, the $GABA_B$R antagonist CGP 35348 had no significant effects on the C-fiber-induced nociceptive flexion withdrawal reflex [166]. However, $GABA_BR$ B1 or B2 subunit knockout mice do exhibit hyperalgesia [54,163]. Without an effect on the protein level, injury-related sensory input may affect trafficking of $GABA_BRs$ and dissociate the $GABA_BR$ heterodimer, thus altering its responsiveness to the endogenous ligand [96]. Following peripheral inflammation, there is a loss of $GABA_BR$-mediated inhibition of C-fiber transmission in the spinal cord [168]. The enhanced glutamatergic miniature EPSCs and the amplitude of monosynaptic EPSCs evoked from the dorsal root in rats with diabetic neuropathy is most likely due to reduced inhibition by presynaptic $GABA_BRs$ [198]. Further, $GABA_BR$ may promote disinhibition of spinal sensory processing by mediating presynaptic inhibition of glycinergic IPSCs [27].

Changing Role of Primary Afferent Depolarization

Some spinal GABAergic interneurons receiving Aβ input produce PAD of fine primary afferents through axoaxonic synapses to gate nociceptive input. It is possible that, under pathological conditions such as those after injury, PAD would be intensified to an extent that it actually triggers action potentials in nociceptive afferent terminals to excite postsynaptic dorsal horn nociceptive neurons. In this scenario, Aβ-fiber input could induce pain instead of touch sensation [20,149]. The $GABA_BR$ does not appear to be involved in this process. Consistent with this model, sensitization of dorsal horn nociceptive-specific neurons can be reversed by low doses of $GABA_AR$ antagonists that reduce the novel low-threshold responses after application of capsaicin or mustard oil to the receptive fields [50]. Bicuculline also dose-dependently blocks Aβ-evoked wind-up of nociceptive withdrawal reflexes in rats with inflamed knee joints [199].

Enhanced PAD of peripheral terminals may also lead to increased pain sensitivity. $GABA_AR$ β_2/β_3 and α_1 subunits are localized to unmyelinated nerve terminals in the glabrous skin of the cat paw [15]. Local peripheral application of muscimol produced antinociception at a low dose and hyperalgesia at a high dose. These effects were prevented by bicuculline [15]. The effect of muscimol at a low dose is likely related to inhibition by peripheral PAD, and the hyperalgesic response to muscimol with a high dose may be due to increased PAD that led to activation of nociceptive dorsal horn neurons.

Shift in Anion Equilibrium Potential in Dorsal Horn Neurons

Spinal GABAergic/glycinergic interneurons normally hyperpolarize postsynaptic pain transmission neurons. Peripheral nerve or tissue injury may convert this inhibitory control by inducing a shift in the anionic equilibrium potential in nociceptive neurons [30]. The shift in anion gradient is related to injury-induced regulation of cation-chloride cotransporters NKCC1 (sodium-potassium-chloride cotransporter 1) and KCC2 (potassium-chloride cotransporter 2), which regulate Cl^- homeostasis [149]. Under normal physiological conditions, KCC2 exports one Cl^- and one K^+ ion and NKCC1 transports two Cl^- ions into the cell, with cotransport of one Na^+ and one K^+. Although KCC2 and NKCC1 are electroneutral transporters, their activity may alter the chloride equilibrium

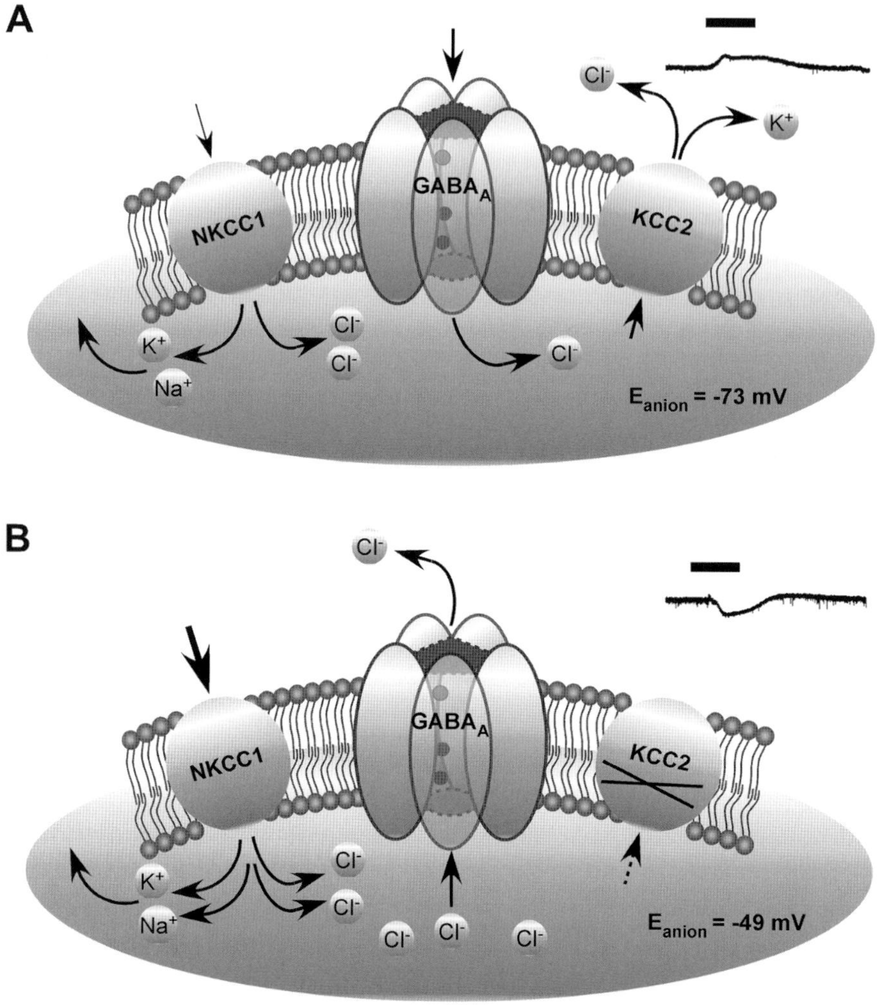

Fig. 4. The anionic equilibrium potential hypothesis of persistent pain. (A) Under normal physiological conditions, the potassium-chloride cotransporter 2 (KCC2) exports one Cl^- and one K^+ ion, and the sodium-potassium-chloride cotransporter 1 (NKCC1) transports two Cl^- ions into the cell with cotransport of one Na^+ and one K^+. The K^+ gradient established by Na^+/K^+-ATPase (not shown) helps KCC2 to extrude Cl^-. KCC2 helps to maintain an anion gradient that favors hyperpolarizing currents, indicated by inflow of Cl^- through the γ-aminobutyric acid A receptor ($GABA_AR$) channel. The Na^+ gradient allows uptake of Cl^- through NKCC1. The net effect of NKCC1 transport is an increase in intracellular Cl^-, which favors depolarization when $GABA_AR$ channels are open. In naive rats, the anion reversal potential (E_{anion}) is −73 mV [30], which is more negative than the resting membrane potential (≈60 mV). Stimulation of $GABA_AR$ by GABA (horizontal bar) will induce an outward hyperpolarizing current, as illustrated to the right. (B) Peripheral injury alters cation-chloride-cotransporter function. When there is an increase in NKCC1 activity (thicker arrow) and a reduction or loss of KCC2 function (cross, dashed arrow) due to injury, Cl^- accumulates in the cell. This change of anion gradient results in a significantly less negative E_{anion} (−49 mV) [30]. Thus, GABA will induce an inward depolarizing current, carried by outgoing Cl^-, in injured animals, as illustrated to the right. The switch from inhibition to excitation of GABAergic synaptic activity presumably contributes to increased pain.

and its reversal potential, which in turn affects the outcome of $GABA_AR$ channel activity. In general, reduced KCC2 and excessive NKCC1 activity results in a buildup of intracellular Cl^- and a less negative reversal potential, thus favoring membrane depolarization and neuronal excitation (Fig. 4).

A number of studies show a decrease in KCC2 expression [30,120,215] and an increase in NKCC1 in the spinal dorsal horn [127] after nerve or tissue injury. Blocking NKCC1 with bumetanide suppressed referred allodynia in the visceral hyperalgesia mouse model [144]. In homozygote NKCC1 knockout mice, the GABA equilibrium potential was significantly more negative, and little or no net GABA-evoked current was observed at the resting membrane potential in DRG neurons, suggesting a lack of intracellular Cl^- accumulation due to elimination of NKCC1 [177]. NKCC1 knockout mice showed an increase in tail-flick latencies and a reduction of the duration of pain behavior induced by intradermal capsaicin, along with reduced touch-evoked hyperalgesia [97].

Consistent with the above hypothesis, in rats exhibiting neuropathic pain behavior, GABA induces a novel bicuculline-sensitive, depolarizing current at resting membrane potential, and this GABA-induced synaptic current can lead to action potentials in lamina I neurons [30]. These findings indicate that nerve injury converts postsynaptic GABAergic inhibition to excitation via an effect on the anionic equilibrium potential in superficial dorsal horn neurons (Fig. 4). Further studies show that (1) brain-derived neurotrophic factor (BDNF) released from ATP-stimulated microglia can mimic the effects of nerve injury on the anionic equilibrium potential and pain sensitivity [29]; (2) BDNF facilitates the K^+-stimulated release of GABA from the dorsal horn [141]; and (3) dorsal root injury induces a BDNF-dependent increase in the density of GABAergic interneuronal processes in the spinal dorsal horn [169]. These findings suggest a role of glia-neuronal signaling and BDNF in altering spinal GABAergic function and pain transmission. Additionally, the pro-inflammatory cytokine interferon-γ, a regulator of glial activation, may induce excitatory GABAergic transmission in the dorsal horn [195].

The change in polarity of the effect of GABAergic transmission after inflammation is consistent with the anionic equilibrium potential hypothesis. In naive rats, muscimol increased nociceptive threshold and the $GABA_AR$ antagonist gabazine decreased it [5]. After inflammation, the effects of these compounds were reversed: low doses of muscimol exacerbated the inflammation-induced mechanical allodynia, and gabazine increased nociceptive threshold. The increase in GABA during the formalin test [194] and after inflammation [18,128], together with facilitation of Fos protein expression by midazolam, a benzodiazepine agonist, in monoarthritic rats [16], may also be interpreted as support for an excitatory role of GABAergic transmission in increased pain. However, some studies apparently conflict with the anionic equilibrium potential hypothesis. In response to inflammation and arthritis, NKCC1 expression was decreased in DRG neurons and KCC2 was increased in the superficial dorsal horn [127]. Finally, KCC2-deficient mice showed reduced sensitivity to tactile and noxious thermal stimuli in von Frey, hot-plate, and tail-flick tests [187].

Interactions of Glutamate and GABA Receptors in Pain Transmission

GABAergic synaptic activity clearly modulates spinal glutamatergic transmission associated with primary afferent input. Blocking $GABA_AR$ with bicuculline leads to repetitive, long-lasting, polysynaptic EPSCs and ERK activation that can be blocked by an NMDAR antagonist [8]. Similarly, spinal administration of the $GABA_AR$ and $GABA_BR$ antagonists augmented C-fiber-stimulation-induced polysynaptic field potentials in the spinal cord, and an NMDAR antagonist blocked these effects [14]. In normal rats, AMPARs mediate responses of a population of lamina I neurons to high-threshold, but not low-threshold, primary afferent stimulation [165]. These AMPAR-dependent responses to high-threshold input, particularly those related to Aδ-fiber input, are controlled by $GABA_ARs$, as shown by bicuculline-produced facilitation. The benzodiazepine site agonist, midazolam, attenuated the expression and function of spinal AMPARs through activation of spinal $GABA_ARs$ in rats following nerve injury [105].

Spinal GABAergic transmission can also be modulated by glutamatergic activity associated with primary afferent input. All subtypes of iGluRs are expressed in GABAergic terminals in the rat superficial dorsal horn, as determined by colocalization with GABA and GAD65 immunoreactivity [111,173]. This localization provides a structural basis for regulation of inhibitory synaptic transmission by iGluRs. With regard to AMPARs, the majority of GABAergic interneurons in the spinal cord exhibit GluR1 but not GluR2/3 immunoreactivity [173], suggesting that these AMPARs are permeable to Ca^{2+}. Presynaptic AMPARs, including Ca^{2+}-permeable ones, enhance spontaneous GABA and glycine release onto lamina I NK1R-containing neurons and lamina II neurons [39]. These Ca^{2+}-permeable AMPARs may synaptically activate GABAergic neurons to induce inhibition, which could explain JSTx-induced facilitation of C-fiber-evoked responses of dorsal horn neurons in rats [175].

However, presynaptic AMPARs also inhibit GABA and glycine release onto lamina I NK1R-containing neurons [39], suggesting that interactions between spinal glutamatergic and GABAergic synapses could facilitate pain transmission via disinhibition. Enhanced nociceptive input suppresses GABAergic IPSCs via iGluRs and group II/III mGluRs on GABAergic interneurons [218]. Interestingly, presynaptic KARs on terminals of dorsal horn interneurons may produce a subtle facilitation of nociceptive transmission. In a model based on recordings from primary dorsal horn neuronal cultures and adult rat spinal cord slices, activation of presynaptic KARs evoked GABA release [87], which is consistent with activation of GABAergic interneurons by a non-NMDA type of iGluRs [42]. Further studies confirmed that ATPA facilitated GABAergic and glycinergic sIPSCs of substantia gelatinosa neurons in mouse spinal slices [205]. GABA released in this fashion would diffuse back to the same presynaptic terminal and activate $GABA_BRs$ on the same presynaptic site where the KARs are located. Feedback activation of $GABA_BR$ will inhibit release of inhibitory transmitters including GABA [87]. Thus, in this model, KARs promote GABAergic inhibition but at the same time reduce this effect via activation of presynaptic $GABA_BRs$. When there is an enhanced primary afferent drive due to injury, the inhibitory action of $GABA_BRs$ in this circuitry may dominate, resulting in reduced activation of postsynaptic GABAergic and glycinergic interneurons. This effect would facilitate pain transmission and generate hyperalgesia. The nociceptive input-mediated inhibition of GABAergic synapses implies active removal of inhibition and provides an additional mechanism underlying the disinhibition theory of hyperalgesia.

Clinical Perspectives and Concluding Remarks

Chronic pain conditions are often resistant to regular analgesics. Based on information gathered from animal studies, antagonism or activation of subtypes of glutamate or GABA receptors at the spinal level may provide alternative approaches for the management of chronic pain. Drugs that target glutamate and GABA receptors have been tested on humans in clinical settings [34,41,56,60]. For example, Kristensen et al. [94] showed that the wind-up-like component of an intractable neurogenic pain was eliminated after intrathecal administration of the competitive NMDAR antagonist CPP. Interestingly, CPP only inhibited the spread of pain outside of the territory of the injured nerve and left the thermal pain threshold unchanged. Dextromethorphan has shown certain efficacy against postoperative hyperalgesia [57] and painful diabetic neuropathy [159]. Ketamine, a noncompetitive NMDAR antagonist, has shown efficacy in alleviating opiate-induced hyperalgesia (for review, see [109]). The AMPAR antagonist LY293558 is efficacious against acute migraine [160]. The GABAergic agents have shown analgesic properties, but they have limited usage in pain management due to their complex actions on the nervous system [41]. These clinical observations are consistent with findings from animal studies and indicate the involvement of excitatory and inhibitory amino acids and their receptors in pain hypersensitivity. To date, the side effects of the glutamatergic and GABAergic agents have hampered their use in pain control, although the development of subunit specific antagonists with a reduced aversive profile is promising [34,56,91]. The second-generation memantine derivatives, nitromemantines, target both the nitrosylation site on the NR2 subunit and the NMDAR channel and may be developed into NMDAR antagonists with acceptable side-effect profiles [24].

In conclusion, glutamatergic and GABAergic synapses are dominant excitatory and inhibitory signaling machinery, respectively, in the spinal pain transmission circuitry. The sophisticated interactions between receptors occur at multiple synaptic sites, and the input can come from primary afferents, interneurons, and supraspinal neurons. In the event of peripheral injury, synaptic plasticity develops and signal processing is altered, leading to amplification of afferent input and hyperalgesia. Studies in this area have exposed numerous potential targets for the analgesic drug development (see Chapter 17 by Dray and Perkins). Notably, and beyond the scope of this chapter, non-neuronal components such as glia and related chemical mediators have also been recognized as important modulators in pain transmission. Injury-activated glial cells can release inflammatory cytokines such as interleukin-1β and affect glutamatergic transmission via signal coupling to NMDAR phosphorylation [154]. This glial contribution further broadens the spectrum of analgesic targets.

Acknowledgments

The authors' work is supported by NIH grants DE11964, NS060735, and NS059028.

References

[1] Abe T, Matsumura S, Katano T, Mabuchi T, Takagi K, Xu L, Yamamoto A, Hattori K, Yagi T, Watanabe M, et al. Fyn kinase-mediated phosphorylation of NMDA receptor NR2B subunit at Tyr1472 is essential for maintenance of neuropathic pain. Eur J Neurosci 2005;22:1445–54.

[2] Adwanikar H, Karim F, Gereau RW 4th. Inflammation persistently enhances nocifensive behaviors mediated by spinal group I mGluRs through sustained ERK activation. Pain 2004;111:125–35.

[3] Ali DW, Salter MW. NMDA receptor regulation by Src kinase signalling in excitatory synaptic transmission and plasticity. Curr Opin Neurobiol 2001;11:336–42.

[4] Alvarez FJ, Kavookjian AM, Light AR. Synaptic interactions between GABA-immunoreactive profiles and the terminals of functionally defined myelinated nociceptors in the monkey and cat spinal cord. J Neurosci 1992;12:2901–17.

[5] Anseloni VC, Gold MS. Inflammation-induced shift in the valence of spinal GABA-A receptor-mediated modulation of nociception in the adult rat. J Pain 2008;9:732–8.

[6] Azkue JJ, Liu XG, Zimmermann M, Sandkühler J. Induction of long-term potentiation of C fibre-evoked spinal field potentials requires recruitment of group I, but not group II/III metabotropic glutamate receptors. Pain 2003;106:373–9.

[7] Baba H, Doubell TP, Moore KA, Woolf CJ. Silent NMDA receptor-mediated synapses are developmentally regulated in the dorsal horn of the rat spinal cord. J Neurophysiol 2000;83:955–62.

[8] Baba H, Ji RR, Kohno T, Moore KA, Ataka T, Wakai A, Okamoto M, Woolf CJ. Removal of GABAergic inhibition facilitates polysynaptic A fiber-mediated excitatory transmission to the superficial spinal dorsal horn. Mol Cell Neurosci 2003;24:818–30.

[9] Bernard A, Ferhat L, Dessi F, Charton G, Represa A, Ben-Ari Y, Khrestchatisky M. Q/R editing of the rat GluR5 and GluR6 kainate receptors in vivo and in vitro: evidence for independent developmental, pathological and cellular regulation. Eur J Neurosci 1999;11:604–16.

[10] Berthele A, Boxall SJ, Urban A, Anneser JM, Zieglgänsberger W, Urban L, Tölle TR. Distribution and developmental changes in metabotropic glutamate receptor messenger RNA expression in the rat lumbar spinal cord. Brain Res Dev Brain Res 1999;112:39–53.

[11] Bhave G, Karim F, Carlton SM, Gereau RW 4th. Peripheral group I metabotropic glutamate receptors modulate nociception in mice. Nat Neurosci 2001;4:417–23.

[12] Boxall SJ, Berthele A, Tölle TR, Zieglgänsberger W, Urban L. mGluR activation reveals a tonic NMDA component in inflammatory hyperalgesia. Neuroreport 1998;9:1201–3.

[13] Brenner GJ, Ji RR, Shaffer S, Woolf CJ. Peripheral noxious stimulation induces phosphorylation of the NMDA receptor NR1 subunit at the PKC-dependent site, serine-896, in spinal cord dorsal horn neurons. Eur J Neurosci 2004;20:375–84.

[14] Buesa I, Ortiz V, Aguilera L, Torre F, Zimmermann M, Azkue JJ. Disinhibition of spinal responses to primary afferent input by antagonism at GABA receptors in urethane-anaesthetised rats is dependent on NMDA and metabotropic glutamate receptors. Neuropharmacology 2006;50:585–94.

[15] Carlton SM, Zhou S, Coggeshall RE. Peripheral $GABA_A$ receptors: evidence for peripheral primary afferent depolarization. Neuroscience 1999;93:713–22.

[16] Castro AR, Bowery N, Castro-Lopes JM. Baclofen and midazolam alter c-fos induction by peripheral noxious or innocuous stimulation in the spinal cord of normal and monoarthritic rats. Neuropharmacology 1999;38:1775–88.

[17] Castro AR, Pinto M, Lima D, Tavares I. Secondary hyperalgesia in the monoarthritic rat is mediated by GABAB and NK1 receptors of spinal dorsal horn neurons: a behavior and c-fos study. Neuroscience 2006;141:2087–95.

[18] Castro-Lopes JM, Tavares I, Tölle TR, Coito A, Coimbra A. Increase in GABAergic cells and GABA levels in the spinal cord in unilateral inflammation of the hindlimb in the rat. Eur J Neurosci 1992;4:296–301.

[19] Caudle RM, Perez FM, Del Valle-Pinero AY, Iadarola MJ. Spinal cord NR1 serine phosphorylation and NR2B subunit suppression following peripheral inflammation. Mol Pain 2005;1:25.

[20] Cervero F, Laird JM. Mechanisms of touch-evoked pain (allodynia): a new model. Pain 1996;68:13–23.

[21] Chapman V, Dickenson AH. Time-related roles of excitatory amino acid receptors during persistent noxiously evoked responses of rat dorsal horn neurones. Brain Res 1995;703:45–50.

[22] Chatterton JE, Awobuluyi M, Premkumar LS, Takahashi H, Talantova M, Shin Y, Cui J, Tu S, Sevarino KA, Nakanishi N, et al. Excitatory glycine receptors containing the NR3 family of NMDA receptor subunits. Nature 2002;415:793–8.

[23] Chebib M. GABAC receptor ion channels. Clin Exp Pharmacol Physiol 2004;31:800–4.

[24] Chen HS, Lipton SA. The chemical biology of clinically tolerated NMDA receptor antagonists. J Neurochem 2006;97:1611–26.

[25] Chen SR, Pan HL. Distinct roles of group III metabotropic glutamate receptors in control of nociception and dorsal horn neurons in normal and nerve-injured Rats. J Pharmacol Exp Ther 2005;312:120–6.

[26] Cheng HT, Suzuki M, Hegarty DM, Xu Q, Weyerbacher AR, South SM, Ohata M, Inturrisi CE. Inflammatory pain-induced signaling events following a conditional deletion of the N-methyl-d-aspartate receptor in spinal cord dorsal horn. Neuroscience 2008;155:948–58.

[27] Choi IS, Cho JH, Jeong SG, Hong JS, Kim SJ, Kim J, Lee MG, Choi BJ, Jang IS. $GABA_B$ receptor-mediated presynaptic inhibition of glycinergic transmission onto substantia gelatinosa neurons in the rat spinal cord. Pain 2008;138:330–42.

[28] Collingridge GL, Olsen RW, Peters J, Spedding M. A nomenclature for ligand-gated ion channels. Neuropharmacology 2009;56:2–5.

[29] Coull JA, Beggs S, Boudreau D, Boivin D, Tsuda M, Inoue K, Gravel C, Salter MW, De Koninck Y. BDNF from microglia causes the shift in neuronal anion gradient underlying neuropathic pain. Nature 2005;438:1017–21.

[30] Coull JA, Boudreau D, Bachand K, Prescott SA, Nault F, Sík A, De Koninck P, De Koninck Y. Trans-synaptic shift in anion gradient in spinal lamina I neurons as a mechanism of neuropathic pain. Nature 2003;424:938–42.

[31] Curtis DR, Phillis JW, Watkins JC. The depression of spinal neurones by gamma-amino-n-butyric acid and beta-alanine. J Physiol 1959;146:185–203.

[32] Dickenson AH, Chapman V, Green GM. The pharmacology of excitatory and inhibitory amino acid-mediated events in the transmission and modulation of pain in the spinal cord. Gen Pharmacol 1997;28:633–8.

[33] Dmitrieva N, Rodríguez-Malaver AJ, Pérez J, Hernández L. Differential release of neurotransmitters from superficial and deep layers of the dorsal horn in response to acute noxious stimulation and inflammation of the rat paw. Eur J Pain 2004;8:245–52.

[34] Dray A. Neuropathic pain: emerging treatments. Br J Anaesth 2008;101:48–58.

[35] Drdla R, Sandkühler J. Long-term potentiation at C-fibre synapses by low-level presynaptic activity in vivo. Mol Pain 2008;4:18.

[36] Dubner R, Ruda MA. Activity-dependent neuronal plasticity following tissue injury and inflammation. Trends Neurosci 1992;15:96–103.

[37] Eaton MJ, Plunkett JA, Karmally S, Martinez MA, Montanez K. Changes in GAD- and GABA-immunoreactivity in the spinal dorsal horn after peripheral nerve injury and promotion of recovery by lumbar transplant of immortalized serotonergic precursors. J Chem Neuroanat 1998;16:57–72.

[38] Engelman HS, Allen TB, MacDermott AB. The distribution of neurons expressing calcium-permeable AMPA receptors in the superficial laminae of the spinal cord dorsal horn. J Neurosci 1999;19:2081–9.

[39] Engelman HS, Anderson RL, Daniele C, Macdermott AB. Presynaptic alpha-amino-3-hydroxy-5-methyl-4-isoxazole-propionic acid (AMPA) receptors modulate release of inhibitory amino acids in rat spinal cord dorsal horn. Neuroscience 2006;139:539–553.

[40] Engle MP, Gassman M, Sykes KT, Bettler B, Hammond DL. Spinal nerve ligation does not alter the expression or function of GABA(B) receptors in spinal cord and dorsal root ganglia of the rat. Neuroscience 2006;138:1277–87.

[41] Enna SJ, McCarson KE. The role of GABA in the mediation and perception of pain. Adv Pharmacol 2006;54:1–27.

[42] Evans RH, Long SK. Primary afferent depolarization in the rat spinal cord is mediated by pathways utilising NMDA and non-NMDA receptors. Neurosci Lett 1989;100:231–6.

[43] Fang L, Wu J, Zhang X, Lin Q, Willis WD. Increased phosphorylation of the GluR1 subunit of spinal cord alpha-amino-3-hydroxy-5-methyl-4-isoxazole propionate receptor in rats following intradermal injection of capsaicin. Neuroscience 2003;122:237–45.

[44] Ferrini F, Salio C, Vergnano AM, Merighi A. Vanilloid receptor-1 (TRPV1)-dependent activation of inhibitory neurotransmission in spinal substantia gelatinosa neurons of mouse. Pain 2007;129:195–209.

[45] Florenzano F, De Luca B. Nociceptive stimulation induces glutamate receptor down-regulation in the trigeminal nucleus. Neuroscience 1999;90:201–7.

[46] Frazao R, Nogueira MI, Wässle H. Colocalization of synaptic $GABA_C$-receptors with $GABA_A$-receptors and glycine-receptors in the rodent central nervous system. Cell Tissue Res 2007;330:1–15.

[47] Gabra BH, Kessler FK, Ritter JK, Dewey WL, Smith FL. Decrease in N-methyl-D-aspartic acid receptor-NR2B subunit levels by intrathecal short-hairpin RNA blocks group I metabotropic glutamate receptor-mediated hyperalgesia. J Pharmacol Exp Ther 2007;322:186–94.

[48] Galan A, Laird JM, Cervero F. In vivo recruitment by painful stimuli of AMPA receptor subunits to the plasma membrane of spinal cord neurons. Pain 2004;112:315–23.

[49] Gao X, Kim HK, Chung JM, Chung K. Enhancement of NMDA receptor phosphorylation of the spinal dorsal horn and nucleus gracilis neurons in neuropathic rats. Pain 2005;116:62–72.

[50] Garcia-Nicas E, Laird JM, Cervero F. GABAA-Receptor blockade reverses the injury-induced sensitization of nociceptor-specific (NS) neurons in the spinal dorsal horn of the rat. J Neurophysiol 2006;96:661–70.

[51] Garraway SM, Xu Q, Inturrisi CE. Design and evaluation of small interfering RNAs that target expression of the N-methyl-D-aspartate receptor NR1 subunit gene in the spinal cord dorsal horn. J Pharmacol Exp Ther 2007;322:982–8.

[52] Garry EM, Moss A, Delaney A, O'Neill F, Blakemore J, Bowen J, Husi H, Mitchell R, Grant SG, Fleetwood-Walker SM. Neuropathic sensitization of behavioral reflexes and spinal NMDA receptor/CaM kinase II interactions are disrupted in PSD-95 mutant mice. Curr Biol 2003;13:321–8.

[53] Garry EM, Moss A, Rosie R, Delaney A, Mitchell R, Fleetwood-Walker SM. Specific involvement in neuropathic pain of AMPA receptors and adapter proteins for the GluR2 subunit. Mol Cell Neurosci 2003;24:10–22.

[54] Gassmann M, Shaban H, Vigot R, Sansig G, Haller C, Barbieri S, Humeau Y, Schuler V, Müller M, Kinzel B, et al. Redistribution of GABAB(1) protein and atypical GABAB responses in GABAB(2)-deficient mice. J Neurosci 2004;24:6086–97.

[55] Gerber G, Randić M. Excitatory amino acid-mediated components of synaptically evoked input from dorsal roots to deep dorsal horn neurons in the rat spinal cord slice. Neurosci Lett 1989;106:211–9.

[56] Gogas KR. Glutamate-based therapeutic approaches: NR2B receptor antagonists. Curr Opin Pharmacol 2006;6:68–74.

[57] Gordon SM, Dubner R, Dionne RA. Antihyperalgesic effect of the N-methyl-D-aspartate receptor antagonist dextromethorphan in the oral surgery model. J Clin Pharmacol 1999;39:139–46.

[58] Goudet C, Chapuy E, Alloui A, Acher F, Pin JP, Eschalier A. Group III metabotropic glutamate receptors inhibit hyperalgesia in animal models of inflammation and neuropathic pain. Pain 2008;137:112–4.

[59] Guo H, Huang LY. Alteration in the voltage dependence of NMDA receptor channels in rat dorsal horn neurones following peripheral inflammation. J Physiol 2001;537:115–23.

[60] Guo W, Dubner R, Ren K. Spinal N-methyl-D-aspartate receptor mechanisms of central sensitization and persistent pain following tissue injury. In: Mao JR, editor. Translational pain research. New York: Nova Science; 2006. p. 45–78.

[61] Guo W, Wei F, Zou S, Robbins MT, Sugiyo S, Ikeda T, Tu JC, Worley PF, Dubner R, Ren K. Group I metabotropic glutamate receptor NMDA receptor coupling and signaling cascade mediate spinal dorsal horn NMDA receptor 2B tyrosine phosphorylation associated with inflammatory hyperalgesia. J Neurosci 2004;24:9161–73.

[62] Guo W, Zou S, Guan Y, Ikeda T, Tal M, Dubner R, Ren K. Tyrosine phosphorylation of the NR2B subunit of the NMDA receptor in the spinal cord during the development and maintenance of inflammatory hyperalgesia. J Neurosci 2002;22:6208–17.

[63] Guo W, Zou S, Ikeda T, Dubner R, Ren K. Rapid and lasting increase in serine phosphorylation of rat spinal cord NMDAR1 and GluR1 subunits after peripheral inflammation. Thalamus Relat Syst 2005;3:9–18.

[64] Guo W, Zou S, Tal M, Ren K. Activation of spinal kainate receptors after inflammation: behavioral hyperalgesia and subunit gene expression. Eur J Pharmacol 2002;452:309–18.

[65] Gwak YS, Crown ED, Unabia GC, Hulsebosch CE. Propentofylline attenuates allodynia, glial activation and modulates GABAergic tone after spinal cord injury in the rat. Pain 2008;138:410–22.

[66] Gwak YS, Kang J, Leem JW, Hulsebosch CE. Spinal AMPA receptor inhibition attenuates mechanical allodynia and neuronal hyperexcitability following spinal cord injury in rats. J Neurosci Res 2007;85:2352–9.

[67] Hanley JG. PICK1: a multi-talented modulator of AMPA receptor trafficking. Pharmacol Ther 2008;118:152–60.

[68] Harris JA, Corsi M, Quartaroli M, Arban R, Bentivoglio M. Upregulation of spinal glutamate receptors in chronic pain. Neuroscience 1996;74:7–12.

[69] Hartmann B, Ahmadi S, Heppenstall PA, Lewin GR, Schott C, Borchardt T, Seeburg PH, Zeilhofer HU, Sprengel R, Kuner R. The AMPA receptor subunits GluR-A and GluR-B reciprocally modulate spinal synaptic plasticity and inflammatory pain. Neuron 2004;44:637–50.

[70] Heinke B, Sandkühler J. Signal transduction pathways of group I metabotropic glutamate receptor-induced long-term depression at sensory spinal synapses. Pain 2005;118:145–54.

[71] Heinke B, Sandkühler J. Group I metabotropic glutamate receptor-induced Ca^{2+}-gradients in rat superficial spinal dorsal horn neurons. Neuropharmacology 2007;52:1015–23.

[72] Huettner JE. Glutamate receptor channels in rat DRG neurons: activation by kainate and quisqualate and blockade of desensitization by Con A. Neuron 1990;5:255–66.

[73] Ibuki T, Hama AT, Wang XT, Pappas GD, Sagen J. Loss of GABA-immunoreactivity in the spinal dorsal horn of rats with peripheral nerve injury and promotion of recovery by adrenal medullary grafts. Neuroscience 1997;76:845–58.

[74] Isaac JT, Nicoll RA, Malenka RC. Evidence for silent synapses: implications for the expression of LTP. Neuron 1995;15:427–34.

[75] Iyadomi M, Iyadomi I, Kumamoto E, Tomokuni K, Yoshimura M. Presynaptic inhibition by baclofen of miniature EPSCs and IPSCs in substantia gelatinosa neurons of the adult rat spinal dorsal horn. Pain 2000;85:385–93.

[76] Jacob TC, Moss SJ, Jurd R. GABA(A) receptor trafficking and its role in the dynamic modulation of neuronal inhibition. Nat Rev Neurosci 2008;9:331–43.

[77] Jasmin L, Rabkin SD, Granato A, Boudah A, Ohara PT. Analgesia and hyperalgesia from GABA-mediated modulation of the cerebral cortex. Nature 2003;424:316–20.

[78] Ji RR, Befort K, Brenner GJ, Woolf CJ. ERK MAP kinase activation in superficial spinal cord neurons induces prodynorphin and NK-1 upregulation and contributes to persistent inflammatory pain hypersensitivity. J Neurosci 2002;22:478–85.

[79] Ji Y, Traub RJ. Differential effects of spinal CNQX on two populations of dorsal horn neurons responding to colorectal distension in the rat. Pain 2002;99:217–22.

[80] Jin HC, Keller AJ, Jung JK, Subieta A, Brennan TJ. Epidural tezampanel, an AMPA/kainate receptor antagonist, produces postoperative analgesia in rats. Anesth Analg 2007;105:1152–9.

[81] Jones CK, Alt A, Ogden AM, Bleakman D, Simmons RM, Iyengar S, Dominguez E, Ornstein PL, Shannon HE. Antiallodynic and antihyperalgesic effects of selective competitive GLUK5 (GluR5) ionotropic glutamate receptor antagonists in the capsaicin and carrageenan models in rats. J Pharmacol Exp Ther 2006;319:396–404.

[82] Jung CY, Choi HS, Ju JS, Park HS, Kwon TG, Bae YC, Ahn DK. Central metabotropic glutamate receptors differentially participate in interleukin-1beta-induced mechanical allodynia in the orofacial area of conscious rats. J Pain 2006;7:747–56.

[83] Jung SJ, Kim SJ, Park YK, Oh SB, Cho K, Kim J. Group I mGluR regulates the polarity of spike-timing dependent plasticity in substantia gelatinosa neurons. Biochem Biophys Res Commun 2006;347:509–16.

[84] Kalia LV, Pitcher GM, Pelkey KA, Salter MW. PSD-95 is a negative regulator of the tyrosine kinase Src in the NMDA receptor complex. EMBO J 2006;25:4971–82.

[85] Karlsson U, Sjödin J, Angeby Möller K, Johansson S, Wikström L, Nässtrom J. Glutamate-induced currents reveal three functionally distinct NMDA receptor populations in rat dorsal horn: effects of peripheral nerve lesion and inflammation. Neuroscience 2002;112:861–8.

[86] Kawasaki Y, Kohno T, Zhuang ZY, Brenner GJ, Wang H, Van Der Meer C, Befort K, Woolf CJ, Ji RR. Ionotropic and metabotropic receptors, protein kinase A, protein kinase C, and Src contribute to C-fiber-induced ERK activation and cAMP response element-binding protein phosphorylation in dorsal horn neurons, leading to central sensitization. J Neurosci 2004;24:8310–21.

[87] Kerchner GA, Wang GD, Qiu CS, Huettner JE, Zhuo M. Direct presynaptic regulation of GABA/glycine release by kainate receptors in the dorsal horn: an ionotropic mechanism. Neuron 2001;32:477–88.

[88] Kerr RC, Maxwell DJ, Todd AJ. GluR1 and GluR2/3 subunits of the AMPA-type glutamate receptor are associated with particular types of neurone in laminae I-III of the spinal dorsal horn of the rat. Eur J Neurosci 1998;10:324–33.

[89] Kew JN. Positive and negative allosteric modulation of metabotropic glutamate receptors: emerging therapeutic potential. Pharmacol Ther 2004;104:233–44.

[90] Kew JN, Kemp JA. Ionotropic and metabotropic glutamate receptor structure and pharmacology. Psychopharmacology (Berl) 2005;179:4–29.

[91] Knabl J, Witschi R, Hösl K, Reinold H, Zeilhofer UB, Ahmadi S, Brockhaus J, Sergejeva M, Hess A, Brune K, Fritschy JM, Rudolph U, Möhler H, Zeilhofer HU. Reversal of pathological pain through specific spinal $GABA_A$ receptor subtypes. Nature 2008;451:330–4.

[92] Ko S, Zhao MG, Toyoda H, Qiu CS, Zhuo M. Altered behavioral responses to noxious stimuli and fear in glutamate receptor 5 (GluR5)- or GluR6-deficient mice. J Neurosci 2005;25:977–84.

[93] Kovacs G, Kocsis P, Tarnawa I, Horvath C, Szombathelyi Z, Farkas S. NR2B containing NMDA receptor dependent windup of single spinal neurons. Neuropharmacology 2004;46:23–30.

[94] Kristensen JD, Svensson B, Gordh T Jr. The NMDA-receptor antagonist CPP abolishes neurogenic 'wind-up pain' after intrathecal administration in humans. Pain 1992;51:249–53.

[95] Kyrozis A, Goldstein PA, Heath MJ, MacDermott AB. Calcium entry through a subpopulation of AMPA receptors desensitized neighbouring NMDA receptors in rat dorsal horn neurons. J Physiol 1995;485:373–81.

[96] Laffray S, Tan K, Dulluc J, Bouali-Benazzouz R, Calver AR, Nagy F, Landry M. Dissociation and trafficking of rat GABAB receptor heterodimer upon chronic capsaicin stimulation. Eur J Neurosci 2007;25:1402–16.

[97] Laird JM, García-Nicas E, Delpire EJ, Cervero F. Presynaptic inhibition and spinal pain processing in mice: a possible role of the NKCC1 cation-chloride co-transporter in hyperalgesia. Neurosci Lett 2004;361:200–3.

[98] Lalo U, Pankratov Y, Kirchhoff F, North RA, Verkhratsky A. NMDA receptors mediate neuron-to-glia signaling in mouse cortical astrocytes. J Neurosci 2006;26:2673–83.

[99] Larson AA, Giovengo SL, Shi Q, Velázquez RA, Kovacs KJ. Zinc in the extracellular area of the central nervous system is necessary for the development of kainic acid-induced persistent hyperalgesia in mice. Pain 2000;86:177–84.

[100] Lea PM 4th, Faden AI. Metabotropic glutamate receptor subtype 5 antagonists MPEP and MTEP. CNS Drug Rev 2006;12:149–66.

[101] Lee CJ, Kong H, Manzini MC, Albuquerque C, Chao MV, MacDermott AB. Kainate receptors expressed by a subpopulation of developing nociceptors rapidly switch from high to low Ca2+ permeability. J Neurosci 2001;21:4572–81.

[102] Lee MK, Choi BY, Yang GY, Jeon HJ, Kyung HM, Kwon OW, Park HS, Bae YC, Mokha SS, Ahn DK. Low doses of cannabinoids enhance the antinociceptive effects of intracisternally administered mGluRs groups II and III agonists in formalin-induced TMJ nociception in rats. Pain 2008;139:367–75.

[103] Li P, Kerchner GA, Sala C, Wei F, Huettner JE, Sheng M, Zhuo M. AMPA receptor-PDZ interactions in facilitation of spinal sensory synapses. Nat Neurosci 1999;2:972–7.

[104] Li P, Zhuo M. Silent glutamatergic synapses and nociception in mammalian spinal cord. Nature 1998;393:695–8.

[105] Lim J, Lim G, Sung B, Wang S, Mao J. Intrathecal midazolam regulates spinal AMPA receptor expression and function after nerve injury in rats. Brain Res 2006;1123:80–8.

[106] Lin Q, Peng YB, Willis WD. Role of GABA receptor subtypes in inhibition of primate spinothalamic tract neurons: difference between spinal and periaqueductal gray inhibition. J Neurophysiol 1996;75:109–23.

[107] Liu H, Mantyh PW, Basbaum AI. NMDA-receptor regulation of substance P release from primary afferent nociceptors. Nature 1997;386:721–4.

[108] Lodge D. The history of the pharmacology and cloning of ionotropic glutamate receptors and the development of idiosyncratic nomenclature. Neuropharmacology 2009;56:6–21.

[109] Lois F, De Kock M. Something new about ketamine for pediatric anesthesia? Curr Opin Anaesthesiol 2008;21:340–4.

[110] Lorrain DS, Correa L, Anderson J, Varney M. Activation of spinal group I metabotropic glutamate receptors in rats evokes local glutamate release and spontaneous nociceptive behaviors: effects of 2-methyl-6-(phenylethynyl)-pyridine pretreatment. Neurosci Lett 2002;327:198–202.

[111] Lu CR, Willcockson HH, Phend KD, Lucifora S, Darstein M, Valtschanoff JG, Rustioni A. Ionotropic glutamate receptors are expressed in GABAergic terminals in the rat superficial dorsal horn. J Comp Neurol 2005;486:169–78.

[112] Lucifora S, Willcockson HH, Lu CR, Darstein M, Phend KD, Valtschanoff JG, Rustioni A. Presynaptic low- and high-affinity kainate receptors in nociceptive spinal afferents. Pain 2006;120:97–105.

[113] Maione S, Marabese I, Leyva J, Palazzo E, de Novellis V, Rossi F. Characterisation of mGluRs which modulate nociception in the PAG of the mouse. Neuropharmacology 1998;37:1475–83.

[114] Malan TP, Mata HP, Porreca F. Spinal $GABA_A$ and $GABA_B$ receptor pharmacology in a rat model of neuropathic pain. Anesthesiology 2002;96:1161–7.

[115] Mandolesi G, Cesa R, Autuori E, Strata P. An orphan ionotropic glutamate receptor: the delta2 subunit. Neuroscience 2009;158:67–77.

[116] McCarson KE, Duric V, Reisman SA, Winter M, Enna SJ. $GABA_B$ receptor function and subunit expression in the rat spinal cord as indicators of stress and the antinociceptive response to antidepressants. Brain Res 2006;1068:109–17.
[117] McGowan MK, Hammond DL. Intrathecal GABAB antagonists attenuate the antinociception produced by microinjection of L-glutamate into the ventromedial medulla of the rat. Brain Res 1993;607:39–46.
[118] Meller ST, Dykstra CL, Gebhart GF. Acute mechanical hyperalgesia is produced by coactivation of AMPA and metabotropic glutamate receptors. Neuroreport 1993;4:879–82.
[119] Miletic G, Draganic P, Pankratz MT, Miletic V. Muscimol prevents long-lasting potentiation of dorsal horn field potentials in rats with chronic constriction injury exhibiting decreased levels of the GABA transporter GAT-1. Pain 2003;105:347–53.
[120] Miletic G, Miletic V. Loose ligation of the sciatic nerve is associated with TrkB receptor-dependent decreases in KCC2 protein levels in the ipsilateral spinal dorsal horn. Pain 2007;137:532–9.
[121] Millan MJ. The induction of pain: an integrative review. Prog Neurobiol 1999;57:1–164.
[122] Millan MJ, Seguin L. (+)-HA 966, a partial agonist at the glycine site coupled to NMDA receptors, blocks formalin-induced pain in mice. Eur J Pharmacol 1993;238:445–7.
[123] Mills CD, Johnson KM, Hulsebosch CE. Group I metabotropic glutamate receptors in spinal cord injury: roles in neuroprotection and the development of chronic central pain. J Neurotrauma 2002;19:23–42.
[124] Mitchell EA, Gentet LJ, Dempster J, Belelli D. $GABA_A$ and glycine receptor-mediated transmission in rat lamina II neurones: relevance to the analgesic actions of neuroactive steroids. J Physiol 2007;583:1021–40.
[125] Momiyama A. Distinct synaptic and extrasynaptic NMDA receptors identified in dorsal horn neurones of the adult rat spinal cord. J Physiol 2000;523:621–8.
[126] Moore KA, Kohno T, Karchewski LA, Scholz J, Baba H, Woolf CJ. Partial peripheral nerve injury promotes a selective loss of GABAergic inhibition in the superficial dorsal horn of the spinal cord. J Neurosci 2002;22:6724–31.
[127] Morales-Aza BM, Chillingworth NL, Payne JA, Donaldson LF. Inflammation alters cation chloride cotransporter expression in sensory neurons. Neurobiol Dis 2004;17:62–9.
[128] Nahin RL, Hylden JL. Peripheral inflammation is associated with increased glutamic acid decarboxylase immunoreactivity in the rat spinal cord. Neurosci Lett 1991;128:226–30.
[129] Naisbitt S, Kim E, Tu JC, Xiao B, Sala C, Valtschanoff J, Weinberg RJ, Worley PF, Sheng M. Shank, a novel family of postsynaptic density proteins that binds to the NMDA receptor/PSD-95/GKAP complex and cortactin. Neuron 1999;23:569–82.
[130] Nakazawa T, Komai S, Tezuka T, Hisatsune C, Umemori H, Semba K, Mishina M, Manabe T, Yamamoto T. Characterization of Fyn-mediated tyrosine phosphorylation sites on GluR epsilon 2 (NR2B) subunit of the N-methyl-D-aspartate receptor. J Biol Chem 2001;276:693–9.
[131] Neugebauer V. Glutamate receptor ligands. Handb Exp Pharmacol 2007;177:217–49.
[132] Neugebauer V, Chen PS, Willis WD. Role of metabotropic glutamate receptor subtype mGluR1 in brief nociception and central sensitization of primate STT cells. J Neurophysiol 1999;82:272–82.
[133] Nicoll RA, Tomita S, Bredt DS. Auxiliary subunits assist AMPA-type glutamate receptors. Science 2006;311:1253–6.
[134] Nishiyama T. Interaction between a NMDA receptor antagonist, AP-5 and an AMPA receptor antagonist, YM 872 in antinociception in the spinal cord. Acta Anaesthesiol Scand 2008;52:493–8.
[135] Pan HL, Wu ZZ, Zhou HY, Chen SR, Zhang HM, Li DP. Modulation of pain transmission by G-protein-coupled receptors. Pharmacol Ther 2008;117:141–61.
[136] Paoletti P, Ascher P, Neyton J. High-affinity zinc inhibition of NMDA NR1-NR2A receptors. J Neurosci 1997;17:5711–25.
[137] Paoletti P, Neyton J. NMDA receptor subunits: function and pharmacology. Curr Opin Pharmacol 2007;7:39–47.
[138] Park JS, Higashi H, Nagata K, Yoshimura M. Bicuculline-resistant, Cl-dependent GABA response in the rat spinal dorsal horn. Neurosci Res 1999;33:261–8.
[139] Patel S, Naeem S, Kesingland A, Froestl W, Capogna M, Urban L, Fox A. The effects of GABA(B) agonists and gabapentin on mechanical hyperalgesia in models of neuropathic and inflammatory pain in the rat. Pain 2001;90:217–26.
[140] Pedersen LH, Blackburn-Munro G. Pharmacological characterisation of place escape/avoidance behaviour in the rat chronic constriction injury model of neuropathic pain. Psychopharmacology (Berl) 2006;185:208–17.
[141] Pezet S, Cunningham J, Patel J, Grist J, Gavazzi I, Lever IJ, Malcangio M. BDNF modulates sensory neuron synaptic activity by a facilitation of GABA transmission in the dorsal horn. Mol Cell Neurosci 2002;21:51–62.
[142] Pezet S, Marchand F, D'Mello R, Grist J, Clark AK, Malcangio M, Dickenson AH, Williams RJ, McMahon SB. Phosphatidylinositol 3-kinase is a key mediator of central sensitization in painful inflammatory conditions. J Neurosci 2008;28:4261–70.
[143] Pinheiro P, Mulle C. Kainate receptors. Cell Tissue Res 2006;326:457–82.
[144] Pitcher MH, Price TJ, Entrena JM, Cervero F. Spinal NKCC1 blockade inhibits TRPV1-dependent referred allodynia. Mol Pain 2007;3:17.
[145] Poisbeau P, Patte-Mensah C, Keller AF, Barrot M, Breton JD, Luis-Delgado OE, Freund-Mercier MJ, Mensah-Nyagan AG, Schlichter R. Inflammatory pain upregulates spinal inhibition via endogenous neurosteroid production. J Neurosci 2005;25:11768–76.
[146] Polgár E, Watanabe M, Hartmann B, Grant SG, Todd AJ. Expression of AMPA receptor subunits at synapses in laminae I-III of the rodent spinal dorsal horn. Mol Pain 2008;4:5.
[147] Popratiloff A, Weinberg RJ, Rustioni A. AMPA receptor subunits underlying terminals of fine-caliber primary afferent fibers. J Neurosci 1996;16:3363–72.
[148] Popratiloff A, Weinberg RJ, Rustioni A. AMPA receptors at primary afferent synapses in substantia gelatinosa after sciatic nerve section. Eur J Neurosci 1998;10:3220–30.

[149] Price TJ, Cervero F, de Koninck Y. Role of cation-chloride-cotransporters (CCC) in pain and hyperalgesia. Curr Top Med Chem 2005;5:547–55.
[150] Procter MJ, Houghton AK, Faber ES, Chizh BA, Ornstein PL, Lodge D, Headley PM. Actions of kainate and AMPA selective glutamate receptor ligands on nociceptive processing in the spinal cord. Neuropharmacology 1998;37:1287–97.
[151] Rahman W, Sikandar S, Suzuki R, Hunt SP, Dickenson AH. Superficial NK1 expressing spinal dorsal horn neurones modulate inhibitory neurotransmission mediated by spinal $GABA_A$ receptors. Neurosci Lett 2007;419:278–83.
[152] Ransom RW, Stec NL. Cooperative modulation of [^{3}H]MK-801 binding to the N-methyl-D-aspartate receptor-ion channel complex by L-glutamate, glycine, and polyamines. J Neurochem 1988;51:830–6.
[153] Reis GM, Duarte ID. Involvement of chloride channel coupled $GABA_C$ receptors in the peripheral antinociceptive effect induced by $GABA_C$ receptor agonist cis-4-aminocrotonic acid. Life Sci 2007;80:1268–73.
[154] Ren K, Dubner R. Neuron-glia crosstalk gets serious: role in pain hypersensitivity. Curr Opin Anesthesiol 2008;21:570–9.
[155] Riley RC, Trafton JA, Chi SI, Basbaum AI. Presynaptic regulation of spinal cord tachykinin signaling via $GABA_B$ but not $GABA_A$ receptor activation. Neuroscience 2001;103:725–37.
[156] Rozzo A, Armellin M, Franzot J, Chiaruttini C, Nistri A, Tongiorgi E. Expression and dendritic mRNA localization of $GABA_C$ receptor rho1 and rho2 subunits in developing rat brain and spinal cord. Eur J Neurosci 2002;15:1747–58.
[157] Sahara Y, Noro N, Iida Y, Soma K, Nakamura Y. Glutamate receptor subunits GluR5 and KA-2 are coexpressed in rat trigeminal ganglion neurons. J Neurosci 1997;17:6611–20.
[158] Sakurada K, Masu M, Nakanishi S. Alteration of Ca^{2+} permeability and sensitivity to Mg^{2+} and channel blockers by a single amino acid substitution in the N-methyl-D-aspartate receptor. J Biol Chem 1993;268:410–5.
[159] Sang CN, Booher S, Gilron I, Parada S, Max MB. Dextromethorphan and memantine in painful diabetic neuropathy and postherpetic neuralgia: efficacy and dose-response trials. Anesthesiology 2002;96:1053–61.
[160] Sang CN, Ramadan NM, Wallihan RG, Chappell AS, Freitag FG, Smith TR, Silberstein SD, Johnson KW, Phebus LA, Bleakman D, et al. LY293558, a novel AMPA/GluR5 antagonist, is efficacious and well-tolerated in acute migraine. Cephalalgia 2004;24:596–602.
[161] Schlichter R, Keller AF, De Roo M, Breton JD, Inquimbert P, Poisbeau P. Fast nongenomic effects of steroids on synaptic transmission and role of endogenous neurosteroids in spinal pain pathways. J Mol Neurosci 2006;28:33–51.
[162] Schoffnegger D, Ruscheweyh R, Sandkühler J. Spread of excitation across modality borders in spinal dorsal horn of neuropathic rats. Pain 2008;135:300–10.
[163] Schuler V, Lüscher C, Blanchet C, Klix N, Sansig G, Klebs K, Schmutz M, Heid J, Gentry C, Urban L, et al. Epilepsy, hyperalgesia, impaired memory, and loss of pre- and postsynaptic $GABA_B$ responses in mice lacking $GABA_B$1. Neuron 2001;31:47–58.
[164] Scotland PE, Coderre TJ. Enhanced 3,5-dihydroxyphenylglycine-induced sustained nociceptive behaviors in rats with neuropathy or chronic inflammation. Behav Brain Res 2007;184:150–6.
[165] Seagrove LC, Suzuki R, Dickenson AH. Electrophysiological characterisations of rat lamina I dorsal horn neurones and the involvement of excitatory amino acid receptors. Pain 2004;108:76–87.
[166] Sivilotti L, Woolf CJ. The contribution of GABAA and glycine receptors to central sensitization: disinhibition and touch-evoked allodynia in the spinal cord. J Neurophysiol 1994;72:169–79.
[167] Sluka KA, Audette KM. Activation of protein kinase C in the spinal cord produces mechanical hyperalgesia by activating glutamate receptors, but does not mediate chronic muscle-induced hyperalgesia. Mol Pain 2006;2:13.
[168] Sokal DM, Chapman V. Spinal $GABA_B$-receptor antagonism increases nociceptive transmission in vivo. Neuroreport 2001;12:3247–50.
[169] Soril LJ, Ramer LM, McPhail LT, Kaan TK, Ramer MS. Spinal brain-derived neurotrophic factor governs neuroplasticity and recovery from cold-hypersensitivity following dorsal rhizotomy. Pain 2007;138:98–110.
[170] Sorkin LS, Yaksh TL, Doom CM. Mechanical allodynia in rats is blocked by a Ca^{2+} permeable AMPA receptor antagonist. Neuroreport 1999;10:3523–6.
[171] Sorkin LS, Yaksh TL, Doom CM. Pain models display differential sensitivity to Ca^{2+}-permeable non-NMDA glutamate receptor antagonists. Anesthesiology 2001;95:965–73.
[172] South SM, Kohno T, Kaspar BK, Hegarty D, Vissel B, Drake CT, Ohata M, Jenab S, Sailer AW, Malkmus S, et al. A conditional deletion of the NR1 subunit of the NMDA receptor in adult spinal cord dorsal horn reduces NMDA currents and injury-induced pain. J Neurosci 2003;23:5031–40.
[173] Spike RC, Kerr R, Maxwell DJ, Todd AJ. GluR1 and GluR2/3 subunits of the AMPA-type glutamate receptor are associated with particular types of neurone in laminae I-III of the spinal dorsal horn of the rat. Eur J Neurosci 1998;10:324–33.
[174] Stanfa LC, Dickenson AH. The role of non-N-methyl-D-aspartate ionotropic glutamate receptors in the spinal transmission of nociception in normal animals and animals with carrageenan inflammation. Neuroscience 1999;93:1391–8.
[175] Stanfa LC, Hampton DW, Dickenson AH. Role of Ca2+-permeable non-NMDA glutamate receptors in spinal nociceptive transmission. Neuroreport 2000;11:3199–202.
[176] Stepanović-Petrović RM, Tomić MA, Vucković SM, Kocev N, Ugresić ND, Prostran MS, Bosković B. GABAergic mechanisms are involved in the antihyperalgesic effects of carbamazepine and oxcarbazepine in a rat model of inflammatory hyperalgesia. Pharmacology 2008;82:53–8.
[177] Sung KW, Kirby M, McDonald MP, Lovinger DM, Delpire E. Abnormal GABAA receptor-mediated currents in dorsal root ganglion neurons isolated from Na-K-2Cl cotransporter null mice. J Neurosci 2000;20:7531–8.
[178] Tachibana M, Wenthold RJ, Morioka H, Petralia RS. Light and electron microscopic immunocytochemical localization of AMPA-selective glutamate receptors in the rat spinal cord. J Comp Neurol 1994;344:431–54.
[179] Tan PH, Yang LC, Shih HC, Lan KC, Cheng JT. Gene knockdown with intrathecal siRNA of NMDA receptor NR2B subunit reduces formalin-induced nociception in the rat. Gene Ther 2005;12:59–66.

[180] Tao F, Skinner J, Su Q, Johns RA. New role for spinal Stargazin in alpha-amino-3-hydroxy-5-methyl-4-isoxazolepropionic acid receptor-mediated pain sensitization after inflammation. J Neurosci Res 2006;84:867–73.

[181] Tao YX, Huang YZ, Mei L, Johns RA. Expression of PSD-95/SAP90 is critical for N-methyl-D-aspartate receptor-mediated thermal hyperalgesia in the spinal cord. Neuroscience 2000;98:201–6.

[182] Tao YX, Rumbaugh G, Wang GD, Petralia RS, Zhao C, Kauer FW, Tao F, Zhuo M, Wenthold RJ, Raja SN, et al. Impaired NMDA receptor-mediated postsynaptic function and blunted NMDA receptor-dependent persistent pain in mice lacking postsynaptic density-93 protein. J Neurosci 2003;23:6703–12.

[183] Tingley WG, Ehlers MD, Kameyama K, Doherty C, Ptak JB, Riley CT, Huganir RL. Characterization of protein kinase A and protein kinase C phosphorylation of the N-methyl-D-aspartate receptor NR1 subunit using phosphorylation site-specific antibodies. J Biol Chem 1997;272:5157–66.

[184] Tölle TR, Berthele A, Zieglgänsberger W, Seeburg PH, Wisden W. The differential expression of 16 NMDA and non-NMDA receptor subunits in the rat spinal cord and in periaqueductal gray. J Neurosci 1993;13:5009–28.

[185] Tölle TR, Berthele A, Zieglgänsberger W, Seeburg PH, Wisden W. Flip and Flop variants of AMPA receptors in the rat lumbar spinal cord. Eur J Neurosci 1995;7:1414–9.

[186] Tong CK, MacDermott AB. Both Ca^{2+}-permeable and -impermeable AMPA receptors contribute to primary synaptic drive onto rat dorsal horn neurons. J Physiol 2006;575:133–44.

[187] Tornberg J, Voikar V, Savilahti H, Rauvala H, Airaksinen MS. Behavioural phenotypes of hypomorphic KCC2-deficient mice. Eur J Neurosci 2005;21:1327–37.

[188] Torsney C, MacDermott AB. Disinhibition opens the gate to pathological pain signaling in superficial neurokinin 1 receptor-expressing neurons in rat spinal cord. J Neurosci 2006;26:1833–43.

[189] Traynelis SF, Burgess MF, Zheng F, Lyuboslavsky P, Powers JL. Control of voltage-independent zinc inhibition of NMDA receptors by the NR1 subunit. J Neurosci 1998;18:6163–75.

[190] Traynelis SF, Hartley M, Heinemann SF. Control of proton sensitivity of the NMDA receptor by RNA splicing and polyamines. Science 1995;268:873–6.

[191] Tu JC, Xiao B, Naisbitt S, Yuan JP, Petralia RS, Brakeman P, Doan A, Aakalu VK, Lanahan AA, Sheng M, Worley PF. Coupling of mGluR/Homer and PSD-95 complexes by the Shank family of postsynaptic density proteins. Neuron 1999;23:583–92.

[192] Varty GB, Grilli M, Forlani A, Fredduzzi S, Grzelak ME, Guthrie DH, Hodgson RA, Lu SX, Nicolussi E, Pond AJ, et al. The antinociceptive and anxiolytic-like effects of the metabotropic glutamate receptor 5 (mGluR5) antagonists, MPEP and MTEP, and the mGluR1 antagonist, LY456236, in rodents: a comparison of efficacy and side-effect profiles. Psychopharmacology (Berl) 2005;179:207–17.

[193] Vergnano AM, Salio C, Merighi A. NK1 receptor activation leads to enhancement of inhibitory neurotransmission in spinal substantia gelatinosa neurons of mouse. Pain 2004;112:37–47.

[194] Viggiano A, Monda M, Viggiano A, Chiefari M, Aurilio C, De Luca B. Evidence that GABAergic neurons in the spinal trigeminal nucleus are involved in the transmission of inflammatory pain in the rat: a microdialysis and pharmacological study. Eur J Pharmacol 2004;496:87–92.

[195] Vikman KS, Duggan AW, Siddall PJ. Interferon-gamma induced disruption of GABAergic inhibition in the spinal dorsal horn in vivo. Pain 2007;133:18–28.

[196] Vikman KS, Rycroft BK, Christie MJ. Switch to Ca2+-permeable AMPA and reduced NR2B NMDA receptor-mediated neurotransmission at dorsal horn nociceptive synapses during inflammatory pain in the rat. J Physiol 2008;586:515–27.

[197] Vissel B, Royle GA, Christie BR, Schiffer HH, Ghetti A, Tritto T, Perez-Otano I, Radcliffe RA, Seamans J, Sejnowski T, Wehner JM, Collins AC, O'Gorman S, Heinemann SF. The role of RNA editing of kainate receptors in synaptic plasticity and seizures. Neuron 2001;29:217–27.

[198] Wang XL, Zhang HM, Chen SR, Pan HL. Altered synaptic input and GABAB receptor function in spinal superficial dorsal horn neurons in rats with diabetic neuropathy. J Physiol 2007;579:849–61.

[199] Weng HR, Laird JM, Cervero F, Schouenborg J. $GABA_A$ receptor blockade inhibits A beta fibre evoked wind-up in the arthritic rat. Neuroreport 1998;9:1065–9.

[200] Willis WD, Coggeshall RE. Sensory mechanisms of the spinal cord, 3rd ed. Vol. 1. New York: Kluwer Academic/Plenum; 2004.

[201] Wood PL, Mahmood SA, Moskal JR. Antinociceptive action of GLYX-13: an N-methyl-D-aspartate receptor glycine site partial agonist. Neuroreport 2008;19:1059–61.

[202] Woolf CJ, Salter MW. Neuronal plasticity: increasing the gain in pain. Science 2000;288:1765–9.

[203] Woolf CJ, Thompson SW. The induction and maintenance of central sensitization is dependent on N-methyl-D-aspartic acid receptor activation; implications for the treatment of post-injury pain hypersensitivity states. Pain 1991;44:293–9.

[204] Wu LJ, Ko SW, Zhuo M. Kainate receptors and pain: from dorsal root ganglion to the anterior cingulate cortex. Curr Pharm Des 2007;13:1597–605.

[205] Xu H, Wu LJ, Zhao MG, Toyoda H, Vadakkan KI, Jia Y, Pinaud R, Zhuo M. Presynaptic regulation of the inhibitory transmission by GluR5-containing kainate receptors in spinal substantia gelatinosa. Mol Pain 2006;2:29.

[206] Yamamoto T, Hirasawa S, Wroblewska B, Grajkowska E, Zhou J, Kozikowski A, Wroblewski J, Neale JH. Antinociceptive effects of N-acetylaspartylglutamate (NAAG) peptidase inhibitors ZJ-11, ZJ-17 and ZJ-43 in the rat formalin test and in the rat neuropathic pain model. Eur J Neurosci 2004;20:483–94.

[207] Yang L, Zhang FX, Huang F, Lu YJ, Li GD, Bao L, Xiao HS, Zhang X. Peripheral nerve injury induces trans-synaptic modification of channels, receptors and signal pathways in rat dorsal spinal cord. Eur J Neurosci 2004;19:871–83.

[208] Ye Z, Westlund KN. Ultrastructural localization of glutamate receptor subunits (NMDAR1, AMPA GluR1 and GluR2/3) and spinothalamic tract cells. Neuroreport 1996;7:2581–5.

[209] Youn DH, Randic M. Modulation of excitatory synaptic transmission in the spinal substantia gelatinosa of mice deficient in the kainate receptor GluR5 and/or GluR6 subunit. J Physiol 2004;555:683–98.
[210] Youn DH, Royle G, Kolaj M, Vissel B, Randić M. Enhanced LTP of primary afferent neurotransmission in AMPA receptor GluR2-deficient mice. Pain 2008;136:158–67.
[211] Young MR, Blackburn-Munro G, Dickinson T, Johnson MJ, Anderson H, Nakalembe I, Fleetwood-Walker SM. Antisense ablation of type I metabotropic glutamate receptor mGluR1 inhibits spinal nociceptive transmission. J Neurosci 1998;18:10180–8.
[212] Yung KK. Localization of glutamate receptors in dorsal horn of rat spinal cord. Neuroreport 1998;9:1639–44.
[213] Zahn PK, Pogatzki-Zahn EM, Brennan TJ. Spinal administration of MK-801 and NBQX demonstrates NMDA-independent dorsal horn sensitization in incisional pain. Pain 2005;114:499–510.
[214] Zeilhofer HU, Zeilhofer UB. Spinal dis-inhibition in inflammatory pain. Neurosci Lett 2008;437:170–4.
[215] Zhang W, Liu LY, Xu TL. Reduced potassium-chloride co-transporter expression in spinal cord dorsal horn neurons contributes to inflammatory pain hypersensitivity in rats. Neuroscience 2008;152:502–10.
[216] Zhang X, Wu J, Lei Y, Fang L, Willis WD. Protein phosphatase modulates the phosphorylation of spinal cord NMDA receptors in rats following intradermal injection of capsaicin. Brain Res Mol Brain Res 2005;138:264–72.
[217] Zhang X, Wu J, Lei Y, Fang L, Willis WD. Protein phosphatase 2A regulates central sensitization in the spinal cord of rats following intradermal injection of capsaicin. Mol Pain 2006;2:9.
[218] Zhou HY, Zhang HM, Chen SR, Pan HL. Increased nociceptive input rapidly modulates spinal GABAergic transmission through endogenously released glutamate. J Neurophysiol 2007;97:871–82.
[219] Zhou Q, Imbe H, Zou S, Dubner R, Ren K. Selective upregulation of the flip-flop splice variants of AMPA receptor subunits in the rat spinal cord after hindpaw inflammation. Mol Brain Res 2001;88:186–93.
[220] Zou X, Lin Q, Willis WD. Role of protein kinase A in phosphorylation of NMDA receptor 1 subunits in dorsal horn and spinothalamic tract neurons after intradermal injection of capsaicin in rats. Neuroscience 2002;115:775–86.

Correspondence to: Ke Ren, MD, PhD, Department of Neural and Pain Sciences, Dental School, University of Maryland, 650 W. Baltimore Street, Baltimore, MD 21201-1586, USA. Email: kren@umaryland.edu.

Dopamine Pathways and Receptors in Nociception and Pain

11

Francisco Pellicer, J. Manuel Ortega-Legaspi, Alberto López-Avila, Ulises Coffeen, and Orlando Jaimes

Ramón de la Fuente National Institute of Psychiatry, Neuroscience Division, Mexico City, Mexico

"Nociception" is the term used to name a number of defense mechanisms that help protect animals from harm. This alarm system is present in organisms as simple as protozoa [47]. Moreover, humans, as well as other highly evolved species, exhibit the concept of "pain." This second construct implies, in addition to nociceptive mechanisms, more complex memory, learning, cognitive, and affective processes related to real or potential harm. We now know that many of the physiological mechanisms related to nociception and pain were early acquired in evolution and have been preserved along the phylogenetic line [32]. A good example is the fact that neurotransmitters and neuromodulators, including dopamine, have actions related to harm-avoidance behaviors in invertebrates [66].

In 1817, James Parkinson described a disease characterized by "shaking palsy." Afterwards, Charcot was the first to notice a relationship between altered pain perception and what was later known as Parkinson's disease [15]. In 1957, dopamine was described by Carlsson and was later attributed to the etiology of this disease [8,20,29]. Patients with Parkinson's disease not only have motor abnormalities, but also have an altered perception of pain [61].

The actions of the dopaminergic system can be divided into two major categories. The first is an effector system involved in carrying out functions such as motor, cardiovascular, and neuroendocrine control. The second is a system related to cognition that encompasses reward, learning, memory, and addiction; this system can also control

Pharmacology of Pain
edited by Pierre Beaulieu, David Lussier, Frank Porreca, and Anthony H. Dickenson
IASP Press, Seattle, © 2010

the effector system. There are four main supraspinal dopaminergic pathways (Fig. 1A). The first is the tuberoinfundibular pathway, which is closely related to neuroendocrine control; it originates in the nucleus arcuatus of the hypothalamus and projects to dopaminergic neurons located in the intermediate lobe of the hypophysis. These neurons constitute melanotrophs, which regulate proopiomelanocortin release, and lactotrophs, which regulate prolactin [9,13]. The second pathway is the nigrostriatal pathway, related to motor control, which projects from the substantia nigra (pars compacta or A9) in the midbrain to the dorsal striatum in the basal ganglia complex. Dysfunction of this pathway is associated with Parkinsonism [16]. The other two pathways—the mesolimbic and mesocortical pathways—have a common origin in the ventral tegmental area (VTA) or A10. The mesolimbic pathway innervates the ventral striatum (which comprises the nucleus accumbens and the olfactory tuberculum), as well as structures that constitute the limbic system such as the septum, amygdala, and piriform cortex, which all play a role in motivation, positive reinforcement, and addiction processes. On the other hand, the mesocortical pathway projects to areas related to the affective and cognitive spheres—the cingulate, frontal, and entorhinal cortices [48].

All four dopaminergic pathways thus constitute separate entities, the first two being defined by movement and endocrine control, and the last two being linked to the modulation of cognition and affect. Clinical evidence shows that a malfunction of any of these pathways can disrupt pain processing [2,57,59,61,72].

Dopamine Pathways within the Pain Matrix

The term "pain matrix" is used to name the nuclei and pathways related to pain perception. This matrix consists mainly of the spinal cord, the thalamus, the amygdala, the VTA, the periaqueductal gray, and the basal ganglia, as well as the cerebellar, insular, posterior parietal, prefrontal, anterior cingulate, supplementary motor, and primary and secondary somatosensory cortices. Pain perception is known to be integrated in these structures, which rely on several neurotransmission systems [10,24,43,52,63].

In order to elicit its specific effects within the pain matrix, dopamine binds to its receptors. These receptors are part of the superfamily of metabotropic receptors with seven transmembrane-spanning domains. The dopaminergic system has two receptor families, known as the D1 and D2 families; both are coupled to G-protein mechanisms. The first family, which includes the D1 and D5 receptor subtypes, is coupled to a Gs protein, therefore exerting an excitatory effect, whereas the second family comprises the D2, D3, and D4 receptor subtypes and is related to an inhibitory G protein [19,33] (Fig. 1B). Even though the two families of dopaminergic receptors activate different intracellular signalling mechanisms, the concomitant stimulation of D1 and D2 receptors is required under normal conditions for many actions of dopamine. This phenomenon is often referred to as "D1/D2 synergism." The combined response of these receptors to a pharmacological agent exceeds the algebraic sum of their separate responses [19].

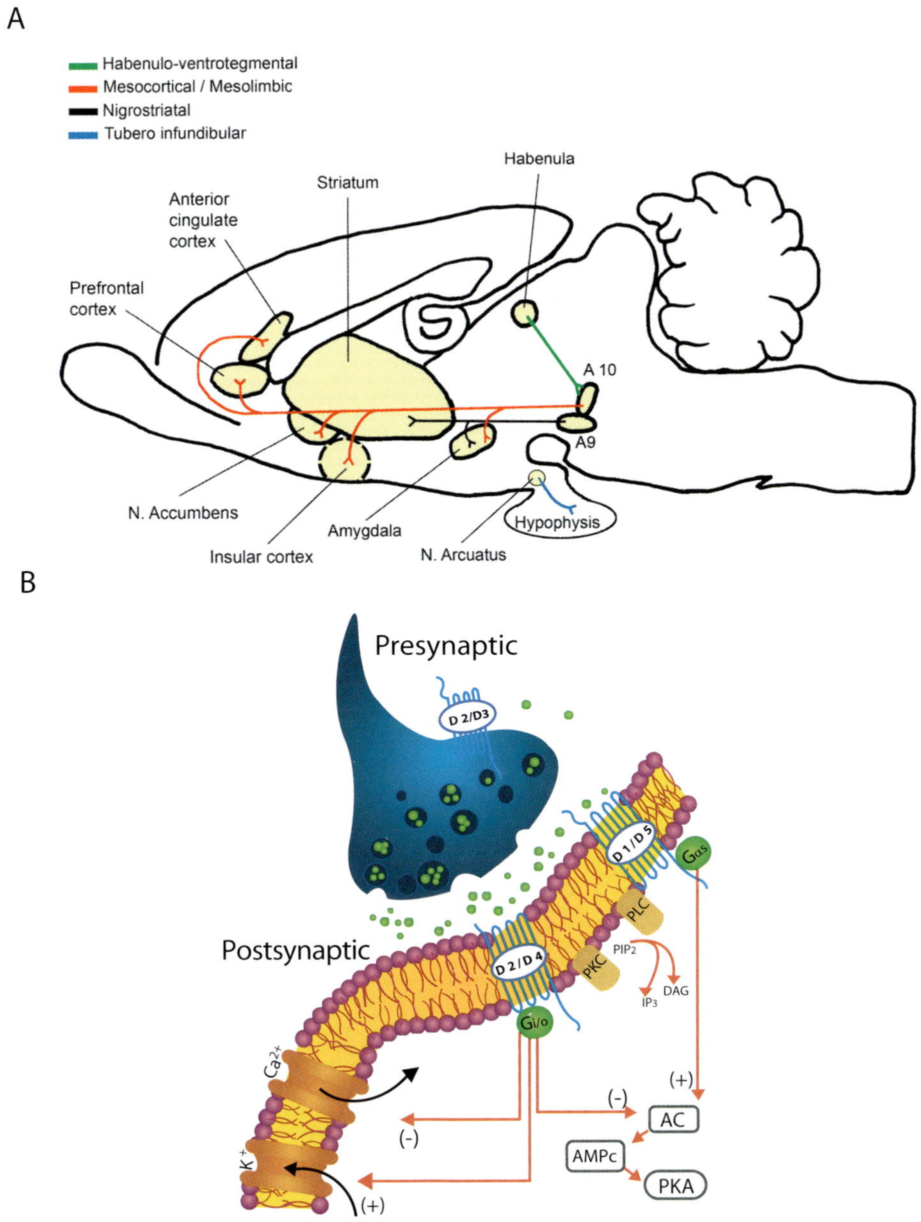

Fig. 1. (A) This figure depicts the origin of the mesocortical and mesolimbic pathways (shown in red) in the ventral tegmental area (VTA or A10), which sends projections to the amygdala, nucleus accumbens, and the insular, prefrontal, and anterior cingulate cortices. These constitute the main affective and cognitive pain-related dopaminergic pathways. The habenulo-ventrotegmental pathway (shown in green) is involved in the activation by substance P on dopaminergic neurons in the VTA. The nigrostriatal pathway (shown in black) goes from A9 or the substantia nigra to the striatum and amygdala and is involved in the motor control sphere. Another dopaminergic pathway is the tuberoinfundibular (shown in blue), which plays a role in neuroendocrine control. (B) The figure shows the five subtypes of dopaminergic receptors, their general neuronal localization, and their mechanism of action. Dopamine D1 and D5 receptors are postsynaptic; they activate a Gs protein, therefore stimulating adenylate cyclase (AC) in order to increase cyclic adenosine monophosphate (cAMP) and ultimately phosphokinase A (PKA). Dopamine D2, D3, and D4 receptors activate a G_i protein that inhibits AC. D3 is localized presynaptically, D4 postsynaptically, and D2 both pre- and postsynaptically.

The most important and best-studied nuclei that are dopaminergic or receive dopaminergic projections will be analyzed in the following sections.

Anterior Cingulate Cortex

The anterior cingulate cortex (ACC) is a region that has traditionally been related to the affective component of pain [1]. It receives dopaminergic input directly from the VTA via the medial forebrain bundle [18,70]. It is known that dopamine can modulate the functions of the ACC and that it is a major site of nociceptive modulation, but there is very little experimental evidence on either of these issues. One study found that a single microinjection of dopamine into the ACC in an animal neuropathic pain model significantly reduced neurectomy-induced nociception, measured as autotomy behavior, for 25 days. Moreover, amantadine, an NMDA antagonist [34] that also has dopamine release properties [28], can diminish chronic nociception and has an effect similar to that of dopamine in the ACC. Microinjection of this compound into the ACC produced a decrease in neuropathic nociception (Fig. 2A). To test whether dopamine release triggered by the action of amantadine is responsible for this compound's antinociceptive effect, a combination of dopamine D1- and D2-receptor antagonists together with amantadine was microinjected into the ACC in the same animal model of neuropathic pain. The results of this experiment show that the blockade of dopaminergic receptors abolishes the antinociceptive effect of amantadine [38]. More recent evidence shows that intraperitoneal administration of amantadine not only diminishes neuropathic nociception induced by denervation but also increases levels of dopamine in the ACC, as measured with high-performance liquid chromatography (Fig. 2B) [37]. This evidence highlights the role of the dopaminergic system as a modulator of nociception within the ACC and encourages further experimental studies. There is also clinical evidence of the effectiveness of amantadine in neuropathic pain. The oral administration of amantadine for 2 weeks can reduce pain for 5 months in a patient with neuropathic pain [21].

Insular Cortex

The anterior insular cortex, and more specifically the rostral agranular region, receives somatic afferent input and has been related to nociceptive input. Clinical evidence in pathologies related to abnormal central pain modulation, such as asymbolia for pain and pseudothalamic pain syndrome, along with evidence from functional imaging studies, has allowed researchers to establish a relationship between the processing of pain and the insular cortex [5,17,58]. However, these studies do not reveal the nature of the neurotransmission systems involved. Jasmin et al. have studied diverse neurotransmission systems such as the opioidergic, GABAergic, and dopaminergic systems in acute and inflammatory nociception in relation to the functional anatomy of the insular cortex in the rat [6,7,30,31,49].

The rostral agranular insular cortex (RAIC) has a close relationship with the mesolimbic dopaminergic system and receives projections from the ventral tegmental area

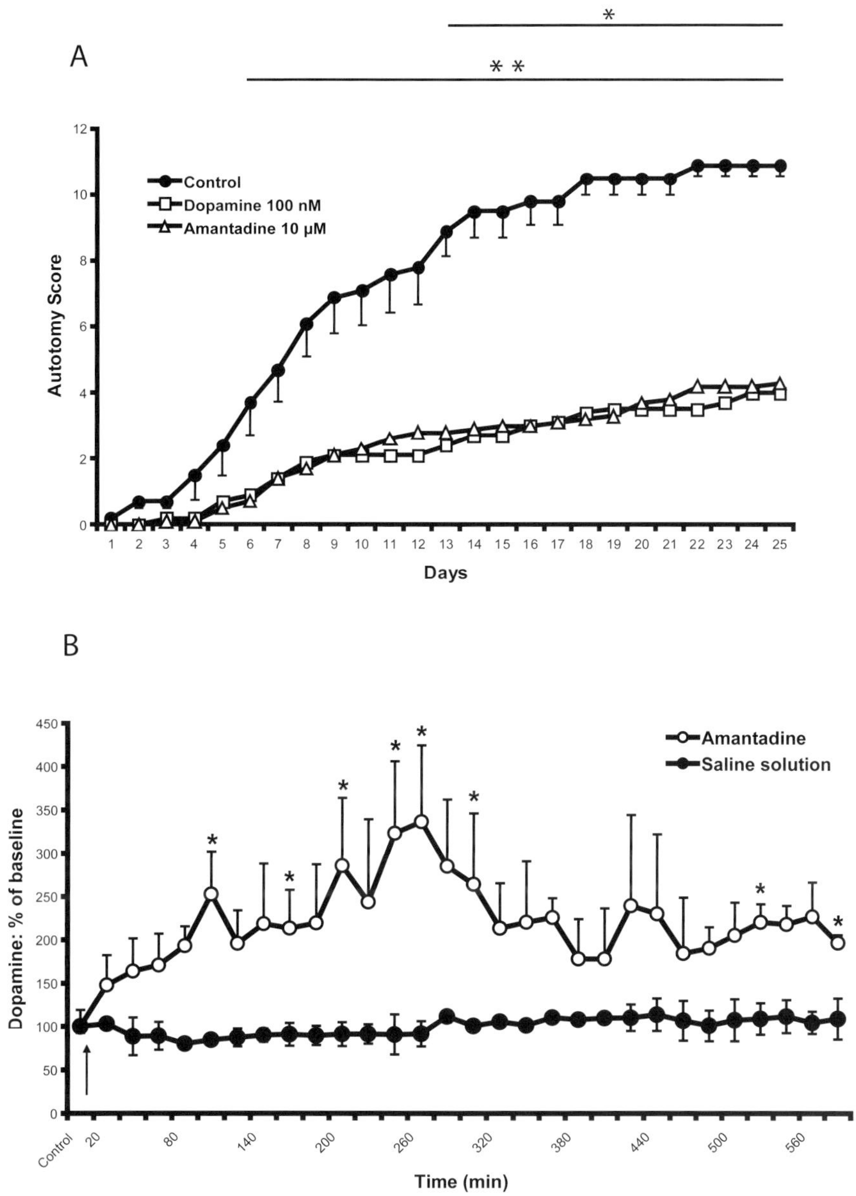

Fig. 2. (A) The figure shows the effect of a microinjection of dopamine and amantadine into the anterior cingulate cortex (ACC) on chronic nociception, measured as autotomy behavior over 25 days. All groups were subjected to a nociceptive process (the rat's right hindpaw was immersed in 55°C water for 20 seconds), and a right sciatic denervation was performed 30 minutes afterwards, followed by a 2-μL microinjection of saline solution 0.9% for the control, dopamine 100 nM, or amantadine 10 μM, respectively, into the ACC. A significant decrease in autotomy score was observed in both treatment groups when compared to the control group (repeated-measures ANOVA, $P < 0.05$). The significance of differences between groups each day was established by a post hoc Tukey test ($P < 0.05$) (** dopamine 100 nM and * amantadine 10 μM). Modified from [38]. (B) This figure depicts a dopamine increase in the ACC after the systemic administration of amantadine (90 mg/kg). The measurement was obtained using a high-performance liquid chromatography system from a dialysate taken every 20 minutes for 10 hours. The amantadine group shows an immediate increase in dopamine levels, with significance 100 minutes after the injection (arrow). The maximum increase (236%, $F = 15.836$, $P < 0.001$) was obtained at 260 minutes. The control group (injected with saline solution) shows no change along the same time frame.

through the medial forebrain bundle [49]. In a rat study focusing on afferent and efferent connections of the RAIC with sites implicated in nociceptive processing, an increased dopaminergic tone produced by the use of a dopamine uptake inhibitor increased the thermonociceptive threshold [30]. Also, the presence of dopamine D1 and D2 receptors in the RAIC has been documented [27,53]. Results obtained by our group using a neuropathic pain model (thermonociception followed by denervation) [11] show that dopamine D2-receptor activation with a selective agonist (TNPA), as well as selective dopamine D1-receptor blockade with an antagonist (SCH-23390) in the insular cortex, both diminish the incidence of nociceptive behavior (autotomy score) (Fig. 3A) and delay its onset. In contrast, in an experimental approach in which nociception was not enhanced with thermonociception prior to denervation, the administration of a dopamine D1 agonist increased autotomy behavior, whereas the use of an antagonist diminished it (Fig. 3B). This evidence suggests that there is a differential modulation between dopamine D1 and D2 receptors in the insular cortex regarding chronic nociception [12].

Clinical and experimental evidence highlights the insular cortex as an important locus in which sensory input and perceptual processes converge [26]. In this context, all these data demonstrate the functional differences between dopamine D1 and D2 receptors within the RAIC in relation to the genesis and maintenance of neuropathic nociception. We have shown evidence of the pronociceptive role of the dopamine D1 receptor as well as the antinociceptive role of dopamine D2 receptors in an animal model of chronic pain [12].

Nucleus Accumbens

The nucleus accumbens has traditionally been related to pleasure, addiction, sexual behavior, and food intake. Nevertheless, it has also been ascribed a role in pain modulation. This nucleus is a target for dopaminergic fibers that come from the VTA and that are activated by substance P and opioid agonists; this system has shown an important effect in tonic pain [3,25]. Also, dopamine neurons play a key role in the suppression of tonic, but not phasic, pain [41]; this evidence supports a role of this system in long-lasting pain. In this context, dopamine agonists such as cocaine, amphetamine, apomorphine, and quinpirole induce analgesia in the formalin test for tonic pain. The analgesic effect of cocaine in this test is blocked by pretreatment with either the nonselective dopamine receptor antagonist, chlorpromazine, the selective D1-like dopamine receptor antagonist, SCH 23390, or the selective D2-like dopamine receptor antagonist, eticlopride. In contrast, when tests for phasic pain (e.g., the tail-flick test) are employed, dopamine agonists such as amphetamine, cocaine, bromocriptine, and apomorphine either have no effect on the latency of withdrawal responses, or they elicit hyperalgesia (i.e., enhanced responsiveness to pain) [3]. Also, Wood has proposed tonic/phasic models of mesolimbic dopamine activity. Briefly, phasic dopamine release occurs as a consequence of burst-firing dopamine neurons and has a short duration due to dopamine transporters. Tonic dopamine corresponds to the low concentration of dopamine in the extracellular space that results from spontaneous

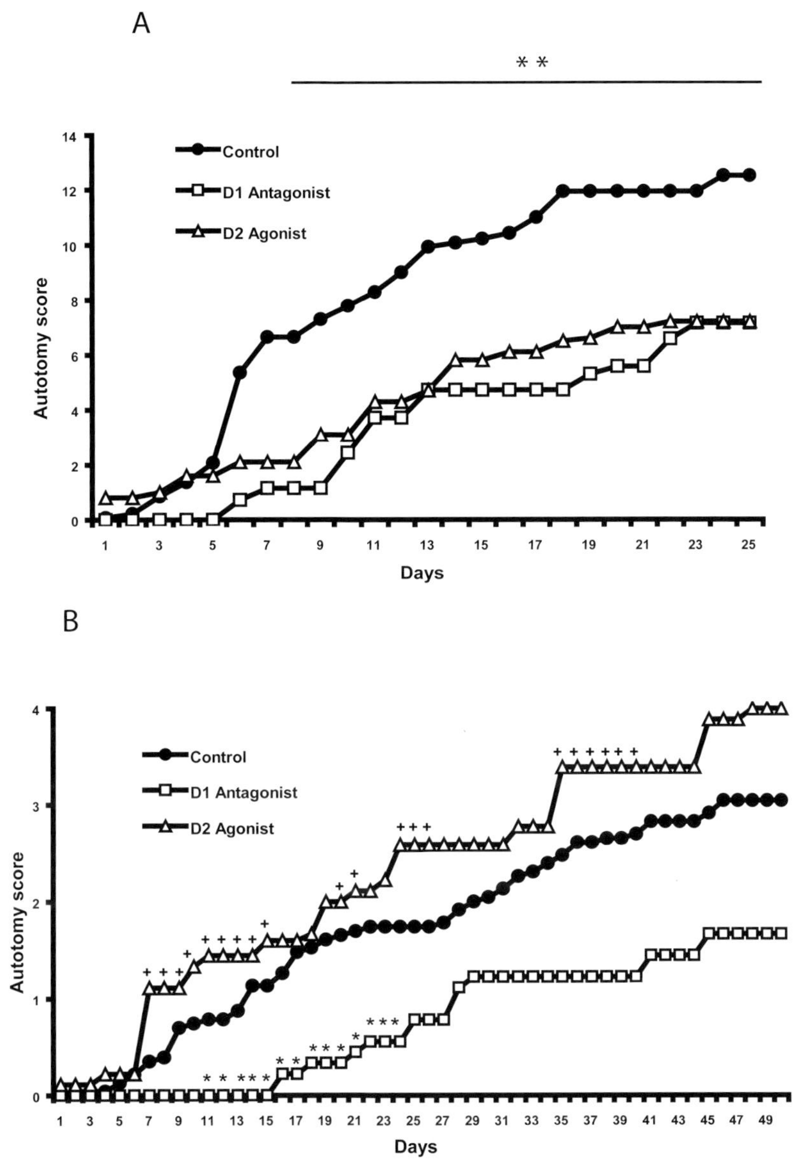

Fig. 3. (A) Behavioral nociceptive response measured as autotomy score during 25 days for groups of rats with either a dopamine D1 antagonist (SCH-23390) or a D2 agonist (TNPA) microinjected into the rostral agranular insular cortex (RAIC). Both the experimental and control groups had a right sciatic denervation performed 30 minutes after thermonociception (hindpaw immersed in 55°C water for 20 seconds) and were microinjected with 1 μL of 0.9% saline solution for the control group, SCH-23390 at 30 nM for the D1 antagonist group, or TNPA at 250 nM for the D2 agonist group. Both the D1 antagonist and D2 agonist groups showed a significant decrease in autotomy score as compared to the control group, with significance from day 6 to day 25 (**, Kruskal-Wallis test, $P < 0.05$). (B) The effect on chronic nociception (induced by right sciatic denervation only), measured as autotomy behavior over 50 days, for groups of rats with a dopamine D1 agonist or antagonist microinjected into the RAIC. The control group was microinjected with 0.9% saline solution into the RAIC. The experimental groups were microinjected with SCH-23390 (D1 antagonist group) at 30 nM and with SKF-38393 (D1 agonist group) at 300 nM. Note the diminished autotomy score when a dopamine D1 antagonist is microinjected; conversely, autotomy score increases when an agonist is used, as compared to control. There are significant differences in behavior between groups: control vs. D1 antagonist group (*) and D1 agonist group vs. D1 antagonist group (+) (Kruskal-Wallis test, $P < 0.05$). Modified from [12].

firing of dopamine neurons in response to glutamatergic input from the hippocampus to the nucleus accumbens. The increase in inhibitory dopamine D2 autoreceptor activity attenuates phasic activity [71].

Furthermore, the activation of the VTA by nitrous oxide (N_2O) causes dopamine release in the accumbens with an antinociceptive effect. When raclopride, a D2-receptor antagonist, is microinjected into the shell of this nucleus, it inhibits the antinociceptive effect of N_2O. This evidence confirms the role of dopamine D2 receptors in the nucleus accumbens regarding nociception [35].

Thus, in addition to evidence of the role that the nucleus accumbens plays in reward behaviors, it is clear that this region is also involved in pain processing [3]. This functional overlap may explain why people associate pain with these behaviors. Another line of evidence suggests that the genesis of fibromyalgia comes from unavoidable stress that decreases dopaminergic tone in the nucleus accumbens shell. This hypothesis cannot disregard the participation of other neurotransmitter systems (e.g., the serotonergic system) that stabilize the proalgesic and analgesic effects of stress [73].

The Ventral Tegmental Area and Dopaminergic Integration of Nociception

One supraspinal system that clearly plays a role in the modulation of nociceptive input is the dopaminergic system. The key dopaminergic nucleus that projects to the pain matrix is the VTA (A10) [3,59,73]. This nucleus projects monosynaptically to the anterior and medial thalamus, hippocampus, amygdala, nucleus accumbens, and the insular and anterior cingulate cortices [48]. Some of the first evidence to implicate the VTA in pain modulation was provided by Albe-Fessard and colleagues, who proved the analgesic effect of self-stimulation of the VTA in deafferented rats [55]. This structure participates in various neural circuits that are involved in analgesia induced by electrical stimulation [44,45,51], stress [65], morphine [46], and also electroacupuncture [40]. Moreover, it has been suggested that the VTA participates in what is sometimes called dissociative analgesia [25], in which the affective component of pain is lost.

Furthermore, the importance of the VTA as a nociceptive modulator has emerged in animal experimental models of neuropathic pain [54,55]. From another experimental point of view, the induction of long-lasting inflammatory nociception (induced by a carrageenan injection into the hindpaw) triggers a quantifiable self-injury behavior [39]. The suppression of VTA output by a radiofrequency lesion enhances the occurrence of self-injury behavior, while the electrical activation of the same area after the induction of the nociceptive stimulus, but not before, facilitates analgesic processes by diminishing this behavior. These results help to clarify the role of the VTA in the processing and modulation of persistent nociceptive information [62]. Also, there is evidence that the neurochemical lesion caused by administering 6-hydroxy-dopamine into the VTA can modulate nociceptive responses. Subacute and chronic models of nociception (the formalin test and neurectomy-induced nociception) can be modified with this approach, whereas there is no effect in an acute pain model (the tail-flick test) [46,54].

We have presented evidence regarding the dopaminergic pathways and nuclei that are involved in the pain matrix. The nucleus that seems to respond to noxious stimuli and subsequently activate the dopaminergic mesolimbic and mesocortical pathways is the ventral tegmental area. Recent evidence has shown that two different types of dopaminergic neurons emerge from the VTA, both with well-defined targets. One family is the mesocorticolimbic dopaminergic system, with unconventional fast-firing properties (20–60 Hz), which selectively projects to the prefrontal cortex and nucleus accumbens core and shell as well as to the basolateral amygdala. In contrast, slow-firing (<10 Hz) dopaminergic midbrain neurons only project to the lateral shell of the nucleus accumbens and the dorsolateral striatum. These new findings underline the high complexity and specificity of affective and cognitive information [36]. From our point of view, we can assume that there are two separate systems with the same origin that drive different types of information. One of them is closely related to cognition (the mesocortical system) and the other one to affect (the mesolimbic system).

In addition, electrophysiological and morphological evidence from Ungless and colleagues [69] has shown that dopaminergic neurons within the VTA are inhibited by acute noxious stimuli, whereas nondopaminergic ones are activated. While this result may appear to be the opposite of what we have described in this chapter, their findings are described in acute stimulation. This evidence may be explained by a normal acute inhibition of dopaminergic neurons in the VTA, with a gradually increasing firing rate under long-lasting nociceptive conditions. We hypothesize that the increase in dopamine is a response to a chronic nociceptive state; when this dopaminergic action is insufficient, then chronic pain is perceived, such as in patients with Parkinson's disease [61].

The activation of the VTA by peripheral nociceptive stimuli was first established in pioneer studies by Cuello and colleagues [14], who showed that an important percentage of the fibers that arrive to the VTA come from the habenula via the habenulo-interpeduncular-ventrotegmental tract (Fig. 1A). The medial neurons of the habenula contain substance P and project mainly to the VTA (habenulo-ventrotegmental). More recent evidence [3,4] has shown that the activation of the VTA by substance P agonism increases dopamine or its metabolites in mesolimbic structures such as the nucleus accumbens.

A relevant anatomical fact is that the VTA projects monosynaptically to three limbic structures that belong to the pain matrix—the nucleus accumbens and the insular and anterior cingulate cortices. There is plenty of evidence that dopamine in these three nuclei inhibits nociception [3,6,42,49,56,60,64]. More specifically, the activation of dopamine D2 receptors in both the ACC and insular cortex diminishes chronic nociception in animals [12,38].

Another important relationship is that of the VTA and insular cortex. Studies focusing on this relationship have provided insight into the etiology of neurological pathologies such as asymbolia for pain or pseudothalamic pain syndrome [5,17,23,58,67,68]. Nevertheless, these studies do not reveal the nature of the neurotransmission systems involved.

Recent evidence highlights the role of dopamine D2 receptors in this cortex in the modulation of neuropathic nociception [12].

Final Remarks

In this chapter, we have tried to assemble abundant lines of evidence related to dopamine, its pathways and receptors, and neuropathic pain that manifests as hyperalgesia, allodynia, and phantom limb pain.

Dopamine is not only highly relevant in cognitive and affective disorders, which are closely involved in mental health, but is also a key neurotransmitter in long-lasting pain or nociception. In fact, the administration of L-dopa can diminish behavioral nociceptive responses in animals [50] as well as in humans [22].

The data presented in this chapter indicate that a global increase in dopaminergic tone inhibits long-lasting pain. In support of this idea, there is clinical evidence that the disruption of supraspinal dopaminergic pathways, apart from those that emerge from the VTA, can also involve increased perception of pain. Examples of these pathways are the nigrostriatal pathway, which is implicated in Parkinson's disease [57,59,61,72], and the tuberoinfundibular pathway, implicated in prolactinemia [2]. This insight provides a new perspective for investigating the dopaminergic modulation of pain by other dopaminergic pathways that have specific defined roles but may also be involved in pain modulation.

Acknowledgments

Some data presented in this chapter are from work partially supported by CONACyT FP-62433 and by the Instituto Nacional de Psiquiatría Ramón de la Fuente grant 3230. We would like to thank Raúl Cardoso, José Luis Calderón, and Karina Bucio for image editing.

References

[1] Abbott FV, Melzack R. Analgesia produced by stimulation of limbic structures and its relation to epileptiform after-discharges. Exp Neurol 1978;62:720–34.

[2] Afzal KI, Briones DF, DeVargas C. Risperidone-induced polydipsia and polyphagia associated with galactorrhea, abdominal pain, and rapid weight gain in an adolescent Hispanic female. CNS Spectr 2007;12:818–20.

[3] Altier N, Stewart J. The role of dopamine in the nucleus accumbens in analgesia. Life Sci 1999;65:2269–87.

[4] Bannon MJ, Elliott PJ, Alpert JE, Goedert M, Iversen SD, Iversen LL. Role of endogenous substance P in stress-induced activation of mesocortical dopamine neurones. Nature 1983;306:791–2.

[5] Berthier M, Starkstein S, Leiguarda R. Asymbolia for pain: a sensory-limbic disconnection syndrome. Ann Neurol 1988;24:41–9.

[6] Burkey AR, Carstens E, Jasmin L. Dopamine reuptake inhibition in the rostral agranular insular cortex produces antinociception. J Neurosci 1999;19:4169–79.

[7] Burkey AR, Carstens E, Wenniger JJ, Tang J, Jasmin L. An opioidergic cortical antinociception triggering site in the agranular insular cortex of the rat that contributes to morphine antinociception. J Neurosci 1996;16:6612–23.

[8] Carlsson A, Lindqvist M, Magnusson T. 3,4-Dihydroxyphenylalanine and 5-hydroxytryptophan as reserpine antagonists. Nature 1957;180:1200.

[9] Caron MG, Beaulieu M, Raymond V, Gagne B, Drouin J, Lefkowitz RJ, Labrie F. Dopaminergic receptors in the anterior pituitary gland. Correlation of [^{3}H]dihydroergocryptine binding with the dopaminergic control of prolactin release. J Biol Chem 1978;253:2244–53.

[10] Casey KL. Forebrain mechanisms of nociception and pain: analysis through imaging. Proc Natl Acad Sci USA 1999;96:7668–74.

[11] Coderre TJ, Melzack R. Procedures which increase acute pain sensitivity also increase autotomy. Exp Neurol 1986;92:713–22.
[12] Coffeen U, Lopez-Avila A, Ortega-Legaspi JM, del Angel R, Lopez-Munoz FJ, Pellicer F. Dopamine receptors in the anterior insular cortex modulate long-term nociception in the rat. Eur J Pain 2008;12:535–43.
[13] Cote TE, Eskay RL, Frey EA, Grewe CW, Munemura M, Stoof JC, Tsuruta K, Kebabian JW. Biochemical and physiological studies of the beta-adrenoceptor and the D-2 dopamine receptor in the intermediate lobe of the rat pituitary gland: a review. Neuroendocrinology 1982;35:217–24.
[14] Cuello AC, Emson PC, Paxinos G, Jessell T. Substance P containing and cholinergic projections from the habenula. Brain Res 1978;149:413–29.
[15] Charcot JM. Lectures on the diseases of the nervous system, Vol. 1. New Syndenham Society; 1877.
[16] Chase TN, Oh JD, Blanchet PJ. Neostriatal mechanisms in Parkinson's disease. Neurology 1998;51:S30–5.
[17] Derbyshire SW, Jones AK, Gyulai F, Clark S, Townsend D, Firestone LL. Pain processing during three levels of noxious stimulation produces differential patterns of central activity. Pain 1997;73:431–45.
[18] Devinsky O, Morrell MJ, Vogt BA. Contributions of anterior cingulate cortex to behaviour. Brain 1995;118:279–306.
[19] Dziedzicka-Wasylewska M. Brain dopamine receptors: research perspectives and potential sites of regulation. Pol J Pharmacol 2004;56:659–71.
[20] Ehringer H, Hornykiewicz O. Distribution of noradrenaline and dopamine (3-hydroxytyramine) in the human brain and their behavior in diseases of the extrapyramidal system. Klin Wochenschr 1960;38:1236–9.
[21] Eisenberg E, Pud D. Can patients with chronic neuropathic pain be cured by acute administration of the NMDA receptor antagonist amantadine? Pain 1998;74:337–9.
[22] Ertas M, Sagduyu A, Arac N, Uludag B, Ertekin C. Use of levodopa to relieve pain from painful symmetrical diabetic polyneuropathy. Pain 1998;75:257–9.
[23] Fairhurst M, Wiech K, Dunckley P, Tracey I. Anticipatory brainstem activity predicts neural processing of pain in humans. Pain 2007;128:101–10.
[24] Forss N, Raij TT, Seppa M, Hari R. Common cortical network for first and second pain. Neuroimage 2005;24:132–42.
[25] Franklin KB. Analgesia and the neural substrate of reward. Neurosci Biobehav Rev 1989;13:149–54.
[26] Frot M, Magnin M, Mauguiere F, Garcia-Larrea L. Human SII and posterior insula differently encode thermal laser stimuli. Cereb Cortex 2007;17:610–20.
[27] Gaspar P, Bloch B, Le Moine C. D1 and D2 receptor gene expression in the rat frontal cortex: cellular localization in different classes of efferent neurons. Eur J Neurosci 1995;7:1050–63.
[28] Gordon I, Weizman R, Rehavi M. Modulatory effect of agents active in the presynaptic dopaminergic system on the striatal dopamine transporter. Eur J Pharmacol 1996;298:27–30.
[29] Hornykiewicz O. L-DOPA: from a biologically inactive amino acid to a successful therapeutic agent. Amino Acids 2002;23:65–70.
[30] Jasmin L, Burkey AR, Granato A, Ohara PT. Rostral agranular insular cortex and pain areas of the central nervous system: a tract-tracing study in the rat. J Comp Neurol 2004;468:425–40.
[31] Jasmin L, Rabkin SD, Granato A, Boudah A, Ohara PT. Analgesia and hyperalgesia from GABA-mediated modulation of the cerebral cortex. Nature 2003;424:316–20.
[32] Kavaliers M. Evolutionary and comparative aspects of nociception. Brain Res Bull 1988;21:923–31.
[33] Kebabian JW, Calne DB. Multiple receptors for dopamine. Nature 1979;277:93–6.
[34] Kornhuber J, Quack G, Danysz W, Jellinger K, Danielczyk W, Gsell W, Riederer P. Therapeutic brain concentration of the NMDA receptor antagonist amantadine. Neuropharmacology 1995;34:713–21.
[35] Koyanagi S, Himukashi S, Mukaida K, Shichino T, Fukuda K. Dopamine D2-like receptor in the nucleus accumbens is involved in the antinociceptive effect of nitrous oxide. Anesth Analg 2008;106:1904–9.
[36] Lammel S, Hetzel A, Hackel O, Jones I, Liss B, Roeper J. Unique properties of mesoprefrontal neurons within a dual mesocorticolimbic dopamine system. Neuron 2008;57:760–73.
[37] Lopez-Avila A, Coffeen U, Ortega-Legaspi JM, del Angel R, Jaimes O, Pellicer F. Amantadine modulates nociception by dopamine increase in the anterior cingulate cortex in the rat. Work presented at: Dopamine 50 years. Göteborg; 2007.
[38] Lopez-Avila A, Coffeen U, Ortega-Legaspi JM, del Angel R, Pellicer F. Dopamine and NMDA systems modulate long-term nociception in the rat anterior cingulate cortex. Pain 2004;111:136–43.
[39] Lopez-Avila A, Rodriguez-Manzo G, Coffeen U, del Angel R, Pellicer F. Self-injury behaviour induced by intraplantar carrageenan infiltration: a model of tonic nociception. Brain Res Brain Res Protoc 2004;13:37–44.
[40] Ma QP, Zhou Y, Han JS. Electroacupuncture accelerated the expression of c-Fos protooncogene in dopaminergic neurons in the ventral tegmental area of the rat. Int J Neurosci 1993;70:217–22.
[41] Manning BH, Morgan MJ, Franklin KB. Morphine analgesia in the formalin test: evidence for forebrain and midbrain sites of action. Neuroscience 1994 ;63:289–94.
[42] Marinelli S, Pascucci T, Bernardi G, Puglisi-Allegra S, Mercuri NB. Activation of TRPV1 in the VTA excites dopaminergic neurons and increases chemical- and noxious-induced dopamine release in the nucleus accumbens. Neuropsychopharmacology 2005;30:864–70.
[43] May A. Neuroimaging: visualising the brain in pain. Neurol Sci 2007;28:S101–7.
[44] Mayer DJ, Liebeskind JC. Pain reduction by focal electrical stimulation of the brain: an anatomical and behavioral analysis. Brain Res 1974;68:73–93.
[45] Mayer DJ, Price DD. Central nervous system mechanisms of analgesia. Pain 1976;2:379–404.
[46] Morgan MJ, Franklin KB. 6-Hydroxydopamine lesions of the ventral tegmentum abolish D-amphetamine and morphine analgesia in the formalin test but not in the tail flick test. Brain Res 1990;519:144–9.

[47] Naitoh Y. Protozoa. In: Shelton GAB, editor. Electrical conduction and behaviour in "simple" invertebrates. Oxford: Clarendon Press; 1982. p. 1–48.
[48] Oades RD, Halliday GM. Ventral tegmental (A10) system: neurobiology. 1. Anatomy and connectivity. Brain Res 1987;434:117–65.
[49] Ohara PT, Granato A, Moallem TM, Wang BR, Tillet Y, Jasmin L. Dopaminergic input to GABAergic neurons in the rostral agranular insular cortex of the rat. J Neurocytol 2003;32:131–41.
[50] Paalzow GH. L-dopa induces opposing effects on pain in intact rats: (-)-sulpiride, SCH 23390 or alpha-methyl-DL-p-tyrosine methylester hydrochloride reveals profound hyperalgesia in large antinociceptive doses. J Pharmacol Exp Ther 1992;263:470–9.
[51] Pellicer F, Torres-López E, Sotres-Bayón F, Lopez-Avila A, Coffeen U, Ortega-Legaspi JM. The affective and cognitive dimension of nociception in an animal model: the role of the anterior cingulate cortex. In: Lucas A, editor. Frontiers in pain research. Nova Science; 2006.
[52] Peyron R, Garcia-Larrea L, Gregoire MC, Convers P, Richard A, Lavenne F, Barral FG, Mauguiere F, Michel D, Laurent B. Parietal and cingulate processes in central pain. A combined positron emission tomography (PET) and functional magnetic resonance imaging (fMRI) study of an unusual case. Pain 2000;84:77–87.
[53] Richfield EK, Young AB, Penney JB. Comparative distributions of dopamine D-1 and D-2 receptors in the cerebral cortex of rats, cats, and monkeys. J Comp Neurol 1989;286:409–26.
[54] Saade NE, Atweh SF, Bahuth NB, Jabbur SJ. Augmentation of nociceptive reflexes and chronic deafferentation pain by chemical lesions of either dopaminergic terminals or midbrain dopaminergic neurons. Brain Res 1997;751:1–12.
[55] Sarkis D, Souteyrand JP, Albe-Fessard D. Self-stimulation in the ventral tegmental area suppresses self-mutilation in rats with forelimb deafferentation. Neurosci Lett 1984;44:199–204.
[56] Scott DJ, Heitzeg MM, Koeppe RA, Stohler CS, Zubieta JK. Variations in the human pain stress experience mediated by ventral and dorsal basal ganglia dopamine activity. J Neurosci 2006;26:10789–95.
[57] Schestatsky P, Kumru H, Valls-Sole J, Valldeoriola F, Marti MJ, Tolosa E, Chaves ML. Neurophysiologic study of central pain in patients with Parkinson disease. Neurology 2007;69:2162–9.
[58] Schmahmann JD, Leifer D. Parietal pseudothalamic pain syndrome. Clinical features and anatomic correlates. Arch Neurol 1992;49:1032–7.
[59] Schott GD. Pain in Parkinson's disease. Pain 1985;22:407–11.
[60] Shih YY, Chang C, Chen JC, Jaw FS. BOLD fMRI mapping of brain responses to nociceptive stimuli in rats under ketamine anesthesia. Med Eng Phys 2008;30:953–8.
[61] Silva EG, Viana MA, Quagliato EM. Pain in Parkinson's disease: analysis of 50 cases in a clinic of movement disorders. Arq Neuropsiquiatr 2008;66:26–9.
[62] Sotres-Bayon F, Torres-Lopez E, Lopez-Avila A, del Angel R, Pellicer F. Lesion and electrical stimulation of the ventral tegmental area modify persistent nociceptive behavior in the rat. Brain Res 2001;898:342–9.
[63] Symonds LL, Gordon NS, Bixby JC, Mande MM. Right-lateralized pain processing in the human cortex: an FMRI study. J Neurophysiol 2006;95:3823–30.
[64] Taylor BK, Joshi C, Uppal H. Stimulation of dopamine D2 receptors in the nucleus accumbens inhibits inflammatory pain. Brain Res 2003;987:135–43.
[65] Thierry AM, Tassin JP, Blanc G, Glowinski J. Selective activation of mesocortical DA system by stress. Nature 1976;263:242–4.
[66] Tobin DM, Bargmann CI. Invertebrate nociception: behaviors, neurons and molecules. J Neurobiol 2004;61:161–74.
[67] Treede RD, Kenshalo DR, Gracely RH, Jones AK. The cortical representation of pain. Pain 1999;79:105–11.
[68] Treede RD, Vogel H, Rios M, Krauss G, Lesser RP, Lenz FA. Pain-related evoked potentials from parasylvian cortex in humans. Electroencephalogr Clin Neurophysiol Suppl 1999;49:250–4.
[69] Ungless MA, Magill PJ, Bolam JP. Uniform inhibition of dopamine neurons in the ventral tegmental area by aversive stimuli. Science 2004;303:2040–2.
[70] Vogt BA, Finch DM, Olson CR. Functional heterogeneity in cingulate cortex: the anterior executive and posterior evaluative regions. Cereb Cortex 1992;2:435–43.
[71] Wood PB. Mesolimbic dopaminergic mechanisms and pain control. Pain 2006;120:230–4.
[72] Wood PB. Role of central dopamine in pain and analgesia. Expert Rev Neurother 2008;8:781–97.
[73] Wood PB. Stress and dopamine: implications for the pathophysiology of chronic widespread pain. Med Hypotheses 2004;62:420–4.

Correspondence to: Francisco Pellicer, MD, PhD, Instituto Nacional de Psiquiatría Ramón de la Fuente, Calzada Mexico-Xochimilco 101, Colonia San Lorenzo Huipulco, Mexico City 14370, México. Email: pellicer@imp.edu.mx.

12

Neurotrophic Factors, Neuropeptides, and Nitric Oxide: Therapeutic Targets in Chronic Pain Mechanisms

Amelia A. Staniland,[a] Jean-Sébastien Walczak,[b] and Stephen B. McMahon[a]

[a]Wolfson Centre for Age-Related Diseases, King's College London, London, United Kingdom; [b]Anesthesia Research Unit, Faculty of Medicine, Faculty of Dentistry, and Alan-Edwards Centre for Research on Pain, McGill University, Montreal, Quebec, Canada

Neurotrophic factors and neuropeptides comprise structurally unrelated families of endogenous peptides that exert profound and varied effects on many aspects of neuronal activity, including pain signaling. Both groups can be further divided into subfamilies containing several related members whose effects are exerted through interaction with a range of receptor targets. While there is a degree of specificity in these peptide-receptor interactions, there is also a level of promiscuity associated with their binding. This promiscuity, coupled with the variety of intracellular signaling pathways that can be initiated following receptor activation, results in the diverse effects these neuroactive compounds have on pain signaling. This chapter describes several of the key members of both the neurotrophic factor and neuropeptide families, with particular focus on their roles in nociception and pain signaling and their potential as therapeutic targets. Evidence for the involvement of the small signaling molecule nitric oxide in pain signaling and its potential role as an analgesic in combination therapies will also be reviewed.

Neurotrophic Factors

Neurotrophic factors determine the long-term survival and differentiated function of neurons expressing appropriate neurotrophic receptors. There are a number of neurotrophic factor families, but here we will consider the neurotrophins, which bind tropomyosin-receptor kinase (trk) receptors, and the glial cell line-derived neurotrophic factor (GDNF)

Pharmacology of Pain
edited by Pierre Beaulieu, David Lussier, Frank Porreca, and Anthony H. Dickenson
IASP Press, Seattle, © 2010

family of ligands. Receptors for neurotrophic factors are expressed throughout the central and peripheral nervous systems; during development, the production of specific neurotrophic factors by target tissues selectively promotes the survival of the subpopulation of neurons innervating that tissue that express the complementary receptor profiles [118]. However, neurotrophic factors are not exclusively involved in developmental cell survival, and the neurotrophins in particular have prominent roles in the adult organism. One such role is regulation of the sensitivity of nociceptive nerve fibers to noxious stimuli. This process can occur through both rapid phosphorylation of ion channels and receptors on the cell membrane and also via long-term alterations in gene expression that occur as a result of retrograde transport of internalized neurotrophin-receptor complexes to the cell nucleus [134].

Neurotrophins

The mammalian neurotrophin family contains four members: nerve growth factor (NGF), brain-derived neurotrophic factor (BDNF), neurotrophin 3 (NT-3) and neurotrophin 4/5 (NT-4/5). All four neurotrophins are synthesized as precursors that are cleaved intra- or extracellularly by proteases, such as the matrix metalloproteases, to produce mature neurotrophins [3]. The actions of the neurotrophins are mediated through two different receptor types. The pan-neurotrophin receptor $p75^{NTR}$ is a low-affinity receptor that binds all four members of the neurotrophin family with approximately equal strength [125]. The other neurotrophin receptor class, as mentioned above, is the trk receptor family. Three different subtypes of this tyrosine kinase receptor family exist, each with different affinities for the different neurotrophins: trkA primarily associates with NGF, trkB with BDNF and NT-4/5, and trkC with NT-3 [125] (Fig. 1). Mature neurotrophins exist as homodimers and are able to bind to two trk receptors, enabling transphosphorylation of residues in their intracellular domains. This property leads to the activation of several different signaling pathways, including mitogen-activated protein kinase (MAPK), phosphatidyl inositide-3 kinase (PI3K), and phospholipase C (PLC), thereby promoting cell survival, differentiation, and synaptic plasticity [3,118]. Activation of the $p75^{NTR}$ leads to the activation of nuclear factor-κB (NF-κB) and Jun N-terminal kinase (JNK), which can promote apoptosis [118], particularly in the absence of trk. Of the four identified mammalian neurotrophins, NGF and BDNF appear to have the strongest pronociceptive function, as described below.

Nerve Growth Factor

NGF was the first neurotrophin to be identified, following research in 1948 that demonstrated penetration of sensory nerve fibers from chick embryo dorsal root ganglia (DRG) into implanted mouse sarcoma cells [25]. Evidence from human conditions involving dysfunction of NGF signaling demonstrates the importance of this neurotrophic factor in nociceptive processing. Firstly, mutations of the trkA receptor gene have been identified in patients diagnosed with congenital insensitivity to pain with anhidrosis (CIPA), and the pain insensitivity observed in these patients is thought to result from a loss of NGF-sensitive neurons during embryogenesis [59]. Additionally, increased NGF levels have been observed in affected tissues from patients with painful inflammatory disorders such as interstitial cystitis and osteoarthritis [83,57].

Peripheral inflammation in the rat causes upregulation of NGF in the skin, and administration of NGF leads to rapid-onset thermal hyperalgesia and a slower-onset mechanical hyperalgesia [78]. Cytokines and growth factors released following injury are thought to evoke NGF secretion from keratinocytes and fibroblasts [171]. In addition, mast cells express trkA receptors and also contain NGF, so NGF release can be amplified by NGF-mediated activation of mast cells [76]. Activated mast cells also release a range of other proinflammatory mediators and therefore provide an indirect mechanism by which NGF can evoke nociceptor sensitization [150]. More directly, NGF causes phosphorylation of a thermosensitive ion channel that is expressed in nociceptors, the transient receptor potential vanilloid 1 (TRPV1) receptor, thereby reducing the thermal threshold for channel activation [180]. This molecular mechanism is thought to manifest as the rapid-onset thermal hyperalgesia described above. Slower-onset, long-term changes in nociceptor function arise through alterations in gene expression. NGF is known to increase production of a number of neuropeptides involved in nociceptive signaling, such as substance P and calcitonin gene-related peptide (CGRP), and it can also increase expression and trafficking of nociceptive ion channels and receptors, such as the chemoreceptors TRPV1 and TRPA1, the acid-sensing ion channel ASIC3, the voltage-gated sodium channel $Na_V1.8$, bradykinin, and the purinergic receptor $P2X_3$ [180,90,29,108,123,117].

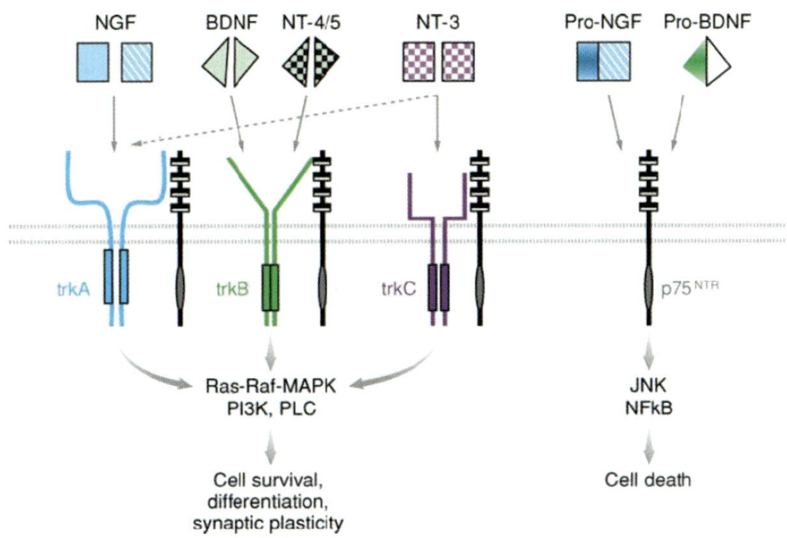

Fig. 1. Neurotrophin receptors and the intracellular pathways activated downstream of their activation. BDNF, brain-derived neurotrophic factor; JNK, Jun N-terminal kinase; NGF, nerve growth factor; NT, neurotrophin; MAPK, mitogen-activated protein kinase; NFκB, nuclear factor kappa-light-chain-enhancer of activated B cells; PI3K, phosphoinositide 3-kinase. Reproduced with permission from [118].

Evidence for the involvement of endogenous NGF in inflammatory pain hypersensitivity includes the ability of NGF-sequestering molecules to prevent the hyperalgesia that accompanies carrageenan-induced inflammation [94]. There is strong evidence for a proalgesic role of NGF in inflammatory pain [118], and NGF has been shown to be both proalgesic and neuroprotective in models of neuropathic pain. Indeed, the clinical use of NGF for the treatment of diabetic neuropathy has had limited success due to the low doses required to avoid induction of hyperalgesia [118]. These observations in patients mirror findings using a transgenic mouse strain overexpressing NGF, which was shown to have enhanced hyperalgesia and sympathetic nerve sprouting after peripheral nerve injury [124]. The idea that anti-NGF treatment could alleviate neuropathic pain has been validated in rodent models of peripheral neuropathy and bone cancer pain using anti-NGF antibodies and NGF-receptor antagonists [43,132,111]. Interestingly, recently presented clinical data show considerable promise for anti-NGF therapies in the treatment of pain associated with osteoarthritis [130]. Tanezumab, a humanized monoclonal antibody directed against NGF, significantly reduced walking knee pain over 16 weeks versus placebo control and is now entering phase III trials [130].

Brain-Derived Neurotrophic Factor

BDNF was originally isolated from porcine brain following a search for neurotrophic factors that could promote the survival of NGF-insensitive neurons. It is produced by the cell bodies of small- and medium-diameter (nociceptive) peptidergic neurons, which also express the trkA receptor [98], and is then transported to the central terminals of these primary afferents, from where it is released in response to depolarization [106]. Binding of BDNF to trkB receptors expressed by spinal cord neurons leads to extracellular receptor kinase (ERK) activation and *N*-methyl-D-aspartate (NMDA) receptor phosphorylation, thus enhancing the excitability of the postsynaptic membrane [140]. BDNF and trkB receptors are also expressed in ascending and descending fibers and in supraspinal centers [97].

Whilst sequestration of BDNF does not alter normal nociceptive processing, intrathecal administration of exogenous BDNF can lead to thermal and mechanical hypersensitivity [106]. However, BDNF is thought to be most important in the context of inflammatory pain signaling. Following inflammation, BDNF synthesis is markedly upregulated, and a major factor driving this increase is NGF, which is itself rapidly produced following tissue damage, as described above [106]. In support of this theory, intraplantar administration of NGF antibody prevented the inflammation-induced upregulation of BDNF mRNA in the DRG and also relieved the behavioral nociceptive responses observed in models of inflammatory pain [20,66]. Direct evidence for the pronociceptive role of endogenous BDNF comes from the use of the BDNF-scavenging protein trkB-immunoglobulin G and the use of BDNF antisense. Intrathecal delivery of either of these tools attenuates inflammatory hyperalgesia in mice [36,79]. In addition to BDNF upregulation, expression of the trkB receptor by second-order neurons in the dorsal horn is also increased following inflammation, providing an additional mechanism by which the BDNF signaling pathway can amplify nociceptive transmission in the presence of tissue damage [91].

BDNF expression undergoes complex regulation following nerve injury, with strong temporal variations that are dependent on the exact nature of the experimental injury performed [21]. BDNF levels can be up- or downregulated depending on the size and injury status of the neuronal population examined. For example, de novo expression of BDNF occurs in medium- to large-diameter uninjured neurons, while small-diameter injured neurons have reduced levels of BDNF [184]. Application of anti-BDNF antibody intrathecally or directly to the DRG of injured sensory nerve fibers reduces injury-evoked thermal hyperalgesia and mechanical allodynia [178,121]. Moreover, these behavioral pain correlates were also reduced in heterozygote BDNF knockout mice [178], suggesting that at the level of the primary afferent and spinal cord, BDNF is pronociceptive in the presence of nerve injury.

A further interesting dimension in the role of BDNF in pain signaling is its role as a mediator of neuroimmune communication. Spinal cord glial cells are activated following nerve injury and contribute to the development and maintenance of neuropathic pain through release of various neuroactive compounds, such as BDNF. In vitro activation of microglia with adenosine triphosphate (ATP) evokes release of BDNF and thus alters the electrophysiological characteristics of lamina I neuronal membranes in such a way that the anion reversal potential is depolarized and γ-aminobutyric acid (GABA) can become excitatory [23]. The mechanism underlying this alteration in the electrical properties of the projection neurons is proposed to involve downregulation of the potassium-chloride cotransporter KCC2, a change that may be mediated by BDNF.

Neurotrophin-3

Injection of NT-3 into the rat hindpaw does not evoke the thermal hyperalgesia or C-fiber sensitization that is observed following administration of either of the trkB-receptor agonists BDNF or NT-4/5 [135]. Moreover, in the context of neuropathic pain, NT-3 apparently plays an analgesic role, opposing the function of NGF. This analgesia is mediated through attenuation of neuropathy-induced upregulation of expression of nociceptive sodium channels, TRPV1 channels, and the neuropeptide galanin [168,170,169]. In the brachial plexus avulsion model of neuropathic pain, pretreatment with NT-3 antibody was able to reduce mechanical hypernociception [121], and in a model of inflammatory pain, local administration of NT-3 after inflammation reduced hyperalgesia, supporting the idea that NT-3 opposes the proalgesic functions of NGF [160].

Neurotrophin-4/5

NT-4/5 also binds preferentially to the trkB receptor subtype and has been shown to evoke nociceptor sensitization when applied in a skin-nerve preparation [127]. Furthermore, injection of NT-4/5 into a rodent hindpaw causes thermal hyperalgesia, the behavioral correlate of this nociceptor sensitization [135].

GDNF Family of Ligands

The GDNF family of ligands includes GDNF, artemin, neurturin and persephin, and these neurotrophic factors activate a receptor complex containing RET (rearranged during transfection) receptor tyrosine kinase. Instead of directly associating with the RET receptor, these neurotrophic factors associate with a subtype-specific coreceptor, the GDNF family receptor (GFR) [9]. GDNF has the highest affinity for the GFRα_1 subtype, neurturin to GFRα_2, artemin to GFRα_3, and persephin to GFRα_4, although other signaling pathways have also been described [9].

While GDNF has shown some promise in clinical trials for the treatment of Parkinson's disease, both GDNF and artemin have also been implicated as therapeutic targets for chronic pain [9,89]. The artemin receptor subtype is predominantly expressed in nociceptive neurons, and artemin expression is upregulated in a rodent model of peripheral inflammation [89]. Artemin, GDNF and neurturin are all able to sensitize nociceptive primary afferents in vitro [89]. Moreover, intraplantar administration of any one of these three neurotrophic factors causes thermal hyperalgesia in vivo [89].

Neuropeptides

Neuropeptides are defined as short-chain (3–100-amino-acid) peptides found in neural tissue, and so far over 100 have been identified [49]. Their effects are normally mediated through binding to specific G-protein-coupled receptors (GPCRs), of which there are a multitude of subtypes that activate a wide range of intracellular signaling pathways (Table I). These receptors are not only important for interneuronal communication but may also act as autoreceptors. Furthermore, a significant proportion of neuropeptide activity results from the release of these molecules by the peripheral terminals of primary afferent fibers, where they can interact with neuropeptide receptors expressed on non-neuronal tissue.

Many neuronal subpopulations coexpress both classical neurotransmitters and neuropeptides [49] (Fig. 2). Compared to many "canonical" neurotransmitters, neuropeptides evoke prolonged excitatory postsynaptic potentials that are thought to modulate neuronal signaling. Neuropeptides are synthesized as precursors and are stored in large dense-core vesicles that require sustained neuronal activation for release [49], in contrast to classical neurotransmitters, which are stored in light vesicles and are released in response to less electrical activity. Furthermore, whereas classical neurotransmitters often alter membrane excitability through depolarization or hyperpolarization, neuropeptides have many diverse effects, including alterations in gene expression, glial cell morphology, blood flow, and synaptogenesis.

The broad range of neuropeptides, receptors, and intracellular signaling cascades provides a wide scope for modulation of this signaling system during inflammation or nerve damage, with the possibility of differential regulation of some or many of the key components of these pain-signaling pathways (Fig. 3). Importantly, this complex system also provides many potential therapeutic targets for the treatment of chronic pain.

Table I
Summary of neuropeptides involved in pain signaling

Neuropeptide	Size	Receptor	Intracellular Signaling	Function
SST	14/18 amino acids	SST_{1-5} (isoforms 2a, 2b)	$G_{i/o}$: inhibition of AC/cAMP/PKA	–
SP	11 amino acids	NK1	G_q: PLC/IP_3/PIP_2 and DAG	+
CGRPα, CGRPβ	37 amino acids	CLR and RAMP1	G_s: AC/cAMP/PKA	+
VIP	28 amino acids	$VPAC_1$, $VPAC_2$, PAC_1	G_s: AC/cAMP/PKA	+
PACAP	27/38 amino acids	PAC_1, $VPAC_1$, $VPAC_2$	G_s: AC/cAMP/PKA	+/–
NPY	36 amino acids	Y_{1-5}	$G_{i/o}$: inhibition of AC/cAMP/PKA	–
GAL	29 amino acids	$GalR_{1-3}$	$G_{i/o}$: inhibition of AC ($GalR_{1,3}$); G_q: PLC/IP_3/PIP_2 and DAG ($GalR_2$)	+/–

Abbreviations and symbols: +, enhancement of pain signaling; –, inhibition of pain signaling; AC, adenylate cyclase; cAMP, cyclic adenosine monophosphate; CGRP, calcitonin gene-related peptide; CLR, calcitonin receptor-like receptor; DAG, diacylglycerol; GAL, galanin; GalR, galanin receptor; IP_3, inositol triphosphate; NK1, neurokinin receptor 1; NPY, neuropeptide Y; PACAP, pituitary adenylate cyclase-activating peptide; PIP_2, phosphatidylinositol 4,5-bisphosphate; PKA, protein kinase A; PLC, phospholipase C; RAMP1, receptor activity-modifying protein 1; SP, substance P; SST, somatostatin; VIP, vasoactive intestinal polypeptide.

Substance P

Substance P is an 11-amino-acid peptide that was first identified due to its hypotensive properties, which result from its ability to cause peripheral vasodilation. Substance P belongs to the tachykinin family of neuropeptides, which also includes neurokinin A and neurokinin B [86]. Three tachykinin receptor subtypes are endogenously expressed, and substance P shows most affinity for the neurokinin 1 receptor (NK1R) subtype [86,40]. Substance P is expressed by small-diameter, unmyelinated, nociceptive primary afferents and is transported to both the peripheral and central terminals of these neurons [6]. Substance P immunoreactivity is often used as a marker for a subpopulation of nociceptive afferents known as "peptidergic" fibers, which also express the neuropeptide CGRP and the NGF receptor trkA, but do not bind the plant lectin IB4 or express purinergic P2X3 receptors [55]. A subset of these peptidergic afferents are also positive for the capsaicin-sensitive receptor TRPV1 [38]. Almost half of lamina I projection neurons express the NK1 receptor, and furthermore, NK1R immunoreactivity is observed in 80% of lamina I neurons receiving inputs from substance P-positive primary afferents [152]. Receptor signaling is mediated through activation of G_q, causing increased phospholipase C activity and mobilization of calcium from intracellular stores, enhancing neuronal excitability [68].

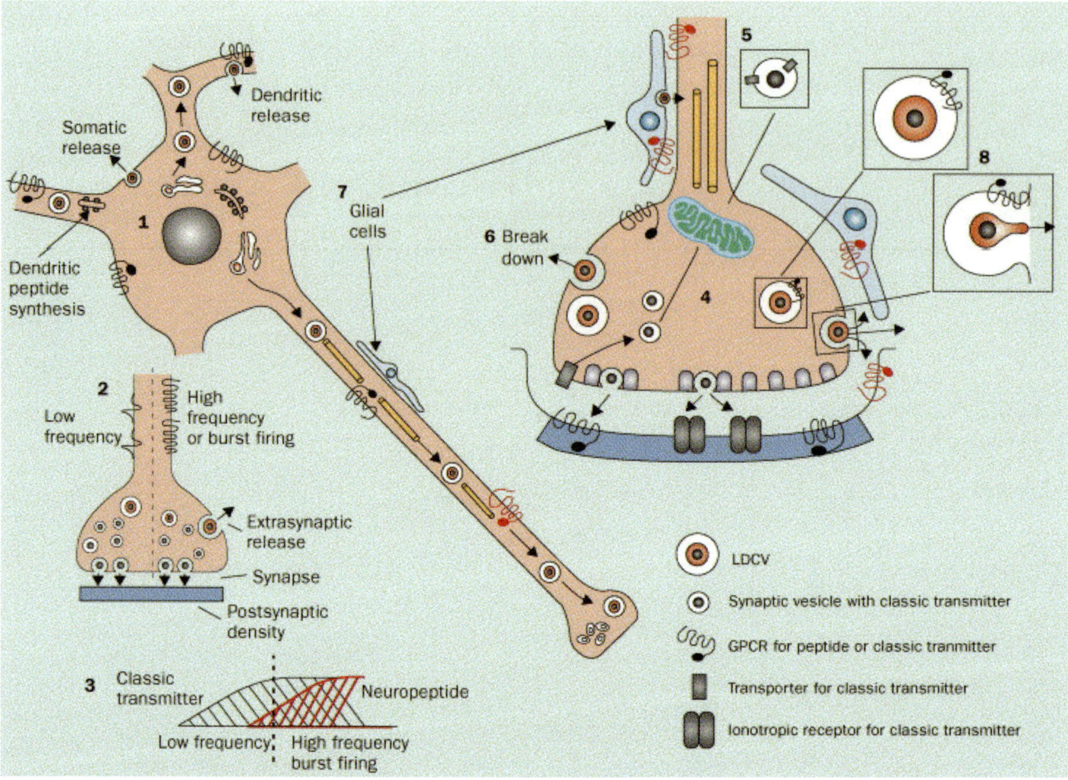

Fig. 2. Neuropeptides are produced ribosomally in the cell body and, to a lesser extent, in dendrites, and then they are packaged in large dense-core vesicles (LDCVs) that are transported into axons and dendrites (1). LDCVs can contain classic transmitters (1, 2, 4). LDCVs contain processing enzymes (convertases) that release the bioactive peptide from the precursor. The peptides can be released not only from nerve endings but also from dendrites and cell soma (1, 2, 4); in fact, dendritic release can be independent from axon terminal release. The peptide receptors are G-protein-coupled receptors (GPCRs) with seven transmembrane-spanning regions and are present on cell soma, dendrites, axons, and nerve endings (1, 4). Peptides are preferentially released (mainly outside the synapse) under burst or high-frequency firing, whereas the classic transmitters, stored in clear synaptic vesicles, are released into the synaptic cleft during low-frequency activity (2–4). Classic transmitters act on ionotropic receptors and GPCRs in the synaptic cleft, whereas peptide receptors are mostly found outside the synapse (4). Classic transmitters can be produced in all parts of the neurons, including the nerve endings, because the synthesizing enzymes are present throughout the neuron (4). Moreover, classic transmitters, in contrast with peptides, have reuptake mechanisms (transporter molecules) at both the cell and the vesicle membrane (5), leading to termination of the action as well as allowing recycling (4). In contrast, peptides are broken down by extracellular peptidases (6), and replacement must occur via axonal transport. There is evidence that one peptide can inhibit peptidase breakdown of another peptide (6). Also, glial cells can produce peptides and their receptors (7). Receptors are mostly processed via the constitutive pathway, are transported in small vesicles, and are inserted into the cell membrane, but there is evidence that δ-opioid receptors are localized in the membrane of LDCVs (8). Reproduced with permission from [49].

Following nerve injury, substance P expression is downregulated in nociceptive C fibers, and this alteration is claimed to contribute to the loss of C-fiber-associated pain in models of neuropathy [153]. However, in nerve-injured animals, Aβ-fiber stimulation causes release of substance P into the dorsal horn, suggesting de novo expression of substance P in these fibers as a result of peripheral neuropathy [88]. After inflammation, levels of substance P in afferent nerve fibers and the dorsal horn are increased [75,65]. Substance

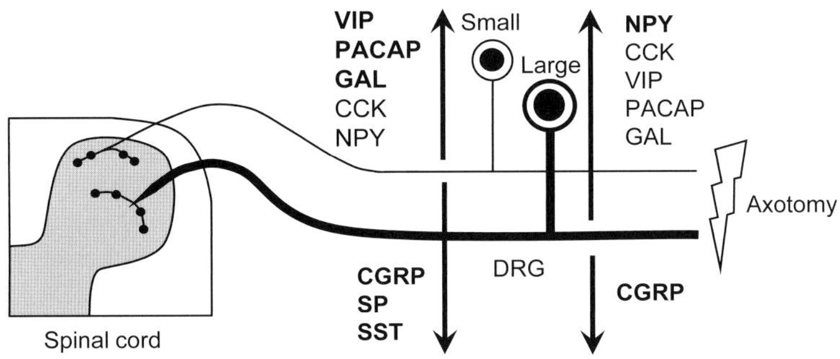

Fig. 3. Schematic drawing of a small and a large primary sensory neuron in a dorsal root ganglion (DRG) sending a central branch to the dorsal horn of the spinal cord and with a peripheral branch that has been sectioned (axotomy). The changes occurring in levels of peptides are indicated by arrows. Thus, in small, unmyelinated DRG neurons, calcitonin-gene-related peptide (CGRP), substance P (SP), and somatostatin (SST) are downregulated, whereas vasoactive intestinal peptide (VIP), pituitary adenylate cyclase-activating polypeptide (PACAP), galanin (GAL), cholecystokinin (CCK), and neuropeptide Y (NPY) are upregulated. In the large, myelinated neurons, CGRP is downregulated, whereas NPY, CCK, VIP, PACAP, and GAL are upregulated. Bold letters indicate pronounced changes; normal typeface denotes modest changes. Modified with permission from [48].

P signaling in chronic pain can also be modulated through alterations in NK1R expression after peripheral nerve damage or inflammation. In experimental models of both chronic inflammatory and neuropathic pain, immunoreactivity for the NK1R is significantly increased in superficial laminae of the dorsal horn [1]. These findings provide a basis for the involvement of substance P and the NK1R in chronic pain signaling. However, studies on mice with null mutations for substance P or NK1R do not reinforce this view, and clinical trials with NK1R antagonists have not supported a prominent role for substance P in a variety of clinical pain states.

A popular technique used to study the role of the substance P-NK1R signaling pathway in nociceptive processing involves selective ablation of NK1R-expressing projection neurons using a substance P-saporin conjugate [166]. Saporin is a cytotoxic ribosome-inactivating protein that is internalized into NK1R-expressing neurons as part of the substance P-NK1R complex, leading to cell death. While loss of this NK1R-positive neuronal population does not significantly alter acute pain processing, hypersensitivity evoked by inflammation or nerve injury is completely abolished in the absence of this receptor complex [93,167]. These data suggest that the substance P signaling pathway is integral to the development of sensory hyperalgesia. Transgenic mice lacking the NK1R also had normal responses to acute nociceptive stimuli combined with reduced nocifensive behavior following formalin injection and showed attenuated mechanical, but not thermal, hypersensitivity after nerve injury [69,92]. These findings were supported by electrophysiological analysis of deep dorsal horn neurons in these knockout mice, which showed reduced wind-up of these fibers in response to both mechanical and thermal stimuli [146]. However, NK1R antagonists disappointingly showed minimal analgesic efficacy when moved into human clinical trials, raising a question mark over the validity of preclinical studies in predicting analgesic efficacy, particularly in the field of neuropeptides [45]. Several theories have been proposed for this failure, including species differences in substance P physiology and also the potential confusion between pain- and stress-related behavior in animal models [45]. Interestingly, NK1R antagonists were successful as antiemetics, demonstrating that neuropeptides do represent feasible clinical targets [128].

Calcitonin Gene-Related Peptide

CGRP is a 37-amino-acid peptide produced by alternative processing of RNA transcripts from the calcitonin gene. This form of CGRP is more correctly termed CGRPα, as another form of CGRP exists: CGRPβ, which is highly homologous to CGRPα but is transcribed from a different gene [102]. CGRP is produced by neuronal tissue, and in the rat the CGRPα subtype is more highly expressed in sensory neurons than CGRPβ [102]. CGRPα and substance P are strongly coexpressed in the peptidergic population of primary afferent nociceptors, which account for approximately 40% of adult rat DRG neurons [8].

The CGRP receptor belongs to the GPCR subfamily B1, which also includes the receptors for vasoactive intestinal polypeptide (VIP) and pituitary adenylate cyclase-activating peptide (PACAP). However, the CGRP receptor is unusual as it is actually a heterodimer of a classical seven-transmembrane GPCR, the calcitonin receptor-like receptor, and the single transmembrane protein receptor activity-modifying protein 1 (RAMP1) [22]. CGRP-receptor signaling is further complicated by the potential existence of two CGRP-receptor subtypes ($CGRP_1$ and $CGRP_2$), although the molecular identity of the $CGRP_2$ receptor remains unclear [41,122].

Binding of CGRP to the CGRP receptor complex activates cyclic adenosine monophosphate (cAMP), increasing neuronal excitability [22]. However, in addition to directly enhancing neuronal excitability, CGRP can also modulate pain processing through alterations in ion channel expression (e.g., P2X3) in a mechanism involving protein kinase A (PKA), cAMP response element binding protein (CREB), mitogen activated protein kinase, and ERK [4,138]. In cultured trigeminal neurons, CGRP enhances trafficking of P2X3 receptors and increases P2X3-receptor gene transcription, potentiating the response of these neurons to extracellular ATP and possibly contributing to the pain associated with migraine [138]. Similar effects on gene transcription have also been observed in primary afferent fibers expressing CGRP receptors, which may act as autoreceptors for CGRP released from neurons in response to tissue injury, causing upregulation of proteins involved in nociceptive signaling [4]. In spinal dorsal horn neurons, NK1-receptor expression is increased by CGRP, demonstrating an important synergy between CGRP and substance P [133].

Peripheral noxious thermal, mechanical, or chemical stimulation causes release of CGRP from the central terminals of primary afferent fibers. Intrathecal injection of CGRP led to the development of mechanical hyperalgesia, whereas intrathecal administration of the CGRP antagonist CGRP8-37 (an inactive truncated form of the peptide) alleviated mechanical and thermal hyperalgesia in a rat model of chronic central neuropathic pain [145,7]. The induction of mechanical hyperalgesia following intrathecal CGRP is thought to be mediated by sensitization of wide-dynamic-range neurons in the deep lamina of the spinal cord dorsal horn in a PKA-and PKC-dependent mechanism [145]. CGRP levels are also increased in models of inflammatory pain, particularly arthritis, where dorsal horn neuron excitability is enhanced due to increased CGRP-evoked excitatory postsynaptic potentials [12].

As observed for substance P, CGRP is also a potent vasodilator. Antidromic stimulation of peptidergic nerve fibers causes the release of CGRP from their peripheral terminals, where it can act with substance P on blood vessels to cause vasodilation and protein extravasation, in a process known as neurogenic inflammation [50]. This effect of CGRP, in addition to its neuromodulatory actions, may underlie its involvement in two chronic pain conditions: complex regional pain syndrome and migraine [13,30]. The first oral nonpeptide CGRP antagonist, telcagepant, has entered into phase III clinical trials for the treatment of migraine, with promising results reported so far. Interestingly, there appears to be a substantial genetic component to the role of CGRP in nociceptive transmission, particularly with respect to thermal sensitivity [100].

Somatostatin

Somatostatin (SST) is an inhibitory neuropeptide secreted by the hypothalamus that prevents release of growth hormone from the pituitary gland. The precursor preprosomatostatin is cleaved to produce two bioactive forms, SST-14 and SST-28, and the actions of these peptides are mediated through binding with one of five SST receptors (sst_{1-5}), which are expressed in both the central and peripheral nervous systems [131]. All five SST GPCR subtypes couple to the G_i subunit, and therefore SST binding leads to inhibition of adenylate cyclase and a reduction in neuronal excitability [131]. This inhibitory function of SST is potentiated through inhibition of voltage-gated calcium channels and activation of G-protein-coupled inwardly rectifying potassium (GIRK) channels [112].

Release of SST into the dorsal horn of the spinal cord can occur from the central terminals of small diameter, unmyelinated afferent fibers, local spinal interneurons or the terminals of descending axons [87]. Activation of dorsal horn projection neurons by SST, particularly through binding to the sst_2 splice variant sst_{2a}, inhibits firing of these fibers and thereby impedes the transmission of nociceptive signals from the periphery [64]. Indeed, an analgesic role for SST and its synthetic analogue octreotide has been demonstrated in humans after central administration (i.e., intrathecal, epidural, or intracerebroventricular), which provides effective relief from pain in a wide range of clinical conditions (e.g., postoperative pain, intractable cancer pain, osteoarthritis, rheumatoid arthritis, migraine, and visceral pain) [87]. However, the benefits of the SST signaling pathway as a novel analgesic target have been limited by the necessity for central administration in addition to the short half-life and low selectivity of SST (both improved with octreotide) and neurotoxicity following bolus intrathecal dosing [87].

SST receptors have also been identified in primary afferent fibers [5]. Interestingly, up to a third of TRPV1-positive nociceptive primary afferent neurons are also immunoreactive for sst_{2a}, and approximately 60% of sst_{2a}-positive neurons colocalize with TRPV1 [19], suggesting a role for this receptor family in peripheral nociceptive signaling. Indeed, in a rat model of unilateral antigen-induced arthritis, sst_{2a} immunostaining (but not mRNA levels) was reduced in lumbar DRG neurons after injury, suggesting that attenuated sst_{2a}-mediated SST inhibition of neuronal function may be a contributing factor to the pain associated with arthritis in this model [5].

These immunological findings are supported by pharmacological evidence demonstrating that intra-articular injection of either SST or octreotide diminished noxious and non-noxious movement-evoked discharges from fine afferent fibers innervating the knee joint [116]. In addition, peripherally-administered SST analogues are also efficacious in several behavioral models of acute and chronic pain in rodents. For example, intraplantar injection of octreotide was effective in reducing formalin- and capsaicin-evoked nociceptive behavior and decreasing C-fiber responses to noxious activation in rats [19]. The sst_4-selective agonist TT-232 reduced mechanical hyperalgesia when administered 7 days after partial sciatic nerve injury and also ameliorated nocifensive behavior in both phases of the formalin test, reduced the thermal sensitization evoked by intraplantar injection of the capsaicin analogue resiniferatoxin, and inhibited mechanical allodynia in a rat model of diabetes [147,119]. Another analogue selective for the sst_4 receptor subtype, J-2156, also shows analgesic activity when administered intraperitoneally, as demonstrated by reduction of pain-like behavior in the second phase of the formalin test and by decreased mechanical allodynia and hyperalgesia in models of inflammatory and neuropathic pain, respectively [129]. The sst_2 agonist SCR007 also reduced formalin- and capsaicin-evoked nociceptive activity when given via either intraplantar or intraperitoneal injection, and although this nonpeptide analogue has the potential to cross the blood-brain barrier, the authors proposed a peripheral mechanism of action for its analgesic effects in these models [63].

Vasoactive Intestinal Polypeptide and Pituitary Adenylate Cyclase-Activating Peptide

VIP is a 28-amino-acid polypeptide with a broad range of biological functions that was originally isolated from porcine small intestine. PACAP occurs in two forms (PACAP-27 and PACAP-38), both of which have high homology with the N-terminal domain of VIP. PACAP was initially isolated from ovine hypothalamus, and its first known function was to increase adenylate cyclase activity in rat pituitary cells.

VIP/PACAP signaling is mediated through one of three receptors: $VPAC_1$, $VPAC_2$, or PAC_1, the latter having a higher affinity for PACAP than for VIP [27]. These receptors associate strongly with G_s, and so their activation leads to stimulation of the cAMP/PKA pathway and a general increase in neuronal excitability [84,143]. All three receptor subtypes are expressed in laminae II–IV of the dorsal horn, with $VPAC_1$ being the most widely expressed [28]. Interestingly, significant modulation of receptor expression profiles has been observed in rodent models of chronic pain. In a rat model of neuropathic pain,

$VPAC_1$ expression in laminae III–IV was decreased, whereas $VPAC_2$ levels were increased, and in a model of inflammatory pain in which complete Freund's adjuvant was applied unilaterally to the hindpaw, PACAP expression was upregulated in L5 DRG neurons [58,181].

Intrathecal administration of VIP has been shown to enhance flexor reflexes in rats [24]. However, intrathecal application of a VIP antagonist was unable to attenuate C-fiber-induced sensitization in normal animals, suggesting that endogenous VIP is not necessary for normal pain processing [175]. The effects of PACAP are slightly more complex, potentially due to its ability to interact with all three receptor subtypes. When applied to single dorsal horn neurons, PACAP is always excitatory, and intrathecal application can enhance formalin-evoked pain behavior and cause a dose-dependent decrease in tail-flick latency [174,103,28]. However, intrathecal application can also suppress C-fiber-evoked reflexes and formalin-induced nocifensive behavior, suggesting that in some circumstances PACAP may be antinociceptive [183,179,182]. In naive animals, $VPAC_1$ and PAC_1 antagonists reduced responses of dorsal horn neurons to innocuous and noxious stimuli, whereas a $VPAC_2$ antagonist was specifically antinociceptive [28]. In neuropathic animals, $VPAC_1$ and PAC_1 antagonists reduced cold allodynia, whereas all three receptors appear to mediate mustard oil hypersensitivity in these animals [28]. In a model of visceral inflammation (cystitis), expression of both PACAP and PAC_1 increased, and moreover, PACAP evoked release of the algogen ATP from bladder urothelial cells, further contributing to the inflammatory pain [35].

Together, these data suggest that this family of peptides may be involved in nociceptive processing, both in naive animals and in the presence of injury or inflammation. However, the complex alterations in receptor expression and the differing affinities of PACAP and VIP for different receptor subtypes suggest that elucidating specific functions of these peptides is likely to be challenging.

Neuropeptide Y

Neuropeptide Y (NPY) is a 36-amino-acid peptide that was first isolated from the porcine hypothalamus. The actions of NPY and the other members of its family (neuropeptide YY and pancreatic polypeptide) are mediated through binding to one of five GPCRs (Y_1–Y_5) [136]. NPY and its receptors are distributed throughout the peripheral and central nervous systems on both pre- and postsynaptic neuronal cell membranes [46]. In fibers associated with pain signaling, the Y_1 and Y_2 receptor subtypes are the most prominently expressed [15].

Peptide binding to NPY receptors leads to activation of $G_{i/o}$ subunits and inhibition of cAMP production from ATP [136]. Conversely, NPY can also enhance neuronal excitability through increased intracellular calcium via mobilization of calcium from intracellular stores and through activation or inhibition of voltage-gated calcium channel function [144,159]. The Y_1 receptor can also activate GIRK channels and thereby reduce membrane excitability [144]. This complex array of downstream signaling mechanisms is likely to underlie the range of behavioral and electrophysiological findings that demonstrate both inhibition and excitation of nociceptive signaling in response to NPY exposure.

Intrathecal application of Y_2-receptor agonists inhibits thermal nociception in naive animals, and this analgesic effect is thought to be mediated through reduced release of excitatory mediators from the presynaptic primary afferent membrane, in much the same way as opioid analgesia is achieved [52,101]. Expression of Y_2 receptors in the spinal cord is limited to the central terminals of primary afferent fibers, supporting this mechanism of action [16]. However, some studies have found no alteration in response to exogenous NPY or have even found a pronociceptive effect that may be dose dependent [15].

In models of peripheral inflammation, intrathecal NPY reduced thermal hyperalgesia, but, interestingly, this reduction was almost completely abolished by concomitant treatment with Y_1-receptor agonists, suggesting that this subtype may be more important than Y_2 in the context of inflammatory pain [148]. Nocifensive activity and increased c-fos expression evoked by formalin injection were also abolished following intrathecal NPY [60]. The proposed mechanism for this analgesia is thought to involve presynaptically mediated disinhibition of inhibitory (GABAergic) interneurons, or alternatively postsynaptic inhibition of excitatory interneurons (through GIRK activation), both of which would reduce the excitability of dorsal horn projection neurons [142,99].

After peripheral nerve injury, NPY expression is upregulated in DRG and spinal cord neurons [81]. Y_1-receptor knockout mice have enhanced allodynia after nerve injury, and intrathecal NPY reduced neuropathic pain behavior and upregulation of c-fos [104,60]. The latter findings were inhibited by both Y_1- and Y_2-receptor antagonists, suggesting that both receptor subtypes may be important targets in the treatment of neuropathic pain [60].

Interestingly, activation of peripheral Y_1 receptors can attenuate mechanical allodynia evoked by peripheral capsaicin injection, potentially due to direct inhibition of TRPV1-positive fibers [34]. Another possible mechanism for NPY signaling in pain is "cross-excitation" between DRG cell bodies, which have been shown to express both Y_1 and Y_2 receptors [15].

Galanin

Galanin is a 29-amino-acid (30 in humans) polypeptide that was originally isolated from the porcine intestine. Galanin is proteolytically released from a propeptide along with a 59- or 60-amino-acid fragment known as galanin message-associated peptide (GMAP) [73]. While both galanin and GMAP are involved in nociceptive processing, another member of the galanin peptide family, galanin-like peptide (GALP), has not been shown to play any such role [107]. Galanin and its related peptides interact with one of three GPCRs: GalR1–3 [73]. Binding to GalR1 or GalR3 inhibits adenylate cyclase through $G_{i/o}$ stimulation and also activates GIRK, whereas GalR2 binding promotes phospholipase C activity [70,141]. These diverse intracellular signaling pathways provide a mechanism by which galanin can both enhance and inhibit nociceptive processing.

Expression of galanin in adult DRG neurons is low, with only 2–3% of naive rat DRG cells showing galanin-like immunoreactivity [47]. However, galanin synthesis is rapidly upregulated after peripheral nerve damage in both small and large DRG neurons

[47,72]. In the spinal cord, galanin is found in lamina II inhibitory GABAergic interneurons and in the peripheral terminals of primary afferent fibers [139,137]. Galanin receptors are expressed in both the peripheral and central nervous systems, with the GalR2 subtype being most highly expressed in small-diameter, nociceptive, peptidergic primary sensory afferents [105,18]. The GalR1 subtype is exclusively expressed in nervous tissue, and GalR3 mRNA is broadly distributed throughout many neuronal and non-neuronal tissues, but at a lower level than the other two subunits [161].

Behavioral studies using intrathecal administration of exogenous galanin showed both facilitation and inhibition of pain signaling in an apparently dose- and modality-dependent fashion [24,120,71]. These biphasic effects were reproduced in electrophysiological paradigms, where low doses caused facilitation while high doses caused depression of nociceptive activity, supporting the behavioral findings [163,164]. Only moderate alterations in nociceptive thresholds were observed in naive animals, suggesting that galanin does not represent a pharmacological target for the development of drugs to treat acute pain [173].

Interestingly, in the context of spinal cord hyperexcitability, intrathecal galanin was antinociceptive and prevented the activity-dependent increase in nocifensive reflex activity [176,164,177]. The mechanism underlying this function is likely to involve reduced release of pronociceptive neuropeptides, such as substance P, from the primary afferent terminals in the dorsal horn [54]. Following intraplantar formalin administration, intrathecal galanin was able to reduce the nocifensive activity in the second phase of the test and also potentiated the analgesic effects of morphine and of the NMDA-receptor antagonist AP-5, possibly through interactions with GalR1 [165,53]. However, following nerve injury, intrathecal treatment with a galanin receptor antagonist or galanin antisense reduced autotomy, and galanin knockout mice had reduced thermal and mechanical allodynia after nerve injury, suggesting that endogenous galanin is pronociceptive in the context of neuropathic pain [155,67]. In contrast, behavioral allodynia was reduced by addition of exogenous galanin after nerve injury, and galanin overexpressing mice also demonstrate reduced neuropathic pain-like behavior, indicating that this peptide has an antinociceptive role through inhibition of pain signaling [39,56]. These contrasting findings may be a result of the different experimental models used, but they are also likely to reflect the complex downstream signaling systems evoked by galanin binding and also differences in peptide and receptor expression profiles after injury. Indeed, it has been proposed that the analgesic effects of galanin may be mediated through the GalR1-receptor subtype, whereas GalR2 could be responsible for galanin's hyperalgesic effects [82]. These differences provide scope for selectivity in drug development, making galanin and its receptors interesting pharmacological targets for the treatment of chronic pain.

Other Neuropeptides

The neuropeptides described above should not be considered a comprehensive list. Indeed, other chapters describe the importance of dynorphin (see Chapter 5 by Marvizon et al.) and cholecystokinin (see Chapter 20 by Goffaux et al.) in pain. Other neuropeptides of particular interest in the context of pain include corticotrophin-releasing hormone [42], neurokinins A and C [44,33], and neuropeptides B and W [51]. Much remains to be discovered about the role of these neuropeptides in pain, and they are likely to present further diverse targets for the development of drugs to treat chronic pain.

Nitric Oxide

Nitric oxide (NO) is a highly diffusible free radical that acts as a biological messenger [17] but has also been shown to play a role in inflammation and pain signaling. It is produced from the substrate L-arginine by an enzymatic reaction (Fig. 4) involving one of three subtypes of the enzyme nitric oxide synthase (NOS): neuronal NOS (nNOS), inducible NOS (iNOS), or endothelial NOS (eNOS). Expression of nNOS and eNOS is constitutive, and activation of these enzymes is regulated by intracellular calcium via calmodulin binding. In contrast, iNOS expression is induced in many cells after exposure to different stimuli, including bacterial lipopolysaccharide and proinflammatory cytokines. Activation of iNOS leads to a massive production of NO that exceeds levels produced by the other two isoforms. Under some physiological or pathological circumstances, NO can also be formed from nitrites (NO_2^-) and nitrates (NO_3^-) in a mechanism that is independent of NOS (see [10] for a detailed review).

The NO molecule is small enough to cross cell membranes, but as it has a short half-life in the extracellular space, its biological effect is spatially limited. Therefore, NO is mostly produced on demand. Intracellularly, NO reacts with the ferric atom of soluble guanylate cyclase. This reaction stimulates the production of cyclic guanosine monophosphate (cGMP), which in turn acts as a second messenger in the cell through activation of the cGMP-dependent protein kinase (PKG) (Fig. 5) [10]. The production of cGMP plays a

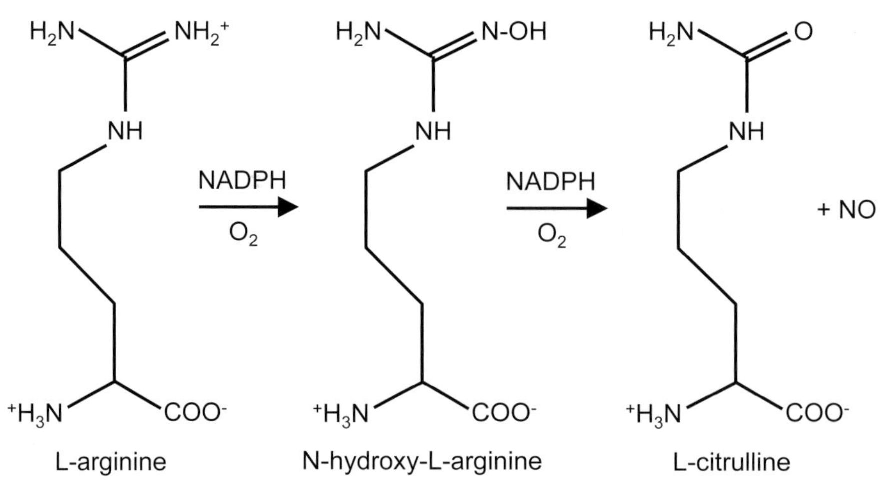

Fig. 4. Synthesis of nitric oxide (NO) by the enzymatic action of NO synthase. NADPH = the reduced form of nicotinamide adenine dinucleotide phosphate.

role in vasodilation, neuronal transmission, platelet activation and aggregation, leukocyte differentiation, and cytokine production [158].

The pro- or antinociceptive role of NO is still a controversial subject, with the exact nature of the effects of NO apparently determined by the location in which the NO-cGMP-PKG pathway is activated.

Pronociceptive Effects

In the central nervous system, NO plays a role in synaptic plasticity and long-term potentiation. As seen in Fig. 5, NO can be produced postsynaptically and can act as a retrograde transmitter to enhance presynaptic activity through the activation of soluble guanylate cyclase. This mechanism is thought to underlie the maintenance of thermal hyperalgesia, because intrathecal administration of L-arginine produces thermal hyperalgesia, whereas

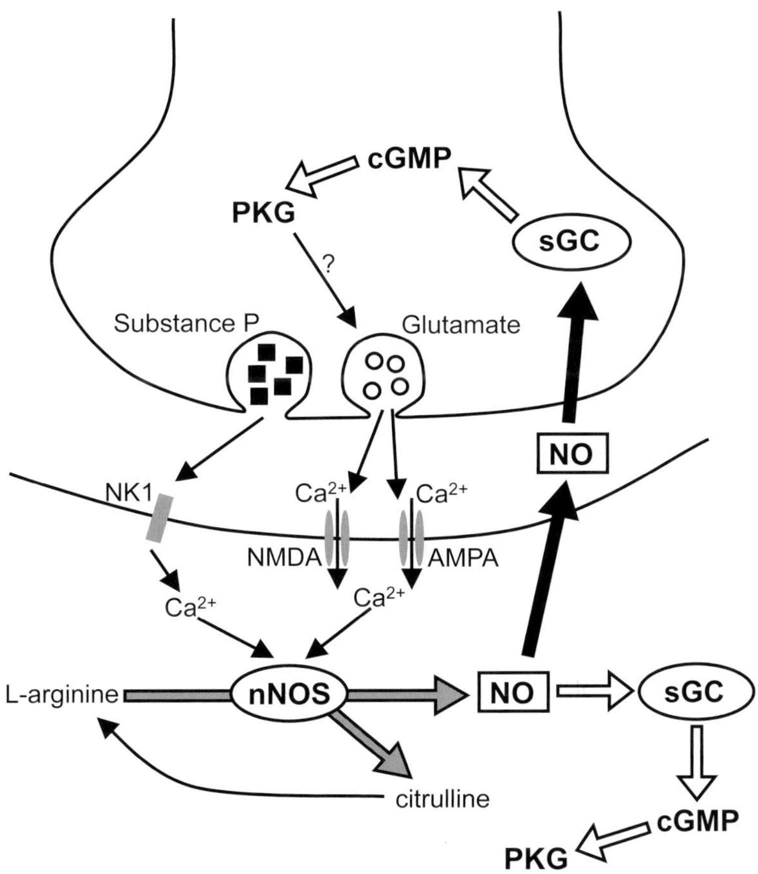

Fig. 5. Molecular effect of nitric oxide (NO) on synaptic transmission. The increase in intracellular calcium by activation of N-methyl-D-aspartate (NMDA) or α-amino-3-hydroxy-5-methyl-4-isoxazole propionate (AMPA) glutamate receptors or the activation of neurokinin NK1 receptors activates neuronal NO synthase (nNOS), which produces NO, which in turn activate soluble guanylate cyclase (sGC) to produce cyclic guanosine monophosphate (cGMP), which then activates protein kinase G (PKG). NO can easily diffuse through plasma membrane to act on the presynaptic terminal to enhance synaptic transmission, possibly via the cGMP-PKG pathway.

intrathecal administration of the nonselective NOS blocker L-NAME reverses thermal hyperalgesia and blocks ectopic mechanically elicited discharges of the sciatic nerve in a model of neuropathic pain [95,77].

In the DRG, nNOS is normally found only in a small proportion of lumbar DRG neurons, but its expression is increased in this location after peripheral nerve injury [37,48]. Genetic knockdown and selective pharmacological blockade of nNOS have shown a role of this isoform in mechanical hypersensitivity after nerve injury [37]. A similar role has also been observed for iNOS [149]. The latter study suggests that in addition to its actions via the cGMP-PKG pathway, NO activity is also mediated through the NO-peroxynitrites, which are formed by combination of NO and superoxide [149]. The constitutively expressed eNOS has also been shown to mediate thermal hypersensitivity after peripheral lesion of the sciatic nerve [77].

All three NOS isoforms also have pronociceptive effects in models of inflammatory pain. When complete Freund's adjuvant was administered to knockout mice lacking either nNOS, iNOS, or eNOS, all three strains demonstrated deficiencies in pain signaling [14]. Mice deficient in nNOS showed reduced thermal hyperalgesia and no mechanical allodynia, whereas the two other knockout strains showed a more rapid recovery from thermal hyperalgesia compared to wild-type mice [14]. Expression of all three isoforms is increased in rats following injection of capsaicin into the craniofacial muscle [74].

Finally, the NO-cGMP pathway has a role in primary headaches, such as migraine. NO is an important molecule for the control of cerebral and cranial blood flow, and NO donors such as glyceryl trinitrate are known to induce headache in healthy volunteers. Evidence demonstrates that blockade of NOS is successful in the treatment of headache types such as migraine without aura, chronic tension-type headache, and cluster headache [11,109,110].

Antinociceptive Effects

Despite the pronociceptive effects described above, some studies show a potential analgesic effect of NO in different pathological conditions. For example, topical administration of glyceryl trinitrate via patches relieves the pain of Achilles tendinopathy [113,114]. In addition to its vascular effect, NO may have some effects on nerve endings in tendinopathy, which is now classified as a degenerative neuronal-induced inflammation [162].

The analgesic effect of nitrous oxide (N_2O) is antagonized by blockade of NO production [61,80], and many studies report the involvement of the NO-cGMP pathway in the explanation of mechanisms of analgesic drugs. Accordingly, the peripheral (local) NO-cGMP-PKG pathway has been shown to play a role in the antinociceptive effects of different classes of drug such as opioids or coxibs in different models of pain, including inflammatory and bone cancer pain models. This pathway would facilitate the opening of the ATP-sensitive K^+ channel in the periphery [96,26]. The analgesic effect of sildenafil has been described using the same pathway in different models of inflammatory pain [62,115,154]. However, the effect of morphine and related analgesics can be either enhanced or reduced by NO [151].

During osteoarthritis it appears that NO can have catabolic or protective effects, and it seems that the effect of NO is dependent on concentration and/or time. The beneficial effects of NO in osteoarthritis would involve an improvement of blood flow to the affected joint (thus reducing ischemic pain) and activation of the opioid pathway or of an anti-inflammatory pathway [2]. It has been proposed that coupling the beneficial effects of NO and anti-inflammatory drugs would help in the treatment of osteoarthritis [85].

Nitric Oxide Donor Drugs

A recent strategy regarding the use of NO in pharmacological treatment of pain consists of coupling a classical drug with an NO donor. Hence, various anti-inflammatory drugs have been coupled to an NO-releasing moiety to create cyclooxygenase-inhibiting NO donors (CINODs) such as nitroacetaminophen (nitroparacetamol), nitroaspirin, and combinations of NO donors with other nonspecific nonsteroidal anti-inflammatory drugs (NSAIDs) such as naproxen, ketoprofen, ibuprofen, and diclofenac [32]. The initial concept was to improve the gastrointestinal safety of NSAIDs because the NO released from these molecules enhances the microcirculation of the gastric mucosa and reduces leukocyte/endothelial cell adhesion [31,156]. In addition to this protective effect, it seems that these molecules are more effective analgesics than their parent compounds [126]. To date, the most promising CINOD is Naproxcinod, based on naproxen, which is in the late stage of phase III trials involving patients with osteoarthritis. The main benefits appear to be gastrointestinal protection and a decrease in systolic blood pressure compared to naproxen or placebo [157]. These properties would help to protect from the cardiovascular risks associated with long-term NSAIDs treatment.

The same strategy has been applied to gabapentin, with the molecule NCX-8001, which seemed to have interesting properties in preclinical models of neuropathic pain [172], but no further studies have been published so far to confirm the potential benefit of coupling gabapentin to an NO donor moiety.

Nitric oxide is involved in many physiological systems in the body, and its role in nociception is still a matter of debate. However, it appears that it has a more pronounced pronociceptive role in the central nervous system, while it can have antinociceptive effects in the periphery. Research on the beneficial potential of NO in pain is currently focusing on the combination of NO with other analgesic drugs, especially NSAIDs.

Conclusion

In this chapter we have shown that many factors can contribute to or modulate pain processing, even within the category of peptides and neurotrophic factors. Some of these factors appear to act as peripheral pain mediators, released from damaged or diseased tissues and able to activate nociceptor populations. Examples include NGF and bradykinin. Some act as central modulators, released from primary sensory neurons in normal (e.g., substance P, CGRP) or pathological states (e.g., galanin). Others also have central modulatory roles, but are released from second- or higher-order neurons or even from non-neuronal cells (e.g., BDNF). Since the role of the central neurons releasing these factors is unknown, there is still some uncertainty regarding their mechanism of action.

This chapter also illustrates some of the opportunities and difficulties in developing analgesic drugs. The vast majority of currently used analgesic drugs belong to just two long-known drug categories (opioids and NSAIDs). Some of the factors discussed here have been targets of drug development programs. The failure of NK1-receptor antagonists to function as effective analgesics demonstrates the difficulty in translating some of the preclinical findings. On the other hand, the early clinical findings with anti-NGF molecules offer the hope of new classes of analgesics being available to patients soon.

Acknowledgments

One of the authors (S.B. McMahon) regularly undertakes consultancy work for multiple pharmaceutical companies. None of the author's research described in this article is funded by grants from the pharmaceutical industry.

References

[1] Abbadie C, Brown JL, Mantyh PW, Basbaum AI. Spinal cord substance P receptor immunoreactivity increases in both inflammatory and nerve injury models of persistent pain. Neuroscience 1996;70:201–9.
[2] Abramson SB. Nitric oxide in inflammation and pain associated with osteoarthritis. Arthritis Res Ther 2008;10:S2.
[3] Allen SJ, Dawbarn D. Clinical relevance of the neurotrophins and their receptors. Clin Sci 2006;110:175–91.
[4] Anderson LE, Seybold VS. Calcitonin gene-related peptide regulates gene transcription in primary afferent neurons. J Neurochem 2004;91:1417–29.
[5] Bar KJ, Schurigt U, Scholze A, von Segond BG, Stopfel N, Brauer R, Halbhuber KJ, Schaible HG. The expression and localization of somatostatin receptors in dorsal root ganglion neurons of normal and monoarthritic rats. Neuroscience 2004;127:197–206.
[6] Basbaum AI. Spinal mechanisms of acute and persistent pain. Reg Anesth Pain Med 1999;24:59–67.
[7] Bennett AD, Chastain KM, Hulsebosch CE. Alleviation of mechanical and thermal allodynia by CGRP8-37 in a rodent model of chronic central pain. Pain 2000;86:163–75.
[8] Bennett DL, Dmietrieva N, Priestley JV, Clary D, McMahon SB. trkA, CGRP and IB4 expression in retrogradely labelled cutaneous and visceral primary sensory neurones in the rat. Neurosci Lett 1996;206:33–6.
[9] Bespalov MM, Saarma M. GDNF family receptor complexes are emerging drug targets. Trends Pharmacol Sci 2007;28:68–74.
[10] Bian K, Murad F. Nitric oxide (NO): biogeneration, regulation, and relevance to human diseases. Front Biosci 2003;8:d264–78.
[11] Bigal ME, Rapoport AM, Hargreaves R. Advances in the pharmacologic treatment of tension-type headache. Curr Pain Headache Rep 2008;12:442–6.
[12] Bird G, Han J, Fu Y, Adwanikar H, Willis W, Neugebauer V. Pain-related synaptic plasticity in spinal dorsal horn neurons: role of CGRP. Mol Pain 2006;2:31.
[13] Birklein F, Schmelz M. Neuropeptides, neurogenic inflammation and complex regional pain syndrome (CRPS). Neurosci Lett 2008;437:199–202.
[14] Boettger MK, Uceyler N, Zelenka M, Schmitt A, Reif A, Chen Y, Sommer C. Differences in inflammatory pain in nNOS-, iNOS- and eNOS-deficient mice. Eur J Pain 2007;11:810–8.
[15] Brumovsky P, Shi TS, Landry M, Villar MJ, Hokfelt T. Neuropeptide tyrosine and pain. Trends Pharmacol Sci 2007;28:93–102.
[16] Brumovsky P, Stanic D, Shuster S, Herzog H, Villar M, Hokfelt T. Neuropeptide Y2 receptor protein is present in peptidergic and nonpeptidergic primary sensory neurons of the mouse. J Comp Neurol 2005;489:328–48.
[17] Bryan NS, Bian K, Murad F. Discovery of the nitric oxide signaling pathway and targets for drug development. Front Biosci 2009;14:1–18.
[18] Burgevin MC, Loquet I, Quarteronet D, Habert-Ortoli E. Cloning, pharmacological characterization, and anatomical distribution of a rat cDNA encoding for a galanin receptor. J Mol Neurosci 1995;6:33–41.

[19] Carlton SM, Zhou S, Du J, Hargett GL, Ji G, Coggeshall RE. Somatostatin modulates the transient receptor potential vanilloid 1 (TRPV1) ion channel. Pain 2004;110:616–27.
[20] Cho HJ, Kim SY, Park MJ, Kim DS, Kim JK, Chu MY. Expression of mRNA for brain-derived neurotrophic factor in the dorsal root ganglion following peripheral inflammation. Brain Res 1997;749:358–62.
[21] Cho HJ, Kim JK, Park HC, Kim JK, Kim DS, Ha SO, Hong HS. Changes in brain-derived neurotrophic factor immunoreactivity in rat dorsal root ganglia, spinal cord, and gracile nuclei following cut or crush injuries. Exp Neurol 1998;154:224–30.
[22] Conner AC, Simms J, Barwell J, Wheatley M, Poyner DR. Ligand binding and activation of the CGRP receptor. Biochem Soc Trans 2007;35:729–32.
[23] Coull JAM, Beggs S, Boudreau D, Boivin D, Tsuda M, Inoue K, Gravel C, Salter MW, De Koninck Y. BDNF from microglia causes the shift in neuronal anion gradient underlying neuropathic pain. Nature 2005;438:1017–21.
[24] Cridland RA, Henry JL. Effects of intrathecal administration of neuropeptides on a spinal nociceptive reflex in the rat: VIP, galanin, CGRP, TRH, somatostatin and angiotensin II. Neuropeptides 1988;11:23–32.
[25] Dawbarn D, Allen SJ. Neurotrophins and neurodegeneration. Neuropathol Appl Neurobiol 2003;29:211–30.
[26] Deciga-Campos M, Lopez-Munoz FJ. Participation of the L-arginine-nitric oxide-cyclic GMP-ATP-sensitive K^+ channel cascade in the antinociceptive effect of rofecoxib. Eur J Pharmacol 2004;484:193–9.
[27] Dickinson T, Fleetwood-Walker SM. VIP and PACAP: very important in pain? Trends Pharmacol Sci 1999;20:324–9.
[28] Dickinson T, Mitchell R, Robberecht P, Fleetwood-Walker SM. The role of VIP/PACAP receptor subtypes in spinal somatosensory processing in rats with an experimental peripheral mononeuropathy. Neuropharmacology 1999;38:167–80.
[29] Diogenes A, Akopian AN, Hargreaves KM. NGF up-regulates TRPA1: implications for orofacial pain. J Dent Res 2007;86:550–5.
[30] Doods H, Arndt K, Rudolf K, Just S. CGRP antagonists: unravelling the role of CGRP in migraine. Trends Pharmacol Sci 2007;28:580–7.
[31] Fiorucci S, Del SP. NO-aspirin: mechanism of action and gastrointestinal safety. Dig Liver Dis 2003;35:S9–19.
[32] Fiorucci S, Santucci L, Distrutti E. NSAIDs, coxibs, CINOD and H2S-releasing NSAIDs: what lies beyond the horizon. Dig Liver Dis 2007;39:1043–51.
[33] Gerspacher M. Selective and combined neurokinin receptor antagonists. Prog Med Chem 2005;43:49–103.
[34] Gibbs JL, Flores CM, Hargreaves KM. Attenuation of capsaicin-evoked mechanical allodynia by peripheral neuropeptide Y Y1 receptors. Pain 2006;124:167–74.
[35] Girard BM, Wolf-Johnston A, Braas KM, Birder LA, May V, Vizzard MA. PACAP-Mediated ATP release from rat urothelium and regulation of PACAP/VIP and receptor mRNA in micturition pathways after cyclophosphamide (CYP)-induced cystitis. J Mol Neurosci 2008;36:310–20.
[36] Groth R, Aanonsen L. Spinal brain-derived neurotrophic factor (BDNF) produces hyperalgesia in normal mice while antisense directed against either BDNF or trkB, prevent inflammation-induced hyperalgesia. Pain 2002;100:171–81.
[37] Guan Y, Yaster M, Raja SN, Tao YX. Genetic knockout and pharmacologic inhibition of neuronal nitric oxide synthase attenuate nerve injury-induced mechanical hypersensitivity in mice. Mol Pain 2007;3:29.
[38] Guo A, Vulchanova L, Wang J, Li X, Elde R. Immunocytochemical localization of the vanilloid receptor 1 (VR1): relationship to neuropeptides, the P2X3 purinoceptor and IB4 binding sites. Eur J Neurosci 1999;11:946–58.
[39] Hao JX, Shi TJ, Xu IS, Kaupilla T, Xu XJ, Hokfelt T, Bartfai T, Wiesenfeld-Hallin Z. Intrathecal galanin alleviates allodynia-like behaviour in rats after partial peripheral nerve injury. Eur J Neurosci 1999;11:427–32.
[40] Harrison S, Geppetti P. Substance P. Int J Biochem Cell Biol 2001;33:555–76.
[41] Hay DL. What makes a CGRP2 receptor? Clin Exp Pharmacol Physiol 2007;34:963–71.
[42] Hemley CF, McCluskey A, Keller PA. Corticotropin releasing hormone: a GPCR drug target. Curr Drug Targets 2007;8:105–15.
[43] Herzberg U, Eliav E, Dorsey JM, Gracely RH, Kopin IJ. NGF involvement in pain induced by chronic constriction injury of the rat sciatic nerve. Neuroreport 1997;8:1613–8.
[44] Hill RG, Oliver KR. Neuropeptide and kinin antagonists. Handb Exp Pharmacol 2007;181–216.
[45] Hill R. NK1 (substance P) receptor antagonists: why are they not analgesic in humans? Trends Pharmacol Sci 2000;21:244–6.
[46] Hokfelt T, Brumovsky P, Shi T, Pedrazzini T, Villar M. NPY and pain as seen from the histochemical side. Peptides 2007;28:365–72.
[47] Hokfelt T, Wiesenfeld-Hallin Z, Villar M, Melander T. Increase of galanin-like immunoreactivity in rat dorsal root ganglion cells after peripheral axotomy. Neurosci Lett 1987;83:217–20.
[48] Hokfelt T, Zhang X, Wiesenfeld-Hallin Z. Messenger plasticity in primary sensory neurons following axotomy and its functional implications. Trends Neurosci 1994;17:22–30.
[49] Hokfelt T, Bartfai T, Bloom F. Neuropeptides: opportunities for drug discovery. Lancet Neurol 2003;2:463–72.
[50] Holzer P. Neurogenic vasodilatation and plasma leakage in the skin. Gen Pharmacol 1998;30:5–11.
[51] Hondo M, Ishii M, Sakurai T. The NPB/NPW neuropeptide system and its role in regulating energy homeostasis, pain, and emotion. Results Probl Cell Differ 2008;46:239–56.
[52] Hua XY, Boublik JH, Spicer MA, Rivier JE, Brown MR, Yaksh TL. The antinociceptive effects of spinally administered neuropeptide Y in the rat: systematic studies on structure-activity relationship. J Pharmacol Exp Ther 1991;258:243–8.
[53] Hua XY, Hayes CS, Hofer A, Fitzsimmons B, Kilk K, Langel U, Bartfai T, Yaksh TL. Galanin acts at GalR1 receptors in spinal antinociception: synergy with morphine and AP-5. J Pharmacol Exp Ther 2004;308:574–82.
[54] Hua XY, Salgado KF, Gu G, Fitzsimmons B, Kondo I, Bartfai T, Yaksh TL. Mechanisms of antinociception of spinal galanin: how does galanin inhibit spinal sensitization? Neuropeptides 2005;39:211–6.
[55] Hunt SP, Mantyh PW. The molecular dynamics of pain control. Nat Rev Neurosci 2001;2:83–91.

[56] Hygge-Blakeman K, Brumovsky P, Hao JX, Xu XJ, Hokfelt T, Crawley JN, Wiesenfeld-Hallin Z. Galanin over-expression decreases the development of neuropathic pain-like behaviors in mice after partial sciatic nerve injury. Brain Res 2004;1025:152–8.

[57] Iannone F, De BC, Dell'Accio F, Covelli M, Patella V, Lo BG, Lapadula G. Increased expression of nerve growth factor (NGF) and high affinity NGF receptor (p140 TrkA) in human osteoarthritic chondrocytes. Rheumatology (Oxford) 2002;41:1413–8.

[58] Inagaki N, Yoshida H, Mizuta M, Mizuno N, Fujii Y, Gonoi T, Miyazaki J, Seino S. Cloning and functional characterization of a third pituitary adenylate cyclase-activating polypeptide receptor subtype expressed in insulin-secreting cells. Proc Natl Acad Sci USA 1994;91:2679–83.

[59] Indo Y. Molecular basis of congenital insensitivity to pain with anhidrosis (CIPA): mutations and polymorphisms in TRKA (NTRK1) gene encoding the receptor tyrosine kinase for nerve growth factor. Hum Mutat 2001;18:462–71.

[60] Intondi AB, Dahlgren MN, Eilers MA, Taylor BK. Intrathecal neuropeptide Y reduces behavioral and molecular markers of inflammatory or neuropathic pain. Pain 2008;137:352–65.

[61] Ishikawa M, Quock RM. Role of nitric-oxide synthase isoforms in nitrous oxide antinociception in mice. J Pharmacol Exp Ther 2003;306:484–9.

[62] Jain NK, Patil CS, Singh A, Kulkarni SK. Sildenafil-induced peripheral analgesia and activation of the nitric oxide-cyclic GMP pathway. Brain Res 2001;909:170–8.

[63] Ji GC, Zhou ST, Shapiro G, Reubi JC, Jurczyk S, Carlton SM. Analgesic activity of a non-peptide imidazolidinedione somatostatin agonist: in vitro and in vivo studies in rat. Pain 2006;124:34–49.

[64] Jiang N, Furue H, Katafuchi T, Yoshimura M. Somatostatin directly inhibits substantia gelatinosa neurons in adult rat spinal dorsal horn in vitro. Neurosci Res 2003;47:97–107.

[65] Kantner RM, Kirby ML, Goldstein BD. Increase in substance P in the dorsal horn during a chemogenic nociceptive stimulus. Brain Res 1985;338:196–9.

[66] Kerr BJ, Bradbury EJ, Bennett DL, Trivedi PM, Dassan P, French J, Shelton DB, McMahon SB, Thompson SW. Brain-derived neurotrophic factor modulates nociceptive sensory inputs and NMDA-evoked responses in the rat spinal cord. J Neurosci 1999;19:5138–48.

[67] Kerr BJ, Cafferty WB, Gupta YK, Bacon A, Wynick D, McMahon SB, Thompson SW. Galanin knockout mice reveal nociceptive deficits following peripheral nerve injury. Eur J Neurosci 2000;12:793–802.

[68] Khawaja AM, Rogers DF. Tachykinins: receptor to effector. Int J Biochem Cell Biol 1996;28:721–38.

[69] King TE, Heath MJ, Debs P, Davis MB, Hen R, Barr GA. The development of the nociceptive responses in neurokinin-1 receptor knockout mice. Neuroreport 2000;11:587–91.

[70] Kolakowski LF Jr, O'Neill GP, Howard AD, Broussard SR, Sullivan KA, Feighner SD, Sawzdargo M, Nguyen T, Kargman S, Shiao LL, et al. Molecular characterization and expression of cloned human galanin receptors GALR2 and GALR3. J Neurochem 1998;71:2239–51.

[71] Kuraishi Y, Kawamura M, Yamaguchi T, Houtani T, Kawabata S, Futaki S, Fujii N, Satoh M. Intrathecal injections of galanin and its antiserum affect nociceptive response of rat to mechanical, but not thermal, stimuli. Pain 1991;44:321–4.

[72] Landry M, Holmberg K, Zhang X, Hokfelt T. Effect of axotomy on expression of NPY, galanin, and NPY Y1 and Y2 receptors in dorsal root ganglia and the superior cervical ganglion studied with double-labeling in situ hybridization and immunohistochemistry. Exp Neurol 2000;162:361–84.

[73] Lang R, Gundlach AL, Kofler B. The galanin peptide family: receptor pharmacology, pleiotropic biological actions, and implications in health and disease. Pharmacol Ther 2007;115:177–207.

[74] Lee JS, Zhang Y, Ro JY. Involvement of neuronal, inducible and endothelial nitric oxide synthases in capsaicin-induced muscle hypersensitivity. Eur J Pain 2008; Epub Dec 10.

[75] Lembeck F, Donnerer J, Colpaert FC. Increase of substance P in primary afferent nerves during chronic pain. Neuropeptides 1981;1:175–80.

[76] Leon A, Buriani A, Dal TR, Fabris M, Romanello S, Aloe L, Levi-Montalcini R. Mast cells synthesize, store, and release nerve growth factor. Proc Natl Acad Sci USA 1994;91:3739–43.

[77] Levy D, Tal M, Hoke A, Zochodne DW. Transient action of the endothelial constitutive nitric oxide synthase (ecNOS) mediates the development of thermal hypersensitivity following peripheral nerve injury. Eur J Neurosci 2000;12:2323–32.

[78] Lewin GR, Ritter AM, Mendell LM. Nerve growth factor-induced hyperalgesia in the neonatal and adult rat. J Neurosci 1993;13:2136–48.

[79] Li CQ, Xu JM, Liu D, Zhang JY, Dai RP. Brain derived neurotrophic factor (BDNF) contributes to the pain hypersensitivity following surgical incision in the rats. Mol Pain 2008;4:27.

[80] Li S, Bieber AJ, Quock RM. Antagonism of nitrous oxide antinociception in mice by antisense oligodeoxynucleotide directed against neuronal nitric oxide synthase enzyme. Behav Brain Res 2004;152:361–3.

[81] Li WP, Xian C, Rush RA, Zhou XF. Upregulation of brain-derived neurotrophic factor and neuropeptide Y in the dorsal ascending sensory pathway following sciatic nerve injury in rat. Neurosci Lett 1999;260:49–52.

[82] Liu HX, Brumovsky P, Schmidt R, Brown W, Payza K, Hodzic L, Pou C, Godbout C, Hokfelt T. Receptor subtype-specific pronociceptive and analgesic actions of galanin in the spinal cord: selective actions via GalR1 and GalR2 receptors. Proc Natl Acad Sci USA 2001;98:9960–4.

[83] Lowe EM, Anand P, Terenghi G, Williams-Chestnut RE, Sinicropi DV, Osborne JL. Increased nerve growth factor levels in the urinary bladder of women with idiopathic sensory urgency and interstitial cystitis. Br J Urol 1997;79:572–7.

[84] Lutz EM, Sheward WJ, West KM, Morrow JA, Fink G, Harmar AJ. The VIP2 receptor: molecular characterisation of a cDNA encoding a novel receptor for vasoactive intestinal peptide. FEBS Lett 1993;334:3–8.

[85] Mackenzie IS, Rutherford D, MacDonald TM. Nitric oxide and cardiovascular effects: new insights in the role of nitric oxide for the management of osteoarthritis. Arthritis Res Ther 2008;10:S3.

[86] Maggi CA. The mammalian tachykinin receptors. Gen Pharmacol 1995;26:911–44.
[87] Malcangio M. GDNF and somatostatin in sensory neurones. Curr Opin Pharmacol 2003;3:41–5.
[88] Malcangio M, Ramer MS, Jones MG, McMahon SB. Abnormal substance P release from the spinal cord following injury to primary sensory neurons. Eur J Neurosci 2000;12:397–9.
[89] Malin SA, Molliver DC, Koerber HR, Cornuet P, Frye R, Albers KM, Davis BM. Glial cell line-derived neurotrophic factor family members sensitize nociceptors in vitro and produce thermal hyperalgesia in vivo. J Neurosci 2006;26:8588–99.
[90] Mamet J, Lazdunski M, Voilley N. How nerve growth factor drives physiological and inflammatory expressions of acid-sensing ion channel 3 in sensory neurons. J Biol Chem 2003;278:48907–13.
[91] Mannion RJ, Costigan M, Decosterd I, Amaya F, Ma QP, Holstege JC, Ji RR, Acheson A, Lindsay RM, Wilkinson GA, et al. Neurotrophins: peripherally and centrally acting modulators of tactile stimulus-induced inflammatory pain hypersensitivity. Proc Natl Acad Sci USA 1999;96:9385–90.
[92] Mansikka H, Sheth RN, DeVries C, Lee H, Winchurch R, Raja SN. Nerve injury-induced mechanical but not thermal hyperalgesia is attenuated in neurokinin-1 receptor knockout mice. Exp Neurol 2000;162:343–9.
[93] Mantyh PW, Rogers SD, Honore P, Allen BJ, Ghilardi JR, Li J, Daughters RS, Lappi DA, Wiley RG, Simone DA. Inhibition of hyperalgesia by ablation of lamina I spinal neurons expressing the substance P receptor. Science 1997;278:275–9.
[94] McMahon SB, Bennett DL, Priestley JV, Shelton DL. The biological effects of endogenous nerve growth factor on adult sensory neurons revealed by a trkA-IgG fusion molecule. Nat Med 1995;1:774–80.
[95] Meller ST, Gebhart GF. Nitric oxide (NO) and nociceptive processing in the spinal cord. Pain 1993;52:127–36.
[96] Menendez L, Juarez L, Garcia V, Hidalgo A, Baamonde A. Involvement of nitric oxide in the inhibition of bone cancer-induced hyperalgesia through the activation of peripheral opioid receptors in mice. Neuropharmacology 2007;53:71–80.
[97] Merighi A, Salio C, Ghirri A, Lossi L, Ferrini F, Betelli C, Bardoni R. BDNF as a pain modulator. Prog Neurobiol 2008;85:297–317.
[98] Michael GJ, Averill S, Nitkunan A, Rattray M, Bennett DL, Yan Q, Priestley JV. Nerve growth factor treatment increases brain-derived neurotrophic factor selectively in TrkA-expressing dorsal root ganglion cells and in their central terminations within the spinal cord. J Neurosci 1997;17:8476–90.
[99] Miyakawa A, Furue H, Katafuchi T, Jiang N, Yasaka T, Kato G, Yoshimura M. Action of neuropeptide Y on nociceptive transmission in substantia gelatinosa of the adult rat spinal dorsal horn. Neuroscience 2005;134:595–604.
[100] Mogil JS, Miermeister F, Seifert F, Strasburg K, Zimmermann K, Reinold H, Austin JS, Bernardini N, Chesler EJ, Hofmann HA, et al. Variable sensitivity to noxious heat is mediated by differential expression of the CGRP gene. Proc Natl Acad Sci USA 2005;102:12938–43.
[101] Moran TD, Colmers WF, Smith PA. Opioid-like actions of neuropeptide Y in rat substantia gelatinosa: Y1 suppression of inhibition and Y2 suppression of excitation. J Neurophysiol 2004;92:3266–75.
[102] Muddhrry PK, Ghatki MA, Spokks RA, Jonhs PM, Pierson AM, Hamid QA, Kanse S, Amara SG, Burrik JM, Legon S, Polak JM, Bloom SR. Differential expression of α-CGRP and β-CGRP by primary sensory neurons and enteric autonomic neurons of the rat. Neuroscience 1988;25:195–205.
[103] Narita M, Dun SL, Dun NJ, Tseng LF. Hyperalgesia induced by pituitary adenylate cyclase-activating polypeptide in the mouse spinal cord. Eur J Pharmacol 1996;311:121–6.
[104] Naveilhan P, Hassani H, Lucas G, Blakeman KH, Hao JX, Xu XJ, Wiesenfeld-Hallin Z, Thoren P, Ernfors P. Reduced antinociception and plasma extravasation in mice lacking a neuropeptide Y receptor. Nature 2001;409:513–7.
[105] O'Donnell D, Ahmad S, Wahlestedt C, Walker P. Expression of the novel galanin receptor subtype GALR2 in the adult rat CNS: distinct distribution from GALR1. J Comp Neurol 1999;409:469–81.
[106] Obata K, Noguchi K. BDNF in sensory neurons and chronic pain. Neurosci Res 2006;55:1–10.
[107] Ohtaki T, Kumano S, Ishibashi Y, Ogi K, Matsui H, Harada M, Kitada C, Kurokawa T, Onda H, Fujino M. Isolation and cDNA cloning of a novel galanin-like peptide (GALP) from porcine hypothalamus. J Biol Chem 1999;274:37041–5.
[108] Okuse K, Chaplan SR, McMahon SB, Luo ZD, Calcutt NA, Scott BP, Akopian AN, Wood JN. Regulation of expression of the sensory neuron-specific sodium channel SNS in inflammatory and neuropathic pain. Mol Cell Neurosci 1997;10:196–207.
[109] Olesen J. The role of nitric oxide (NO) in migraine, tension-type headache and cluster headache. Pharmacol Ther 2008;120:157–71.
[110] Olesen J, Tfelt-Hansen P, Ashina M. Finding new drug targets for the treatment of migraine attacks. Cephalalgia 2009; Epub Feb 25.
[111] Owolabi JB, Rizkalla G, Tehim A, Ross GM, Riopelle RJ, Kamboj R, Ossipov M, Bian D, Wegert S, Porreca F, Lee DK. Characterization of antiallodynic actions of ALE-0540, a novel nerve growth factor receptor antagonist, in the rat. J Pharmacol Exp Ther 1999;289:1271–6.
[112] Pan HL, Wu ZZ, Zhou HY, Chen SR, Zhang HM, Li DP. Modulation of pain transmission by G-protein-coupled receptors. Pharmacol Ther 2008;117:141–61.
[113] Paoloni JA, Appleyard RC, Nelson J, Murrell GA. Topical glyceryl trinitrate treatment of chronic noninsertional Achilles tendinopathy. A randomized, double-blind, placebo-controlled trial. J Bone Joint Surg Am 2004;86:916–22.
[114] Paoloni JA, Murrell GA. Three-year followup study of topical glyceryl trinitrate treatment of chronic noninsertional Achilles tendinopathy. Foot Ankle Int 2007;28:1064–8.
[115] Patil CS, Jain NK, Singh VP, Kulkarni SK. Cholinergic-NO-cGMP mediation of sildenafil-induced antinociception. Indian J Exp Biol 2004;42:361–7.
[116] Pawlak M, Schmidt RF. Octreotide, a somatostatin analogue, attenuates movement evoked discharges of fine afferent units from inflamed knee joints of rats. Neurosci Lett 2004;361:180–3.

[117] Petersen M, Segond von BG, Heppelmann B, Koltzenburg M. Nerve growth factor regulates the expression of bradykinin binding sites on adult sensory neurons via the neurotrophin receptor p75. Neuroscience 1998;83:161–8.
[118] Pezet S, McMahon SB. Neurotrophins: mediators and modulators of pain. Annu Rev Neurosci 2006;29:507–38.
[119] Pinter E, Helyes Z, Nemeth J, Porszasz R, Petho G, Than M, Keri G, Horvath A, Jakab B, Szolcsanyi J. Pharmacological characterisation of the somatostatin analogue TT-232: effects on neurogenic and non-neurogenic inflammation and neuropathic hyperalgesia. Naunyn Schmiedebergs Arch Pharmacol 2002;366:142–50.
[120] Post C, Alari L, Hokfelt T. Intrathecal galanin increases the latency in the tail-flick and hot-plate test in mouse. Acta Physiol Scand 1988;132:583–4.
[121] Quintao NLM, Santos ARS, Campos MM, Calixto JB. The role of neurotrophic factors in genesis and maintenance of mechanical hypernociception after brachial plexus avulsion in mice. Pain 2008;136:125–33.
[122] Quirion R, Van RD, Dumont Y, St-Pierre S, Fournier A. Characterization of CGRP1 and CGRP2 receptor subtypes. Ann NY Acad Sci 1992;657:88–105.
[123] Ramer MS, Bradbury EJ, McMahon SB. Nerve growth factor induces P2X3 expression in sensory neurons. J Neurochem 2001;77:864–75.
[124] Ramer MS, Kawaja MD, Henderson JT, Roder JC, Bisby MA. Glial overexpression of NGF enhances neuropathic pain and adrenergic sprouting into DRG following chronic sciatic constriction in mice. Neurosci Lett 1998;251:53–6.
[125] Reichardt LF. Neurotrophin-regulated signalling pathways. Philos Trans R Soc Lond B Biol Sci 2006;361:1545–64.
[126] Romero-Sandoval EA, Curros-Criado MM, Gaitan G, Molina C, Herrero JF. Nitroparacetamol (NCX-701) and pain: first in a series of novel analgesics. CNS Drug Rev 2007;13:279–95.
[127] Rueff A, Mendell LM. Nerve growth factor NT-5 induce increased thermal sensitivity of cutaneous nociceptors in vitro. J Neurophysiol 1996;76:3593–6.
[128] Rupniak NM, Kramer MS. Discovery of the antidepressant and anti-emetic efficacy of substance P receptor (NK1) antagonists. Trends Pharmacol Sci 1999;20:485–90.
[129] Sandor K, Elekes K, Szabo A, Pinter E, Engstrom M, Wurster S, Szolcsanyi J, Helyes Z. Analgesic effects of the somatostatin sst4 receptor selective agonist J-2156 in acute and chronic pain models. Eur J Pharmacol 2006;539:71–5.
[130] Schnitzer T, Lane N, Smith M, Brown M. Efficacy and safety of PF04383119 for moderate to severe pain due to osteoarthritis (OA) of the knee: a randomized trial. 12th World Congress on Pain, Glasgow, 2008. Abstract PT214.
[131] Selmer I, Schindler M, Allen JP, Humphrey PP, Emson PC. Advances in understanding neuronal somatostatin receptors. Regul Pept 2000;90:1–18.
[132] Sevcik MA, Ghilardi JR, Peters CM, Lindsay TH, Halvorson KG, Jonas BM, Kubota K, Kuskowski MA, Boustany L, Shelton DL, Mantyh PW. Anti-NGF therapy profoundly reduces bone cancer pain and the accompanying increase in markers of peripheral and central sensitization. Pain 2005;115:128–41.
[133] Seybold VS, McCarson KE, Mermelstein PG, Groth RD, Abrahams LG. Calcitonin gene-related peptide regulates expression of neurokinin1 receptors by rat spinal neurons. J Neurosci 2003;23:1816–24.
[134] Shu XQ, Mendell LM. Neurotrophins and hyperalgesia. Proc Natl Acad Sci USA 1999;96:7693–6.
[135] Shu X-Q, Llinas A, Mendell LM. Effects of trkB and trkC neurotrophin receptor agonists on thermal nociception: a behavioral and electrophysiological study. Pain 1999;80:463–70.
[136] Silva AP, Cavadas C, Grouzmann E. Neuropeptide Y and its receptors as potential therapeutic drug targets. Clin Chim Acta 2002;326:3–25.
[137] Simmons DR, Spike RC, Todd AJ. Galanin is contained in GABAergic neurons in the rat spinal dorsal horn. Neurosci Lett 1995;187:119–22.
[138] Simonetti M, Giniatullin R, Fabbretti E. Mechanisms mediating the enhanced gene transcription of P2X3 receptor by calcitonin gene-related peptide in trigeminal sensory neurons. J Biol Chem 2008;283:18743–52.
[139] Skofitsch G, Jacobowitz DM. Galanin-like immunoreactivity in capsaicin sensitive sensory neurons and ganglia. Brain Res Bull 1985;15:191–5.
[140] Slack SE, Pezet S, McMahon SB, Thompson SW, Malcangio M. Brain-derived neurotrophic factor induces NMDA receptor subunit one phosphorylation via ERK and PKC in the rat spinal cord. Eur J Neurosci 2004;20:1769–78.
[141] Smith KE, Walker MW, Artymyshyn R, Bard J, Borowsky B, Tamm JA, Yao WJ, Vaysse PJ, Branchek TA, Gerald C, Jones KA. Cloned human and rat galanin GALR3 receptors. Pharmacology and activation of G-protein inwardly rectifying K^+ channels. J Biol Chem 1998;273:23321–6.
[142] Smith PA, Moran TD, Abdulla F, Tumber KK, Taylor BK. Spinal mechanisms of NPY analgesia. Peptides 2007;28:464–74.
[143] Spengler D, Waeber C, Pantaloni C, Holsboer F, Bockaert J, Seeburg PH, Journot L. Differential signal transduction by five splice variants of the PACAP receptor. Nature 1993;365:170–5.
[144] Sun QQ, Huguenard JR, Prince DA. Neuropeptide Y receptors differentially modulate G-protein-activated inwardly rectifying K^+ channels and high-voltage-activated Ca^{2+} channels in rat thalamic neurons. J Physiol 2001;531:67–79.
[145] Sun RQ, Tu YJ, Lawand NB, Yan JY, Lin Q, Willis WD. Calcitonin gene-related peptide receptor activation produces PKA- and PKC-dependent mechanical hyperalgesia and central sensitization. J Neurophysiol 2004;92:2859–66.
[146] Suzuki R, Hunt SP, Dickenson AH. The coding of noxious mechanical and thermal stimuli of deep dorsal horn neurones is attenuated in NK1 knockout mice. Neuropharmacology 2003;45:1093–100.
[147] Szolcsanyi J, Bolcskei K, Szabo A, Pinter E, Petho G, Elekes K, Borzsei R, Almasi R, Szuts T, Keri G, et al. Analgesic effect of TT-232, a heptapeptide somatostatin analogue, in acute pain models of the rat and the mouse and in streptozotocin-induced diabetic mechanical allodynia. Eur J Pharmacol 2004;498:103–9.
[148] Taiwo OB, Taylor BK. Antihyperalgesic effects of intrathecal neuropeptide Y during inflammation are mediated by Y1 receptors. Pain 2002;96:353–63.

[149] Tanabe M, Nagatani Y, Saitoh K, Takasu K, Ono H. Pharmacological assessments of nitric oxide synthase isoforms and downstream diversity of NO signaling in the maintenance of thermal and mechanical hypersensitivity after peripheral nerve injury in mice. Neuropharmacology 2009;56:702–8.
[150] Thacker MA, Clark AK, Marchand F, McMahon SB. Pathophysiology of peripheral neuropathic pain: immune cells and molecules. Anesth Analg 2007;105:838–47.
[151] Toda N, Kishioka S, Hatano Y, Toda H. Modulation of opioid actions by nitric oxide signaling. Anesthesiology 2009;110:166–81.
[152] Todd AJ, Puskar Z, Spike RC, Hughes C, Watt C, Forrest L. Projection neurons in lamina I of rat spinal cord with the neurokinin 1 receptor are selectively innervated by substance p-containing afferents and respond to noxious stimulation. J Neurosci 2002;22:4103–13.
[153] Ueda H. Molecular mechanisms of neuropathic pain-phenotypic switch and initiation mechanisms. Pharmacol Ther 2006;109:57–77.
[154] Vale ML, Rolim DE, Cavalcante IF, Ribeiro RA, Souza MH. Role of NO/cGMP/KATP pathway in antinociceptive effect of sildenafil in zymosan writhing response in mice. Inflamm Res 2007;56:83–8.
[155] Verge VM, Xu XJ, Langel U, Hokfelt T, Wiesenfeld-Hallin Z, Bartfai T. Evidence for endogenous inhibition of autotomy by galanin in the rat after sciatic nerve section: demonstrated by chronic intrathecal infusion of a high affinity galanin receptor antagonist. Neurosci Lett 1993;149:193–7.
[156] Wallace JL, Ignarro LJ, Fiorucci S. Potential cardioprotective actions of NO-releasing aspirin. Nat Rev Drug Discov 2002;1:375–82.
[157] Wallace JL, Viappiani S, Bolla M. Cyclooxygenase-inhibiting nitric oxide donators for osteoarthritis. Trends Pharmacol Sci 2009;30:112–7.
[158] Walter U, Gambaryan S. cGMP and cGMP-dependent protein kinase in platelets and blood cells. Handb Exp Pharmacol 2009;533–48.
[159] Wang SJ. Activation of neuropeptide Y Y1 receptors inhibits glutamate release through reduction of voltage-dependent Ca^{2+} entry in the rat cerebral cortex nerve terminals: suppression of this inhibitory effect by the protein kinase C-dependent facilitatory pathway. Neuroscience 2005;134:987–1000.
[160] Watanabe M, Endo Y, Kimoto K, Katoh-Semba R, Arakawa Y. Inhibition of adjuvant-induced inflammatory hyperalgesia in rats by local injection of neurotrophin-3. Neurosci Lett 2000;282:61–4.
[161] Waters SM, Krause JE. Distribution of galanin-1, -2 and -3 receptor messenger RNAs in central and peripheral rat tissues. Neuroscience 2000;95:265–71.
[162] Webborn AD. Novel approaches to tendinopathy. Disabil Rehabil 2008;30:1572–7.
[163] Wiesenfeld-Hallin Z, Villar MJ, Hokfelt T. The effects of intrathecal galanin and C-fiber stimulation on the flexor reflex in the rat. Brain Res 1989;486:205–13.
[164] Wiesenfeld-Hallin Z, Xu XJ, Villar MJ, Hokfelt T. The effect of intrathecal galanin on the flexor reflex in rat: increased depression after sciatic nerve section. Neurosci Lett 1989;105:149–54.
[165] Wiesenfeld-Hallin Z, Xu XJ, Villar MJ, Hokfelt T. Intrathecal galanin potentiates the spinal analgesic effect of morphine: electrophysiological and behavioural studies. Neurosci Lett 1990;109:217–21.
[166] Wiley RG. Substance P receptor-expressing dorsal horn neurons: lessons from the targeted cytotoxin, substance P-saporin. Pain 2008;136:7–10.
[167] Wiley RG, Kline RH, Vierck CJ, Jr. Anti-nociceptive effects of selectively destroying substance P receptor-expressing dorsal horn neurons using [Sar^9,$Met(O_2)^{11}$]-substance P-saporin: behavioral and anatomical analyses. Neuroscience 2007;146:1333–45.
[168] Wilson-Gerwing TD, Verge VMK. Neurotrophin-3 attenuates galanin expression in the chronic constriction injury model of neuropathic pain. Neuroscience 2006;141:2075–85.
[169] Wilson-Gerwing TD, Dmyterko MV, Zochodne DW, Johnston JM, Verge VMK. Neurotrophin-3 suppresses thermal hyperalgesia associated with neuropathic pain and attenuates transient receptor potential vanilloid receptor-1 expression in adult sensory neurons. J Neurosci 2005;25:758–67.
[170] Wilson-Gerwing TD, Stucky CL, McComb GW, Verge VMK. Neurotrophin-3 significantly reduces sodium channel expression linked to neuropathic pain states. Exp Neurol 2008;213:303–14.
[171] Woolf CJ, Allchorne A, Safieh-Garabedian B, Poole S. Cytokines, nerve growth factor and inflammatory hyperalgesia: the contribution of tumour necrosis factor alpha. Br J Pharmacol 1997;121:417–24.
[172] Wu WP, Hao JX, Ongini E, Impagnatiello F, Presotto C, Wiesenfeld-Hallin Z, Xu XJ. A nitric oxide (NO)-releasing derivative of gabapentin, NCX 8001, alleviates neuropathic pain-like behavior after spinal cord and peripheral nerve injury. Br J Pharmacol 2004;141:65–74.
[173] Xu XJ, Hokfelt T, Wiesenfeld-Hallin Z. Galanin and spinal pain mechanisms: where do we stand in 2008? Cell Mol Life Sci 2008;65:1813–9.
[174] Xu XJ, Wiesenfeld-Hallin Z. Intrathecal pituitary adenylate cyclase activating polypeptide facilitates the spinal nociceptive flexor reflex in the rat. Neuroscience 1996;72:801–4.
[175] Xu XJ, Wiesenfeld-Hallin Z. An analogue of growth hormone releasing factor (GRF), (Ac-Try1, D-Phe2)-GRF-(1-29), specifically antagonizes the facilitation of the flexor reflex induced by intrathecal vasoactive intestinal peptide in rat spinal cord. Neuropeptides 1991;18:129–35.
[176] Xu XJ, Wiesenfeld-Hallin Z, Hokfelt T. Intrathecal galanin blocks the prolonged increase in spinal cord flexor reflex excitability induced by conditioning stimulation of unmyelinated muscle afferents in the rat. Brain Res 1991;541:350–3.
[177] Xu XJ, Wiesenfeld-Hallin Z, Villar MJ, Fahrenkrug J, Hokfelt T. On the role of galanin, substance P and other neuropeptides in primary sensory neurons of the rat: studies on spinal reflex excitability and peripheral axotomy. Eur J Neurosci 1990;2:733–43.

[178] Yajima Y, Narita M, Usui A, Kaneko C, Miyatake M, Narita M, Yamaguchi T, Tamaki H, Wachi H, Seyama Y, et al. Direct evidence for the involvement of brain-derived neurotrophic factor in the development of a neuropathic pain-like state in mice. J Neurochem 2005;93:584–94.
[179] Yamamoto T, Tatsuno I. Antinociceptive effect of intrathecally administered pituitary adenylate cyclase activating polypeptide (PACAP) on the rat formalin test. Neurosci Lett 1995;184:32–5.
[180] Zhang X, Huang J, McNaughton PA. NGF rapidly increases membrane expression of TRPV1 heat-gated ion channels. EMBO J 2005;24:4211–23.
[181] Zhang Y, Danielsen N, Sundler F, Mulder H. Pituitary adenylate cyclase-activating peptide is upregulated in sensory neurons by inflammation. Neuroreport 1998;9:2833–6.
[182] Zhang Y, Malmberg AB, Sjolund B, Yaksh TL. The effect of pituitary adenylate cyclase activating peptide (PACAP) on the nociceptive formalin test. Neurosci Lett 1996;207:187–90.
[183] Zhang YZ, Sjolund B, Moller K, Hakanson R, Sundler F. Pituitary adenylate cyclase activating peptide produces a marked and long-lasting depression of a C-fibre-evoked flexion reflex. Neuroscience 1993;57:733–7.
[184] Zhou X-F, Chie ET, Deng Y-S, Zhong J-H, Xue Q, Rush RA, Xian CJ. Injured primary sensory neurons switch phenotype for brain-derived neurotrophic factor in the rat. Neuroscience 1999;92:841–53.

Correspondence to: Stephen B. McMahon, PhD, London Pain Consortium, Wolfson CARD, King's College London, Guy's Campus, London SE1 1UL, United Kingdom. Email: stephen.mcmahon@kcl.ac.uk.

13

Cytokines, Chemokines, and Pain

Claudia Sommer[a] and Fletcher White[b]

[a]Department of Neurology, University of Würzburg, Würzburg, Germany; [b]Departments of Cell Biology, Neurobiology and Anatomy, and Anesthesiology, Loyola University, Chicago, Illinois, USA

Cytokines and Chemokines: Basic Data

Cytokines are extracellular signaling proteins phylogenetically related to opioid peptides. They are mostly water-soluble molecules ranging between 8 and 30 kDa. Their synthesis is activated by mitogen-activated protein kinases (MAPK), which in turn are stimulated by cell stressors such as heat, ultraviolet light, or inflammatory molecules via toll-like receptors (TLRs). Cytokines were originally found to mediate activation of the immune system and inflammatory responses; it was later discovered that they can be produced in many cell types and that they provide a means of communication between the immune system and the nervous system. In the broader sense, cytokines comprise the interleukins (IL, consecutively numbered from IL-1 to, at present, IL-35), the tumor necrosis factors (TNF), the chemokines (CXC, CC, and other subfamilies, consecutively numbered), the interferons (IFN), and the mesenchymal growth factors, transforming growth factor β (TGF-β) and others. Cytokines are labeled "proinflammatory" or "Th1," others "anti-inflammatory" or "Th2," depending on their effects on immune cells, in particular on lymphocytes. However, certain cytokines may have pro- or anti-inflammatory actions, influenced by the particular microenvironment.

This chapter will discuss those cytokines and chemokines that have been studied in the context of pain. Within the group of proinflammatory cytokines, data on pain are available for IL-1, IL-2, IL-6, IL-17, and TNF. Among the cytokines considered anti-inflammatory,

Pharmacology of Pain
edited by Pierre Beaulieu, David Lussier, Frank Porreca, and Anthony H. Dickenson
IASP Press, Seattle, © 2010

IL-4, IL-10, IL-13, and TGF-β have been investigated in the context of pain. In the group of chemokines and chemokine receptors, there are several candidate factors that may influence nociception either from the onset or during the maintenance of chronic nociception. These include fractalkine/CX3CL1, SDF-1 (stromal cell-derived factor-1)/CXCL12, MCP-1 (monocyte chemoattractant protein-1)/CCL2, MIP-1α (macrophage inflammatory protein-1a)/CCL3, RANTES (regulated on activation normal T-cell expressed and secreted)/CCL5, and their respective receptors, CX3CR1, CXCR4, CCR2, CCR1, and CCR5.

Interleukins and Tumor Necrosis Factor

Interleukin-1

IL-1 is present as IL-1α and IL-1β, which are products of two different genes. In the context of pain, mostly IL-1β has been studied. Both are synthesized as 31–33 kDa, variably glycosylated pro-cytokines that share 22% amino acid identity over their mature segments. IL-1α and IL-1β act on the same receptors, IL-1RI and IL-1RII. IL-RI is considered the active receptor, while IL-1RII lacks a transduction molecule and is a functional antagonist. The IL-1 receptor antagonist (IL-1Ra) is another naturally occurring antagonist [30]. IL-1β is rapidly increased in tissues after trauma or in inflammation.

Applied by intraplantar (i.pl.) injection in rats, IL-1β reduces mechanical nociceptive thresholds [38]. Further studies confirmed the induction of mechanical hyperalgesia by IL-1. IL-1β given intraperitoneally (i.p.) reduced tail-flick latency to noxious heat between 10 and 55 minutes after the injection, and IL-1Ra blocked lipopolysaccharide- and lithium-induced hyperalgesia [72,140]. When injected directly into a peripheral nerve, low doses of IL-1β in the picogram range induce hyperalgesia, whereas higher doses have no effect [153]. In the central nervous system (CNS), large doses of IL-1α in the nanogram range administered into the cerebral ventricles (i.c.v.) had analgesic effects [85]. A dose of 10 pg to 1 ng/kg i.c.v. of IL-1β reduced paw-licking latency in the hot-plate test, indicating hyperalgesia, and enhanced the response of wide-dynamic-range (WDR) neurons in the trigeminal nucleus caudalis to noxious pinch [90]. Since the cytokine system is extremely complex and tightly regulated at various levels, this biphasic effect of IL-1 in pain is as yet incompletely understood. One possibility may be the development of tolerance after application of higher doses through toll-like receptor signaling [37].

Antagonizing endogenous IL-1β applied either locally or intrathecally in nerve injury models reduces pain behavior [116,148]. Mice deficient in the IL-1 receptor do not develop hyperalgesia after nerve injury; they also have reduced spontaneous activity in dorsal root axons compared to wild-type mice [149].

Interleukin-2

IL-2 is a 15-kDa protein that is primarily produced by CD4+ T cells. It acts via three class I receptors with low, intermediate, and high affinity to IL-2. The intracellular signaling uses the JAK/STAT pathway (for review see [68]). An interaction of the opioid-like peptide IL-2 with μ-opioid receptors is assumed [118]. Both pro- and analgesic effects have been described for IL-2. IL-2 is elevated in the serum of rats after a sciatic nerve crush lesion [142]. Although in vitro studies indicate a proinflammatory role of IL-2, i.pl. injection of IL-2 and IL-2 gene therapy produced antihyperalgesia [152]. Central application of IL-2 in the locus ceruleus also inhibited pain behavior [45]. Further studies are needed to clarify the role of IL-2 in pain processing. Interestingly, IL-2 was one of the first cytokines observed to induce pain in humans, as a side effect of drugs used in anti-tumor trials [137].

Interleukin-6

Interleukin-6 (IL-6) is a variably glycosylated, 22–27 kDa secreted glycoprotein. It is a prototypic pleiotropic cytokine with an evolutionary structural relationship with IL-4, leukemia inhibiting factor, erythropoietin, and ciliary neurotrophic factor. IL-6 needs IL-6 receptor-α (IL-6R) and the gp130 subunit, members of the class I cytokine receptor superfamily, to exert its actions. IL-6 is expressed at low levels in astrocytes and possibly neurons of the normal brain and is upregulated in disease. IL-6 has a hyperalgesic effect in the hotplate test when given i.c.v. [91]. Data from IL-6 knockout mice are discrepant, with reduced pain responses in some but not in all studies. The results must be interpreted with care because IL-6 knockout mice have a markedly increased production of TNF.

Tumor Necrosis Factor

Tumor necrosis factor (TNF) is a pleiotropic proinflammatory cytokine produced by a wide variety of cells. The structurally related peptide lymphotoxin-α (LTα, formerly TNF-β) binds to the same receptors, TNFR1 and TNFR2. TNF exists in a 26-kDa transmembrane and in a 17-kDa secreted form, both of which are biologically active [3]. Several other structurally related proteins belong to the TNF family. TNF is regulated at various levels, and the second messenger pathways are complex. TNF mRNA can be detected in the normal mouse, rat, and human CNS and in normal and lesioned peripheral nerves.

TNF has been extensively studied in animal models of pain (see [114] for review). Injections of TNF with doses in the picogram range induce hyperalgesia. Higher doses have a lesser or even an inhibitory effect. Intracerebroventricular injections of TNF at doses of 10 pg, 100 pg, and 1 ng reduced paw-withdrawal latency in the hotplate test, with a maximal response at a dose of 10 pg that peaked 60 minutes after injection. In rats, TNF injected into muscle induces pressure hyperalgesia and a pain-related loss in muscle strength, which can be antagonized by drugs used in neuropathic pain. TNF induces pain and hypersensitivity when applied to a normal dorsal root ganglion (DRG), an effect that is further enhanced in a compressed DRG. In vitro perfusion of TNF to DRG elicits neuronal discharges in both A and C fibers. The firing frequency is markedly higher and the discharge longer-lasting after nerve injury, indicating an increased sensitivity of injured afferent neurons to TNF. Injection or perfusion of TNF into or onto rat DRG in vivo induces allodynia. Subthreshold quantities of TNF injected into a DRG when its spinal nerve is ligated results in faster onset of allodynia and increased spontaneous pain behavior. Mice overexpressing TNF in astrocytes have increased mechanical allodynia after L5 spinal nerve transection [27]. In contrast, thermal hyperalgesia is reduced in mice deficient in TNFR1, but not in those lacking TNFR2 [134]. TNF signaling also contributes to the development of nociceptive sensitization in a tibia fracture model of complex regional pain syndrome type I [105].

When the function of endogenous TNF is inhibited, either by blocking its synthesis, its release, or its reaction with its receptors, pain behavior is reduced in animal models of inflammatory and neuropathic pain. Although in some models TNF inhibition had to occur before the injury in order to have an effect, in others, even established hyperalgesia could be attenuated by TNF inhibition [117]. TNF inhibition also shows efficacy in models of low back pain.

Interleukin-17

The cytokine originally named IL-17, now IL-17A, is a prototypic IL-17 family member, a disulfide-linked homodimeric glycoprotein consisting of 155 amino acids. It exerts its actions as a homodimer with a molecular weight of around 35 kDa. IL-17A is mainly produced by CD4 T-lymphocytes. It can induce expression of a variety of other cytokines and chemokines. In a model of neuropathic pain (chronic constriction injury, CCI) of the sciatic nerve in mice, IL-17A displayed a monophasic expression in degenerating nerves at day 7 after CCI, whereas transcripts for the IL-17A regulatory cytokines IL-23 and IL-15 peaked earlier. RAG-1 (recombination-activating gene-1) knockout mice lacking functional T lymphocytes did not express IL-17A mRNA in distal nerve segments following CCI and had less thermal hyperalgesia, indicating a role for this cytokine and its downstream mediators in pain [62].

Interleukin-4

The 15-kDa glycoprotein IL-4 is a pleiotropic anti-inflammatory (Th-2) cytokine produced by activated CD4 T lymphocytes, mast cells, eosinophils and basophils. IL-4 affects T and B lymphocytes, natural killer cells, mast cells, synoviocytes and endothelial cells. It activates and supports the growth of B cells and triggers the production of IgG and IgE. IL-4 inhibits macrophage activation and directs the T-helper cell differentiation to the Th2 side. IL-4 acts via two receptors, the classical and alternative IL-4 receptor. The alternative IL-4 receptor is also shared by IL-13. The signaling involves the JAK family and STAT6 (for review see [92]).

Animal studies unequivocally show an analgesic action of IL-4 [23]. IL-4 reduces the acetic acid-induced writhing response in mice and the zymosan-induced knee-joint incapacitance in rats [132]. IL-4 gene therapy attenuates mechanical allodynia and thermal hyperalgesia induced by spinal nerve ligation in mice [46].

Interleukin-10

IL-10 is an approximately 18-kDa nonglycosylated polypeptide. It was originally described as "cytokine synthesis inhibitory factor," because it inhibits production of cytokines by activated T-cells and macrophages, and thus it belongs to the anti-inflammatory (Th2) cytokines. It is synthesized in immune cells and in neuroendocrine and neural tissues. The production of IL-10 is inhibited by several cytokines including IL-4, IL-13, and interferon gamma (IFN-γ) and through autoregulation by IL-10 itself. The IL-10 receptor belongs to the class II cytokine receptor family, like receptors for the interferons, and binding of the ligand activates the JAK/STAT pathway in interaction with other signaling pathways (for review see [32]). IL-10 pretreatment reduces hyperalgesic responses to i.pl. injections of carrageenan, IL-1β, IL-6, and TNF [99] and to nerve injury [136]. The intrathecal injection of IL-10 protein, of IL-10 DNA via viral vectors, and of naked DNA attenuates hyperalgesia after CCI [80].

Chemokines

Immune cells, when activated in response to infection, inflammation, or trauma, typically migrate to the source of injury via the presence of specific factors called chemotactic cytokines or chemokines. The expression of chemokines and their receptors is heterogeneous and is not restricted to the function of attracting hematopoietic cells. Chemokine receptor signaling serves the nervous system under both normal and pathological conditions [144]. Chemokine/receptor expression in the nervous system can be constitutive or inducible, but may also be downregulated by exposure to a ligand or to activating and differentiating stimuli (Fig. 1).

Monocyte Chemoattractant Protein-1 (MCP-1/CCL2)

MCP-1 is a highly inducible C-C chemokine with a molecular weight of ~9.3 kD that falls under the category of inflammatory chemokines. Although largely conserved across species, the murine MCP-1 (the product of the *JE* gene) is not a complete ortholog of human

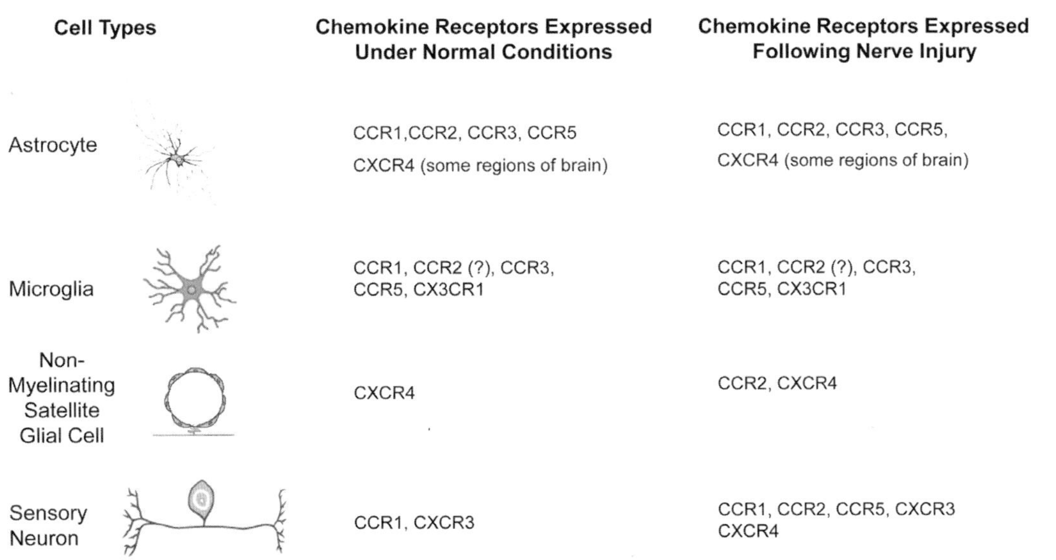

Fig. 1. Many types of neurons and glial cells release proinflammatory chemokines constitutively or following activity and may modulate pain processing by affecting presynaptic release of neurotransmitters and/or postsynaptic excitability.

MCP-1 because it exhibits a 49 amino acid C-terminus extension. MCP-1 is the high-affinity chemokine for CCR2 and is a potent chemoattractant and activator of monocytes, activated T cells, natural killer cells, and eosinophils. Mice deficient in MCP-1 or CCR2 have normal lifespans and normal numbers of monocytes. However, mouse mutations for either ligand or receptor cannot attract monocytes following inflammatory stimuli, despite otherwise normal signs of inflammation, and do not develop inflammatory lesions in CNS models of demyelinating diseases [18]. In contrast, transgenic expression of MCP-1 produces a number of effects that are dependent on the promoter. These effects include a high level of expression of MCP-1 in several organs without the presence of cellular infiltrates, perivascular cuffing (accumulation of inflammatory cells around blood vessels) in the CNS, and only subtle thymic infiltration by monocytes [42].

It is clear that MCP-1 is central to inflammation associated with disease or injury, so it is perhaps not surprising that MCP-1 also contributes to elements of both inflammatory and chronic pain states [144]. Following peripheral nerve compression injury, MCP-1/CCR2 signaling is known to directly excite subsets of sensory neurons [122,146]. Occurring in the peripheral nervous system (PNS) only after injury [122,146], this chemokine/receptor neuronal excitation is most likely due to transactivation of TRPV1 and/or TRPA1 present on sensory nerves [57]. Interestingly, mice deficient in CCR2 exhibit an impaired neuropathic pain response following spared nerve injury [1], and glial overexpression of MCP-1 leads to enhanced nociceptive responses [77]. Perhaps more importantly, a CCR2-receptor antagonist reverses tactile hypernociception following peripheral nerve injury, further demonstrating a link between chemokines/receptors and chronic nociceptive behavior [12].

Although some reports suggest that the focus of nociceptive chemokine/receptor action is within the dorsal horn of the spinal cord via CCR2-positive microglial cells [1,154], there is very little direct evidence to directly support this ligand-receptor interaction in the spinal cord [35].

Stromal-Derived Factor 1 (SDF-1/CXCL12)

SDF-1a is a chemokine with an amino acid sequence that contains four cysteine residues conserved by most CXC chemokines. The N-terminus of SDF-1 is particularly important for activity. The chemokine is highly conserved between mice and humans, is widely expressed throughout the body, and exhibits a broad range of actions affecting stromal cell migration, leukocyte chemotaxis, vascularization of multiple organ systems, metastatic tumor formation, and neural development [79]. SDF-1 (also known as CXCL12) and its receptor CXCR4 are essential for fetal development because mice with mutations for either SDF-1$^{-/-}$ or CXCR4$^{-/-}$ die in utero due to incomplete heart development, defects in intestinal vascularization, and malformations within the cerebellum [79]. Applied by i.pl. injection, SDF-1 produces tactile allodynia in the adult rat [89]. SDF-1α signaling via the T-tropic HIV coreceptor, CXCR4, has been implicated in HIV-1-associated and toxic antiretroviral neuropathies [12,13].

The monomer form of SDF-1 is known to produce CXCR4 internalization, intracellular Ca^{2+} mobilization, and chemotaxis. Recent studies using nuclear magnetic resonance structure analysis of the SDF-1:CXCR4-N-domain complex have also determined that the structural basis of the recognition of receptor residues by the chemokine is indicative of a constitutively active dimeric form of SDF-1. Importantly, this dimeric form serves only to activate intracellular Ca^{2+} mobilization [133]. The differential effects on CXCR4-bearing cells by either the monomeric or dimeric forms reveal the latter to be a potent partial agonist [133]. Perhaps the least promiscuous of the chemokines, SDF-1α also reportedly signals through the former orphan chemokine receptor, RDC-1 (also known as CXCR7) [125].

Regulated upon Activation, Normal T-Cell Expressed, and Secreted (RANTES/CCL5)

RANTES is a CC chemokine with an amino acid sequence that contains four cysteine residues conserved by most CC chemokines. Like SDF-1, the N-terminus of RANTES is essential for activity. The chemotaxic effects of RANTES extend to a variety of leukocytes that include monocytes, macrophages, microglia, T cells, eosinophils, basophils, and developing DRG neurons via the chemokine receptors CCR1, CCR3, and CCR5 [15]. RANTES can also produce rapid release of histamine from basophils and elicit intracellular Ca^{2+} mobilization in rat hippocampal neurons [78]. Of particular interest for HIV-1-associated painful peripheral neuropathies is the ability of both RANTES and the viral coat protein for HIV-1, gp120, to produce intracellular Ca^{2+} fluxes within sensory neurons through the M-tropic HIV-1 coreceptor, CCR5 [12,13,89].

Macrophage Inflammatory Protein-1α (MIP-1α/CCL3)

MIP-1α is an 8-kD member of the CC chemokine family. MIP-1α, an inducible chemokine, has been implicated in a wide range of acute and chronic inflammatory conditions initiated by bacterial, viral, fungal and parasitic pathogens. MIP-1α functions to regulate cellular recruitment, trafficking of leukocytes and host response. MIP-1α binds with high affinity to the chemokine receptors CCR1, CCR3, and CCR5 [106]. The action of MIP-1α through chemokine receptors produces intracellular Ca^{2+} mobilization in astrocytes and neurons, in addition to leukocytes [89]. Two additional studies demonstrated that MIP-1α acting through CCR1 desensitizes DRG and PAG neurons to μ-opioid receptor agonists, presumably by reducing membranal μ-opioid receptors [156]. This effect was also observed with RANTES (CCL5) and SDF-1 (CXCL12) [123]. Perhaps more importantly, Zhang and colleagues demonstrated that activation of chemokine receptors during inflammation enhances the sensitivity of TRPV1, thereby promoting hyperalgesia [156]. Similar actions on TRPV1 and TRPA1 are observed with the chemokine MCP-1 [57].

Fractalkine/CX3CL1

Fractalkine is the only member of the CX3C chemokine family, a subgroup of the chemokines that exhibit three amino acids between the initial pair of cysteines and only one intervening amino acid in CXC chemokines; hence the nomenclature, CX3CL1. Fractalkine is a large cytokine protein of 373 amino acids with an extended mucin-like stalk and a chemokine domain on top. Unlike other chemokines, fractalkine was discovered using an expressed sequence tabs (EST) sequence from a human brain DNA library [9]. The murine form of fractalkine exhibits a high degree of homology in the chemokine and intracellular domain. There is less cross-species homology within the hydrophobic membrane-spanning domain for the mucin stalk. Fractalkine is expressed by endothelial cells, by a subpopulation of macrophages and dendritic cells, and by nearly all sensory and dorsal horn neurons [81]. Functional signaling with fractalkine occurs following release of the chemokine from the cell surface by metalloproteinase-dependent cleavage, generating a soluble molecule that functions as a chemoattractant for T cells, monocytes, natural killer T cells, and microglia that bear the fractalkine receptor, CX3CR1 [81].

Fractalkine function is not limited to non-neuronal cells because the chemokine has been reported to mediate calcium signaling in hippocampal and neonatal sensory neurons [78,89]. Functional significance of the fractalkine/CX3CR1 signaling in the spinal cord or periaqueductal gray (PAG) following intrathecal administration reportedly produces mechanical allodynia and thermal hyperalgesia [81]. In sharp contrast, intraneural administration of fractalkine inhibits nociceptive behavior following spared nerve injury (SNI), and CX3CR1 knockout mice, when compared with control mice, display greatly increased allodynia after SNI [81].

Mechanisms of Cytokine/Chemokine-Related Pain

Sensitization of Nociceptors

Actions on Na^+ and K^+ Channels and Modulation of Neuronal Activity

Changes in pain behavior after cytokine application in experimental animals are paralleled by changes in ectopic activity or sensitivity of nerve fibers. TNF applied to peripheral nerve fibers lowers mechanical activation thresholds in C nociceptors, rapidly evokes ongoing activity in C fibers, increases plasma permeability and extravasation, and elicits mechanical allodynia [58,119] (Fig. 2). Intraplantar injection of IL-1β rapidly induces transient spontaneous discharges and hyperalgesia [43]. Deletion of the IL-1 receptor type I and transgenic overexpression of the IL-1 receptor antagonist reduce spontaneous ectopic activity following spinal nerve injury [149]. IL-1β also sensitizes abdominal visceral afferents of cats to ischemia and histamine [41].

In vitro perfusion of DRG with TNF elicits electrical activity in both A and C fibers, with lower concentrations needed and higher firing frequencies after nerve injury or prior compression of the DRG [110,155]. The same treatment in vivo induces allodynia in experimental animals [50,110]. Application of nucleus pulposus from spinal disks to the DRG induces spontaneous firing in dorsal horn WDR neurons, which can be blocked by TNF antagonists, implying that the activity is TNF-mediated [21]. Application of

TNF directly to the dorsal root also evoked spontaneous discharges in dorsal horn WDR neurons [93].

At the spinal cord level, TNF levels rise following peripheral or spinal injury because of increased local synthesis in glial cells, increased transport across the blood brain barrier, and local increases in ADAM-17, a molecule that cleaves membrane-bound TNF (mTNF) to its soluble form [98]. Intrathecal administration of TNF enhances responses to C-fiber stimulation and increases both wind-up and the postdischarge response of deep dorsal horn neurons [102]. Local spinal increases in mTNF are associated with hyperalgesia, and local viral vector production of a TNF antagonist reduced spinal mTNF and elicited a concomitant reduction in pain behavior [47]. At the spinal level, TNF and IL-1β enhanced AMPA- or NMDA-induced currents, and IL-1β and IL-6 suppressed GABA- and glycine-induced currents in lamina II nociceptors, clearly indicating that these proinflammatory cytokines shift the balance toward an increased excitability of the neurons [61].

It is now becoming clearer how cytokines act on ion channels at the molecular level. TNF was shown to rapidly enhance tetrodotoxin-resistant Na^+ currents in DRG neurons via activation of TNFR1 and p38 MAPK [56]. p38 MAPK, in turn, is colocalized with the Na^+ channel subtype $Na_V1.8$ in DRG neurons, and direct phosphorylation of Na_V 1.8 causes an increase in current density, which may contribute to inflammatory and neuropathic pain [52]. In capsaicin-sensitive trigeminal ganglion neurons, prolonged IL-1β exposure for 24 hours increased total Na^+ current without specific effects on tetrodotoxin (TTX)-resistant channels [69].

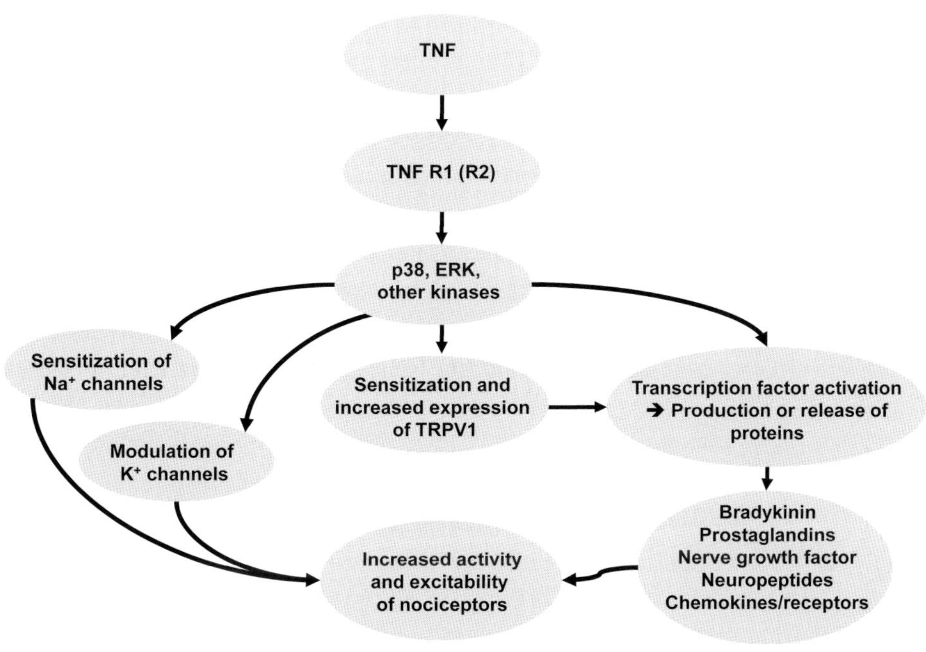

Fig. 2. Simplified diagram of peripheral mechanisms by which tumor necrosis factor (TNF) induces pain and hyperalgesia. ERK = extracellular regulated kinase; TNF R1 = TNF receptor 1.

Increased excitability may also be caused by a decrease in K^+ currents. Direct TNF-induced modulation of K^+ currents has not been studied in the context of pain, but data from other experimental systems may be of relevance. For instance, application of TNF reduces the outward K^+ current in *Aplysia* neurons [108], in retinal ganglion cells [29], and in cortical neurons [51]. In cultured cortical astrocytes, TNF induces a protein-kinase C-dependent reduction in K^+ conductance (inward rectifying K^+ currents), which affects the capacity of glial cells to buffer extracellular K^+ and to take up glutamate released by neuronal firing, resulting in increased neuronal vulnerability [63]. Variable actions of IL-1β on K^+ currents have been shown in different cell systems.

Actions on TRPV Channels

TNF enhances TRPV1-mediated currents in DRG neurons [86]. In a skin-nerve in vitro preparation, brief exposure of the skin to TNF or IL-1β facilitated heat-evoked calcitonin gene-related peptide (CGRP) release [94] from peptidergic neurons, which was a direct effect independent of changes in gene expression or receptor upregulation. Brief application of IL-1β to DRG yielded a potentiation of heat-activated inward currents and a shift of activation thresholds toward lower temperatures, mediated by activation of protein kinases [88]. Further, TNF increases the proportion of DRG neurons expressing TRPV1 via the TNFR1 receptor and activation of extracellular regulated kinase [48].

Chemokines as Neurotransmitters

A multitude of chemokine/receptors are present in the naive CNS, including CCR1, CCR2, CCR5, CXCR3, CXCR4, and CX3CR1 [145]. As such, chemokine/receptor signaling within the adult nervous system may, in addition to its injury or disease-related roles, be defined as the ability to regulate synaptic activity, modulate transmission and evoke second messenger systems within neurons and glia [144].

Prime examples of functional roles for chemokines in the CNS are the chemokine receptor-regulated neurotransmission effects by interferon-γ producing protein-10 (IP-10/CXCL10) acting via CXCR3 on the intracellular Ca^{2+} dynamics and production of electrical activity in hippocampal neurons [26], and the dose-dependent ability of SDF1/CXCL12 to reduce the amplitude of evoked excitatory postsynaptic currents in Purkinje neurons [26]. Neurons of the rodent hippocampus and cerebellum also exhibit Ca^{2+} transients following stimulation with growth-related gene product alpha (GROα)/CXCL2, IL-8/CXCL8, RANTES/CCL5, macrophage-derived chemokine (MDC/CCL22), and fractalkine/CX3CL1 [78]. Chemokines such as SDF1/CXCL12 acting via CXCR4 on neurons and/or astrocytes are also thought to affect the release of glutamate, potentially affecting neuronal excitability [11,67] and/or neuronal apoptosis [7]. In addition, the chemokine GROα/CXCL2 is thought to provoke the release of gamma-aminobutyric acid (GABA) at central synapses [44], and MCP-1/CCL2 negatively modulates GABA-induced currents and/or facilitates excitotoxic events in the neonatal rat CNS [79].

Chemokine induction of excitatory effects in rodent neurons is not limited to cells in the CNS, because chemokines have also been shown to produce changes in intracellular Ca^{2+} dynamics of acutely dissociated sensory neurons and peripheral glia derived from uninjured animals [144].

Heterologous Desensitization of Chemokine/Opioid Receptors

Another means by which chemokines potentially alter neuronal signaling in the nervous system is via heterologous desensitization between chemokines and opioids. This phenomenon was first discovered in vitro and confirmed in vivo [123,156]. Injections of the individual chemokines RANTES/CCL5, SDF1a/CXCL12 and fractalkine/CX3CL1, but not MCP-1/CCL2 into the PAG 30 minutes prior to morphine or DAMGO administration effectively blocked the expected analgesic effect on a rodent tail subjected to a cold water bath. These authors further determined that the effects of the chemokines were both dose- and time-dependent. As the receptor for MCP-1/CCL2, CCR2, is not found normally in the PAG (whereas those for the other aforementioned chemokine receptors are present), a distinct lack of opioid receptor cross-desensitization by MCP-1/CCL2 prior to morphine administration comes as no surprise [123].

Actions on Glutamate Transporters and Receptors

TNF may alter the excitability of CNS neurons via its effects on glutamate transporters. TNF decreases expression of the glutamate transporter gene EAAT2/GLT-1 [113] and glutamate uptake by other glial transporters such as glutamate-aspartate transporter (GLAST) [65]. Reduced glutamate uptake via these transporters has been associated with increased pain behavior because of changes in spinal processing [87].

In hippocampal neurons, TNF increases cell surface expression of the amino-3-hydroxy-5-methyl-4-isoxazolepropionate (AMPA) receptor subunit GluR1 [10]. This process is accompanied by a decrease in membrane GluR2 and is thought to be the result of rapid insertion of Ca^{2+}-permeable AMPA/kainate channels and decreased Ca^{2+}-impermeable AMPA receptors into the membrane. The increase in AMPA receptor surface expression is mediated by TNFR1 and requires phosphoinositide 3-kinase (PI3K) activity [121]. Changes in AMPA-receptor subtype density induced by glial TNF release may be involved in synaptic scaling, i.e., adjustments in the strength of all synapses on a neuron.

Opioid Tolerance

Opioids are the primary treatment for pain management in cancer patients reporting moderate to severe pain, and are being increasingly used for noncancer chronic pain. However, prolonged administration of opioids is associated with significant problems, including the development of antinociceptive tolerance, wherein higher doses of the drug are required over time to elicit the same amount of analgesia (see Chapter 18 by Simonnet and Le Moal). These higher doses are also thought to be increasing pain sensitivity, known as opioid-induced tactile hyperalgesia (OIH). This increased pain is usually experienced at a different location separate from the original site [95].

OIH has previously been shown to be blocked by a number of different methods such as glutamate antagonism [17,66]. The involvement of glutamate receptors is not surprising because the long-lasting effects that are witnessed in OIH would require neural plasticity, changes that likely require glutamate receptors. However, the ability of glutamate blockade to effectively treat OIH is questioned because neural plastic changes that occur in OIH affect not only the sensitivity of the glutamate receptor, but also the perceived decreased responsiveness of the μ-opioid receptor. Blockade of the glutamate receptor would transiently reverse the nociceptive behavior; however, it would not address the changes that have occurred in the μ-opioid-receptor-bearing cell [74].

Very little is known about the interaction between chemokine receptors and the μ-opioid receptor. However, a potentially key discovery is the documented interaction between μ-opioid receptor agonists and lymphocytes. In this set of experiments, Steele and colleagues [120] determined that exposure of monocytes and lymphocytes to μ-opioid receptor agonists produced an increase in the expression of the HIV viral coat protein coreceptors, CCR5 and CXCR4, respectively. The pragmatic outcome of such an experiment is that intravenous heroin users, in addition to risky lifestyle choices (sharing needles and having unprotected sex [33]), are more susceptible to HIV infection as a result of the effects of heroin on chemokine receptor upregulation. Taken together, these observations lead us to the question of whether exposure to opioids and subsequent increases in chemokine/receptor signaling are central to opioid-induced hyperalgesia. Moreover, if increased chemokine signaling is a central feature of opioid-induced hyperalgesia, which cell type is more important in the initiation of the paradoxical nociceptive behavior—the glial cell or the neuron?

Any cell type within the nervous system may that bears the μ-opioid receptor can conceivably serve as a potential source of chemokine receptor signaling following chronic morphine treatment, including non-neuronal cells [144]. Candidate non-neuronal cells include leukocytes, fibroblasts, and endothelial cells [145]. However, CXCR4-receptor-bearing cells in the CNS are largely restricted to neurogenic regions [126]. Peripheral nervous system expression of either of the HIV-1 coreceptors is restricted to CXCR4 [13]. Bhangoo and colleagues [13] further demonstrated that the chemokine receptor CXCR4 and its cognate ligand, SDF1, is restricted to nonmyelinating satellite glial cells in the naive DRG. Following chronic morphine treatment and subsequent induction of OIH, the same group demonstrated that the CXCR4-receptor antagonist can completely attenuate tactile hypernociceptive behavior [147].

A confounding factor regarding opioid-induced increases in chemokine production and release by glial cells is the complete lack of opioid receptors on glia [16]. Possible exceptions to this rule exist in the form of recently discovered non-classical opioid receptors. Recent investigations by Watkins and her group have discovered that opioids can cause direct glial activation (astrocytes and microglial cells) in a nonclassical opioid receptor fashion via the bacterial endotoxin (lipopolysaccharide) receptor, toll-like receptor 4 (TLR4) [53]. This is a remarkable finding because TLR4 normally enables innate immune cells and many glial cells in both the CNS [139] and PNS [19,138] to respond to bacterial infection by releasing proinflammatory cytokines and chemokines [139]. Two recent reports even implicate sensory neurons as bearers of TLR4 [2,135]. Whether neuron cells respond to opioids via TLR4, like their glial cell counterparts in the CNS (astrocytes), is unknown.

The Inflammatory Cascade

Beside direct actions on nerve endings and ion channels, cytokines may exert their effects through several other pain mediators. These interactions are not completely understood, but there is evidence for an important role of cytokines as initiators of several downstream cascades.

Neuropeptides

Substance P acts as a neurotransmitter, neuromodulator, or trophic factor via its G-protein-linked neurokinin receptor type 1. Calcitonin gene-related peptide (CGRP) is a potent vasodilatator and is also involved in the induction of pain. The secretion of both substance P and CGRP can be induced by cytokines. IL-1β induces increased release of substance P [73] and CGRP [43], and IL-6 contributes to the expression of substance P in sensory neurons [43]. TNF induces the production of substance P in sympathetic ganglia [31]. As mentioned above, TNF and IL-1β facilitate heat-evoked CGRP release [94]. Intramuscular injection of TNF increases CGRP levels in muscle tissue [111]. Interestingly, endogenous TNF, which is produced in injured nerves, is transported anterogradely to muscle, where it might induce CGRP release.

There is also considerable overlap between the neuropeptides CGRP and substance P and the chemokine MCP-1 given that large dense-core vesicles present in sensory neurons colocalize with CGRP following peripheral injury [57,101]. There is also evidence of neuronal secretion of MCP-1 concurrent with CGRP or substance P release [57,101].

Bradykinin

Bradykinin, formed from kininogens by cleavage of kallikrein and acting via two receptors, the kinin B1 and B2 receptors, is one of the most potent algesic peptides. The increased expression of bradykinin receptors plays a major role in inflammatory hyperalgesia. This upregulation is facilitated by cytokines such as IL-1β [75]. IL-1β but not TNF-α induces B1 receptors, which then mediate thermal hyperalgesia [97]. Recently, the B2 receptor was shown to be responsible for inflammatory hyperalgesia mediated by TNF and IL-1β [24]. In turn, bradykinin induces the secretion of TNF and IL-1β from macrophages [124].

Prostaglandins

TNF, IL-1β, and IL-6 are potent inducers of prostaglandins. The i.pl. injection of IL-1β, for instance, leads to reduced paw-withdrawal latencies in a prostaglandin-dependent manner [38]. TNF also induces the release of prostaglandins [22]. A TNF-induced increase in capsaicin sensitivity in rat DRG neurons was also shown to be mediated by prostaglandins [86].

Nerve Growth Factor

TNF and IL-1β induce NGF in inflamed tissue. IL-1β triggers the secretion of NGF from macrophages. Intramuscular injection of TNF also upregulates NGF [111], which is excitatory to mechanosensitive group IV muscle afferents [49].

Opioid Peptides

Under inflammatory conditions, opioid peptides are produced in increased amounts in the DRG and are axonally transported to the periphery [83]. Similarly, the synthesis of opioid receptors is increased, and these receptors are also transported peripherally. This effect can be produced by i.pl. injection of IL-1β [100]. In vitro, IL-1β induces the secretion of opioid peptides from lymphocytes, and the injection of IL-1β into the inflamed paw of a rat has hypoalgesic effects [109]. In vivo, the release of opioid peptides is enhanced by IL-1β, IL-6, and TNF, which leads to peripheral analgesia [25]. Chemokines may increase the number of leukocytes in inflamed tissue that carry opioid peptides and may thus contribute to analgesia [104].

Painful Disorders with a Presumed Role of Cytokines or Chemokines

Many studies show correlative data between cytokine/chemokine levels and human painful disorders (see Table I). In some of them, a causative role for cytokines in both the disease and the associated pain seems likely, given the results of treatment directed at reduction of the inflammatory mediators.

Rheumatoid Arthritis

Rheumatoid arthritis is a prototypic disease in which both disease progression and pain are determined by proinflammatory cytokines. TNF and IL-1β levels in synovial fluid of affected joints correlate with patients' symptoms and disability, and both TNF- and IL-1 inhibitors are clinically effective in reducing disease progression, inflammation, and pain [6]. The TNF antagonists etanercept and infliximab are now widely used in patients with rheumatoid arthritis refractory to other treatments, as well as in other chronic inflammatory diseases.

Chemokines, not unlike cytokines, are thought to be a central influence in the disease progress by attracting a variety of cell types to inflamed tissue. Whether chemokines or their receptors modulate the pain associated with rheumatoid arthritis is largely unknown.

Table I
Examples of human painful disorders involving cytokines or chemokines

Disorder	Cytokines	Refs.
Rheumatoid arthritis	TNF, IL-1β, IL-6, CCL2	[34,103]
Craniomandibular dysfunction	IL-1β, IL-6, TNF	[70]
Leprosy	TNF, IL-1β	[107]
Peripheral neuropathies	TNF, IL-2	[129]
Complex regional pain syndrome	TNF, IL-2, IL-6, CCL2	[4,127]
Fibromyalgia syndrome	IL-4, IL-10*	[129]
Chronic pelvic pain syndrome	CCL2, CCL3	[28]

Abbreviations: IL = interleukin, TNF = tumor necrosis factor.
* Reduced levels.

Craniomandibular Dysfunction

Painful temporomandibular joint dysfunction or craniomandibular dysfunction is another condition with a well-established role for cytokines (for review, see [70]). IL-1β, IL-6, and TNF have been found in the joint fluid, and TNF levels correlated with tenderness on palpation, indicating a contribution to local hyperalgesia (for review, see [64]). Elevated cytokine levels were associated with worse outcome. On the other hand, a deficiency of the anti-inflammatory mediators IL-1 receptor antagonist (IL-1ra), IL-10, and TGF-β1 was found in affected joints, and the presence of IL-1ra was associated with lower pain intensity. Arthrocentesis is regarded as a therapeutic measure to reduce inflammatory mediators from the temporomandibular joint fluid [59].

Leprosy and Other Neuropathies

A striking correlation between cytokine levels and neuropathic pain was observed in patients with leprosy, where a subgroup of patients with elevated serum levels of TNF and IL-1β suffer from excruciating pain [107]. Treatment of leprosy with thalidomide reduces TNF-α secretion in peripheral blood mononuclear cells by >90% and greatly reduces pain in these patients [8]. Despite its deleterious side effects, thalidomide is still used in the clinic for the treatment of various painful TNF-mediated diseases. Recently, treatment with infliximab was reported to completely abolish symptoms of erythema nodosum leprosum [36].

In other human neuropathies, preliminary data also point to a correlation between cytokine expression and pain. In a series of sural nerve biopsies, cytokine levels were increased more often in patients with painful neuropathies. Recently, it was shown that patients with peripheral neuropathies display a certain proinflammatory cytokine blood profile (increased IL-2 and TNF, lowered IL-10 and IL-4) that seems to be associated with pain [128]. Occasionally, TNF inhibitors have been used to treat inflammatory neuropathies, but data on pain are lacking in these reports.

Complex Regional Pain Syndrome (CRPS)

The phenotype of CRPS is suggestive of inflammation, and so the involvement of the cytokine system has been assumed (see Chapter 16). Studies on systemic changes in cytokine expression have given conflicting results, with elevated or unchanged protein levels of proinflammatory cytokines in the serum and cerebrospinal fluid of patients with CRPS. However, the local production of proinflammatory cytokines is elevated in the affected extremity [54,112], and this increase even outlasts the clinical symptoms [84]. Recently we found an increase of TNF and IL-2 mRNA and protein levels in the blood of patients with CRPS, along with reduced levels of the anti-inflammatory cytokines IL-4 and IL-10 [127]. Interestingly, there are reports about an improvement of symptoms in patients with CRPS after treatment with TNF-α inhibitors, such as thalidomide and infliximab [20,55].

Fibromyalgia Syndrome

In chronic widespread pain and fibromyalgia, the results of the different studies analyzing local or systemic cytokine expression are divergent, mostly due to varying methodology and the heterogeneity of the patient group investigated. We examined a group of 40 patients and age- and gender-matched healthy controls with regard to their blood mRNA and serum protein levels of selected pro- and anti-inflammatory cytokines. In our cohort, the proinflammatory cytokines TNF, IL-2, and IL-8 did not differ between patients and controls. However, patients with chronic widespread pain had reduced levels of the anti-inflammatory cytokines IL-4 and IL-10 [129]. Evidence for a potential chemokine role in fibromyalgia has recently been described; however, whether there is a link between pain and chemokines is unknown [157].

Human Immunodeficiency Virus

Neuropathic pain is a topic of great concern for individuals with autoimmune or life-threatening diseases because the pain syndromes are difficult to treat and significantly detract from the quality of life. A prime example is the pain syndrome called distal symmetrical polyneuropathy, which affects as many as one-third of all HIV-infected individuals [143]. This painful sensory neuropathy frequently begins with paresthesias in the fingers and toes progressing over weeks to months, followed by the development of pain, often of a burning and lancinating nature, which can make walking very difficult. Measurements of pain hypersensitivity have demonstrated allodynia and hyperalgesia in HIV-1 infected individuals. Interestingly, as mentioned above in the context of HIV-1-associated effects on the CNS, there is no productive infection of peripheral neurons by the virus. Thus, indirect effects of HIV-1 must lead to the development of this pain state (e.g., gp120 binding to either CCR5 or CXCR4).

There are at least two ways in which HIV-1-induced distal symmetrical polyneuropathy may occur: (1) viral protein shedding in the PNS enables gp120 to indirectly produce painful neuropathy via glial/neuronal signaling in the DRG and/or spinal cord or (2) gp120 directly activates sensory neurons. Support for the indirect effect of gp120 includes the observation that perineural gp120 exposure is accompanied by nerve pathology (decreased fiber density and axonal swelling) and an upregulation of proinflammatory cytokines [143]. Injury site-induced changes following direct injection of gp120 into the rat hindpaw may also be responsible for acute tactile hyperalgesia in this model [89]. Another set of studies suggest that sensory neuron cultures subjected to gp120 exhibit neuritic degeneration and apoptosis through Schwann cell activity, which could be blocked with CXCR4 and CCR5 chemokine receptor blockers [143]. In contrast, few studies have examined the direct role of gp120-induced nociception via chemokine receptors. One such study provides evidence that exposing neonatal sensory neuron cultures to gp120 elicits neural activity [89]. A follow-up study of these initial observations suggests that perineural activation by gp120 is dependent on MCP-1/CCR2 signaling [13].

Perhaps complicating matters further, AIDS patients who are treated with highly active anti-retroviral therapeutic (HAART) agents can also develop a painful sensory neuropathy. Intriguingly, the symptoms of this syndrome are clinically indistinguishable from those of HIV-induced distal symmetrical polyneuropathy, including a burning sensation in the hands and feet and hypersensitivity to pain. The fact that the two syndromes are usually seen in association with one another makes diagnosis more difficult.

Recent studies in rats and mice by Bhangoo and colleagues [14] have shed new light on the mechanisms of HAART-induced distal symmetrical polyneuropathy. These investigators found that the HAART drug, 2',3'-dideoxycytidine (zalcitabine or ddC), produced neuropathic pain behavior, increased CXCR4 mRNA expression in the DRG, and significantly increased SDF1/CXCL12-dependent neuronal activation. Moreover, ddC-induced rodent pain behavior could be attenuated using the highly specific CXCR4 antagonist, AMD3100 [14].

Despite the aforementioned findings, little effort has been made to determine what potential interactions may occur between the neuropathology of NRTIs and gp120. In order to study this interaction, a model was developed in which the sciatic nerve was first exposed to the HIV1 viral coat glycoprotein, gp120, after which an injection of NRTI, 2'3'-dideoxycytidine (ddC), was administered [13]. Interestingly, the results of these experiments suggest that tactile hypernociception in gp120-treated animals is reversed following treatment with a CCR2 receptor antagonist, whereas the hypernociceptive behavior produced by a combination of both gp120 injury followed 14 days later by injection of ddC is effectively reversed by only the CXCR4 antagonist, AMD3100 [13]. These studies indicate that the functional upregulation of CCR2 and CXCR4 signaling systems following a combination of gp120/ddc injury are central to distal symmetrical polyneuropathy and may serve as potential therapeutic targets.

Drugs Targeting Cytokines and Chemokines and Their Possible Role in Analgesia

Glucocorticoids

Glucocorticoids have been in clinical usage for decades. Their mechanism of action in the context of cytokines is mainly assumed to involve inhibition of NF-κB, which is crucial for regulation of proinflammatory cytokine and chemokine gene expression. Glucocorticoids have antihyperalgesic effects in animal models of neuropathic pain, concomitant with reductions in cytokine levels [39,151]. In humans glucocorticoids are the first-line treatment in painful diseases such as acute CRPS and radiculopathies [76], where cytokines are assumed to be involved in the generation of pain.

Chemokines associated with inflammatory process are typically thought to be NF-κB-dependent. It follows that glucocorticoids directly or indirectly modulate chemokine expression in many tissue types. Despite ample experimental evidence that glucocorticoids modulate chemokine expression in targets external to the nervous system, there have been relatively few investigations on the effects of corticosteroids on levels of chemokines in the nervous system and none that address issues of pathological pain.

Thalidomide

Thalidomide was banned from the medical market because of severe teratogenic effects, but it was later rediscovered as a therapeutic option in otherwise incurable dermatological conditions, cancer, and gastrointestinal diseases. The discovery that thalidomide can inhibit TNF production, degrade TNF mRNA, and recruit IL-10-producing macrophages made it an interesting candidate as a potential analgesic drug. Indeed, the application of thalidomide reduced hyperalgesia in CCI [115] and had an antinociceptive effect on zymosan-induced articular incapacitation in rats [131]. Today thalidomide is the first-line treatment in painful erythema nodosum leprosum.

Thalidomide also has a profound ability to modulate chemokine expression under both experimental and clinical conditions. Again, the impact of thalidomide on chemokines/receptors in the nervous system remains to be explored. Current reports on teratogenic cases after treatment with thalidomide show that great caution is still necessary and that equally effective but less toxic derivatives are needed [96].

Pentoxifylline

Pentoxifylline was initially used to ameliorate blood circulation in patients with vascular diseases. Additionally, it is a nonspecific cytokine inhibitor that reduces levels of proinflammatory cytokines such as TNF-α, IL-2 and IFN-γ and increases IL-10 levels in experiments in vitro. The analgesic potential of pentoxifylline has been demonstrated in different animal models [130,150]. In clinical studies, pentoxifylline was beneficial in postoperative pain and lessened morphine consumption with a concomitant reduction of serum proinflammatory cytokine levels [71,150].

Specific TNF and IL-1 Inhibitors

Currently three TNF inhibitors are in clinical usage, mostly in different types of painful arthritis. Etanercept is a p75 TNF receptor/immunoglobulin G-fusion protein that prevents the interaction of TNF with its physiological receptors. It is successfully used in patients with rheumatoid arthritis, where several randomized controlled trials have shown its effectiveness [82]. Further TNF inhibitors are the chimeric anti-TNF antibody infliximab, and adalimumab, a completely human monoclonal anti-TNF antibody [60,141]. Anakinra is an IL-1 receptor antagonist already in clinical use in painful rheumatoid arthritis [40].

Further Cytokine Modulators

The analgesic properties of anti-inflammatory cytokines have been increasingly recognized through findings from animal experiments [46,80] and in patients [129]. Drugs that restore the balance between pro- and anti-inflammatory cytokines might be helpful in chronic painful conditions. Many drugs influence the cytokine system as a "side effect" [5], and their potential remains to be explored. Whether gene therapy for neuropathic pain will become a clinical reality, as suggested by experimental data [152], remains to be shown.

References

[1] Abbadie C, Lindia JA, Cumiskey AM, Peterson LB, Mudgett JS, Bayne EK, DeMartino JA, MacIntyre DE, Forrest MJ. Impaired neuropathic pain responses in mice lacking the chemokine receptor CCR2. Proc Natl Acad Sci USA 2003;100:7947–52.

[2] Acosta C, Davies A. Bacterial lipopolysaccharide regulates nociceptin expression in sensory neurons. J Neurosci Res 2008;86:1077–86.

[3] Aggarwal BB. Signalling pathways of the TNF superfamily: a double-edged sword. Nat Rev Immunol 2003;3:745–56.

[4] Alexander GM, Perreault MJ, Reichenberger ER, Schwartzman RJ. Changes in immune and glial markers in the CSF of patients with Complex Regional Pain Syndrome. Brain Behav Immun 2007;21:668–76.

[5] Alkharfy KM, Kellum JA, Matzke GR. Unintended immunomodulation: part II. Effects of pharmacological agents on cytokine activity. Shock 2000;13:346–60.

[6] Arend WP, Dayer JM. Cytokines and cytokine inhibitors or antagonists in rheumatoid arthritis. Arthritis Rheum 1990;33:305–15.

[7] Bajetto A, Bonavia R, Barbero S, Schettini G. Characterization of chemokines and their receptors in the central nervous system: physiopathological implications. J Neurochem 2002;82:1311–29.

[8] Barnes PF, Chatterjee D, Brennan PJ, Rea TH, Modlin RL. Tumor necrosis factor production in patients with leprosy. Infect Immun 1992;60:1441–6.

[9] Bazan JF, Bacon KB, Hardiman G, Wang W, Soo K, Rossi D, Greaves DR, Zlotnik A, Schall TJ. A new class of membrane-bound chemokine with a CX3C motif. Nature 1997;385:640–4.

[10] Beattie EC, Stellwagen D, Morishita W, Bresnahan JC, Ha BK, Von Zastrow M, Beattie MS, Malenka RC. Control of synaptic strength by glial TNFalpha. Science 2002;295:2282–5.

[11] Bezzi P, Domercq M, Vesce S, Volterra A. Neuron-astrocyte cross-talk during synaptic transmission: physiological and neuropathological implications. Prog Brain Res 2001;132:255–65.

[12] Bhangoo S, Ren D, Miller RJ, Henry KJ, Lineswala J, Hamdouchi C, Li B, Monahan PE, Chan DM, Ripsch MS, White FA. Delayed functional expression of neuronal chemokine receptors following focal nerve demyelination in the rat: a mechanism for the development of chronic sensitization of peripheral nociceptors. Mol Pain 2007;3:38.

[13] Bhangoo S, Ripsch MS, Miller RJ, White FA. Increased chemokine signaling in a rodent model of HIV-associated painful neuropathy. 38th Society for Neuroscience Annual Meeting. Washington, DC; 2008.

[14] Bhangoo SK, Ren D, Miller RJ, Chan DM, Ripsch MS, Weiss C, McGinnis C, White FA. CXCR4 chemokine receptor signaling mediates pain hypersensitivity in association with antiretroviral toxic neuropathy. Brain Behav Immun 2007;21:581–91.

[15] Bolin LM, Murray R, Lukacs NW, Strieter RM, Kunkel SL, Schall TJ, Bacon KB. Primary sensory neurons migrate in response to the chemokine RANTES. J Neuroimmunol 1998;81:49–57.

[16] Börner C, Stumm R, Hollt V, Kraus J. Comparative analysis of mu-opioid receptor expression in immune and neuronal cells. J Neuroimmunol 2007;188:56–63.

[17] Celerier E, Rivat C, Jun Y, Laulin JP, Larcher A, Reynier P, Simonnet G. Long-lasting hyperalgesia induced by fentanyl in rats: preventive effect of ketamine. Anesthesiology 2000;92:465–72.

[18] Charo IF, Ransohoff RM. The many roles of chemokines and chemokine receptors in inflammation. N Engl J Med 2006;354:610–21.

[19] Cheng C, Qin Y, Shao X, Wang H, Gao Y, Cheng M, Shen A. Induction of TNF-alpha by LPS in Schwann cell is regulated by MAPK activation signals. Cell Mol Neurobiol 2007;27:909–21.

[20] Ching DW, McClintock A, Beswick F. Successful treatment with low-dose thalidomide in a patient with both Behcet's disease and complex regional pain syndrome type I: case report. J Clin Rheumatol 2003;9:96–8.

[21] Cuellar JM, Montesano PX, Carstens E. Role of TNF-alpha in sensitization of nociceptive dorsal horn neurons induced by application of nucleus pulposus to L5 dorsal root ganglion in rats. Pain 2004;110:578–87.

[22] Cunha F, Poole S, Lorenzetti B, Ferreira S. The pivotal role of tumor necrosis factor alpha in the development of inflammatory hyperalgesia. Br J Pharmacol 1992;107:660–4.

[23] Cunha FQ, Poole S, Lorenzetti BB, Veiga FH, Ferreira SH. Cytokine-mediated inflammatory hyperalgesia limited by interleukin-4. Br J Pharmacol 1999;126:45–50.

[24] Cunha TM, Verri WA, Jr., Fukada SY, Guerrero AT, Santodomingo-Garzon T, Poole S, Parada CA, Ferreira SH, Cunha FQ. TNF-alpha and IL-1beta mediate inflammatory hypernociception in mice triggered by B1 but not B2 kinin receptor. Eur J Pharmacol 2007;573:221–9.

[25] Czlonkowski A, Stein C, Herz A. Peripheral mechanisms of opioid antinociception in inflammation: involvement of cytokines. Eur J Pharmacol 1993;242:229–35.

[26] de Haas AH, van Weering HR, de Jong EK, Boddeke HW, Biber KP. Neuronal chemokines: versatile messengers in central nervous system cell interaction. Mol Neurobiol 2007;36:137–51.

[27] DeLeo JA, Rutkowski MD, Stalder AK, Campbell IL. Transgenic expression of TNF by astrocytes increases mechanical allodynia in a mouse neuropathy model. Neuroreport 2000;11:599–602.

[28] Desireddi NV, Campbell PL, Stern JA, Sobkoviak R, Chuai S, Shahrara S, Thumbikat P, Pope RM, Landis JR, Koch AE, Schaeffer AJ. Monocyte chemoattractant protein-1 and macrophage inflammatory protein-1alpha as possible biomarkers for the chronic pelvic pain syndrome. J Urol 2008;179:1857–61; discussion 1861–2.

[29] Diem R, Meyer R, Weishaupt JH, Bahr M. Reduction of potassium currents and phosphatidylinositol 3-kinase- dependent AKT phosphorylation by tumor necrosis factor-(alpha) rescues axotomized retinal ganglion cells from retrograde cell death in vivo. J Neurosci 2001;21:2058–66.

[30] Dinarello CA. Interleukin-1 family [IL-1F1, F2]. In: Thomson AW, Lotze MT, editors. The cytokine handbook. London: Academic Press; 2004. p. 643–68.

[31] Ding M, Hart RP, Jonakait GM. Tumor necrosis factor-alpha induces substance P in sympathetic ganglia through sequential induction of interleukin-1 and leukemia inhibitory factor. J Neurobiol 1995;28:445–54.

[32] Ding YZ, Fu S, Zamarin D, Bromberg J. Interleukin 10. In: Thomson AW, Lotze MT, editors. The cytokine handbook. 4th ed. London: Academic Press; 2004. p. 603–25.

[33] Donahoe RM, Vlahov D. Opiates as potential cofactors in progression of HIV-1 infections to AIDS. J Neuroimmunol 1998;83:77–87.

[34] Ellingsen T, Buus A, Stengaard-Pedersen K. Plasma monocyte chemoattractant protein 1 is a marker for joint inflammation in rheumatoid arthritis. J Rheumatol 2001;28:41–6.

[35] Eltayeb S, Berg AL, Lassmann H, Wallstrom E, Nilsson M, Olsson T, Ericsson-Dahlstrand A, Sunnemark D. Temporal expression and cellular origin of CC chemokine receptors CCR1, CCR2 and CCR5 in the central nervous system: insight into mechanisms of MOG-induced EAE. J Neuroinflammation 2007;4:14.

[36] Faber WR, Jensema AJ, Goldschmidt WF. Treatment of recurrent erythema nodosum leprosum with infliximab. N Engl J Med 2006;355:739.

[37] Fan H, Cook JA. Molecular mechanisms of endotoxin tolerance. J Endotoxin Res 2004;10:71–84.

[38] Ferreira S, Lorenzetti B, Bristow A, Poole S. Interleukin-1β as a potent hyperalgesic agent antagonized by a tripeptide analogue. Nature 1988;334:698–700.

[39] Ferreira SH, Cunha FQ, Lorenzetti BB, Michelin MA, Perretti M, Flower RJ, Poole S. Role of lipocortin-1 in the antihyperalgesic actions of dexamethasone. Br J Pharmacol 1997;121:883–8.

[40] Fleischmann RM, Schechtman J, Bennett R, Handel ML, Burmester GR, Tesser J, Modafferi D, Poulakos J, Sun G. Anakinra, a recombinant human interleukin-1 receptor antagonist (r-metHuIL-1ra), in patients with rheumatoid arthritis: a large, international, multicenter, placebo-controlled trial. Arthritis Rheum 2003;48:927–34.

[41] Fu LW, Longhurst JC. Interleukin-1beta sensitizes abdominal visceral afferents of cats to ischaemia and histamine. J Physiol (Lond) 1999;521:249–60.

[42] Fuentes ME, Durham SK, Swerdel MR, Lewin AC, Barton DS, Megill JR, Bravo R, Lira SA. Controlled recruitment of monocytes and macrophages to specific organs through transgenic expression of monocyte chemoattractant protein-1. J Immunol 1995;155:5769–76.

[43] Fukuoka H, Kawatani M, Hisamitsu T, Takeshige C. Cutaneous hyperalgesia induced by peripheral injection of interleukin-1β in the rat. Brain Res 1994;657:133–40.

[44] Giovannelli A, Limatola C, Ragozzino D, Mileo AM, Ruggieri A, Ciotti MT, Mercanti D, Santoni A, Eusebi F. CXC chemokines interleukin-8 (IL-8) and growth-related gene product alpha (GROalpha) modulate Purkinje neuron activity in mouse cerebellum. J Neuroimmunol 1998;92:122–32.

[45] Guo H, Zhao ZQ. Inhibition of nociceptive withdrawal reflex by microinjection of interleukin 2 into rat locus coeruleus. Neuropeptides 2000;34:216–20.
[46] Hao S, Mata M, Glorioso JC, Fink DJ. HSV-mediated expression of interleukin-4 in dorsal root ganglion neurons reduces neuropathic pain. Mol Pain 2006;2:6.
[47] Hao S, Mata M, Glorioso JC, Fink DJ. Gene transfer to interfere with TNFalpha signaling in neuropathic pain. Gene Ther 2007;14:1010–6.
[48] Hensellek S, Brell P, Schaible HG, Brauer R, Segond von Banchet G. The cytokine TNFalpha increases the proportion of DRG neurones expressing the TRPV1 receptor via the TNFR1 receptor and ERK activation. Mol Cell Neurosci 2007;36:381–91.
[49] Hoheisel U, Unger T, Mense S. Excitatory and modulatory effects of inflammatory cytokines and neurotrophins on mechanosensitive group IV muscle afferents in the rat. Pain 2005;114:168–76.
[50] Homma Y, Brull SJ, Zhang JM. A comparison of chronic pain behavior following local application of tumor necrosis factor alpha to the normal and mechanically compressed lumbar ganglia in the rat. Pain 2002;95:239–46.
[51] Houzen H, Kikuchi S, Kanno M, Shinpo K, Tashiro K. Tumor necrosis factor enhancement of transient outward potassium currents in cultured rat cortical neurons. J Neurosci Res 1997;50:990–9.
[52] Hudmon A, Choi JS, Tyrrell L, Black JA, Rush AM, Waxman SG, Dib-Hajj SD. Phosphorylation of sodium channel $Na_V1.8$ by p38 mitogen-activated protein kinase increases current density in dorsal root ganglion neurons. J Neurosci 2008;28:3190–201.
[53] Hutchinson MR, Bland ST, Johnson KW, Rice KC, Maier SF, Watkins LR. Opioid-induced glial activation: mechanisms of activation and implications for opioid analgesia, dependence, and reward. ScientificWorldJournal 2007;7:98–111.
[54] Huygen FJ, De Bruijn AG, De Bruin MT, Groeneweg JG, Klein J, Zijistra FJ. Evidence for local inflammation in complex regional pain syndrome type 1. Mediators Inflamm 2002;11:47–51.
[55] Huygen FJ, Niehof S, Zijlstra FJ, van Hagen PM, van Daele PL. Successful treatment of CRPS 1 with anti-TNF. J Pain Symptom Manage 2004;27:101–3.
[56] Jin X, Gereau RW. Acute p38-mediated modulation of tetrodotoxin-resistant sodium channels in mouse sensory neurons by tumor necrosis factor-alpha. J Neurosci 2006;26:246–55.
[57] Jung H, Toth PT, White FA, Miller RJ. Monocyte chemoattractant protein-1 functions as a neuromodulator in dorsal root ganglia neurons. J Neurochem 2008;104:254–63.
[58] Junger H, Sorkin LS. Nociceptive and inflammatory effects of subcutaneous TNFalpha. Pain 2000;85:145–51.
[59] Kaneyama K, Segami N, Nishimura M, Sato J, Fujimura K, Yoshimura H. The ideal lavage volume for removing bradykinin, interleukin-6, and protein from the temporomandibular joint by arthrocentesis. J Oral Maxillofac Surg 2004;62:657–61.
[60] Karppinen J, Korhonen T, Malmivaara A, Paimela L, Kyllonen E, Lindgren KA, Rantanen P, Tervonen O, Niinimaki J, Seitsalo S, et al. Tumor necrosis factor-alpha monoclonal antibody, infliximab, used to manage severe sciatica. Spine 2003;28:750–3; discussion 753–4.
[61] Kawasaki Y, Zhang L, Cheng JK, Ji RR. Cytokine mechanisms of central sensitization: distinct and overlapping role of interleukin-1beta, interleukin-6, and tumor necrosis factor-alpha in regulating synaptic and neuronal activity in the superficial spinal cord. J Neurosci 2008;28:5189–94.
[62] Kleinschnitz C, Hofstetter HH, Meuth SG, Braeuninger S, Sommer C, Stoll G. T cell infiltration after chronic constriction injury of mouse sciatic nerve is associated with interleukin-17 expression. Exp Neurol 2006;200:480–5.
[63] Koller H, Allert N, Oel D, Stoll G, Siebler M. TNF alpha induces a protein kinase C-dependent reduction in astroglial K+ conductance. Neuroreport 1998;9:1375–8.
[64] Kopp S, Sommer C. Inflammatory mediators in temporomandibular joint pain. In: Türp J, Sommer C, Hugger A, editors. The puzzle of orofacial pain: integrating research into clinical management. Basel: Karger; 2007. p. 28–43.
[65] Korn T, Magnus T, Jung S. Autoantigen specific T cells inhibit glutamate uptake in astrocytes by decreasing expression of astrocytic glutamate transporter GLAST: a mechanism mediated by tumor necrosis factor-alpha. Faseb J 2005;19:1878–80.
[66] Laulin JP, Larcher A, Celerier E, Le Moal M, Simonnet G. Long-lasting increased pain sensitivity in rat following exposure to heroin for the first time. Eur J Neurosci 1998;10:782–5.
[67] Limatola C, Ciotti MT, Mercanti D, Vacca F, Ragozzino D, Giovannelli A, Santoni A, Eusebi F, Miledi R. The chemokine growth-related gene product beta protects rat cerebellar granule cells from apoptotic cell death through alpha-amino-3-hydroxy-5-methyl-4-isoxazolepropionate receptors. Proc Natl Acad Sci USA 2000;97:6197–201.
[68] Lin JX, Leonard WJ. Interleukin-2. In: Thomson AW, Lotze MT, editors. The cytokine handbook. London: Academic Press; 2004. p. 167–88.
[69] Liu L, Yang TM, Liedtke W, Simon SA. Chronic IL-1beta signaling potentiates voltage-dependent sodium currents in trigeminal nociceptive neurons. J Neurophysiol 2006;95:1478–90.
[70] Lobbezoo F, Drangsholt M, Peck C, Sato H, Kopp S, Svensson P. Topical review: new insights into the pathology and diagnosis of disorders of the temporomandibular joint. J Orofac Pain 2004;18:181–91.
[71] Lu CH, Chao PC, Borel CO, Yang CP, Yeh CC, Wong CS, Wu CT. Preincisional intravenous pentoxifylline attenuating perioperative cytokine response, reducing morphine consumption, and improving recovery of bowel function in patients undergoing colorectal cancer surgery. Anesth Analg 2004;99:1465–71.
[72] Maier SF, Wiertelak EP, Martin D, Watkins LR. Interleukin-1 mediates the behavioral hyperalgesia produced by lithium chloride and endotoxin. Brain Res 1993;623:321–4.
[73] Malcangio M, Bowery NG, Flower RJ, Perretti M. Effect of interleukin-1 beta on the release of substance P from rat isolated spinal cord. Eur J Pharmacol 1996;299:113–8.
[74] Mao J, Price DD, Mayer DJ. Mechanisms of hyperalgesia and morphine tolerance: a current view of their possible interactions. Pain 1995;62:259–74.

[75] Marceau F. Kinin B1 receptors: a review. Immunopharmacology 1995;30:1–26.

[76] McLain RF, Kapural L, Mekhail NA. Epidural steroids for back and leg pain: mechanism of action and efficacy. Cleve Clin J Med 2004;71:961–70.

[77] Menetski J, Mistry S, Lu M, Mudgett JS, Ransohoff RM, Demartino JA, Macintyre DE, Abbadie C. Mice overexpressing chemokine ligand 2 (CCL2) in astrocytes display enhanced nociceptive responses. Neuroscience 2007;149:706–14.

[78] Meucci O, Fatatis A, Simen AA, Bushell TJ, Gray PW, Miller RJ. Chemokines regulate hippocampal neuronal signaling and gp120 neurotoxicity. Proc Natl Acad Sci USA 1998;95:14500–5.

[79] Miller RJ, Banisadr G, Bhattacharyya BJ. CXCR4 signaling in the regulation of stem cell migration and development. J Neuroimmunol 2008;198:31–8.

[80] Milligan ED, Sloane EM, Langer SJ, Hughes TS, Jekich BM, Frank MG, Mahoney JH, Levkoff LH, Maier SF, Cruz PE, et al. Repeated intrathecal injections of plasmid DNA encoding interleukin-10 produce prolonged reversal of neuropathic pain. Pain 2006;126:294–308.

[81] Milligan ED, Sloane EM, Watkins LR. Glia in pathological pain: a role for fractalkine. J Neuroimmunol 2008;198:113–120.

[82] Moreland LW, Baumgartner SW, Schiff MH, Tindall EA, Fleischmann RM, Weaver AL, Ettlinger RE, Cohen S, Koopman WJ, Mohler K, et al. Treatment of rheumatoid arthritis with a recombinant human tumor necrosis factor receptor (p75)-Fc fusion protein. N Engl J Med 1997;337:141–7.

[83] Mousa SA, Zhang Q, Sitte N, Ji R, Stein C. Beta-Endorphin-containing memory-cells and mu-opioid receptors undergo transport to peripheral inflamed tissue. J Neuroimmunol 2001;115:71–8.

[84] Munnikes RJ, Muis C, Boersma M, Heijmans-Antonissen C, Zijlstra FJ, Huygen FJ. Intermediate stage complex regional pain syndrome type 1 is unrelated to proinflammatory cytokines. Mediators Inflamm 2005;2005:366–72.

[85] Nakamura H, Nakanishi K, Kita A, Kadokawa T. Interleukin-1 induces analgesia in mice by a central action. Eur J Pharmacol 1988;149:49–54.

[86] Nicol GD, Lopshire JC, Pafford CM. Tumor necrosis factor enhances the capsaicin sensitivity of rat sensory neurons. J Neurosci 1997;17:975–82.

[87] Niederberger E, Schmidtko A, Coste O, Marian C, Ehnert C, Geisslinger G. The glutamate transporter GLAST is involved in spinal nociceptive processing. Biochem Biophys Res Commun 2006;346:393–9.

[88] Obreja O, Rathee PK, Lips KS, Distler C, Kress M. Intermediate stage complex regional pain syndrome type 1 is unrelated to proinflammatory cytokines. FASEB J 2002;16:1497–503.

[89] Oh SB, Tran PB, Gillard SE, Hurley RW, Hammond DL, Miller RJ. Chemokines and glycoprotein120 produce pain hypersensitivity by directly exciting primary nociceptive neurons. J Neurosci 2001;21:5027–35.

[90] Oka T, Aou S, Hori T. Intracerebroventricular injection of interleukin-1β induces hyperalgesia in rats. Brain Res 1993;624:61–8.

[91] Oka T, Oka K, Hosoi M, Hori T. Intracerebroventricular injection of interleukin-6 induces thermal hyperalgesia in rats. Brain Res 1995;692:123–8.

[92] Okada H, Banchereau J, Lotze MT. Interleukin 4. In: Thomson AW, Lotze MT, editors. The cytokine handbook, 4th ed. London: Academic Press; 2003. p. 227–62.

[93] Onda A, Hamba M, Yabuki S, Kikuchi S. Exogenous tumor necrosis factor-alpha induces abnormal discharges in rat dorsal horn neurons. Spine 2002;27:1618–24.

[94] Opree A, Kress M. Involvement of the proinflammatory cytokines tumor necrosis factor-alpha, IL-1beta, and IL-6 but not IL-8 in the development of heat hyperalgesia: effects on heat-evoked calcitonin gene-related peptide release from rat skin. J Neurosci 2000;20:6289–93.

[95] Ossipov MH, Lai J, King T, Vanderah TW, Malan TP, Jr., Hruby VJ, Porreca F. Antinociceptive and nociceptive actions of opioids. J Neurobiol 2004;61:126–48.

[96] Paumgartten FJ, Chahoud I. Thalidomide embryopathy cases in Brazil after 1965. Reprod Toxicol 2006;22:1–2.

[97] Perkins MN, Kelly D. Interleukin-1β induced desArg9 bradykinin-mediated thermal hyperalgesia in the rat. Neuropharmacology 1994;33:657–60.

[98] Plumb J, Cross AK, Surr J, Haddock G, Smith T, Bunning RA, Woodroofe MN. ADAM-17 and TIMP3 protein and mRNA expression in spinal cord white matter of rats with acute experimental autoimmune encephalomyelitis. J Neuroimmunol 2005;164:1–9.

[99] Poole S, Cunha FQ, Selkirk S, Lorenzetti BB, Ferreira SH. Cytokine-mediated inflammatory hyperalgesia limited by interleukin-10. Br J Pharmacol 1995;115:684–8.

[100] Puehler W, Zollner C, Brack A, Shaqura MA, Krause H, Schafer M, Stein C. Rapid upregulation of mu opioid receptor mRNA in dorsal root ganglia in response to peripheral inflammation depends on neuronal conduction. Neuroscience 2004;129:473–9.

[101] Qin X, Wan Y, Wang X. CCL2 and CXCL1 trigger calcitonin gene-related peptide release by exciting primary nociceptive neurons. J Neurosci Res 2005;82:51–62.

[102] Reeve AJ, Patel S, Fox A, Walker K, Urban L. Intrathecally administered endotoxin or cytokines produce allodynia, hyperalgesia and changes in spinal cord neuronal responses to nociceptive stimuli in the rat. Eur J Pain 2000;4:247–57.

[103] Ridderstad A, Abedi-Valugerdi M, Moller E. Cytokines in rheumatoid arthritis. Ann Med 1991;23:219–23.

[104] Rittner HL, Brack A, Stein C. The other side of the medal: how chemokines promote analgesia. Neurosci Lett 2008;437:203–8.

[105] Sabsovich I, Guo TZ, Wei T, Zhao R, Li X, Clark DJ, Geis C, Sommer C, Kingery WS. TNF signaling contributes to the development of nociceptive sensitization in a tibia fracture model of complex regional pain syndrome type I. Pain 2008;137:507–19.

[106] Saeki T, Naya A. CCR1 chemokine receptor antagonist. Curr Pharm Des 2003;9:1201–8.

[107] Sarno EN, Grau GE, Vieira LM, Nery JA. Serum levels of tumour necrosis factor-alpha and interleukin-1 beta during leprosy reactional states. Clin Exp Immunol 1991;84:103–8.
[108] Sawada M, Hara N, Maeno T. Tumor necrosis factor reduces the ACh-induced outward current in identified *Aplysia* neurons. Neurosci Lett 1991;131:217–20.
[109] Schäfer M, Carter L, Stein C. Interleukin 1 beta and corticotropin-releasing factor inhibit pain by releasing opioids from immune cells in inflamed tissue. Proc Natl Acad Sci USA 1994;91:4219–23.
[110] Schäfers M, Lee DH, Brors D, Yaksh TL, Sorkin LS. Increased sensitivity of injured and adjacent uninjured rat primary sensory neurons to exogenous tumor necrosis factor-alpha after spinal nerve ligation. J Neurosci 2003;23:3028–38.
[111] Schäfers M, Sorkin LS, Sommer C. Intramuscular injection of tumor necrosis factor-alpha induces muscle hyperalgesia in rats. Pain 2003;104:579–88.
[112] Schinkel C, Gaertner A, Zaspel J, Zedler S, Faist E, Schuermann M. Inflammatory mediators are altered in the acute phase of posttraumatic complex regional pain syndrome. Clin J Pain 2006;22:235–9.
[113] Sitcheran R, Gupta P, Fisher PB, Baldwin AS. Positive and negative regulation of EAAT2 by NF-kappaB: a role for N-myc in TNFalpha-controlled repression. EMBO J 2005;24:510–20.
[114] Sommer C. Cytokines and pain. In: Aminoff MJ, Boller F, Swaab DF, editors. Handbook of clinical neurology. Edinburgh: Elsevier; 2006. p. 231–48.
[115] Sommer C, Marziniak M, Myers RR. The effect of thalidomide treatment on vascular pathology and hyperalgesia caused by chronic constriction injury of rat nerve. Pain 1998;74:83–91.
[116] Sommer C, Petrausch S, Lindenlaub T, Toyka KV. Neutralizing antibodies to interleukin 1-receptor reduce pain associated behavior in mice with experimental neuropathy. Neurosci Lett 1999;270:25–8.
[117] Sommer C, Schäfers M, Marziniak M, Toyka KV. Etanercept reduces hyperalgesia in experimental painful neuropathy. J Peripher Nerv Syst 2001;6:67–72.
[118] Song P, Lie-Cheng W, Wang GD, Zhou Z, Zhao ZQ. Interleukin-2 regulates membrane potentials and calcium channels via mu opioid receptors in rat dorsal root ganglion neurons. Neuropharmacology 2002;43:1324–9.
[119] Sorkin LS, Xiao WH, Wagner R, Myers RR. Tumour necrosis factor-alpha induces ectopic activity in nociceptive primary afferent fibres. Neuroscience 1997;81:255–62.
[120] Steele AD, Henderson EE, Rogers TJ. Mu-opioid modulation of HIV-1 coreceptor expression and HIV-1 replication. Virology 2003;309:99–107.
[121] Stellwagen D, Beattie EC, Seo JY, Malenka RC. Differential regulation of AMPA receptor and GABA receptor trafficking by tumor necrosis factor-alpha. J Neurosci 2005;25:3219–28.
[122] Sun JH, Yang B, Donnelly DF, Ma C, LaMotte RH. MCP-1 enhances excitability of nociceptive neurons in chronically compressed dorsal root ganglia. J Neurophysiol 2006;96:2189–99.
[123] Szabo I, Chen XH, Xin L, Adler MW, Howard OM, Oppenheim JJ, Rogers TJ. Heterologous desensitization of opioid receptors by chemokines inhibits chemotaxis and enhances the perception of pain. Proc Natl Acad Sci USA 2002;99:10276–81.
[124] Tiffany CW, Burch RM. Bradykinin stimulates tumor necrosis factor and interleukin-1 release from macrophages. FEBS Lett 1989;247:189–92.
[125] Tiveron MC, Cremer H. CXCL12/CXCR4 signalling in neuronal cell migration. Curr Opin Neurobiol 2008;18:237–44.
[126] Tran PB, Banisadr G, Ren D, Chenn A, Miller RJ. Chemokine receptor expression by neural progenitor cells in neurogenic regions of mouse brain. J Comp Neurol 2007;500:1007–33.
[127] Üçeyler N, Eberle T, Rolke R, Birklein F, Sommer C. Differential expression patterns of cytokines in complex regional pain syndrome. Pain 2007;132:195–205.
[128] Üçeyler N, Rogausch JP, Toyka KV, Sommer C. Differential expression of cytokines in painful and painless neuropathies. Neurology 2007;69:42–9.
[129] Üçeyler N, Valenza R, Stock M, Schedel R, Sprotte G, Sommer C. Reduced levels of antiinflammatory cytokines in patients with chronic widespread pain. Arthritis Rheum 2006;54:2656–64.
[130] Vale ML, Benevides VM, Sachs D, Brito GA, da Rocha FA, Poole S, Ferreira SH, Cunha FQ, Ribeiro RA. Antihyperalgesic effect of pentoxifylline on experimental inflammatory pain. Br J Pharmacol 2004.
[131] Vale ML, Cunha FQ, Brito GA, Benevides VM, Ferreira SH, Poole S, Ribeiro RA. Anti-nociceptive effect of thalidomide on zymosan-induced experimental articular incapacitation. Eur J Pharmacol 2006;536:309–17.
[132] Vale ML, Marques JB, Moreira CA, Rocha FA, Ferreira SH, Poole S, Cunha FQ, Ribeiro RA. Antinociceptive effects of interleukin-4, -10, and -13 on the writhing response in mice and zymosan-induced knee joint incapacitation in rats. J Pharmacol Exp Ther 2003;304:102–8.
[133] Veldkamp CT, Seibert C, Peterson FC, De la Cruz NB, Haugner JC 3rd, Basnet H, Sakmar TP, Volkman BF. Structural basis of CXCR4 sulfotyrosine recognition by the chemokine SDF-1/CXCL12. Sci Signal 2008;1:ra4.
[134] Vogel C, Stallforth S, Sommer C. Altered pain behavior and regeneration after nerve injury in TNF receptor deficient mice. J Peripher Nerv Syst 2006;11:294–303.
[135] Wadachi R, Hargreaves KM. Trigeminal nociceptors express TLR-4 and CD14: a mechanism for pain due to infection. J Dent Res 2006;85:49–53.
[136] Wagner R, Janjigian M, Myers RR. Anti-inflammatory interleukin-10 therapy in CCI neuropathy decreases thermal hyperalgesia, macrophage recruitment, and endoneurial TNF-alpha expression. Pain 1998;74:35–42.
[137] Wallace DJ, Margolin K, Waller P. Fibromyalgia and interleukin-2 therapy for malignancy. Ann Intern Med 1988;108:909.
[138] Wang JG, Strong JA, Xie W, Zhang JM. Local inflammation in rat dorsal root ganglion alters excitability and ion currents in small-diameter sensory neurons. Anesthesiology 2007;107:322–32.
[139] Watkins LR, Hutchinson MR, Milligan ED, Maier SF. "Listening" and "talking" to neurons: implications of immune activation for pain control and increasing the efficacy of opioids. Brain Res Rev 2007;56:148–69.

[140] Watkins LR, Wiertelak EP, Goehler LE, Smith KP, Martin D, Maier SF. Characterization of cytokine-induced hyperalgesia. Brain Res 1994;654:15–26.

[141] Weinblatt ME, Keystone EC, Furst DE, Moreland LW, Weisman MH, Birbara CA, Teoh LA, Fischkoff SA, Chartash EK. Adalimumab, a fully human anti-tumor necrosis factor alpha monoclonal antibody, for the treatment of rheumatoid arthritis in patients taking concomitant methotrexate: the ARMADA trial. Arthritis Rheum 2003;48:35–45.

[142] Wells MR, Racis SP Jr, Vaidya U. Changes in plasma cytokines associated with peripheral nerve injury. J Neuroimmunol 1992;39:261–8.

[143] White FA, Bhangoo SK, Miller RJ. Chemokines: integrators of pain and inflammation. Nat Rev Drug Discov 2005;4:834–44.

[144] White FA, Jung H, Miller RJ. Chemokines and the pathophysiology of neuropathic pain. Proc Natl Acad Sci USA 2007;104:20151–8.

[145] White FA, Monahan P, LaMotte RH. Chemokines and their receptors in the nervous system: a link to neuropathic pain. In: Watkins LA, DeLeo JA, Sorkin L, editors. Immune and glial activation in pain. Seattle: IASP Press; 2007.

[146] White FA, Sun J, Waters SM, Ma C, Ren D, Ripsch M, Steflik J, Cortright DN, Lamotte RH, Miller RJ. Excitatory monocyte chemoattractant protein-1 signaling is up-regulated in sensory neurons after chronic compression of the dorsal root ganglion. Proc Natl Acad Sci USA 2005;102:14092–7.

[147] Wilson NM, Jung H, Ripsch MS, Miller RJ, White FA. Opioid-induced tactile hypernociception is attenuated by the CXCR4 antagonist AMD3100. Soc Neurosci Abstr 2008;270.14.

[148] Winkelstein BA, Rutkowski MD, Sweitzer SM, Pahl JL, DeLeo JA. Nerve injury proximal or distal to the DRG induces similar spinal glial activation and selective cytokine expression but differential behavioral responses to pharmacologic treatment. J Comp Neurol 2001;439:127–39.

[149] Wolf G, Gabay E, Tal M, Yirmiya R, Shavit Y. Genetic impairment of interleukin-1 signaling attenuates neuropathic pain, autotomy, and spontaneous ectopic neuronal activity, following nerve injury in mice. Pain 2006;120:315–24.

[150] Wordliczek J, Szczepanik AM, Banach M, Turchan J, Zembala M, Siedlar M, Przewlocki R, Serednicki W, Przewlocka B. The effect of pentoxifylline on post-injury hyperalgesia in rats and postoperative pain in patients. Life Sci 2000;66:1155–64.

[151] Xie W, Luo S, Xuan H, Chou C, Song G, Lv R, Jin Y, Li W, Xu J. Betamethasone affects cerebral expressions of NF-kappaB and cytokines that correlate with pain behavior in a rat model of neuropathy. Ann Clin Lab Sci 2006;36:39–46.

[152] Yao MZ, Gu JF, Wang JH, Sun LY, Liu H, Liu XY. Adenovirus-mediated interleukin-2 gene therapy of nociception. Gene Ther 2003;10:1392–9.

[153] Zelenka M, Schäfers M, Sommer C. Intraneural injection of interleukin-1beta and tumor necrosis factor-alpha into rat sciatic nerve at physiological doses induces signs of neuropathic pain. Pain 2005;116:257–63.

[154] Zhang J, Shi XQ, Echeverry S, Mogil JS, De Koninck Y, Rivest S. Expression of CCR2 in both resident and bone marrow-derived microglia plays a critical role in neuropathic pain. J Neurosci 2007;27:12396–406.

[155] Zhang JM, Li H, Liu B, Brull SJ. Acute topical application of tumor necrosis factor alpha evokes protein kinase A-dependent responses in rat sensory neurons. J Neurophysiol 2002;88:1387–92.

[156] Zhang N, Rogers TJ, Caterina M, Oppenheim JJ. Proinflammatory chemokines, such as C-C chemokine ligand 3, desensitize mu-opioid receptors on dorsal root ganglia neurons. J Immunol 2004;173:594–9.

[157] Zhang Z, Cherryholmes G, Mao A, Marek C, Longmate J, Kalos M, Amand RP, Shively JE. High plasma levels of MCP-1 and eotaxin provide evidence for an immunological basis of fibromyalgia. Exp Biol Med (Maywood) 2008;233:1171–80.

Correspondence to: Prof. Dr. Claudia Sommer, Department of Neurology, University of Würzburg, Josef-Schneider-Str. 11, D-97080 Würzburg, Germany. Tel: +49-931-201-23763; fax: +49-931-201-23697; email: sommer@uni-wuerzburg.de.

14

Adenosine Triphosphate and Adenosine Receptors and Pain

Geoffrey Burnstock[a] and Jana Sawynok[b]

[a]Autonomic Neuroscience Centre, Royal Free and University College Medical School, London, United Kingdom; [b]Department of Pharmacology, Dalhousie University, Halifax, Nova Scotia, Canada

The concept of purinergic signaling was proposed in 1972 following early hints of potent extracellular actions of purines in the heart and peripheral ganglia, the demonstration of the release of adenosine 5'-triphosphate (ATP) during antidromic stimulation of sensory nerve collaterals, and evidence that ATP was the transmitter in nonadrenergic, noncholinergic nerves in the gut and bladder [17]. It is now recognized that ATP is a cotransmitter in nerves in both the peripheral and central nervous systems [25] and that receptors for purines and pyrimidines are widely expressed on non-neuronal as well as nerve cells [29]. Two types of purinoceptor, identified as P1 (for adenosine) and P2 (for adenosine triphosphate or diphosphate) were proposed in 1978 [18], but it was not until 1985 that a pharmacological basis was established for distinguishing two types of P2 receptors (P2X and P2Y) [28]. Currently, seven P2X ionotropic receptor subunits and eight P2Y metabotropic receptor subtypes are recognized, and these include receptors that are sensitive to pyrimidines as well as purines [26,128] (see Table I). Four subtypes of P1 receptors have been cloned—A1, A2A, A2B, and A3 (see Table II)—all of which couple to G proteins and have seven transmembrane (TM) domains, with an extracellular NH_2 terminus and a cytoplasmic COOH terminus [50]. $P2X_{1-7}$-receptor subunits show a subunit topology of intracellular NH_2 and COOH termini, two TM-spanning regions (the first gates the ion channel and the second lines the ion pore), and a large extracellular loop. P2X-receptor subunits can combine to form either homomultimers or heteromultimers [121]. Metabotropic P2Y receptors ($P2Y_1$, $P2Y_2$, $P2Y_4$, $P2Y_6$, $P2Y_{11}$, $P2Y_{12}$, $P2Y_{13}$, and $P2Y_{14}$) have an extracellular NH_2 terminus and intracellular COOH terminus and seven TM-spanning regions [1]. Until recently, apart from vesicular release from nerves, it was usually assumed that the only source of extracellular ATP acting on purinoceptors was damaged or dying cells, but it is now recognized that ATP release from healthy cells is a physiological mechanism. In fact, ATP is released from many non-neuronal cell types during mechanical deformation in response to shear stress, stretch, or osmotic swelling, as well as hypoxia and stimulation by various agents [15]. After release, ATP and other nucleotides undergo rapid enzymatic degradation by ectonucleotidases to result in the formation of adenosine [189].

There were early hints that ATP might be involved in pain, including the demonstration of pain produced by injection of ATP into human skin blisters [13], ATP involvement in migraine [19], and ATP participation in pain pathways in the spinal cord [80]. A significant advance was made in 1995 when the $P2X_3$ ionotropic ion channel purinergic receptor was cloned and shown to be localized predominantly on small nociceptive sensory neurons in dorsal root ganglia (DRG) together with $P2X_{2/3}$ heteromultimer receptors [33,101]. A unifying purinergic hypothesis for the initiation of pain was proposed in 1996 [21]; this proposal has been followed by an increasing number of papers expanding on the concept [23,24,45]. A schematic illustrating the initiation of nociception in the periphery and purinergic relay pathways in the spinal cord is shown in Fig. 1a. While $P2X_3$ and $P2X_{2/3}$ receptors expressed in sensory neurons were the predominant P2 receptor subtypes recognized to be involved in initiating pain, it has become apparent that P2Y receptors are also present on sensory afferents [137] and that these receptors are also involved in modulating pain transmission [54].

A role for adenosine in nociception first appeared in the 1970s with the use of methylxanthines (first as inhibitors of phosphodiesterase, then as adenosine receptor antagonists) in combination with morphine [70], along with the demonstration of antinociception by systemic administration of an analogue of adenosine [172]. During the 1980s, the spinal cord became a prominent site of investigation following the demonstration that spinal administration of methylxanthines inhibited systemic effects of morphine [85],

Fig. 1. (a) Hypothetical schematic of the roles of purine nucleotide and nucleoside receptors in pain pathways. At peripheral sensory nerve terminals, $P2X_3$ and $P2X_{2/3}$ receptors are the main P2X purinoceptors; $P2Y_1$ and possibly $P2Y_2$ receptors are present on a subpopulation of $P2X_3$ receptor-immunopositive fibers. Other P2X-receptor subtypes (1–7) are also expressed at low levels in dorsal root ganglia. Adenosine (ADO) also acts on sensory terminals: A1 receptors lead to suppression of pain signaling, while A2A receptors lead to pain facilitation. In the dorsal spinal cord, ATP acts postsynaptically through $P2X_2$, $P2X_4$, and/or $P2X_6$ receptor subtypes; after breakdown to ADO, it acts as a presynaptic inhibitor of transmission through P1 (A1) receptors. ATP and glutamate are cotransmitters in primary afferent central nerve terminals. $P2X_4$ and $P2X_7$ receptors on activated microglia have been implicated in neuropathic pain. Yellow dots, molecules of ATP; blue dots, molecules of ADO. (Modified from [30] with permission from Elsevier). (b) Purinergic mechanosensory transduction. Schematic representation of hypothesis for purinergic mechanosensory transduction in tubes (e.g., ureter, vagina, salivary and bile ducts, gut) and sacs (e.g., urinary and gall bladders, lungs). It is proposed that mechanical distension leads to release of ATP from the epithelium lining the tube or sac, which then acts on $P2X_3$ and/or $P2X_{2/3}$ receptors on subepithelial sensory nerves to convey sensory/nociceptive information to the CNS. (From [22] with permission from Blackwell.) →

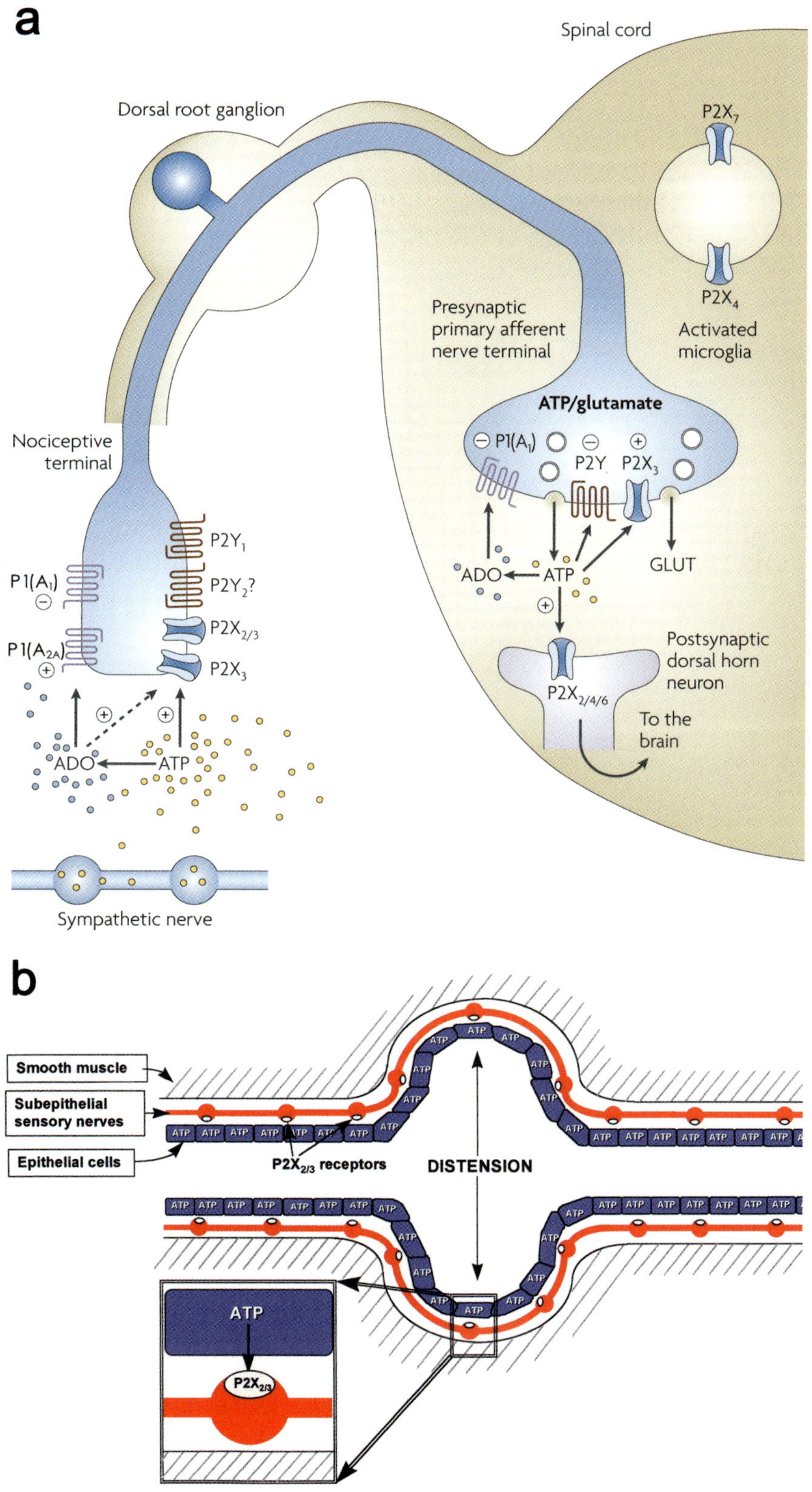
a
Spinal cord
Dorsal root ganglion
P2X7
P2X4
Activated microglia
Presynaptic primary afferent nerve terminal
ATP/glutamate
P1(A1)
P2Y
P2X3
ADO
ATP
GLUT
Postsynaptic dorsal horn neuron
P2X2/4/6
To the brain
Nociceptive terminal
P2Y1
P2Y2?
P1(A1)
P2X2/3
P1(A2A)
P2X3
ADO
ATP
Sympathetic nerve
b
Smooth muscle
Subepithelial sensory nerves
Epithelial cells
P2X2/3 receptors
DISTENSION
ATP
P2X2/3

Table I
Characteristics of P2 receptors

Receptor	Main Distribution	Main Functions
$P2X_1$	Smooth muscle, platelets, cerebellum, dorsal horn spinal neurons	Smooth muscle contraction, platelet activation
$P2X_2$	Smooth muscle, CNS, retina, chromaffin cells, autonomic and sensory ganglia	Sensory transmission and modulation of synaptic function
$P2X_3$	Sensory neurons, NTS, some sympathetic neurons	Mediates sensory transmission; facilitates glutamate release in CNS
$P2X_4$	CNS, testes, colon	Modulates chronic inflammatory and neuropathic pain
$P2X_5$	Proliferating cells in skin, gut, bladder, thymus, spinal cord	Inhibits proliferation and increase differentiation
$P2X_6$	CNS, motor neurons in spinal cord	Functions as a heteromeric channel in combination with $P2X_2$ and $P2X_4$ subunits
$P2X_7$	Apoptotic cells, e.g., immune cells, pancreas, skin	Mediates apoptosis, cell proliferation and proinflammatory cytokine release
$P2Y_1$	Epithelial and endothelial cells, platelets, immune cells, osteoclasts, glial cells	Smooth muscle relaxation and mitogenic actions; platelet shape change and aggregation; bone resorption
$P2Y_2$	Immune cells, epithelial and endothelial cells, kidney tubules, osteoblasts, astrocytes	Vasodilatation via endothelium and vasoconstriction via smooth muscle; mitogenic actions; mediates surfactant secretion; epithelial cell Cl^- secretion; bone remodeling
$P2Y_4$	Endothelial and endothelial cells, intestine, pituitary, brain (low levels in liver and bone marrow)	Regulates epithelial chloride transport; vasodilatation via endothelium; mitogenic actions
$P2Y_6$	Some epithelial cells, placenta, T cells, thymus, spleen, kidney, activated microglia	NaCl secretion in colonic epithelium; role in epithelial proliferation
$P2Y_{11}$	Spleen, intestine, brain, granulocytes	Role in maturation and migration of dendritic cells; granulocytic differentiation
$P2Y_{12}$	Platelets, glial cells, spinal cord	Platelet aggregation; role in dense granule secretion
$P2Y_{13}$	Spleen, brain, lymph nodes, bone marrow, liver, pancreas, heart	Platelet aggregation; role in dense granule secretion; function largely unknown, but present in both immune system and brain
$P2Y_{14}$	Placenta, adipose tissue, stomach, intestine, discrete brain regions, spleen, lung, heart, bone marrow, peripheral immune cells	Chemoattractant receptor in bone marrow hematopoietic stem cells; dendritic cell activation

Source: Reproduced from [27] by courtesy of the Nature Publishing Group.
Abbreviations: CNS, central nervous system; NTS, nucleus tractus solitarius.

while spinal administration of adenosine analogues produced antinociception [127]. Further studies showed that spinal methylxanthines inhibit antinociception by spinal morphine [41,163] and that morphine directly releases adenosine from the spinal cord [163]. Adenosine, with actions mediated by several receptor subtypes, is now known to be involved in pain signaling at peripheral, spinal, and supraspinal sites (see the next section), and several reviews of the actions of adenosine in relation to nociception have been published [43,140,141].

This chapter highlights key functions of ATP and adenosine in relation to pain signaling and considers the potential for pharmaceuticals and approaches based on these mediators to contribute to pain management.

Table II
Characteristics of P1 (adenosine) receptors

Receptor	Main Distribution	Main Functions
A_1	Brain, spinal cord, testes, heart, autonomic nerve terminals	Prejunctional neuromodulation of neurotransmitter release; behavioral effects (sedation, anticonvulsive, anxiolytic); cardiac depression
A_{2A}	Brain, heart, lungs, spleen	Facilitates neurotransmission; smooth muscle relaxation
A_{2B}	Large intestine, bladder	Role in allergic and inflammatory disorders; vasodilatation
A_3	Lung, liver, brain, testes, heart	Facilitates release of allergic mediators; cardioprotective and cytoprotective

Source: Reproduced from [27] by courtesy of the Nature Publishing Group.

Role of ATP and Adenosine in Pain Signaling

ATP and Pain Signaling

The Periphery

P2X receptors in sensory neurons, including those from dorsal root, trigeminal, nodose, and petrosal ganglia, have been characterized extensively [25]. All P2X-receptor subtypes are found on sensory neurons, although the $P2X_3$ receptor has the highest level of expression (both mRNA and protein) [91]. $P2X_3$ and $P2X_{2/3}$ receptors are expressed on isolectin B_4 (IB_4)-binding subpopulations of small nociceptive neurons [16]. $P2Y_1$, $P2Y_2$, $P2Y_4$, and $P2Y_6$ receptor mRNA is also expressed on neurons of DRG, nodose, and trigeminal ganglia, and receptor protein for the $P2Y_1$ receptor is localized mainly (over 80%) on small neurons; double immunolabeling reveals that ~80% of $P2X_3$-receptor-positive neurons also stain for $P2Y_1$ receptors, while ~30% also stain for $P2Y_4$ receptors [137].

A hypothesis has been proposed that purinergic mechanosensory transduction occurs in visceral tubes and sacs (including ureter, bladder, and gut), whereby ATP released from epithelial cells during distension acts on $P2X_3$ homomeric and $P2X_{2/3}$ heteromeric receptors on subepithelial sensory nerves initiating impulses in pain pathways (Fig. 1b) [22]. Evidence supporting this hypothesis is as follows. (a) Mice lacking $P2X_3$ receptors exhibit reduced inflammatory pain and marked urinary bladder hyporeflexia [35]. (b) ATP is released from urothelial cells during distension; activity in pelvic sensory nerves is mimicked by ATP and α,β-methylene ATP (α,β-meATP) and attenuated by $P2X_3$ antagonists and in $P2X_3$ knockout mice; $P2X_3$ receptors are localized on suburothelial sensory nerve fibers [173]. (c) Botulinum toxin A, which has antinociceptive effects in interstitial cystitis, inhibits distension-mediated urothelial release of ATP in conditions of bladder inflammation [32,107]. (d) Ureteric colic induced by the passage of a kidney stone causes severe pain. Immunostaining of $P2X_3$ receptors in sensory nerves in the subepithelial region has been reported [99]; distension of the ureter results in ATP release from the urothelium [92], and distension of the ureter results in increased afferent nerve discharge which is mimicked by intraluminal ATP or α,β-meATP and attenuated by 2',3'-O-(2,4,6-trinitrophenyl)-ATP (TNP-ATP) [135]. (e) In the gut, purinergic mechanosensory transduction initiates physiological reflex modulation of peristalsis via intrinsic sensory fibers and nociception via extrinsic sensory fibers [23,180]. Distension of the colorectum led to pressure-dependent increase in release of ATP from mucosal epithelial cells and also evoked pelvic nerve excitation, which was mimicked by ATP and α,β-meATP and attenuated by TNP-ATP and pyridoxalphosphate-6-azonphenyl-2',4'-disulphonic acid (PPADS). Inflammatory mediators augment $P2X_3$-receptor-mediated responses on pelvic afferent fibers in the rat colorectum [179], and $P2X_3$-receptor-mediated responses are enhanced in a model of colitis [178]. (f) It is possible that tissue stress or damage in the uterine cervix during late pregnancy and parturition may lead to ATP release and sensory signaling via $P2X_3$ receptors [125].

ATP and α,β-meATP activate nociceptive sensory nerve terminals in the skin [188], and these responses are increased in inflammatory conditions [65]. Skin cell damage causes action potential firing and inward currents in nociceptive fibers, and this response is eliminated by enzymatic degradation of ATP or blockade of P2X receptors, implicating release of cytosolic ATP [37]. Inflammation upregulates $P2X_2$ and $P2X_3$ receptors on DRG neurons [182]. $P2Y_2$ receptors on the terminals of sensory neurons in mice mediate nociceptive transmission, and P2Y signaling may contribute to mechanotransduction in low-threshold Aβ fibers [160]. A pathogenic role for keratinocyte-derived ATP in irritant dermatitis has been proposed [118]. It has been reported recently that cutaneous sensory neurons expressing a family of G-protein-coupled receptors, named mas-related G-protein-coupled receptors (Mrgprd receptors), sense extracellular ATP and are putative nociceptors [48].

ATP is also implicated in sensory signaling in several other systems. $P2X_3$ and $P2X_{2/3}$ receptors on sensory afferents in tooth pulp appear to mediate nociception [4,132], perhaps from ATP released by mechanical distension or inflammation of odontoblasts. $P2X_2$, $P2X_3$, and $P2Y_1$ receptors are abundant on sensory nerve terminals in the tongue [14]. ATP and α,β-meATP were shown to excite trigeminal lingual nerve terminals of rats in an in vitro preparation, mimicking nociceptive responses to noxious mechanical stimulation and high temperature and suggesting the involvement of purinergic mechanosensory transduction [136].

Pain related to the musculoskeletal system (myofascial pain) is common, and ATP has been claimed to excite or sensitize myofascial nociceptors [12]. Nociceptive information arising from the orofacial region via $P2X_3$ receptors on afferent fibers are carried to trigeminal brainstem sensory nuclei [91]. ATP stimulates group IV receptors in mechanically sensitive muscle afferents [131]. It enhances the muscle pressor response evoked by mechanically sensitive muscle stretch; this response was attenuated by PPADS [102]. ATP induces sustained facilitation of cranial nociception through P2X receptors on neck muscle nociceptors in mice [109]. ATP acting on $P2X_3$ receptors in sensory nerve fibers in masseter muscle plays an important role in pressure pain and mechanical hyperalgesia caused by excessive muscular contraction [154]. ATP is a stimulant of articular nociceptors in the knee joint via $P2X_3$ receptors [47,145]. $P2Y_2$-receptor mRNA is expressed in both cultured normal and osteoarthritic chondrocytes taken from human knee joints, and ATP is released by mechanical stimulation [117]. When monoarthritis was induced by injection of complete Freund's adjuvant into the unilateral temporomandibular joint of the rat, the nociception produced was associated with an increase in $P2X_3$-receptor-positive small neurons in the trigeminal ganglion [153]. Activation of P2X receptors in rat temporomandibular joint induces nociception, and blockage by PPADS decreases carrageenan-induced inflammatory hyperalgesia [124]. Oxidized ATP inhibits inflammatory pain in arthritic rats by inhibiting the $P2X_7$ receptor for ATP localized in nerve terminals [42].

The Spinal Cord

Excitation of dorsal horn neurons by ATP was recognized early [52,80] and described in more detail later (see [25]). ATP-evoked increases in intracellular calcium were demonstrated in both neurons and glia of the dorsal spinal cord [138]. Salter and Hicks later showed that the ATP-evoked release of Ca^{2+} from astrocytes was via the phospholipase C-β/inositol triphosphate pathway, suggesting mediation via a P2Y receptor. ATP was shown to inhibit slow depolarization via P2Y receptors in substantia gelatinosa neurons [185]. A recent study has identified $P2Y_1$- and $P2Y_4$-receptor mRNA in subpopulations of dorsal horn neurons, whereas motor neurons in the ventral horn expressed $P2Y_4$- and $P2Y_6$-receptor mRNA [93]. This study also showed that astrocytes in the gray matter expressed mRNA for $P2Y_1$ receptors, and that microglia throughout the spinal cord expressed mRNA for $P2Y_{12}$ receptors. Messenger RNA for $P2X_2$, $P2X_4$, and $P2X_6$ receptors has been identified within spinal motor nuclei [36].

$P2X_3$ immunoreactivity is present on the axon terminals of DRG neurons that extend across the entire mediolateral extent of inner lamina II of the dorsal horn [16,59]. The immunolabeled nerve profiles in lamina II for $P2X_3$ receptors are located largely on terminals with ultrastructural characteristics of sensory afferent terminals [105]. In contrast, although $P2X_2$ immunoreactivity is most prominent in lamina II, it is also seen in deeper layers, and only rarely overlaps with $P2X_3$ immunoreactivity [174]. At central terminals of primary afferent neurons, ATP has been shown to act either presynaptically (facilitating glutamate release) [60] or postsynaptically [9]. P2X receptors are also expressed on glycinergic presynaptic nerve terminals [81]. Distinct subtypes of P2X receptors are functionally expressed at pre- and postsynaptic sites in lamina V neurons in the rat dorsal spinal cord, and it was suggested that purinergic signaling in deep dorsal horn neurons becomes more important during postnatal development [155]. In addition to acting as a fast excitatory synaptic transmitter, ATP facilitates excitatory transmission by increasing glutamate release and enhances inhibitory neurotransmission mediated by both γ-aminobutyric acid (GABA) and glycine [73,133]. $P2X_3$ receptors are involved in transient modulation of glutamate release in lamina II of the spinal cord, but a different P2X-receptor subtype (perhaps $P2X_{1/5}$ or $P2X_{4/6}$) was involved in long-lasting modulation in lamina V [120].

Activation of P2X receptors in the spinal cord elicits allodynia, and in a seminal study published in *Nature* in 2004, $P2X_4$ receptors on spinal cord microglia were implicated in neuropathic pain using $P2X_4$ antisense oligonucleotides [168]. This latter study has led to an explosion of work focused on purinergic signaling in neuropathic pain (see the section below on ATP and neuropathic pain).

Adenosine and Pain Signaling

The Periphery

Adenosine A1, A2A, A2B, and A3 receptors (ARs) are all present at peripheral sites either directly on sensory afferent nerve terminals (A1R and A2ARs) or on adjacent cell types that can potentially influence nociception under certain conditions (A2AR, A2BR, and A3Rs) (Fig. 1a). A1Rs have been visualized directly in sensory afferent neurons using immunohistochemistry [31,144]. In functional studies, peripheral administration of A1R agonists leads to antinociception against mechanical hyperalgesia [5,164] and thermal hyperalgesia (but not mechanical allodynia) following nerve injury [104]. In vitro studies indicate that A1Rs lead to reduced Ca^{2+} entry [64], decreased cyclic AMP (cAMP) generation, and decreased peptide release in sensory neurons [31]. Changes in G proteins, cAMP, and protein kinase A (PKA) activity are implicated in antinociception by A1R agonists [90]. A2ARs are also present in DRG [86]. In functional studies, local peripheral administration of A2AR agonists leads to mechanical hyperalgesia [164] and increased flinching with formalin [44,89]. Hyperalgesia is mediated by increases in cAMP in the sensory nerve terminal, activation of PKA, phosphorylation of Na^+ channels, increased inward currents, and sensory afferent activation [57]. A2ARs also mediate anti-inflammatory and immunosuppressive effects [66,96], and such actions may contribute indirectly to reduced pain signaling in inflammatory states.

Adenosine A2B and A3 receptors have not been identified directly on sensory neurons, but their localization on mast cells and ability to contribute to aspects of inflammation make them potential indirect contributors to inflammatory pain via release of mediators from such cells. Systemic administration of A2BR antagonists produced antinociception in the hotplate test, and this effect was attributed to a peripheral site of action because an analogue that did not cross the blood-brain barrier had the same effect [2]. Furthermore, local administration of a selective A2BR antagonist (PSB-1115) inhibited pain behaviors and paw edema produced by formalin [11], and this finding also supports a pronociceptive and pro-inflammatory role of A2BRs. Adenosine A3Rs are present on several types of immune and inflammatory cells, and they exert complex pro- and anti-inflammatory effects.

Administered acutely to uninjured animals, A3R agonists promote mast cell degranulation and release of mediators that increase nociception [142]. Mice lacking A3Rs exhibit reduced hyperalgesia in response to carrageenan, and this finding is consistent with an involvement of A3Rs in inflammatory pain [177]. In a recent study, local administration of a selective A3R antagonist (PSB-10) inhibited paw edema but had no effect on pain behaviors produced by formalin [11].

The Central Nervous System

Adenosine receptors, particularly A1Rs, also contribute to pain regulation by actions at central sites. The spinal cord is a prominent site at which A1Rs produce antinociception in models of physiological pain (as revealed by sensory thresholds in the uninjured state), inflammatory pain (in several models of inflammation), and neuropathic pain (produced by various forms of injury to the peripheral nerve) [43,140,141]. A1Rs are concentrated in laminae I and II of the dorsal horn of the spinal cord and are present on intrinsic dorsal horn neurons [144]. Increased K^+ conductance and hyperpolarization of dorsal horn neurons [95,126] are implicated in spinal antinociception by adenosine. While A1Rs have not been directly identified at presynaptic sites on sensory nerve terminals in the dorsal spinal cord, presynaptic actions and inhibition of neuropeptide and glutamate release from such terminals has been demonstrated, suggesting the presence and functional actions of A1Rs contributing to antinociception at such sites [31,103,111,139]. The ability of A1R agonists to inhibit wind-up (a progressive increase in response following repeated stimulation) within the spinal cord has been emphasized, along with their ability to contribute to antinociception in the normal state, following inflammation, and following neuropathy [39,161].

A1Rs also are widely expressed at other sites throughout the CNS, including several areas involved in transmission and regulation of pain. The microinjection of adenosine A1R agonists into the periaqueductal gray (PAG) region produces antinociception (in thermal threshold and formalin tests) and alters ON- and OFF-cell activity in the rostroventral medulla, recognized as sites of supraspinal nociceptive circuitry [108]. Inhibition of both glutamate and GABA transmission within the PAG may contribute to such actions [7]. Supraspinal actions may contribute to antinociception following systemic delivery of A1R agonists that readily access the CNS, and studies in spinalized animals provide direct support for this involvement [130].

There is less information on the role of central A2ARs, A2BRs, and A3Rs in nociception. Microglia are involved in chronic and neuropathic pain, express most adenosine receptor subtypes, including A2ARs, A2BRs, and A3Rs [40], and potentially could contribute to AR-mediated nociception. The spinal administration of selective agonists for A2ARs and A3Rs produces antinociception in the formalin model [183], while spinal administration of selective antagonists for A2ARs, A2BRs, and A3Rs inhibits the action of adenosine in this model [184]. However, it is not known whether these actions reflect effects on neurons or on other types of cells.

Purines and Neuropathic Pain

ATP and Neuropathic Pain

Neuropathic pain, which results from damage to peripheral nerves or injury to the CNS, is difficult to treat clinically. Thus, while several classes of drugs are currently in clinical use, they are limited by partial efficacy and adverse effects. Neuropathic pain involves neurons, immune cells, and glia [143]. In addition to $P2X_3$ receptors on neurons, $P2X_4$, $P2X_7$, and $P2Y_{12}$ receptors on microglia in the spinal cord are implicated in neuropathic pain; the location of such receptors in relation to pain signaling is depicted schematically in Fig. 2.

$P2X_3$ and $P2X_{2/3}$ Receptors

There is considerable evidence that $P2X_3$ receptors are involved in neuropathic pain; the literature includes evidence of peripheral receptors located on sensory afferent nerves, as well as central receptors on primary afferent nerve terminals in the spinal cord [176] and in the trigeminal brainstem sensory nuclei [91]. Nerve injury can lead to complex effects on $P2X_3$-receptor expression in DRG neurons, as there are reports of both increases [122] and decreases [16,87] in receptors following various forms of nerve injury. Some of this difference may reflect the state of the nerve, because when the investigators distinguished between injured and uninjured neurons (using the transcription factor ATF3), $P2X_3$ receptors were reduced in injured DRG neurons but increased in uninjured neurons [171]. Functional studies reveal enhanced pain signaling in response to local application of ATP and/or α,β-meATP into the hindpaw following nerve injury [115]. Some of the increased functional response may reflect increased translocation of the $P2X_3$ receptor to the cell membrane [110]. In the spinal cord, $P2X_3$ receptors on

Fig. 2. Purinergic signaling in the spinal cord. Presynaptic primary afferent nerve terminals in the dorsal horn of the spinal cord are depicted releasing both glutamate (GLUT) and adenosine triphosphate (ATP) as cotransmitters by exocytosis. ATP acts postsynaptically on $P2X_2$, $P2X_4$, and $P2X_6$ receptors and on various P2Y-receptor subtypes. Glutamate acts postsynaptically on α-amino-3-hydroxy-5-methyl-4-isoxazole propionic acid receptors (AMPARs) and *N*-methyl-D-aspartate receptors (NMDARs). ATP is broken down by ectonucleotidase to adenosine (ADO), which acts as a presynaptic inhibitory modulator via P1 (A1) receptors, but ATP itself also can act presynaptically to inhibit the release of transmitter through P2Y receptors or to enhance release of glutamate through $P2X_3$ receptors. ATP is also released from astrocytes (and probably also microglia) together with glutamate to participate in glial-neuron interactions. Both P2X- and P2Y-receptor subtypes are expressed by astrocytes. Leukemia-inhibiting factor (LIF) released by astrocytes in response to ATP promotes myelination in oligodendrocytes and remyelination through $P2Y_1$ receptors. $P2X_7$ receptors on oligodendrocytes mediate apoptosis. Resting microglia express $P2X_4$ and $P2X_7$ receptors involved in neuropathic pain. ATP, through $P2X_7$ receptors, promotes interleukin 1β (IL-1β) release. Activation of $P2X_4$ receptors leads to release of brain-derived neurotrophic factor (BDNF), which acts on tropomyosin-related kinase B (TrkB) receptors on neurons in the pain pathway. Activation of $P2X_7$ receptors (via extracellular regulated kinase [ERK] and/or nuclear factor of activated T cells [NFAT]) activates transcription factor cyclic AMP response element-binding protein (CREB), whereas $P2Y_1$ receptors activate CREB through p38 signaling. $P2Y_{12}$ receptors on resting microglia mediate cell migration after injury, whereas $P2Y_6$ receptors on activated ameboid microglia mediate phagocytosis of debris at the site of damage. Inhibitory interneurons co-release γ-aminobutyric acid (GABA), glycine, and ATP and also modulate nociception. (From [27] with permission of Nature Publishing Group.) →

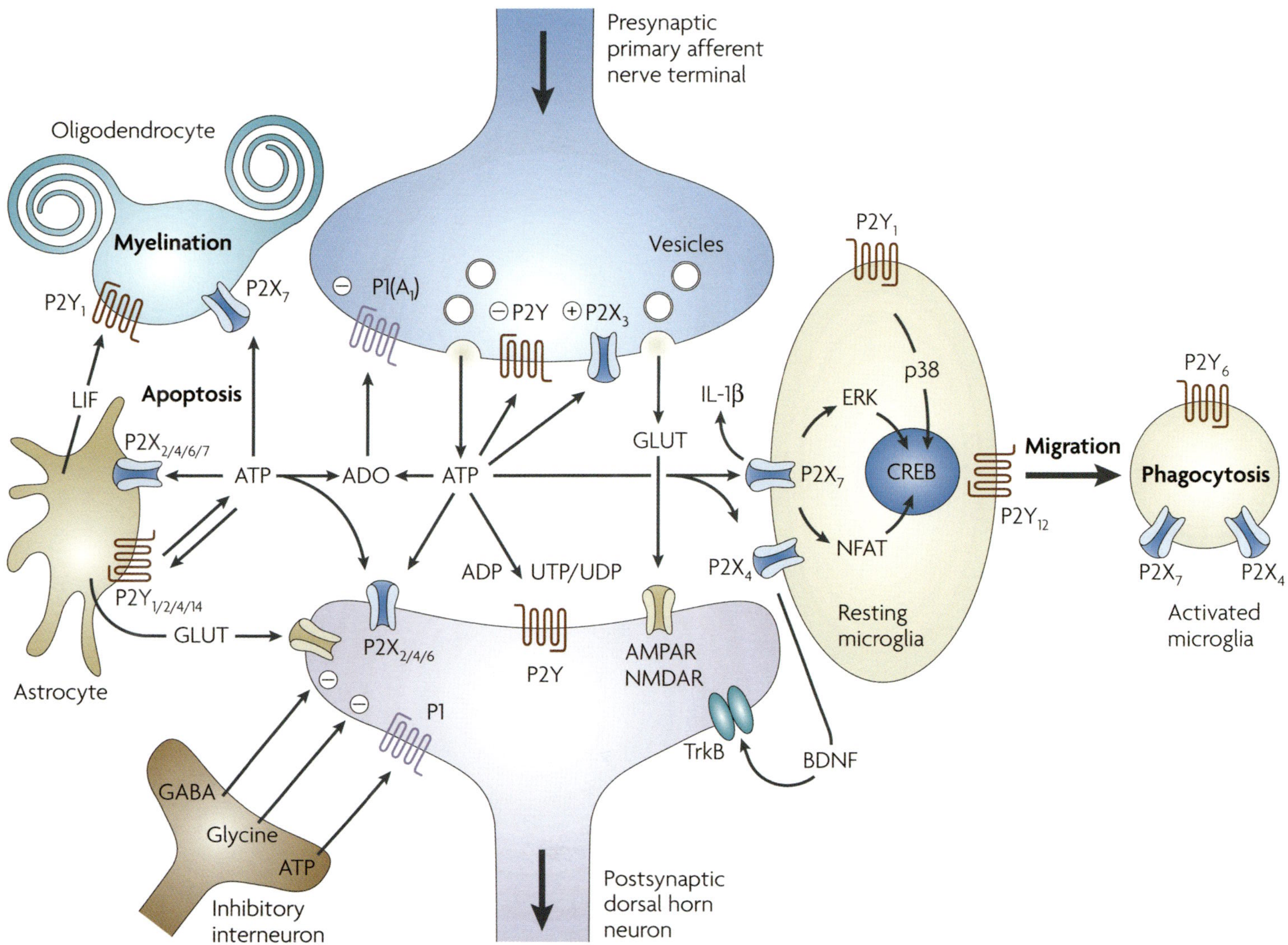

Presynaptic
primary afferent
nerve terminal
Oligodendrocyte
Myelination
P2Y1
P2X7
Vesicles
P1(A1)
P2Y
P2X3
LIF
Apoptosis
P2X2/4/6/7
ATP
ADO
ATP
GLUT
IL-1β
P2Y1
ERK
p38
P2X7
CREB
NFAT
P2Y12
Migration
P2Y6
Phagocytosis
P2X7
P2X4
Activated
microglia
P2X4
Resting
microglia
P2Y1/2/4/14
ADP
UTP/UDP
GLUT
P2X2/4/6
P2Y
AMPAR
NMDAR
Astrocyte
P1
TrkB
BDNF
GABA
Glycine
ATP
Inhibitory
interneuron
Postsynaptic
dorsal horn
neuron

terminals of primary afferent nerves in the inner lamina of the dorsal spinal cord mediate facilitation of glutamate release [60]. Furthermore, ATP co-released with GABA in spinal interneurons is probably involved in modulation of nociceptive pathways [84]. Curiously, supraspinal $P2X_3$ and $P2X_{2/3}$ receptors may play an inhibitory role in pain transmission [51].

Functional studies using receptor antagonists and antisense oligonucleotides have revealed a prominent role of $P2X_3$ receptors in pain regulation in nerve injury states. Thus, selective receptor antagonists produce antinociceptive actions in behavioral [113] and electrophysiological paradigms [149] in several nerve injury models. Downregulation of $P2X_3$ receptors using antisense oligonucleotides revealed a significant role for these receptors in neuropathic pain [71]. A recent study indicates that $P2X_3$ receptors mediate thermal hyperalgesia in a rat model of trigeminal neuropathic pain [152].

One particular condition in which ATP may contribute prominently to neuropathic pain is in sympathetically maintained pain states. Normally, the sympathetic nervous system does not interact directly with sensory nerves; however, after nerve injury, a sympathetic-afferent interaction can occur whereby sympathetic activity can enhance pain [82]. This interaction results from sprouting of sympathetic nerves in response to growth factors and cytokines and has been demonstrated directly in DRG. Different nerve injury models lead to different time courses and patterns of sympathetic-sensory coupling, which can reflect different origins and mechanisms of sprouting at DRG vs. peripheral sites [98]. Several growth factors cause upregulation of $P2X_3$ receptors in DRG neurons [16,129]. ATP is co-released with norepinephrine and neuropeptide Y from sympathetic nerves [20]. Norepinephrine potentiates pain behaviors induced by local administration of α,β-meATP into the hindpaw, as well as excitatory responses of ATP/α,β-meATP on DRG neurons in vitro [175]; this potentiation is particularly prominent following nerve injury [110,115]. Adrenergic regulation of $P2X_3$ receptors involves α_1-adrenergic receptors and intracellular signaling via PKC [110,116]. Adrenergic-purinergic interactions on sensory nerves are depicted schematically in Fig. 3. While neuropeptide Y is co-released with norepinephrine and ATP from sympathetic nerves and can augment vascular effects of norepinephrine and ATP [75], its role in regulating peripheral sympathetic influences on pain has not been elaborated.

$P2X_4$ Receptors

A number of papers have described the role of $P2X_4$ receptors on spinal microglia in neuropathic pain following the initial discovery by Tsuda and colleagues in 2003 (see [77]). Microglial $P2X_4$ receptors were upregulated and microglial reactivity was produced during allodynia in rats with experimental autoimmune neuritis [187]. Brain-derived neurotrophic factor is released from microglia by the stimulation of $P2X_4$ receptors [38]. The involvement of increased levels of spinal fibronectin/integrin following peripheral nerve injury in upregulation of microglial $P2X_4$ receptors and neuropathic pain has been considered [169]. Ligands for toll-like receptors and nucleotide-binding oligomerization domain 2 receptors stimulate microglial $P2X_4$-receptor upregulation, suggesting that microglia sense the presence of inflammatory stimulation using multiple recognition systems [62]. A recent study showed that Lyn tyrosine kinase plays an important role in the pathogenesis of neuropathic pain and is required to mediate nerve-injury-induced upregulation of $P2X_4$ receptors [170]. In rats displaying allodynia, the level of p38 was increased in microglia. Intraspinal administration of the p38 inhibitor, SB203580, suppressed allodynia, suggesting that neuropathic pain hypersensitivity depends on the activation of the p38 signaling pathway in microglia. Platelet activating factor, which is released from activated microglia, is a potent inducer of tactile allodynia and thermal hyperalgesia after intrathecal injection into the spinal cord, and this response is mediated by ATP [119]. The possible mechanisms that underlie the role of $P2X_4$ receptors in neuropathic pain and the involvement of inflammatory cytokines have been discussed [76,167].

$P2X_7$ Receptors

$P2X_7$ receptors were shown to be expressed in a mouse microglial cell line in 1997 (see [29]) and subsequently on microglia in rat brain [186]. The $P2X_7$-receptor antagonist oxidized ATP relieves inflammation-induced mechanical hyperalgesia in rats [42]. Both

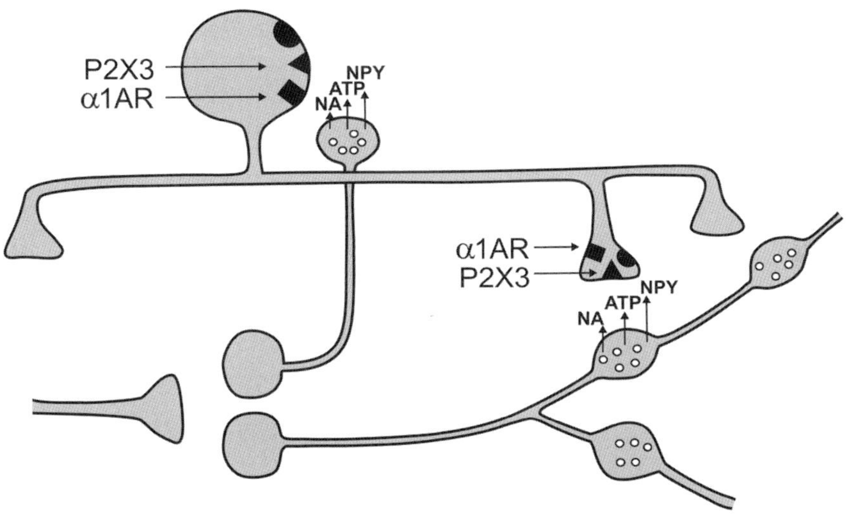

Fig. 3. Schematic depicting sympathetic innervation of dorsal root ganglion (DRG) cell bodies and peripheral aspects of sensory afferent nerves by sympathetic nerves. Following nerve injury, growth factors and cytokines cause sympathetic nerve sprouting, leading to abnormal sympathetic terminal arborizations around some DRG neurons. Different nerve injury models lead to different time courses and patterns of sympathetic-sensory coupling at the two sites, which can reflect actions in distinct populations of sympathetic nerves (releasing NA, ATP, and neuropeptide Y [NPY] as cotransmitters) and different mechanisms of sprouting. Norepinephrine (noradrenaline, NA) augments ATP and/or α,β-meATP responses at $P2X_3$ receptors at peripheral sites (following local drug application to the rat hindpaw) and on DRG cell bodies (following drug application to isolated DRG neurons). Alpha-1 adrenergic receptors (α_1-ARs) are implicated in adrenergic augmentation of $P2X_3$-receptor-mediated responses at both sites, and intracellular signaling involves protein kinase C.

inflammatory pain and neuropathic pain were abolished in $P2X_7$ knockout mice [34]. $P2X_4$ and $P2X_7$ receptor knockout mice share a common pain phenotype, but this phenotype appears to be conferred via different mechanisms [74].

P2Y Receptors

The contributions of the metabotropic P2Y receptors to normal and pathological pain have been less well examined compared to P2X receptors [54]. However, the expression of $P2Y_1$, $P2Y_2$, $P2Y_4$, and $P2Y_6$ mRNA in DRG neurons suggests that these receptors may be involved in peripheral somatosensory transmission [25]. Activation of uridine 5'-triphosphate (UTP)-sensitive $P2Y_2$ and/or $P2Y_4$ receptors and the uridine diphosphate (UDP)-sensitive $P2Y_6$ receptor, in contrast to P2X receptors, inhibits spinal pain transmission [123]. $P2Y_1$ and $P2Y_4$ receptors were identified on predominantly small-diameter sensory neurons in a subpopulation that were colocalized with $P2X_3$ receptors [137]. Activation of $P2Y_1$ receptors on DRG neurons modulates currents generated through *N*-type calcium channels and $P2X_3$ receptors [54]. Indeed, activation of *N*-type calcium channels in cultured DRG neurons was inhibited by ATP and even more potently by the $P2Y_{1,12,13}$-receptor agonist ADP. The effects of ATP were blocked by the selective $P2Y_1$-receptor antagonist MRS 2179. The outcome of these $P2Y_1$-related inhibitions is likely to result in a decreased release of nociceptive transmitters into the spinal cord [25]. $P2Y_1$ receptor mRNA is upregulated in the lumbar DRG after peripheral axotomy [181]. In the isolated skin-nerve preparation, 54% of cutaneous C fibers and 12% of A-mechanoreceptors responded to UTP (approximately 70–80% were capsaicin-sensitive) [160]. However, an additional 22–26% of large-diameter Aβ fibers responded to UTP, suggesting that $P2Y_2$ receptors also may be directly involved in the transmission of low-threshold mechanical inputs to the spinal cord. It is also possible that activation of the hetero-oligomeric $P2Y_2$/A1 receptor complex [162] may also negatively modulate the antinociceptive effects of A1-receptor agonists [45]. The rostral ventromedial medulla serves as a critical link in bulbospinal nociceptive modulation, and it has been suggested that while ON-cells preferentially express P2X receptors, OFF-cells express P2Y receptors in this region [146]. Activation of P2Y receptors inhibits $P2X_3$-receptor channels via G-protein-dependent facilitation of their desensitization [55]. It has been reported recently that $P2Y_{12}$ receptors expressed on microglia [68] are required for neuropathic pain after peripheral nerve injury [166].

Adenosine and Neuropathic Pain

Interest in the role of adenosine in treating neuropathic pain developed following a clinical report that spinal delivery, by intrathecal injection, of an A1R agonist produced long-lasting relief of neuropathic pain [88], as well as a preclinical report that intrathecal adenosine analogues, particularly A1R agonists, were very effective in relieving hypersensitivity responses (mechanical allodynia) after spinal nerve ligation in rats [100]. Subsequent preclinical studies confirmed the efficacy of spinal A1R agonists (or adenosine itself) in the spinal nerve ligation model [97], the chronic constriction model [157], and a model of central pain [158]. Following safety evaluation, intrathecal adenosine was shown to reduce neuropathic pain in humans [10,49].

Several mechanisms have been implicated in spinal analgesia by A1Rs following nerve injury. These include: (a) inhibition of release of glutamate from sensory afferent nerves [103], (b) interactions with spinal noradrenergic systems [8,58], and (c) inhibition of spinal wind-up processes [39,161]. Other effects implicated in nociceptive mechanisms in general, such as inhibition of neuropeptide release from sensory afferents and increased K^+ conductance and postsynaptic inhibition, have not specifically been examined following nerve injury but are still presumed to potentially contribute to spinal analgesia.

Several clinical studies have also examined effects of intravenous (i.v.) infusions of adenosine for neuropathic pain, and the authors reported pain reductions following treatment [106,156]. However, Eisenach et al. [49] reported reduced allodynia in neuropathic pain following intrathecal, but not i.v., administration of adenosine. Clinical reports and studies of adenosine in neuropathic pain, in several experimental pain models in humans, and in other clinical situations have been reviewed recently [67]. The analgesic action of i.v. adenosine is not fully understood due to the short half-life of adenosine in the blood, but it has been presumed to reflect a spinal site of action for A1Rs; contributions from supraspinal and peripheral actions at adenosine A1Rs are also possible.

Potential Clinical Applications

Clinical Applications of ATP Agents

There is increasing interest in developing P2 receptor antagonists for the treatment of chronic and neuropathic pain [24,27,45,56,134]. Towards this end, an active search is ongoing for selective $P2X_3$, $P2X_{2/3}$, $P2X_4$, $P2X_7$, and $P2Y_{12}$ receptor antagonists that are orally bioavailable, can cross the blood-brain barrier, and are metabolically stable as potential novel therapeutics for the treatment of pain.

$P2X_3$-Receptor Antagonists

TNP-ATP is a potent $P2X_3$-receptor antagonist; it has a low nanomolar affinity for $P2X_3$ receptors but also a high affinity for $P2X_1$ receptors [79]. This compound is rapidly degraded in situ [121], and in vivo studies have been limited to intrathecal administration [83] or direct administration into a site of peripheral tissue damage [83]. Several non-nucleotide small-molecule $P2X_3$ antagonists have been developed. A-317491 has nanomolar affinity for blocking both $P2X_3$ and $P2X_{2/3}$ receptors [113]; while it is generally stable and shows high systemic bioavailability following subcutaneous administration, it lacks oral bioavailability. A recent paper reported that intraplantar injection of A-317491 improved experimental cystitis in rats [78]. Systemic administration of A-317491 reduced nociception in inflammatory and neuropathic pain models [113]. A-317491 also blocked persistent pain in formalin and acetic acid abdominal constriction tests, but it was inactive in models of acute noxious stimulation [113]. RO-3 is another antagonist that potently blocks $P2X_3$

receptors; it has lower protein binding compared with A-317491 (48% versus 99%) and good CNS penetration [56]. RO-3 reduced nociceptive sensitivity in several animal pain models [56].

Antisense oligonucleotides also have been used to downregulate $P2X_3$ receptors. In models of neuropathic and inflammatory pain, this approach has been shown to relieve hypersensitivity responses [71]. $P2X_3$ antisense oligonucleotides (and antagonists) appear to be less effective for treating diskogenic pain (of the lumbar intervertebral disks) than for cutaneous tissue pain [6]. Combined antisense and RNA interference-mediated treatment for specific inhibition of the recombinant rat $P2X_3$ receptor appears to be promising for pain therapy [69]. $P2X_3$ double-stranded short interfering RNA relieves chronic neuropathic pain and opens up new avenues for therapeutic pain strategies in humans [46].

$P2X_4$-Receptor Antagonists

The lack of selective $P2X_4$-receptor antagonists has hindered the pharmacological validation of the role for $P2X_4$ receptors in pain. However, 5-(3-bromophenyl)-1,3-dihydro-2*H*-benzofuro-[3,2-e]-1,4-diazepin-2-one was recently shown to block $P2X_4$-receptor-mediated currents expressed in Chinese hamster ovary cells [45], and may prove to be useful in this regard. A series of benzofuro-1,4-diazepin-2-ones have been reported to be effective $P2X_4$ antagonists in a Bayer Health Care, AG patent [151]. Antidepressants have been shown to be effective in relieving neuropathic pain [114] and a recent communication [77] suggests that paroxetine is a $P2X_4$-receptor antagonist, but this needs to be confirmed and tested clinically.

$P2X_7$-Receptor Antagonists

Several $P2X_7$-receptor antagonists have been developed recently including oxidized ATP, Brilliant Blue G, the tyrosine derivatives KN-62 and KN-04, cyclic imides, adamantane and benzamide derivatives [61], compound 4g [134], chelerythrine and other benzophenanthridine alkaloids [150], U73122 and U73343 [165] and compounds such as cyanoguanidines and aminotetrazoles [151]. Direct support for a role of $P2X_7$ receptors in pain modulation has been provided by studies using such selective antagonists. Thus, systemic administration of the $P2X_7$-receptor-selective antagonists, A-438079 and A-740003, produced dose-dependent antinociceptive effects in models of neuropathic and inflammatory pain [45].

P2Y-Receptor Antagonists

2-Methylthio-ADP is a potent agonist of mammalian $P2Y_1$ receptors and N^6-methyl-2'-deoxyadenosine 3',5'-bisphosphate (MRS2179) and MRS2500 have been identified as selective antagonists [72]. At $P2Y_2$ and $P2Y_4$ receptors in the rat, ATP and UTP are equipotent, but the two receptors can be distinguished with antagonists. MRS2578 appears to be a selective antagonist at $P2Y_6$ receptors and there are a number of selective antagonists to the $P2Y_{12}$ receptor, including ARL-66096, INS-4266, and AZ-6140 [26]. Intrathecal administration of a $P2Y_{12}$-receptor antagonist, AR-C69931MX, has been shown to prevent the development of tactile allodynia [166].

Other Approaches

Other therapeutic approaches to pain management using ATP systems are being considered, including development of agents that control expression of ATP receptors and those that inhibit ATP breakdown by selective inhibition of ectonucleotidases. In the meantime, while it is now clear that many different cell types release ATP physiologically in response to mechanical distortion, hypoxia, and various agents, we still await clear understanding of the mechanisms that underlie ATP transport. When this functioning becomes clearer, agents can be developed that can enhance or inhibit ATP release, another potential way forward as a therapeutic strategy. At this time, there are no publications to date describing clinical evaluations of P2-receptor antagonists and related purinergic compounds for the relief of pain. However, clinical trials for some compounds are in progress [56].

Clinical Applications of Adenosine Agents

The preclinical profile of adenosine A1R agonists in nociception, whereby selective agonists have inhibited pain in several inflammatory and neuropathic pain conditions, appeared promising. Based on these findings, several novel selective A1R agonists have been developed. However, the orally active A1R agonist SDZ WAG 994 did not produce analgesia in postoperative dental pain [147]. Similarly, GR79236X, which exhibited antinociceptive actions in a preclinical model and was well tolerated, also lacked analgesic effects following third molar dental extractions [159]. It remains to be seen if these agents exhibit analgesic properties in other pain conditions.

In addition to direct effects on neurons, adenosine A2A, A2B, and A3 receptors can have widespread effects on immune and inflammatory cells, and potentially they could contribute to antinociception via such indirect actions. Recent reviews describing progress in the development of adenosine receptor ligands as anti-inflammatory drugs are available [3,96].

An additional line of exploration of potential adenosine-based agents for pain has been in developing inhibitors of adenosine metabolism via adenosine kinase [94,112]. Several selective compounds have emerged (ABT-702, A134974); these agents exhibit a spectrum of antinociceptive actions in inflammatory and neuropathic pain models following systemic spinal and local administration; they also exhibit a wider separation between antinociceptive actions and (adverse) hypomotor and cardiovascular effects than do A1R agonists [112]. However, despite these promising preclinical observations, these agents have not undergone clinical development.

One area of clinical application of adenosine for pain management that has been explored has been potential use for postoperative pain; this line of research was based on early reports of anesthetic and analgesic sparing effects of i.v. adenosine [67]. A recent systematic review of such studies reported on eight randomized, double-blind, placebo-controlled parallel-group studies between 1996 and 2006 [53]. In three trials, i.v. infusions of adenosine during surgery led to anesthetic sparing and some analgesic sparing effects, and in two trials, i.v. adenosine was superior to remifentanil for pain relief and reduced opioid analgesia requirements following surgery. Two trials reported no beneficial effects of i.v. adenosine in the perioperative setting, while one trial reported no analgesia from intrathecal adenosine prior to anesthesia. While such studies suggest that adenosine is worthy of further investigation, some caution is necessary. (1) Methodological issues were identified in trials that showed anesthetic and analgesic sparing effects [53]. (2) The strongest support for analgesic properties of i.v. adenosine was from trials in which this treatment was compared to remifentanil. However, remifentanil can increase postoperative pain and increase analgesic requirements due to acute opioid tolerance [63], and this hyperalgesic action may account for the observed differences between groups. (3) A recent study administered adequate doses of adenosine intrathecally—both early and late, to test for possible preemptive as well as analgesic effects—and found no analgesic effects of adenosine [148]. Further studies will need to resolve these issues.

Conclusions and Future Directions

Multiple P2 receptor subtypes are involved in pain pathways, where they serve both as initiators and modulators of pain transmission. Peripheral homomeric $P2X_3$ receptors on sensory afferent neurons probably contribute to acute nociception and to some aspects of acute inflammatory pain [25,45], whereas heteromeric $P2X_{2/3}$ receptors appear to modulate longer-lasting nociceptive sensitivity associated with nerve injury or chronic inflammation [83]. Furthermore, under conditions of persistent nociceptive input activation, $P2X_4$, $P2X_7$, and $P2Y_{12}$ receptors on microglia may serve to maintain nociceptive sensitivity through complex neural-glial cell interactions or via sensitization (via $P2Y_2$) of other nociceptive receptors such as TRPV1 channels. There is still an urgent need to understand mechanisms underlying the successful application of $P2X_3$, $P2X_4$, $P2X_7$, and $P2Y_{12}$ receptor antagonists for the treatment of neuropathic pain.

With respect to adenosine systems, the preclinical literature demonstrates widespread antinociceptive actions of A1R agonists and inhibitors of adenosine metabolism (particularly via adenosine kinase) in models of inflammatory and neuropathic pain, potentially reflecting spinal, supraspinal, and peripheral actions. However, there are no convincing reports of analgesia in clinical trials using A1R agonists or adenosine kinase inhibitors. The largest body of clinical evidence relates to perioperative i.v. adenosine for pain management, and while studies of adenosine in comparison with remifentanil appeared promising, the reported differences in pain outcomes could reflect an acute opioid tolerance with remifentanil rather than an analgesic action of adenosine. Intrathecal adenosine does not produce either pre-emptive or postoperative analgesia in clinical trials. The most promising area for investigation of adenosine and its analogs is for neuropathic pain, where there are several reports of pain relief following both i.v. and intrathecal adenosine, and this area merits further exploration.

Acknowledgment

We would like to thank Dr. Gillian E. Knight for her brilliant editorial assistance.

References

[1] Abbracchio MP, Burnstock G, Boeynaems J-M., Barnard EA, Boyer JL, Kennedy C, Knight GE, Fumagalli M, Gachet C, Jacobson KA, et al. International Union of Pharmacology LVIII: update on the P2Y G protein-coupled nucleotide receptors: from molecular mechanisms and pathophysiology to therapy. Pharmacol Rev 2006;58:281–341.
[2] Abo-Salem OM, Hayallah AM, Bilkei-Gorso A, Filipek B, Zimmer A, Müller CE. Antinociceptive effects of novel A2B adenosine receptor antagonists. J Pharmacol Exp Ther 2004;308:358–66.
[3] Akkari R, Burbiel JC, Hockemeyer J, Müller CE. Recent progress in the development of adenosine receptor ligands as anti-inflammatory drugs. Curr Top Med Chem 2006;6:1375–99.
[4] Alavi AM, Dubyak GR, Burnstock G. Immunohistochemical evidence for ATP receptors in human dental pulp. J Dent Res 2001;80476–83.
[5] Aley KO, Green PG, Levine JD. Opioid and adenosine peripheral antinociception are subject to tolerance and withdrawal. J Neurosci 1995;15:8031–8.
[6] Aoki Y, Ohtori S, Takahashi K, Ino H, Ozawa T, Douya H, Chiba T, Moriya H. $P2X_3$-immunoreactive primary sensory neurons innervating lumbar intervertebral disc in rats. Brain Res 2003;989:214–20.
[7] Bagley EE, Vaughan CW, Christie MJ. Inhibition by adenosine receptor agonists of synaptic transmission in rat periaqueductal grey neurons. J Physiol 1999;516:219–25.
[8] Bantel C, Li X, Eisenach JC. Intraspinal adenosine induces spinal cord norepinephrine release in spinal nerve-ligated rats but not in normal or sham controls. Anesthesiology 2003;98:1461–6.
[9] Bardoni R, Goldstein PA, Lee CJ, Gu JG, MacDermott AB. ATP P2X receptors mediate fast synaptic transmission in the dorsal horn of the rat spinal cord. J Neurosci 1997;17:5297–304.
[10] Belfrage M, Segerdahl M, Arnér S, Sollevi A. The safety and efficacy of intrathecal adenosine in patients with chronic neuropathic pain. Anesth Analg 1999;89:136–42.
[11] Bilkei-Gorzo A, Abo-Salem OM, Hayallah AM, Michel K, Müller CE, Zimmer A. Adenosine receptor subtype-selective antagonists in inflammation and hyperalgesia. Naunyn Schmiedebergs Arch Pharmacol 2008;377:65–76.
[12] Bland-Ward PA, Humphrey PPA. Acute nociception mediated by hindpaw P2X receptor activation in the rat. Br J Pharmacol 1997;122:365–71.
[13] Bleehen T, Keele CA. Observations on the algogenic actions of adenosine compounds on human blister base preparation. Pain 1977;3:367–77.
[14] Bo X, Alavi A, Xiang Z, Oglesby I, Ford A, Burnstock G. Localization of ATP-gated $P2X_2$ and $P2X_3$ receptor immunoreactive nerves in rat taste buds. Neuroreport 1999;10:1107–11.
[15] Bodin P, Burnstock G. Purinergic signalling: ATP release. Neurochem Res 2001;26:959–69.
[16] Bradbury EJ, Burnstock G, McMahon SB. The expression of $P2X_3$ purinoceptors in sensory neurons: effects of axotomy and glial-derived neurotrophic factor. Mol Cell Neurosci 1998;12:256–68.
[17] Burnstock G. Purinergic nerves. Pharmacol Rev 1972;24:509–81.
[18] Burnstock G. A basis for distinguishing two types of purinergic receptor. In: Straub RW, Bolis L, editors. Cell membrane receptors for drugs and hormones: a multidisciplinary approach. New York: Raven Press; 1978. p. 107–18.
[19] Burnstock G. Pathophysiology of migraine: a new hypothesis. Lancet 1981;317:1397–9.
[20] Burnstock G. Noradrenaline and ATP: cotransmitters and neuromodulators. J Physiol Pharmacol 1995;46:365–84.
[21] Burnstock G. A unifying purinergic hypothesis for the initiation of pain. Lancet 1996;347:1604–5.
[22] Burnstock G. Release of vasoactive substances from endothelial cells by shear stress and purinergic mechanosensory transduction. J Anat 1999;194:335–42.
[23] Burnstock G. Purine-mediated signalling in pain and visceral perception. Trends Pharmacol Sci 2001;22:2–188.
[24] Burnstock G. Purinergic P2 receptors as targets for novel analgesics. Pharmacol Ther 2006;110:433–54.
[25] Burnstock G. Physiology and pathophysiology of purinergic neurotransmission. Physiol Rev 2007;87:659–797.
[26] Burnstock G. Purine and pyrimidine receptors. Cell Mol Life Sci 2007;64:71–1483.
[27] Burnstock G. Purinergic signalling and disorders of the central nervous system. Nat Rev Drug Discov 2008;7:575–90.
[28] Burnstock G, Kennedy C. Is there a basis for distinguishing two types of P2-purinoceptor? Gen Pharmacol 1985;16:433–40.
[29] Burnstock G, Knight GE. Cellular distribution and functions of P2 receptor subtypes in different systems. Int Rev Cytol 2004;240:31–304.
[30] Burnstock G, Wood JN. Purinergic receptors: their role in nociception and primary afferent neurotransmission. Curr Opin Neurobiol 1996;6:526–32.
[31] Carruthers AM, Sellers LA, Jenkins DW, Jarvie EM, Feniuk W, Humphrey PPA. Adenosine A1 receptor-mediated inhibition of protein kinase A-induced calcitonin gene-related peptide release from rat trigeminal neurons. Mol Pharmacol 2001;59:1533–41.
[32] Chancellor MB, Fowler CJ, Apostolidis A, de Groat WC, Smith CP, Somogyi GT, Roger AK. Drug Insight: biological effects of botulinum toxin A in the lower urinary tract. Nat Clin Pract Urol 2008;5:319–28.

[33] Chen CC, Akopian AN, Sivilotti L, Colquhoun D, Burnstock G, Wood JN. A P2X purinoceptor expressed by a subset of sensory neurons. Nature 1995;377:428–31.
[34] Chessell IP, Hatcher JP, Bountra C, Michel AD, Hughes JP, Green P, Egerton J, Murfin M, Richardson J, Peck WL, et al. Disruption of the $P2X_7$ purinoceptor gene abolishes chronic inflammatory and neuropathic pain. Pain 2005;114:386–96.
[35] Cockayne DA, Hamilton SG, Zhu Q-M, Dunn PM, Zhong Y, Novakovic S, Malmberg AB, Cain G, Berson A, Kassotakis L, et al. Urinary bladder hyporeflexia and reduced pain-related behaviour in $P2X_3$-deficient mice. Nature 2000;407:1011–5.
[36] Collo G, North RA, Kawashima E, Merlo-Pich E, Neidhart S, Surprenant A, Buell G. Cloning of $P2X_5$ and $P2X_6$ receptors and the distribution and properties of an extended family of ATP-gated ion channels. J Neurosci 1996;16:2495–507.
[37] Cook SP, McCleskey EW. Cell damage excites nociceptors through release of cytosolic ATP. Pain 2002;95:1–47.
[38] Coull JA, Beggs S, Boudreau D, Boivin D, Tsuda M, Inoue K, Gravel C, Salter MW, De Koninck Y. BDNF from microglia causes the shift in neuronal anion gradient underlying neuropathic pain. Nature 2005;438:1017–21.
[39] Curros-Criado MM, Herrero JF. The antinociceptive effects of systemic adenosine A1 receptor agonist CPA in the absence and in the presence of spinal cord sensitization. Pharmacol Biochem Behav 2005;82:721–6.
[40] Daré E, Schulte G, Karovic O, Hammerberg C, Fredholm BB. Modulation of glial cell functions by adenosine receptors. Physiol Behav 2007;92:15–20.
[41] De Lander GE, Hopkins CJ. Spinal adenosine modulates descending antinociceptive pathways stimulated by morphine. J Pharmacol Exp Ther 1986;239:88–93.
[42] Dell'Antonio G, Quattrini A, Cin ED, Fulgenzi A, Ferrero ME. Relief of inflammatory pain in rats by local use of the selective $P2X_7$ ATP receptor inhibitor, oxidized ATP. Arthritis Rheum 2002;46:3378–85.
[43] Dickenson AH, Suzuki R, Reeve AJ. Adenosine as a potential analgesic target in inflammatory and neuropathic pains. CNS Drugs 2000;13:77–85.
[44] Doak G, Sawynok J. Complex role of peripheral adenosine in the genesis of response to subcutaneous formalin in the rat. Eur J Pharmacol 1995;281:311–8.
[45] Donnelly-Roberts DL, McGaraughty S, Shieh CC, Honore P, Jarvis MF. Painful purinergic receptors. J Pharmacol Exp Ther 2008;324:409–15.
[46] Dorn G, Patel S, Wotherspoon G, Hemmings-Mieszczak M, Barclay J, Natt FJ, Martin P, Bevan S, Fox A, Ganju P, et al. siRNA relieves chronic neuropathic pain. Nucleic Acids Res 2004;32:e49.
[47] Dowd E, McQueen DS, Chessell IP, Humphrey PPA. P2X receptor-mediated excitation of nociceptive afferents in the normal and arthritic rat knee joint. Br J Pharmacol 1998;125:341–6.
[48] Dussor G, Zylka MJ, Anderson DJ, McCleskey EW. Cutaneous sensory neurons expressing the Mrgprd receptor sense extracellular ATP and are putative nociceptors. J Neurophysiol 2008;99:1581–9.
[49] Eisenach JC, Rauck RL, Curry R. Intrathecal, but not intravenous adenosine reduces allodynia in patients with neuropathic pain. Pain 2003;105:65–70.
[50] Fredholm BB, Ijzerman AP, Jacobson KA, Klotz KN, Linden J. International Union of Pharmacology. XXV. Nomenclature and classification of adenosine receptors. Pharmacol Rev 2001;53:527–52.
[51] Fukui M, Nakagawa T, Minami M, Satoh M, Kaneko S. Inhibitory role of supraspinal $P2X_3/P2X_{2/3}$ subtypes on nociception in rats. Mol Pain 2006;2:19.
[52] Fyffe REW, Perl ER. Is ATP a central synaptic mediator for certain primary afferent fibres from mammalian skin? Proc Natl Acad Sci USA 1984;81:6890–3.
[53] Gan TJ, Habib AS. Adenosine as a non-opioid analgesic in the perioperative setting. Anesth Analg 2007;105:487–94.
[54] Gerevich Z, Illes P. P2Y receptors and pain transmission. Purinerg Signal 2004;1:3–10.
[55] Gerevich Z, Zadori Z, Müller C, Wirkner K, Schröder W, Rubini P, Illes P. Metabotropic P2Y receptors inhibit $P2X_3$ receptor-channels via G protein-dependent facilitation of their desensitization. Br J Pharmacol 2007;151:226–36.
[56] Gever J, Cockayne DA, Dillon MP, Burnstock G, Ford APDW. Pharmacology of P2X channels. Pflugers Arch 2006;452:513–7.
[57] Gold MS, Reichling DB, Shuster MJ, Levine JD. Hyperalgesic agents increase a tetrodotoxin-resistant Na^+ current in nociceptors. Proc Natl Acad Sci USA 1996;93:1108–12.
[58] Gomes JA, Li X, Pan HL, Eisenach JC. Intrathecal adenosine interacts with a spinal noradrenergic system to produce antinociception in nerve-injured rats. Anesthesiology 1999;91:1072–9.
[59] Gu JG, Heft MW. P2X receptor-mediated purinergic sensory pathways to the spinal cord dorsal horn. Purinerg Signal 2004;1:11–6.
[60] Gu JG, MacDermott AB. Activation of ATP P2X receptors elicits glutamate release from sensory neuron synapses. Nature 1997;389:749–53.
[61] Gunosewoyo H, Coster MJ, Kassiou M. Molecular probes for $P2X_7$ receptor studies. Curr Med Chem 2007;14:1505–23.
[62] Guo LH, Guo KT, Wendel HP, Schluesener HJ. Combinations of TLR and NOD2 ligands stimulate rat microglial P2X4R expression. Biochem Biophys Res Commun 2006;349:1156–62.
[63] Guignard B, Bossard AE, Coste C, Sessler DI, Lebrault C, Alfonsi P, Fletcher D, Chauvin M. Acute opioid tolerance: intraoperative remifentanil increases postoperative pain and morphine requirement. Anesthesiology 2000;93:409–17.
[64] Haas HL, Selbach O. Functions of neuronal adenosine receptors. Naunyn-Schmiedebergs Arch Pharmacol 2000;362:375–81.
[65] Hamilton SG, McMahon SB, Lewin GR. Selective activation of nociceptors by P2X receptor agonists in normal and inflamed rat skin. J Physiol 2001;534:437–45.

[66] Haskó G, Pacher P. A2A receptors in inflammation and injury: lessons learned from transgenic animals. J Leukocyte Biol 2008;83:1–9.
[67] Hayashida M, Fukuda KI, Fukunaga A. Clinical application of adenosine and ATP for pain control. J Anesth 2005;19:225–35.
[68] Haynes SE, Hollopeter G, Yang G, Kurpius D, Dailey ME, Gan WB, Julius D. The $P2Y_{12}$ receptor regulates microglial activation by extracellular nucleotides. Nat Neurosci 2006;9:1512–9.
[69] Hemmings-Mieszczak M, Dorn G, Natt FJ, Hall J, Wishart WL. Independent combinatorial effect of antisense oligonucleotides and RNAi-mediated specific inhibition of the recombinant rat $P2X_3$ receptor. Nucleic Acids Res 2003;31:2117–26.
[70] Ho IK, Loh HH, Way EL. Cyclic adenosine monophosphate antagonism of morphine analgesia. J Pharmacol Exp Ther 1973;185:336–46.
[71] Honore P, Kage K, Mikusa J, Watt AT, Johnston JF, Wyatt JR, Faltynek CR, Jarvis MF, Lynch K. Analgesic profile of intrathecal $P2X_3$ antisense oligonucleotide treatment in chronic inflammatory and neuropathic pain states in rats. Pain 2002;99:11–9.
[72] Houston D, Costanzi S, Jacobson KA, Harden TK. Development of selective high affinity antagonists, agonists, and radioligands for the P2Y1 receptor. Comb Chem High Throughput Screen 2008;11:410–9.
[73] Hugel S, Schlichter R. Presynaptic P2X receptors facilitate inhibitory GABAergic transmission between cultured rat spinal cord dorsal horn neurons. J Neurosci 2000;20:2121–30.
[74] Hughes JP, Hatcher JP, Chessell IP. The role of $P2X_7$ in pain and inflammation. Purinerg Signal 2007;3:163–9.
[75] Huidobro-Toro JP, Donoso MV. Sympathetic co-transmission: the coordinated action of ATP and noradrenaline and their modulation by neuropeptide Y in human vascular neuroeffector junctions. Eur J Pharmacol 2004;500:27–35.
[76] Inoue K. The function of microglia through purinergic receptors: neuropathic pain and cytokine release. Pharmacol Ther 2006;109:210–26.
[77] Inoue K. P2 receptors and chronic pain. Purinerg Signal 2007;3:135–44.
[78] Ito K, Iwami A, Katsura H, Ikeda M. Therapeutic effects of the putative $P2X_3/P2X_{2/3}$ antagonist A-317491 on cyclophosphamide-induced cystitis in rats. Naunyn Schmiedebergs Arch Pharmacol 2008;377:483–90.
[79] Jacobson KA, Jarvis MF, Williams M. Purine and pyrimidine (P2) receptors as drug targets. J Med Chem 2002;45:4057–93.
[80] Jahr CE, Jessell TM. ATP excites a subpopulation of rat dorsal horn neurones. Nature 1983;304:730–3.
[81] Jang IS, Rhee JS, Kubota H, Akaike N, Akaike N. Developmental changes in P2X purinoceptors on glycinergic presynaptic nerve terminals projecting to rat substantia gelatinosa neurones. J Physiol 2001;536:505–19.
[82] Jänig W, Levine JD, Michaelis M. Interactions of sympathetic and primary afferent neurons following nerve injury and tissue trauma. Prog Brain Res 1996;113:161–84.
[83] Jarvis MF. Contributions of $P2X_3$ homomeric and heteromeric channels to acute and chronic pain. Expert Opin Ther Targets 2003;7:513–22.
[84] Jo YH, Schlichter R. Synaptic corelease of ATP and GABA in cultured spinal neurons. Nat Neurosci 1999;2:241–5.
[85] Jurna I. Cyclic nucleotides and aminophylline produce different effects on nociceptive motor and sensory responses in the rat spinal cord. Naunyn Schmiedebergs Arch Pharmacol 1984;327:23–30.
[86] Kaelin-Lang A, Lauterburg T, Burgunder JM. Expression of adenosine A2A receptor gene in rat dorsal root and autonomic ganglia. Neurosci Lett 1998;246:21–4.
[87] Kage K, Niforatos W, Zhu CZ, Lynch KJ, Honore P, Jarvis MF. Alteration of dorsal root ganglion $P2X_3$ receptor expression and function following spinal nerve ligation in the rat. Exp Brain Res 2002;147:511–9.
[88] Karlsten R, Gordh T. An A1-selective adenosine agonist abolishes allodynia elicited by vibration and touch after intrathecal injection. Anesth Analg 1995;80:844–7.
[89] Karlsten R, Gordh T, Post C. Local antinociceptive and hyperalgesic effects in the formalin test after peripheral administration of adenosine analogues in mice. Pharmacol Toxicol 1992;70:434–8.
[90] Khasar SG, Wang JF, Taiwo YO, Heller PH, Green PG, Levine JD. Mu-opioid agonist enhancement of prostaglandin-induced hyperalgesia in the rat: a G-protein beta gamma subunit-mediated effect? Neuroscience 1995;67:189–95.
[91] Kim YS, Paik SK, Cho YS, Shin HS, Bae JY, Moritani M, Yoshida A, Ahn DK, Valtschanoff J, Hwang SJ, et al. Expression of $P2X_3$ receptor in the trigeminal sensory nuclei of the rat. J Comp Neurol 2008;506:627–39.
[92] Knight GE, Bodin P, De Groat WC, Burnstock G. ATP is released from guinea pig ureter epithelium on distension. Am J Physiol Renal Physiol 2002;282:F281–8.
[93] Kobayashi K, Fukuoka T, Yamanaka H, Dai Y, Obata K, Tokunaga A, Noguchi K. Neurons and glial cells differentially express P2Y receptor mRNAs in the rat dorsal root ganglion and spinal cord. J Comp Neurol 2006;498:443–54.
[94] Kowaluk EA, Jarvis MF. Therapeutic potential of adenosine kinase inhibitors. Exp Opin Invest Drugs 2000;9:551–64.
[95] Lao LJ, Kumamoto E, Luo C, Furue H, Yoshimura M. Adenosine inhibits excitatory transmission to substantia gelatinosa neurons of the adult rat spinal cord through the activation of presynaptic A1 adenosine receptors. Pain 2001;94:315–24.
[96] Lappas CM, Sullivan GW, Linden J. Adenosine A2A agonists in development for the treatment of inflammation. Expert Opin Invest Drugs 2005;14:797–806.
[97] Lavand'homme PM, Eisenach JC. Exogenous and endogenous adenosine enhance the spinal antiallodynic effects of morphine in a rat model of neuropathic pain. Pain 1999;80:31–6.
[98] Lee BH, Yoon YW, Chung K, Chung JM. Comparison of sympathetic sprouting in sensory ganglia in three animal models of neuropathic pain. Exp Brain Res 1998;120:432–8.
[99] Lee HY, Bardini M, Burnstock G. Distribution of P2X receptors in the urinary bladder and the ureter of the rat. J Urol 2000;163:2002–7.

[100] Lee YW, Yaksh TL. Pharmacology of the spinal adenosine receptor which mediates the antiallodynic action of intrathecal adenosine agonists. J Pharmacol Exp Ther 1996;277:1642–8.
[101] Lewis C, Neidhart S, Holy C, North RA, Buell G, Surprenant A. Coexpression of $P2X_2$ and $P2X_3$ receptor subunits can account for ATP-gated currents in sensory neurons. Nature 1995;377:432–5.
[102] Li J, Sinoway LI. ATP stimulates chemically sensitive and sensitizes mechanically sensitive afferents. Am J Physiol Heart Circ Physiol 2002;283:H2636–43.
[103] Li X, Eisenach JC. Adenosine reduces glutamate release in rat spinal synaptosomes. Anesthesiology 2005;103:1060–5.
[104] Liu XJ, Sawynok J. Peripheral antihyperalgesic effects by adenosine A1 receptor agonists and inhibitors of adenosine metabolism in a rat neuropathic pain model. Analgesia 2000;5:19–29.
[105] Llewellyn-Smith IJ, Burnstock G. Ultrastructural localization of $P2X_3$ receptors in rat sensory neurons. Neuroreport 1998;9:2245–50.
[106] Lynch ME, Clark AJ, Sawynok J. Intravenous adenosine alleviates neuropathic pain: a double blind placebo controlled crossover trial using an enriched enrolment design. Pain 2003;103:111–7.
[107] MacKenzie I, Burnstock G, Dolly JO. The effects of purified botulinum neurotoxin type A on cholinergic, adrenergic and non-adrenergic, atropine-resistant autonomic neuromuscular transmission. Neuroscience 1982;7:997–1006.
[108] Maione S, de Novellis V, Cappellacci L, Plaasso E, Vita D, Luongo L, Stella L, Franchetti P, Marabese I, Rossi F, et al. The antinociceptive effect of 2-chloro-2'-C-methyl-N6-cyclopentyladenosine (2'-Me-CCPA), a highly selective adenosine A1 receptor agonist, in the rat. Pain 2007;131:281–92.
[109] Makowska A, Panfil C, Ellrich J. ATP induces sustained facilitation of craniofacial nociception through P2X receptors on neck muscle nociceptors in mice. Cephalalgia 2006;26:697–706.
[110] Maruo K, Yamamoto H, Yamamoto S, Nagata T, Fujikawa H, Kamo T, Yaguchi T, Maruo S, Yoshiya S, Nishizaki T. Modulation of P2X receptors via adrenergic pathways in rat dorsal root ganglion neurons after sciatic nerve injury. Pain 2006;120:106–12.
[111] Mauborgne A, Poliénor H, Hamon M, Cesselin F, Bourgoin S. Adenosine receptor-mediated control of in vitro release of pain-related neuropeptides from the rat spinal cord. Eur J Pharmacol 2002;441:47–55.
[112] McGaraughty S, Cowart M, Jarvis MF, Berman RF. Anticonvulsant and antinociceptive actions of novel adenosine kinase inhibitors. Curr Top Med Chem 2005;5:43–58.
[113] McGaraughty S, Wismer CT, Zhu CZ, Mikusa J, Honore P, Chu KL, Lee CH, Faltynek CR, Jarvis MF. Effects of A-317491, a novel and selective $P2X_3/P2X_{2/3}$ receptor antagonist, on neuropathic, inflammatory and chemogenic nociception following intrathecal and intraplantar administration. Br J Pharmacol 2003;140:1381–8.
[114] McQuay HJ, Tramer M, Nye BA, Carroll D, Wiffen PJ, Moore RA. A systematic review of antidepressants in neuropathic pain. Pain 1996;68:217–27.
[115] Meisner JG, Reid AR, Sawynok J. Adrenergic regulation of $P2X_3$ and TRPV1 receptors: differential effects of spared nerve injury. Neurosci Lett 2008;444:172–5.
[116] Meisner JG, Waldron JB, Sawynok J. $Alpha_1$-adrenergic receptors augment $P2X_3$ receptor-mediated nociceptive responses in the uninjured state. J Pain 2007;8:556–62.
[117] Millward-Sadler SJ, Wright MO, Flatman PW, Salter DM. ATP in the mechano-transduction pathway of normal human chondrocytes. Biorheology 2004;41:567–75.
[118] Mizumoto N, Mummert ME, Shalhevet D, Takashima A. Keratinocyte ATP release assay for testing skin-irritating potentials of structurally diverse chemicals. J Invest Dermatol 2003;121:1066–72.
[119] Morita K, Morioka N, Abdin J, Kitayama S, Nakata Y, Dohi T. Development of tactile allodynia and thermal hyperalgesia by intrathecally administered platelet-activating factor in mice. Pain 2004;111:351–9.
[120] Nakatsuka T, Tsuzuki K, Ling JX, Sonobe H, Gu JG. Distinct roles of P2X receptors in modulating glutamate release at different primary sensory synapses in rat spinal cord. J Neurophysiol 2003;89:3243–52.
[121] North RA. Molecular physiology of P2X receptors. Physiol Rev 2002;82:1013–67.
[122] Novakovic SD, Kassotakis LC, Oglesby IB, Smith JAM, Eglen RM, Ford APDW, Hunter JC. Immunocytochemical localization of $P2X_3$ purinoceptors in sensory neurons in naïve rats following neuropathic injury. Pain 1999;80:273–82.
[123] Okada M, Nakagawa T, Minami M, Satoh M. Analgesic effects of intrathecal administration of P2Y nucleotide receptor agonists UTP and UDP in normal and neuropathic pain model rats. J Pharmacol Exp Ther 2002;303:66–73.
[124] Oliveira MC, Parada CA, Veiga MC, Rodrigues LR, Barros SP, Tambeli CH. Evidence for the involvement of endogenous ATP and P2X receptors in TMJ pain. Eur J Pain 2005;9:87–93.
[125] Papka RE, Hafemeister J, Storey-Workley M. P2X receptors in the rat uterine cervix, lumbosacral dorsal root ganglia, and spinal cord during pregnancy. Cell Tissue Res 2005;321:35–44.
[126] Patel MK, Pinnock RD, Lee K. Adenosine exerts multiple effects in dorsal horn neurones of the adult rat spinal cord. Brain Res 2001;920:19–26.
[127] Post C. Antinociceptive effects in mice after intrathecal injection of 5'-N-ethylcarboxamide adenosine. Neurosci Lett 1984;51:325–30.
[128] Ralevic V, Burnstock G. Receptors for purines and pyrimidines. Pharmacol Rev 1998;50:413–92.
[129] Ramer MS, Bradbury EJ, McMahon SB. Nerve growth factor induces $P2X_3$ expression in sensory neurons. J Neurochem 2001;77:864–75.
[130] Ramos-Zepeda G, Schröder W, Rosenow S, Herro JF. Spinal vs supraspinal antinociceptive activity of the adenosine A1 receptor agonist cyclopentyl-adenosine in rats with inflammation. Eur J Pharmacol 2004;499:247–56.
[131] Reinöhl J, Hoheisel U, Unger T, Mense S. Adenosine triphosphate as a stimulant for nociceptive and non-nociceptive muscle group IV receptors in the rat. Neurosci Lett 2003;338:25–8.
[132] Renton T, Yiangou Y, Baecker PA, Ford AP, Anand P. Capsaicin receptor VR1 and ATP purinoceptor $P2X_3$ in painful and nonpainful human tooth pulp. J Orofac Pain 2003:17:245–50.

[133] Rhee JS, Wang ZM, Nabekura J, Inoue K, Akaike N. ATP facilitates spontaneous glycinergic IPSC frequency at dissociated rat dorsal horn interneuron synapses. J Physiol 2000;524:471–83.
[134] Romagnoli R, Baraldi PG, Cruz-Lopez O, Lopez-Cara C, Preti D, Borea PA, Gessi S. The $P2X_7$ receptor as a therapeutic target. Expert Opin Ther Targets 2008;12:647–61.
[135] Rong W, Burnstock G. Activation of ureter nociceptors by exogenous and endogenous ATP in guinea pig. Neuropharmacology 2004;47:1093–101.
[136] Rong W, Burnstock G, Spyer KM. P2X purinoceptor-mediated excitation of trigeminal lingual nerve terminals in an in vitro intra-arterially perfused rat tongue preparation. J Physiol 2000;524:891–902.
[137] Ruan H-Z, Burnstock G. Localisation of P2Y 1 and P2Y4 receptors in dorsal root, nodose and trigeminal ganglia of the rat. Histochem Cell Biol 2003;120:415–26.
[138] Salter MW, Hicks JL. ATP-evoked increases in intracellular calcium in neurons and glia from the dorsal spinal cord. J Neurosci 1994;14:1563–75.
[139] Santicioli P, Del Bianco E, Maggi CA. Adenosine A1 receptors mediate the presynaptic inhibition of calcitonin gene-related peptide release by adenosine in the rat spinal cord. Eur J Pharmacol 1993;231:139–42.
[140] Sawynok J. Adenosine receptor activation and nociception. Eur J Pharmacol 1998;347:1–11.
[141] Sawynok J, Liu XJ. Adenosine in the spinal cord and periphery: release and regulation of pain. Prog Neurobiol 2003;69:313–40.
[142] Sawynok J, Zarrindast MR, Reid AR, Doak G. Adenosine A3 receptor activation produced nociceptive behaviour and edema by release of histamine and 5-hydroxytryptamine. Eur J Pharmacol 1997;333:1–7.
[143] Scholz J, Woolf CJ. The neuropathic pain triad: neurons, immune cells and glia. Nat Neurosci 2007;10:1361–8.
[144] Schulte G, Robertson B, Fredholm BB, DeLander GE, Shortland P, Molander C. Distribution of antinociceptive adenosine A1 receptors in the spinal cord dorsal horn, and relationship to primary afferents and neuronal subpopulations. Neuroscience 2003;121:907–16.
[145] Seino D, Tokunaga A, Tachibana T, Yoshiya S, Dai Y, Obata K, Yamanaka H, Kobayashi K, Noguchi, K. The role of ERK signaling and the P2X receptor on mechanical pain evoked by movement of inflamed knee joint. Pain 2006;123:193–203.
[146] Selden NR, Carlson JD, Cetas J, Close LN, Heinricher MM. Purinergic actions on neurons that modulate nociception in the rostral ventromedial medulla. Neuroscience 2007;146:1808–16.
[147] Seymour RA, Hawkesford JE, Hill CM, Frame J, Andrews C. The efficacy of a novel adenosine agonist (WAG 994) in postoperative dental pain. Br J Clin Pharmacol 1999;47:675–80.
[148] Sharma M, Mohta M, Chawla R. Efficacy of intrathecal adenosine for postoperative pain relief. Eur J Anaesthesiol 2006;23:449–53.
[149] Sharp CJ, Reeve AJ, Collins SD, Martindale JC, Summerfield SG, Sargent BS, Bate ST, Chessell IP. Investigation into the role of $P2X_3/P2X_{2/3}$ receptors in neuropathic pain following chronic constriction injury in the rat: an electrophysiological study. Br J Pharmacol 2006;148:845–52.
[150] Shemon AN, Sluyter R, Conigrave AD, Wiley JS. Chelerythrine and other benzophenanthridine alkaloids block the human $P2X_7$ receptor. Br J Pharmacol 2004;142:1015–9.
[151] Shieh CC, Jarvis MF, Lee H, Perner RJ. P2X receptor ligands and pain. Exp Opin Ther Patents 2006;16:1113–27.
[152] Shinoda M, Kawashima K, Ozaki N, Asai H, Nagamine K, Sugiura Y. $P2X_3$ receptor mediates heat hyperalgesia in a rat model of trigeminal neuropathic pain. J Pain 2007;8:588–97.
[153] Shinoda M, Ozaki N, Asai H, Nagamine K, Sugiura Y. Changes in $P2X_3$ receptor expression in the trigeminal ganglion following monoarthritis of the temporomandibular joint in rats. Pain 2005;116:42–51.
[154] Shinoda M, Ozaki N, Sugiura Y. Involvement of ATP and its receptors on nociception in rat model of masseter muscle pain. Pain 2008;134:148–57.
[155] Shiokawa H, Nakatsuka T, Furue H, Tsuda M, Katafuchi T, Inoue K, Yoshimura M. Direct excitation of deep dorsal horn neurones in the rat spinal cord by the activation of postsynaptic P2X receptors. J Physiol 2006;573:753–63.
[156] Sjölund KF, Belfrage M, Karlsten R, Segerdahl M, Arnér S, Gordh T, Sollevi A. Systemic adenosine infusion reduces the area of tactile allodynia in neuropathic pain following peripheral nerve injury: a multi-centre, placebo-controlled study. Eur J Pain 2001;5:199–207.
[157] Sjölund KF, Sollevi A, Segerdahl M, Hansson P, Lundeberg T. Intrathecal and systemic R-isopropyl-adenosine reduces scratching behaviour in a rat mononeuropathic model. NeuroReport 1996;7:1856–69.
[158] Sjölund KF, von Heijne M, Hao JX, Xu XJ, Sollevi A, Wiesenfeld-Hallin Z. Intrathecal administration of the adenosine A1 receptor agonist R-isophenylpropyl adenosine reduced presumed pain behaviour in a rat model of central pain. Neurosci Lett 1998;243:89–92.
[159] Sneyd JR, Langton JA, Allan LG, Peacock JE, Rowbotham DJ. Multicentre evaluation of the adenosine agonist GR79236X in patients with dental pain after third molar extraction. Br J Anaesth 2007;98:672–6.
[160] Stucky CL, Medler KA, Molliver DC. The P2Y agonist UTP activates cutaneous afferent fibers. Pain 2004;109:36–44.
[161] Suzuki R, Gale A, Dickenson A. Altered effects of an A1 adenosine receptor agonist on the evoked responses of spinal dorsal horn neurons in a rat model of mononeuropathy. J Pain 2000;1:99–110.
[162] Suzuki T, Hide I, Matsubara A, Hama C, Harada K, Miyano K, Andra M, Matsubayashi H, Sakai N, Kohsaka S, et al. Microglial α7 nicotinic acetylcholine receptors drive a phospholipase C/IP3 pathway and modulate the cell activation toward a neuroprotective role. J Neurosci Res 2006;83:1461–70.
[163] Sweeney MI, White TD, Sawynok J. Involvement of adenosine in the spinal antinociceptive effects of morphine and noradrenaline. J Pharmacol Exp Ther 1987;243:657–65.
[164] Taiwo YO. Levine JD. Direct cutaneous hyperalgesia induced by adenosine. Neuroscience 1990;38:757–62.

[165] Takenouchi T, Ogihara K, Sato M, Kitani H. Inhibitory effects of U73122 and U73343 on Ca^{2+} influx and pore formation induced by the activation of $P2X_7$ nucleotide receptors in mouse microglial cell line. Biochim Biophys Acta 2005;1726:177–86.

[166] Tozaki-Saitoh H, Tsuda M, Miyata H, Ueda K, Kohsaka S, Inoue K. $P2Y_{12}$ receptors in spinal microglia are required for neuropathic pain after peripheral nerve injury. J Neurosci 2008;28:4949–56.

[167] Trang T, Beggs S, Salter MW. Purinoceptors in microglia and neuropathic pain. Pflugers Arch 2006;452:645–52.

[168] Tsuda M, Shigemoto-Mogami Y, Koizumi S, Mizokoshi A, Kohsaka S, Salter MW, Inoue K. $P2X_4$ receptors induced in spinal microglia gate tactile allodynia after nerve injury. Nature 2003;424:778–83.

[169] Tsuda M, Toyomitsu E, Komatsu T, Masuda T, Kunifusa E, Nasu-Tada K, Koizumi S, Yamamoto K, Ando J, Inoue K. Fibronectin/integrin system is involved in $P2X_4$ receptor upregulation in the spinal cord and neuropathic pain after nerve injury. Glia 2008;56:579–85.

[170] Tsuda M, Tozaki-Saitoh H, Masuda T, Toyomitsu E, Tezuka T, Yamamoto T, Inoue K. Lyn tyrosine kinase is required for $P2X_4$ receptor upregulation and neuropathic pain after peripheral nerve injury. Glia 2008;56:50–8.

[171] Tsuzuki K, Kondo E, Fukuoka T, Yi D, Tsujino H, Sakagami M, Noguchi K. Differential regulation of $P2X_3$ mRNA expression by peripheral nerve injury in intact and injured neurons in rat sensory ganglia. Pain 2001;91:351–60.

[172] Vapaatalo H, Onken D, Neuvonen PJ, Westermann E. Stereospecificity in some central and circulatory effects of phenylisopropyladenosine (PIA). Arzneimittelforschung 1975;25:407–10.

[173] Vlaskovska M, Kasakov L, Rong W, Bodin P, Bardini M, Cockayne DA, Ford APDW, Burnstock G. $P2X_3$ knockout mice reveal a major sensory role for urothelially released ATP. J Neurosci 2001;21:5670–7.

[174] Vulchanova L, Riedl M, Shuster SJ, Buell G, Surprenant A, North RA, Elde R. Immunocytochemical study of the $P2X_2$ and $P2X_3$ receptor subunits in rat and monkey sensory neurons and their central terminals. Neuropharmacology 1997;36:1229–42.

[175] Waldron JB, Sawynok J. Peripheral P2X receptors and nociception: interactions with biogenic amine systems. Pain 2004;110:79–89.

[176] Wirkner K, Sperlagh B, Illes P. $P2X_3$ receptor involvement in pain states. Mol Neurobiol 2007;36:165–83.

[177] Wu WP, Hao JX, Halldner-Henricksson L, Xu XJ, Jacobson MA, Wiesenfeld-Hallin Z, Fredholm BB. Decreased inflammatory pain due to reduced carrageenan-induced inflammation n mice lacking adenosine A3 receptors. Neuroscience 2002;114:523–7.

[178] Wynn G, Bei M, Ruan H-Z, Burnstock G. Purinergic component of mechanosensory transduction is increased in a rat model of colitis. Am J Physiol Gastrointest Liver Physiol 2004;287:G647–57.

[179] Wynn G, Burnstock G. Adenosine 5'-triphosphate and its relationship with other mediators that activate pelvic afferent neurons in the rat colorectum. Purinerg Signal 2006;2:517–26.

[180] Wynn G, Rong W, Xiang Z, Burnstock G. Purinergic mechanisms contribute to mechanosensory transduction in the rat colorectum. Gastroenterology 2003;125:1398–409.

[181] Xiao HS, Huang QH, Zhang FX, Bao L, Lu YJ, Guo C, Yang L, Huang WJ, Fu G, Xu SH, et al. Identification of gene expression profile of dorsal root ganglion in the rat peripheral axotomy model of neuropathic pain. Proc Natl Acad Sci USA 2002;99:8360–5.

[182] Xu GY, Huang LY. Peripheral inflammation sensitizes P2X receptor-mediated responses in rat dorsal root ganglion neurons. J Neurosci 2002;22:93–102.

[183] Yoon MH, Bae HB, Choi JI. Antinociception of intrathecal adenosine receptor subtype agonists in rat formalin test. Anesth Analg 2005;101:1417–21.

[184] Yoon MH, Bae HB, Choi JI, Kim SJ, Chung ST, Kim CM. Roles of adenosine receptor subtypes in the antinociceptive effect of intrathecal adenosine in a rat formalin test. Pharmacology 2006;78:21–6.

[185] Yoshida K, Nakagawa T, Kaneko S, Akaike A, Satoh M. Adenosine 5'-triphosphate inhibits slow depolarization induced by repetitive dorsal root stimulation via P2Y purinoceptors in substantia gelatinosa neurons of the adult rat spinal cord slices with the dorsal root attached. Neurosci Lett 2002;320:121–4.

[186] Yu Y, Ugawa S, Ueda T, Ishida Y, Inoue K, Kyaw NA, Umemura A, Mase M, Yamada K, Shimada S. Cellular localization of $P2X_7$ receptor mRNA in the rat brain. Brain Res 2008;1194:45–55.

[187] Zhang Z, Zhang ZY, Fauser U, Schluesener HJ. Mechanical allodynia and spinal up-regulation of $P2X_4$ receptor in experimental autoimmune neuritis rats. Neuroscience 2008;152:495–501.

[188] Zhong Y, Banning AS, Cockayne DA, Ford APDW, Burnstock G, McMahon SB. Bladder and cutaneous sensory neurons of the rat express different functional P2X receptors. Neuroscience 2003;120:667–75.

[189] Zimmermann H. Ectonucleotidases: some recent developments and a note on nomenclature. Drug Dev Res 2001;52:44–56.

Correspondence to: Prof. Geoffrey Burnstock, PhD, Autonomic Neuroscience Centre, Royal Free and University College Medical School, Rowland Hill Street, London NW3 2PF, United Kingdom. Tel: +44 20 7830 2948; fax: +44 20 7830 2949; email: g.burnstock@ucl.ac.uk.

15

The Transient Receptor Potential (TRP) Family in Pain and Temperature Sensation

Gehoon Chung,[a] Sung Jun Jung,[b] and Seog Bae Oh[a]

[a]National Research Laboratory for Pain, Dental Research Institute, and Department of Physiology, School of Dentistry, Seoul National University, Seoul, Korea; [b]Department of Physiology, College of Medicine, Kangwon National University, Chunchon, Korea

Transient receptor potential (TRP) channels, a large family of receptor channel proteins, initially attracted researchers in the pain field as key molecules in nociception, but later they became known as more general transducer molecules for various physical stresses. In this chapter, we will discuss their roles in temperature and mechanical sensation, and then consider their contribution to physiological and pathological nociceptive pain, finally describing various analgesic strategies targeting these channels.

TRP Channels

TRP channels are one of the most extensively studied protein families in neuroscience. They were first described in 1969 in mutant *Drosophila*, and were given their name because this mutant lacked sustained photoreceptor activity and showed only transient receptor potential [35]. TRP channels were not on the main stage of pain study, however, until 1997, when Caterina et al. cloned a vanilloid receptor and found that its structure was closely related to TRP channels [25]. Sensitivity to capsaicin, the hot ingredient of capsicum peppers, was believed to be one of the key features of nociceptors, and the protein responsible had been long sought. The vanilloid receptor found in this study was activated not only by capsaicin but also by noxious heat, which made it a perfect fit with the nociceptor-related protein. Since then, a tremendous amount of pain-related study has been dedicated to the vanilloid receptor and other TRP channels.

Pharmacology of Pain
edited by Pierre Beaulieu, David Lussier, Frank Porreca, and Anthony H. Dickenson
IASP Press, Seattle, © 2010

Currently the mammalian TRP channels include over 30 members that are classified into six subfamilies: TRPC (canonical), TRPV (vanilloid), TRPM (melastatin), TRPP (polycystin), TRPML (mucolipin), and TRPA (ankyrin) [23]. Although their amino acids do not share very many common sequences, their overall structure is the same: four subunits join to form a functional channel, and each subunit contains six transmembrane domains, with a pore-forming region between the fifth and sixth transmembrane domains and large amino and carboxyl termini on the cytosolic side [32,103]. Of all the mammalian TRP channels, six channels have been of particular interest in the study of transduction of nociception related to temperature and stretch: TRPV1, TRPV2, TRPV3, TRPV4, TRPA1, and TRPM8 (Fig. 1).

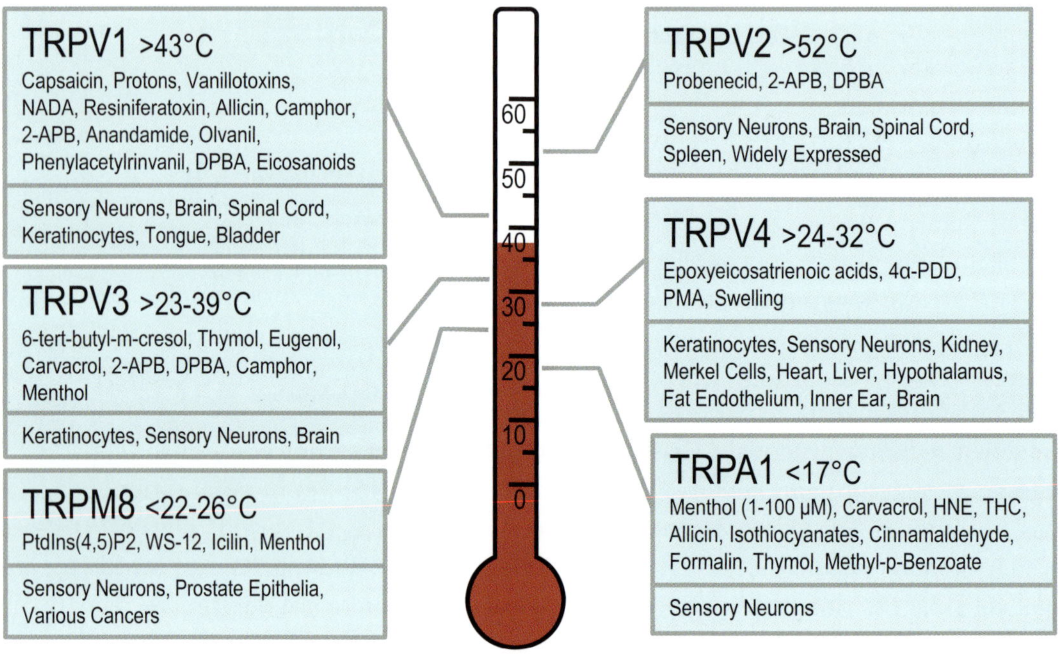

Fig. 1. Temperature thresholds, chemical agonists, and tissue distribution of six temperature-sensitive TRP channels. NADA, *N*-arachidonoyl-dopamine; 2-APB, 2-aminoethoxydiphenyl borate; DPBA, diphenylboronic anhydride; 4α-PDD, 4α-phorbol 12,13-didecanoate; PMA, phorbol 12-myristate 13-acetate; PtdIns(4,5) P2, phosphatidylinositol 4,5-bisphosphate; HNE, 4-hydroxynonenal; THC, tetrahydrocannabinol. (The thermometer diagram was adapted from Fig. 2 of [130].)

TRP Channels in Physiological Nociception

Heat Receptors

TRPV1

Exposure to capsaicin evokes a painful burning sensation, and thus sensitivity to capsaicin has long been believed to be an important feature of nociceptive neurons, even before its specific receptor was known. However, a prolonged exposure to capsaicin desensitizes neurons and diminishes nociception, contrary to the painful sensation of the initial exposure. This paradoxical phenomenon was exploited in many analgesic drugs targeting physiological or pathological pain conditions, from herpes zoster to diabetic neuropathies [22,73,103]. The receptor protein of capsaicin was the subject of intensive study because it was obvious that capsaicin sensitivity and nociceptive neurons were closely related.

In 1997, Caterina et al. isolated and cloned the capsaicin receptor gene, by expressing various subdivisions of rodent dorsal root ganglion (DRG) cDNA on HEK293 cells and verifying the calcium response to capsaicin. They named the receptor vanilloid receptor subtype 1 (VR1) after the active vanilloid moiety of capsaicin [25]; it was later renamed TRPV1 for simplification of the pedigree [93]. According to their report, TRPV1 showed a robust inward current and fast desensitization to capsaicin, with a half-maximal effective concentration (EC_{50}) of 39.1 nM, and the capsaicin-evoked inward current was reversibly blocked by the competitive vanilloid receptor antagonist capsazepine, with a half-maximal inhibitory concentration (IC_{50}) of 283.5 nM. The current-voltage relationship curve was outwardly rectifying with the characteristics of a nonselective cation current. Testing with an ion-substituted bath solution revealed that calcium permeability was about 10 times higher than sodium permeability. The cloned receptor was also activated by noxious thermal stimuli above 43°C or by an acidic environment of pH 5.4 [25,131].

In addition to its sensitivity to various pain-inducing stimuli such as capsaicin, heat, and protons, TRPV1 has many features that a receptor related to nociception is supposed to have, such as its preferential distribution within small to medium-sized DRG and trigeminal ganglion (TG) neurons, which are believed to serve as nociceptive neurons. Phosphatidylinositol 4,5-bisphosphate (PIP_2) bound to the C-terminus inactivates TRPV1, suggesting that conditions that remove or degrade PIP_2, such as activation of phospholipase C (PLC) during inflammation, can also activate or potentiate TRPV1. TRPV1 is also activated by an alkaline environment [39] and by various chemical stimulants including resiniferatoxin, vanillotoxins, phenylacetylrinvanil, olvanil, anandamide, camphor, allicin, eicosanoids, *N*-arachidonoyl-dopamine, 2-aminoethoxydiphenyl borate (2-APB), diphenylboronic anhydride (DPBA), nitric oxide, diacylglycerol (DAG), spider toxins, and eugenol [3,143]. It is potentiated by ethanol and modulated by extracellular cations. But the most important aspect of TRPV1 is that it can integrate all of these noxious stimuli and inflammatory mediators to modulate its threshold of activation [34,74,131].

Thus, it is not surprising that TRPV1 has been a promising target in the field of pain research. Understanding how TRPV1 transduces various physical and noxious chemical stimuli into an electrical potential in the peripheral endings of nociceptive neurons could lead to better understanding of the nature of nociception, and blocking the activation of TRPV1 could be a very effective analgesic strategy [103].

TRPV2

TRPV2 is widely expressed in neuronal cells (mostly Aδ fibers and a small portion of C fibers) and non-neuronal cells [66,75,121,137]. It is activated by temperature above 52°C, a threshold higher than that of TRPV1 and close to that of Aδ fibers; therefore, it was initially believed to be a nociceptive receptor dealing with higher temperatures. However, its role in nociception has been debated because it is not sensitive to capsaicin or protons, and nociceptors lacking both TRPV1 and TRPV2 showed normal heat responses in ex vivo recordings, suggesting that mechanisms other than TRPV1 and TRPV2 might be more important in the intact physiological environment [140]. Recently, a possible role of TRPV2 in inflammatory hyperalgesia has been reported, in which TRPV2 protein level in medium-sized DRG neurons was increased by intraplantar injection of complete Freund's adjuvant (CFA) [114]. TRPV2 has not been studied as intensively as TRPV1 because of its high threshold and differential distribution. A few chemical agonists known to activate TRPV2 include probenecid, 2-APB, and DPBA [3]. Evidence from in vivo studies is also lacking because TRPV2-knockout mice have not been produced.

TRPV3 and TRPV4

Two other TRPV members, TRPV3 and TRPV4, can be activated at warm temperatures, which can hardly be perceived as nociceptive. TRPV3 is activated at 32–39°C and shows an increased response to higher temperature or repetitive stimuli. It shares 40–50% homology with TRPV1 and has certain common features such as activation and sensitization by camphor and 2-APB. Other agonists of TRPV3 include 6-tert-butyl-*m*-cresol, carvacrol, eugenol, thymol, menthol, and DPBA. TRPV4 has an even lower threshold of 27–34°C and has a variety of chemical ligands, such as phorbol esters 4-alpha-phorbol 12,13-didecanoate (4α-PDD) and phorbol 12-myristate 13-acetate (PMA), low pH, citrate, endocannabinoids, arachidonic acid metabolites, nitric oxide, and bisandrographolide A, the active compound of the Chinese herb *Andrographis paniculata*. It is interesting to note that TRPV4 is not activated by 2-APB, unlike TRPV1, TRPV2, and TRPV3 [3,74].

Both TRPV3 and TRPV4 are expressed most extensively in skin keratinocytes, providing the possibility that keratinocytes may signal to sensory neurons, instead of the direct transduction of thermal information by neurons. Accordingly, camphor activates keratinocytes but not sensory neurons in mice. Moreover, TRPV3-deleted mice lack camphor-induced activation of keratinocytes and exhibit strong deficits in response to innocuous and noxious heat. Thus, TRPV3 expressed in skin keratinocytes may have an important role in mammalian thermosensation [94].

There are no reports of these channels being involved in nociceptive thermosensation in the nervous system, except for sensitization of TRPV3 upon repeated noxious heat stimuli. TRPV4 is more likely to be involved in pain related to mechanical stretch, which will be discussed in detail below.

TRPM2, TRPM4, and TRPM5

Three more TRP channels were found to be temperature sensitive in non-neuronal tissue unrelated to nociception. TRPM2, which plays an important role in secreting insulin from the pancreas, can be activated by cyclic ADP ribose only when temperature is above 35°C [129]. Heat activation of TRPM5 in taste receptor cells is shown to modulate the sensitivity of sweet taste, and a similar temperature activation was observed in TRPM4 [127].

Cold Receptors

Psychophysical studies in humans report that temperatures of around and below 15°C are perceived as pain [95], but unlike the discrete temperature threshold of hot nociception, the transition from cool to painfully cold is less well defined [45]. Subpopulations of both Aδ- and C-fiber neurons are responsive to cooling, although there is no consensus on the proportion of neurons capable of this response. Calcium imaging experiments showed that only 7% of DRG neurons and 14% of TG neurons were responsive to cooling to 18°C [89], which was similar to the proportions reported from skin-nerve preparation studies in the rat [50]. However, whole-cell electrophysiological recordings of rats suggest that almost all nociceptive neurons are sensitive to cold, although some are activated at temperature as low as 0°C, which might be due to a nonspecific response following tissue damage from freezing [45].

TRPM8

Just as the search for the hot capsaicin receptor led to the discovery of the heat-sensitive TRPV subfamily, the search for the cold receptor began with menthol, the cool chemical found in mint. The cooling sensation of menthol was established as early as 1951 [54], and researchers found that both cooling and menthol were able to evoke a nonselective cation current in DRG neurons [110,111].

Two independent groups cloned and characterized a cold- and menthol-sensitive TRP channel, TRPM8 [89,105], which had been found in the prostate without a known function. TRPM8 is mostly expressed in small DRG and TG neurons. It is activated by temperatures below 25°C and by various chemicals including menthol, menthone, eucalyptol, spearmint, and icilin [130]. There seems to be an interaction between these activators, such as an increase in temperature threshold from 25°C to 30°C by subthreshold concentrations of menthol, which is somewhat similar to the lowering of the temperature threshold of TRPV1 in acidic conditions [131]. Similar to TRPV1, the current-voltage relationship of TRPM8 is outwardly rectifying, and calcium permeates more easily than sodium. However, unlike TRPV1, the expression of TRPM8 does not overlap with that of other nociception-related markers [37], except for a 10–20% overlap with TRPV1 [37,126].

Several studies of independently derived lines of TRPM8-null mice have shown deficient response behaviors to moderately cool temperatures [11,38], but the contribution of TRPM8 to the response to noxious cold temperature was difficult to determine. Thus, although TRPM8 may contribute to the transduction of innocuous cool temperature [82], it is not clear whether or how this receptor is involved in nociception [40,45,74,88,109]. Moreover, there are populations of neurons that are sensitive to cold but not to menthol [9,97].

TRPA1

Given that the features of TRPM8 were insufficient to explain the mechanisms of cold sensation, other TRP channels were reviewed. The receptor ANKTM1, later renamed TRPA1 after its rich ankyrin repeat domains in the N-terminal, was found to be cold sensitive [122]. It is activated at temperatures below 17°C, which is lower than the temperature threshold of TRPM8 and close to the cold temperature known to initiate nociception. While TRPM8 is expressed in a different subset of neurons that do not express TRPV1, most of the expression of TRPA1 overlaps with that of TRPV1. Thus, it seemed reasonable to link TRPA1 to cold nociception.

However, two groups reported that TRPA1 was irrelevant to noxious cold in vitro [10,99], leaving controversies as to whether TRPA1 was responsible for noxious cold sensation. Different age and sex of the animals and differences in experimental conditions might have led to mixed results. Moreover, a study showing that increased intracellular calcium is sufficient to activate TRPA1 [145] opened up more questions about the gating of this receptor by cold stimuli. Recently, Karashima et al. clarified the cold sensitivity of TRPA1 with three sets of findings: (1) heterologously expressed TRPA1 is activated by cold in calcium-independent manner, (2) the TRPA1-deleted mice they developed lacked a specific subset of cold-sensitive TG neurons, and (3) these transgenic mice showed impaired behavioral responses to a cold plate at a temperature of 0°C [65].

Several thermosensitive TRP channels involved in nociception can also be activated by chemical stimuli. TRPA1 can be activated by icilin, a synthetic compound that induces intense cold sensations when applied to human mucous membranes [138]. It has a slightly different action from menthol, such as its requirement of elevated cytosolic calcium for activation and its different target residues of TRPM8 [29]. Pungent cysteine-reactive chemicals, such as isothiocyanates (horseradish, mustard), cinnamaldehyde (cinnamon), and allicin (garlic), activate TRPA1 through covalent modification of cysteine, regardless of their overall structures [55,80,103]. Other chemicals that activate TRPA1 include thymol, carvacrol, Δ_9-tetrahydrocannabinol (THC), formalin, the highly reactive aldehyde 4-hydroxy-2-nonenal (4-HNE), methyl-p-hydroxybenzoate, the fatty acid amide hydrolase inhibitor URB597, 15-deoxy-12,14-prostaglandin J_2, and reactive oxygen and nitrogen species [3,103]. An alkaline environment [46] and menthol [64] were recently added to the list. It is noteworthy, however, that TRPA1 is insensitive to capsaicin and that its activation is inhibited by application of a high concentration of menthol [64,81]. TRPA1 is specifically expressed, unlike TRPM8, in neurons with the nociceptive markers calcitonin gene-related peptide (CGRP) and substance P, and it is frequently coexpressed with TRPV1. This coexpression might explain why an extremely cold stimulus may cause a paradoxical hot sensation [130].

Mechanical Receptors

TRPV1

Besides its major role as a hot temperature sensor, a few reports have implicated a role for TRPV1 in mechanical stretch sensitive receptors, such as those related to stretch sensitivity to regulate bladder voiding [18,19]. The organum vasculosum lamina terminalis (OVLT) is a part of the brain that is responsible for sensing the osmolarity of cerebrospinal fluid, in which TRPV4 has been shown to play key roles. However, TRPV1 is also expressed in the region, and mice lacking TRPV1 exhibited reduced water intake during a systemic hyperosmotic condition [31]. Also, reports suggest a role for TRPV1 in irritable bowel syndrome [62,91]. Afferent nerve firing recorded in vivo from the experimentally distended colon was reduced in capsazepine-treated or TRPV1-deficient mice, implying that TRPV1 is also somehow linked to mechanical stretch stimulus. A more recent study reported that stress-induced colonic hypersensitivity in maternally separated rats was reduced by treatment with capsazepine [134].

However, Cavanaugh et al. provided evidence that TRPV1 is not related to mechanical sensation by showing that the mechanical threshold of rats with chemically ablated TRPV1 channels was no different from that of control animals. On the contrary, ablation of a distinct set of nociceptive neurons that do not express TRPV1 (i.e., neurons positive for Mas-related G-protein-coupled receptor D) reduced behavioral responses to noxious mechanical stimuli [26].

TRPV4

Although TRPV4 has been discussed earlier in this chapter as a receptor activated by moderately warm temperatures, it was initially identified and more often referred to as an osmotic pressure sensor protein. It is activated by a decrease in osmolarity of as little as 30 milliosmoles and is expressed in many tissues in which mechanosensitivity is critical, such as cochlear hair cells, vibrissal Merkel cells, sensory ganglia, and keratinocytes, as well as cutaneous A- and C-fiber terminals [74]. This distribution suggests that TRPV4 is a more general stretch-activated receptor channel rather than being limited to osmotic pressure. This notion is supported by a study showing that this channel's nonmammalian homologue, Osm9, serves as an osmotic and mechanical sensor in *Caenorhabditis elegans* and that disrupted functions from mutations of Osm9 can be restored by transgenic expression of TRPV4 [78]. A recent study demonstrated that mechanosensory responses of colonic afferents were reduced by deletion of TRPV4 and enhanced by a TRPV4 agonist [21].

Agonists of TRPV4 promote the release of substance P and CGRP from central terminals of primary afferent neurons, which suggests that TRPV4 is involved in nociception [52]. However, it seems to contribute only to mechanical nociception, because mice lacking TRPV4 showed an increased mechanical nociceptive threshold, but their response to innocuous low-threshold mechanical stimuli and noxious heat was normal [74,123].

TRPA1

The role of TRPA1 in mechanical transduction is also controversial, as in thermal transduction. At first, this channel was believed to be a solid candidate for a molecular entity responsible for mechanical transduction for several reasons: (1) its *Drosophila* homologue, *painless*, contributes to mechanical nociception; (2) its functional properties fit the description of mechanosensory channels in inner ear hair cells; and (3) its tandem ankyrin-repeat may form a spring to act as a mechanoreceptor [33,74]. However, behavioral studies in two independent lines of TRPA1$^{-/-}$ mice have created a controversy. Transgenic mice created by Kwan et al. showed a higher threshold and reduced response to suprathreshold mechanical stimuli [72], whereas those engineered by Bautista et al. did not show any difference in threshold compared to wild-type mice [10].

TRPC1 and TRPC6

The stretch-activated cation channel (SAC), first recognized more than 20 years ago in the skeletal muscles of chicks, is present in most eukaryotic cells [27,53,104]. The molecular identity of the SAC was initially attributed to the cytoskeleton, but later immunological and electrophysiological studies suggested that TRPC1 is the channel protein responsible for the stretch-activating current. Furthermore, in *Xenopus* oocytes, the endogenous and background activity of SAC was upregulated by heterologous expression of human TRPC1 and reduced by TRPC1-specific antisense RNA [87]. However, the possible role of TRPC1 as a SAC was contradicted by studies in TRPC1$^{-/-}$ mice, which exhibited no change in phenotype [41]. It is possible that the role of deleted TRPC1 may have been replaced by another SAC, such as TRPA1. TRPA1 is also suggested to be an important SAC in hair cells of the inner ear, but this supposition is rebutted by the normal phenotype of TRPA1$^{-/-}$ mice.

TRPC6, a close relative of TRPC1, is also proposed to be a SAC protein. TRPC6 is mainly distributed in smooth muscle-enriched tissues such as the stomach, colon, esophagus, and myometrium [12]. A study focusing on arterial smooth muscle suggested that TRPC6 may contribute to the tight regulation of blood pressure within arteries [139]. An interesting recent study described that a newly developed spider toxin (GsMTx-4), which is known to inhibit TRPC6 from activation by DAG, can also block stretch activation of TRPC6, suggesting a common pathway of ligand activation and stretch activation of TRPC6 [118].

TRP Channels in Pathological Pain

Although unpleasant, nociception is in fact helpful to maintenance of life. More problematic are hyperalgesia and allodynia, which cause patients to experience exaggerated nociception to stimuli that are not particularly noxious or are even innocuous. The pathological conditions associated with hyperalgesia and allodynia are divided into inflammatory and neuropathic according to their contributing causes.

TRPV1

As described earlier in this chapter, TRPV1 was initially considered to be a simple receptor that reacts to nociceptive heat because its threshold temperature is close to what humans perceive as pain. As expected, TRPV1-deleted mice had diminished behavioral responses to acute thermal stimuli and did not respond to capsaicin, and their sensory neurons had no response to capsaicin, resiniferatoxin, protons, or noxious temperatures below 50°C [74]. Surprisingly, however, the mice also lacked thermal hypersensitivity in the inflammatory setting. Unlike their wild-type counterparts, these animals did not show decreased threshold or withdrawal latency to thermal stimuli after application of CFA, carrageenan or inflammatory mediators like bradykinin, nerve growth factor, or adenosine triphosphate. The knockout mice only showed mechanical hypersensitivity. This finding led to the idea that inflammatory mediators might sensitize TRPV1, to the extent that normal body temperature could activate nociceptors [20,24,30,36,96]. However, nocifensive behavior to formalin were normal [74]. In fact, it was TRPA1 that was later shown to be a dominant player in formalin-induced pain [90].

Several mechanisms by which inflammatory mediators can influence TRPV1 have been proposed. Inflammatory mediators, such as bradykinin, can increase the membrane expression of TRPV1 [61,144], phosphorylate TRPV1 [92,107], reverse the inhibition of TRPV1 by PIP_2 [14,30], or act on other G-protein-coupled receptors or tyrosine kinase pathways to release arachidonic acid metabolites, which are believed to act as endogenous ligands [59,115]. Activation of protein kinase C (PKC) also contributes to inflammatory hyperalgesia through TRPV1 because the PKC activator, phorbol 12-myristate 13-acetate (PMA), cannot induce inflammatory hyperalgesia in mice lacking TRPV1. Moreover, protease-activated receptor 2, or PAR2, can also sensitize TRPV1 during inflammation through PKA and PKD as well as PKCε [5,6].

The role of TRPV1 has also been investigated in various neuropathy models. TRPV1 plays an important role in chemical and thermal hyperalgesia in a diabetic neuropathy model [44,56,63], and several reports have described increased expression of TRPV1 in nerve trauma models [47,58]. The role of TRPV1 in peripheral neuropathy seems more complicated. While cold allodynia produced by sciatic nerve ligation was reduced with the silencer RNA for TRPV1, both mechanical and heat hyperalgesia were about the same in both genotypes. However, TRPV1 antisense oligodeoxynucleotides were successful in reducing mechanical hyperalgesia induced by spinal nerve ligation [28,74].

TRPV1 is also proposed to act as a mechanical transducer, and study of its influence on mechanical allodynia has created much controversy. While TRPV1$^{-/-}$ mice showed reduced mechanical hyperalgesia to mild heat injury [20], they exhibited normal mechanical hyperalgesia to carrageenan injection [20,106]. Reaction to CFA is more complex. Caternia et al. reported that mechanical hyperalgesia in TRPV1$^{-/-}$ mice after 1 day of CFA was similar to wild-type mice [24], but Szabo et al. reported that after 16 days of CFA, mechanical hyperalgesia was attenuated in TRPV1$^{-/-}$ mice [124]. These results suggest that the role of TRPV1 in developing inflammation may differ with different stages [74]. However, a recent study denied the role of TRPV1 as a mechanical transducer by showing that mechanosensitive and thermosensitive neurons are two different subsets with little overlap [26].

In summary, although a more detailed explanation is yet to come, it is clear that TRPV1 is not only a transducer of hot temperature, but also a more complex gateway through which numerous factors and inflammatory mediators are integrated in the mechanisms of physiological and pathological pain. Thus, blocking its activation would provide a very promising treatment, and it is not surprising that there have been numerous attempts to develop specific blockers for TRPV1.

TRPV4

Studies conducted in TRPV4-deleted mice have revealed that TRPV4 is related to the development of acute inflammatory mechanical hyperalgesia [1,74]. Both PKA and PKCε can engage TRPV4 in hyperalgesia to mechanical and osmotic changes, a process that requires a certain amount of cyclic adenosine monophosphate (cAMP) produced by a concerted action of inflammatory mediators. In addition to inflammatory mediators such as prostaglandin E_2 or serotonin, protease-activated receptor 2 can also activate the second-messenger pathways and sensitize TRPV4 to release substance P and CGRP, leading to TRPV4-mediated mechanical hyperalgesia. Recently, TRPV4 was also shown to contribute to inflammatory thermal hyperalgesia because TRPV4-deleted mice showed reduced responses when capsaicin or carrageenan was injected [128].

When the mitotic inhibitor paclitaxel, generally used for cancer treatment, induced chemotherapy-induced neuropathy in rats, nociceptive behavioral responses to mechanical and hypotonic stimulation of the hindpaw were increased. When TRPV4 antisense oligodeoxynucleotides were administered, however, the mechanical hyperalgesia was reversed and osmotic hyperalgesia was reduced [2]. Several subsequent studies discovered that the paclitaxel-induced TRPV4-mediated hyperalgesia depends on the integrin/Src tyrosine kinase pathway [43], along with PKCε and PKA [42]. Mechanical allodynia induced by direct activation of PKA or PKCε was absent in mice lacking TRPV4 and was reduced in mice treated with TRPV4 antisense oligodeoxynucleotides [74].

TRPM8

TRPM8 is unique in its reversing effect on inflammatory or neuropathic hyperalgesia. Activation of TRPM8 by icilin or menthol elicited analgesia in three models of pain: neuropathic pain caused by chronic constriction injury, inflammatory pain induced by CFA, and a peripheral demyelination model [108]. The icilin/menthol-induced analgesia was abolished when TRPM8 antisense oligonucleotides was applied, even though the expression of TRPM8 was upregulated by chronic constriction injury. Evidence suggests that TRPM8 is correlated to metabotropic glutamate receptors, so it is possible that TRPM8 has a protective role in neuropathic pain, in which glutamate released from nociceptive afferents may activate TRPM8 to reduce the exaggerated pain. TRPM8-mediated analgesia was also reported after painful tissue damage from formalin administration. These findings provide the rationale for applying moderately cool dressings to injured or inflamed wounds [38,103].

However, inflammatory cellular events that activate other TRP channels, such as activation of PLC and PKC, release of arachidonic acid, and depletion of PIP_2, are reported to inhibit TRPM8, and cold and menthol responses in DRG neurons are reduced following administration of bradykinin and prostaglandin E_2 [79]. Acidic environment (pH below

6.3), which is common in inflammatory sites, also inhibits TRPM8 [8]. In summary, activation of TRPM8 provides analgesia, but inflammation inhibits the activation of TRPM8, which makes the overall outcome unpredictable. Studies with TRPM8-deleted mice would be interesting to see which role of TRPM8 would predominate.

TRPA1

Increased expression of TRPA1 is necessary to induce cold hyperalgesia after inflammation and nerve injury [101]. TRPA1 is activated by the inflammatory mediator bradykinin, in addition to pungent compounds. Activation of G-protein-coupled bradykinin receptor 2 can activate TRPA1 via PLC and PKA pathway, which means that TPRA1 could mediate the firing of nociceptive neurons in an inflammatory environment. Accordingly, two independent lines of TRPA1$^{-/-}$ mice showed reduced or impaired cellular and behavioral responses to bradykinin injection [10,72]. However, TRPA1 is always coexpressed with TRPV1, and TRPV1$^{-/-}$ mice also showed reduced responses to bradykinin, leaving the possibility of an interaction between TRPV1 and TRPA1 in response to bradykinin. For example, bradykinin activates TRPV1 via PLC, and elevated calcium opens TRPA1 [10]. In contrast, TRPA1 is the principal site of action of formalin-induced pain [90], to which TRPV1 does not contribute [74]. Although a contribution of TRPA1 in inflammatory pain is more than probable, the exact mechanism of action needs further investigation.

TRP Channels and Analgesia

There have been numerous attempts to antagonize the activation of TRP channels involved in nociception because, unlike traditional means of analgesia such as nonsteroidal anti-inflammatory drugs, sodium channel blockers, and opioids, targeting TRP channels for analgesia will block nociception from where it begins [103]. Most of these pharmaceutical studies are aimed at TRPV1 because this channel has the most concrete evidence so far. However, preclinical tests on TRPA1, TRPV3, and TRPV4 antagonists are also ongoing.

Capsaicin as an Analgesic Agent

Capsaicin is a unique compound in that it stimulates nociceptive neurons on initial exposure, but it causes a long-lasting refractory period, as if it desensitizes the neurons. This prolonged effect of blocking nociceptive stimuli has been adopted in many analgesic drugs such as capsaicin-containing creams, patches, and site-specific injections used for diabetic polyneuropathy, postherpetic neuralgia, and arthritis [125,70,73].

TRPV1 Antagonists

The large collection of TRPV1 antagonists includes capsazepine, ruthenium red, 5′-iodoresiniferatoxin, and 6-iodo-nordihydrocapsaicin [3,22,73,103]. Capsazepine is the oldest and most widely used antagonist in the laboratory environment [132], whereas ruthenium red is a more general TRP channel blocker.

Several synthetic antagonists are now in clinical trials. For example, MK2295 and NGD 8243 are in Phase II trials for postoperative pain after tooth extraction [34]. Some trials have been terminated, however. For example, trials of GRC-6211 for osteoarthritis, dental pain, and neuropathic pain were discontinued for undisclosed reasons [73], and a clinical trial of AMG 517 for inflammatory pain in dental patients was discontinued due to long-lasting hyperthermia above 40°C [49,103]. It is reported that tonically active TRPV1 is involved in regulation of body temperature [48,67,113], and the unpredicted hyperthermia could be attributed to suppression of this function [49]. The hyperthermia caused by a peripherally administered TRPV1 antagonist suggests that the site of tonically active TRPV1 in the regulation of body temperature is outside the blood-brain barrier, probably in the abdominal viscera [103,120]. However, other TRPV1 antagonists, such as AMG-8562 and SB-705498, studied in phase II trials for migraine, are not reported to cause hyperthermia, which suggests a compensatory mechanism to the inhibition of tonically active TRPV1 [103]. More thorough understanding of the function and modulation of TRPV1 is required.

A New Approach

A brilliant new approach to analgesia was published in late 2007. In complete contrast to previous attempts, which were mainly intended to block initiation of nociceptive transduction by TRPV1, this strategy uses activation of TRPV1 to achieve nociception-specific anesthesia. Lidocaine is a widely used local anesthetic agent that works by blocking activation of voltage-gated sodium channels. It features many advantages for use as a local anesthetic agent, such as reversible blockade, easy degradation, rare systemic complications, and a hydrophobic, nonpolar molecular structure. The only drawback of lidocaine is that it works on all kinds of nerve fibers that conduct nerve impulses via voltage-gated sodium channels. This property of lidocaine sometimes produces undesirable effects because normal sensory, motor, and autonomic nerve fibers are also anesthetized.

To be clinically important, the most important feature of a local anesthetic agent is a hydrophobic nonpolar molecular structure, because the lidocaine-binding site of the sodium channel is in the cytosolic side, and the local anesthetic agent must gain access to the binding site through the membrane. Therefore, only hydrophobic molecules have been used as clinical local anesthetic agents. However, Binshtok et al. delivered a hydrophilic polar derivative of lidocaine, QX-314, into the cell through the large pore of the TRPV1 channel by coadministration with capsaicin, and showed that only nociceptors expressing TRPV1 were blocked while those without TRPV1 were still unaffected [16,17].

Capsaicin, however, is not an ideal TRPV1 agonist for clinical use because of its pungent, irritating nature. An agonist that provokes less of a burning sensation would be better, such as eugenol, which activates TRPV1 [143] but does not trigger an action potential, probably due to sodium channel inactivation [102]. Recently, lidocaine has been reported to be a TRPV1 agonist, and therefore it can be used instead of capsaicin [17]. Moreover, other nociceptive-specific channels, such as TRPA1 or $P2X_{2/3}$ heteromers that could be dilated with appropriate agonists [136], might be used as the additional transporting route because TRPV1 is not expressed in all nociceptors [103].

TRP Channels in the Central Nervous System

Interestingly, TRPV1 is highly expressed in central termini of primary sensory neurons as well as in higher brain centers [4,133]. However, its function in these areas is poorly understood, because exogenous compounds such as capsaicin can hardly reach them and their temperature cannot rise above 42°C. For these reasons, the function of TRPV1 in the central nervous system (CNS) is more generally proposed as modulating neuronal activity such as anxiety and synaptic plasticity rather than acting as a sensory receptor [4,51,119]. Understanding the role of TRPV1 in the brain will not only provide new insights into how the brain works, but also help researchers to anticipate possible undesirable side effects of TRPV1 antagonists being developed for analgesia.

TRPV1 is found in various areas in brain, such as hippocampal pyramidal neurons in areas CA1 and CA3, the dentate gyrus, the thalamic and hypothalamic nuclei, the locus ceruleus, periaqueductal gray, cerebellum, central amygdala, caudate putamen, and substantia nigra pars compacta [119]. Although less intensively studied, TRPV2, TRPV3, and TRPV4 are also found in the CNS [23,67]. TRPV2 is found coexpressed with TRPV1 in layers IV, V, and VI of the cerebral cortex [76,135]. TRPV3 is expressed in the cortex, thalamus, striatum, hippocampal pyramidal neurons, and cerebellum [71,117,142]. TRPV4 is found in the lamina terminalis in the medial preoptic area, the optic chiasm, the subfornical organ, anterior hypothalamic structures, cerebellum, basal ganglia, ependymal cells of the choroid plexus in the lateral ventricles, and hippocampal pyramidal neurons [71,77,98,100]. TRPV channels are also found in glial and microglial populations and may be upregulated in gliomas [7,13,68].

Given the role of TRPV1 as the primary temperature-sensing molecule in the periphery, it is natural to suspect the same function in the CNS. The temperature-sensing function of TRPV1 in the CNS area was shown nearly 40 years ago in a study in which capsaicin injected to the rat hypothalamus caused rapid hypothermia; repeated administration caused desensitization, and the animal became unable to regulate its body temperature [60]. However, brain temperature cannot rise above the threshold of TRPV1 under normal circumstances. Therefore, the possibility of tonic activation of TRPV1 within physiological range has been proposed [67], such as by decreasing the threshold of TRPV1 with PKC and anandamide [107,116] or cAMP-dependent kinase [15]. Tonic activation of TRPV1 could also be possible by a supply of lipid agonists in the CNS region [67] or by heteromerization with another TRP channel to form a different channel [112].

In the CNS region, lipid ligands may trigger TRPV1 more often than temperature changes [67]. Activation of TRPV1 by lipid ligands is proposed to cause long-term depression in such a way that glutamate released from high-frequency stimulation of the presynaptic neuron activates postsynaptic mGlu1/5 receptors, which in turn leads to the activation of PLC, and then arachidonic acid is converted to 12-(S)-HPETE by 12-lipoxygenase. 12-(S)-HPETE is reported to cross the synapse to activate presynaptic TRPV1, through which calcium entry depresses glutamate release [51].

TRPV1 has been reported to enhance synaptic transmission, such that application of capsaicin increased the frequency of miniature excitatory postsynaptic currents in the spinal cord [116], periaqueductal gray [141], substantia nigra [83], dopamine neurons of ventral tegmental area [85], and the locus ceruleus [86]. N-arachidonoyl-dopamine, an endogenous substance with a similar chemical structure and potency to capsaicin [57], was shown to increase synaptic activity of dopaminergic neurons in the substantia nigra [84]. All of these synaptic increases might result from calcium entry through presynaptic TRPV1 [67], as recently demonstrated by Kim et al. [69]. TRPV1 on the central presynaptic terminals of nociceptive neurons is coupled to mGluR5 in a membrane-delimited manner. Thus, mGluR5 could be activated by glutamate that spills over the synaptic cleft following excessive release from central terminals of nociceptive neurons under pathological conditions such as peripheral inflammation and nerve injury. The subsequent calcium influx via TRPV1 induced by mGluR5 activation may lead to further glutamate release from central terminals, thereby contributing to the modulation of nociceptive synaptic transmission in the substantia gelatinosa neurons of the spinal cord. This line of reasoning suggests that, whereas TRPV1 is a thermal and chemical sensor in the peripheral nervous system, TRPV1 in the CNS might have a more important role as a modulator of multiple G-protein-coupled receptor signals by regulating calcium influx [69] (Fig. 2).

Perspectives

Although molecular and electrophysiological approaches are frequently adopted to study receptors involved in nociception, behavioral animal studies are mandatory in the end. However, more often than not, the results from in vivo studies with genetically modified animals do not match those from in vitro experiments. Numerous factors can cause these inconsistencies, such as duplicated receptor proteins that can substitute for the deleted TRP channels or different physiological conditions between invasive in vitro and conservative in vivo settings, not to mention the discrepancies in age, gender, and species used in each experiment.

Nonetheless, it seems certain that TRP channels are intricately involved in physiological and pathological pain. Understanding the mechanism and modality of the activation and modulation of TRP channels will provide invaluable insights into nociception. Pain research related to these channels, including their possible roles as modulators of neuronal calcium signaling, has progressed rapidly over the last 10 years, and it seems likely that in the not too distant future we may see clinical TRP channel antagonists available for pain control. In the meantime, better understanding of the role of TRP channels in the CNS will help clinical researchers to predict and screen for possible side effects. Recent approaches using TRP channels as a drug delivery system are also promising and may provide an efficient means of nociception-specific analgesia.

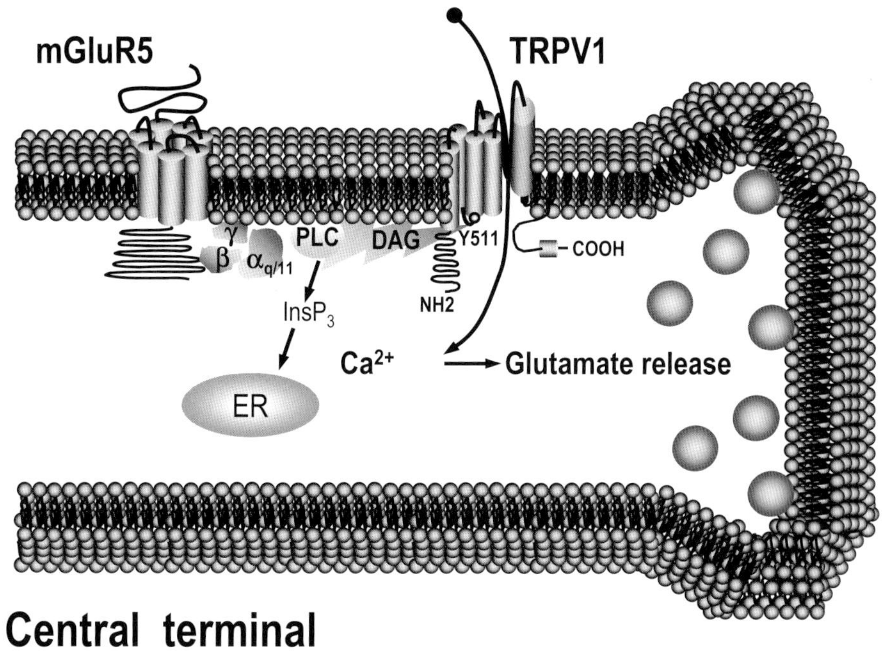

Fig. 2. Schematic diagram that depicts a working hypothesis of central presynaptic TRPV1 in nociceptors (for details, see the text and ref. [69]). DAG, diacylglycerol; ER, endoplasmic reticulum; InsP3, inositol 1,4,5-triphosphate; mGluR5, metabotropic glutamate receptor 5; PLC, phospholipase C; TRPV1, transient receptor potential vanilloid 1.

Acknowledgments

This work was supported by a grant (R0A-2008-000-20101-0) from the National Research Laboratory Program and a grant (2009K001256) from Brain Research Center of the 21st Century Frontier Research Program, funded by the Ministry of Education, Science and Technology, the Republic of Korea.

References

[1] Alessandri-Haber N, Dina OA, Joseph EK, Reichling D, Levine JD. A transient receptor potential vanilloid 4-dependent mechanism of hyperalgesia is engaged by concerted action of inflammatory mediators. J Neurosci 2006;26:3864–74.

[2] Alessandri-Haber N, Dina OA, Yeh JJ, Parada CA, Reichling DB, Levine JD. Transient receptor potential vanilloid 4 is essential in chemotherapy-induced neuropathic pain in the rat. J Neurosci 2004;24):4444–52.

[3] Alexander SP, Mathie A, Peters JA. Guide to receptors and channels (GRAC), 3rd ed. Br J Pharmacol 2008;153(Suppl 2):S1–209.

[4] Alter BJ, Gereau RW. Hotheaded: TRPV1 as mediator of hippocampal synaptic plasticity. Neuron 2008;57:629–31.

[5] Amadesi S, Cottrell GS, Divino L, Chapman K, Grady EF, Bautista F, Karanjia R, Barajas-Lopez C, Vanner S, Vergnolle N, Bunnett NW. Protease-activated receptor 2 sensitizes TRPV1 by protein kinase C epsilon- and A-dependent mechanisms in rats and mice. J Physiol 2006;575(Pt 2):555–71.

[6] Amadesi S, Grant AD, Cottrell GS, Vaksman N, Poole DP, Rozengurt E, Bunnett NW. Protein kinase D isoforms are expressed in rat and mouse primary sensory neurons and are activated by agonists of protease-activated receptor 2. J Comp Neurol 2009;516:141–56.

[7] Amantini C, Mosca M, Nabissi M, Lucciarini R, Caprodossi S, Arcella A, Giangaspero F, Santoni G. Capsaicin-induced apoptosis of glioma cells is mediated by TRPV1 vanilloid receptor and requires p38 MAPK activation. J Neurochem 2007;102:977–90.

[8] Andersson DA, Chase HW, Bevan S. TRPM8 activation by menthol, icilin, and cold is differentially modulated by intracellular pH. J Neurosci 2004;24:5364–9.

[9] Babes A, Zorzon D, Reid G. A novel type of cold-sensitive neuron in rat dorsal root ganglia with rapid adaptation to cooling stimuli. Eur J Neurosci 2006;24(3):691–8.

[10] Bautista DM, Jordt SE, Nikai T, Tsuruda PR, Read AJ, Poblete J, Yamoah EN, Basbaum AI, Julius D. TRPA1 mediates the inflammatory actions of environmental irritants and proalgesic agents. Cell 2006;124:1269–82.

[11] Bautista DM, Siemens J, Glazer JM, Tsuruda PR, Basbaum AI, Stucky CL, Jordt SE, Julius D. The menthol receptor TRPM8 is the principal detector of environmental cold. Nature 2007;448:204–8.

[12] Beech DJ, Muraki K, Flemming R. Non-selective cationic channels of smooth muscle and the mammalian homologues of *Drosophila* TRP. J Physiol 2004;559(Pt 3):685–706.

[13] Benfenati V, Amiry-Moghaddam M, Caprini M, Mylonakou MN, Rapisarda C, Ottersen OP, Ferroni S. Expression and functional characterization of transient receptor potential vanilloid-related channel 4 (TRPV4) in rat cortical astrocytes. Neuroscience 2007;148:876–92.

[14] Bhave G, Gereau RW. Posttranslational mechanisms of peripheral sensitization. J Neurobiol 2004;61:88–106.

[15] Bhave G, Zhu W, Wang H, Brasier DJ, Oxford GS, Gereau RW. cAMP-dependent protein kinase regulates desensitization of the capsaicin receptor (VR1) by direct phosphorylation. Neuron 2002;35:721–31.

[16] Binshtok AM, Bean BP, Woolf CJ. Inhibition of nociceptors by TRPV1-mediated entry of impermeant sodium channel blockers. Nature 2007;449:607–10.

[17] Binshtok AM, Gerner P, Oh SB, Puopolo M, Suzuki S, Roberson DP, Herbert T, Wang C-F, Kim D, Chung G, et al. Coapplication of lidocaine and the permanently charged sodium channel blocker QX-314 produces a long-lasting nociceptive blockade in rodents. Anesthesiology 2009;111:127–37.

[18] Birder LA, Kanai AJ, De Groat WC, Kiss S, Nealen ML, Burke NE, Dineley KE, Watkins S, Reynolds IJ, Caterina MJ. Vanilloid receptor expression suggests a sensory role for urinary bladder epithelial cells. Proc Natl Acad Sci USA 2001;98:13396–401.

[19] Birder LA, Nakamura Y, Kiss S, Nealen ML, Barrick S, Kanai AJ, Wang E, Ruiz G, De Groat WC, Apodaca G, et al. Altered urinary bladder function in mice lacking the vanilloid receptor TRPV1. Nat Neurosci 2002;5:856–60.

[20] Bölcskei K, Helyes Z, Szabó A, Sándor K, Elekes K, Németh J, Almási R, Pintér E, Petho G, Szolcsányi J. Investigation of the role of TRPV1 receptors in acute and chronic nociceptive processes using gene-deficient mice. Pain 2005;117:368–76.

[21] Brierley SM, Page AJ, Hughes PA, Adam B, Liebregts T, Cooper NJ, Holtmann G, Liedtke W, Blackshaw LA. Selective role for TRPV4 ion channels in visceral sensory pathways. Gastroenterology 2008;134:2059–69.

[22] Broad LM, Mogg AJ, Beattie RE, Ogden AM, Blanco MJ, Bleakman D. TRP channels as emerging targets for pain therapeutics. Expert Opin Ther Targets 2009;13:69–81.

[23] Caterina MJ. Transient receptor potential ion channels as participants in thermosensation and thermoregulation. Am J Physiol Regul Integr Comp Physiol 2007;292:R64–76.

[24] Caterina MJ, Leffler A, Malmberg AB, Martin WJ, Trafton J, Petersen-Zeitz KR, Koltzenburg M, Basbaum AI, Julius D. Impaired nociception and pain sensation in mice lacking the capsaicin receptor. Science 2000;288:306–13.

[25] Caterina MJ, Schumacher MA, Tominaga M, Rosen TA, Levine JD, Julius D. The capsaicin receptor: a heat-activated ion channel in the pain pathway. Nature 1997;389:816–24.

[26] Cavanaugh DJ, Lee H, Lo L, Shields SD, Zylka MJ, Basbaum AI, Anderson DJ. Distinct subsets of unmyelinated primary sensory fibers mediate behavioral responses to noxious thermal and mechanical stimuli. Proc Natl Acad Sci USA 2009;106:9075–80.

[27] Christensen A, Corey D. TRP channels in mechanosensation: direct or indirect activation? Nat Rev Neurosci 2007;8:510–21.

[28] Christoph T, Gillen C, Mika J, Grünweller A, Schäfer MK, Schiene K, Frank R, Jostock R, Bahrenberg G, Weihe E, et al. Antinociceptive effect of antisense oligonucleotides against the vanilloid receptor VR1/TRPV1. Neurochem Int 2007;50:281–90.

[29] Chuang HH, Neuhausser WM, Julius D. The super-cooling agent icilin reveals a mechanism of coincidence detection by a temperature-sensitive TRP channel. Neuron 2004;43:859–69.

[30] Chuang HH, Prescott ED, Kong H, Shields S, Jordt SE, Basbaum AI, Chao MV, Julius D. Bradykinin and nerve growth factor release the capsaicin receptor from PtdIns(4,5)P2-mediated inhibition. Nature 2001;411:957–62.

[31] Ciura S, Bourque C. Transient receptor potential vanilloid 1 is required for intrinsic osmoreception in organum vasculosum lamina terminalis neurons and for normal thirst responses to systemic hyperosmolality. J Neurosci 2006;26:9069–75.

[32] Clapham DE. TRP channels as cellular sensors. Nature 2003;426:517–24.

[33] Corey D, García-Añoveros J, Holt JR, Kwan KY, Lin SY, Vollrath MA, Amalfitano A, Cheung EL, Derfler BH, Duggan A, et al. TRPA1 is a candidate for the mechanosensitive transduction channel of vertebrate hair cells. Nature 2004;432:723–30.

[34] Cortright DN, Krause JE, Broom DC. TRP channels and pain. Biochim Biophys Acta 2007;1772:978–88.

[35] Cosens DJ, Manning A. Abnormal electroretinogram from a *Drosophila* mutant. Nature 1969;224:285–7.

[36] Davis JB, Gray J, Gunthorpe MJ, Hatcher JP, Davey PT, Overend P, Harries MH, Latcham J, Clapham C, Atkinson K, et al. Vanilloid receptor-1 is essential for inflammatory thermal hyperalgesia. Nature 2000;405:183–7.
[37] Dhaka A, Earley TJ, Watson J, Patapoutian A. Visualizing cold spots: TRPM8-expressing sensory neurons and their projections. J Neurosci 2008;28:566–75.
[38] Dhaka A, Murray AN, Mathur J, Earley TJ, Petrus MJ, Patapoutian A. TRPM8 is required for cold sensation in mice. Neuron 2007;54:371–8.
[39] Dhaka A, Uzzell V, Dubin AE, Mathur J, Petrus M, Bandell M, Patapoutian A. TRPV1 is activated by both acidic and basic pH. J Neurosci 2009;29:153–8.
[40] Dhaka A, Viswanath V, Patapoutian A. TRP ion channels and temperature sensation. Annu Rev Neurosci 2006;29:135–61.
[41] Dietrich A, Kalwa H, Storch U, Mederos y Schnitzler M, Salanova B, Pinkenburg O, Dubrovska G, Essin K, Gollasch M, Birnbaumer L, Gudermann T. Pressure-induced and store-operated cation influx in vascular smooth muscle cells is independent of TRPC1. Pflugers Arch 2007;455:465–77.
[42] Dina OA, Chen X, Reichling D, Levine JD. Role of protein kinase Cepsilon and protein kinase A in a model of paclitaxel-induced painful peripheral neuropathy in the rat. Neuroscience 2001;108:507–15.
[43] Dina OA, Parada CA, Yeh J, Chen X, McCarter GC, Levine JD. Integrin signaling in inflammatory and neuropathic pain in the rat. Eur J Neurosci 2004;19:634–42.
[44] Facer P, Casula MA, Smith GD, Benham CD, Chessell IP, Bountra C, Sinisi M, Birch R, Anand P. Differential expression of the capsaicin receptor TRPV1 and related novel receptors TRPV3, TRPV4 and TRPM8 in normal human tissues and changes in traumatic and diabetic neuropathy. BMC Neurol 2007;7:11.
[45] Foulkes T, Wood JN. Mechanisms of cold pain. Channels (Austin) 2007;1:154–60.
[46] Fujita F, Uchida K, Moriyama T, Shima A, Shibasaki K, Inada H, Sokabe T, Tominaga M. Intracellular alkalization causes pain sensation through activation of TRPA1 in mice. J Clin Invest 2008;118:4049–57.
[47] Fukuoka T, Tokunaga A, Tachibana T, Dai Y, Yamanaka H, Noguchi K. VR1, but not $P2X_3$, increases in the spared L4 DRG in rats with L5 spinal nerve ligation. Pain 2002;99:111–20.
[48] Gavva NR, Bannon AW, Surapaneni S, Hovland DN, Lehto SG, Gore A, Juan T, Deng H, Han B, Klionsky L, et al. The vanilloid receptor TRPV1 is tonically activated in vivo and involved in body temperature regulation. J Neurosci 2007;27:3366–74.
[49] Gavva NR, Treanor JJ, Garami A, Fang L, Surapaneni S, Akrami A, Alvarez F, Bak A, Darling M, Gore A, et al. Pharmacological blockade of the vanilloid receptor TRPV1 elicits marked hyperthermia in humans. Pain 2008;136:202–10.
[50] Gee MD, Lynn B, Basile S, Pierau FK, Cotsell B. The relationship between axonal spike shape and functional modality in cutaneous C-fibres in the pig and rat. Neuroscience 1999;90:509–18.
[51] Gibson HE, Edwards JG, Page RS, Van Hook MJ, Kauer JA. TRPV1 channels mediate long-term depression at synapses on hippocampal interneurons. Neuron 2008;57:746–59.
[52] Grant AD, Cottrell GS, Amadesi S, Trevisani M, Nicoletti P, Materazzi S, Altier C, Cenac N, Zamponi GW, Bautista-Cruz F, et al. Protease-activated receptor 2 sensitizes the transient receptor potential vanilloid 4 ion channel to cause mechanical hyperalgesia in mice. J Physiol 2007;578(Pt 3):715–33.
[53] Guharay F, Sachs F. Stretch-activated single ion channel currents in tissue-cultured embryonic chick skeletal muscle. J Physiol 1984;352:685–701.
[54] Hensel H, Zotterman Y. The effect of menthol on the thermoreceptors. Acta Physiol Scand 1951;24:27–34.
[55] Hinman A, Chuang HH, Bautista DM, Julius D. TRP channel activation by reversible covalent modification. Proc Natl Acad Sci USA 2006;103:19564–8.
[56] Hong S, Wiley JW. Early painful diabetic neuropathy is associated with differential changes in the expression and function of vanilloid receptor 1. J Biol Chem 2005;280:618–27.
[57] Huang SM, Bisogno T, Trevisani M, Al-Hayani A, De Petrocellis L, Fezza F, Tognetto M, Petros TJ, Krey JF, Chu CJ, et al. An endogenous capsaicin-like substance with high potency at recombinant and native vanilloid VR1 receptors. Proc Natl Acad Sci USA 2002;99:8400–5.
[58] Hudson LJ, Bevan S, Wotherspoon G, Gentry C, Fox A, Winter J. VR1 protein expression increases in undamaged DRG neurons after partial nerve injury. Eur J Neurosci 2001;13:2105–14.
[59] Hwang SW, Cho H, Kwak J, Lee SY, Kang CJ, Jung J, Cho S, Min KH, Suh YG, Kim D, OH U. Direct activation of capsaicin receptors by products of lipoxygenases: endogenous capsaicin-like substances. Proc Natl Acad Sci USA 2000;97:6155–60.
[60] Jancsó-Gábor A, Szolcsányi J, Jancsó N. Stimulation and desensitization of the hypothalamic heat-sensitive structures by capsaicin in rats. J Physiol 1970;208:449–59.
[61] Ji RR, Samad TA, Jin SX, Schmoll R, Woolf CJ. p38 MAPK activation by NGF in primary sensory neurons after inflammation increases TRPV1 levels and maintains heat hyperalgesia. Neuron 2002;36:57–68.
[62] Jones RC, Xu L, Gebhart GF. The mechanosensitivity of mouse colon afferent fibers and their sensitization by inflammatory mediators require transient receptor potential vanilloid 1 and acid-sensing ion channel 3. J Neurosci 2005;25:10981–9.
[63] Kamei J, Zushida K, Morita K, Sasaki M, Tanaka S. Role of vanilloid VR1 receptor in thermal allodynia and hyperalgesia in diabetic mice. Eur J Pharmacol 2001;422:83–6.
[64] Karashima Y, Damann N, Prenen J, Talavera K, Segal A, Voets T, Nilius B. Bimodal action of menthol on the transient receptor potential channel TRPA1. J Neurosci 2007;27:9874–84.
[65] Karashima Y, Talavera K, Everaerts W, Janssens A, Kwan KY, Vennekens R, Nilius B, Voets T. TRPA1 acts as a cold sensor in vitro and in vivo. Proc Natl Acad Sci USA 2009;106:1273–8.

[66] Kashiba H, Uchida Y, Takeda D, Nishigori A, Ueda Y, Kuribayashi K, Ohshima M. TRPV2-immunoreactive intrinsic neurons in the rat intestine. Neurosci Lett 2004;366:193–6.
[67] Kauer JA, Gibson HE. Hot flash: TRPV channels in the brain. Trends Neurosci 2009;32:215–24.
[68] Kim SR, Kim SU, Oh U, Jin BK. Transient receptor potential vanilloid subtype 1 mediates microglial cell death in vivo and in vitro via Ca^{2+}-mediated mitochondrial damage and cytochrome C release. J Immunol 2006;177:4322–9.
[69] Kim YH, Park C, Back SK, Lee CJ, Hwang S, Bae Y, Na HS, Kim JS, Jung SJ, Oh SB. Membrane-delimited coupling of TRPV1 and mGluR5 on presynaptic terminals of nociceptive neurons. J Neurosci 2009;29:10000–9.
[70] Knotkova H, Pappagallo M, Szallasi A. Capsaicin (TRPV1 agonist) therapy for pain relief: farewell or revival? Clin J Pain 2008;24:142–54.
[71] Kunert-Keil C, Bisping F, Krüger J, Brinkmeier H. Tissue-specific expression of TRP channel genes in the mouse and its variation in three different mouse strains. BMC Genomics 2006;7:159.
[72] Kwan KY, Allchorne AJ, Vollrath MA, Christensen A, Zhang DS, Woolf CJ, Corey D. TRPA1 contributes to cold, mechanical, and chemical nociception but is not essential for hair-cell transduction. Neuron 2006;50:277–89.
[73] Lazar J, Gharat L, Khairathkar-Joshi N, Blumberg PM, Szallasi A. Screening TRPV1 antagonists for the treatment of pain: lessons learned over a decade. Expert Opin Drug Dis 2009;4:159–80.
[74] Levine JD, Alessandri-Haber N. TRP channels: targets for the relief of pain. Biochim Biophys Acta 2007;1772:989–1003.
[75] Lewinter RD, Skinner K, Julius D, Basbaum AI. Immunoreactive TRPV-2 (VRL-1), a capsaicin receptor homolog, in the spinal cord of the rat. J Comp Neurol 2004;470:400–8.
[76] Liapi A, Wood JN. Extensive co-localization and heteromultimer formation of the vanilloid receptor-like protein TRPV2 and the capsaicin receptor TRPV1 in the adult rat cerebral cortex. Eur J Neurosci 2005;22:825–34.
[77] Liedtke W, Choe Y, Martí-Renom MA, Bell AM, Denis CS, Sali A, Hudspeth AJ, Friedman JM, Heller S. Vanilloid receptor-related osmotically activated channel (VR-OAC), a candidate vertebrate osmoreceptor. Cell 2000;103:525–35.
[78] Liedtke W, Tobin DM, Bargmann CI, Friedman JM. Mammalian TRPV4 (VR-OAC) directs behavioral responses to osmotic and mechanical stimuli in *Caenorhabditis elegans.* Proc Natl Acad Sci USA 2003;100(Suppl 2):14531–6.
[79] Linte RM, Ciobanu C, Reid G, Babes A. Desensitization of cold- and menthol-sensitive rat dorsal root ganglion neurones by inflammatory mediators. Exp Brain Res 2007;178:89–98.
[80] Macpherson LJ, Dubin AE, Evans MJ, Marr F, Schultz PG, Cravatt BF, Patapoutian A. Noxious compounds activate TRPA1 ion channels through covalent modification of cysteines. Nature 2007;445:541–5.
[81] Macpherson LJ, Hwang SW, Miyamoto T, Dubin AE, Patapoutian A, Story GM. More than cool: promiscuous relationships of menthol and other sensory compounds. Mol Cell Neurosci 2006;32:335–43.
[82] Madrid R, Donovan-Rodríguez T, Meseguer V, Acosta MC, Belmonte C, Viana F. Contribution of TRPM8 channels to cold transduction in primary sensory neurons and peripheral nerve terminals. J Neurosci 2006;26:12512–25.
[83] Marinelli S, Di Marzo V, Berretta N, Matias I, Maccarrone M, Bernardi G, Mercuri NB. Presynaptic facilitation of glutamatergic synapses to dopaminergic neurons of the rat substantia nigra by endogenous stimulation of vanilloid receptors. J Neurosci 2003;23:3136–44.
[84] Marinelli S, Di Marzo V, Florenzano F, Fezza F, Viscomi MT, Van Der Stelt M, Bernardi G, Molinari M, Maccarrone M, Mercuri NB. N-arachidonoyl-dopamine tunes synaptic transmission onto dopaminergic neurons by activating both cannabinoid and vanilloid receptors. Neuropsychopharmacology 2007;32:298–308.
[85] Marinelli S, Pascucci T, Bernardi G, Puglisi-Allegra S, Mercuri NB. Activation of TRPV1 in the VTA excites dopaminergic neurons and increases chemical- and noxious-induced dopamine release in the nucleus accumbens. Neuropsychopharmacology 2005;30:864–70.
[86] Marinelli S, Vaughan CW, Christie MJ, Connor M. Capsaicin activation of glutamatergic synaptic transmission in the rat locus coeruleus in vitro. J Physiol 2002;543(Pt 2):531–40.
[87] Maroto R, Raso A, Wood T, Kurosky A, Martinac B, Hamill O. TRPC1 forms the stretch-activated cation channel in vertebrate cells. Nat Cell Biol 2005;7:179–85.
[88] McKemy DD. How cold is it? TRPM8 and TRPA1 in the molecular logic of cold sensation. Mol Pain 2005;1:16.
[89] McKemy DD, Neuhausser WM, Julius D. Identification of a cold receptor reveals a general role for TRP channels in thermosensation. Nature 2002;416:52–8.
[90] McNamara CR, Mandel-Brehm J, Bautista DM, Siemenst J, Deranian KL, Zhao M, Hayward NJ, Chong JA, Julius D, Moran MM, Fanger CM. TRPA1 mediates formalin-induced pain. Proc Natl Acad Sci USA 2007;104:13525–30.
[91] Miranda A, Nordstrom E, Mannem A, Smith C, Banerjee B, Sengupta JN. The role of transient receptor potential vanilloid 1 in mechanical and chemical visceral hyperalgesia following experimental colitis. Neuroscience 2007;148:1021–32.
[92] Mohapatra DP, Nau C. Desensitization of capsaicin-activated currents in the vanilloid receptor TRPV1 is decreased by the cyclic AMP-dependent protein kinase pathway. J Biol Chem 2003;278:50080–90.
[93] Montell C, Birnbaumer L, Flockerzi V, Bindels RJ, Bruford EA, Caterina MJ, Clapham DE, Harteneck C, Heller S, Julius D, et al. A unified nomenclature for the superfamily of TRP cation channels. Mol Cell 2002;9:229–31.
[94] Moqrich A, Hwang SW, Earley TJ, Petrus MJ, Murray AN, Spencer KS, Andahazy M, Story GM, Patapoutian A. Impaired thermosensation in mice lacking TRPV3, a heat and camphor sensor in the skin. Science 2005;307:1468–72.
[95] Morin C, Bushnell MC. Temporal and qualitative properties of cold pain and heat pain: a psychophysical study. Pain 1998;74:67–73.
[96] Moriyama T, Iida T, Kobayashi K, Higashi T, Fukuoka T, Tsumura H, Leon C, Suzuki N, Inoue K, Gachet C, Noguchi K, Tominaga M. Possible involvement of P2Y2 metabotropic receptors in ATP-induced transient receptor potential vanilloid receptor 1-mediated thermal hypersensitivity. J Neurosci 2003;23:6058–62.
[97] Munns C, Al Qatari M, Koltzenburg M. Many cold sensitive peripheral neurons of the mouse do not express TRPM8 or TRPA1. Cell Calcium 2007;41:331–42.

[98] Mutai H, Heller S. Vertebrate and invertebrate TRPV-like mechanoreceptors. Cell Calcium 2003;33:471–8.
[99] Nagata K, Duggan A, Kumar G, García-Añoveros J. Nociceptor and hair cell transducer properties of TRPA1, a channel for pain and hearing. J Neurosci 2005;25:4052–61.
[100] Nilius B, Vriens J, Prenen J, Droogmans G, Voets T. TRPV4 calcium entry channel: a paradigm for gating diversity. Am J Physiol Cell Physiol 2004;286:C195–205.
[101] Obata K, Katsura H, Mizushima T, Yamanaka H, Kobayashi K, Dai Y, Fukuoka T, Tokunaga A, Tominaga M, Noguchi K. TRPA1 induced in sensory neurons contributes to cold hyperalgesia after inflammation and nerve injury. J Clin Invest 2005;115:2393–401.
[102] Park CK, Kim K, Jung SJ, Kim MJ, Ahn DK, Hong SD, Kim JS, Oh SB. Molecular mechanism for local anesthetic action of eugenol in the rat trigeminal system. Pain 2009;144:84–94.
[103] Patapoutian A, Tate S, Woolf CJ. Transient receptor potential channels: targeting pain at the source. Nat Rev Drug Discover 2009;8:55–68.
[104] Pedersen SF, Nilius B. Transient receptor potential channels in mechanosensing and cell volume regulation. Methods Enzymol 2007;428:183–207.
[105] Peier A, Moqrich A, Hergarden AC, Reeve AJ, Andersson DA, Story GM, Earley TJ, Dragoni I, McIntyre P, Bevan S, Patapoutian A. A TRP channel that senses cold stimuli and menthol. Cell 2002;108(5):705–15.
[106] Pogatzki-Zahn EM, Shimizu I, Caterina M, Raja SN. Heat hyperalgesia after incision requires TRPV1 and is distinct from pure inflammatory pain. Pain 2005;115:296–307.
[107] Premkumar LS, Ahern GP. Induction of vanilloid receptor channel activity by protein kinase C. Nature 2000;408:985–90.
[108] Proudfoot CJ, Garry EM, Cottrell DF, Rosie R, Anderson H, Robertson DC, Fleetwood-Walker SM, Mitchell R. Analgesia mediated by the TRPM8 cold receptor in chronic neuropathic pain. Curr Biol 2006;16:1591–605.
[109] Reid G. ThermoTRP channels and cold sensing: what are they really up to? Pflugers Arch 2005;451:250–63.
[110] Reid G, Babes A, Pluteanu F. A cold- and menthol-activated current in rat dorsal root ganglion neurones: properties and role in cold transduction. J Physiol 2002;545(Pt 2):595–614.
[111] Reid G, Flonta ML. Ion channels activated by cold and menthol in cultured rat dorsal root ganglion neurones. Neurosci Lett 2002;324:164–8.
[112] Schaefer M. Homo- and heteromeric assembly of TRP channel subunits. Pflugers Arch 2005;451:35–42.
[113] Sharif-Naeini R, Ciura S, Bourque C. TRPV1 gene required for thermosensory transduction and anticipatory secretion from vasopressin neurons during hyperthermia. Neuron 2008;58:179–85.
[114] Shimosato G, Amaya F, Ueda M, Tanaka Y, Decosterd I, Tanaka M. Peripheral inflammation induces up-regulation of TRPV2 expression in rat DRG. Pain 2005;119:225–32.
[115] Shin J, Cho H, Hwang SW, Jung J, Shin CY, Lee SY, Kim SH, Lee MG, Choi YH, Kim J, et al. Bradykinin-12-lipoxygenase-VR1 signaling pathway for inflammatory hyperalgesia. Proc Natl Acad Sci USA 2002;99:10150–5.
[116] Sikand P, Premkumar LS. Potentiation of glutamatergic synaptic transmission by protein kinase C-mediated sensitization of TRPV1 at the first sensory synapse. J Physiol 2007;581(Pt 2):631–47.
[117] Smith GD, Gunthorpe MJ, Kelsell RE, Hayes PD, Reilly P, Facer P, Wright JE, Jerman JC, Walhin JP, Ooi Let al. TRPV3 is a temperature-sensitive vanilloid receptor-like protein. Nature 2002;418:186–90.
[118] Spassova MA, Hewavitharana T, Xu W, Soboloff J, Gill DL. A common mechanism underlies stretch activation and receptor activation of TRPC6 channels. Proc Natl Acad Sci USA 2006;103:16586–91.
[119] Starowicz K, Cristino L, Di Marzo V. TRPV1 receptors in the central nervous system: potential for previously unforeseen therapeutic applications. Curr Pharm Des 2008;14:42–54.
[120] Steiner AA, Turek VF, Almeida MC, Burmeister JJ, Oliveira DL, Roberts JL, Bannon AW, Norman MH, Louis JC, Treanor JJ, et al. Nonthermal activation of transient receptor potential vanilloid-1 channels in abdominal viscera tonically inhibits autonomic cold-defense effectors. J Neurosci 2007;27:7459–68.
[121] Stokes AJ, Wakano C, Del Carmen KA, Koblan-Huberson M, Turner H. Formation of a physiological complex between TRPV2 and RGA protein promotes cell surface expression of TRPV2. J Cell Biochem 2005;94:669–83.
[122] Story GM, Peier A, Reeve AJ, Eid SR, Mosbacher J, Hricik TR, Earley TJ, Hergarden AC, Andersson DA, Hwang SW, et al. ANKTM1, a TRP-like channel expressed in nociceptive neurons, is activated by cold temperatures. Cell 2003;112:819–29.
[123] Suzuki M, Mizuno A, Kodaira K, Imai M. Impaired pressure sensation in mice lacking TRPV4. J Biol Chem 2003;278:22664–8.
[124] Szabó A, Helyes Z, Sándor K, Bite A, Pintér E, Németh J, Bánvölgyi A, Bölcskei K, Elekes K, Szolcsányi J. Role of transient receptor potential vanilloid 1 receptors in adjuvant-induced chronic arthritis: in vivo study using gene-deficient mice. J Pharmacol Exp Ther 2005;314:111–9.
[125] Szallasi A, Blumberg PM. Vanilloid (capsaicin) receptors and mechanisms. Pharmacol Rev 1999;51:159–212.
[126] Takashima Y, Daniels RL, Knowlton W, Teng J, Liman ER, McKemy DD. Diversity in the neural circuitry of cold sensing revealed by genetic axonal labeling of transient receptor potential melastatin 8 neurons. J Neurosci 2007;27:14147–57.
[127] Talavera K, Yasumatsu K, Voets T, Droogmans G, Shigemura N, Ninomiya Y, Margolskee RF, Nilius B. Heat activation of TRPM5 underlies thermal sensitivity of sweet taste. Nature 2005;438:1022–5.
[128] Todaka H, Taniguchi J, Satoh J, Mizuno A, Suzuki M. Warm temperature-sensitive transient receptor potential vanilloid 4 (TRPV4) plays an essential role in thermal hyperalgesia. J Biol Chem 2004;279:35133–8.
[129] Togashi K, Hara Y, Tominaga T, Higashi T, Konishi Y, Mori Y, Tominaga M. TRPM2 activation by cyclic ADP-ribose at body temperature is involved in insulin secretion. EMBO J 2006;25:1804–15.
[130] Tominaga M, Caterina MJ. Thermosensation and pain. J Neurobiol 2004;61:3–12.
[131] Tominaga M, Caterina MJ, Malmberg AB, Rosen TA, Gilbert H, Skinner K, Raumann BE, Basbaum AI, Julius D. The cloned capsaicin receptor integrates multiple pain-producing stimuli. Neuron 1998;21:531–43.

[132] Urban L, Dray A. Capsazepine, a novel capsaicin antagonist, selectively antagonises the effects of capsaicin in the mouse spinal cord in vitro. Neurosci Lett 1991;134:9–11.
[133] Valtschanoff JG, Rustioni A, Guo A, Hwang SJ. Vanilloid receptor VR1 is both presynaptic and postsynaptic in the superficial laminae of the rat dorsal horn. J Comp Neurol 2001;436:225–35.
[134] van den Wijngaard RM, Klooker TK, Welting O, Stanisor OI, Wouters MM, van der Coelen D, Bulmer DC, Peeters PJ, Aerssens J, de Hoogt R, et al. Essential role for TRPV1 in stress-induced (mast cell-dependent) colonic hypersensitivity in maternally separated rats. Neurogastroenterol Motil 2009;21:1107–e94.
[135] Venkatachalam K, Montell C. TRP channels. Annu Rev Biochem 2007;76:387–417.
[136] Virginio C, MacKenzie A, Rassendren FA, North RA, Surprenant A. Pore dilation of neuronal P2X receptor channels. Nat Neurosci 1999;2:315–21.
[137] Wainwright A, Rutter AR, Seabrook GR, Reilly K, Oliver KR. Discrete expression of TRPV2 within the hypothalamo-neurohypophysial system: implications for regulatory activity within the hypothalamic-pituitary-adrenal axis. J Comp Neurol 2004;474:24–42.
[138] Wei ET, Seid DA. AG-3-5: a chemical producing sensations of cold. J Pharm Pharmacol 1983;35:110–2.
[139] Welsh DG, Morielli AD, Nelson MT, Brayden JE. Transient receptor potential channels regulate myogenic tone of resistance arteries. Circ Res 2002;90:248–50.
[140] Woodbury CJ, Zwick M, Wang S, Lawson JJ, Caterina MJ, Koltzenburg M, Albers KM, Koerber HR, Davis BM. Nociceptors lacking TRPV1 and TRPV2 have normal heat responses. J Neurosci 2004;24:6410–5.
[141] Xing J, Li J. TRPV1 receptor mediates glutamatergic synaptic input to dorsolateral periaqueductal gray (dl-PAG) neurons. J Neurophysiol 2007;97:503–11.
[142] Xu H, Ramsey IS, Kotecha SA, Moran MM, Chong JA, Lawson D, Ge P, Lilly J, Silos-Santiago I, Xie Y, et al. TRPV3 is a calcium-permeable temperature-sensitive cation channel. Nature 2002;418:181–6.
[143] Yang BH, Piao ZG, Kim YB, Lee CH, Lee JK, Park K, Kim JS, Oh SB. Activation of vanilloid receptor 1 (VR1) by eugenol. J Dent Res 2003;82:781–5.
[144] Zhang X, Huang J, McNaughton PA. NGF rapidly increases membrane expression of TRPV1 heat-gated ion channels. EMBO J 2005;24:4211–23.
[145] Zurborg S, Yurgionas B, Jira JA, Caspani O, Heppenstall PA. Direct activation of the ion channel TRPA1 by Ca^{2+}. Nat Neurosci 2007;10:277–9.

Correspondence to: Seog Bae Oh, DDS, PhD, National Research Lab for Pain, Department of Physiology, School of Dentistry, Seoul National University, 28 Yeongun, Jongno, Seoul, 110-749, Korea. Tel: +82-2-740-8656; fax: +82-2-762-5107; email: odolbae@snu.ac.kr.

16

Adrenergic and Cholinergic Targets in Pain Pharmacology

Ralf Baron and Wilfrid Jänig

Department of Neurological Pain Research and Therapy, Neurological Clinic, University Hospital Schleswig Holstein, Campus Kiel, and Department of Physiology, Christian-Albrechts University of Kiel, Kiel, Germany

For almost a century it has been assumed that in certain clinical syndromes that are characterized by severe pain, such as causalgia and reflex sympathetic dystrophy, activity in the sympathetic nervous system may be involved in the generation of pain. This assumption is based mainly upon two observations: (1) the pain is spatially correlated with signs of autonomic dysfunction, i.e., with abnormalities in blood flow and sweating, as well as with trophic changes; and (2) blocking the efferent sympathetic supply to the affected extremity relieves the pain.

In 1995, the terminology of these pain syndromes was changed. The term "reflex sympathetic dystrophy" was thought to be inappropriate as a clinical designation because it has been used to describe a much more extensive range of clinical presentations than was originally intended. Moreover, since the pathophysiological mechanisms underlying these syndromes are poorly understood, it is probably premature to use the terms "reflex" and "sympathetic." Therefore, the new terminology is based entirely on elements of history, symptoms, and findings on clinical examination with no implied pathophysiological mechanism [128]. According to the International Association for the Study of Pain (IASP) *Classification of Chronic Pain,* reflex sympathetic dystrophy and causalgia are now called complex regional pain syndromes (CRPS). In CRPS type I (reflex sympathetic dystrophy), minor injuries at the limb or lesions in remote body areas precede the onset of symptoms. CRPS type II (causalgia) develops after injury of a major peripheral nerve [90].

Pharmacology of Pain
edited by Pierre Beaulieu, David Lussier, Frank Porreca, and Anthony H. Dickenson
IASP Press, Seattle, © 2010

This chapter summarizes both animal experiments and clinical observations that address the role of the sympathetic nervous system in the generation of pain in CRPS and related pain syndromes. This subject is of considerable clinical interest. Conceptually, it must be looked at in the context of how the cellular processes that lead to ongoing and evoked inflammatory, neuropathic, or generalized pain are orchestrated by the brain in the continuous protection of the body against agents from outside as well as from within the body [54,55,60].

The Role of the Autonomic Nervous System in the Generation of Pain: Sympathetically Maintained Pain

Interruption of the efferent sympathetic nerve supply to the affected extremity has been used to treat certain pain syndromes for many years. These syndromes include CRPS-I, CRPS-II, post-traumatic neuralgia, phantom limb pain, and to a certain extent acute herpes zoster. René Leriche was the first who reported that sympathectomy dramatically relieves causalgia (CRPS-II) [77]. (It should be noted that sympathectomy performed by Leriche consisted of periarterial stripping of large arteries based on the erroneous belief that sympathetic fibers to blood vessels in extremities pass along the blood vessels and not through the gray rami and peripheral nerves [53]. It is puzzling how this intervention led to pain relief.) This notion was supported by several large clinical series, primarily in wounded soldiers. Richards [113] described the clinical features of causalgia and the effect of sympatholytic interventions in hundreds of cases, and he was emphatic about the dramatic response of causalgia to sympathetic blockade. He stated: "One of the outstanding surgical lessons that was learned during World War II was that interruption of the appropriate sympathetic nerve fibers is almost invariably effective in the treatment of causalgia. When the sympathetic chain is blocked by a local anesthetic, complete relief occurs almost immediately if the injection has been correctly placed, and the dramatic change in the patient's appearance and attitude is remarkable." The finding that sympatholysis relieves causalgic pain gave rise to the concept of sympathetically maintained pain.

Mitchell [95], Livingston [83] (in particular Chapters 5, 6, 14, and 15), and Bonica [18] (Chapter 28) are not only of historical interest (discussing the literature before 1953), but provide a wealth of carefully reported clinical observations. The ideas developed on the basis of these clinical observations are still quite modern, showing that the progress in this field is not as impressive as it appears to be.

In CRPS types I and II, clinical experience and uncontrolled studies in hundreds of patients show a beneficial effect of sympatholytic procedures. Therefore, many authors believe that a sympathetic component of the pain is a characteristic feature of these syndromes, and a successful symptomatic blockade was considered necessary for the diagnosis of CRPS [17]. The concept that the sympathetic nervous system may be actively involved in the generation of pain is controversial, however, mainly because the techniques and results of sympathetic blockade have rarely been adequately evaluated, and in most cases the studies were not placebo-controlled [136,137] (but see [8,107,121]).

On the basis of experience and recent studies, the following change was suggested that is now generally accepted [128]: patients with chronic pain presenting with exactly the same clinical signs and symptoms can clearly be divided into two groups by the negative or positive effect of sympathetic blockade [4,108]. The pain component that is relieved by specific sympatholytic procedures is considered "sympathetically maintained pain" (SMP). Thus, SMP is now defined as a symptom and not as a clinical entity. The positive effect of a sympathetic blockade is not essential for the diagnosis of CRPS. On the other hand, the only possible way to differentiate between SMP and "sympathetically independent pain" (SIP) is the efficacy of a correctly applied sympatholytic intervention.

Pathophysiology of Sympathetic-Afferent Coupling: A Concept

There is no obvious indication for direct or indirect coupling between the efferent sympathetic systems and the afferent systems in the peripheral tissues leading to pain, discomfort, or other sensations maintained by the sympathetic outflow. This situation may change after trauma with or without a nerve lesion. Activity in sympathetic neurons may now lead to SMP. The concept is shown schematically in Fig. 1. During inflammation or following nerve lesion, the efferent (noradrenergic) innervation of the affected tissue may feed back to the primary afferent neurons and activate them, enhancing their ongoing activity or increasing their responsiveness to mechanical or thermal stimuli. This in turn would amplify physiological impulse transmission in the spinal or trigeminal dorsal horn (sensitization of dorsal horn neurons) or would enhance the hyperexcitability of these neurons after a nerve lesion [54].

Crosstalk from sympathetic postganglionic (noradrenergic) neurons may occur in several forms (for details see [54] and below). The physiological changes in the dorsal horn following peripheral inflammation or nerve injury are also dependent on supraspinal control (the CNS loop in Fig. 1) of nociceptive impulse transmission in the dorsal horn. Thus, SMP in patients is not simply a function of the sympathetic feedback loop.

Evidence for Sympathetically Maintained Pain from Animal Models

Behavioral Animal Models Involving Nerve Lesions

Several rat models for inflammatory pain conditions (intact but sensitized peripheral nociceptors), as well as behavioral models for neuropathic pain involving controlled nerve lesions, have been used to determine the contribution of the sympathetic nervous system to neuropathic or inflammatory pain (Tables I and II). The interventions performed were surgical or chemical sympathectomy, systemic or local application of adrenoceptor blockers such as phentolamine (α_1, α_2), prazosin (α_1), or yohimbine (α_2), or of adrenoceptor agonists such as clonidine (α_2), or intraperitoneal application of guanethidine (which is taken up by the noradrenergic terminals and depletes norepinephrine).

Partial Lesion of the Sciatic Nerve

Partial ligation (one-third to one-half) of the rat sciatic nerve leads to signs of spontaneous pain, thermal hyperalgesia, and mechanical allodynia and hyperalgesia [124]. Chemical sympatholysis with intraperitoneal guanethidine prevented thermal hyperalgesia but caused very little change in mechanical hyperalgesia [127]. When performed months after nerve lesion, sympatholysis by guanethidine alleviated all sensory disorders. Similarly, norepinephrine injected locally into the affected paw exacerbated mechanical and thermal hyperalgesic behavior. However, surgical sympathectomy performed 1 week after partial sciatic nerve lesion had no significant effects on mechanical and cold allodynia or ongoing pain [70]. The interpretation of these results depends heavily on the interpretation of the pharmacological interventions.

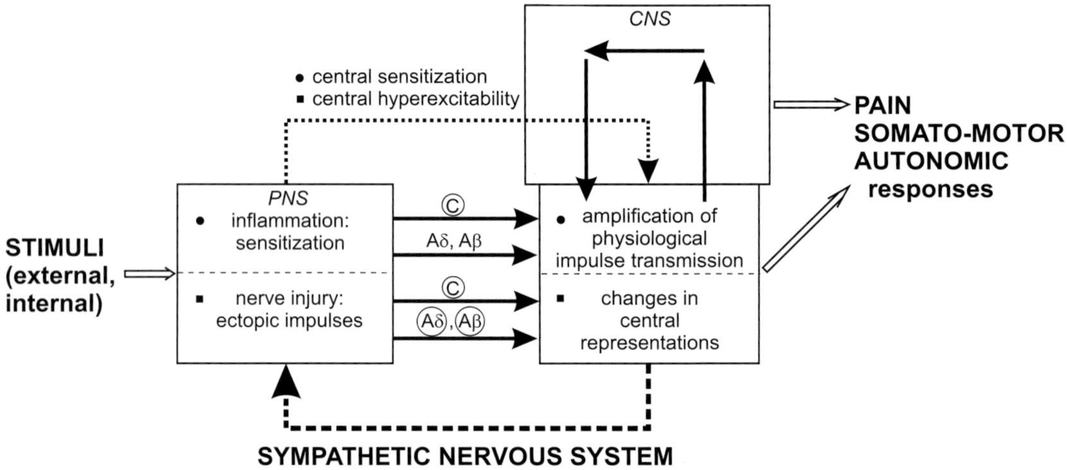

Fig. 1. The generation of peripheral and central hyperexcitability during inflammatory pain and neuropathic pain involving the sympathetic nervous system. The pain is always associated with motor, autonomic, and endocrine responses. The upper interrupted arrow indicates that the central changes are generated (and possibly maintained) (a) by persistent activation of nociceptors with unmyelinated (C) fibers (e.g., during chronic inflammation), called here "central sensitization," or (b) after trauma with nerve lesion by ectopic activity in myelinated (Aδ, Aβ) and C afferents and other changes in the lesioned afferent neurons, called here "central hyperexcitability." The lower interrupted arrow indicates the efferent feedback via the sympathetic nervous system (including the sympathoadrenal system). The transmission of nociceptive impulses is under multiple control of the brain (upper right, CNS). Primary afferent nociceptive neurons (in particular those with C fibers) are sensitized during inflammation. After nerve lesion, *all* lesioned primary afferent neurons (unmyelinated as well as myelinated) undergo biochemical, physiological, and morphological changes that become irreversible with time. These peripheral changes entail changes of the central representations (of the somatosensory system), which become irreversible if no regeneration of primary afferent neurons to their target tissue occurs. The central functional changes, induced by persistent activity in afferent nociceptive neurons during chronic inflammation or by ectopic activity in afferent neurons after nerve lesion, are also reflected in the sympathetic efferent feedback system that may establish positive feedback loops to the primary afferent neurons. CNS, central nervous system; PNS, peripheral nervous system.

Table I
Influence of sympathetic activity or catecholamines on primary afferents or neuropathic pain behavior after nerve lesion (animal experiments)

Species	Sympathetic Intervention	Nerve Lesion	Variable Affected	Effect	Receptor	Refs.
Rat	Adr i.v.	Complete nerve lesion, neuroma	Discharge in A fibers	+		119
Rat	Adr i.a.	Complete nerve lesion, neuroma	Discharge in A fibers	+		74
Rat	Electr. stim. ST, Adr i.v.	Complete nerve lesion, neuroma	Discharge in A fibers	+	α	37
Rat	Adr i.v., hypoxia	Complete nerve lesion, neuroma	Discharge in A fibers	+	α	23
Cat	Electr. stim. ST, NAd i.v.	Complete nerve lesion, neuroma	Discharge in A and C fibers	+		16
Cat	electr. stim. ST (1–5 Hz), Adr i.v., hypoxia	Complete nerve lesion, regeneration	Discharge in C fibers	+	α	48
Rabbit	Electr. stim. ST, NAd, Adr i.a.	Partial nerve lesion	Discharge in skin C nociceptors	+	α_2	100, 117
Rat	Guanethidine s.c.	Partial nerve lesion	Spontaneous pain Mechanical HA Thermal HA	 Ø +		97
Rat	Guanethidine i.p.	Partial nerve lesion	Mechanical HA, Heat HA	+ Ø		127
Rat	Sympathectomy, phentolamine i.v., guanethidine i.v.	SNL	Mechanical HA Heat HA	+ +		69, 70*
Rat	Sympathectomy	CCI, partial nerve lesion	Mechanical HA	Ø		70
Rat	Electr. stim. of ST, Adr i.v.	Complete nerve lesion	Discharge in spontaneously active large DRG neurons	+	α_2	26, 37, 93
Rat	Electr. stim. of ST, morphology	Complete nerve lesion SNL	Sprouting of symp. fibers around DRG somata	+	α	29, 30, 87
Rat	Sympathectomy	CCI	Spontaneous pain Mechanical HA Thermal HA	Ø Ø +		35
Rat	Sympathectomy	SNL	Mechanical HA	Ø		114*

Abbreviations and symbols: +, positive effect of sympathectomy or pharmacological intervention on afferent neurons; Ø, no effect on afferent neurons; Adr, epinephrine; CCI, chronic constriction injury of the sciatic nerve; DRG, dorsal root ganglion; electr. stim., electrical stimulation; HA, hyperalgesia; i.a., intraarterial; i.c., intracutaneous; i.p., intraperitoneal; i.v., intravenous; NAd, norepinephrine; SNL, spinal nerve ligation (of L5/L6 or L5); ST, sympathetic trunk.

* Ringkamp et al. [114] could not reproduce the results of Kim et al. [69,70].

Table II
Influence of sympathetic activity or catecholamines on intact but sensitized primary afferents in animals and pain perception in humans after tissue inflammation

Species	Sympathetic Intervention	Primary Afferent Sensitization	Variable Affected	Effect	Receptor	Refs.
Rabbit	Electr. stim. of ST	Noxious heat	Discharge in single C nociceptors	Ø		125
Rat	Electr. stim. of ST, NA i.a.	Compound algogenic substance	Discharge in single C nociceptors	+		51
Rat	Electr. stim of ST, NAd i.a.	Freund's adjuvant	Discharge in single C nociceptors	+	α_2	118
Rat	Sympathectomy	Bradykinin	Mechanical HA	+		64*
Rat	Removal or denervation of adrenal medulla	Bradykinin	Mechanical HA	+	β_2	65, 66
Rat	Sympathectomy	Bradykinin	Sensitization of C nociceptors to heat	Ø		73
Rat	Sympathectomy guanethidine i.v.	NGF i.c.	Heat HA	+		3
Rat	Guanethidine neonatal	Freund's adjuvant NGF	Heat HA Mechanical HA	+ +		88, 146
Human	NAd-iontophoresis, skin	Capsaicin iontophoresis, skin	Heat HA	+		38
Human	Phentolamine s.c.	Capsaicin i.c.	Spontaneous pain Mechanical HA	+ +		72
Human	Phentolamine i.v.	Capsaicin i.c.	Spontaneous pain Mechanical dynamic HA Mechanical pinprick HA	Ø + Ø		81
Human	Tonic sympathetic reflexes	Capsaicin i.c. topical, skin	Spontaneous pain Mechanical dynamic HA Mechanical pinprick HA	Ø Ø Ø		7
Human	Phasic sympathetic reflexes	Mustard oil topical, skin	Discharge in single C nociceptors	Ø		44
Human	Tonic sympathetic reflexes	Capsaicin i.m., muscle	Spontaneous pain Referred pain	Ø Ø		142

Abbreviations and symbols: +, positive effect of sympathectomy or pharmacological intervention on afferent neurons; Ø, no effect on afferent neurons; electr. stim., electrical stimulation; HA, hyperalgesia; i.a., intraarterial; i.c., intracutaneous; i.v., intravenous; NAd, norepinephrine; NGF, nerve growth factor; s.c., subcutaneous; ST, sympathetic trunk.

* Bradykinin-induced mechanical hyperalgesic behavior was dependent on the innervation of skin by sympathetic postganglionic neurons but *not* on activity in these neurons.

Chronic Constriction Injury of the Sciatic Nerve

Chronic constriction injury of the sciatic nerve generates mechanical and thermal hyperalgesic behavior [9]. Both surgical sympathectomy and depletion of sympathetic transmitters by guanethidine result in a reduction of thermal hyperalgesia, with little or no effect on mechanical hyperalgesia and spontaneous pain behavior [35]. Self-mutilating behavior and spontaneous pain behavior were not changed after guanethidine or surgical sympathectomy, respectively. However, only a slight (statistically nonsignificant) reduction of mechanical and cold allodynia was found after surgical sympathectomy by others [70].

Spinal Nerve Lesion

Ligation and transection of spinal nerves L5 and L6 or L5 alone is followed by mechanical hyperalgesia and allodynia as well as thermal hyperalgesia [28,68]. These pain behaviors were permanently reversed by surgical lumbar sympathectomy, were prevented by surgical sympathectomy prior to spinal nerve lesion, or were temporarily attenuated by intraperitoneal injection of phentolamine or guanethidine [69]. Thus, in this model a coupling between the somatic and sympathetic nervous system appeared to be critical not only for the development but also for the maintenance of the behavioral changes. However, this spinal nerve lesion model is subject to considerable differences between rat strains and substrains in the development of signs of mechanical allodynia and heat hyperalgesia and in the dependence of mechanical allodynic behavior on adrenoceptors [148]. More importantly, the dependence of mechanical allodynic behavior on the sympathetic supply could not be reproduced in an extensive experimental study conducted by two groups using two different strains of rat (Sprague-Dawley, Wistar) and two different testing procedures with von Frey hairs of different strengths (to measure the frequency and threshold of paw withdrawal) [114].

Reduced Animal Models with Nerve Lesions in Vivo and in Vitro

After *complete nerve injury* in experimental animals, surviving cutaneous afferents may develop noradrenergic sensitivity (Fig. 2). Some myelinated and unmyelinated afferents innervating the stump neuroma can be excited by epinephrine or by stimulation of sympathetic efferents that have regenerated into the neuroma [16,23,36,119]. However, in mature neuromata, catecholamine sensitivity is weak and activation of afferent fibers requires rather high (nonphysiological) frequencies of stimulation of the sympathetic supply [16]. As late as 1 year after complete section and re-anastomosis of peripheral nerves, electrical stimulation of the sympathetic trunk at physiological frequencies remained capable of activating regenerated C fibers, probably with nociceptive functions [48]. Furthermore, unmyelinated afferent fibers terminating in old neuromata may be excited by stimulation of postganglionic fibers at a low frequency of 0.5–4 Hz, but this activation was mediated by a nonadrenergic mechanism [52].

Within 2 weeks of a *partial nerve lesion,* electrical stimulation of the sympathetic trunk and injections of catecholamines can activate or sensitize C-fiber nociceptors in the partially injured nerve, including those in continuity with their peripheral targets [100,117] (Fig. 2). More recent in vitro neurophysiological studies, using a primate skin-nerve preparation, have demonstrated that uninjured cutaneous C-fiber nociceptors that innervate skin partially denervated by a spinal nerve ligation have a higher incidence of adrenergic sensitivity than nociceptive afferents from normal skin [1]. Recent histological studies on rat skin show that following partial nerve lesion, postganglionic sympathetic fibers may sprout into the upper dermis, where they are normally absent. These plastic changes of innervation of the upper dermis may favor interaction between regenerating sympathetic and afferent fibers [115,147].

In addition to these peripheral interactions, coupling of sympathetic and afferent neurons may also occur within the dorsal root ganglion (DRG; Fig. 2). After a complete nerve lesion, some DRG somata with Aβ fibers and a few with C fibers develop ectopic activity. Electrical stimulation of sympathetic efferents innervating the DRG may lead to an α_2-adrenoceptor mediated increase of this spontaneous activity [26,37,93]. This increased adrenergic sensitivity is paralleled by morphological changes within the DRG (Fig. 2). After the nerve lesion, sympathetic postganglionic fibers that normally innervate blood vessels within the DRG sprout to form basket-like terminals around large primary afferent somata that project into the injured nerve [29,30,87]. However, the relationship of this DRG sprouting to pain is uncertain. The relevant findings are summarized as follows: (1) In the first 2–3 weeks after nerve lesion, most A-fiber neurons with spontaneous activity and very few silent A-fiber neurons are excited. At later time periods, when

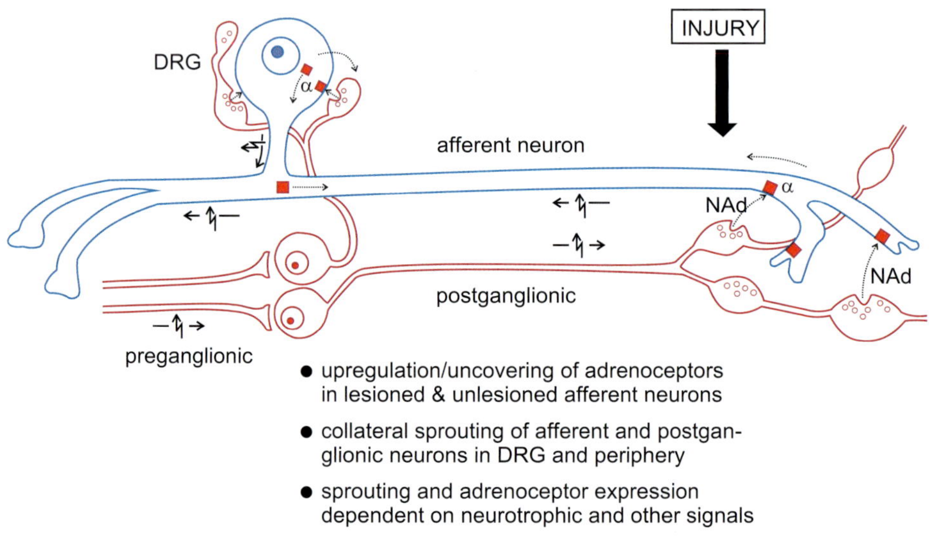

Fig. 2. Influence of sympathetic activity and catecholamines on primary afferent neurons following nerve injury. Sympathetic and afferent neurons start to sprout in the periphery and dorsal root ganglion (DRG; only afferent neurons with C fibers). Afferent neurons express adrenoceptors in their membranes. The sympathetic-afferent coupling is located in the periphery and in the DRG. It occurs in lesioned and possibly unlesioned afferent neurons. It is mediated by norepinephrine (noradrenaline; NAd) released from sympathetic postganglionic neurons and by α-adrenoreceptors expressed at the plasma membrane of afferent neurons. The type of adrenoceptor is mainly α_2 in rats and possibly α_1 in humans.

the catecholaminergic sprouting in the DRG is more prominent, most spontaneously active A-fiber neurons are inhibited during stimulation of the sympathetic supply and are rarely excited. (2) Very few afferent neurons with unmyelinated axons respond to electrical stimulation of the sympathetic trunk; most of them are inhibited in their activity [37,87,93]. (3) The coupling from sympathetic postganglionic fibers to the afferent cell bodies in the DRG probably occurs only with spontaneously active muscle afferent neurons containing Aδ fibers [94]. (4) Activation of the afferent neurons, via the DRG, requires high-frequency stimulation of the sympathetic neurons at 5 to 20 Hz. Sympathetic pre- and postganglionic neurons rarely discharge at these frequencies under physiological conditions. (5) Mechanical allodynic and hyperalgesic behavior shown by rats with L5 spinal nerve injury (transection and ligation) is not dependent on the innervation of the DRG by sympathetic neurons [114]. The rate of ectopic activity originating in the DRG, 15 to 45 days after spinal nerve injury, is not maintained by activity in sympathetic neurons [82]. (6) Afferent neurons in the DRG may be activated indirectly by ischemia generated by decrease of blood flow during vasoconstriction in the DRG following electrical stimulation of the sympathetic trunk and not directly via adrenoceptors expressed in the DRG cells [49]. (7) Axotomized medium- to large-diameter DRG neurons express α_{2A}-adrenoceptors after sciatic nerve injury [14]. However, these upregulated adrenoceptors disappear after several weeks as perineural catecholaminergic sprouting develops, and only small depolarizations can be generated by high concentrations of norepinephrine in axotomized DRG somata [34].

Adrenoceptors Involved in Sympathetic-Afferent Coupling Following Nerve Lesion

The excitation and depression of axotomized DRG cells and the excitation of afferent terminals in neuromas generated by activation of the sympathetic innervation are suggested to be mediated by α-adrenoceptors. Any hypothesis about this chemical norepinephrine-mediated coupling between sympathetic and afferent neurons would have to explain how functional adrenoceptors appear on the surface of nociceptive and other afferent neurons as a consequence of a nerve lesion or infection. The cellular mechanisms underlying the increased sensitivity are unknown. An obvious explanation is the novel expression or upregulation of adrenoceptors. Alternatively, the receptors may normally be present on primary nociceptive afferents but not be functional; they may become uncovered and effective during the response to damage or infection. This possibility is consistent with the finding that adrenoceptor mRNA is normally constitutively present in DRG cells [99,106]. The affinity for ligands or the effectiveness of the subsequent cellular transduction may change in injured nociceptive and non-nociceptive afferent neurons. These possibilities are not mutually exclusive, and it is possible that several mechanisms contribute simultaneously to the expression of sympathetically mediated afferent excitation.

Based on experiments on polymodal nociceptors following partial nerve lesion, it was proposed that expression or upregulation of adrenoceptors in primary afferent neurons is related to the sympathetic denervation of the target tissue [103,117], analogous to the development of the "denervation supersensitivity" that is observed in blood vessels following their denervation [45]. This suggestion appears to be supported by experiments showing that cutaneous nociceptive C fibers in the rabbit ear may develop adrenoceptor sensitivity following surgical sympathectomy [20]. However, we question this mechanism for the following reasons: (1) The percentage of afferents excited and the number of impulses in the responding afferents to close-arterial injection of norepinephrine are small. (2) The concentration of the close-arterially injected norepinephrine was high (1 μM) compared to the concentration of circulating norepinephrine. (3) In the dermis, sympathetic and afferent fibers terminate separately.

Knowledge about the subtypes of α-adrenoreceptor involved in the sympathetic-afferent coupling following nerve trauma is important for an understanding of the underlying neural mechanism, and it may be useful in the design of more specific treatment modalities for neuropathic pain conditions involving sympathetic efferent activity. Excitation and sensitization of polymodal nociceptors in rabbit ear skin generated by electrical stimulation of the sympathetic supply, or by norepinephrine after partial lesion of the auricular nerve, is largely mediated by α_2-adrenoceptors [117]. Investigations of sympathetic-sensory coupling at the site of experimental nerve injury in neuromas and at the cell bodies of axotomized afferent neurons using type-selective agonists and antagonists have shown that this transmission is also largely mediated by α_2-adrenoreceptors [26]. Recordings from primate cutaneous C-fiber nociceptors after an L6 spinal nerve ligation, however, showed a significantly higher incidence of response to both the selective α_1- and α_2-adrenergic agonists, phenylephrine and brimonidine, respectively [1]. In normal (uninjured) DRG neurons mRNAs for α_{2A}-adrenoceptors and particularly α_{2B}-adrenoceptors are present, whereas mRNA for α_1-adrenoceptors is either absent or present in very low levels [106]. After nerve lesion, mRNA for α_{2A}-adrenoceptors is clearly upregulated in DRG neurons [126]. Furthermore, immunohistochemistry with polyclonal antibodies supports the upregulation of α_{2A}-receptors after partial nerve lesion in 15–20% of mainly large-diameter afferent neurons. Importantly, injured as well as uninjured neurons showed this phenotypic switch. However, these changes only lasted for up to 72 days, arguing that this noradrenergic sensitivity is very unlikely to be relevant for the chronic changes seen in patients. Moreover, there may be species differences as far as the expression of adrenoceptors following trauma is concerned.

In conclusion, the behavioral and reduced animal models, in vivo and in vitro, show that sympathetic-afferent coupling can occur under pathophysiological conditions, involving expression of functional adrenoceptors by the lesioned or infected afferent neurons and plastic changes of both sympathetic and afferent neurons. However, the data from these models are inconsistent with observations of SMP in patients. The experimental interventions used in the animal models to date (e.g., frequency of stimulation of sympathetic neurons, concentrations of applied adrenoceptor agonists) seem out of proportion to what happens under biological conditions. Therefore, the experimental data must be considered with the utmost care with regard to the human situation.

The Link between Sympathetic Neurons, Inflammation, and Nociception

In some patients with CRPS, sympatholytic procedures can ameliorate not only pain but also inflammation and edema. Accordingly, animal studies have demonstrated that the sympathetic nervous system can influence the intensity of an inflammatory process [61,78,91,92,104]. Furthermore, it has been shown that acute inflammation leads to nociceptor sensitization, with an enhanced response to adrenergic substances [51] (Table III). The question arises as to whether the sympathetic nervous system might be involved in the inflammatory process in CRPS and whether it might also interact with immune cells.

Under normal conditions, catecholamines act via β_2-adrenoceptors on immune cells to inhibit the production and release of proinflammatory cytokines. These immune cells do not express α-adrenoceptors under basal conditions. However, the situation can dramatically change with chronic inflammation, as immune cells downregulate their expression of

Table III
Influence of sympathetic activity or catecholamines on pain perception in neuropathic pain in humans

Sympathetic Intervention	Nerve Lesion	Variable Affected	Effect	Refs.
Electr. stim. of ST intraoperatively	Causalgia	Spontaneous pain	+	139
Electr. stim. of ST intraoperatively	Causalgia	Spontaneous pain	+	144
Adr injection, perineuromal	Phantom limb pain	Spontaneous pain	+	25
NAd injection, skin	Causalgia	Spontaneous pain Mechanical HA	+ +	133
Adr i.c., phenylephrine i.c.	Postherpetic neuralgia	Spontaneous pain Mechanical HA	+ +	27
NAd injection, skin	CRPS I, II	Spontaneous pain Mechanical HA	+ +	2
Tonic sympathetic reflexes	CRPS I	Spontaneous pain Mechanical dynamic HA Mechanical punctate HAa	+ + +	8
NAd iontophoresis, skin	Polyneuropathy	Spontaneous pain Mechanical dynamic HA Thermal HA	Ø Ø	120
Phasic sympathetic reflexes	Nerve entrapment syndrome	Spontaneous pain Mechanical dynamic HA Thermal HA	Ø Ø +	Schatt-schneider et al. (unpubl.)

Abbreviations and symbols: +, positive effect of sympathectomy or pharmacological intervention on afferent neurons; Ø, no effect on afferent neurons; Adr, epinephrine; CRPS, complex regional pain syndrome; electr. stim., electrical stimulation; HA, hyperalgesia; i.c., intracutaneous; NAd, norepinephrine;. ST, sympathetic trunk.

β_2-adrenoceptors and upregulate their expression of α_1-adrenoceptors over time [46]. In contrast to β_2-adrenoceptors, α_1-adrenoceptors stimulate the production and release of proinflammatory cytokines. If α_1-adrenoceptors were to be expressed by the resident

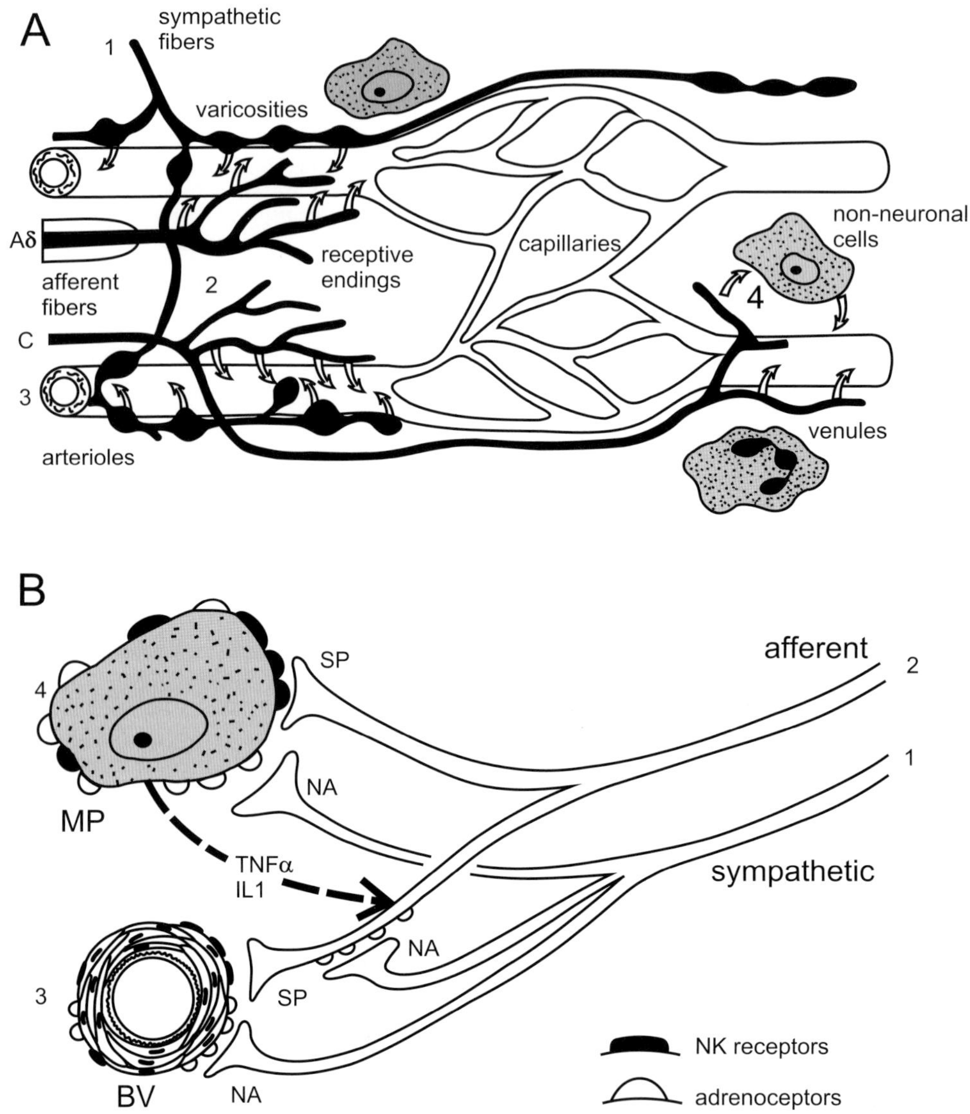

Fig. 3. Hypothetical relationship between sympathetic noradrenergic nerve fibers (1), peptidergic afferent nerve fibers (2), blood vessels (3), and macrophages (4). The activated and sensitized afferent nerve fibers activate macrophages (via substance P [SP] release). The immune cells start to release cytokines, such as tumor necrosis factor α (TNF-α) and interleukin 1 (IL1), which further activate afferent fibers by enhancing sodium influx into the cells. Substance P (and calcitonin gene-related peptide [CGRP]) released from the afferent nerve fibers react with neurokinin 1 (NK1) receptors (CGRP receptors) in the blood vessels (leading to arteriolar vasodilation, venular plasma extravasation, and neurogenic inflammation). The sympathetic nerve fibers interact with this system on three levels: (1) via adrenoceptors (mainly α) on the blood vessels (vasoconstriction); (2) via adrenoceptors (mainly β) on macrophages (further release of cytokines), and (3) via adrenoceptors (mainly α) on afferents (further sensitization of these fibers). BV, blood vessel; MP, macrophage; NA, norepinephrine. From [57], with permission.

and/or recruited immune or immunocompetent cells of the CRPS-affected extremity, then sympathetic activation would be predicted to cause pain and other inflammatory signs via cytokine release.

Summarizing the hypothetical ideas described above, Fig. 3 illustrates the possible interactions between sympathetic fibers, afferent fibers, blood vessels, and nonneural cells related to the immune system (e.g., macrophages) that theoretically lead to the inflammatory changes observed in CRPS patients. Four groups of rat behavioral experiments support the notion that sympathetic postganglionic neurons may be involved in the sensitization of nociceptors and therefore in hyperalgesia during inflammation.

Cytokines and Inflammatory Painful Behavior

Behavioral experiments conducted in rats (studying mechanical hyperalgesic behavior) have shown that tissue injury generated by inflammatory stimuli (e.g., antigens, carrageenan, or lipopolysaccharide) leads to sensitization of nociceptors and subsequently to hyperalgesic behavior. Pharmacological interventions using blockers of inflammatory or proinflammatory mediators indicate that various proinflammatory cytokines are involved in the sensitization of nociceptors under these experimental conditions. Pathogenic stimuli lead to activation of resident cells (lymphocytes, macrophages, mast cells, and dendritic cells) and cause the release of inflammatory mediators (e.g., bradykinin). The inflammatory mediators and the pathogenic stimuli themselves activate immune and immune-related cells that release tumor necrosis factor alpha (TNF-α). TNF-α generates sensitization of nociceptors by two possible pathways (Fig. 4) [116]: (1) Interleukin 1β (IL-1β) and IL-6 are produced by immune cells, with IL-6 enhancing the production of IL-1β. These interleukins stimulate cyclooxygenase 2 (COX 2) and the production of prostaglandins (PGE_2, PGI_2), which in turn react with the nociceptive terminal via E-type receptors. (2) IL-8 released from endothelial cells and macrophages reacts with the sympathetic terminals that are thought to mediate sensitization of nociceptive afferent terminals by release of norepinephrine to act via β-adrenoceptors. (IL-8 is a chemotactic cytokine and therefore belongs to the chemokines. Other chemokines, such as keratinocyte-derived chemokines or chemokine-induced neutrophil chemoattractant-1, may also be involved in this function mediated by sympathetic terminals [138].) These two peripheral pathways by which nociceptive afferents can be sensitized involving cytokines are under inhibitory control of circulating glucocorticoids (indicated by asterisks in Fig. 4) and of other, anti-inflammatory, interleukins (e.g., IL-4 and IL-10, indicated by # in Fig. 4) (for review, see [31,138]).

Nerve Growth Factor and Inflammatory Painful Behavior

Systemic injection of nerve growth factor (NGF) is followed by a transient thermal and mechanical hyperalgesia in rats [79,80] and humans [105]. During experimental inflammation (evoked by Freund's adjuvant in the rat hindpaw), NGF increases in the inflamed tissue, and these increases are paralleled by the development of thermal and mechanical hyperalgesia. Both are prevented by anti-NGF antibodies [80]. The mechanisms responsible are sensitization of nociceptors via high-affinity NGF receptors (trkA receptors) and an increased synthesis of calcitonin gene-related peptide (CGRP) and substance P in the afferent cell bodies, induced by NGF taken up by the afferent terminals and transported to the cell bodies. The NGF-induced sensitization of nociceptors seems to be at least partly mediated indirectly by the sympathetic postganglionic terminals. In rats, heat and mechanical hyperalgesic behavior generated by local injection of NGF into the skin are prevented or significantly reduced after chemical or surgical sympathectomy [146]. These experiments suggest that NGF released during inflammation by inflammatory cells acts on the sympathetic terminals via high-affinity trkA receptors, inducing the release of inflammatory mediators (the source of which is unknown) and subsequently the sensitization of

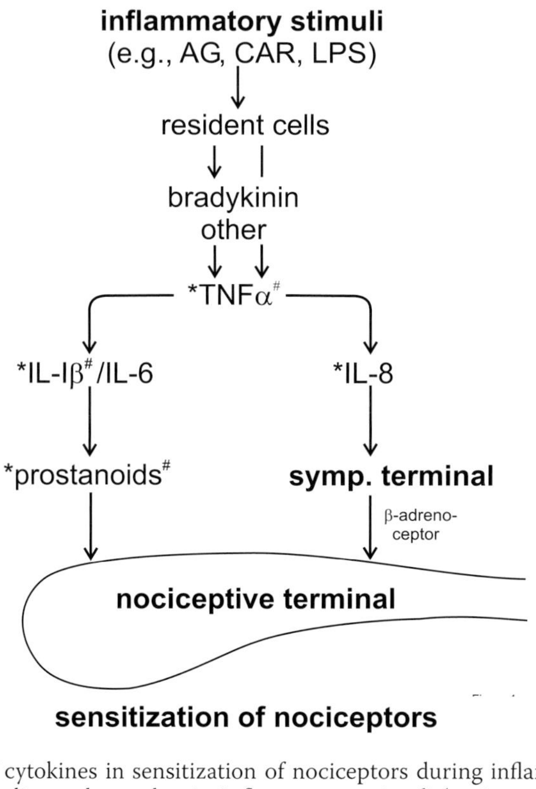

Fig. 4. Hypothetical role of cytokines in sensitization of nociceptors during inflammation and the underlying putative mechanisms leading to hyperalgesia. Inflammatory stimuli (antigens [AG], carrageenan [CAR], and lipopolysaccharide [LPS]) activate resident cells and lead to release of inflammatory mediators (such as bradykinin). Pro-inflammatory cytokines are synthesized and released by macrophages and other immune or immune-related cells. Nociceptors are postulated to be sensitized by two pathways involving the cytokines: (1) Tumor necrosis factor α (TNF-α) induces synthesis and release of interleukin 1β (IL-1β) and IL-6, which, in turn, induces the release of prostanoids (prostaglandin E_2 and I_2 [PGE_2, PGI_2]) by activating cyclooxygenase-2 (COX-2). (2) TNF-α induces synthesis and release of IL-8. IL-8 activates sympathetic terminals that sensitize nociceptors via β-adrenoceptors (possibly $β_2$). Glucocorticoids inhibit the synthesis of the cytokines and the activation of COX-2 (indicated by asterisks). Anti-inflammatory cytokines (such as IL-4 and IL-10) that are also synthesized and released by immune cells inhibit the synthesis and release of pro-inflammatory cytokines (indicated by #). This scheme is fully dependent on behavioral experiments and pharmacological interventions. After Verri et al. [138].

nociceptors to mechanical or heat stimuli [58,88,146]. It is unclear whether this sensitization of nociceptors, mediated by terminal sympathetic nerve fibers, (1) is dependent on activity in the sympathetic neurons, on the release of norepinephrine, and on the expression of adrenoceptors in the nociceptive afferent neurons or (2) is independent of neural activity and release of norepinephrine.

Bradykinin-Induced Mechanical Hyperalgesic Behavior

Withdrawal threshold to mechanical stimulation of the rat hindpaw decreases dose-dependently after intradermal injection of the inflammatory mediator bradykinin. Following a single injection of bradykinin, this decrease lasts for more than 1 hour [58,62,63]). In normal rats, this behavior is blocked by the cyclooxygenase inhibitor indomethacin and is therefore mediated by a prostaglandin (probably PGE_2) that sensitizes nociceptors to mechanical stimulation. However, in rats that had either been vagotomized at least 7 days beforehand [64] or sound-stressed for 4 days [67], indomethacin has almost no effect on this bradykinin-induced hyperalgesic behavior; thus, the hyperalgesia may not be mediated by prostanoids in these experimental conditions. In neurophysiological experiments, sensitization to mechanical stimulation by bradykinin has only been demonstrated convincingly for afferent fibers innervating the cat knee joint [98] or the cat skeletal muscle [89]. Manning et al. [85] demonstrated in humans that intradermal injection of bradykinin (100 ng to 10 μg) generates hyperalgesia to heat stimulation but not to mechanical stimulation.

The decrease in paw-withdrawal threshold to mechanical stimulation generated by intradermal injection of bradykinin is significantly reduced after surgical sympathectomy. However, decentralization of the lumbar paravertebral sympathetic ganglia (denervation of the postganglionic neurons by cutting the preganglionic sympathetic axons leaving the postganglionic neurons intact) is *not* followed by attenuation of the bradykinin-induced mechanical hyperalgesic behavior. This finding indicates that the sensitizing effect of bradykinin is *not* dependent on activity in the sympathetic neurons innervating skin and therefore does not depend on the release of norepinephrine [64]. It shows that bradykinin stimulates the release of prostaglandin from the sympathetic terminals or from other cells in association with the sympathetic terminals in the skin.

Mechanical hyperalgesic behavior generated by intracutaneous injection of bradykinin and its dependence on the sympathetic innervation of the skin is an interesting phenomenon. However, to explain this hyperalgesic behavior by prostanoids sensitizing nociceptors because indomethacin prevents it appears to be too simplistic, the main reasons being that (1) sympathetic fibers mediate this hyperalgesia independent of neural activity and release of norepinephrine and (2) indomethacin does not block this behavior under conditions of chronic subdiaphragmatic vagotomy or chronic sound stress (see above). These points argue that the dependence of bradykinin-induced cutaneous mechanical behavior on the sympathetic innervation must be reinvestigated using a rigorous experimental approach.

Sympathoadrenal System and Nociceptor Sensitization

In rats, activation of the sympathoadrenal system (e.g., by release of the central sympathetic circuits—connected to preganglionic neurons that innervate the adrenal medulla—from vagal inhibition) generates mechanical hyperalgesia and enhances bradykinin-induced mechanical hyperalgesia (a decrease of paw-withdrawal threshold to mechanical stimulation of the skin). Activation of the sympathoneural system does not have the same effect (compare closed circles with open triangles in Fig. 5A). Both

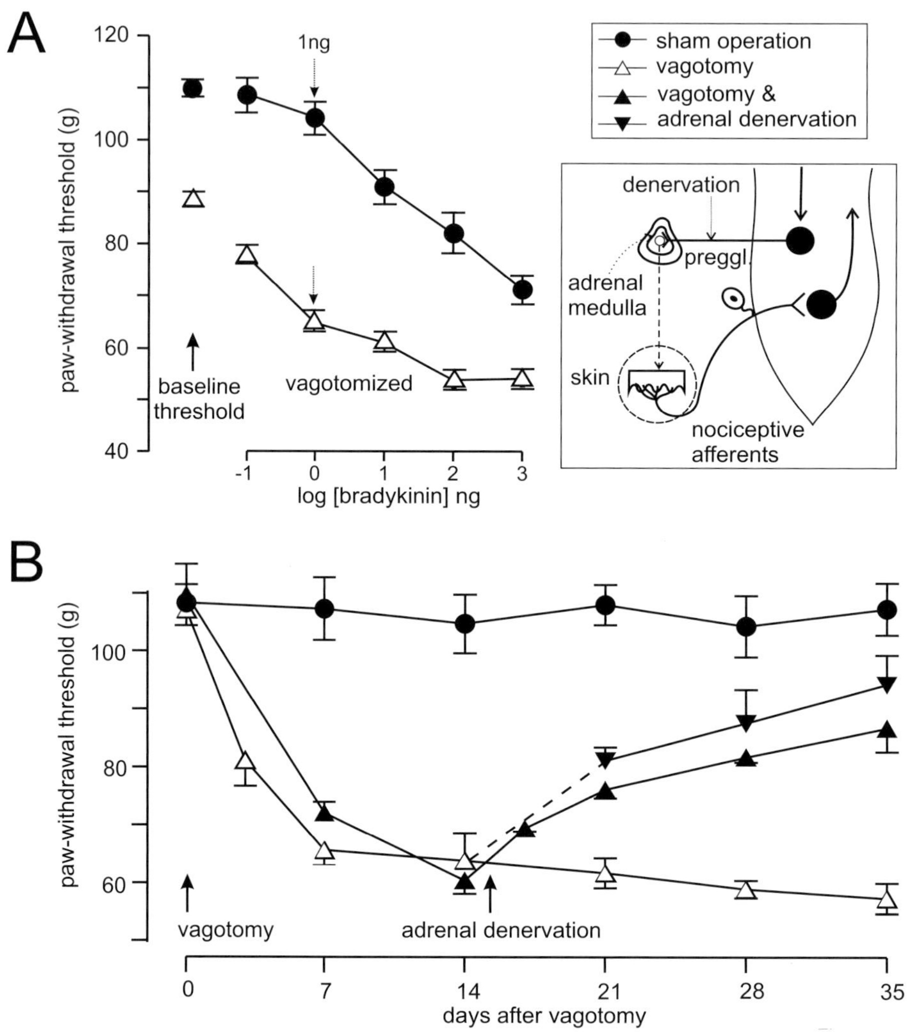

Fig. 5. Long-term enhancement of bradykinin-induced behavioral mechanical hyperalgesia by epinephrine released by the adrenal medulla (AM). (A) Bradykinin-induced hyperalgesia (decrease of paw-withdrawal threshold) in sham-operated rats (closed circles; n = 6 hindpaws) and in vagotomized rats (open triangles; n = 16 hindpaws). Bradykinin was injected intracutaneously at the site of mechanical stimulation and at the dose indicated (abscissa scale) in volumes of 2.5 μL. Subdiaphragmatic vagotomy performed 7 days before the experiments led to activation of the AM (probably by removal of central inhibition) and release of epinephrine. Paw-withdrawal thresholds (baseline and after bradykinin) decreased significantly. (B) Paw-withdrawal threshold to intracutaneous injection of 1 ng bradykinin over 14 days after subdiaphragmatic vagotomy and

types of hyperalgesia develop slowly over 7–14 days following activation of the adrenal medullae (induced by vagotomy) and are maintained over 5 weeks of testing (open triangles in Fig. 5B). They are reversed slowly after denervation of the adrenal medullae performed 14 days after vagotomy (closed triangles and inverse triangles in Fig. 5B [64,65]). Application of epinephrine through a minipump over 3–14 days slowly enhances the development of mechanical hyperalgesia. Furthermore, continuous application of a β_2-adrenoceptor blocker over 7–14 days by way of a minipump prevents the enhancement of bradykinin-induced hyperalgesic behavior generated by activation of the adrenal medullae [66].

The results of this experiment are interpreted in the following way. Epinephrine released by persistent activation of the adrenal medullae sensitizes cutaneous nociceptors to mechanical stimuli. This sensitization of nociceptors and its reversal are slow, taking several days to develop. The slow time course implies that the nociceptor sensitization cannot be acutely blocked by an adrenoceptor antagonist given intracutaneously. Epinephrine probably does not act directly on the cutaneous nociceptors but acts on cells in the microenvironment of the nociceptors, inducing slow cellular and subcellular changes that result in nociceptor sensitization. Candidate cells may be mast cells, macrophages, or keratinocytes, which then release substances that generate sensitization [58,59,65]. The change in sensitivity of a population of nociceptors generated by epinephrine released by the adrenal medullae, which is regulated by the brain, would be a novel mechanism of sensitization. This mechanism would be different from mechanisms that lead to activation and/or sensitization of nociceptors by sympathetic-afferent coupling, as discussed above.

This novel mechanism of pain and hyperalgesia involving the sympathoadrenal system may operate in ill-defined pain syndromes such as irritable bowel syndrome, functional dyspepsia, fibromyalgia, and chronic fatigue syndrome [22,32,86,145]. The conclusions regarding the long-term sensitization of nociceptors for mechanical stimulation by epinephrine are indirect and rely completely on behavioral experiments. Neurophysiological experiments in vivo on primary afferent nociceptive neurons are required to test whether all or only a subpopulation of nociceptors are sensitized.

its attenuation after denervation of the AM 14 days after vagotomy. Paw-withdrawal threshold in response to intradermal injection of 1 ng bradykinin in rats before and 3 to 35 days after vagotomy (open triangles, $n = 6$), before and 7 to 35 days after sham-vagotomy (closed circles, $n = 8$; control) and in rats that received AM denervation 14 days after vagotomy (see inset in (A) right), in which measurements were taken for up to 35 days after initial surgery. The latter group of animals consisted of two subgroups: rats that were tested after vagotomy and after additional denervation of the AM (closed triangles, $n = 6$) and rats which were only tested after additional denervation of the AM (closed inverted triangles, $n = 4$). Intradermal injection of 1 ng bradykinin did not significantly decrease paw-withdrawal threshold to mechanical stimulation in control rats (see A). Ordinate scale is threshold in grams. Data of the sham-vagotomy and the vagotomy group of rats are significantly different 7 days after vagotomy ($P < 0.01$). Data from vagotomized rats with denervated AM and rats that were only vagotomized are significantly different on days 28 and 35 ($P < 0.01$). Data from sham-vagotomized rats and vagotomized rats with denervated AM were not significantly different on days 28 and 35 (Fisher's protected least significant difference post hoc test). Ordinate scale, change of baseline threshold and threshold to intracutaneous bradykinin together. Modified from [64,65].

Conclusions

It is important to emphasize that the mechanisms involving NGF, proinflammatory cytokines, epinephrine, and sympathetic postganglionic fibers in the sensitization of nociceptive afferents have been deduced on the basis of behavioral and pharmacological experiments. Proof of these interactions must be obtained by directly measuring the activity in nociceptive neurons in vivo and in vitro with electrophysiological techniques.

Data for Sympathetically Maintained Pain from Human Pain Models and Patients

Influence of Sympathetic Activity and Catecholamines on Intact Primary Afferents after Tissue Inflammation

In healthy subjects, physiological activation of sympathetic neurons innervating skin by arousal and thermal stimuli did not change cutaneous sensations, thermal detection thresholds, or discharge patterns of microneurographically recorded myelinated cutaneous afferents [7,43]. Furthermore, when sympathetic cutaneous vasoconstrictor or sudomotor activity was modulated within physiological range by thermoregulatory stress, it did not measurably influence capsaicin-induced cutaneous pain [7,141]. Accordingly, activation of skin sympathetic vasoconstrictor neurons by forced mental arithmetic did not change the irritant-induced discharge of single microneurographically recorded cutaneous C-nociceptors [44]. Similar results were reported when sympathetic muscle vasoconstrictor activity was altered physiologically and the intensity of pain after capsaicin injection into the muscle was quantified. Muscle pain did not change in this experiment [142]. Finally, cutaneous ongoing pain and heat hyperalgesia in subjects with an experimental cutaneous heat injury are not altered by sympathetic blocks with bupivacaine [102,109]. These negative experimental data appear to be at variance with experiments showing that heat hyperalgesia developing after topical application of capsaicin to the skin of human volunteers was enhanced following iontophoresis of norepinephrine [38] and that norepinephrine-induced pain and mechanical hyperalgesia in capsaicin-sensitized skin were attenuated by phentolamine, a mixed α_1 and α_2 antagonist [81]. However, changes in blood flow may account for the norepinephrine-enhanced cutaneous sensitivity seen in capsaicin-induced hyperalgesic skin, particularly because the changes observed were very small [39,41]. These negative data obtained in humans are furthermore at variance with experiments conducted on rats showing directly and indirectly that sensitization of Aδ- and C-fiber afferents innervating the plantar skin is dependent, at least in part, on activity in the sympathetic innervation of skin involving α_1-adrenoceptors [80a,112a,139a].

Influence of Sympathetic Activity of Primary Afferents and Catecholamines in Patients with Neuropathic Pain

Amputation Pain

Long after limb amputation, injection of epinephrine around a stump neuroma is reported to be intensely painful [25]. Recent studies also demonstrate that the perineuromal administration of physiological doses of norepinephrine induces more pain than saline injections [110].

Postherpetic Neuralgia

In some patients with postherpetic neuralgia, spontaneous pain and mechanical hyperalgesia are enhanced after intramuscular injection of epinephrine or phenylephrine [27].

Polyneuropathy

In patients with painful and nonpainful polyneuropathy of different origins, spontaneous pain was quantified and heat pain thresholds were measured on the dorsum of the foot before and after iontophoresis of norepinephrine and saline. No differences could be demonstrated in the decrease in heat pain thresholds in both groups and controls. There was no change in spontaneous pain perception. Thus, in human polyneuropathy, adrenergic mechanisms are obviously not involved in the generation of pain [120].

Nerve Entrapment Syndromes

In a subgroup of patients with a nerve entrapment syndrome, clinical signs of peripheral nociceptor sensitization (heat hyperalgesia) are present. This heat hyperalgesia is enhanced during tonic activation of the sympathetic neurons supplying skin by whole body cooling showing that the sympathetic nervous system contributes to nociceptor sensitization in these patients but without heat hyperalgesia. Furthermore, they did not exhibit changes of heat pain threshold during sympathetic activation (J. Schattschneider and R. Baron, unpublished data).

Post-Traumatic Neuralgia and Complex Regional Pain Syndrome Type II

CRPS-II is characterized by a demonstrable lesion of a peripheral nerve. Therefore, it is by definition a neuropathic disorder. Intraoperative stimulation of the sympathetic chain induces an increase of spontaneous pain in patients with CRPS-II, but not in patients with hyperhidrosis [144]. In addition, intravenous phentolamine, but not propranolol, relieves pain in these patients [4,106]. In these patients, pain relief following local anesthetic sympathetic ganglion block by an anesthetic was highly correlated with pain relief during a phentolamine infusion.

In CRPS-II and post-traumatic neuralgia, intracutaneous application of norepinephrine into a symptomatic area rekindles spontaneous pain and mechanical allodynia that had been relieved by sympathetic blockade, supporting the idea that noradrenergic sensitivity of human nociceptors is present after partial nerve lesion [133]. Ali et al. confirmed these data [2], showing that intradermal injection of norepinephrine in physiologically relevant doses in patients with SMP evokes greater pain in the affected regions than in the contralateral unaffected limb or in control subjects. Most patients who had an increase in pain after injection of norepinephrine in the affected extremity also reported a decrease in pain with systemic administration of phentolamine. Rekindling of spontaneous and evoked pain, or enhancement of both by norepinephrine injected into the area of skin that was painful before sympathetic block or before successful treatment, took 10 minutes or longer to develop. This long latency indicates that norepinephrine may not act directly on the afferent fiber terminals, but may act by some unknown mechanism via changes in the micromilieu of the nociceptors [133].

Topical application of the α_2-adrenoceptor agonist clonidine relieves hyperalgesia at the site of application in SMP, but not SIP patients [33]. This effect was considered to be secondary to a reduction in the release of norepinephrine via activation of the α_2-adrenergic autoreceptor on the sympathetic terminal. Injection of norepinephrine and the α_1-adrenoceptor agonist, phenylephrine, into the clonidine-treated area produced marked pain and hyperalgesia.

In further support of the concept, quantitative autoradiographic studies indicate that the number of α_1-adrenoceptors in hyperalgesic skin of patients with SMP is significantly higher than in the skin of normal subjects [44]. Finally, an increase in venous α-adrenoceptor responsiveness has been observed in patients with CRPS-I [5].

Complex Regional Pain Syndrome Type I

In CRPS-I patients, no demonstrable nerve lesion is present per definition. Therefore, it is questionable that CRPS-I is a neuropathic disorder. In the acute stage in particular, it is likely that different mechanisms underlying pain and SMP operate in CRPS-I as compared with syndromes associated with nerve lesions (e.g., CRPS-II).

Tonic sympathetic activation can enhance pain sensations. In patients with CRPS-I with identified SMP, spontaneous pain and mechanical hyperalgesia were augmented when sympathetic cutaneous vasoconstrictor neurons were activated physiologically by cold stress [8] (Fig. 6). In these patients, sympathetic blocks with a local anesthetic (leading to an increase of the skin temperature of the hand to 35°C) led to a significant decrease of spontaneous pain and mechanical allodynia; thus, there was a high correlation between pain relief during sympathetic blocks and augmentation of pain during thermoregulatory cold stress. Patients with CRPS-I who had SIP served as controls. In those patients, thermoregulatory cold stress did not augment spontaneous pain or mechanical allodynia, nor was the pain relieved after sympathetic blocks. This experiment in human CRPS patients does not indicate whether the experimentally evoked SMP is generated by direct or indirect coupling between sympathetic fibers and afferent fibers. These results are supported by Drummond et al. [42], who showed that ongoing pain increased in 70% of patients with CRPS-I during phasic reflex activation of the sympathetic neurons innervating skin. However, in this study, the pain increased within seconds of the stimulation, the pain increase was minimal, and no distinction was made between patients with or without SMP.

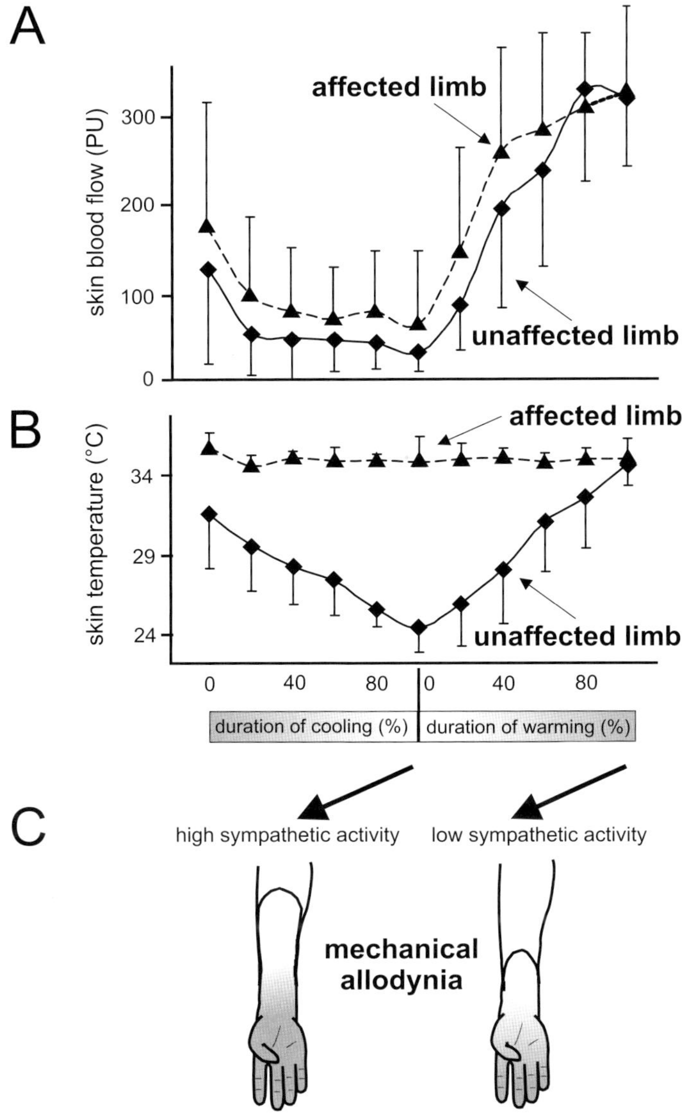

Fig. 6. Modulation of mechanical allodynia by activity in cutaneous vasoconstrictor neurons in 13 patients with complex regional pain syndrome, type I (CRPS-I), with sympathetically maintained pain (SMP). With the help of a thermal suit, whole-body cooling and warming were performed to alter sympathetic skin nerve activity. The subjects were lying in a suit supplied by tubes, in which running water of 12°C and 50°C, respectively (inflow temperature), was used to cool or warm the whole body. By these means, activity in cutaneous vasoconstrictor neurons can be switched on and off (A, B). Cooling of the patients lowers core temperature and increases activity in cutaneous vasoconstrictor neurons with decrease of skin temperature (closed diamonds in B) and skin blood flow (hand; closed triangles and diamonds in A). Warming of the patients increases core temperature, with a decrease of activity in cutaneous vasoconstrictor neurons and an increase in skin temperature (closed diamonds in B) and skin blood flow (closed triangles and diamonds in A). On the affected side, the forearm temperature was clamped at 35°C by a feedback-controlled heat lamp to exclude temperature effects on the sensory receptors. Measurements of blood flow and skin temperature were taken at 5-minute intervals (mean + SD), thus the whole cycle lasted 50 minutes. (C) Effect of cutaneous vasoconstrictor activity on mechanical allodynia in one CRPS-I patient with SMP. Activation of sympathetic neurones (during cooling) leads to an increase in the area of mechanical allodynia. Modified from [8].

The experimental setup used in the above study (Fig. 6) selectively alters sympathetic cutaneous vasoconstrictor activity without influencing other sympathetic systems innervating the extremities—muscle vasoconstrictor neurons and sympathetic neurons innervating other deep somatic structures such as bones, tendons, and ligaments. Therefore, the interaction of sympathetic and afferent neurons measured here is likely to be located within the skin, as predicted by the pain-enhancing effect of intracutaneous norepinephrine injections [2,133].

Interestingly, the relief of spontaneous pain after sympathetic blockade was significantly more pronounced than changes in spontaneous pain that could be induced experimentally by sympathetic activation (Figs. 6, 7). Complete sympathetic block affects all sympathetic outflow channels projecting to the affected extremity. Therefore, it is likely that sympathetic-afferent coupling is more prominent in deep somatic tissues such as bones, skeletal muscles, or joints. The fact that these structures are extremely painful in some cases with CRPS lends support to this view [6]. Furthermore, there may be patients who are characterized by a selective or predominant sympathetic-afferent interaction in deep somatic tissues, sparing the skin [140].

As mentioned above, there is no overt nerve lesion in CRPS-I patients. It is, therefore, very likely that different mechanisms may be involved in SMP in these patients compared to CRPS-II patients. One possible explanation is that the acute inflammatory component of this disorder is influenced by sympathetic activity. The idea that CRPS-I patients undergo inflammatory processes in the affected extremity, in particular in the deep somatic tissues, including bones, has been suggested repeatedly, starting with Sudeck [15,130,131]. Fig. 3 illustrates the possible interactions between sympathetic fibers, afferent fibers, blood vessels, and nonneural cells related to the immune system (e.g., macrophages), leading theoretically to the inflammatory changes observed in CRPS-I patients [57].

Clinical Data from Sympatholytic Interventions in Patients with Neuropathic Pain

The important question for clinical practice is whether these findings obtained in animal and human models and in patients can be translated for therapeutic interventions in patients with neuropathic pain. As mentioned above, longstanding but nonquantitative clinical observations indicate that the interruption of the efferent sympathetic nerve supply can relieve pain in several neuropathic pain states, including CRPS, acute herpetic neuralgia, and phantom limb pain. However, this effect was found only in subgroups of patients.

Currently, two therapeutical techniques to block sympathetic activity are used: (1) injections of a local anesthetic around sympathetic paravertebral ganglia that project to the affected body part (mostly the extremities; sympathetic ganglion blocks) and (2) regional intravenous application of guanethidine, bretylium, or reserpine (which all deplete norepinephrine in the postganglionic axon) to an isolated extremity blocked with a tourniquet (intravenous regional sympatholysis [IVRS]).

There are many uncontrolled surveys in the literature reviewing the effect of sympathetic interventions in CRPS. About 70% of patients report a full or partial response [24]. The efficacy of these procedures is, however, still debated and has been questioned in the past [71,101,122,123,136,137]. In fact, the specificity of the procedures, the long-term results, and the techniques used have rarely been adequately evaluated.

One controlled study in patients with CRPS-I has shown that sympathetic ganglion blocks with a local anesthetic have the same immediate effect on pain as a control injection with saline [107]. However, after 24 hours, pain was significantly reduced in patients of the local anesthetic group but not in control patients, indicating that nonspecific (placebo) effects occur initially and that the efficacy of sympatholytic interventions must be measured after 24 hours. With these data in mind, the uncontrolled studies mentioned above must be interpreted cautiously. Only a few studies have assessed the long-term effects of sympathetic blocks [54,55]. Unraveling the mechanisms underlying these long-term effects is a key and essential issue of research in animal models and patients. Results obtained in this type of (basic) research will change our concepts in this field. The results of studies using IVRS with reserpine, guanethidine, or bretylium are still inconsistent. Most studies, however, show negative results [50].

Caveats in the Interpretation of Sympathetic Blocks

From the aforementioned data, it is clear that we desperately need further controlled studies to scientifically evaluate the efficacy of sympathetic interventions. However, there are some inherent problems with the interpretation of such interventions.

Unreliability of Sympatholytic Interventions

Some authors claim that interventions that block sympathetic activity lack specificity. They argue that the techniques and results of sympathetic blockade have rarely been adequately evaluated and in most cases are not placebo-controlled, as discussed earlier. Therefore, *false-positive* results have been attributed to placebo effects or stress-induced analgesia. There is some merit to such arguments, although they cannot explain the long-lasting effect (days to weeks) of sympathetic blocks.

False-positive results have two possible causes. (1) Sympatholytic interventions do not exclusively block the sympathetic system. Sympathetic ganglion blocks may be associated with spread of the local anesthetic to somatic nerves, and local anesthetics may have systemic analgesic effects. Moreover, guanethidine also has local anesthetic properties. Therefore, the possibility merits consideration that a pain-relieving effect of local anesthetic "sympathetic" blocks or guanethidine application is not related specifically to sympatholysis. (2) Many patients with CRPS-II and post-traumatic neuralgia have cold allodynia, i.e., pain to normally innocuous cold stimuli. Complete blocking of the sympathetic outflow to the affected extremity leads to skin vasodilatation and warming and could therefore relieve cold allodynia. In this case, the effect of the sympathetic block is not mediated by a direct interaction of norepinephrine and afferents but rather by the increase in skin temperature.

On the other hand, a problem inherent in the evaluation of sympatholytic procedures is the high potential for *false-negative* results. Several factors could contribute to this problem. (1) Blockade of sympathetic activity may be technically inadequate because of either anatomical maldistribution or inadequate concentration of the drug at the site of action. (2) Anatomical variability of the sympathetic chain may be present. (3) When stellate ganglion blocks are performed, neurons as far caudal as T2 that contribute to the upper limb innervation may escape the block (although conduction of their axons should be blocked because they pass the stellate ganglion). (4) A proximal location of the sympathetic-afferent interaction (e.g., in the DRG or in the nerve) may escape IVRS. It is not possible to completely rule out false-negative results and, therefore, the percentage of patients that could benefit from sympatholytic interventions may even be underestimated. Even careful monitoring of Horner's syndrome and cutaneous vasodilatation during a sympathetic block does not ensure that the sympathetic innervation of deep tissues, the DRG, or both, has been blocked.

To establish the effectiveness and specificity of sympatholytic procedures, several types of blocks and careful controls are necessary. Because few studies have done so, proof of the effectiveness of sympatholysis is still lacking.

No Correlation between Pain and Sympathetic Dysfunction

Several clinical observations have shown that there is no consistent correlation between pain and sympathetic dysfunction. A similar degree of pain can occur in CRPS, whatever the vascular state of the affected region. Moreover, some patients with CRPS or zoster pain have no evidence of sympathetic dysfunction other than an apparent pain response to sympathetic blockade. These observations have led some authors to conclude that the sympathetic nervous system is not involved in the generation of pain. It is important to point out, however, that a *normally* functioning sympathetic efferent system could elicit pain if its target effectors (e.g., nociceptors) are abnormal. Many sympathetic neurons show a characteristic tonic activity. Given the existence of a pathological coupling between sympathetic and nociceptive neurons, this normal ongoing sympathetic activity would lead to persistent SMP.

No Correlation between Onset of Pain Relief and Sympathetic Blockade

The pain relief that occurs after sympathetic blockade often does not correlate with the time of onset, duration, or degree of the sympatholytic effect observed. Sometimes, relief is described well before the increase in skin temperature. Even more striking is the observation that sympathetic blocks may relieve pain in acute CRPS, although the cutaneous sympathetic outflow to the affected limb is already significantly inhibited (see above). However, both of the clinical characteristics that indicate sympathetic blockade (i.e., an increase in skin temperature and a decrease in sweat production) are cutaneous measures. Furthermore, studies that have demonstrated an inhibition of sympathetic activity have only analyzed neurons innervating the skin. It is therefore possible that while the cutaneous sympathetic outflow is inhibited or blocked, the sympathetic innervation of deeper tissues such as blood vessels, muscles, the periosteum, or even the DRG (Fig. 2) is unaffected. Experimental studies in animals indicate that different functional channels of the sympathetic nervous system exist that can be activated and probably also blocked selectively and independently, e.g., the cutaneous or muscle vasoconstrictor outflow [53]. The pathological interaction of sympathetic fibers and nociceptive afferents that forms the basis for SMP might therefore involve sympathetic neurons innervating deep tissues rather than cutaneous sympathetic neurons [8,121]. Evidence for the involvement of deep tissues includes abnormalities in the three-phase bone scan and the appearance of the spontaneous pain that characteristically is located deep within the affected extremity. Furthermore, in CRPS, the inciting events often include trauma to deep somatic structures.

In conclusion, there is a desperate need for controlled studies that assess the acute as well as the long-term effect of sympathetic blockade and IVRS on pain and other CRPS symptoms, in particular motor function. Well-performed sympathetic ganglion blocks should be performed rather than IVRS [50,107].

Changes in the SMP Component in the Course of CRPS

The percentage of the pain that depends on sympathetic activity steadily declines during the course of the disease. After 24 months there is only a very small chance that sympathetic interventions might be successful. This finding is supported by studies that analyzed the effect of sympathetic blockade as well as cutaneous injections of norepinephrine in a group of patients with acute CRPS and in the same patients after up to 10 years [121,133]. Most patients with chronic pain did not respond to sympathetic blockade, and the pain did not change after norepinephrine injection, although this subgroup had demonstrated favorable effects in the acute phase. These findings argue that patients with acute CRPS should be assigned to diagnostic and if applicable to therapeutic sympathetic interventions as soon as possible to achieve the highest degree of pain relief in order to facilitate physiotherapy and have a better chance of full rehabilitation. Bonica vigorously recommended this therapeutic regimen [19].

As mentioned above, by using the technique of thermoregulation to modulate sympathetic activity to the affected extremity in combination with sympathetic blocks, it is possible to distinguish between SMP that depends on the cutaneous sympathetic innervation and SMP that depends on the deep somatic sympathetic innervation. Complete sympathetic blocks affect all sympathetic outflow channels projecting to the affected extremity (deep and cutaneous), whereas thermoregulatory modulation exclusively alters the cutaneous sympathetic channel. Thus, in addition to a coupling in the skin, a sympathetic-afferent coupling is also very likely to occur in deep somatic tissues (bone, muscle or joints). Fig. 7 illustrates the different components of the pain: the component that depends on sympathetic activity (SMP) and the component that is independent of the sympathetic innervation (SIP) during the course of the disease.

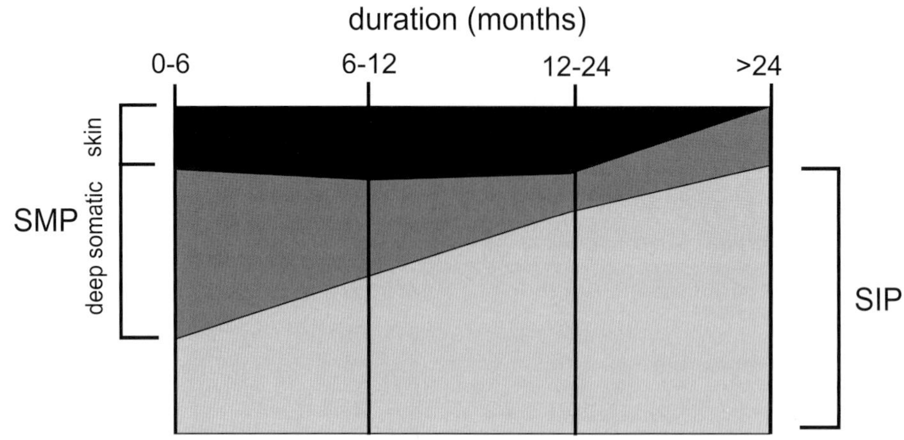

Fig. 7. Different components of sympathetic maintained pain (SMP). The component of pain that depends on the cutaneous sympathetic innervation (skin SMP), the component that depends on the deep somatic sympathetic innervation (deep SMP), and the component that is not maintained by sympathetic activity, i.e., sympathetically independent pain (SIP) during the course of the disease in 13 patients with complex regional pain syndrome (CRPS). Note that SMP decreases with time after the initiating event leading to CRPS. From [121], with permission.

Interpretation of the Clinical and Experimental Data Obtained in Humans

Although studies in pain patients are the basis for the belief that the sympathetic nervous system is involved in the generation of pain, they do not reveal which mechanisms are involved. Several conclusions can be drawn from the clinical observations (Fig. 1):

1) Primary afferent nociceptors are excited and possibly sensitized by norepinephrine released by the sympathetic fibers.

2) Either the primary afferent nociceptive neurons have expressed adrenoceptors and/or their increased excitability is generated indirectly, i.e., via the vascular bed (e.g., by changes in blood flow) or other components, such as inflammatory cells in the environment of the nociceptive neurons which may have a permissive effect on sympathetic to nociceptor coupling or are modulated directly by sympathetic postganglionic neurons.

3) Sympathetically maintained spontaneous and evoked activity in nociceptive neurons may generate a state of central sensitization/hyperexcitability, e.g., in dorsal horn neurons.

4) Central sensitization leads to spontaneous pain and to pain evoked by stimulation of mechanoreceptors, thermoreceptors, or nociceptors (mechanical and thermal allodynia and hyperalgesia).

5) Finally, it is very likely that sympathetic coupling to non-nociceptive afferent neurons may turn out to be a peripheral mechanism underlying SMP. Sympathetically maintained activity in these afferent neurons may activate sensitized second-order neurons, leading to pain.

The most important question, however, is still unsolved: *What factors determine adrenergic sensitivity in different human neuropathies?* As shown above, human peripheral painful neuropathies differ considerably concerning the development of adrenergic sensitivity, although all peripheral neuropathies are characterized by lesions of peripheral nerves. Furthermore, only subgroups of patients with an identical disorder (e.g., CRPS-I) develop noradrenergic sensitivity. Finally, the SMP component tends to decline in individual patients during the course of the disorder. There are disorders that are also characterized by peripheral nerve lesion that never develop adrenergic sensitivity (e.g., polyneuropathies). Thus, additional factors that are responsible for adrenergic sensitivity and SMP besides nerve damage per se must be postulated as follows.

1) The etiology of the lesion might determine the expression of adrenoceptors on afferent neurons. For example, there is evidence that virus infection triggers adrenoreceptor expression on afferent neurons. This particular mechanism might be responsible for the catecholamine response demonstrated in patients with zoster-associated pain [27].

2) Type and severity of nerve lesion might be important. Phantom limb pain is characterized by a *severance of all nerves* supplying one extremity, whereas in CRPS-I *no major nerve lesion* is demonstrable at all. These differences indicate that different mechanisms of adrenergic sensitivity exist.

3) One feature of most polyneuropathies, which is distinct from the aforementioned norepinephrine-sensitive syndromes, is the fact that the underlying disease, such as diabetes mellitus or chronic alcoholism, is an ongoing process. This chronic process leads to neuronal degeneration and regeneration occurring in parallel, a phenomenon that might account for the absence of norepinephrine sensitivity.

4) There is evidence that acute CRPS and acute mechanical nerve lesions are associated with a profound inflammatory reaction [15,84]. Acute inflammation leads to nociceptor sensitization with an enhanced response to adrenergic substances (Fig. 4) [51]. This adrenergic component emerging during inflammatory reactions is thought to be time dependent. Accordingly, clinical data show that a subgroup of patients with acute CRPS (SMP patients) responds well to sympathetic blocks, but that the effect is diminished over time [133]. A decline of the inflammatory component in the course of the disease [15] may be followed by a reduction of the SMP component. Thus, it is possible that patients with long-standing CRPS have lost the SMP component over time.

5) We have learned from animal models that considerable differences appear to exist in the dependence of sympathetically maintained allodynic behavior between rat strains with spinal nerve lesion. These results point to genetic differences and predispositions that might determine the expression of adrenoceptors or the function of these receptors on afferent neurons in human neuropathies.

6) Finally, based on clinical observations and experiments, we have put forward the hypothesis that CRPS is a disease of the central nervous system [55–57]. How are the peripheral changes observed in CRPS patients (sympathetic-afferent coupling, edema, and inflammation) related to the central changes?

In summary, it seems to be obvious from animal and human research that afferent neurons may develop adrenergic sensitivity after trauma, infection, or inflammation.

Therefore, the efferent sympathetic nervous system is clearly involved in pain processing. The exact mechanisms underlying adrenergic sensitivity of afferent neurons in human neuropathies of different etiologies, their time course during the disease process, and the genetic predisposition for the development of adrenergic sensitivity must be established in future research.

The Role of Cholinergic Mechanisms in the Generation of Pain

Acetylcholine and its receptors (nicotinic and muscarinic) in afferent and autonomic neurons may be important in the modulation of the excitability of peripheral nociceptive neurons. Here we will briefly discuss this aspect and concentrate on afferent nociceptive neurons and autonomic neurons. We will not discuss the cholinergic anti-inflammatory pathway acting via efferent vagal (parasympathetic) neurons and mainly nicotinic acetylcholine receptors on macrophages and other cytokine-producing cells. Activation of this pathway (by electrical stimulation of the vagus nerve) leads to inhibition of these cells' release of proinflammatory cytokines (such as TNF-α, IL-1, IL-6, and IL-8) but not their expression of inhibitory cytokines [134,135]. This neural inhibition of cytokine activity reduces inflammation and should therefore also decrease the activation and sensitization of nociceptive afferent neurons, resulting in decreased pain. However, this effect of activity in cholinergic parasympathetic neurons on nociceptive neurons is indirect. Furthermore, the concept of the cholinergic anti-inflammatory pathway as propagated by Tracey [134,135] is still rather hypothetical and needs experimental verification.

Acetylcholine Receptors on Nociceptive Afferent Fibers

Behavioral experiments on rats and rabbits and experiments on humans show that acetylcholine is an algogenic agent in the skin and elsewhere (for review, see [75]). Using the skin-nerve preparation or the cornea, neurophysiological investigations have shown that only C fibers (and practically no A fibers) are excited by acetylcholine or its analogue carbachol [129,132]. About 50% of cutaneous C fibers with nociceptive function are excited by carbachol, exhibit weak enhanced responses to heat stimuli, and show desensitization to mechanical stimulation [129]. These neurophysiological data correlate with the finding that nicotinic and muscarinic acetylcholine receptors are expressed by small-diameter DRG cells and by unmyelinated afferent fibers in peripheral nerves [10,21].

Neurophysiological investigations conducted more recently show that nicotine dose-dependently activates about 80% of cutaneous nociceptive C fibers and induces a mild sensitization of the responses to heat stimuli, but not to mechanical stimuli [11]. Muscarine activates nociceptive C fibers only weakly or not at all, but it leads to a marked desensitization of the C fibers to mechanical or heat stimulation. The relatively selective muscarinic receptor M2 agonist arecaidine has the same effect. The responses elicited by the muscarinic agonists can be prevented by scopolamine or by the M2 antagonist gallamine [11]. These experimental neurophysiological findings are strongly supported by three groups of measurements: (1) Cutaneous nociceptive C fibers in knockout mice for the muscarinic M2 receptor subtype did not exhibit desensitization to muscarine for mechanical or heat stimuli, but nociceptive C fibers in knockout mice for the muscarinic M4 receptor showed normal responses [13]. (2) Thin epidermal afferent nerve fibers in rat hairy skin express the muscarinic M2 receptor but not the muscarinic M3 receptor [13]. (3) CGRP released from isolated (but innervated) rat hairy skin during heat stimulation is inhibited by the muscarinic M2 agonist arecaidine [12].

These experiments show that the excitability of nociceptive C fibers may be controlled via the muscarinic M2 receptor by acetylcholine released extraneurally in the dermis and epidermis. Acetylcholine is synthesized and released by keratinocytes in the epidermis, and possibly by other cells such as fibroblasts or immune cells (for discussion see [76,143]). These muscarinic M2 subtype acetylcholine receptors in the nociceptive neurons may turn out to be a peripheral target for specific analgesics.

Acetylcholine, the Sympathetic Nervous System, and Pain

Besides norepinephrine, acetylcholine is also used as a neurotransmitter in the autonomic nervous system. Synaptic transmission in autonomic ganglia between the pre- and postganglionic sympathetic and parasympathetic neurons is mediated exclusively by acetylcholine. Furthermore, at the postganglionic level, all parasympathetic and sympathetic sudomotor neurons and some other functional types of sympathetic neurons contain acetylcholine [53]. Animal experimental studies examining the influence of this neuron system on nociceptive transmission are sparse; however, several clinical studies have addressed this issue.

In the facial area, sympathetic and parasympathetic neurons innervate the same blood vessels. Following a chronic constriction injury of the mental nerve (a branch of the trigeminal nerve), cutaneous sprouting of adrenergic and cholinergic fibers was observed [47,111]. These findings indicate that as a result of autonomic sprouting, remaining intact nociceptive fibers may potentially develop sensitivity to activation of sympathetic or parasympathetic postganglionic neurons, which may play a role in the generation of abnormal pain following nerve injury.

According to these findings, there is anecdotal evidence for the efficacy of local anesthetic blocks of the spheno- or pterygopalatine ganglion in primary headache syndromes and facial pain [96]. In extremity pain syndromes such as CRPS, an interaction between sympathetic vasoconstrictor neurons and nociceptors via adrenoceptors has been proposed as an underlying mechanism of SMP (see above). Alternatively, a cholinergic coupling of sympathetic sudomotor neurons and nociceptors is theoretically possible.

In one study, the effect of cutaneous sympathetic sudomotor activity on pain induced by primary afferent C-nociceptor activation with capsaicin was analyzed in healthy humans [141]. After injection of capsaicin into the forearm skin, sympathetic sudomotor skin activity was altered by whole-body temperature changes with a thermal suit. By altering whole-body temperature from a moderately warm to an intensely warm state, sympathetic sudomotor activity is modulated selectively in the widest range that can be achieved physiologically while sympathetic vasoconstrictor activity is continuously inhibited. The intensity and spatial distribution of capsaicin-evoked ongoing pain and dynamic and punctate mechanical hyperalgesia were not significantly different during the presence of high and low sympathetic sudomotor discharge, indicating that there is no interaction between both systems under these experimental conditions. These negative results are not surprising in view of the fact that the cutaneous nociceptive fibers and the sudomotor fibers terminate in separate layers of the skin (sudomotor fibers subcutaneously around the sweat glands and nociceptive fibers in the dermis and epidermis).

Botulinum toxin mainly blocks the release of acetylcholine at cholinergic synapses, thereby inhibiting neuronal activity for up to 3 months. A recent study showed that intradermal application of botulinum toxin relieves spontaneous pain and allodynia in patients with neuropathic pain [112]. It is proposed that the mechanism of action does not involve an interaction of cholinergic and afferent fibers but is characterized by a direct effect of the toxin on nociceptive afferents.

Botulinum toxin was also used in sympathetic ganglion blocks. In patients with CRPS, the duration of pain relief lasted considerably longer if the patients were treated with a mixture of botulinum toxin and local anesthetic as compared with the local anesthetic alone [23a].

Acknowledgments

Supported by the Deutsche Forschungsgemeinschaft (DFG Ba 1921/1-3, Jä 240/19-1), the German Ministry of Research and Education, German Research Network on Neuropathic Pain (BMBF, 01EM01/04) and an unrestricted educational grant from Pfizer, Germany.

References

[1] Ali Z, Ringkamp M, Hartke TV, Chien HF, Flavahan NA, Campbell JN, Meyer RA. Uninjured C-fiber nociceptors develop spontaneous activity and alpha-adrenergic sensitivity following L6 spinal nerve ligation in monkey. J Neurophysiol 1999;81:455–66.

[2] Ali Z, Raja SN, Wesselmann U, Fuchs PN, Meyer RA, Campbell JN. Intradermal injection of norepinephrine evokes pain in patients with sympathetically maintained pain. Pain 2000;88:161–8.

[3] Andreev NY, Dimitrieva N, Koltzenburg M, McMahon SB. Peripheral administration of nerve growth factor in the adult rat produces a thermal hyperalgesia that requires the presence of sympathetic post-ganglionic neurones. Pain 1995;63:109–15.

[4] Arnér S. Intravenous phentolamine test: diagnostic and prognostic use in reflex sympathetic dystrophy. Pain 1991;46:17–22.

[5] Arnold JM, Teasell RW, MacLeod AP, Brown JE, Carruthers SG. Increased venous alpha-adrenoceptor responsiveness in patients with reflex sympathetic dystrophy. Ann Intern Med 1993;118:619–21.

[6] Baron R, Wasner G. Complex regional pain syndromes. Curr Pain Headache Rep 2001;5:114–23.

[7] Baron R, Wasner G, Borgstedt R, Hastedt E, Schulte H, Binder A, Kopper F, Rowbotham M, Levine JD, Fields HL. Effect of sympathetic activity on capsaicin-evoked pain, hyperalgesia, and vasodilatation. Neurology 1999;52:923–32.

[8] Baron R, Schattschneider J, Binder A, Siebrecht D, Wasner G. Relation between sympathetic vasoconstrictor activity and pain and hyperalgesia in complex regional pain syndromes: a case-control study. Lancet 2002;359:1655–60.

[9] Bennett GJ, Xie YK. A peripheral mononeuropathy in rat that produces disorders of pain sensation like those seen in man. Pain 1988;33:87–107.

[10] Bernardini N, de Stefano ME, Tata AM, Biagioni S, Augusti-Tocco G. Neuronal and non-neuronal cell populations of the avian dorsal root ganglia express muscarinic acetylcholine receptors. Int J Dev Neurosci 1998;16:365–77.

[11] Bernardini N, Sauer SK, Haberberger R, Fischer MJ, Reeh PW. Excitatory nicotinic and desensitizing muscarinic (M2) effects on C-nociceptors in isolated rat skin. J Neurosci 2001;21:3295–302.
[12] Bernardini N, Reeh PW, Sauer SK. Muscarinic M2 receptors inhibit heat-induced CGRP release from isolated rat skin. Neuroreport 2001;12:2457–60.
[13] Bernardini N, Roza C, Sauer SK, Gomeza J, Wess J, Reeh PW. Muscarinic M2 receptors on peripheral nerve endings: a molecular target of antinociception. J Neurosci 2002;22:RC229.
[14] Birder LA, Perl ER. Expression of alpha2-adrenergic receptors in rat primary afferent neurones after peripheral nerve injury or inflammation. J Physiol 1999;515:533–42.
[15] Birklein F, Schmelz M, Schifter S, Weber M. The important role of neuropeptides in complex regional pain syndrome. Neurology 2001;57:2179–84.
[16] Blumberg H, Jänig W. Discharge pattern of afferent fibers from a neuroma. Pain 1984;20:335–53.
[17] Blumberg H, Hoffmann U, Mohadjer M, Scheremet R. Clinical phenomenology and mechanisms of reflex sympathetic dystrophy: emphasis on edema. In: Gebhart GF, Hammond DL, Jensen TS, editors. Proceedings of the 7th World Congress on Pain. Seattle: IASP Press; 1994. p. 455–81.
[18] Bonica JJ. Causalgia and other reflex sympathetic dystrophies. In: Bonica JJ, editor. Management of pain. Philadelphia: Lea and Febiger; 1953. p. 913–78.
[19] Bonica JJ. Causalgia and other reflex sympathetic dystrophies. In: Bonica JJ, editor. The management of pain. Philadelphia: Lea and Febiger; 1990. p. 220–43.
[20] Bossut DF, Shea VK, Perl ER. Sympathectomy induces adrenergic excitability of cutaneous C-fiber nociceptors. J Neurophysiol 1996;75:514–7.
[21] Boyd RT, Jacob MH, McEachern AE, Caron S, Berg DK. Nicotinic acetylcholine receptor mRNA in dorsal root ganglion neurons. J Neurobiol 1991;22:1–14.
[22] Bradesi S, Mayer EA, Schwetz I. Irritable bowel syndrome. In: Basbaum AI, Bushnell MC, editors. Science of pain. San Diego: Academic Press; 2009. p. 571-8.
[23] Burchiel KJ. Effects of electrical and mechanical stimulation on two foci of spontaneous activity which develop in primary afferent neurons after peripheral axotomy. Pain 1984;18:249–65.
[23a] Carroll I, Clark JD, Mackey S. Sympathetic block with botulinum toxin to treat complex regional pain syndrome. Ann Neurol 2009 65:348–51.
[24] Cepeda MS, Lau J, Carr DB. Defining the therapeutic role of local anesthetic sympathetic blockade in complex regional pain syndrome: a narrative and systematic review. Clin J Pain 2002;18:216–33.
[25] Chabal C, Jacobson L, Russell LC, Burchiel KJ. Pain response to perineuromal injection of normal saline, epinephrine, and lidocaine in humans. Pain 1992;49:9–12.
[26] Chen Y, Michaelis M, Jänig W, Devor M. Adrenoreceptor subtype mediating sympathetic-sensory coupling in injured sensory neurons. J Neurophysiol 1996;76:3721–30.
[27] Choi B, Rowbotham MC. Effect of adrenergic receptor activation on post-herpetic neuralgia pain and sensory disturbances. Pain 1997;69:55–63.
[28] Choi Y, Yoon YW, Na HS, Kim SH, Chung JM. Behavioral signs of ongoing pain and cold allodynia in a rat model of neuropathic pain. Pain 1994;59:369–76.
[29] Chung K, Lee BH, Yoon YW, Chung JM. Sympathetic sprouting in the dorsal root ganglia of the injured peripheral nerve in a rat neuropathic pain model. J Comp Neurol 1996;376:241–52.
[30] Chung K, Yoon YW, Chung JM. Sprouting sympathetic fibers form synaptic varicosities in the dorsal root ganglion of the rat with neuropathic injury. Brain Res 1997;751:275–80.
[31] Cunha TM, Verri WA Jr, Poole S, Parada CA, Cunha FQ, Ferreira SH. Pain facilitation by proinflammatory cytokine actions at peripheral nerve terminals. In: DeLeo JA, Sorkin LS, Watkins LR, editors. Immune and glial regulation of pain. Seattle: IASP Press; 2007. p. 67–83.
[32] Clauw DJ, Chrousos GP. Chronic pain and fatigue syndromes: overlapping clinical and neuroendocrine features and potential pathogenic mechanisms. Neuroimmunomodulation 1997;4:134–53.
[33] Davis KD, Treede RD, Raja SN, Meyer RA, Campbell JN. Topical application of clonidine relieves hyperalgesia in patients with sympathetically maintained pain. Pain 1991;47:309–17.
[34] de Armentia ML, Leeson AH, Stebbing MJ, Urban L, McLachlan EM. Responses to sympathomimetics in rat sensory neurones after nerve transection. Neuroreport 2003;14:9–13.
[35] Desmeules JA, Kayser V, Weil-Fuggaza J, Bertrand A, Guilbaud G. Influence of the sympathetic nervous system in the development of abnormal pain-related behaviours in a rat model of neuropathic pain. Neuroscience 1995;67:941–51.
[36] Devor M, Jänig W. Activation of myelinated afferents ending in a neuroma by stimulation of the sympathetic supply in the rat. Neurosci Lett 1981;24:43–7.
[37] Devor M, Jänig W, Michaelis M. Modulation of activity in dorsal root ganglion neurons by sympathetic activation in nerve-injured rats. J Neurophysiol 1994;71:38–47.
[38] Drummond PD. Noradrenaline increases hyperalgesia to heat in skin sensitized by capsaicin. Pain 1995;60:311–5.
[39] Drummond PD. Independent effects of ischaemia and noradrenaline on thermal hyperalgesia in capsaicin-treated skin. Pain 1996;67:129–33.
[40] Drummond PD, Finch PM, Gibbins I. Innervation of hyperalgesic skin in patients with complex regional pain syndrome. Clin J Pain 1996;12:222–31.
[41] Drummond PD. Enhancement of thermal hyperalgesia by alpha-adrenoceptors in capsaicin-treated skin. J Auton Nerv Syst 1998;69:96–102.
[42] Drummond PD, Finch PM, Skipworth S, Blockey P. Pain increases during sympathetic arousal in patients with complex regional pain syndrome. Neurology 2001;57:1296–303.

[43] Elam M, Macefield VG. Does sympathetic nerve discharge affect the firing of myelinated cutaneous afferents in humans? Auton Neurosci 2004;111:116–26.

[44] Elam M, Olausson B, Skarphedinsson JO, Wallin BG. Does sympathetic nerve discharge affect the firing of polymodal C-fibre afferents in humans? Brain 1999;122:2237–44.

[45] Fleming WW, Westfall D. Adaptive supersensitivity. In: Trendelenburg U, Weiner N, editors. Catecholamines. Handbook of experimental pharmacology, Vol. 90. New York: Springer Verlag; 1988. p. 509–59.

[46] Gazda LS, Milligan ED, Hansen MK, Twining CM, Poulos NM, Chacur M, O'Connor KA, Armstrong C, Maier SF, Watkins LR, Myers RR. Sciatic inflammatory neuritis (SIN): behavioral allodynia is paralleled by peri-sciatic proinflammatory cytokine and superoxide production. J Peripher Nerv Syst 2001;6:111–29.

[47] Grelik C, Bennett GJ, Ribeiro-da-Silva A. Autonomic fibre sprouting and changes in nociceptive sensory innervation in the rat lower lip skin following chronic constriction injury. Eur J Neurosci 2005;21:2475–87.

[48] Häbler HJ, Jänig W, Koltzenburg M. Activation of unmyelinated afferents in chronically lesioned nerves by adrenaline and excitation of sympathetic efferents in the cat. Neurosci Lett 1987;82:35–40.

[49] Häbler H-J, Eschenfelder S, Liu X-G, Jänig W. Sympathetic-sensory coupling after L5 spinal nerve lesion in the rat and its relation to changes in dorsal root ganglion blood flow. Pain 2000;87:335–45.

[50] Hord ED, Oaklander AL. Complex regional pain syndrome: a review of evidence-supported treatment options. Curr Pain Headache Rep 2003;7:188–96.

[51] Hu SJ, Zhu J. Sympathetic facilitation of sustained discharges of polymodal nociceptors. Pain 1989;38:85–90.

[52] Jänig W. Activation of afferent fibers ending in an old neuroma by sympathetic stimulation in the rat. Neurosci Lett 1990;111:309–14.

[53] Jänig W. The integrative action of the autonomic nervous system. Neurobiology of homeostasis. Cambridge: Cambridge University Press; 2006.

[54] Jänig W. Autonomic nervous system and pain. In: Basbaum AI, Bushnell MC, editors. Science of pain. San Diego: Academic Press; 2009. p. 193-26.

[55] Jänig W. Autonomic nervous system dysfunction. In: Mayer EA, Bushnell MC, editors. Functional pain syndromes: presentation and pathophysiology. Seattle: IASP Press; 2009. p. 265–300.

[56] Jänig W, Baron R. Complex regional pain syndrome is a disease of the central nervous system. Clin Auton Res 2002;12:150–64.

[57] Jänig W, Baron R. Complex regional pain syndrome: mystery explained? Lancet Neurol 2003;2:687–97.

[58] Jänig W, Häbler HJ. Sympathetic nervous system: contribution to chronic pain. Prog Brain Res 2000;129:451–68.

[59] Jänig W, Levine JD. Autonomic-neuroendocrine-immune responses in acute and chronic pain. In: McMahon SB, Koltzenburg M, editors. Wall & Melzack's textbook of pain, 5th ed. Edinburgh: Elsevier Churchill Livingstone; 2006. p. 205–18.

[60] Jänig W, Khasar SG, Levine JD, Miao FJP. The role of vagal visceral afferents in the control of nociception. Prog Brain Res 2000;122:273–87.

[61] Jänig W, Levine JD, Michaelis M. Interactions of sympathetic and primary afferent neurons following nerve injury and tissue trauma. Prog Brain Res 1996;112:161–84.

[62] Khasar SG, Green PG, Levine JD. Comparison of intradermal and subcutaneous hyperalgesic effects of inflammatory mediators in the rat. Neurosci Lett 1993;153:215–8.

[63] Khasar SG, Miao FJP, Levine JD. Inflammation modulates the contribution of receptor-subtypes to bradykinin-induced hyperalgesia in the rat. Neurosci 1995;69:685–90.

[64] Khasar SG, Miao JP, Jänig W, Levine JD. Modulation of bradykinin-induced mechanical hyperalgesia in the rat by activity in abdominal vagal afferents. Eur J Neurosci 1998;10:435–44.

[65] Khasar SG, Miao FJP, Jänig W, Levine JD. Vagotomy-induced enhancement of mechanical hyperalgesia in the rat is sympathoadrenal-mediated. J Neurosci 1998;18:3043–9.

[66] Khasar SG, Green PG, Miao FJ, Levine JD. Vagal modulation of nociception is mediated by adrenomedullary epinephrine in the rat. Eur J Neurosci 2003;17:909–15.

[67] Khasar SG, Green PG, Levine JD. Repeated sound stress enhances inflammatory pain in the rat. Pain 2005;116:79–86.

[68] Kim SH, Chung JM. An experimental model for peripheral neuropathy produced by segmental spinal nerve ligation in the rat. Pain 1992;50:355–63.

[69] Kim SH, Na HS, Sheen K, Chung JM. Effects of sympathectomy on a rat model of peripheral neuropathy. Pain 1993;55:85–92.

[70] Kim KJ, Yoon YW, Chung JM. Comparison of three rodent neuropathic pain models. Exp Brain Res 1997;113:200–6.

[71] Kingery WS. A critical review of controlled clinical trials for peripheral neuropathic pain and complex regional pain syndromes. Pain 1997;73:123–39.

[72] Kinnman E, Nygards EB, Hansson P. Peripheral alpha-adrenoreceptors are involved in the development of capsaicin induced ongoing and stimulus evoked pain in humans. Pain 1997;69:79–85.

[73] Koltzenburg M, Kress M, Reeh PW. The nociceptor sensitization by bradykinin does not depend on sympathetic neurons. Neurosci 1992;46:465–73.

[74] Korenman EM, Devor M. Ectopic adrenergic sensitivity in damaged peripheral nerve axons in the rat. Exp Neurol 1981;72:63–81.

[75] Kress M, Reeh P. Chemical excitation and sensitization in nociceptors. In: Belmonte C, Cervero F, editors. Neurobiology of nociceptors. Oxford: Oxford University Press; 1996. p. 258–97.

[76] Kurzen H, Wessler I, Kirkpatrick CJ, Kawashima K, Grando SA. The non-neuronal cholinergic system of human skin. Horm Metab Res 2007;39:125–35.

[77] Leriche R. De la causalgie envisagée comme une névrite du sympathique et son traitement par la dénudation et l'excision des plexus nerveux périartériels [On causalgia as a neuritis of the sympathetic system and its treatment by stripping and excision of the periarterial nerve plexus]. La Presse Med 1916;178–80.
[78] Levine JD, Dardick SJ, Basbaum AI, Scipio E. Reflex neurogenic inflammation. I. Contribution of the peripheral nervous system to spatially remote inflammatory responses that follow injury. J Neurosci 1985;5:1380–6.
[79] Lewin GR, Ritter AM, Mendell LM. Nerve growth factor-induced hyperalgesia in the neonatal and adult rat. J Neurosci 1993;13:2136–48.
[80] Lewin GR, Rueff A, Mendell LM. Peripheral and central mechanisms of NGF-induced hyperalgesia. Eur J Neurosci 1994;6:1903–12.
[80a] Lin Q, Wu J, Willis WD. Effects of protein kinase a activation on the responses of primate spinothalamic tract neurons to mechanical stimuli. J Neurophysiol 2002;88:214–21.
[81] Liu M, Max MB, Parada S, Rowan JS, Bennett GJ. The sympathetic nervous system contributes to capsaicin-evoked mechanical allodynia but not pinprick hyperalgesia in humans. J Neurosci 1996;16:7331–5.
[82] Liu X, Eschenfelder S, Blenk KH, Jänig W, Häbler H. Spontaneous activity of axotomized afferent neurons after L5 spinal nerve injury in rats. Pain 2000;84:309–18.
[83] Livingston WK. Pain mechanisms. A physiological interpretation of causalgia and related states. Reprinted by Plenum Press; 1976 (originally published in 1943).
[84] Manning DC. Immunomodulatory therapies for complex regional pain syndrome: thalidomide and beyond. In: DeLeo JA, Sorkin LS, Watkins LR, editors. Immune and glial regulation of pain. Seattle: IASP Press; 2007. p. 407–16.
[85] Manning DC, Raja SN, Meyer RA, Campbell JN. Pain and hyperalgesia after intradermal injection of bradykinin in humans. Clin Pharmacol Ther 1991;50:721–9.
[86] Mayer EM, Bushnell MC, editors. Functional pain syndromes: presentation and pathophysiology. Seattle: IASP Press; 2009.
[87] McLachlan EM, Jänig W, Devor M, Michaelis M. Peripheral nerve injury triggers noradrenergic sprouting within dorsal root ganglia. Nature 1993;363:543–6.
[88] McMahon SB. NGF as a mediator of inflammatory pain. Philos Trans R Soc Lond B Biol Sci 1996;351:431–40.
[89] Mense S, Meyer H. Bradykinin-induced modulation of the response behaviour of different types of feline group III and IV muscle receptors. J Physiol (Lond) 1988;398:49–63.
[90] Merskey H, Bogduk N. Classification of chronic pain: descriptions of chronic pain syndromes and definition of pain terms. Seattle: IASP Press; 1994.
[91] Miao FJP, Green PG, Coderre TJ, Jänig W, Levine JD. Sympathetic-dependence in bradykinin-induced synovial plasma extravasation is dose-related. Neurosci Lett 1996;205:165–8.
[92] Miao FJP, Jänig W, Levine JD. Role of sympathetic postganglionic neurons in synovial plasma extravasation induced by bradykinin. J Neurophysiol 1996;75:715–24.
[93] Michaelis M, Devor M, Jänig W. Sympathetic modulation of activity in rat dorsal root ganglion neurons changes over time following peripheral nerve injury. J Neurophysiol 1996;76:753–63.
[94] Michaelis M, Liu X, Jänig W. Axotomized and intact muscle afferents but no skin afferents develop ongoing discharges of dorsal root ganglion origin after peripheral nerve lesion. J Neurosci 2000;20:2742–8.
[95] Mitchell SW. Injuries of nerves and their consequences. Philadelphia: J.P. Lippincott; 1872.
[96] Narouze S, Kapural L, Casanova J, Mekhail N. Sphenopalatine ganglion radiofrequency ablation for the management of chronic cluster headache. Headache 2009;49:571–7.
[97] Neil A, Attal N, Guilbaud G. Effects of guanethidine on sensitization to natural stimuli and self-mutilating behaviour in rats with a peripheral neuropathy. Brain Res 1991;565:237–46.
98] Neugebauer V, Schaible HG, Schmidt RF. Sensitization of articular afferents to mechanical stimuli by bradykinin. Pflügers Arch 1989;415:330–5.
[99] Nicholas AP, Pieribone VA, Hokfelt T. Cellular localization of messenger RNA for beta-1 and beta-2 adrenergic receptors in rat brain: an in situ hybridization study. Neuroscience 1993;56:1023–39.
[100] O'Halloran KD, Perl ER. Effects of partial nerve injury on the responses of C-fiber polymodal nociceptors to adrenergic agonists. Brain Res 1997;759:233–40.
[101] Ochoa JL. Truths, errors, and lies around "reflex sympathetic dystrophy" and "complex regional pain syndrome." J Neurol 1999;246:875–9.
[102] Pedersen JL, Rung GW, Kehlet H. Effect of sympathetic nerve block on acute inflammatory pain and hyperalgesia. Anesthesiology 1997;86:293–301.
[103] Perl ER. A reevaluation of mechanisms leading to sympathetically related pain. In: Fields HL, Liebeskind JC, editors. Pharmacological approach to the treatment of chronic pain: new concepts and critical issues. Seattle: IASP Press; 1994. p. 129–50.
[104] Perl ER. Cutaneous polymodal receptors: characteristics and plasticity. Prog Brain Res 1996;113:21–37.
[105] Petty BG, Cornblath DR, Adornato BT, Chaudhry V, Flexner C, Wachsman M, Sinicropi D, Burton LE, Peroutka SJ. The effect of systemically administered recombinant human nerve growth factor in healthy human subjects. Ann Neurol 1994;36:244–6.
[106] Pieribone VA, Nicholas AP, Dagerlind A, Hokfelt T. Distribution of alpha 1 adrenoceptors in rat brain revealed by in situ hybridization experiments utilizing subtype-specific probes. J Neurosci 1994;14:4252–68.
[107] Price DD, Long S, Wilsey B, Rafii A. Analysis of peak magnitude and duration of analgesia produced by local anesthetics injected into sympathetic ganglia of complex regional pain syndrome patients. Clin J Pain 1998;14:216–26.
[108] Raja SN, Treede RD, Davis KD, Campbell JN. Systemic alpha-adrenergic blockade with phentolamine: a diagnostic test for sympathetically maintained pain. Anesthesiology 1991;74:691–8.

[109] Raja SN. Role of the sympathetic nervous system in acute pain and inflammation. Ann Med 1995;27:241–6.
[110] Raja SN. Peripheral modulatory effects of catecholamines in inflammatory and neuropathic pain. Adv Pharmacol 1998;42:567–71.
[111] Ramien M, Ruocco I, Cuello AC, St-Louis M, Ribeiro-da-Silva A. Parasympathetic nerve fibers invade the upper dermis following sensory denervation of the rat lower lip skin. J Comp Neurol 2004;469:83–95.
[112] Ranoux D, Attal N, Morain F, Bouhassira D. Botulinum toxin type A induces direct analgesic effects in chronic neuropathic pain. Ann Neurol 2008;64:274–83.
[112a] Ren Y, Zou X, Fang L, Lin Q. Involvement of peripheral purinoceptors in sympathetic modulation of capsaicin-induced sensitization of primary afferent fibers. J Neurophysiol 2006;96:2207–16.
[113] Richards RL. Causalgia. A centennial review. Arch Neurol 1967;16:339–50.
[114] Ringkamp M, Eschenfelder S, Grethel EJ, Häbler HJ, Meyer RA, Jänig W, Raja SN. Lumbar sympathectomy failed to reverse mechanical allodynia- and hyperalgesia-like behavior in rats with L5 spinal nerve injury. Pain 1999;79:143–53.
[115] Ruocco I, Cuello AC, Ribeiro-da-Silva A. Peripheral nerve injury leads to the establishment of a novel pattern of sympathetic fibre innervation in the rat skin. J Comp Neurol 2000;422:287–96.
[116] Sachs D, Cunha FQ, Poole S, Ferreira SH. Tumour necrosis factor-alpha, interleukin-1beta and interleukin-8 induce persistent mechanical nociceptor hypersensitivity. Pain 2002;96:89–97.
[117] Sato J, Perl ER. Adrenergic excitation of cutaneous pain receptors induced by peripheral nerve injury. Science 1991;251:1608–10.
[118] Sato J, Suzuki S, Iseki T, Kumazawa T. Adrenergic excitation of cutaneous nociceptors in chronically inflamed rats. Neurosci Lett 1993;164:225–8.
[119] Scadding JW. Development of ongoing activity, mechanosensitivity, and adrenaline sensitivity in severed peripheral nerve axons. Exp Neurol 1981;73:345–64.
[120] Schattschneider J, Uphoff J, Binder A, Wasner G, Baron R. No adrenergic sensitization of afferent neurons in painful sensory polyneuropathy. J Neurol 2006;253:280–6.
[121] Schattschneider J, Binder A, Siebrecht D, Wasner G, Baron R. Complex regional pain syndromes: the influence of cutaneous and deep somatic sympathetic innervation on pain. Clin J Pain 2006;22:240–4.
[122] Schott GD. Interrupting the sympathetic outflow in causalgia and reflex sympathetic dystrophy. BMJ 1998;316:792–3.
[123] Schott G. Clinical features of algodystrophy: is the sympathetic nervous system involved? Funct Neurol 1989;4:131–4.
[124] Seltzer Z, Dubner R, Shir Y. A novel behavioral model of neuropathic pain disorders produced in rats by partial sciatic nerve injury. Pain 1990;43:205–18.
[125] Shea VK, Perl ER. Failure of sympathetic stimulation to affect responsiveness of rabbit polymodal nociceptors. J Neurophysiol 1985;54:513–9.
[126] Shi TS, Winzer-Serhan U, Leslie F, Hokfelt T. Distribution and regulation of alpha$_2$-adrenoceptors in rat dorsal root ganglia. Pain 2000;84:319–30.
[127] Shir Y, Seltzer Z. Effects of sympathectomy in a model of causalgiform pain produced by partial sciatic nerve injury in rats. Pain 1991;45:309–20.
[128] Stanton-Hicks M, Jänig W, Hassenbusch S, Haddox JD, Boas R, Wilson P. Reflex sympathetic dystrophy: changing concepts and taxonomy. Pain 1995;63:127–33.
[129] Steen KH, Reeh PW. Actions of cholinergic agonists and antagonists on sensory nerve endings in rat skin, in vitro. J Neurophysiol 1993;70:397–405.
[130] Sudeck P. Über die akute (trophoneurotische) Knochenatrophie nach Entzündungen und Traumen der Extremitäten [On acute (trophoneurotic) bone atrophy following inflammation and traumas at the extremities]. Deutsche Med Wschr 1902;28:336–42.
[131] Sudeck P. Die trophische Extremitätenstörung durch periphere (infektiöse und traumatische) Reize [The trophic extremity disturbance induced by peripheral (infectious and traumatic) stimuli]. Deutsche Zeitschr Chirurg 1931;234:596–612.
[132] Tanelian DL. Cholinergic activation of a population of corneal afferent nerves. Exp Brain Res 1991;86:414–20.
[133] Torebjörk HE, Wahren LK, Wallin BG, Hallin R, Koltzenburg M. Noradrenaline-evoked pain in neuralgia. Pain 1995;63:11–20.
[134] Tracey KJ. The inflammatory reflex. Nature 2002;420:853–9.
[135] Tracey KJ. Physiology and immunology of the cholinergic antiinflammatory pathway. J Clin Invest 2007;117:289–96.
[136] Verdugo RJ, Campero M, Ochoa JL. Phentolamine sympathetic block in painful polyneuropathies. II. Further questioning of the concept of 'sympathetically maintained pain'. Neurology 1994;44:1010–4.
[137] Verdugo RJ, Ochoa JL. 'Sympathetically maintained pain.' I. Phentolamine block questions the concept. Neurology 1994;44:1003–10.
[138] Verri WA Jr, Cunha TM, Parada CA, Poole S, Cunha FQ, Ferreira SH. Hypernociceptive role of cytokines and chemokines: targets for analgesic drug development? Pharmacol Ther 2006;112:116–38.
[139] Walker AE, Nulsen F. Electrical stimulation of the upper thoracic portion of the sympathetic chain in man. Arch Neurol Psychiatry 1948;59:559–60.
[139a] Wang J, Ren Y, Zou X, Fang L, Willis WD, Lin Q. Sympathetic influence on capsaicin-evoked enhancement of dorsal root reflexes in rats. J Neurophysiol 2004;92:2017–26.
[140] Wasner G, Heckmann K, Maier C, Baron R. Vascular abnormalities in acute reflex sympathetic dystrophy (CRPS I): complete inhibition of sympathetic nerve activity with recovery. Arch Neurol 1999;56:613–20.
[141] Wasner G, Binder A, Kopper F, Baron R. No effect of sympathetic sudomotor activity on capsaicin-evoked ongoing pain and hyperalgesia. Pain 2000;84:331–8.

[142] Wasner G, Bréchôt A, Schattschneider J, Allardt A, Binder A, Jensen TS, Baron R. Effect of sympathetic muscle vasoconstrictor activity on capsaicin-induced muscle pain. Muscle Nerve 2002;26:113–21.
[143] Wess J, Duttaroy A, Gomeza J, Zhang W, Yamada M, Felder CC, Bernardini N, Reeh PW. Muscarinic receptor subtypes mediating central and peripheral antinociception studied with muscarinic receptor knockout mice: a review. Life Sci 2003;72:2047–54.
[144] White JC, Sweet WH. Pain and the neurosurgeon: a forty year experience. Springfield, IL: Charles C. Thomas, 1969.
[145] Wolfe F, Smythe HA, Yunus MB, et al. The American College of Rheumatology 1990 Criteria for the Classification of Fibromyalgia. Report of the Multicenter Criteria Committee. Arthritis Rheum 1990;33:160–72.
[146] Woolf CJ. Phenotypic modification of primary sensory neurons: the role of nerve growth factor in the production of persistent pain. Philos Trans R Soc Lond B 1996;351:441–8.
[147] Yen LD, Bennett GJ, Ribeiro-da-Silva A. Sympathetic sprouting and changes in nociceptive sensory innervation in the glabrous skin of the rat hind paw following partial peripheral nerve injury. J Comp Neurol 2006;495:679–90.
[148] Yoon YW, Lee DH, Lee BH, Chung K, Chung JM. Different strains and substrains of rats show different levels of neuropathic pain behaviors. Exp Brain Res 1999;129:167–71.

Correspondence to: Prof. Dr. Wilfrid Jänig, Physiologisches Institut, Christian-Albrechts-Universität zu Kiel, Olshausenstr. 40, 24098 Kiel, Germany. Tel: +431/8802036; fax: +431/8805256; email: w.janig@physiologie.uni-kiel.de.

17

New Pain Treatments in Late Development

Andre Dray and Martin N. Perkins

AstraZeneca R&D Montreal, Montreal, Quebec, Canada

Both physiological pain and pathophysiological pain result from the integration of sensory, affective, and cognitive processes, which in the former case are operating normally but in the latter situation are abnormal. The two broad areas of pathophysiological pain are (1) chronic inflammatory pain, exemplified by osteoarthritis (OA), and (2) neuropathic pain, where postherpetic neuralgia (PHN) and diabetic neuropathy are the two largest segments.

Satisfactory chronic pain treatment is recognized as a huge unmet medical need in society today, with the reality that present therapeutic approaches to chronic pain are not fully efficacious. For example, in the case of neuropathic pain only 40% efficacy can be achieved overall in some patient populations. Additionally, the side-effect profiles either severely limit the dose that can be given to obtain relief or reduce, significantly, the quality of life. Nearly 70% of chronic patients taking prescription medication report side effects debilitating enough to have an adverse effect on their daily lives as well as their emotional well-being [3], even to the extent, sadly, of doubling the risk of suicide in chronic pain patients [99]. Furthermore, with an aging population, at least in the developed world, this unmet need is expected to increase. Finally, over 50% of hospitalized patients experience pain in the last days of their lives [94], and 50–75% of terminal cancer patients die in moderate to severe pain [102].

Massive economic costs are associated with chronic pain patients. In the United Kingdom, some 206 million working days a year are lost to pain [29]. In dollar terms, in the

Pharmacology of Pain
edited by Pierre Beaulieu, David Lussier, Frank Porreca, and Anthony H. Dickenson
IASP Press, Seattle, © 2010

United States the annual cost of chronic pain, including health care expenses, lost income, and lost productivity, is estimated to be $100 billion [65]. Concomitantly, the commercial market size for analgesics is projected to grow from the current total of about $20 billion to about $40 billion by 2020.

With both an unmet medical need and a commercially attractive market, it is not surprising, therefore, that there has been considerable investment by big and small pharmaceutical companies in identifying and developing new analgesics. However, despite this therapeutic need and industry effort, there has been a relative lack of success in bringing therapeutic agents directed toward novel targets to the clinic. It is possible to make the case that during the entire 20th century only two or three truly novel mechanisms were exploited, successfully, for pain. One of these, the triptans, was specific for migraine. The others were either a variation of an already established exploitable mechanism—reducing prostaglandin levels with a selective nonsteroidal anti-inflammatory drug (NSAID) or with cyclooxygenase (COX)-2 inhibitors—or exploitation of a therapeutic principle developed for a non-pain indication. The best example of this latter type is gabapentin, which supplanted tricyclic antidepressants, themselves a serendipitous therapy, as the first-line treatment for neuropathic pain. In fact, only in the 21st century is consensus emerging as to what molecular entity gabapentin and its successor, pregabalin, are targeting.

When the current and future prospects for novel analgesic targets are considered, the picture is very mixed. With respect to the preclinical field, a very large number of molecular targets are proposed for the development of novel analgesics with, in all cases, data derived from cellular and animal models of pain supporting a role in nociceptive transmission. However, there are still very few novel principles being evaluated in late-stage (Phase IIb–III) clinical development. This chapter does not cover all the highly novel preclinical targets, but instead will focus on those novel targets that are in, or are believed to be very close to, clinical development.

Opioids

The opioids are probably the best known, certainly the most powerful and, arguably, the oldest analgesics known to humanity. There are three receptor types for opioids, the mu-, delta-, and kappa-opioid receptors, and they are present throughout the peripheral and central nervous systems [109] (see Chapter 5 by Marvizon et al.). It is agonists at the mu-opioid receptor that are the basis for all clinically active opioid analgesics, providing powerful pain relief due to actions at multiple sites throughout the neuraxis. Unfortunately, in all cases the chronic use of opioids is limited by the well-known side effects such as sedation, respiratory depression, and constipation. As most of these side effects are centrally mediated, the possibility of a peripheral mu-opioid-receptor-induced analgesia has been explored. Preclinical studies have shown reduction of peripheral afferent nerve excitability and analgesic effects following either local application of opioids [90] or peripherally restricted mu-receptor agonists, such as loperamide, which is known to be excluded from the central nervous system (CNS) by virtue of being a substrate for the efflux transporter, p-glycoprotein [61]. Several clinical trials of varying size and design have explored the potential for analgesia with intra-articular morphine during knee arthroscopic surgery with mixed results; two meta-analyses of these trials have concluded there is either no or only a mild analgesic effect of morphine via this route [40,82]. Currently, any further development of mu-opioid agonists by the pharmaceutical industry is focused on fixed dose combinations and reformulation of existing mu opioids. For example, Adolor is developing loperamide (ADL-3-1294), formulated for intra-articular administration.

Both the delta- and kappa-opioid receptors are also targeted for development of an analgesic, albeit with a lower level of interest. Delta-receptor agonists, such as SNC80 and DPDPE ([D-Pen2,D-Pen5]-enkephalin), have shown analgesic activity in inflammatory pain models but are less active against acute pain. The only company with delta agonists in development is Adolor, with one delta agonist in Phase I (ADL-5747) and one in Phase II (ADL-5859). A kappa opioid is also in Phase II (CR-845, Cara Therapeutics), with an intravenous formulation.

Prostanoids

The other main class of analgesics in the clinic apart from opioids is the NSAIDs, all of which target the production of prostanoid COX enzyme products (PGE_2, PGD_2, $PGF_{2\alpha}$, thromboxane, and PGI_2) (see Chapter 3 by Vergne-Salle and Beneytout).

PGE_2 is considered to be the main contributor to inflammatory pain. It is not surprising, therefore, that inhibition of the major synthetic enzymes COX-1 and COX-2 and blockade of prostanoid receptors continue to be important approaches for reducing inflammatory pain.

As is now well known, there are, however, significant tolerability and safety concerns associated with the long-term use of NSAIDs. Nonselective and COX-2-selective inhibitors have similar efficacy [15], whereas their side effects differ noticeably. COX-1 selectivity is associated with increased gastrointestinal risk, which may well limit the maximum efficacy attainable in patients with chronic pain. COX-2-selective drugs have less gastrointestinal risk but are associated with increased cardiovascular risk, primarily myocardial infarction, stroke, hypertension, and congestive heart failure [50]. It was the latter concerns that led to the withdrawal of Vioxx (rofecoxib) from the market by Merck in 2004. Several large clinical trials (VIGOR, CLASS, and TARGET) have confirmed an increased risk of serious cardiovascular effects of other COX-2 inhibitors, although the precise mechanism of action for these effects is still not clearly understood (see Chapter 3 by Vergne-Salle and Beneytout). However, the undoubted efficacy of the COX-2-inhibitor class makes this approach attractive, and not all COX-2 inhibitors have been withdrawn. Researchers are still developing COX-2-selective inhibitors (e.g., GW406381, GlaxoSmithKline) with the aim of improving the safety profile. Fixed dose combinations of naproxen and omeprazole (a proton pump inhibitor) (PN400, AstraZeneca) are also being developed as an alternative method of improving NSAID safety.

A possible way to specifically reduce PGE_2 production is to inhibit prostaglandin E synthase (PGES), which converts prostaglandin H_2 to PGE_2 [45]. There are two isoforms of PGES, a cytosolic enzyme (cPGES) and a membrane or microsomal enzyme (mPGES). cPGES is linked with both COX-1 and COX-2 activity and therefore has no obvious advantage as a therapeutic target. However, mPGES has been shown to inhibit PGE_2 production, with no increase in the thromboxane A_2/PGI_2 ratio; it is an increase in this ratio that is thought to contribute to the cardiovascular risk of COX-2 inhibitors. At present, although several pharmaceutical companies have active research programs, there are no mPGES-selective inhibitors in the clinic.

Finally, another approach is to develop antagonists to the receptor for PGE_2—the EP receptor. The challenge here is that there are several subtypes—EP1, 2, 3, and 4—expressed on both peripheral and central neurons. PGE_2 can act on all of them with different effects, both increasing and decreasing neuronal excitability, which suggests a complex interrelationship among subtypes [6]. One EP antagonist is in clinical development, CJ-023,423, an EP4 antagonist from Pfizer.

Kinins

Kinins, of which bradykinin and kallidin are the main forms in humans, are among the first inflammatory mediators formed after injury or trauma. There are two receptors: the constitutively expressed B2 receptor and the inducible B1 receptor. Bradykinin and kallidin are the agonists for the B2 receptor, and the agonists for the B1 receptor are their respective metabolites desArg9bradykinin and desArg10kallidin. The B1 receptor is strongly upregulated following injury or trauma and by inflammatory mediators [28,34,54].

There is a substantial literature showing that activation of both the B2 and B1 receptors is an important mechanism leading to nociceptor activation and sensitization [24,25]. The majority of evidence suggests a role for kinin receptors in inflammatory pain, but increasing evidence suggests a role in neuropathic pain as well [95].

With respect to pharmaceutical development, an initial trial with a peptide antagonist at the B2 receptor, icatibant (HOE140, Sanofi-Aventis), given intra-articularly in OA patients was positive [32], but subsequent larger trials did not confirm this result, and it is believed that development has stopped. No systemic B2 antagonists are known to be in development, which may reflect concerns over a possible cardioprotective action for the B2 receptor. B1 receptor antagonists are believed to be free of such concerns, and there are several programs with compounds in early development, such as AMG379 and SSR240612 from Amgen and Sanofi-Aventis, respectively.

Cannabinoids

There are two major cannabinoid receptors: CB_1 and CB_2. A substantial literature shows that activation of these receptors is antinociceptive in animal models [33] (see Chapter 6 by Guindon et al.). The CB_1 receptor is considered to be the "neuronal" cannabinoid receptor, being expressed widely in the CNS and in peripheral sensory neurons, including the pain pathway, whereas CB_2 receptors are primarily expressed in peripheral tissues, particularly in immunocompetent cells. The receptors are activated by several endogenous cannabinoid ligands or endocannabinoids such as anandamide and 2-arachidonylglycerol [33].

The use of selective CB_1 and CB_2 antagonists (e.g., SR141716A for CB_1 and SR144428 for CB_2) suggests that it is the CB_1 receptor that mediates most of the analgesia [33]. Both peripheral and central sites are involved, but peripheral activation is sufficient to produce therapeutic analgesia. Thus, cannabinoid agonists are still active after genetic deletion of the CB_1 receptor in the CNS [1], and peripherally restricted agonists are analgesic [26,80]. Furthermore, local administration of agonists provides effective analgesia.

The role of CB_2 receptors in nociception is less clearly defined. CB_2-selective agonists (e.g., HU-308, HU-210, CP55940, AM1241, and GW405833) are antinociceptive in animal models [57,103]. If this effect is, indeed, mediated by the CB_2 receptor, then it is probably an indirect effect because CB_2 receptors are seldom found in the CNS or on sensory neurons [92], although they are expressed on glial cells following nerve injury [111], as well as on peripheral immune cells. However, other recent preclinical studies do not support a role for CB_2 receptors, showing that highly selective CB_2-receptor agonists lack efficacy [43]. It is likely that this question will only be resolved when selective cannabinoid agonists are taken into the clinic.

The possibility of effective cannabinoid analgesia, mediated either by peripheral CB_1 receptors or by CB_2 receptors, is of particular importance due to the well-known set of CNS symptoms induced by cannabinoids. Nonselective cannabinoid agonists such as Δ_9-tetrahydrocannabinol (THC) or Sativex (THC plus cannabidiol, GW Pharma) have shown efficacy in reducing neuropathic pain in the clinic [68]. However, these compounds also produce adverse effect such as euphoria, dizziness, and sedation at therapeutic concentrations [8]. These side effects are primarily mediated by CB_1 receptors in the CNS, and they may well prove to be too dose-limiting in chronic pain patients to allow the full efficacy of cannabinoid agonists to be realized.

Currently, therefore, cannabinoids have been limited to patient populations where the side-effect/benefit profile is favorable [8]. For example, Sativex was approved in Canada in 2005 for neuropathic pain associated with multiple sclerosis, and it was approved by the FDA for Phase III trials in the United States for cancer pain.

Clearly, if a peripherally restricted CB_1 agonist with reduced CNS side effects were effective, it would be a major therapeutic advance. Peripherally restricted cannabinoid agonists are being evaluated in humans. CT3 (ajulemic acid) from Indevus has been reported to be effective at a dose without serious CNS side effects [48], and an orally active, peripherally restricted cannabinoid agonist from AstraZeneca (AZD1940) is undergoing early clinical testing.

A few CB_2 agonists are also in Phase II clinical trials for pain, including PRS-211,375 (Cannabinor, Pharmos Corp.) and GW842166 (GlaxoSmithKline). However, a clinical trial with PRS-211,375 showed disappointing effects that were not dose-related. It is not clear if this compound is still in development.

Another possibility for producing cannabinoid-driven analgesia is to increase the levels of the endocannabinoids. One approach to achieve this goal is to inhibit the primary degradative enzymes for endocannabinoids [18], fatty acid amide hydrolase (FAAH) and monoacylglycerol lipase (MGL). Although this concept has found support in several studies in models using knockout mice to test FAAH inhibitors such as URB597 and OL135, or MGL inhibitors such as URB602 [11,19,55], this approach has not yet reached the clinic.

Cytokines and Chemokines

Inflammation and inflammatory pain involve a complexity of interacting humoral inflammatory mediators such as cytokines, chemokines, neurotrophic factors, prostaglandins, and leukotrienes. Prostaglandins have, as discussed above, been therapeutic targets for decades (and, with various historical treatments for pain, an "unknown target" for centuries), but increasingly, other inflammatory mediators are being evaluated for potential efficacy in chronic inflammatory pain.

In many, if not all, cases there is both a direct and indirect sensitizing and activating effect on sensory neurons, either by the mediator acting by itself or via the release of other sensitizing mediators. Cytokines—particularly interleukins IL-1β, IL-6, and IL-8 and tumor necrosis factor-α (TNF-α)—are one such class of mediators able to induce hyperalgesia by direct and indirect actions (see Chapter 13 by Sommer and White). IL-1β can activate nociceptors directly via intracellular kinase activation and can also sensitize them via the production of prostanoids and kinins, as well as by upregulating the kinin B1 receptor [93]. TNF-α acting on TNFR1 and TNFR2 receptors also has direct actions on neuronal excitability as well as indirect effects via cytokine production [72,75].

Both anti-TNF-α and anti-IL-1β human monoclonal antibodies have been trialed in OA patients with mixed results. Abbott reported a reduction in pain with adalimumab (Humira), an antibody to TNF-α, in one clinical trial, but this outcome was not repeated with subsequent open-label use [39,58]. Similarly, with an IL-1 receptor antagonist, anakinra (Kineret, Amgen) given intra-articularly in OA patients, the initial study suggested moderate efficacy, but this outcome was not confirmed with a larger clinical trial [12,13]. Furthermore, Amgen has tested an anti-IL-1 receptor human monoclonal antibody in OA patients, and it also failed to show efficacy [4].

Another important class of inflammatory agents comprises the chemokines, which are both peripheral and central regulators of chronic inflammation. The major chemokines and their respective receptors are MCP1/CCR2, MDC/CCR4, RANTES/CCR5, fractalkine/CX3CR1, and SDF-1-α/CXCR4. Chemokine receptors are expressed throughout the CNS on both primary afferent neurons as well as on the resident immunocompetent cells in the CNS—microglia, astrocytes, and oligodendrocytes [107,112]. Recent studies suggest an involvement of chemokines in brain development, neurodegenerative conditions, and synapse activity.

Chemokines can contribute directly to hyperalgesia by G-protein-coupled sensitization of ligand-gated channels such as transient receptor potential vanilloid 1 (TRPV1), by heterologous desensitization of opioid receptors, and by sensitization of sensory neurons [112,71]. For example, proinflammatory cytokines such as CC chemokine ligand 2 (CCL2) and CCL3 (MIP-1α) sensitize TRPV1 to capsaicin via removal of an intracellular phospholipid inhibitor [112].

CCR2 antagonists have been taken into human trials for treatment of rheumatoid arthritis (INCB3284, Pfizer/Incyte and MK-0812 Merck), but they were not efficacious in either reducing the ongoing inflammation or alleviating pain.

Adrenergic Receptors

Adrenergic receptors play a key role in a particular type of chronic pain disorders termed "sympathetically maintained pain," where release of epinephrine (adrenaline) or norepinephrine (noradrenaline) from sympathetic nerves can lead to pain (see Chapter 16 by Baron and Jänig). Normally, sensory neuron terminals do not express adrenergic receptors, but following nerve injury α_1- and α_2-adrenergic receptors are expressed on sensory neurons or on postganglionic sympathetic terminals [53,89]. Direct activation of sensory neurons by the endogenous release of sympathetic transmitters (via α_1 receptors) has been demonstrated both in animal studies and in humans by intradermal injection of norepinephrine [2]. These interactions between sympathetic and afferent peripheral neurons have been shown to occur in the periphery in neuromas [91] and in the dorsal root ganglion [113].

Another approach is to target pre- and postsynaptic adrenergic receptors in the dorsal horn of the spinal cord with α_2 agonists. This possibility has been explored with α_2 agonists such as clonidine and dexmedetomidine in the clinic. This therapeutic approach is, however, greatly limited by severe target-related side effects, when these agents are given systemically, of sedation and hypotension. The focus for development is to identify ligands with improved α_2-receptor subtype selectivity, to avoid side effects. So far, this effort has not been particularly successful, although there is an α_2 agonist in Phase II development for inflammatory pain and fibromyalgia (AGN 203818, Acadia/Allergan).

Glutamate Regulation and Glutamate Receptors

The excitatory transmitter glutamate plays an important role in the initiation and maintenance of chronic pain (see Chapter 10 by Ren and Dubner). Glutamate acts through a variety of receptors, including the α-amino-3-hydroxy-5-methylisoxazole-4-proprionate

(AMPA)/kainate receptors; ionotropic glutamate receptors (iGluRs); and GPCR-coupled metabotropic glutamate receptors (mGluRs), which can also regulate other ligand-gated ion channels such as NMDA channels. In animal studies, injections of agonists are pronociceptive, and iGluR and mGluR antagonists attenuate pain [66,98].

The pharmaceutical industry has invested heavily in exploiting the glutamatergic system for various therapeutic indications, which represents perhaps the largest investment over the decades for any single target. Target-related side effects have been the main reason for the lack of success in this area.

An AMPA/kainate antagonist has also been taken into the clinic: tezampanel (NGX426: TorreyPines). Given intravenously to overcome poor bioavailability, this agent did show efficacy in several clinical trials [86,87], but it had dose-limiting side effects, including blurred vision and sedation. An orally active prodrug is in development, which will improve bioavailability but may not improve the side-effect profile.

An extensive literature shows that NMDA antagonists inhibit pain behaviors but also induce multiple side effects (sedation, confusion, and motor incoordination) at, or close to, pharmacologically efficacious doses. Consequently, there is no therapeutic margin for these agents. In an attempt to avoid these side effects, specific blockers of NMDA-receptor subtypes (NR1 and NR2) are being developed directed at the strychnine-insensitive glycine B modulatory site. This site modulates the NMDA channel during sustained stimulation of the receptor, which is believed to occur during chronic pain. Animal studies with selective NR1-Gly antagonists have been antinociceptive with reduced side effects [20,78]. However clinical experience has not confirmed this effect yet because GV196771 (Glaxo-Smith-Kline) did not show efficacy, although this result may reflect inadequate CNS exposure [105].

Alternative initiatives have targeted other NMDA-receptor subtypes such as the NR2B receptor, which is specifically expressed in sensory pathways. Blockade of this receptor with ifenprodil or traxoprodil (CP-101,606) has also been claimed to produce antinociception with reduced side effects [100]. Currently, traxoprodil is in a Phase I safety and efficacy study for acute ischemic stroke, but it is not known if pain is being considered as an additional indication. Other NR2B programs targeting pain are also in development, including RGH 896 (Gideon Richter) and EV101 (Evotec) in Phase II for cognition and neuropathic pain [37].

There is also a substantial preclinical literature linking metabotropic glutamate receptors, particularly mGluRs 1 and 5, with central excitability in chronic (but not acute) nociception. For example, spinal administration of selective agonists such as dihydroxy-phenyl-glycine produced allodynia, while mGluR5 has been shown to be significantly over-expressed in some chronic pain models [44]. Peripheral mGluR5 receptors have also been claimed to modulate pain. In keeping with this line of evidence, several mGluR5 antagonists (MPEP, SIB1747) have shown robust efficacy in neuropathic pain models [23,114].

Several compounds have been taken into human trials and have shown efficacy (ADX 10059, ADX 4861), providing good clinical validation of metabotropic glutamate receptors in several pain conditions including migraine and fibromyalgia [76], and other indications are also being explored with agents such as AZD2066 (AstraZeneca). Encouragingly, none of these have yet shown unacceptable side-effect profiles.

Ion Channels

A variety of ligand and membrane voltage-regulated ion channels are involved in pain modulation and have been targeted for development of analgesics [27,110]. Targeting ion channels is extremely attractive for analgesia because many of them are able to modulate the intrinsic hyperexcitability of afferent neurons in chronic pain states and thus have the potential to be effective targets in a wide range of chronic pain conditions, both inflammatory and neuropathic. The challenge, as with many other examples of neuronal targets, is to achieve efficacy without limiting side effects.

Transient Receptor Potential (TRP) Channels

The mammalian TRP channel represents a large receptor family, subdivided into six subfamilies: TRPA, TRPC, TRPM, TRPP, TRPV, and mucolipin (TRPML). Many TRP channels are localized to sensory neurons and play a major role in temperature and mechanical transduction (see Chapter 15 by Chung et al.).

TRPV1 is a nonselective cation channel, gated by capsaicin, noxious heat (>45°C), and acidic conditions (pH <5.3). It could be considered to represent a "final common path" for sensitization of afferent terminals, particularly in inflammatory conditions, as it can be regulated by a variety of inflammatory agents. The therapeutic goal for this target would, therefore, be an antagonist.

Interestingly, there has been another approach to producing analgesia by using agonists, either capsaicin itself in various preparations or capsaicin-like agonists. A particular property of TRPV1 receptors is that strong and/or persistent activation can lead to reversible sensory nerve terminal degeneration caused by prolonged cation influx into the nerve, osmotic damage, and metabolic collapse [97]. This principle has been shown to be effective in the clinic, where a randomized study of intra-articular injections of placebo or capsaicin (ALGRX 4975), prior to knee replacement, found that capsaicin decreased visual analogue scale scores of pain intensity [9].

Topical application of high-dose capsaicin (e.g., Transacin from NeurogesX) has also been shown to be efficacious in a number of neuropathic pain conditions, including Phase III studies in PHN patients [7]. The current focus is on developing TRPV1-channel blockers or selective TRPV1-receptor antagonists [35].

Antagonist approaches can be broadly classed into those that block the effects of capsaicin-, acid-, and heat-mediated channel activation or those that demonstrate a selectivity to capsaicin, such as capsazepine. This is an increasingly competitive field for early clinical development, with several blockers and antagonists in Phase I and II.

Competitive (AMG-9810, AMG628) [36,106] and noncompetitive TRPV1 antagonists (DD161515) [35] block chemical and thermal pain sensitivity. Recent clinical studies in volunteers have shown that oral SB705498 (Glaxo-Smith-Kline) attenuated capsaicin- and ultraviolet radiation-induced pain and hyperalgesia [14], without notable side effects. These studies herald the way for a number of Phase II trials for antagonists (e.g., GRC 6211, Lilly/Glenmark; NDG6243, Merck/Neurogen; AZD1386, AstraZeneca). The most common, and potentially limiting, side effect is hyperthermia, and although this effect has been seen with some antagonists of this class, it does not appear to be a universal finding [36].

Other TRP channels (TRPV3, TRPV4, TRPA1, and TRPM8) may also be involved in pain transduction, particularly when sensitized by a pathophysiological environment. TRPA1 is colocalized with TRPV1 and is activated by capsaicin; like TRPM8, it can also be sensitized by inflammatory mediators and nerve injury to produce cold-induced burning pain [62,70,77]. Studies with antagonists to some of these other TRPs in animal models have shown activity; for example, the TRPA1-selective antagonist HC030031 is antinociceptive [62]. However, no antagonists are currently in clinical development.

Sodium Channels

Voltage-gated sodium channels (Na_Vs) possibly represent one of the best opportunities and at the same time one of the most challenging targets for broad-range analgesics in many chronic pain conditions (see Chapter 7 by Cummins and Waxman).

A number of Na_Vs represent putative pain targets, both tetrodotoxin (TTX) sensitive ($Na_V1.3$, $Na_V1.7$) and insensitive ($Na_V1.8$, $Na_V1.9$), all of which are able to regulate neuronal excitability [27,60]. Broadly, $Na_V1.7$, 1.8, and 1.9 are mainly expressed in the peripheral nervous system (PNS); $Na_V1.1$ and $Na_V1.6$ in the PNS and CNS; and $Na_V1.2$ in the CNS. Perhaps uniquely for this class of ion channels, these particular Na_Vs are not only involved in general hyperexcitability but are activated following nerve injury. Some of them may be a key component of abnormal and ectopic firing in afferents [22].

A unique set of clinical support and validation studies have been published on one of the most interesting Na_Vs—$Na_V1.7$. Genetic studies in individuals with a rare disorder, congenital insensitivity to pain, have established that the cause of this syndrome is a mutation in the gene for $Na_V1.7$, leading to a nonfunctional ion channel. There is complete loss of pain sensation without any other pathology (nonpainful sensations are unaffected). Interestingly, similar ablation of pain sensation has been observed in mice with $Na_V1.7$-deficient sensory neurons [64]. Further clinical support comes from another syndrome, erythromelalgia, characterized by burning pain, which involves a mutation of this sodium channel [28a]. Also, upregulation of $Na_V1.7$ has been demonstrated in human nerves in inflamed tooth pulp [55a].

There is less clinical supporting evidence for the other Na_Vs, although $Na_V1.3$ is overexpressed in large Aβ fibers in chronic pain patients as well as in the spinal cord in animal pain models [17]. Similarly, $Na_V1.8$ is uniquely expressed in small sensory neurons and may be downregulated in small injured axons but upregulated in adjacent uninjured

C fibers and in human peripheral neuropathies [17]. Animal models suggest that $Na_V1.8$ is involved in the generation of spontaneous activity in damaged sensory axons [84], and knockdown of $Na_V1.8$ in models of neuropathic pain reduces pain hypersensitivities [51a]. Recently a $Na_V1.8$-selective compound (A-803467) has been described [46] as having efficacy in chronic, but not acute pain, models, suggesting that this channel makes surprisingly little contribution to physiological nociception.

It is now well established that blockade of Na^+ channels is efficacious in clinical treatment of chronic pain. In OA patients, nonselective Na^+ channel blockade using intra-articular levobupivacaine, the active enantiomer of bupivacaine, reduces pain. However, the systemic administration of local anesthetics, although it provides pain relief for patients with intractable neuropathic pain [49], is accompanied by major adverse side effects. These are, primarily, cardiotoxicity, CNS sedation, and confusion due to blockade of $Na_V1.5$ and $Na_V1.2$ channels.

Two orally active nonselective Na^+ channel blockers are in clinical development: lacosamide (also called Vimpat or harkoseride, Schwarz Pharma) and ralfinamide (NW-1029, Alipamide, Newron Pharma). These agents have activity at both TTX-sensitive and TTX-resistant channels. Lacosamide has shown significant analgesic activity in some Phase III trials, but not in others. Although reportedly well tolerated in the Phase III trials, lacosamide was associated with high rates of adverse events and dropouts in trials in diabetic neuropathic pain.

Ralfinamide is both a Na^+ channel blocker and a monoamine oxidase inhibitor, and the latter may well contribute to its analgesic activity. It is currently in Phase II trials for both neuropathic and nociceptive pain; clinical reports also suggest good tolerability overall, with positive Phase II outcome in a mixed population of neuropathic pain patients [10].

This area is generating a great deal of activity within the pharmaceutical industry, with many companies targeting the Na^+ channel. The focus for future Na^+ channel blockers is selectivity, at least to the extent of lack of activity at $Na_V1.2$ and $Na_V1.5$ in order to gain an acceptable side-effect profile for long-term use in chronic pain.

Calcium Channels

Voltage-gated calcium channels are subdivided into two major categories: low-voltage-activated (T-type) and high-voltage-activated channels. High-voltage-activated channels are further subdivided, based on pharmacology and biophysical characteristics, into L-, N-, R-, P-, and Q-types. Several have been shown to be prominently involved in pain regulation [110] (see Chapter 8 by Ferreira et al.). With respect to calcium channels, N-type channels are unique to neurons and are critical for pain neurotransmission.

Clinical validation of this target for pain comes from trials with the snail conopeptide ziconotide (SNX-111, Prialt, Elan/Esei), a synthetic form of omega-conotoxin, which selectively blocks the N-type channel. Ziconotide is an effective analgesic when given intraspinally [96,108], although clearly, the therapeutic utility of this drug is very limited by the need to dose intrathecally. Building on this concept, small-molecule channel blockers are being developed, although development of one such compound, MK-6721 (Merck/NMED-159), has been halted due to reports that it lacked the required pharmaceutical properties.

High-voltage-activated channels are divided into four subunits: an α_1 subunit and the auxiliary subunits $\alpha_2\delta$, β, and γ. In particular, the $\alpha_2\delta_1$ and $\alpha_2\delta_2$ subunits have been clinically validated as a target because they are the site of action of pregabalin and gabapentin, both clinically effective in neuropathic pain.

The $\alpha_2\delta_1$ subunit is important for channel assembly, and its overexpression in small dorsal root ganglia and spinal neurons has been associated with allodynia in a number of specific pain models [51,56]. It is believed that gabapentin and pregabalin act presynaptically to block Ca^{2+} N-channel-regulated release of neurotransmitters in the pain pathway. Recent evidence suggests that gabapentin is transported into cells via an L-neutral amino acid transporter and then acts to displace an endogenous ligand that regulates the trafficking of $\alpha_2\delta_1$ to the neural membrane [42]. On the clinical side, emerging therapeutic differentiation in terms of bioavailability is claimed for the gabapentin prodrug XP 13512 (Xenoport/Glaxo-Smith-Kline) that is currently in Phase II development.

In addition to the well-established analgesia in neuropathic pain patients, there have been some trials in OA patients, as it has been suggested that there is a neuropathic component to OA pain [83]. Pregabalin was assessed in hip and knee OA in a 12-week, double-blind, placebo-controlled, multicenter study in 296 patients. No response was observed in patients with knee OA, but patients with hip OA experienced improvement in sleep quality and improvements in the Western Ontario and McMaster University Osteoarthritis Index (WOMAC) pain subscale [30].

Neuronal Nicotinic Receptors

Neuronal nicotinic receptors (NNRs) are part of a complex family of ligand-gated ion channels that include 5-HT_3 and $GABA_A$ receptors. NNRs comprise five subunit proteins that form cation-permeable ion channels. Preclinical studies have shown that neuronal injury induces overexpression of key subunits including the α_7 as well as α_4 and α_5 NNR subunits, providing evidence to support a therapeutic potential of NNRs in pain control [21,104]. Activation of these receptors produces antinociception in animal pain models (see Chapter 16 by Baron and Jänig). Epibatidine (ABT-594, Abbott Pharma), which is selective for these subunits, has demonstrated antinociception in several models of pain, including neuropathic pain [63]. Several sites of action have been proposed, including supraspinal sites via descending monoaminergic and muscarinic pathways, as well as actions on peripheral sensory neurons. Earlier clinical evaluation of ABT-594 revealed inadequate tolerability, but more recent compounds such as TC 6499 (Glaxo-Smith-Kline/Targacept) and ABT-894 (Abbott Pharma) are progressing in clinical Phase I and II, respectively, toward a diabetic neuropathy pain indication.

Neurotrophins and Their Receptors

Neurotrophins represent an important family of regulatory proteins essential for sensory nerve development, survival, and the determination of neurochemical phenotype, which is important for the regulation of excitability [85,115] (see Chapter 12 by Staniland et al.). Neurotrophins are formed by cleavage of proneurotrophin precursors by metalloproteinases and plasmin. Neurotrophins identified so far include nerve growth factor (NGF), brain-derived growth factor (BDNF), neurotrophin 3 (NT3), and neurotrophin 4/5 (NT4/5). Each neurotrophin binds with high affinity to a receptor tyrosine kinase (trk): NGF to trkA, BDNF and NT4/5 to trkB, and NT3 to trKC as well as trKA and trKB. Mature neurotrophins also bind to a structurally distinct receptor p75 that is involved in neuronal development.

Levels of NGF are increased in inflammatory situations. NGF is released by immunocompetent cells and Schwann cells and has been shown to sensitize neurons, leading to increases in neuronal excitability. NGF is an important mediator in both injury-induced nociceptive and neuropathic pain [41,81,101], acting on trkA and p75 receptors to activate a number of other kinase pathways. For example, it activates p38 kinase, leading to altered gene transcription and the increased synthesis of sensory neuropeptides (substance P, calcitonin gene-related peptide), ion channels (TRPV1, $Na_V1.8$, ASIC3) [31,47,59], and membrane receptors such as bradykinin and $P2X_3$ [74,79].

NGF can be considered to have good clinical support and validation with respect to pain. Levels of NGF are elevated in various inflammatory conditions in humans, including arthritis, cystitis, prostatitis, and headache as well as ultraviolet burns and surgical injury [5,38,88]. NGF induces pain and thermal and mechanical hyperalgesia in animals and in humans when injected locally, which may involve mast cell degranulation as well as a direct increase in sensory neuronal excitability.

Clinical efficacy has also been shown using humanized monoclonal anti-NGF antibodies. Both RN624 (Tanezumab, Pfizer) and AMG403 (Amgen/Johnson & Johnson) are reported to be efficacious in reducing pain and improved mobility in OA [52], and further indications such as PHN and low back pain are being explored. Other agents are still in the preclinical phase, such as ALE0540 and PD90780, which inhibit NGF binding to TrkA and p75 receptors, respectively, and have shown efficacy in chronic pain models [16,73]. An antibody to TrkA (HuMNAC-12) is also in the preclinical phase.

Another neurotrophin that has been taken to human trials is glial-derived neurotrophic factor (GDNF). GDNF is one of an extensive family of ligands and membrane receptor complexes that play a role in regulating peripheral and central neural phenotypes. Although it does not appear to play a specific role in inflammation, GDNF has been shown, preclinically, to have neuroprotective and restorative properties in a number of neurodegenerative and neuropathic pain states [85]. GDNF has been shown to restore peripheral sensory neuron function, including peptide and ion channel expression patterns, following painful peripheral nerve injury, accompanied by an attenuation of pain behaviors. However, a trial of GDNF given intracerebroventricularly produced unacceptable side effects such as weight loss and allodynia, which has discouraged therapeutic development [69].

Summary and Conclusions

This is undoubtedly an exciting period in the history of developing novel analgesics, driven by the richness of opportunities presented by the emerging pain sciences. Many compounds are in the early stages of clinical development, with many more in the preclinical phase, acting on a wide range of novel molecular targets. Of particular interest is the large number of principles being tested in Phase II, where initial efficacy trials are conducted, and we can expect to see analgesic readouts from these studies being reported over the next few years. What is equally interesting is the growth in biopharmaceuticals for the area of pain and analgesia. Although these agents may, currently at least, have the disadvantage of not being orally available, it is hoped that they will confer other advantages such as reduced adverse-effect profiles.

There is also the prospect of launching novel analgesics, for example cannabinoid agonists or Na^+ channel blockers, that show a much wider spectrum of activity than current therapies, with efficacy in both inflammatory nociceptive and neuropathic pain.

However, there are also areas of continuing concern in that a relatively high proportion of compounds fail in early clinical trials due to lack of efficacy. It is true that an impressive number of compounds have been taken into Phase I and II by the pharmaceutical industry, with approximately 17 novel targets for pain in these two phases of clinical development, a very large increase compared to previous periods in this area. However, the Phase III pipeline is poorly populated. An NMDA-receptor antagonist (Neurodex/Zenvia, Avanir) is under study in neuropathic pain, and norepinephrine/5-hydroxytryptamine reuptake inhibitors (duloxetine, E. Lilly; desvenlafaxine, Wyeth; milnacipran, Forest/Cypress) are being developed for fibromyalgia and are also being evaluated in neuropathic and nociceptive pain. These studies are, essentially, an attempt to broaden the scope for drugs active for depression. A $GABA_B$ agonist, JZP-6 (sodium oxybate, Jazz Pharmaceuticals), already approved for narcolepsy and cataplexy, is also being evaluated for fibromyalgia but not for any other chronic pain indication.

This paucity of novel targets being evaluated in Phase III is not simply due to a timing issue of waiting for compounds currently in the earlier phases to move into Phase III. Quite a few compounds directed at novel targets have moved into Phase III, but their development has been discontinued. The reason for the discontinuation of a compound by the pharmaceutical industry is not always transparent; however, by the time a compound reaches late Phase II or Phase III, the two most common reasons are lack of efficacy and poor tolerability. These two factors are typically interlinked because in order to obtain efficacy, drug exposure may need to be taken to a level that is associated with unacceptable adverse events. Providing clinical compounds with the appropriate safety and pharmacokinetic parameters is essential for evaluation of new mechanisms-based principles for analgesia. This stage, a further critical element in drug development, has been improved with the strengthening of early target validation through rigorous preclinical and clinical translation. This process has been driven by improved pain models (animal and human) and methods (biomarkers). However, a detailed discussion of analgesia translation and target validation is beyond the scope of this chapter.

Potential therapeutic agents targeting the kinin B2, cannabinoid CB_2, CCR2, and AMPA receptors, as well as TNF-α, IL-1β, and Na^+ channels, have all been taken into clinical development and abandoned, or else development has been delayed due to lack of efficacy in early Phase II trials or poor tolerability. Indeed, two early attempts at bringing a novel analgesic to the clinic, antagonists at the NK1 and the NMDA receptors, failed because of lack of efficacy and unacceptable side effects, respectively. Overall, our estimation is that approximately 50% of late-stage clinical development projects for chronic pain currently fail to move forward due to lack of efficacy and/or tolerability. Nevertheless, such attrition can be an acceptable compromise for the successful emergence of new differentiated therapies that will meet the huge unmet needs for patients with chronic pain.

Acknowledgments

Both authors are employees of AstraZeneca Pharmaceuticals.

References

[1] Agarwal N, Pacher P, Tegeder I, et al. Cannabinoid mediated analgesia largely via peripheral type 1 cannabinoid receptors in nociceptors. Nat Neurosci 2007;7:870–9.
[2] Ali Z, Raja SN, Wesselmann U, Fuchs PN, Meyer, RA, Campbell JN. Intradermal injection of norepinephrine evokes pain in patients with sympathetically maintained pain. Pain 2000;88:161–8.
[3] American Chronic Pain Association. Americans living with pain. American Chronic Pain Association; 2004.
[4] Amgen. Amgen investor fact sheet: 3rd quarter 2005. Available at: http://www.amgen.com/pdfs/investors/Fact_Sheet_Investors_2005_Q3.pdf.
[5] Apfel SC. Nerve growth factor for the treatment of diabetic neuropathy: what went wrong, what went right, and what does the future hold? Int Rev Neurobiol 2002;50:393–413.
[6] Bar KJ, Natura G, Telleria-Diaz A, Teschner P, Vogel R, Vasquez E, Schaible HG, Ebersberger A. Changes in the effect of spinal prostaglandin E2 during inflammation: prostaglandin E (EP1-EP4) receptors in spinal nociceptive processing of input from the normal and inflamed knee joint. J. Neurosci 2004;24:642–51.
[7] Bley KR. Recent developments in transient receptor potential vanilloid receptor 1 agonist-based therapies. Expert Opin Investig. Drugs 2004;13:1445–56.
[8] Campbell FA, Tramer MR, Carroll D, Reynolds DJ, Moore RA, McQuay HJ. Are cannabinoids an effective and safe treatment option in the management of pain? A quantitative systematic review. BMJ 2001;323:13–16.
[9] Cantillon M, Vause E, Sykes D, Moon A, Hughes S. Safety, tolerability and efficacy of ALGRX 4975 in osteoarthritis (OA) of the knee. 24th Annual Scientific Meeting of the American Pain Society, Boston, 2005. Abstract 724.
[10] Cattabeni F. Ralfinamide. Newron Pharmaceuticals. IDrugs 2004;10:935–9.
[11] Chang L, Luo L, Palmer JA, Sutton S, Wilson SJ, Barbier AJ, Breitenbucher JG, Chaplan SR, Webb M. Inhibition of fatty acid amide hydrolase produces analgesia by multiple mechanisms. Br J Pharmacol 2006;148:102–13.
[12] Chevalier X, Giraudeau B, Conrozier T, Marliere J, Kiefer P, Goupille P. Safety study of intraarticular injection of interleukin 1 receptor antagonist in patients with painful knee osteoarthritis: a multicenter study. J Rheumatol 2005;32:1317–23.
[13] Chevalier X. Results from a double blind, placebo-controlled, multicenter trial of a single intra-articular injection of anakinra (Kineret) in patients with osteoarthritis of the knee. ACR/ARHP Annual Scientific Meeting, San Diego, 2005. Abstract 1339.

[14] Chizh BA, O'Donnell MB, Napoltano A, Wang J, Brooke AC, Aylott MC, Bullman JN, Gray EJ, Lai RY, Williams PM, et al. The effects of the TRPV1 antagonist SB-705498 on TRPV1 receptor-mediated activity and inflammatory hyperalgesia in humans. Pain 2007;132:132–41.

[15] Chou R, Helfand M, Peterson K, Dana T, Roberts C. Comparative effectiveness and safety of analgesics for osteoarthritis. Comparative effectiveness review no. 4. Agency for Healthcare Research and Quality; 2006. Available at: www.effectivehealthcare.ahrq.gov/reports/final.cfm.

[16] Colquhoun A, Lawrance GM, Shamovsky IL, Riopelle RJ, Ross GM. Differential activity of the nerve growth factor (NGF) antagonist PD90780 [7-(benzoylamino)-4,9-dihydro-4-methyl-9-oxo-pyrazolo-[5,1-b]quinazoline-2-carboxylic acid] suggests altered NGF-p75NTR interactions in the presence of trkA. J Pharmacol Exp Ther 2004;310:505–11.

[17] Coward K, Plumpton C, Facer P, Birch R, Carlstedt T, Tate S, Bountra C, Anand P. Immunolocalization of SNS/PN3 and NaN/SNS2 sodium channels in human pain states. Pain 2000;85:41–50.

[18] Cravatt BF, Lichtman AH. The endogenous cannabinoid system and its role in nociceptive behavior. J Neurobiol 2004;61:149–60.

[19] Cravatt BF, Demarest K, Patricelli MP, Bracey MH, Giang DK, Martin BR, Lichtman AH. Supersensitivity to anandamide and enhanced endogenous cannabinoid signaling in mice lacking fatty acid amide hydrolyse. Proc Natl Acad Sci USA 2001;98:9371–6.

[20] Danysz W, Parsons CG. GlycineB recognition site of NMDA receptors and its antagonists. Amino Acids 1998;14:205–6.

[21] Decker MW, Meyer MD, Sullivan JP. The therapeutic potential of nicotinic acetylcholine receptor agonist for pain control. Expert Opin Investig Drugs 2001;10:1819–30.

[22] Devor M. Sodium channels and mechanisms of neuropathic pain. J Pain 2006;7(Suppl 1):S3–12.

[23] Dogrul A, Ossipov MH, Lai J, Malan TP, Porecca F. Peripheral and spinal antihyperalgesic activity of SIB-1757, a metabotropic glutamate receptor (mGluR5) antagonist, in experimental neuropathic pain in rats. Neurosci Lett 2000;292:115–8.

[24] Dray A. Kinins and their receptors in hyperalgesia. Can J Pharmacol 1997;75:704–12.

[25] Dray A, Perkins MN. Bradykinin and inflammatory pain. Trends Neurosci 1993;16:99–104.

[26] Dyson A, Peacock M, Chen A, Courade JP, Yaqoob M, Groarke A, Brain C, Loong Y, Fox A. Antihyperalgesic properties of the cannabinoid CT-3 in chronic neuropathic and inflammatory pain states in the rat. Pain 2005;116:129–37.

[27] Eglen RM, Hunter JC, Dray A. Ions in the fire: recent ion-channel research and approaches to pain therapy. Trends Pharmacol Sci 1999;8:337–42.

[28] Eisenbarth H, Rukwied R, Petersen M, Schmelz M. Sensitization to bradykinin B1 and B2 receptor activation in UV-B irradiated human skin. Pain 2004;110:197–204.

[28a] Estacion M, Dib-Hajj SD, Benke PJ, te Morsche RHM, Eastman EM, Macala LJ, Drenth JPH, Waxman SG. Nav1.7 Gain-of-function mutations as a continuum: A1632E displays physiological changes associated with erythromelalgia and paroxysmal extreme pain disorder mutations and produces symptoms of both disorders. J Neurosci 2008;28:11079–88.

[29] European Pain Network. European map of pain. Available at: www.europeanpainnetwork.com.

[30] Farrar JT, Young JP Jr, LaMoreaux L, Werth JL, Poole RM. Clinical important of changes in chronic pain intensity measured on an 11-point numerical pain rating scale. Pain 2001:94:149-58.

[31] Fjell J, Cummings TR, Fried K, Black JA, Waxman SG. In vivo NGF deprivation reduces SNS expression and TTX-R sodium currents in IB4-negative DRG neurons. J Neurophysiol 1999;81:803–10.

[32] Flechtenmacher, J. Talke M, Veith D, Heil K, Gebauer A, Schoenharting M. Icatibant induces pain relief in patients with osteoarthritis of the knee. 9th World Congress of the Osteoarthritis Research Society International 2004;12:P332.

[33] Fox A, Bevan S. Therapeutic potential of cannabinoid receptor agonists as analgesic agents. Expert Opin Investig Drugs 2005;14:695–703.

[34] Fox A, Wotherspoon G, McNair K, Hudson L, Patel S, Gentry C, Winter L. Regulation and function of spinal and peripheral neuronal B_1 bradykinin receptors in inflammatory mechanical hyperalgesia. Pain 2003;104:683–91.

[35] García-Martinez C, Humet M, Planells-Cases R, Gomis A, Caprini M, Viana F, De La Pena E, Sanchez-Baeza F, Carbonell T, De Felipe C, et al. Attenuation of thermal nociception and hyperalgesia by VR1 blockers. Proc Natl Acad Sci USA 2002;99:2374–9.

[36] Gavva NR, Tamir R, Qu Y, Klionsky L, Zhang TJ, Immke D, Wang J, Zhu D, Vanderah TW, Porreca F, et al. AMG 9810 [(E)-3-(4-t-butylphenyl)-N-(2,3-dihydrobenzo[b][1,4] dioxin-6-yl)acrylamide], a novel vanilloid receptor 1 (TRPV1) antagonist with antihyperalgesic properties. J Pharmacol Exp Ther 2005;313:473–84.

[37] Gogas K. Glutamate-based therapeutic approaches: NR2B receptor antagonists Curr Opin Pharmacol 2006;6:68–74

[38] Griffin JW. The roles of growth factors in painful length-dependent axonal neuropathies. In: Campbell JN, Basbaum AI, Dray A, Dubner R, Dworkin RH, Sang CN, editors. Emerging strategies for the treatment of neuropathic pain. Seattle: IASP Press; 2006. p. 271–90.

[39] Grunke M, Schulze-Koops H. Successful treatment of inflammatory knee osteoarthritis with tumour necrosis factor blockade. Ann Rheum Dis 2006;65:555–6.

[40] Gupta A, Bodin L, Homstrom B, Berggren L. A systematic review of the peripheral analgesic effect of intraarticular morphine. Anesth Analg 2001;93:761–70.

[41] Hefti FF, Rosenthal A, Walicka PA, Wyatt S, Vergara G, Shelton DL, Davis AM. Novel class of pain drug based on antagonism of NGF. Trends Pharmacol Sci 2006;27:85–91.

[42] Hendrich J, Van Minh AT, Heblich F, Nieto-Rostro M, Watschinger K, Striessnig J, Wratten J, Davies A, Dolphin AC. Pharmacological disruption of calcium channel trafficking by the alpha-2 delta ligand gabapentin. Proc Natl Acad Sci USA 2008;105:3628–33.

[43] Henze DA, Bilodeau M, Burgey C, Della Penna K, Desai R, Karczewski K, Leit M, Lemaire W, Manley P, Nanda K, et al. Highly selective CB2 agonists lack analgesic efficacy. 12th World Congress on Pain 2008; Abstract PW052.

[44] Hudson LJ, Bevan S, McNair K, Gentry C, Fox A, Kuhn R, Winter J. Metabotropic glutamate receptor 5 up-regulation in A-fibers after spinal nerve injury: 2-methyl-6-(phenylethynyl)-pyridine (MPEP) reverses the induced thermal hyperalgesia. J Neurosci 2002;22:2660–8.

[45] Jakobsson PJ, Thoren S, Morgenstern R, Samuelsson B. Identification of human prostaglandin E synthase: a microsomal, glutathione-dependent, inducible enzyme, constituting a potential novel drug target. Proc Natl Acad Sci USA 1999;96:7220–5.

[46] Jarvis MF, Honore P, Shieh CC, Chapman M, Joshi S, Zhang XF, Kort M, Carroll W, Marron B, Atkinson R. A-803467, a potent and selective Nav1.8 sodium channel blocker, attenuates neuropathic and inflammatory pain in the rat. Proc Natl Acad Sci USA 2007;104:8520–5.

[47] Ji RR, Samad TA, Jin SX, Schmoll R, Woolf CJ. P38 MAPK activation by NGF in primary sensory neurons after inflammation increases TRPV1 levels and maintains heat hyperalgesia. Neuron 2002;36:57–68.

[48] Karst M, Salim K, Burstein S, Conrad I, Hoy L, Schneider U. Analgesic effect of the synthetic cannabinoid CT-3 on chronic neuropathic pain: a randomized controlled trial. JAMA 2003;290:1757–62.

[49] Kastrup J, Petersen P, Dejgard A, Angelo FR. Intravenous lidocaine infusion: a new treatment of chronic painful diabetic neuropathy. Pain 1987;28:69–75.

[50] Kearney PM, Baigent C, Godwin J, Halls H, Emberson JR, Patrono C. Do selective cyclo-oxygenase-2 inhibitors and traditional non-steroidal anti-inflammatory drugs increase the risk of atherothrombosis? Meta-analysis of randomised trials, BMJ 2006;332:1302–8.

[51] Kim C, Jun K, Lee T, Kim SS, McEnery MW, Chin H, Kim HL, Park JM, Kim DK, Jung SJ, et al. Altered nociceptive responses in mice deficient in the alpha1δ subunit of the voltage dependent calcium channel. Mol Cell Neurosci 2001;18:235–45.

[51a] Lai J, Gold MS, Kim C-S, Bian Di, Ossipov MH, Hunter JC, Porrecca F. Inhibition of neuropathic pain by decreased expression of the tetrodotoxin-resistant sodium channel, $Na_V1.8$. Pain 2002;95:143–52.

[52] Lane N, Webster L, Shiao-Ping L, et al. RN624 (Anti NGF) improves pain and function in subjects with moderate knee osteoarthritis: a phase 1 study. Arthritis Rheum 2005;52:S461.

[53] Lee DH, Liu X, Kim HT, Chung K, Chung JM. Receptor subtype mediating the adrenergic sensitivity of pain behavior and ectopic discharges in neuropathic Lewis rats. J Neurophysiol 1999;81:2226–33.

[54] Levy D, Zochodne DW. Increased mRNA expression of the B1 and B2 bradykinin receptors and antinociceptive effects of their antagonists in an animal model of neuropathic pain. Pain 2000;86:265–71.

[55] Lichtman AH, Leung D, Shelton CC, Saghatelian A, Hardouin C, Boger DL, Cravatt BJ. Reversible inhibitors of fatty acid amide hydrolase that promote analgesia: evidence for an unprecedented combination of potency and selectivity. J Pharmacol Exp Ther 2004;311:441–8.

[55a] Luo S, Perry GM, Levinson SR, Henry MA. Nav1.7 expression is increased in painful human dental pulp. Mol Pain 2008;4:16.

[56] Luo ZD, Calcutt NA, Higuera ES, Valder CR, Song YH, Svensson CI, Myers RR. Injury type-specific calcium channel alpha-2 delta-1 subunit up-regulation in rat neuropathic pain models correlates with antiallodynic effects of gabapentin. J Pharmacol Exp Ther 2002;303:1199–205.

[57] Malan TP Jr, Ibrahim MM, Lai J, Vanderah TW, Makriyannis A, Porreca F. CB2 cannabinoid receptor agonists: pain relief without psychoactive effects? Curr Opin Pharmacol 2003;3:62–7.

[58] Magnano MD, Chakravarty EF, Broudy C, Chung L, Kelman A, Hillygus J, Genovese MC. A pilot study of tumor necrosis factor inhibition in erosive/inflammatory osteoarthritis of the hands. J Rheumatol 2007;34:1323–7.

[59] Mamet J, Lazdunski M, Voilley N. How nerve growth factor drives physiological and inflammatory expression of acid-sensing ion channels 3 in sensory neurons. J Biol Chem 2003;278:48907–13.

[60] Matzner O, Devor M. Hyperexcitability at sites of nerve injury depends on voltage sensitive sodium channels. J Neurophysiol 1994;72:349–59.

[61] Menendez L, Lastra A, Meana A, Hidalgo A, Baamonde A. Analgesic effects of loperamide in bone cancer pain in mice. Pharmacol Biochem Behav 2005;81:114–2.

[62] McNamara CR, Mandel-Brehm J, Bautista DM, Siemens J, Deranian KL, Zhao M, Hayward NJ, Chong JA, Julius D, Moran MM, et al. TRPA1 mediates formalin-induced pain. Proc Natl Acad Sci USA 2007;104:13525–30.

[63] Meyer MD. Neuronal nicotinic acetylcholine receptors a target for the treatment of neuropathic pain. Drug Level Research 2006;67:355–9.

[64] Nassar MA, Stirling LC, Forlani G, Baker MD, Matthews EA, Dickenson AH, Wood JN. Nociceptor-specific gene deletion reveals a major role for Nav1.7 (PN1) in acute and inflammatory pain. Proc Natl Acad Sci USA 2004;101:12706–11.

[65] National Institutes of Health. NIH guide: new directions in pain research I. National Institutes of Health; 1998.

[66] Neugebauer V. Glutamate receptor ligands. Handb Exp Pharmacol 2007;177:217–49.

[67] Niissalo S. Hukkanen M. Imai S. Tornwall J. Konttinen YT. Neuropeptides in experimental and degenerative arthritis. Ann NY Acad Sci 2002;966:384–99.

[68] Nurmikko TJ, Serpell MG, Hoggart B, Toomey PJ, Morlion BJ, Haines D. Sativex successfully treats neuropathic pain characterized by allodynia: a randomize, double blind, placebo-controlled clinical trial. Pain 2007;133:210–20.

[69] Nutt JG, Burchiel KJ, Comella CL, Jankovic J, Lang AE, Laws ER Jr, Lozano AM, Penn RD, Simpson RK Jr, Stacy M, et al. ICV GDNF Study Group. Implanted intracerebroventricular. Glial cell line-derived neurotrophic factor. Randomized, double-blind trial of glial cell line-derived neurotrophic factor (GDNF) in PD. Neurology 2003;60:69–73.

[70] Obata K, Katsura H, Mizushima T, Yamanaka H, Kobayashi K, Dai Y, Fukuoka T, Tokunaga A, Tominaga M, Noguchi K. TRPA1 induced in sensory neurons contributes to cold hyperalgesia after inflammation and nerve injury. J Clin Invest 2005;115:2393–401.

[71] Oh SB, Tran PB, Gillard SE, Hurley RW, Hammond DL, Miller RJ. Chemokines and glycoprotein 120 produce pain hypersensitivity by directly exciting primary nociceptive neurons. J Neurosci 2001;21:5027–35.
[72] Ohtori S, Takahashi K, Moriya H, Myers RR. TNF-alpha and TNF-alpha receptor type 1 upregulation in glia and neurons after peripheral nerve injury: studies in murine DRG and spinal cord. Spine 2004;29:1082–8.
[73] Owolabi JB, Rizkalla G, Tehim A, Ross GM, Riopelle RJ, Kamboj R, Ossipov M, Bian D, Wegert S, et al. Characterization of antiallodynic actions ALE-0540, a novel nerve growth factor receptor antagonist, in the rat. J Pharmacol Exp Ther 1999;289:1271–6.
[74] Petersen M, Segond von Banchet G, Heppelmann B, Koltzenburg M. Nerve growth factor regulates the expression of bradykinin binding sites on adult sensory neurons via the neurotrophin receptor p75. Neuroscience 1998;83:161–8.
[75] Pollock J, McFarlane SM, Connell MC, Zehavi U, Vandenabeele P, MacEwan DJ, Scott RH. TNF-alpha receptors simultaneously activate Ca^{2+} mobilisation and stress kinases in cultured sensory neurons. Neuropharmacology 2002;42:93–106.
[76] Porter RH, Jaeschke G, Spooren W, Ballard TM, Büttelmann B, Kolczewski S, Peters JU, Prinssen E, Wichmann J, Vieira E, et al. Fenobam: a clinically validated nonbenzodiazepine anxiolytic is a potent, selective, and noncompetitive mGlu5 receptor antagonist with inverse agonist activity. J Pharmacol Exp Ther 2005;315:711–21.
[77] Proudfoot CJ, Garry EM, Cottrell DF, Rosie R, Anderson H, Robertson DC, Fleetwood-Walker SM, Mitchell R. Analgesia mediated by the TRPM8 cold receptor in chronic neuropathic pain. Curr Biol 2006;16:1591–609.
[78] Quartaroli M, Fasdelli N, Bettelini L, Maraia G, Corsi M. GV196771A, an NMDA receptor/glycine site antagonist, attenuates mechanical allodynia in neuropathic rats and reduces tolerance induced by morphine in mice. Eur J Pharmacol 2001;430:219–27.
[79] Ramer MS, Bradbury EJ, McMahon SB. Nerve growth factor induces $P2X_3$ expression in sensory neurons. J Neurochem 2001;77:864–75.
[80] Richardson JD, Kilo S, Hargreaves KM. Cannabinoids reduce hyperalgesia and inflammation via interactions with peripheral CB1 receptors. Pain 1998;75:111–9.
[81] Ro LS, Chen ST, Tang LM, Jacobs JM. Effect of NGF and anti-NGF on neuropathic pain in rats following chronic constriction injury of the sciatic nerve. Pain 1999;79:265–74.
[82] Rosseland LA. No evidence for analgesic effect of intra-articular morphine after knee arthroscopy: a qualitative systematic review. Reg Anesth Pain Med. 2005;30:83–9.
[83] Rowbotham MC, Kidd BL, Porreca F. Role of central sensitization in chronic pain: osteoarthritis and rheumatoid arthritis compared to neuropathic pain. In: Flor H, Kalso E, Dostrovsky J, editors. Proceedings of the 11th World Congress on Pain. Seattle: IASP Press; 2006. p. 231–49.
[84] Roza, Laird JMA, Souslova V, Wood JN, Cervero F. The tetrodotoxin-resistant Na channel NaV1.8 is essential for the expression of spontaneous activity in damaged sensory axons of mice. J Physiol 2003;550.3:921–6.
[85] Sah DWY, Ossipov MH, Porecca F. Neurotrophic factors as novel therapeutics for neuropathic pain. Nat Rev Drug Discov 2003;2:460–72.
[86] Sang CN, Hostetter MP, Gracely RH, Chappell AS, Schoepp DD, Lee G, Whitcup S, Caruso R, Max MB. AMPA/Kainate antagonist LY293558 reduces capsaicin-evoked hyperalgesia but not pain in normal skin in humans. Anesthesiology 1998;89:1060–7.
[87] Sang CN, Ramadan NM, Wallihan RG, Chappell AS, Freitag FG, Smith TR, Silberstein SD, Johnson KW, Phebus LA, Bleakman D, et al. LY293558, a novel AMPA/GluR5 antagonist, is efficacious and well-tolerated in acute migraine. Cephalalgia 2004;24:596–602.
[88] Sarchielli P, Alberti A, Floridi A, Gallai V. Levels of nerve growth factor in cerebrospinal fluid of chronic headache patients. Neurology 2001;57:132–4.
[89] Sato J, Perl ER. Adrenergic excitation of cutaneous pain receptors induced by peripheral nerve injury. Science 1991;251:1608–10.
[90] Sawynok J. Topical and peripherally acting analgesics. Pharmacol Rev 2003;55:1–20.
[91] Shinder V, Govrin-Lippmann R, Cohen S, Belenky M, Ilin P, Fried K, Wilkinson HA, Devor M. Structural basis of sympathetic-sensory coupling in rat and human dorsal root ganglia following peripheral nerve injury. J Neurocytol 1999;28:743–61.
[92] Sokal DM, Elmes SJR, Kendall DA, Chapman V. Intraplantar injection of anandamide inhibits mechanically-evoked responses of spinal neurons via activation of CB2 receptors in anaesthetized rats. Neuropharmacology 2003;45:404–11.
[93] Sommer C, Kress M. Recent findings on how proinflammatory cytokines cause pain: peripheral mechanisms in inflammatory and neuropathic hyperalgesia. Neurosci Lett 2004;361:184–7.
[94] SUPPORT Principal Investigators. A controlled trial to improve care for seriously ill hospitalised patients categorised by DSM-III psychiatric diagnostic criteria. Pain 1986;26:181–97.
[95] Shughrue PJ, Ky B, Austin CP. Localization of B1 bradykinin receptors mRNA in the primate brain and spinal cord: an in situ hybridization study. J Comp Neurol 2003;46:372–84.
[96] Snutch TP. Targeting chronic and neuropathic pain: the N-type calcium channel comes of age. NeuroRx 2005;2:662–70.
[97] Szallasi A, Blumberg PM. Vanilloid (capsaicin) receptors and mechanisms. Pharmacol Rev 1999;51:159–212.
[98] Szekely JI, Torok K, Mate G. The role of ionotropic glutamate receptors in nociception with special regard to the AMPA binding sites. Curr Pharm Des 2002;8:887–912.
[99] Tang N, Crane C. Suicidality in chronic pain: a review of the prevalence, risk factors and psychological links. Psychol Med 2006;36:575–86.
[100] Taniguchi K, Shinjo K, Mizutani M, Shimada K, Ishikawa T, Menniti F, Nagahisa A. Antinociceptive actions of CP-101,606, an NMDA receptor NR2B subunit antagonist. Br J Pharmacol 1997;12:809–12.

[101] Theodosiou M, Rush RA, Zhou XF, Hu D, Walker JS, Tracey DJ. Hyperalgesia due to nerve damage: role of nerve growth factor. Pain 1999;81:245–55.
[102] Weiss SC, Emanuel LL, Fairclough DL, Emanuel EJ. Understanding the experience of pain in terminally ill patients. Lancet 2001;357:1311–15.
[103] Valenzano KJ, Tafesse L, Lee G, Harrison JE, Boulet JM, Gottshall SL, Mark L, Pearson MS, Miller W, Shan S, et al. Pharmacological and pharmacokinetic characterization of the cannabinoid receptor 2 agonist GW405833, utilizing rodent models of acute and chronic pain, anxiety, ataxia and catalepsy. Neuropharmacology 2005;48:658–72.
[104] Vincler M. Neuronal nicotinic receptors as targets for novel analgesics. Expert Opin Investig Drugs 2005;14:1191–8.
[105] Wallace MS, Rowbotham MC, Katz NP, Dworkin RH, Dotson RM, Galer BS, Rauck RL, Backonja MM, Quessy SN, Meisner PD. A randomized, double blind, placebo-controlled trial of a glycine antagonist in neuropathic pain. Neurology 2002;59:1694–1700.
[106] Wang HL, Katon J, Balan C, Bannon AW, Bernard C, Doherty EM, Dominguez C, Gavva NR, Gore V, Ma V, et al. Vanilloid receptor-1 antagonists: 3. the identification of a second-generation clinical candidate with improved physicochemical and pharmacokinetic properties. J Med Chem 2007;50:3528–39.
[107] Watkins LR, Maier S. Beyond neurons: evidence that immune and glial cells contribute to pathological pain states. Physiol Rev 2002;82:981–1011.
[108] Xiao WH, Bennett GJ. Synthetic omega-conopeptides applied to the site of nerve injury suppress neuropathic pains in rats. J Pharmacol Exp Ther 1995;274:666–72.
[109] Yaksh TL. Pharmacology and mechanisms of opioid analgesic activity. Acta Anaesthesiol Scand 1997;41:94–111.
[110] Yaksh TL. Calcium channels as therapeutic targets in neuropathic pain. Pain 2006;7(Suppl 1):S13–30.
[111] Zhang J, Hoffert C, Vu HK, Groblewski T, Ahmad S, O'Donnell D. Induction of CB2 receptor expression in the rat spinal cord of neuropathic but not inflammatory chronic pain models. Eur J Neurosci 2003;17:2750–4.
[112] Zhang N, Inan S, Cowan A, Sun R, Wang JM, Rogers TJ, Caterina M, Oppenheim JJ. A proinflammatory chemokine, CCL3, sensitizes the heat- and capsaicin-gated ion channel TRPV1. Proc Natl Acad Sci USA 2005;102:4536–41.
[113] Zhang JM, LI H, Munir MA. Decreasing sympathetic sprouting in pathological sympathetic ganglia: a new mechanism for treating neuropathic pain using lidocaine. Pain 2004;109:143–9.
[114] Zhu CZ, Wilson SG, Mikusa JP, Wismer CT, Gauvin DM, Lynch JJ 3rd, Wade CL, Decker MW, Honore P. Assessing the role of metabotropic glutamate receptor 5 in multiple nociceptive modalities. Eur J Pharmacol 2004;506:107–18.
[115] Zweifel LS, Kuruvilla R, Ginty DD. Functions and mechanisms of retrograde neurotrophin signaling. Nat Rev Neurosci 2005;6:615–25.

Correspondence to: Martin N. Perkins, PhD, AstraZeneca R&D Montreal, 7171 Frederick Banting Street, Montreal, Quebec, Canada H4S 1Z9. Tel: 1-514-832-3217; fax: 1-514-832-3229; email: martin.perkins@astrazeneca.com.

Part III

Special Topics in the Pharmacology of Pain

18

Vulnerability to Opioid Tolerance, Dependence, and Addiction: an Individual-Centered Versus Drug-Centered Paradigm Analysis

Guy Simonnet[a] and Michel Le Moal[b]

[a]Department of Homeostasis, Allostasis, Pathology and Rehabilitation, Victor Segalen University, Bordeaux, France; [b]Neurocenter Magendie, INSERM U862, Victor Segalen University, and François Magendie Institute, Bordeaux, France

From Physiology to Pathophysiology

Tolerance is commonly considered from a pharmacological viewpoint and is defined as a decreased response to a drug following repeated administration, creating the need for a higher dose to maintain the therapeutic effect. It can be operationally defined as a rightward shift in the function relating drug dose to pharmacological response (Fig. 1A). Therefore, most studies have focused on changes in the opioid receptor signaling cascade at the cellular level. Nevertheless, despite numerous studies showing that tolerance may be easily induced in animals or in vitro by chronic opioid exposure, the question as to whether repeated opioid administration can result in a similar tolerance in humans is more controversial [8]. Indeed, important interindividual variations have been reported in the development of tolerance in humans. It is unclear why some chronic pain patients develop tolerance and hyperalgesia, while the dose of opioids that is required remains constant for years in other patients, suggesting the absence of tolerance. These discrepancies between animal and human studies are intriguing, and they clearly suggest that animal models, especially in vitro cellular models, may not mimic tolerance or dependence as observed in humans.

The word "tolerance" derives from the Latin *tolerare,* which does not mean to decrease or to disappear, but rather to support, to maintain, to live with. This etymological

Pharmacology of Pain
edited by Pierre Beaulieu, David Lussier, Frank Porreca, and Anthony H. Dickenson
IASP Press, Seattle, © 2010

viewpoint suggests that opioid antinociceptive effects could be maintained and would be partially or totally hidden by an active and counteracting process—the activation of a pronociceptive system. According to this concept, and in contrast to the widely accepted pharmacological viewpoint, tolerance can be operationally defined, not as a decrease in opioid effectiveness, but as the result of a leftward shift in the pain sensitivity curve (Fig. 1B).

In most preclinical studies, the results are not considered in relation to the animals' life history but rather in relation to the amount of drug taken, as is typically the case for in vitro studies. However, as suggested by Siegel 20 years ago [110], tolerance observed in humans does not invariably result from repeated opioid administration (the cellular hypothesis) but is displayed only when the drug is administered in the context of the usual drug-predictive cues, because it is these cues that elicit the drug compensatory response that mediates tolerance.

The main purpose of this chapter is to reconcile these two different concepts of tolerance to the analgesic effects of opioids by analyzing pathophysiological, medical aspects of tolerance, dependence, and addiction. In contrast to models of tolerance that do not take into account individual patient history, termed here "ahistorical" models (Fig. 2A), we propose an individual-history model for tolerance (Fig. 2B) that considers pharmacological effects, as well as individual history and environmental components associated with opioid administration.

Although the clinical outcome is similar decreased pain relief, these two tolerance concepts lead to very different approaches from a therapeutic viewpoint. According to the ahistorical model, treatment seeks to restore functioning of the cellular opioid receptor cascade, which is progressively lost after repeated opioid administration. According to the proposed individual-history model, treatment seeks to reduce the paradoxical pain hypersensitivity that develops in an individual following opioid administration. Based on this proposal, new therapeutic perspectives are proposed for improving the use of opioids in humans.

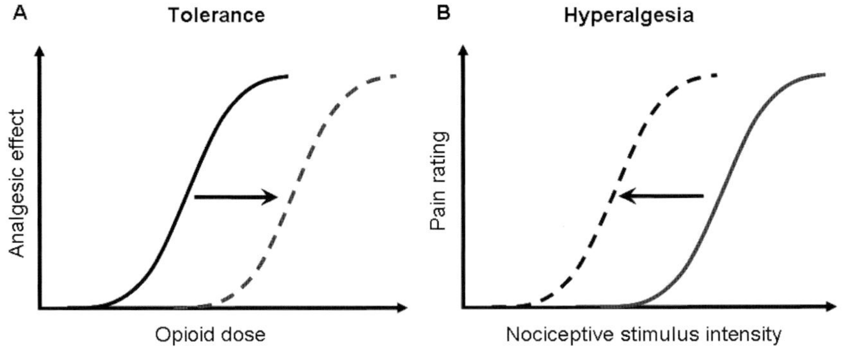

Fig. 1. Operational models of tolerance. (A) Cellular model of tolerance. Tolerance can be operationally defined as a rightward shift in the function relating opioid dose to analgesic effect caused by signaling changes at opioid receptor levels. (B) Adaptive pain hypersensitivity model of tolerance. Tolerance can be operationally defined as a leftward shift in the pain sensitivity curve of an individual, leading to an apparent decrease in opioid analgesic efficacy.

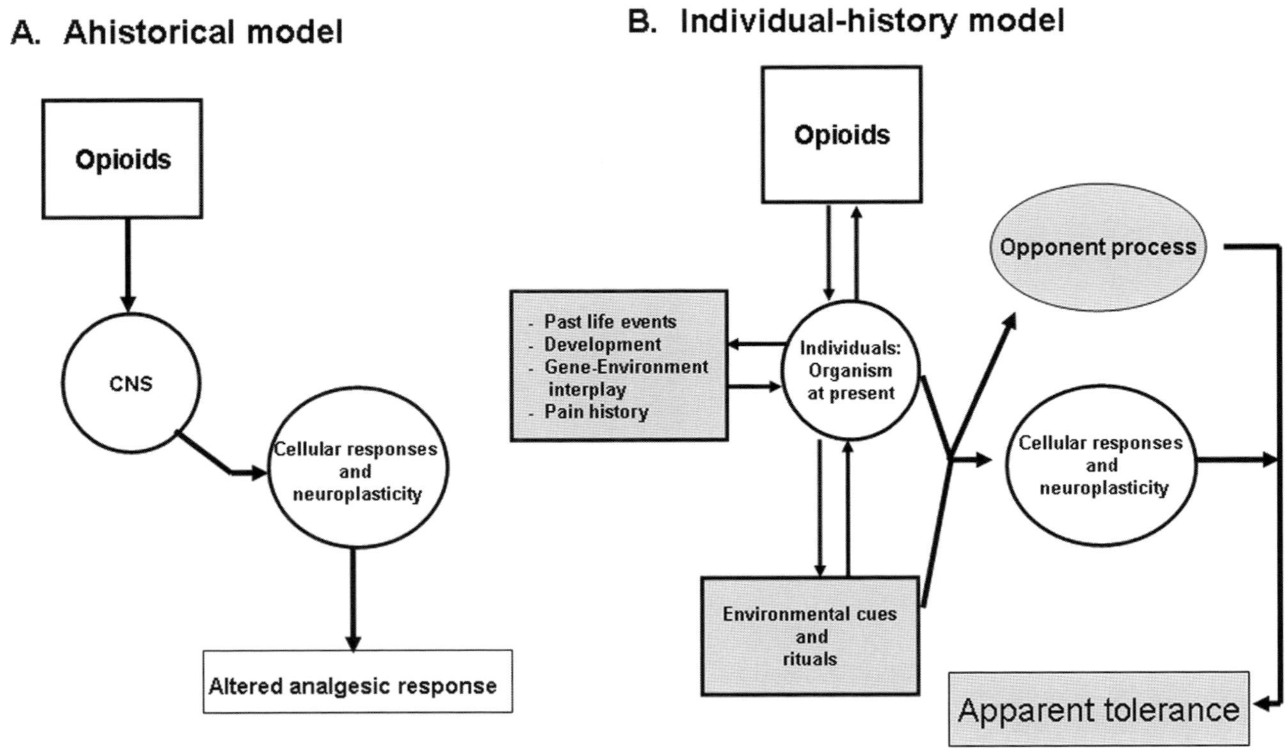

Fig. 2. Comparison of drug- or individual-centered paradigms for tolerance. (A) The ahistorical model: in most preclinical studies and especially in vitro studies, tolerance is mainly examined in relation to the amount of opioid exposure without taking into account the individual patient's life history. CNS = central nervous system. (B) The individual-history model: the patient's medical history and environmental cues or rituals associated with opioid administration are major players for developing apparent tolerance, which appears as an adaptive anticipatory response based on opponent and learning processes (allostatic changes underlying a latent pain sensitization) that modulate the pharmacological effects of opioids. According to this more complex paradigm (adaptive model), it is the shift in pain sensitivity that gives the impression of less opioid analgesia even though analgesic efficacy is unaltered (apparent tolerance).

The Cellular Hypothesis of Tolerance

The μ-opioid receptor (MOR) is critical for the analgesic effect of opioid drugs, and molecular studies have therefore focused on MOR changes induced by opioid treatment. Several recent reviews have documented results in support of the cellular hypothesis [26,56,72,74,75]. Therefore, data from these various studies at the cellular level are only briefly examined in this chapter.

Signaling Changes at the Opioid Receptor Level: Desensitization, Internalization, and Downregulation

"Desensitization" is defined as the progressive loss of receptor function following sustained exposure to an agonist. Numerous studies have indicated the critical role of opioid receptor phosphorylation mediated by different protein kinases such as G-protein-coupled receptor kinases (GRKs), Ca^{2+}/calmodulin-dependent protein kinase II (CaMKII), protein kinase C (PKC), and mitogen-activated kinases (MAPKs). Opioid receptor phosphorylation by GRKs results in changes in receptor conformation and increases the receptors' affinity for cytosolic β-arrestin proteins. Binding to β-arrestin results in the uncoupling of MORs from G proteins and in subsequent receptor internalization mediated by endocytosis. MOR internalization and the associated intracellular degradation result in fewer available MORs at the cell surface, which would contribute to opioid tolerance at the cellular level.

However, recent observations have led scientists to revise this view of tolerance. A key finding was that distinct opioid agonists, all of which produce tolerance, differ in their ability to induce internalization and subsequent downregulation of MORs. Therefore, while endogenous opioids, as well as the potent selective MOR-selective agonists DAMGO and fentanyl, were effective in promoting desensitization and MOR endocytosis, several studies reported that morphine is a poor inducer of GRK-mediated phosphorylation, arrestin binding, and desensitization [6]. Moreover, although numerous in vitro studies support relationships between MOR downregulation and cellular tolerance, chronic in vivo treatment with various opioid receptor agonists results in varying effects on the density of cell surface opioid receptors in the brain [146].

An alternative hypothesis is that instead of relating opioid tolerance directly to desensitization of MOR signaling, the lack of MOR desensitization following morphine treatment results in abnormally prolonged signaling, which exacerbates tolerance [14]. This hypothesis is based on observations indicating that the relative activity of certain opioid drugs in inducing regulatory endocytosis of receptors appears to be inversely correlated with their ability to induce tolerance [76]. These findings gave rise to the theory of "relative activity versus endocytosis" (RA/VE) [137], which assumes that agonist activity and receptor endocytosis have opposite effects on receptor signaling and that the net amount of signaling in the cell is a function of both processes. Interestingly, some studies using in vivo models have shown that administration of morphine with a subanalgesic dose of MOR agonists such as DAMGO (which facilitates morphine-occupied receptor internalization) induced more limited tolerance than morphine injected alone [62]. Taken together, these data do not support a direct correlation between opioid receptor desensitization/internalization/downregulation and tolerance.

Adenylate Cyclase Superactivation

In contrast to the negative aspects of desensitization/internalization/downregulation, certain positive aspects of counteradaptations have been proposed. Collier [28] proposed that opioid dependence and the associated tolerance result from hypertrophy of a neural cyclic adenosine monophosphate (cAMP) system that compensates for the opioid inhibition of adenylate cyclase. Indeed, an increase in adenylate cyclase activity is observable after agonist withdrawal [106]. This phenomenon, termed adenylate cyclase superactivation, is thought to contribute to the development of tolerance at the cellular level by requiring greater adenylate cyclase inhibition via the opioid receptor/G_i-protein-coupled pathway. Several mechanisms have been proposed to explain this counter-regulatory increase. The first is a shift from predominantly $G_{i\alpha}$ inhibitory to $G_{\beta\gamma}$ or Gs stimulatory adenylate cyclase signaling [22,102]. The second proposed mechanism involves a switch from receptor activation of G_i to enhanced receptor interaction with G_s upon chronic receptor activation [3,34]. The third mechanism involves an increase in constitutive receptor activity [23]. Whichever mechanisms underlie adenylate cyclase superactivation, it is interesting to note that it is in agreement with the RA/VE theory, which states that agonists (such as morphine) that do not induce rapid receptor endocytosis cause greater adenylate cyclase superactivation and subsequent tolerance than an agonist such as DAMGO or etorphine that induces rapid receptor endocytosis.

Opioid Receptor Pleiotropy: A Possible Interconversion of Opioid Receptors between Inhibitory and Excitatory Modes

In the late 1980s, Shen and Crain [107] proposed that sustained exposure to opioids induces MOR-G_s coupling, leading to the excitatory effects of opioid agonists. In agreement with the adenylate cyclase superactivation proposal for tolerance, these phenomena are associated with elevated adenylate cyclase activity and increased cAMP levels. Moreover, recent studies have shown that chronic morphine treatment substantially increases the quantity of MOR present in the $G_{s\alpha}$ immunoprecipitate of the rat spinal cord without any corresponding alterations in the quantity of $G_{s\alpha}$ immunoprecipitated [21]. This interconversion of opioid receptors—leading to an exaggerated excitatory effect of opioids—may account for some of the paradoxical effects, including hyperalgesia, observed following opioid withdrawal or naloxone administration.

The Possible Role of Morphine Metabolism

Morphine is metabolized primarily to morphine-3-glucuronide (M3G) and morphine-6-glucuronide (M6G). M6G is more potent than morphine itself, and it probably contributes to morphine's analgesic effect. However, some authors have reported that M3G attenuates the antinociceptive effect of morphine [57], suggesting that it acts as an anti-analgesic. Interestingly, M3G induces hyperalgesia and allodynia in rats [140] and humans [88]. However, this effect of M3G could not be reversed by naloxone and was prevented by *N*-methyl-D-aspartate (NMDA)-receptor antagonists [91]. NMDA receptors are known to play a critical role in tolerance. However, in cancer patients receiving chronic morphine administration, neither the M3G concentration nor the M3G/morphine ratio in the cerebrospinal fluid (CSF) correlated with pain intensity [139]. Therefore, the role of this compound does not appear essential in tolerance during morphine therapy. Moreover, these data do not explain tolerance to the analgesic effects of other opioid compounds used in the clinic.

Limits of the Cellular Hypothesis

Although tolerance could be associated with a decrease in the effectiveness of opioids at the opioid receptor level, two observations from in vivo studies support the idea that tolerance cannot fully be explained by the cellular hypothesis.

The Paradox of Naloxone

Paradoxically, in vivo administration of an opioid receptor antagonist such as naloxone, which is ineffective in drug-naive rats, induces hyperalgesia in tolerant rats [18,73]. These data suggest that MORs remain functional and are activated by exogenous opioids in opioid-tolerant animals. One hypothesis is that stimulation of opioid receptors induces a sustained activation of counteracting systems—antiopioid and/or pronociceptive systems—which oppose the net analgesic effect of the opioid agonist, leading to analgesic tolerance and hyperalgesia when the activity of the opioid is terminated. Taken together, these findings indicate that decreased opioid receptor function at the cellular level may not be necessary for behavioral tolerance. In agreement with this proposal is the recent in vivo data obtained by Kieffer and colleagues [33] showing that tolerance to morphine-induced analgesia does not require MOR desensitization in the periaqueductal gray matter and that somatic signs of morphine withdrawal following naloxone administration do not necessarily involve adenylate cyclase superactivation in the central nervous system (CNS).

Opioid Tolerance as an Associative Process

Initial evidence was based on observations that tolerance to the analgesic effects of opioids is not strictly pharmacologically determined and is to a large extent environmentally dependent and related to individual history (Fig. 2B). Siegel [109] showed that analgesic tolerance is displayed when rats are tested in an environment in which they previously received morphine, but not in an alternative environment. Siegel concluded that "an association between environmental cues and the systemic effects of morphine is crucial to tolerance development." The importance of environmental cues in tolerance to the lethal effects of heroin (diamorphine) has also been validated [111]. Based on this conditioning analysis, tolerance should not invariably result from repeated drug administration. Rather, tolerance should be displayed only when the opioid is administered in the context of the usual drug-predictive cues, because it is these cues that elicit the drug-compensatory response (the conditioned response) that mediates tolerance [110]. Indeed, conditioned responses and the subsequently elicited opposing effects triggered by anticipation would thus counteract the direct pharmacological effect of the opioid, resulting in the appearance of tolerance. Theoretical aspects of this viewpoint are supported by the opponent process theory [116] (see Fig. 3). Unfortunately, although numerous studies have explored associative as well as non-associative processes, these phenomena are always studied separately. Further investigation in this area of study is required.

Based on experimental and clinical data, one can suggest that many pharmacological models, especially in vitro models, have only explored the cellular plasticity induced by a drug, not the tolerance processing mediated by drug-compensatory responses associated with prior life events and drug-predictive cues. One hypothesis is that the primary cause of tolerance is the conditioned response to drug administration for patients or drug intake for addicts. The various cellular events would thus represent the biological substrates of CNS plasticity associated with learning tolerance.

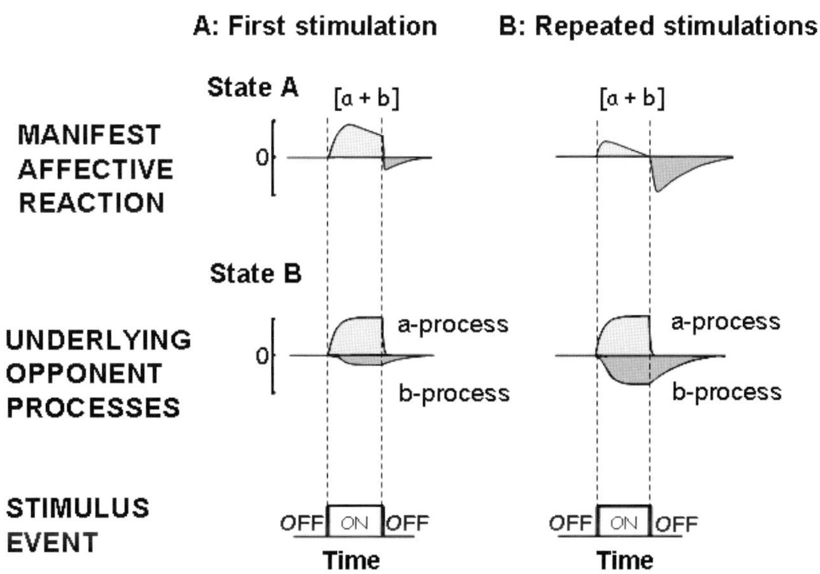

Fig. 3. Opponent-process theory. (A) Following the first exposure to a stimulus, two opposing responses are simultaneously evoked. The observed response results from "a" and "b" processes (a + b). Response "a" is largely predominant following the first exposure, but an opposing effect resulting from activation of the "b" process is observed after cessation of the stimulus event. (B) Following repeated exposure to the stimulus event, the "a" response does not change, but the "b" response is enhanced and lasts longer. The observed response (a + b) is weaker, and after the cessation of the stimulus, the "b" response is more significant. Adapted from [116].

Tolerance: An Adaptive Process Resulting from Pain Sensitization

Considering the critical role of associative learning processes in the development of tolerance, an alternative hypothesis to explain the decrease in opioid efficacy is that repeated opioid administrations provoke compensatory responses that counteract the disturbance to homeostasis produced by the pharmacological effect of the drug. One such compensatory response is hyperalgesia, which may be supported by the progressive development of pain hypersensitivity following repeated opioid administration. Although tolerance and sensitization are two opposite processes and it is difficult to conceive that one drug may have two opposite effects on the same biological process, a growing body of evidence suggests that opioids produce not only analgesia, but also hyperalgesia (Fig. 4). A hyperalgesic response to morphine after chronic administration was reported as early as 1880 by Rossbach, based on clinical observations [103]. A few decades later, in 1943, Andrews noted a definitive lowering of the pain threshold after administration of morphine in 7 out of 57 post-addicts [4]. Results from animal studies are in agreement with these clinical data

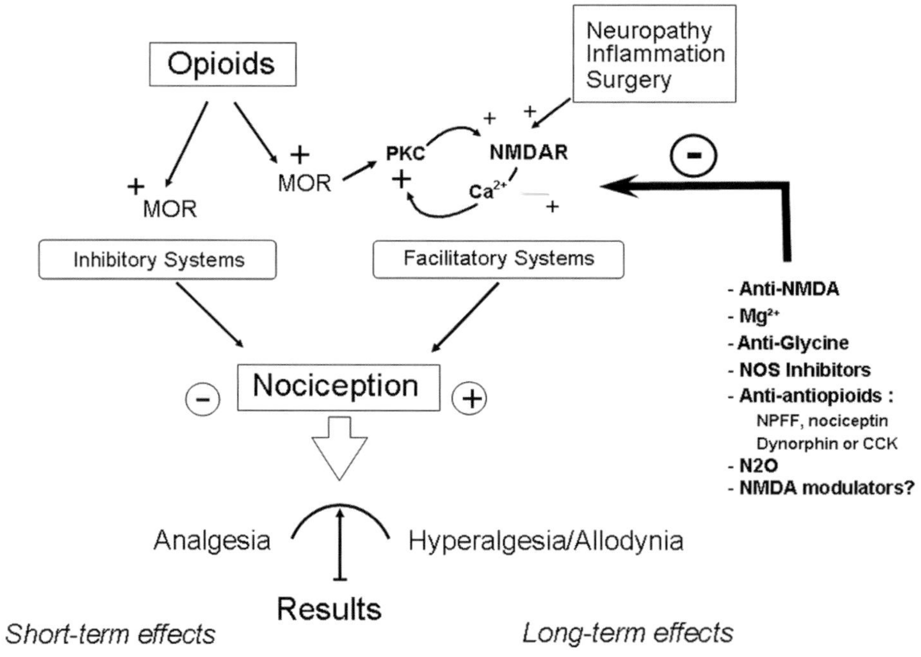

Fig. 4. Dual effects of opioids. Opioids simultaneously activate not only pain inhibitory systems (analgesia) but also *N*-methyl-D-aspartate (NMDA)-dependent pain facilitatory systems, inducing pain hypersensitivity that outlasts opioid analgesia. The analgesic effect of an opioid administration results from these two opposing processes, suggesting that the effect is partially masked as early as the first opioid exposure and that it is followed by hyperalgesia/allodynia. Repeated opioid administration induces a lasting enhancement of glutamate synaptic efficiency in a positive feedback loop leading to an enhancement of the activation level of NMDA-dependent pain facilitatory systems (sensitization), while opioid analgesia is unchanged. This effect leads to an apparent decrease of opioid analgesia (apparent tolerance). CCK = cholecystokinin; NOS = nitric oxide synthase; NPFF = neuropeptide FF; PKC = protein kinase C; MOR= μ-opioid receptor; NMDAR = NMDA receptor. Adapted from [114].

[20,80,143] and with data collected from human studies [2,7,59]. From an adaptive viewpoint, opioid-induced hyperalgesia, termed paradoxical or abnormal pain, may be considered to be a physiological or normal response if opioid-induced analgesia is considered as a perturbance of homeostatic equilibrium. In this context, pain hypersensitivity appears to be an effective response to maintaining a new homeostatic equilibrium, allostasis. This suggestion is in agreement with the opponent process theory [116] (Fig. 3). In contrast to the cellular hypothesis, this concept of tolerance/sensitization suggests that the opioid is no less effective in producing analgesia; rather, the individual is hypersensitive to nociceptive inputs. Therefore, the relationship between pain hypersensitivity and tolerance must be examined in detail.

Analgesia and Hyperalgesia: Two Opposing Processes in Adaptation

There can be little doubt that enhanced pain sensitivity—a greater ability to detect and respond to noxious stimulation—confers an adaptive advantage that promotes the survival of the organism. If the main function of antinociceptive systems is to reduce pain during threatening situations (since pain may compromise defensive behavior), it has been argued that the function of anti-analgesic and pronociceptive systems might be to promote adaptive recuperative behaviors [13,114]. Therefore, it is not surprising that many organisms, especially those with a well-developed CNS such as that found in mammals, have both anti-analgesic and pronociceptive systems. These systems allow the organism to avoid prolonged activation of endogenous analgesic systems, such as opioid systems, which are helpful in conditions of acute danger (defensive behavior) but have deleterious consequences for survival over the long term (recuperative behavior).

Tolerance Associated with Pain Hypersensitivity Induced by Acute and Discontinuous Opioid Administration

In animals, studies have demonstrated that repeated administration of opioids results in analgesia, followed by hyperalgesia [19,79,86,140,143]. Long-lasting heightened pain sensitivity also occurs upon the initial exposure to an opioid such as heroin or fentanyl [20,80]. This phenomenon appears to result from a sensitization of pronociceptive systems because both the magnitude and duration of hyperalgesia increase as a function of subsequent heroin administration [81]. The results of these experiments (Figs. 5, 6, and 8) show that opioid-induced analgesia remains unchanged regardless of the level of pain hypersensitivity induced by opioids. If the shift in nociceptive threshold is not taken into account, one could easily presume the existence of reduced analgesia, i.e., apparent tolerance. This suggestion is confirmed by observations that treatments preventing hyperalgesia induced by acute [81,98] or repeated opioid administration [20,79,112] also prevent apparent tolerance. These observations suggest that tolerance observed after an acute or intermittent opioid administration is the byproduct of a pain sensitization process, i.e., an apparent tolerance [30,114]. Indeed, these data also suggest that it is the enhancement of pain sensitivity that creates the need for a higher dose to maintain the therapeutic effect.

Interestingly, a single administration of fentanyl after tissue injury [98,100] strongly enhances postoperative hyperalgesia for several days, suggesting that such pain hypersensitivity may account for the presence of exaggerated postoperative pain and acute tolerance. Similar observations have been reported in humans [59].

Tolerance Associated with Pain Hypersensitivity during Continuous Delivery of Opioids

It has been argued that opioid-induced hyperalgesia following intermittent opioid administration might be interpreted as a result of repeated episodes of "mini-withdrawals" [60]. Indeed, experimental studies using continuous exposure to opioids (either by constant infusion through an osmotic minipump or by subcutaneous pellet implantation) producing tolerance to the analgesic effects of opioids have shown that pain hypersensitivity was

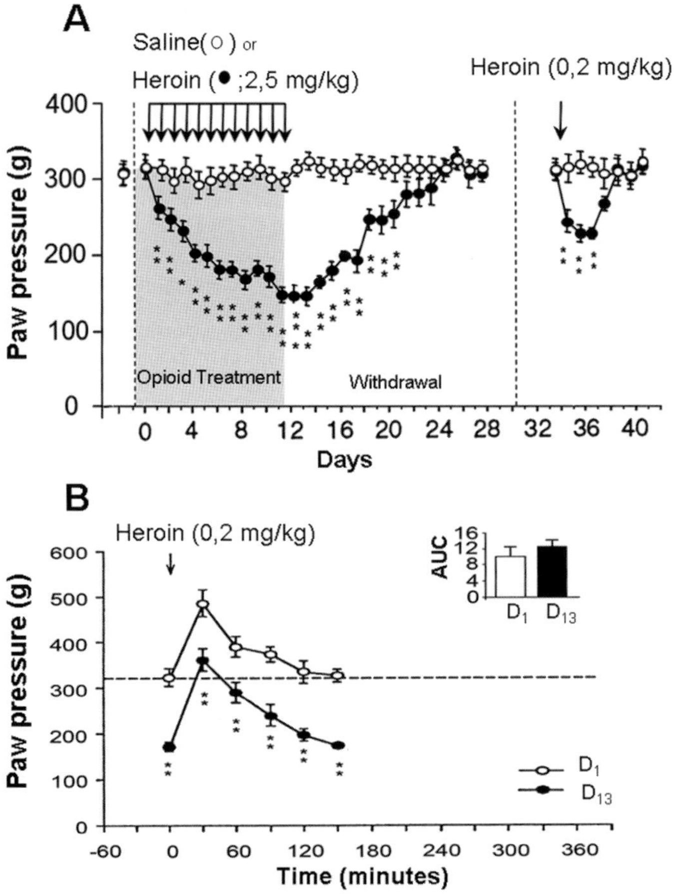

Fig. 5. Changes in pain sensitivity level (paw pressure vocalization test) induced by intermittent heroin (or saline) administrations in rats. (A) After immediate analgesia, the once-daily heroin administration induces a progressive nociceptive threshold decrease (paw pressure vocalization test) indicative of pain hypersensitivity. In this experimental design, the nociceptive threshold was determined just before each once-daily heroin or saline administration, i.e., 24 hours after the last heroin injection. (B) In spite of a dramatic decrease of the nociceptive threshold after 12 once-daily heroin injections, the analgesic index of heroin (represented by the area under the curve [AUC]) is unchanged. It is the shift in pain sensitivity that gives the impression of reduced analgesia (apparent tolerance). From [19].

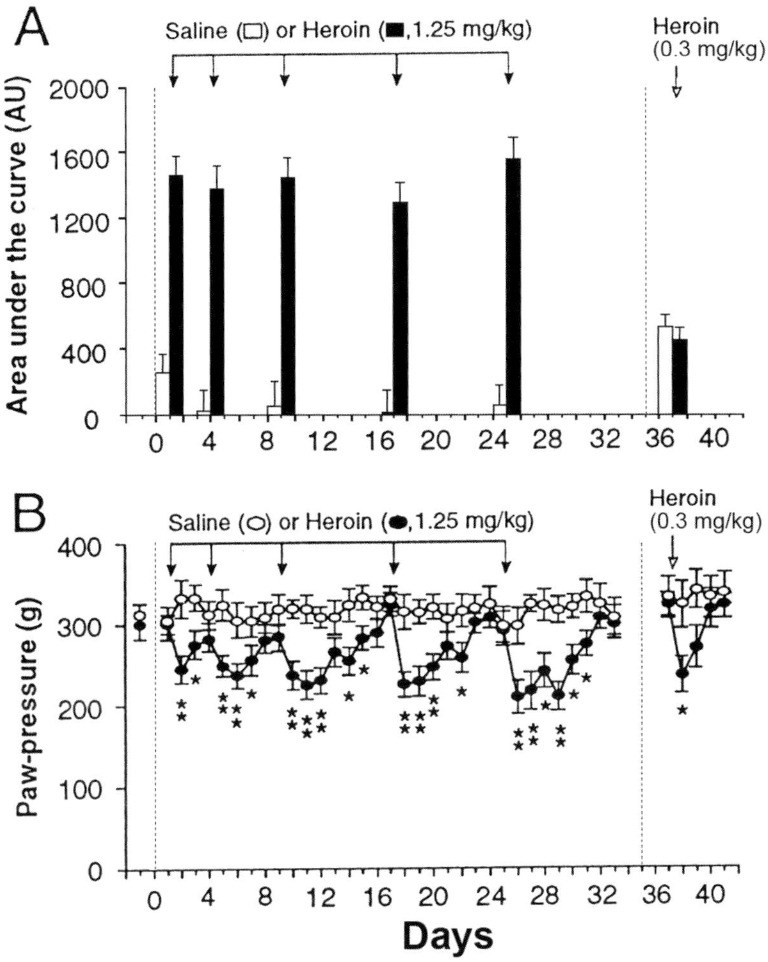

Fig. 6. Long-term effects of intermittent heroin administrations on pain sensitivity in rats. (A) Each heroin administration was performed when the animals' nociceptive threshold (paw pressure vocalization test) was returned to the predrug value. The level of heroin analgesia, estimated by the analgesic index (represented by the area under the curve), is unchanged following repeated administrations. (B) The intermittent heroin administrations progressively enhance both the amplitude and duration of the delayed hyperalgesia (days). The administration of a low heroin dose, which is ineffective for inducing delayed hyperalgesia in rats without prior heroin experience, provokes a sustained hyperalgesia for several days after immediate analgesia in heroin-experienced rats. These findings are indicative of a pain sensitization process induced by repeated heroin administrations. From [19].

present during the continuous delivery of opioids and provide evidence that this hypersensitivity does not reflect a mini-withdrawal state [130]. As suggested by these authors: "As pain may be thought of as a physiological antagonist of antinociception (or analgesia, clinically), opioid-induced increased pain manifests as 'opioid tolerance'" [93]. From an adaptive viewpoint, these data suggest that the hyperalgesia observed following opioid-induced analgesia might be a physiological outcome of opioid administration. Such hyperalgesia might be an anticipatory and compensatory response designed to oppose a homeostatic disequilibrium resulting from the subsequent arrival of an opioid in the body.

It is noteworthy that enhanced responsiveness to noxious stimulation is a reliable sign of opioid withdrawal that appears when the opioid's action is terminated, either by stopping drug administration or by administering an opioid receptor antagonist [18,69,73,79].

Common Mechanisms of Tolerance and Opioid-Induced Hyperalgesia

Based on the concept that opioid-induced hyperalgesia may oppose opioid-induced analgesia and thus plays a critical role in the development of tolerance, it could be proposed that a relationship exists at the neural level between these two opposing processes. This proposal has important clinical implications because treatments capable of preventing the development of pain sensitization leading to hyperalgesia would then be effective in preventing or reducing the development of tolerance to the analgesic effects of opioids (Fig. 1B).

Role of the Central Glutamatergic System via NMDA Receptors

Numerous studies have demonstrated that NMDA receptors play a key role in pain sensitization, leading to hyperalgesia, allodynia, and spontaneous pain [61,87]. It has long been known that activation of NMDA receptors by glutamate results in the sensitization of spinal neurons [84]. First of all, Mao has suggested that hyperalgesia, which develops when animals are rendered tolerant to morphine antinociception, may involve NMDA-dependent mechanisms [86]. Repeated daily intrathecal injections of morphine administered to rats resulted in tolerance to the antinociceptive effect of morphine, which was prevented by concurrent injections of the NMDA-receptor antagonist MK-801. Similar results were obtained with daily heroin administration for several days [19]. These results are in accordance with data from Trujillo and Akil (1991) showing tolerance inhibition by MK-801 [125]. Similarly, the increased pain sensitivity observed for several days in rats following a single exposure to heroin or fentanyl is also prevented by MK-801 [20,80,81]. Interestingly, MK-801 administration enhances the antinociceptive effect of the initial dose of heroin, confirming that the antinociceptive effect is masked by concomitant activation of NMDA-dependent pronociceptive systems.

From a mechanistic viewpoint, electrophysiological studies have demonstrated that MOR stimulation activates intracellular PKC, which reduces Mg^{2+} blocking and thereby activates NMDA receptors [24]. The subsequent increase in the intracellular Ca^{2+} concentration has been suggested to further stimulate PKC activity, leading to a lasting enhancement of glutamatergic synaptic efficiency in a positive feedback loop, a process resembling long-term potentiation [87]. In agreement with the opponent process theory, these findings point to the possible role of NMDA receptors in opioid-induced pain hypersensitivity, which opposes the expression of analgesia, leading to apparent tolerance [116] (Fig. 3).

Role of Antiopioid Peptide Systems

There is now compelling evidence that the CNS synthesizes and releases neuropeptides that function as anti-opioid peptides, acting via specific receptors to attenuate the antinociceptive effects of both endogenous and exogenous opioid receptor ligands. As more opioids are administered, more anti-opioids are released, leading to apparent tolerance. Anti-opioid properties have been attributed to various neuropeptides such as cholecystokinin (CCK), neuropeptide FF (NPFF), and orphanin FQ/nociceptin. Consistent with an anti-opioid role for these neuropeptides, morphine administration induces a dose-dependent release of CCK [11], NPFF [36,144], and orphanin FQ/nociceptin [145] in the spinal cord. These phenomena are associated with the development of tolerance. Numerous studies have demonstrated that coadministration of immunoglobulin G antiserum against these anti-opioids or receptor antagonists does not alter pain sensitivity per se, but prevents the development of tolerance [39,78,123]. Interestingly, coadministration of the compound RF9 with heroin (Fig. 8), a potent and selective NPFF-receptor antagonist, prevents the development of both opioid-induced hyperalgesia and the associated tolerance [112]. Of particular interest is the observation that stimulation of NMDA receptors induces a dose-dependent release of NPFF at the level of the spinal cord [37]. This finding suggests a relationship between the anti-opioid NPFF and NMDA systems in producing pain hypersensitivity associated with the apparent tolerance induced by opioid treatment. Evidence also suggests that dynorphin, which was originally identified as an endogenous κ-opioid ligand, is pronociceptive under certain conditions and promotes the development of tolerance to the opioid's analgesic effects [44]. When injected intracerebroventricularly, dynorphin A1-13 negatively modulates morphine analgesia [49]. Although dynorphin antiserum does not alter the baseline nociceptive threshold, it potentiates morphine analgesia [52] and prevents opioid tolerance [128,129]. Microdialysis studies have demonstrated the dose-dependent release of glutamate and aspartate by exogenous dynorphin, resulting in the activation of NMDA receptors in the spinal cord [115]. Dynorphin has also been shown to enhance the release of substance P from trigeminal nuclear slices; this effect was blocked by the NMDA-receptor antagonist MK-801 [5]. Moreover, sustained morphine exposure induces a dynorphin-dependent enhancement of excitatory transmitter release in the spinal cord from primary afferent fibers, resulting in elevated levels of calcitonin-gene-related peptide (CGRP) [54]. These data reinforce the opioid-induced pain sensitization hypothesis and the critical role of endogenous antiopioid systems in tolerance.

Role of Descending Pain Facilitatory Systems

Several recent studies have demonstrated that opioid-induced hyperalgesia and the associated tolerance may be secondary to neuroplastic changes that result, in part, from an activation of descending pain facilitation mechanisms arising from the rostral ventromedial medulla (RVM). This region is generally described as consisting of three classes of neurons based on response characteristics to nociceptive inputs [45]. Briefly, "ON" cells accelerate firing immediately before the nociceptive reflex occurs; opposite responses have been observed for "OFF" cells. The so-called "NEUTRAL" cells showed no electrophysiological responses to nociception. "ON" cells have been shown to activate the descending facilitation of nociceptive processing, both through local interactions within the RVM and through descending systems projecting to the spinal cord via the dorsolateral funiculus (DLF).

Conversely, activation of "OFF" cells inhibits nociceptive responses. In an elegant study, Vanderah et al. [130] showed, in rats implanted with pellets or osmotic minipumps delivering morphine, that both hyperalgesia and tolerance (Fig.7A) were reversibly blocked via microinjection of lidocaine into the RVM (Fig.7B) or by bilateral lesions in the DLF, which contains bulbospinal projections that mediate both descending pain inhibition and facilitation in the spinal cord. These observations suggest that activation of descending pain facilitatory systems plays a critical role in the development and expression of the component of opioid tolerance associated with opioid-induced hyperalgesia. The antiopioid neuropeptide CCK could be an important player in RVM-mediated descending facilitation because CCK_B-receptor antagonists administered in the RVM block the hyperalgesia observed in rats implanted with morphine pellets [142]. The RVM has been proposed to induce important changes at the level of the spinal cord, leading to upregulation of spinal dynorphin, substance P/NK1 receptors [132], and spinal CGRP in primary afferent fibers [54], and facilitation of NMDA-receptor functioning.

Role of TRPV1 and Mitogen-Activated Protein Kinases

The transient receptor potential vanilloid receptor (TRPV1) acts as an integrator of multiple forms of noxious chemical and thermal stimuli [17] and appears to be critical in inflammatory thermal hyperalgesia [35]. A recent study [131] reported that sustained morphine administration by subcutaneous implantation of morphine pellets elicits hyperalgesia in TRPV1 wild-type mice but not in TRPV1 knockout mice, and that TRPV1 mRNA was

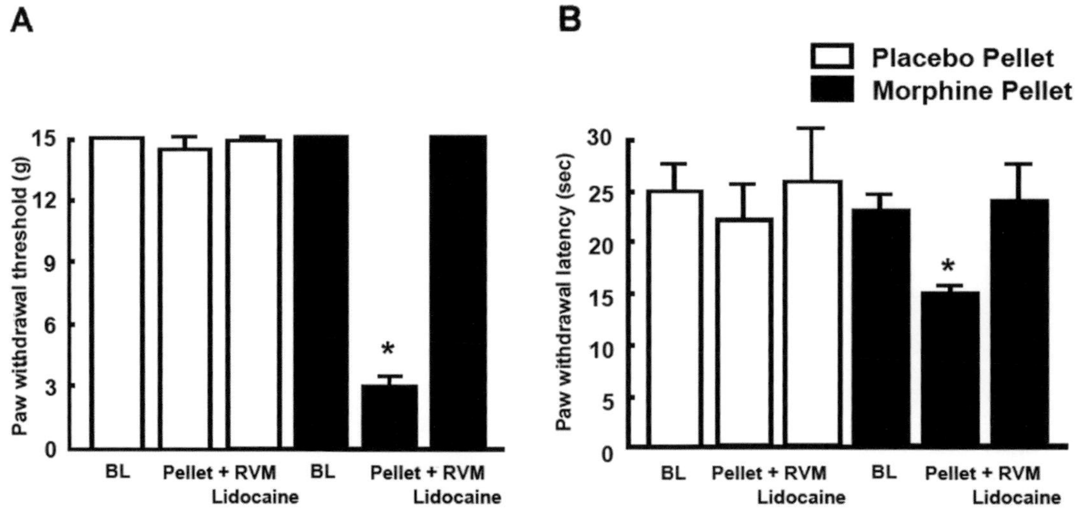

Fig. 7. Tonic descending facilitation from the rostral ventromedial medulla (RVM) mediates opioid-induced hyperalgesia and tolerance in rats. In rats, the 7-day period of constant exposure to morphine pellets results in (A) tactile allodynia (Von Frey's test) and (B) thermal hyperalgesia; placebo pellets do not change nociceptive thresholds. Opioid-induced pain hypersensitivity is observed while morphine delivery continues and while the rats were not in a state of withdrawal. The bilateral microinjection of lidocaine into the RVM on day 7 produces no change in nociceptive thresholds in placebo-pelleted rats but blocks tactile allodynia and thermal hyperalgesia in morphine-pelleted rats. BL = baseline. From [130].

upregulated in the spinal cord but not in the DRG. Intrathecal pretreatment with a selective TRPV1 antagonist attenuated both thermal hyperalgesia and tolerance, suggesting that TRPV1 plays a potential role in opioid tolerance associated with hyperalgesia. Indeed, there is evidence that TRPV1 activation induces the release of glutamate [83] and other

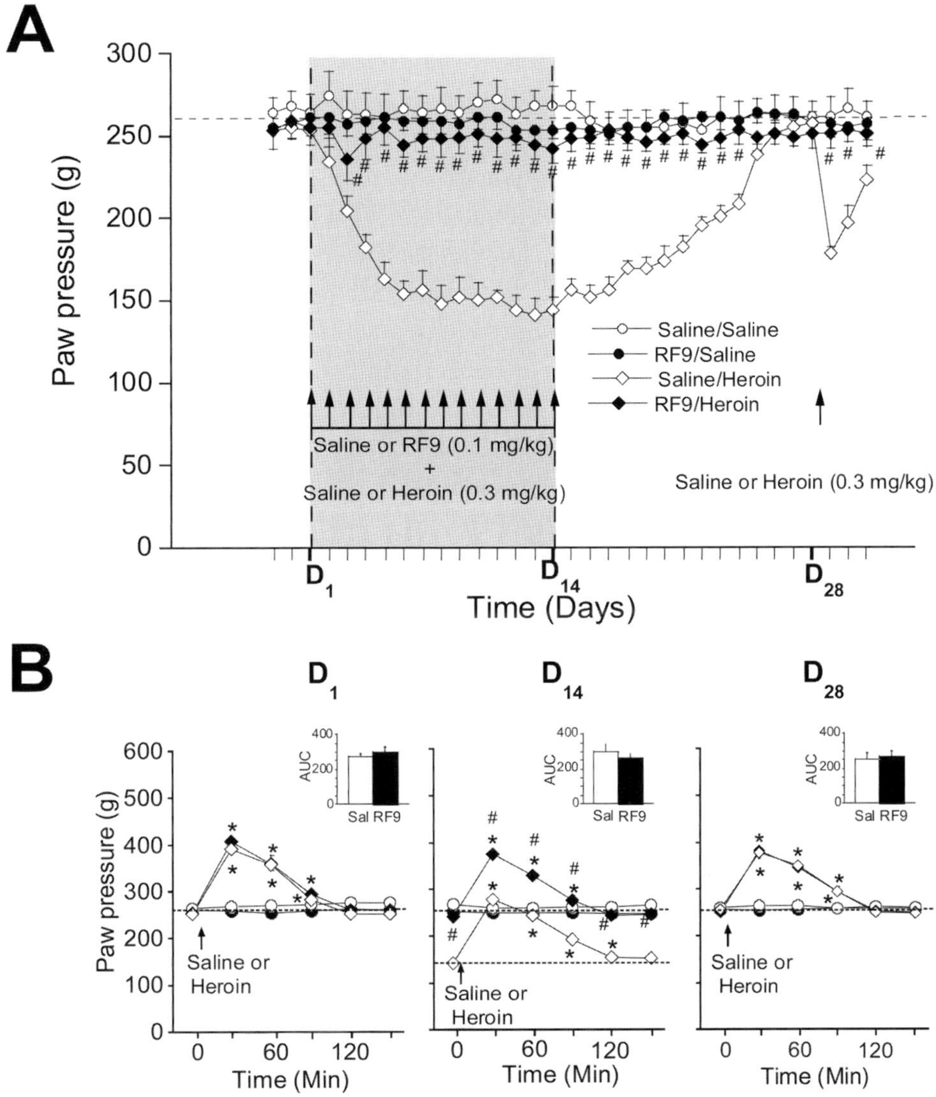

Fig. 8. Prevention of opioid-induced tolerance associated with hyperalgesia by the neuropeptide FF receptor antagonist RF9. (A) After an immediate analgesia, once-daily heroin administration (14 days) induces a progressive decrease in nociceptive threshold (paw pressure vocalization test) indicative of pain hypersensitivity. In this experimental design, the nociceptive threshold was determined just before each once-daily heroin or saline administration, i.e., 24 hours after the last heroin injection. Although RF9 does not shown any effect by itself, the daily coadministration of RF9 with heroin completely blocks the delayed and long-lasting heroin-induced hyperalgesia. (B) In spite of dramatic decrease of the nociceptive threshold after 12 once-daily heroin injections, the analgesic index of heroin (represented by the area under the curve [AUC]) is unchanged. In RF9-treated rats, the shift in pain sensitivity—which gives the impression of reduced analgesia (apparent tolerance)—is suppressed, and the heroin analgesic index is similar to the analgesic index observed in rats without heroin experience. From [112].

neurotransmitters involved in nociception transmission, such as CGRP and substance P [94]. From a mechanistic viewpoint, intrathecal administration of MAPK phosphorylation inhibitors (affecting p38, extracellular signal-regulated kinase, or c-Jun-N-terminal kinase) not only reduces the increases in MAPKs and TRPV1 induced by chronic morphine treatment, but also reduces both morphine tolerance and the associated thermal hyperalgesia [25]. Collectively, these data indicate that the TRPV1 receptor is an essential player in the complex process leading to both opioid-induced hyperalgesia and tolerance.

Role of Glial Cells

Cellular mechanisms involved in pain sensitization processes and tolerance are not limited to neuronal mechanisms. There is mounting evidence that glial cells play a key role in creating exaggerated pain states of diverse etiologies [134]. Indeed, microglia and astrocytes are attractive candidates as mediators of hyperalgesia because activation of these cells causes pain transmission, neuron hyperexcitability, and enhanced release of substance P and excitatory amino acids from presynaptic terminals in the spinal cord [97]. Recently, electrophysiological studies using patch-clamp recordings of lamina II neurons from isolated spinal cord slices showed that centrally produced proinflammatory cytokines in injury conditions induce central sensitization and pain hypersensitivity [68] (see Chapter 13 by Sommer and White). Interestingly, spinal tolerance to morphine analgesia was partially but significantly attenuated when chronic morphine was delivered in combination with fluorocitrate, a specific and reversible inhibitor of glial cells [117]. Taken together, these data suggest that the substances released by glial cells counteract the effects of chronic opioids, and they reinforce the hypothesis that a relationship exists between opioid-induced hyperalgesia and tolerance to the analgesic effects of morphine.

These experimental data indicate that the biochemical events observed at the opioid receptor level, especially with in vitro models, are not the only factors that contribute to the development of tolerance. There is a growing body of evidence that pain hypersensitivity and associative processes play a critical role in triggering neurobiological processes leading to resistance to analgesic effects of opioids (i.e., apparent tolerance), and not to a decrease in opioid efficacy. The idea that drug administration elicits opposing processes appears to make "biological sense" because conditioned opposing processes would seem functionally adaptive in that they limit the disruptive effects of drugs (i.e., unconditioned responses) on the homeostatic equilibrium of biological systems [120]. In agreement with previous suggestions [10,51], we recently proposed that opioids induce a latent pain sensitization, leading to pain vulnerability [99]. We suggest that tolerance might be due, at least partly, to an increased pain response to noxious stimuli in individuals, leading to an escalation of opioid dosing to maintain the therapeutic effect. Recent observations in our laboratory (unpublished data) indicate that non-nociceptive environmental stress that induced immediate analgesia (stress-induced analgesia) provoked both delayed pain vulnerability (pain hypersensitivity) and decreased opioid analgesic efficacy (tolerance). These findings suggest that life history is critical for developing tolerance

(Fig. 2) and would explain why large individual differences for the development of tolerance are observed in humans.

Clinical and Theoretical Implications: Hyperalgesia, Chronic Pain, and Addiction

Difficulties in Evaluating Tolerance

Tolerance after chronic opioid exposure has been demonstrated by several hundred papers using animals, both in vivo and in vitro. However, this issue is more controversial in humans [8]. A common belief regarding the loss of therapeutic action due to tolerance is based on the observation that some chronic pain patients need escalating doses to maintain adequate analgesia in the absence of disease progression [15,89,90]. In this case, some patients received doses as high as 1 g or more of morphine per day, but rarely reported satisfactory analgesia [9]. Paradoxically, cessation of opioid treatment reduced pain intensity. One patient suffering from extensive chordoma began to develop increasing pain after an initial 4–6-month period of spinal opioid infusion [92]; cessation of the morphine infusion brought considerable, though incomplete, pain relief for 2 weeks, at which time pain returned and the subsequent morphine infusion restored a state of analgesia. In contrast, numerous controlled clinical studies reported that the doses required in chronic pain to control either cancer pain or nonmalignant conditions remain constant for years, suggesting an absence of tolerance. In some cases, especially during cancer pain, increased opioid dosing heralds disease progression rather than a real tolerance to the drug [7,29,48,126].

Two other sets of observations are related to the fact that tolerance is difficult to report in clinical settings. First, the differences between analgesia measurements in humans and in animals are considerable. In humans, the measurement is based on assessments of a reported pain sensation, in contrast to the reactive sensation to a nociceptive input that is estimated indirectly in animals using a nociceptive threshold based on a motor response. Studies performed in animals and humans do not evaluate the same biological phenomenon. Second, the opioid dose and the intensity of the noxious stimulus are key factors in the development of tolerance. Interestingly, it has recently been demonstrated that the expression of tolerance to opioids in animals depends to a large extent on the intensity of the noxious stimulus, being maximal and easily observable in response to threshold stimulus intensities but considerably less pronounced with suprathreshold stimulation [1]. Moreover, tolerance in animals—both in vivo and in vitro—generally develops after high doses of opioids, whereas doses are far more moderate in the clinic at the beginning of pain treatment.

In conclusion, there are many contributing factors to dose escalation that lead to worsening pain, from psychopathological processes to alterations in cognition [95]. Dose escalation might not be a robust or valid measurement of tolerance, and little control is maintained over the pain stimulus during its development. In clinical studies, it is difficult to discern what is relevant to a change in pain state and what might be due to real tolerance.

Chronic Pain Management and Hyperalgesia

Long-term use of opioids is frequently associated with the development of an abnormal sensitivity to pain, a latent pain sensitization [10,99]. Many opioid-treated patients develop hyperesthesia associated with allodynia, a state described as being qualitatively different from the original complaint and including body areas not affected by the tissue injury [38,118]. This secondary hyperalgesia involves central hyperexcitability. In the case of postoperative pain, a relationship exists between the importance of the pericicatricial allodynia, the severity of the postoperative pain, and the surface area of the tissue around the scar. Hyperalgesia is predictive of chronic postsurgical pain [43,71]. The combination of neural lesions and of central sensitization is thought to be responsible for the chronicity of postsurgical pain [138]. There are large individual differences among patients with regard to the propensity to develop hyperalgesia [66,119], leading researchers to hypothesize the existence of hyperalgesia-prone phenotypes. Some factors have been identified to facilitate hyperalgesia, such as patients' use of opioids to control previous postoperative pain or a tendency to use these drugs in response to various circumstances. The use of high doses of opioids prior to surgery favors the development of central sensitization [66]. One of the main problems in the near future will be to predict this vulnerability in particular patients for preventing future chronic pain.

Chronic pain conditions are increasing; millions of individuals are partially disabled, and too few large studies have been undertaken to understand why chronic pain persists or to better characterize the complex syndrome in which pain is embedded. The use of opioids is supposed to restore pain physiological system equilibrium, and the appearance of hyperalgesia is in contradiction with this supposition and logically represents a break with homeostasis equilibrium. Even if the potential for abuse currently does not seem to be the main focus in pain treatment, few studies provide clear statistical data on this subject. Furthermore, the causal factors responsible for the transition to abuse have not been elucidated.

Several clinical studies report that tolerance to the analgesic effect of morphine is associated with increased responses to nociceptive stimuli in former drug abusers, including those in a methadone treatment program [31,40,41]. Drug-free ex-addicts and methadone-maintained patients are hypersensitive to cold-pressor pain in comparison to drug-free controls [32,63]. This finding is in accordance with animal experiments showing hyperalgesia while morphine was still being administered and while significant concentrations of the analgesic were present [130]. Moreover, acute tolerance and hyperalgesia following acute opioid administration, as performed for patients undergoing surgery, has been reported in both animal experiments [19,112] and clinical settings [59]. These data suggest that, in humans as well as in animals, tolerance and hyperalgesia following sustained opioid administration might represent two sides of the same adaptive phenomenon [30,114].

Hyperalgesia and Drug Abuse

Hyperalgesia is also observed in the course of drug abstinence or withdrawal; it is a critical component of opioid abstinence syndrome and a reliable measure of the magnitude of dependence [69,124]. Hyperalgesia is observed as plasma opioid levels fall following a simple dose of morphine without naloxone. Somatic pain is a reliable indicator of naloxone-precipitated abstinence after one dose of opioid [73]. Similar changes in pain sensitivity have been observed in pain patients with opioid therapy. This process contributes, as seen above, to the diminishing efficacy of opioid analgesia (apparent tolerance). This process may be the first sign of opioid-induced dependence and, consequently, it indicates the need for opioid dose reduction or for a pharmacological blockade of the circuitry involved in hyperalgesia [93,113,114].

The appearance of hyperalgesia in the course of chronic pain opioid treatment raises the same type of questions as those raised for drug abuse—why does hyperalgesia or drug abuse appear only in some patients? The percentages are roughly similar when considering pain patients who will develop hyperalgesia, pain patients who will develop drug abuse, and individuals in the general population who are free of pain but will develop addiction [47,67]. It is important to understand the inherent or acquired factors that predispose some patients and not others. The level of the dose prescribed is not crucial. Not surprisingly, former addicts treated for chronic pain are prone to exhibit hyperalgesia, which appears during withdrawal and disappears after detoxification. Hyperalgesia is a marker of profound neurobiological changes. It is hypothesized that hyperalgesia is part of a larger syndrome caused by dysregulation of homeostasis, involving new allostatic set points within emotional and reward systems. For example, between 18% and 32% of patients with chronic low back pain have been diagnosed with major depression and/or other psychopathological conditions during the course of treatment, and in this subgroup of patients there is also a high prevalence of substance-abuse disorders [8]. Coexisting mental disorders place pain patients at risk for abusing their pain medication [133]. In many patients, chronic pain is associated with psychiatric comorbidities, including drug abuse [108]. In the field of addiction medicine, it is well documented that those who will succumb to drug abuse demonstrated, prior to drug use, comorbid disorders and emotional suffering [58], and that addiction syndrome is always accompanied by dysphoria, dejection, negative affect, and sadness. These latter characteristics are part of a negative reinforcement process that will precipitate compulsive craving when abstinence begins to be perceived by the body. Allostatic changes also arise in some individuals experiencing chronic pain in the form of depression, anxiety, loss of sleep, various somatic disorders, and emotional distress; these latter symptoms represent a departure from the classic physical dependence symptoms.

From a pharmacological perspective, opioid addiction in pain patients has long been considered as an iatrogenic syndrome [136]. As noted above, discussions in most of the papers blame prescribed doses that are either too high or too low. From another perspective, to draw a parallel with addiction medicine, craving or the motive for compulsive use appears to be similar in chronic pain patients and in individuals entering the process of addiction. Epidemiological data and everyday clinical practice highlight considerable individual differences at each step of the addictive process. Some individuals at risk display an inherent or acquired predisposition to enter into the process or succumb to addiction at one or more stages of the addiction spiral. The various "historical" origins of such a "pro-addictive phenotype" are numerous and intertwined: genetic factors, disrupted development, and stressful life events; age and gender influences; and, importantly, various comorbidities such as personality, behavioral, and psychiatric disorders. Epidemiological studies have demonstrated high prevalence estimates for mood, anxiety, painful effects, and impulse control disorders [82] among those characterized as having a "pro-addictive phenotype."

A new field of research is required to evaluate and predict the risk factors predisposing a segment of the patient population to abuse. A history of drug or alcohol abuse often highlights pain patients at risk for opioid abuse [50]. A recent prospective cohort study [65] of 196 opioid-treated patients with chronic, nonmalignant pain of at least 3 months' duration showed that 62 patients (32% of the sample) engaged in opioid misuse, and 40% of these cases of misuse also involved the use of stimulants [8,47]. It is interesting to consider that, in the case of heroin, the prevalence of dependence or abuse among past-year users was 57% [121]. Chronic pain and negative affect are comorbid [122]. Anxiety, fear avoidance beliefs, social stresses, and psychopathology predict poor outcome of pain treatment [27,42,55,70]. Serial interactions exist between pain, its sensation intensity and unpleasantness, subjective distress, and related secondary affects. More studies are currently being performed to elucidate how brain substrates for pain or hyperalgesia and drug abuse interact with the processing of emotions and negative emotional responses in limbic regions [96].

Pain intensity, drug-induced hyperalgesia, drug abuse, personality traits: which comes first? [53]. Chronic pain patients suffer from a number of comorbid psychiatric conditions far more frequently than do the general population; the comorbidities reported resemble those observed in individuals prone to drug misuse [135]. It remains to be investigated whether the "pain-prone personality" [46], "pro-addictive personality," and "hyperalgesia-prone personality" present common characteristics. Further investigation will be required to study the relationships between a state phenomenon (pain) and a trait phenomenon (personality characteristics) [46]. Recent research has revealed the intimate relationship between addiction medicine and pain management [16,104]. These perspectives represent a paradigmatic change, placing the individual and his or her vulnerability at the center of research on causality (Fig. 2).

New Therapeutic Perspectives

As proposed by Scholz and Woolf [105]: "The notion that there is a class of drug, a universal analgesic, that can intrinsically reduce all pain, is obsolete and has to be abandoned." Relationships between long-lasting pain hypersensitivity and tolerance suggest new approaches for improving opioid treatment in chronic pain patients. It may be clinically more useful to try to prevent the development of central sensitization than to treat chronic pain when it is established [141]. We propose that four types of analgesic therapies could be considered: (1) specific antinociceptive drugs (e.g., acetaminophen/paracetamol); (2) analgesics with hyperalgesic properties, such as opioids; (3) antihyperalgesic drugs, such as NMDA-receptor antagonists and gabapentinoids [64,127]; and (4) drugs with analgesic and antihyperalgesic properties, such as nitrous oxide [12] and certain nonsteroidal anti-inflammatories [77,85]. Recently, polyamine-deficient foods that inhibit NR2B tyrosine phosphorylation enhancement induced by inflammation have been demonstrated to prevent and reduce pain hypersensitivity in various experimental models of hyperalgesia and tolerance induced by opioids, and in animal models of chronic pain [101]. From a tolerance/dependence perspective, a new therapeutic challenge would be to avoid the escalation of opioid dosing for alleviating pain. Rather, restoring opioid effectiveness by reducing pain hypersensitivity induced by opioid treatments could represent the future of pain management. Such "antihyperalgesic" therapies could be a promising and safe strategy for improving the clinical management of pain with opioids.

Acknowledgments

We thank Emilie Laboureyras, Jérémy Chateauraynaud, and Lisa Romero for their expert assistance with word processing and graphics.

References

[1] Adam F, Bonnet F, Le Bars D. Tolerance to morphine analgesia: evidence for stimulus intensity as a key factor and complete reversal by a glycine site-specific NMDA antagonist. Neuropharmacology 2006;51:191–202.

[2] Ali NM. Hyperalgesic response in a patient receiving high concentrations of spinal morphine. Anesthesiology 1986;65:449.

[3] Ammer H, Schulz R. Adenylyl cyclase supersensitivity in opioid-withdrawn NG108-15 hybrid cells requires Gs but is not mediated by the Gs alpha subunit. J Pharmacol Exp Ther 1998;286:855–62.

[4] Andrews HL. The effect of opiates on the pain threshold in post-addicts. J Clin Invest 1943;22:511–6.

[5] Arcaya JL, Cano G, Gomez G, Maixner W, Suarez-Roca H. Dynorphin A increases substance P release from trigeminal primary afferent C-fibers. Eur J Pharmacol 1999;366:27–34.

[6] Arden JR, Segredo V, Wang Z, Lameh J, Sadee W. Phosphorylation and agonist-specific intracellular trafficking of an epitope-tagged mu-opioid receptor expressed in HEK 293 cells. J Neurochem 1995;65:1636–45.

[7] Arner S, Rawal N, Gustafsson LL. Clinical experience of long-term treatment with epidural and intrathecal opioids. A nationwide survey. Acta Anaesthesiol Scand 1988;32:253–9.

[8] Ballantyne JC, LaForge KS. Opioid dependence and addiction during opioid treatment of chronic pain. Pain 2007;129:235–55.

[9] Ballantyne JC, Mao J. Opioid therapy for chronic pain. N Engl J Med 2003;349:1943–53.

[10] Basbaum AI. Insights into the development of opioid tolerance. Pain 1995;61:349–52.

[11] Benoliel JJ, Bourgoin S, Mauborgne A, Legrand JC, Hamon M, Cesselin F. Differential inhibitory/stimulatory modulation of spinal CCK release by mu and delta opioid agonists, and selective blockade of mu-dependent inhibition by kappa receptor stimulation. Neurosci Lett 1991;124:204–7.

[12] Bessiere B, Richebe P, Laboureyras E, Laulin JP, Contarino A, Simonnet G. Nitrous oxide (N_2O) prevents latent pain sensitization and long-term anxiety-like behavior in pain and opioid-experienced rats. Neuropharmacology 2007;53:733–40.

[13] Bolles RC, Fanselow MS. A perceptual-defensive-recuperative model of fear and pain. Behav Brain Sci 1980;3:291–323.

[14] Borgland SL, Connor M, Christie MJ. Nociceptin inhibits calcium channel currents in a subpopulation of small nociceptive trigeminal ganglion neurons in mouse. J Physiol 2001;536:35–47.

[15] Bruera E, Belzile M, Pituskin E, Fainsinger R, Darke A, Harsanyi Z, Babul N, Ford I. Randomized, double-blind, cross-over trial comparing safety and efficacy of oral controlled-release oxycodone with controlled-release morphine in patients with cancer pain. J Clin Oncol 1998;16:3222–9.

[16] Caldeiro R, Malte C, Calsyn D, Baer J, Nichol P, Kivlahan D, Saxon A. The association of persistent pain with outpatient addiction treatment outcomes and service utilization. Addiction 2008;103:1996–2005.
[17] Caterina MJ, Leffler A, Malmberg AB, Martin WJ, Trafton J, Petersen-Zeitz KR, Koltzenburg M, Basbaum AI, Julius D. Impaired nociception and pain sensation in mice lacking the capsaicin receptor. Science 2000;288:306–13.
[18] Célèrier E, Laulin J, Larcher A, Le Moal M, Simonnet G. Evidence for opiate-activated NMDA processes masking opiate analgesia in rats. Brain Res 1999;847:18–25.
[19] Célèrier E, Laulin JP, Corcuff JB, Le Moal M, Simonnet G. Progressive enhancement of delayed hyperalgesia induced by repeated heroin administration: a sensitization process. J Neurosci 2001;21:4074–80.
[20] Célèrier E, Rivat C, Jun Y, Laulin JP, Larcher A, Reynier P, Simonnet G. Long-lasting hyperalgesia induced by fentanyl in rats: preventive effect of ketamine. Anesthesiology 2000;92:465–72.
[21] Chakrabarti S, Regec A, Gintzler AR. Chronic morphine acts via a protein kinase Cγ-Gβ-adenylyl cyclase complex to augment phosphorylation of Gβ and Gβγ stimulatory adenylyl cyclase signaling. Brain Res Mol Brain Res 2005;138:94–103.
[22] Chakrabarti S, Rivera M, Yan SZ, Tang WJ, Gintzler AR. Chronic morphine augments Gβγ/Gsα stimulation of adenylyl cyclase: relevance to opioid tolerance. Mol Pharmacol 1998;54:655–62.
[23] Chavkin C, McLaughlin JP, Celver JP. Regulation of opioid receptor function by chronic agonist exposure: constitutive activity and desensitization. Mol Pharmacol 2001;60:20–5.
[24] Chen L, Huang LY. Sustained potentiation of NMDA-receptor-mediated glutamate responses through activation of protein kinase C by a mu opioid. Neuron 1991;7:319–26.
[25] Chen Y, Geis C, Sommer C. Activation of TRPV1 contributes to morphine tolerance: involvement of the mitogen-activated protein kinase signaling pathway. J Neurosci 2008;28:5836–45.
[26] Christie MJ. Cellular neuroadaptations to chronic opioids: tolerance, withdrawal and addiction. Br J Pharmacol 2008;154:384–96.
[27] Cicero TJ, Lynskey M, Todorov A, Inciardi JA, Surratt HL. Co-morbid pain and psychopathology in males and females admitted to treatment for opioid analgesic abuse. Pain 2008;139:127–35.
[28] Collier HO. Cellular site of opiate dependence. Nature 1980;283:625–9.
[29] Collin E, Poulain P, Gauvain-Piquard A, Petit G, Pichard-Leandri E. Is disease progression the major factor in morphine 'tolerance' in cancer pain treatment? Pain 1993;55:319–26.
[30] Colpaert FC. System theory of pain and of opiate analgesia: no tolerance to opiates. Pharmacol Rev 1996;48:355–402.
[31] Compton MA. Cold-pressor pain tolerance in opiate and cocaine abusers: correlates of drug type and use status. J Pain Symptom Manage 1994;9:462–73.
[32] Compton P, Athanasos P, Elashoff D. Withdrawal hyperalgesia after acute opioid physical dependence in nonaddicted humans: a preliminary study. J Pain 2003;4:511–9.
[33] Contet C, Filliol D, Matifas A, Kieffer BL. Morphine-induced analgesic tolerance, locomotor sensitization and physical dependence do not require modification of mu opioid receptor, cdk5 and adenylate cyclase activity. Neuropharmacology 2008;54:475–86.
[34] Crain SM, Shen KF. Modulation of opioid analgesia, tolerance and dependence by Gs-coupled, GM1 ganglioside-regulated opioid receptor functions. Trends Pharmacol Sci 1998;19:358–65.
[35] Davis JB, Gray J, Gunthorpe MJ, Hatcher JP, Davey PT, Overend P, Harries MH, Latcham J, Clapham C, Atkinson K, et al. Vanilloid receptor-1 is essential for inflammatory thermal hyperalgesia. Nature 2000;405:183–7.
[36] Devillers JP, Labrouche SA, Castes E, Simonnet G. Release of neuropeptide FF, an anti-opioid peptide, in rat spinal cord slices is voltage- and Ca^{2+}-sensitive: possible involvement of P-type Ca^{2+} channels. J Neurochem 1995;64:1567–75.
[37] Devillers JP, Simonnet G. Modulation of neuropeptide FF release from rat spinal cord slices by glutamate. Involvement of NMDA receptors. Eur J Pharmacol 1994;271:185–92.
[38] Devulder J. Hyperalgesia induced by high-dose intrathecal sufentanil in neuropathic pain. J Neurosurg Anesthesiol 1997;9:146–8.
[39] Dourish CT, O'Neill MF, Coughlan J, Kitchener SJ, Hawley D, Iversen SD. The selective CCK-B receptor antagonist L-365,260 enhances morphine analgesia and prevents morphine tolerance in the rat. Eur J Pharmacol 1990;176:35–44.
[40] Doverty M, Somogyi AA, White JM, Bochner F, Beare CH, Menelaou A, Ling W. Methadone maintenance patients are cross-tolerant to the antinociceptive effects of morphine. Pain 2001;93:155–63.
[41] Doverty M, White JM, Somogyi AA, Bochner F, Ali R, Ling W. Hyperalgesic responses in methadone maintenance patients. Pain 2001;90:91–6.
[42] Dufton LM, Konik B, Colletti R, Stanger C, Boyer M, Morrow S, Compas BE. Effects of stress on pain threshold and tolerance in children with recurrent abdominal pain. Pain 2008;136:38–43.
[43] Eisenach JC. Preventing chronic pain after surgery: who, how, and when? Reg Anesth Pain Med 2006;31:1–3.
[44] Faris PL, Komisaruk BR, Watkins LR, Mayer DJ. Evidence for the neuropeptide cholecystokinin as an antagonist of opiate analgesia. Science 1983;219:310–2.
[45] Fields HL, Bry J, Hentall I, Zorman G. The activity of neurons in the rostral medulla of the rat during withdrawal from noxious heat. J Neurosci 1983;3:2545–52.
[46] Fishbain DA, Cole B, Cutler RB, Lewis J, Rosomoff HL, Rosomoff RS. Chronic pain and the measurement of personality: do states influence traits? Pain Med 2006;7:509–29.
[47] Fishbain DA, Cole B, Lewis J, Rosomoff HL, Rosomoff RS. What percentage of chronic nonmalignant pain patients exposed to chronic opioid analgesic therapy develop abuse/addiction and/or aberrant drug-related behaviors? A structured evidence-based review. Pain Med 2008;9:444–59.
[48] Foley KM. Clinical tolerance to opioids. In: Basbaum AI, Besson JM, editors. Towards a new pharmacotherapy of pain. New York: John Wiley & Sons; 1991. p. 181–203.

[49] Friedman HJ, Jen MF, Chang JK, Lee NM, Loh HH. Dynorphin: a possible modulatory peptide on morphine or beta-endorphin analgesia in mouse. Eur J Pharmacol 1981;69:357–60.
[50] Friedman R, Li V, Mehrotra D. Treating pain patients at risk: evaluation of a screening tool in opioid-treated pain patients with and without addiction. Pain Med 2003;4:182–5.
[51] Fry JP, Herz A, Zieglgansberger W. A demonstration of naloxone-precipitated opiate withdrawal on single neurones in the morphine-tolerant/dependent rat brain. Br J Pharmacol 1980;68:585–92.
[52] Fujimoto JM, Arts KS, Rady JJ, Tseng LF. Intracerebroventricular analgesia enhanced by intrathecal (IT) dynorphin A_{1-17} antibody. Prog Clin Biol Res 1990;328:433–6.
[53] Gallagher RM. Pain intensity, emotional state, and personality trait: which comes first? Pain Med 2006;7:471–2.
[54] Gardell LR, Wang R, Burgess SE, Ossipov MH, Vanderah TW, Malan TP Jr, Lai J, Porreca F. Sustained morphine exposure induces a spinal dynorphin-dependent enhancement of excitatory transmitter release from primary afferent fibers. J Neurosci 2002;22:6747–55.
[55] George SZ, Wallace MR, Wright TW, Moser MW, Greenfield WH 3rd, Sack BK, Herbstman DM, Fillingim RB. Evidence for a biopsychosocial influence on shoulder pain: pain catastrophizing and catechol-O-methyltransferase (COMT) diplotype predict clinical pain ratings. Pain 2008;136:53–61.
[56] Gintzler AR, Chakrabarti S. Post-opioid receptor adaptations to chronic morphine: altered functionality and associations of signaling molecules. Life Sci 2006;79:717–22.
[57] Gong QL, Hedner J, Bjorkman R, Hedner T. Morphine-3-glucuronide may functionally antagonize morphine-6-glucuronide induced antinociception and ventilatory depression in the rat. Pain 1992;48:249–55.
[58] Goodman A. Neurobiology of addiction. An integrative review. Biochem Pharmacol 2008;75:266–322.
[59] Guignard B, Bossard AE, Coste C, Sessler DI, Lebrault C, Alfonsi P, Fletcher D, Chauvin M. Acute opioid tolerance: intraoperative remifentanil increases postoperative pain and morphine requirement. Anesthesiology 2000;93:409–17.
[60] Gutstein HB. The effects of pain on opioid tolerance: how do we resolve the controversy? Pharmacol Rev 1996;48:403–7; discussion 9–11.
[61] Haley J, Wilcox GL. Involvement of excitatory amino acids and peptides in the spinal mechanisms underlying hyperalgesia. In: Willis W, editor. Hyperalgesia and allodynia. New York: Raven Press; 1992. p. 281–93.
[62] He L, Fong J, von Zastrow M, Whistler JL. Regulation of opioid receptor trafficking and morphine tolerance by receptor oligomerization. Cell 2002;108:271–82.
[63] Ho A, Dole VP. Pain perception in drug-free and in methadone-maintained human ex-addicts. Proc Soc Exp Biol Med 1979;162:392–5.
[64] Iannetti GD, Zambreanu L, Wise RG, Buchanan TJ, Huggins JP, Smart TS, Vennart W, Tracey I. Pharmacological modulation of pain-related brain activity during normal and central sensitization states in humans. Proc Natl Acad Sci USA 2005;102:18195–200.
[65] Ives TJ, Chelminski PR, Hammett-Stabler CA, Malone RM, Perhac JS, Potisek NM, Shilliday BB, DeWalt DA, Pignone MP. Predictors of opioid misuse in patients with chronic pain: a prospective cohort study. BMC Health Serv Res 2006;6:46.
[66] Joly V, Richebe P, Guignard B, Fletcher D, Maurette P, Sessler DI, Chauvin M. Remifentanil-induced postoperative hyperalgesia and its prevention with small-dose ketamine. Anesthesiology 2005;103:147–55.
[67] Katz NP, Adams EH, Chilcoat H, Colucci RD, Comer SD, Goliber P, Grudzinskas C, Jasinski D, Lande SD, Passik SD, et al. Challenges in the development of prescription opioid abuse-deterrent formulations. Clin J Pain 2007;23:648–60.
[68] Kawasaki Y, Zhang L, Cheng JK, Ji RR. Cytokine mechanisms of central sensitization: distinct and overlapping role of interleukin-1beta, interleukin-6, and tumor necrosis factor-alpha in regulating synaptic and neuronal activity in the superficial spinal cord. J Neurosci 2008;28:5189–94.
[69] Kayan S, Woods LA, Mitchell CL. Morphine-induced hyperalgesia in rats tested on the hot plate. J Pharmacol Exp Ther 1971;177:509–13.
[70] Keeley P, Creed F, Tomenson B, Todd C, Borglin G, Dickens C. Psychosocial predictors of health-related quality of life and health service utilisation in people with chronic low back pain. Pain 2008;135:142–50.
[71] Kehlet H, Jensen TS, Woolf CJ. Persistent postsurgical pain: risk factors and prevention. Lancet 2006;367:1618–25.
[72] Kieffer BL, Evans CJ. Opioid tolerance-in search of the holy grail. Cell 2002;108:587–90.
[73] Kim DH, Fields HL, Barbaro NM. Morphine analgesia and acute physical dependence: rapid onset of two opposing, dose-related processes. Brain Res 1990;516:37–40.
[74] King T, Ossipov MH, Vanderah TW, Porreca F, Lai J. Is paradoxical pain induced by sustained opioid exposure an underlying mechanism of opioid antinociceptive tolerance? Neurosignals 2005;14:194–205.
[75] Koch T, Hollt V. Role of receptor internalization in opioid tolerance and dependence. Pharmacol Ther 2008;117:199–206.
[76] Koch T, Widera A, Bartzsch K, Schulz S, Brandenburg LO, Wundrack N, Beyer A, Grecksch G, Hollt V. Receptor endocytosis counteracts the development of opioid tolerance. Mol Pharmacol 2005;67:280–7.
[77] Koppert W, Schmelz M. The impact of opioid-induced hyperalgesia for postoperative pain. Best Pract Res Clin Anaesthesiol 2007;21:65–83.
[78] Lake JR, Hammond MV, Shaddox RC, Hunsicker LM, Yang HY, Malin DH. IgG from neuropeptide FF antiserum reverses morphine tolerance in the rat. Neurosci Lett 1991;132:29–32.
[79] Laulin JP, Célèrier E, Larcher A, Le Moal M, Simonnet G. Opiate tolerance to daily heroin administration: an apparent phenomenon associated with enhanced pain sensitivity. Neuroscience 1999;89:631–6.
[80] Laulin JP, Larcher A, Célèrier E, Le Moal M, Simonnet G. Long-lasting increased pain sensitivity in rat following exposure to heroin for the first time. Eur J Neurosci 1998;10:782–5.
[81] Laulin JP, Maurette P, Corcuff JB, Rivat C, Chauvin M, Simonnet G. The role of ketamine in preventing fentanyl-induced hyperalgesia and subsequent acute morphine tolerance. Anesth Analg 2002;94:1263–9.

[82] Le Moal M, Koob GF. Drug addiction: pathways to the disease and pathophysiological perspectives. Eur Neuropsychopharmacol 2007;17:377–93.
[83] Li DP, Chen SR, Pan HL. VR1 receptor activation induces glutamate release and postsynaptic firing in the paraventricular nucleus. J Neurophysiol 2004;92:1807–16.
[84] Ma QP, Woolf CJ. Noxious stimuli induce an N-methyl-D-aspartate receptor-dependent hypersensitivity of the flexion withdrawal reflex to touch: implications for the treatment of mechanical allodynia. Pain 1995;61:383–90.
[85] Malmberg AB, Yaksh TL. Antinociceptive actions of spinal nonsteroidal anti-inflammatory agents on the formalin test in the rat. J Pharmacol Exp Ther 1992;263:136–46.
[86] Mao J, Price DD, Mayer DJ. Thermal hyperalgesia in association with the development of morphine tolerance in rats: roles of excitatory amino acid receptors and protein kinase C. J Neurosci 1994;14:2301–12.
[87] Mao J, Price DD, Mayer DJ. Mechanisms of hyperalgesia and morphine tolerance: a current view of their possible interactions. Pain 1995;62:259–74.
[88] Mazoit JX, Butscher K, Samii K. Morphine in postoperative patients: pharmacokinetics and pharmacodynamics of metabolites. Anesth Analg 2007;105:70–8.
[89] McQuay H. Opioids in pain management. Lancet 1999;353:2229–32.
[90] Mercadante S, Bruera E. Opioid switching: a systematic and critical review. Cancer Treat Rev 2006;32:304–15.
[91] Moran TD, Smith PA. Morphine-3beta-D-glucuronide suppresses inhibitory synaptic transmission in rat substantia gelatinosa. J Pharmacol Exp Ther 2002;302:568–76.
[92] Onofrio BM, Yaksh TL, Arnold PG. Continuous low-dose intrathecal morphine administration in the treatment of chronic pain of malignant origin. Mayo Clin Proc 1981;56:516–20.
[93] Ossipov MH, Lai J, Vanderah TW, Porreca F. Induction of pain facilitation by sustained opioid exposure: relationship to opioid antinociceptive tolerance. Life Sci 2003;73:783–800.
[94] Otsuka M, Yoshioka K. Neurotransmitter functions of mammalian tachykinins. Physiol Rev 1993;73:229–308.
[95] Portenoy RK. Management of common opioid side effects during long-term therapy of cancer pain. Ann Acad Med Singapore 1994;23:160–70.
[96] Price DD. Central neural mechanisms that interrelate sensory and affective dimensions of pain. Mol Interv 2002;2:392–403, 339.
[97] Ren K, Dubner R. Neuron-glia crosstalk gets serious: role in pain hypersensitivity. Curr Opin Anaesthesiol 2008;21:570–9.
[98] Richebe P, Rivat C, Laulin JP, Maurette P, Simonnet G. Ketamine improves the management of exaggerated postoperative pain observed in perioperative fentanyl-treated rats. Anesthesiology 2005;102:421–8.
[99] Rivat C, Laboureyras E, Laulin JP, Le Roy C, Richebe P, Simonnet G. Non-nociceptive environmental stress induces hyperalgesia, not analgesia, in pain and opioid-experienced rats. Neuropsychopharmacology 2007;32:2217–28.
[100] Rivat C, Laulin JP, Corcuff JB, Celerier E, Pain L, Simonnet G. Fentanyl enhancement of carrageenan-induced long-lasting hyperalgesia in rats: prevention by the N-methyl-D-aspartate receptor antagonist ketamine. Anesthesiology 2002;96:381–91.
[101] Rivat C, Richebe P, Laboureyras E, Laulin JP, Havouis R, Noble F, Moulinoux JP, Simonnet G. Polyamine deficient diet to relieve pain hypersensitivity. Pain 2008;137:125–37.
[102] Rivera M, Gintzler AR. Differential effect of chronic morphine on mRNA encoding adenylyl cyclase isoforms: relevance to physiological sequela of tolerance/dependence. Brain Res Mol Brain Res 1998;54:165–9.
[103] Rossbach M. Über die Gowöhnung an Gifte. Pfluegers Arc Gesamte Physiol Menschen Tiere 1880;21:213–25.
[104] Samet J, Walley A. Commentary: Can one be an expert in addiction medicine without expertise in pain management? Addiction 2008;103:2006–7.
[105] Scholz J, Woolf CJ. Can we conquer pain? Nat Neurosci 2002;5:1062–7.
[106] Sharma SK, Klee WA, Nirenberg M. Dual regulation of adenylate cyclase accounts for narcotic dependence and tolerance. Proc Natl Acad Sci U S A 1975;72:3092–6.
[107] Shen KF, Crain SM. Cholera toxin-B subunit blocks excitatory effects of opioids on sensory neuron action potentials indicating that GM1 ganglioside may regulate Gs-linked opioid receptor functions. Brain Res 1990;531:1–7.
[108] Sheu R, Lussier D, Rosenblum A, Fong C, Portenoy J, Joseph H, Portenoy RK. Prevalence and characteristics of chronic pain in patients admitted to an outpatient drug and alcohol treatment program. Pain Med 2008;9:911–7.
[109] Siegel S. Morphine analgesic tolerance: its situation specificity supports a Pavlovian conditioning model. Science 1976;193:323–5.
[110] Siegel S. Pharmacological conditioning and drug effects. In: Goudie AJ, Emmett-Oglesby MW, editors. New Jersey: Humana Press; 1989.
[111] Siegel S, Hinson RE, Krank MD, McCully J. Heroin "overdose" death: contribution of drug-associated environmental cues. Science 1982;216:436–7.
[112] Simonin F, Schmitt M, Laulin JP, Laboureyras E, Jhamandas JH, Mactavish D, Matifas A, Mollereau C, Laurent P, Parmentier M, et al. RF9, a potent and selective neuropeptide FF receptor antagonist, prevents opioid-induced tolerance associated with hyperalgesia. Proc Natl Acad Sci USA 2006;103:466–71.
[113] Simonnet G. Preemptive antihyperalgesia to improve preemptive analgesia. Anesthesiology 2008;108:352–4.
[114] Simonnet G, Rivat C. Opioid-induced hyperalgesia: abnormal or normal pain? Neuroreport 2003;14:1–7.
[115] Skilling SR, Sun X, Kurtz HJ, Larson AA. Selective potentiation of NMDA-induced activity and release of excitatory amino acids by dynorphin: possible roles in paralysis and neurotoxicity. Brain Res 1992;575:272–8.
[116] Solomon RL, Corbit JD. An opponent-process theory of motivation. I. Temporal dynamics of affect. Psychol Rev 1974;81:119–45.
[117] Song P, Zhao ZQ. The involvement of glial cells in the development of morphine tolerance. Neurosci Res 2001;39:281–6.

[118] Stillman MJ, Moulin DE, Foley KM. Paradoxical pain following high-dose spinal morphine. Pain 1987;Suppl4:S389.
[119] Stubhaug A, Breivik H, Eide PK, Kreunen M, Foss A. Mapping of punctuate hyperalgesia around a surgical incision demonstrates that ketamine is a powerful suppressor of central sensitization to pain following surgery. Acta Anaesthesiol Scand 1997;41:1124–32.
[120] Subkov AA, Zilov GN. The role of conditioned reflex adaptation in the origin of hyperergic reactions. Bull Biol Med Exp 1937;4:294–6.
[121] Substance Abuse and Mental Health Services Administration. Results from the 2002 National Survey on Drug Use and Health: National Findings. In: National Household Survey on Drug Abuse (NHSDA) Series H-22. Rockville, MD: Office of Applied Statistics; 2003.
[122] Tang NK, Salkovskis PM, Hodges A, Wright KJ, Hanna M, Hester J. Effects of mood on pain responses and pain tolerance: an experimental study in chronic back pain patients. Pain 2008;138:392–401.
[123] Tian J, Han J. Functional studies using antibodies against orphanin FQ/nociceptin. Peptides 2000;21:1047–50.
[124] Tilson HA, Rech RH, Stolman S. Hyperalgesia during withdrawal as a means of measuring the degree of dependence in morphine dependent rats. Psychopharmacologia 1973;28:287–300.
[125] Trujillo KA, Akil H. Inhibition of morphine tolerance and dependence by the NMDA receptor antagonist MK-801. Science 1991;251:85–7.
[126] Twycross RG. Clinical experience with diamorphine in advanced malignant disease. Int J Clin Pharmacol 1974;7:184–98.
[127] Van Elstraete AC, Sitbon P, Mazoit JX, Benhamou D. Gabapentin prevents delayed and long-lasting hyperalgesia induced by fentanyl in rats. Anesthesiology 2008;108:484–94.
[128] Vanderah TW, Gardell LR, Burgess SE, Ibrahim M, Dogrul A, Zhong CM, Zhang ET, Malan TP, Jr., Ossipov MH, Lai J, Porreca F. Dynorphin promotes abnormal pain and spinal opioid antinociceptive tolerance. J Neurosci 2000;20:7074–9.
[129] Vanderah TW, Ossipov MH, Lai J, Malan TP, Jr., Porreca F. Mechanisms of opioid-induced pain and antinociceptive tolerance: descending facilitation and spinal dynorphin. Pain 2001;92:5–9.
[130] Vanderah TW, Suenaga NM, Ossipov MH, Malan TP Jr, Lai J, Porreca F. Tonic descending facilitation from the rostral ventromedial medulla mediates opioid-induced abnormal pain and antinociceptive tolerance. J Neurosci 2001;21:279–86.
[131] Vardanyan A, Wang R, Vanderah TW, Ossipov MH, Lai J, Porreca F, King T. TRPV1 receptor in expression of opioid-induced hyperalgesia. J Pain 2008;4:4.
[132] Vera-Portocarrero LP, Zhang ET, King T, Ossipov MH, Vanderah TW, Lai J, Porreca F. Spinal NK-1 receptor expressing neurons mediate opioid-induced hyperalgesia and antinociceptive tolerance via activation of descending pathways. Pain 2007;129:35–45.
[133] Wasan AD, Butler SF, Budman SH, Benoit C, Fernandez K, Jamison RN. Psychiatric history and psychologic adjustment as risk factors for aberrant drug-related behavior among patients with chronic pain. Clin J Pain 2007;23:307–15.
[134] Watkins LR, Milligan ED, Maier SF. Glial activation: a driving force for pathological pain. Trends Neurosci 2001;24:450–5.
[135] Weisberg JN, Boatwright BA. Mood, anxiety and personality traits and states in chronic pain. Pain 2007;133:1–2.
[136] Weissman DE, Haddox JD. Opioid pseudoaddiction: an iatrogenic syndrome. Pain 1989;36:363–6.
[137] Whistler JL, Chuang HH, Chu P, Jan LY, von Zastrow M. Functional dissociation of mu opioid receptor signaling and endocytosis: implications for the biology of opiate tolerance and addiction. Neuron 1999;23:737–46.
[138] Wilder-Smith OH, Arendt-Nielsen L. Postoperative hyperalgesia: its clinical importance and relevance. Anesthesiology 2006;104:601–7.
[139] Wolff T, Samuelsson H, Hedner T. Concentrations of morphine and morphine metabolites in CSF and plasma during continuous subcutaneous morphine administration in cancer pain patients. Pain 1996;68:209–16.
[140] Woolf CJ. Intrathecal high dose morphine produces hyperalgesia in the rat. Brain Res 1981;209:491–5.
[141] Woolf CJ. A new strategy for the treatment of inflammatory pain. Prevention or elimination of central sensitization. Drugs 1994;47:1–9.
[142] Xie JY, Herman DS, Stiller CO, Gardell LR, Ossipov MH, Lai J, Porreca F, Vanderah TW. Cholecystokinin in the rostral ventromedial medulla mediates opioid-induced hyperalgesia and antinociceptive tolerance. J Neurosci 2005;25:409–16.
[143] Yaksh TL, Harty GJ. Pharmacology of the allodynia in rats evoked by high dose intrathecal morphine. J Pharmacol Exp Ther 1988;244:501–7.
[144] Yang HY, Fratta W, Majane EA, Costa E. Isolation, sequencing, synthesis, and pharmacological characterization of two brain neuropeptides that modulate the action of morphine. Proc Natl Acad Sci USA 1985;82:7757–61.
[145] Yuan L, Han Z, Chang JK, Han JS. Accelerated release and production of orphanin FQ in brain of chronic morphine tolerant rats. Brain Res 1999;826:330–4.
[146] Zadina JE, Kastin AJ, Harrison LM, Ge LJ, Chang SL. Opiate receptor changes after chronic exposure to agonists and antagonists. Ann NY Acad Sci 1995;757:353–61.

Correspondence to: Guy Simonnet, PhD, Université Victor Segalen-Bordeaux 2, CNRS UMR 5227, Homéostasie-Allostasie-Pathology-Réhabilitation, 146, Rue Léo Saignat, 33077 Bordeaux cedex, France. Tel: (33) 557571406; email: gsimonnet@yahoo.com.

19

Pharmacogenetics of Pain Inhibition

Jeffrey S. Mogil

Department of Psychology and Alan Edwards Centre for Research on Pain, McGill University, Montreal, Quebec, Canada

Virtually all drugs exhibit wide interindividual variability in their efficacy, potency, and side effects. This variability can have dramatic implications, resulting in continued suffering in patients not receiving the dose they require, as well as unneeded toxicity in other patients who would have responded to much lower doses. The field of pharmacogenetics/pharmacogenomics is concerned with the inherited basis of such individual differences [29], and the advent of "personalized medicine" is much anticipated. The dream is to be able to adjust doses, or even drug classes, based on a prediction of response suggested by the patient's profile at relevant genetic loci, rather than the current titration approach. In fact, pharmacogenetics (I prefer this less-grandiose term) is rather well advanced compared to most other fields of complex trait genetics, because of the finite number of proteins (and thus genes) involved in drug transport, binding, and metabolism. This is true for analgesics as well: of the commonly used analgesic or antiallodynic drugs, only a small number of genes code for their binding sites (e.g., μ-opioid receptor, κ-opioid receptor, cyclooxygenase-1 and -2, serotonin reuptake protein, norepinephrine reuptake protein, $\alpha_2\delta_1$ calcium channel subunit), phase I and II metabolism (COMT, P450 1A2, P450 2B6, P450 2C8, P450 2C9, P450 2C19, P450 2D6, P450 2E1, P450 3A4, P450 3A5, UGT 2Bs), and outward transport (P-glycoprotein).

Thus, quite a bit of progress has been made in the field of analgesia pharmacogenetics, although it appears that the topic is more complicated than it would first appear.

Pharmacology of Pain
edited by Pierre Beaulieu, David Lussier, Frank Porreca, and Anthony H. Dickenson
IASP Press, Seattle, © 2010

Our own data from the laboratory mouse (see later), for example, suggest that analgesia pharmacogenetics is intimately related to the type of pain being inhibited, such that different genes may be relevant to morphine's inhibition of inflammatory pain than are relevant to its inhibition of thermal pain.

This chapter will discuss evidence for individual differences in, and heritability of, analgesic response to commonly used clinical treatments for pain. In addition, the known and suspected role of individual genes in both pharmacokinetics and pharmacodynamics of analgesia will be discussed. Because this field has been reviewed in depth a number of times in recent years [42,55,56,61,65,72,86,89], I will not attempt to be comprehensive, but rather will focus on clear examples and larger issues.

Individual Differences in Analgesic Response

Human Experimental Studies

In experimental studies with controlled stimuli, analgesics of several classes—including opioids, nonsteroidal anti-inflammatory drugs (NSAIDs), and placebos—produce highly variable effects on pain thresholds, tolerances, and ratings. This variability has been noted for quite some time [99].

Individual Differences in Clinical Opioid Analgesia

The presence of robust interindividual responses in the efficacy, potency, and side effects of analgesics in clinical situations has been asserted in reviews of pain management for many decades. In fact, a perusal of the error bars in data from virtually any clinical trial should convince the reader of the existence of important variability. However, studies specifically analyzing this variability in large and relatively uniform patient populations are quite rare. The largest of these studies was conducted by Aubrun and colleagues [2], who studied intravenous morphine titration requirements in 3,045 postoperative (mostly orthopedic surgery) patients in a postanesthetic care unit. Patients rated their pain on a visual analogue scale (VAS) immediately after tracheal extubation, and when VAS scores exceeded 30 (on a scale of 0–100), they were given intravenous morphine titrated every 5 minutes in 2–3-mg increments, until "pain relief" (VAS $<$ 30) was achieved. An average of four such boluses were required to produce pain relief (mean: 12 $\pm$ 7 mg morphine), but extremes ranged from a single bolus to 20 boluses, a 40-fold range in mg/kg terms [2]. The relationship between initial VAS and the morphine dose required for pain relief was significant but modest. In a chart review of postoperative morphine consumption using patient-controlled analgesia (PCA) in over 10,000 patients, the mean morphine consumption in the first 24 hours was 65.2 mg, but the minimum and maximum consumptions were 2 mg and 345 mg, respectively [57]. There has been much less systematic study of individual differences in opioid responses in chronic pain patients (especially in the absence of malignancy) [58], although there are reports of variable efficacy, adverse events, and abuse [77].

Individual Differences in Responsiveness to Multiple Opioid Drugs

A small number of studies have considered individual differences across multiple opioid drugs. In a study of experimental pain, Chapman and colleagues [15] found that individual differences were greatest for morphine, lowest for alfentanil, and intermediate for fentanyl. In a case study of five patients, dose titration with multiple opioids revealed that each patient was successfully treated by a different opioid while experiencing inadequate relief and intolerable side effects with others [32]. In a head-to-head comparison of PCA-administered morphine, meperidine (pethidine), and fentanyl, it was observed that although overall these drugs were equal in patient satisfaction and side-effect frequency, responses were highly individualized, with some patients tolerating all the drugs, some tolerating none, and some tolerating one but not the others [100].

Individual Differences in Other Analgesics

The first study specifically describing the variable efficacy of NSAIDs was published in 1976 [38], and the topic has been revisited over the next few decades (e.g., refs. [23,74,82]), leading to the concept of individual NSAID "responders" and "nonresponders." Although the concept is still accepted, no recent pharmacogenetic research appears to have been directed at understanding variability in NSAID analgesia (perhaps excepting refs. [94,95]), in contrast to the voluminous literature on the pharmacogenetics of the antiplatelet effects of aspirin.

A particularly important analgesic modality featuring celebrated variability is placebo analgesia, which is said to work in approximately 35% of subjects [3]. A very intriguing study by Amanzio and colleagues [1] suggests that placebo response variability might partially underlie clinical and experimental opioid analgesic variability. Postoperative patients were given either standard ("open") injections of one of four opioid drugs or "hidden" injections. Although both injection procedures actually produced equivalent analgesia, there was twice as much variability in the open-injection groups for each drug. In a follow-up study with volunteers and experimental ischemic pain, the increased variability associated with the open injection was blocked by naloxone, suggesting that variable opioid-mediated placebo responses were responsible for the variability in drug analgesia.

Of the other major classes of clinical analgesics, only triptan drugs for migraine have been systematically evaluated for individual differences in analgesic efficacy (as opposed to pharmacokinetic parameters or side effects). It is well known that 30% of patients are "nonresponders" to any particular triptan, because of either lack of efficacy or intolerable side effects [25]. A number of studies have specifically investigated the shifting of sumatriptan nonresponders to other triptans, with generally positive results [25], implying that sensitivity to each drug is largely independent.

Predictors of Analgesic Sensitivity

Given the extent of the variability, much work has focused on identifying what factors can predict it, in an attempt to guide the choice of initial analgesic doses that can then be titrated. The important influence of age has long been known, with opioid requirements decreasing with advancing age [41,57]. The influence of sex on clinical analgesia has been noted repeatedly, but is highly controversial [22,35]. In general, psychosocial hypotheses have not been consistently supported, and thus genetic explanations for analgesic variability have increasingly been considered likely.

Analgesic Variability in Rodent Studies

Supporting the case that individual differences in analgesia may have a genetic explanation are the multiple demonstrations of highly variable half-maximal effective doses (ED_{50}s) among outbred and especially inbred strains of rats and mice. I and my colleagues have reviewed this literature on multiple occasions [31,48,60,69,71]. Suffice it to say that very robust differences have been noted across multiple drug classes, with ED_{50} values ranging 2-fold to 40-fold depending on the drug [98].

In addition to the simple demonstration of strain differences in ED_{50} values, some very interesting genetic correlations were noted in these studies. First, there is a consistent relationship between analgesic response and initial pain sensitivity, such that strains with higher initial sensitivity to the noxious stimulus display, generally speaking, lower analgesic potency [28,64,98]. Elmer and colleagues [28] have pointed out that higher stimulus intensity requires higher fractional receptor occupancy, and thus lower drug potency. In addition, and somewhat paradoxically, the relationship between pain sensitivity and drug analgesia appears to be specific to the pain modality, but not to the drug class. If the same strains are tested on a different pain test (with independent genetic mediation, presumably), the correlation between pain and analgesia holds, even though completely different mouse strains are sensitive and resistant [16,28]. Gratifyingly, the very same correlation between basal pain thresholds and subsequent opioid analgesia has subsequently been demonstrated in human clinical populations, and might represent a useful predictor of analgesic response [26,27]. Also, we have observed that analgesics of completely different neurochemical classes appear to share genetic determinants (that is, the same strains are sensitive and resistant to each drug), as long as the pain being inhibited by each drug is the same [98]. Such findings strongly challenge the simpleminded notion that drug variability can be explained simply by investigating polymorphisms in the genes coding for each drug's binding site, suggesting instead that the genetic variability lies in common pain-relevant circuitry on which these disparate drugs ultimately exert their actions.

Finally, it is important to note that in both mice and rats, multiple studies have demonstrated an interaction between genotype (strain) and sex in opioid analgesia especially, with sex differences wholly dependent on strain and strain differences often observed in one sex but not the other [44,62,90].

Heritability of Drug Analgesia in Humans and Rodents

The demonstration of individual differences does not automatically imply genetic mediation of that variability. Some variability is inherited, some is not, and some is produced by the interaction between the two. Twin and family studies in humans, and inbred strain surveys and artificial selection projects in animals, can generate estimates of heritability (h^2): the proportion of the overall (trait) variance that is inherited. It is not easy (and has not been considered important enough) to perform twin studies of drug analgesia, and thus we are aware of only one relevant study. Liston and colleagues [54] assessed the analgesic effect of 10 mg/70 kg morphine against ischemic pain in monozygotic twins compared to pairs of unrelated individuals. The results were nondefinitive, because no dizygotic twins were tested and the sample size was limited, but near-significant co-twin concordances were observed. In mouse strain surveys of 10 different analgesic drugs conducted in my laboratory [16,97,98], heritabilities ranged from $h^2 = 0.12$ to 0.49, which are moderate and somewhat lower than those obtained for pain traits per se. It must be noted that estimating heritability is now a somewhat moot point, since techniques exist to identify the sources of genetic variance regardless of how much trait variability they explain.

Techniques for the Identification of Genes Conferring Analgesic Variability

Rapid advances in molecular genetic techniques have allowed the identification of genes, and DNA variants (known as mutations when rare, and polymorphisms when common) within or near genes, responsible for the genetic component of pain and analgesic variability. These techniques have also facilitated the discovery ("cloning") and characterization of genes as relevant to pain and analgesia more generally. It is important to realize, however, that these two tasks are largely achieved by the application of different techniques [66].

Transgenic Knockout Mice

The transgenic "knockout" approach involves the genetic engineering of a null mutation and the placement by homologous recombination of that null mutation onto a murine genetic background, with subsequent testing ("phenotyping") of the mutant mouse line [63]. Although interpretational complexities abound [51], this technique has provided at least suggestive evidence for the involvement of 283 genes in pain-related behavioral traits (according to the Pain Genes Database at the time of writing [47]), including 94 genes whose ablations result in a mouse that is significantly more or less sensitive to some analgesic manipulation compared to its wild-type. This list is presented in Table I. This is important information, of course, but it may be not at all relevant to the issue of analgesic variability, since very few humans (or mice) are likely to be functional "knockouts" (i.e., exhibit no expression or functionality) at the genes in question.

Gene-Expression Profiling

Another exciting current technique is gene-expression profiling, especially as implemented by tissue-specific mRNA hybridization to "gene chip" microarrays [63]. This method

Table I
Null mutants displaying increased or decreased sensitivity to analgesics

Gene	Protein	Analgesic(s)*	Direction†
Abcb1a	ATP-binding cassette, subfamily B (MDR/TAP), member 1A	Alfentanil, DPDPE, fentanyl, methadone, M6G, morphine	▲
Abcc3	ATP-binding cassette, subfamily C (CFTR/MRP), member 3	M6G	▼
Adcy5	Adenylate cyclase 5	Morphine	▼
Adora1	Adenosine 1 receptor	R-PIA	▼
Adora2a	Adenosine A2a receptor	CI-977	▲
		Deltorphin	▼
Adra2a	Adrenergic receptor, alpha 2a	Buprenorphine, tramadol	▲
		Amitriptyline, clonidine, deltorphin, dexmedetomidine, isoflurane, moxonidine, N_2O, UK 14,304	▼
Adra2c	Adrenergic receptor, alpha 2c	Moxonidine	▼
Adrb2	Adrenergic receptor, beta 2	Morphine	▼
Adrbk2	Adrenergic receptor kinase, beta 2	U50,488	▼
Alox12	Arachidonate 12-lipoxygenase	Morphine	▲
Arrb2	Arrestin, beta 2	Morphine, THC, CP55940	▲
Cacna1e	Calcium channel, voltage-dependent, R type, alpha 1E subunit	Morphine	▲
Calca	Calcitonin/calcitonin-related polypeptide, alpha	Nicotine	▲
		Morphine	▼
Cckbr	Cholecystokinin B receptor	Morphine	▲/▼
		RB-101, SIA	▼
Chrm1	Cholinergic receptor, muscarinic 1, CNS	Morphine	▲
Chrm2	Cholinergic receptor, muscarinic 2, cardiac	Oxotremorine, CMI-936, CMI-1145	▼
Chrna4	Cholinergic receptor, nicotinic, alpha polypeptide 4	Epibatidine	▲
		Nicotine	▼
Cnr1	Cannabinoid receptor 1 (brain)	Nicotine	▲
		Acetaminophen, THC, WIN55,212-2	▼
Cnr2	Cannabinoid receptor 2 (macrophage)	GW405833, JWH133	▼
Comt1	Catechol-*O*-methyltransferase 1	SIA	▼
Dbh	Dopamine beta-hydroxylase	Morphine	▼
Drd1a	Dopamine receptor 1A	Morphine	▲
Drd2	Dopamine receptor 2	M6G, morphine, NalBzoH, U50,488	▲
Faah	Fatty acid amide hydrolase	Anandamide, OL135, SR144528	▼
Foxn1	Forkhead box N1	Morphine	▼
Gabrb3	Gamma-aminobutyric acid (GABA-A) receptor, subunit beta 3	Baclofen, gaboxadol	▼
Gja1	gap junction protein, alpha 1	Acupuncture	▼
Gnaz	Guanine nucleotide binding protein, alpha z subunit	Morphine	▼
Gprk5	G-protein-coupled receptor kinase 5	Oxotremorine	▲

Table I
Continued

Gene	Protein	Analgesic(s)*	Direction†
Grasp	GRP1 (general receptor for phosphoinositide 1)-associated scaffold protein	Morphine	▼
Gria2	Glutamate receptor, ionotropic, AMPA2	Isoflurane	▲
Grin2a	Glutamate receptor, ionotropic, NMDA2A (epsilon 1)	Morphine	▲
Hrh1	Histamine receptor H1	Morphine, orexin A	▲
Hrh2	Histamine receptor H2	Orexin A	▲
		Morphine	▼
Il1r	Interleukin 1 receptor	Morphine	▲
		SIA	▲/▼
Il1rap	Interleukin 1 receptor accessory protein	Morphine	▲
Il6	Interleukin 6	Morphine	▼
Itpr1	Inositol 1,4,5-triphosphate receptor 1	Morphine	▼
Kcna1	Potassium voltage-gated channel, shaker-related subfamily, member 1	Morphine	▼
Kcnip	Kv channel interacting protein 3, calsenilin	THC	▼
Kcnj3	Potassium inwardly rectifying channel, subfamily J, member 3	DAMGO, deltorphin, morphine	▼
Kcnj6	Potassium inwardly rectifying channel, subfamily J, member 6	Baclofen, clonidine, DAMGO, deltorphin, ethanol, morphine, oxotremorine, U50,488	▼
Kcnj9	Potassium inwardly rectifying channel, subfamily J, member 9	Clonidine, morphine, WIN55,212-2	▼
Kcnk3	Potassium channel, subfamily K, member 3	WIN55,212-2	▼
Kcnk9	Potassium channel, subfamily K, member 9	WIN55,212-2	▼
Lmx1b	Lim homeobox transcription factor 1	Amitriptyline, DPDPE, duloxetine, fluoxetine, morphine, U50,488	▼
Lyst	Lysosomal trafficking regulator	Bremazocine, DAMGO, DPLPE, morphine, titfluadom, U50,488	▼
Mc1r	Melanocortin 1 receptor	M6G, morphine, U50,488	▲
Mme	Membrane metallo-endopeptidase	HOE140, thiorphan	▼
Nfe2l2	Nuclear factor, erythroid derived 2, like 2	Cobalt protoporphyrin	▼
Nfkb1	Nuclear factor of kappa light chain gene enhancer in B-cells 1, p105	Acupuncture	▲
Nos2	Nitric oxide synthase 2, inducible, macrophage	Acupuncture	▼
Npy1r	Neuropeptide Y receptor Y1	Neuropeptide Y	▼
Ntf5	Neurotrophin 4	Morphine	▼
Ntsr1	Neurotensin receptor 1	Neurotensin-2	▼

Table I
Continued

Gene	Protein	Analgesic(s)*	Direction†
Oprd1	Opioid receptor, delta 1	BW363U86	▲
		Deltorphin, DPDPE	▼/—
		Nortriptyline	▼
Oprk1	Opioid receptor, kappa 1	Salvinorin A, U50,488	▼
Oprl	Opioid receptor-like	Buprenorphine	▲
		Deltorphin II, dynorphin, NalBzoH, [$Nphe^1$]nociceptin(1–13)NH_2, Ro64-6198	▼
		Morphine	▼/—
Oprm1	Opioid receptor, mu	RB-101	▲
		Buprenorphine, endomorphin-1/2, M6G, morphine, SNC80, tramadol	▼
		DPDPE	▼/▲
		Deltorphin, deltorphin II	▲/—
		U50,488	▼/—
Oxt	Oxytocin	SIA	▼
Pcsk2	Proprotein convertase subtilisin/kexin type 2	SIA	▲
Pdyn	Prodynorphin	U50,488, THC	▼/—
Penk1	Preproenkephalin 1	Nicotine, psalmotoxin 1	▼
Plcb1	Phospholipase C, beta 1	Morphine	▼
Plcb3	Phospholipase C, beta 3	Morphine	▲
Plcb4	Phospholipase C, beta 4	AIDA, Et-18-OCH_3, U73122	▼
Pldn	Pallidin	Morphine	▲
Pnoc	Prepronociceptin	N_2O	▼
Pomc1	Pro-opiomelanocortin-alpha	SIA	▼
Ppara	Peroxisome proliferator activated receptor alpha	GW7647, palmitoylethanolamide	▼
Ppp1r9b	Protein phosphatase 1, regulatory subunit 9B	Clonidine	▲
		Fentanyl, methadone, morphine	▼
Prkcc	Protein kinase C, gamma	Fentanyl, naloxone	▲
Prkce	Protein kinase C, epsilon	Morphine	▲
Prkg1	Protein kinase, cGMP-dependent, type 1	8-Br-cGMP	▼
Prlhr	Prolactin-releasing hormone receptor	Morphine	▲
Rabggta	Rab geranylgeranyl transferase, alpha subunit	Morphine	▲
Rgs9	Regulator of G-protein signaling 9	Morphine	▲
Scn10a	Sodium channel, voltage-gated, type X, alpha polypeptide	Lidocaine	▲
Slc6a2	Solute carrier family 6 (neurotransmitter transporter, norepinephrine), member 2	Morphine	▲
Tacr1	Tachykinin receptor 1	Morphine	▼

Table I
Continued

Gene	Protein	Analgesic(s)*	Direction†
Th	Tyrosine hydroxylase	Morphine	▼
Ucp2	Uncoupling protein 2, mitochondrial	Ethanol	▲

Source: Search performed in the *PainGenes Database* (October 22, 2008). See the *PainGenes Database* (http://paingeneticslab.ca/4105/06_02_pain_genetics_database.asp) for details and references.
* *Abbreviations:* AIDA, (RS)-1-aminoindan-1,5-dicarboxylic acid; DAMGO, [D-Ala^2, N-Me-Phe^4-Gly-ol]enkephalin; DPDPE, D-Pen^2, D-Pen^5]enkephalin; M6G, morphine-6 -glucuronide; N_2O, nitrous oxide; NalBzoH, naloxone benzoylhydrazone; R-PIA, R-N6-(2-phenylisopropyl)-adenosine; SIA, stress-induced analgesia; THC, tetrahydrocannabinol.
†▲, Knockout mice displayed *more* analgesia than wild-type mice; ▼, knockout mice displayed *less* analgesia than wild-type mice; —, no significant difference between wild-type and knockout mice. Where more than one symbol is displayed, there is a contradiction in the literature.

can explain inherited variability (e.g., [91]), but mRNA expression levels can vary due to DNA polymorphisms or experiential factors, via transcriptional regulation or epigenetics. One problem with the interpretation of gene-expression profiling studies (in stark contrast to the techniques described below) is the difficulty in distinguishing cause from effect. Gene expression might be up- or downregulated by a drug because the gene is involved in the action of that drug, or as a response to the action of that drug, or as a response to the up- or downregulation of another gene that was itself regulated by the drug. There is often no way to tell the difference between these possibilities, although the incorporation of multiple time points into study designs can help. By contrast, the great value of linkage mapping and association methods (see below) is that they search for DNA variants (rather than mRNA transcripts), and DNA sequences cannot themselves be altered in any way by any event post-conception, and thus are the cause of the inherited trait (or trait change), by definition.

Linkage Mapping

The only surefire ways of identifying genes and variants underlying inherited trait variability are genetic linkage mapping and the genetic association study [50]. Although they rely on similar assumptions (i.e., linkage disequilibrium after generations of breeding), they play a different role in practice. Linkage mapping involves a full-genome search for linkage to broadly spaced DNA "markers" (usually microsatellites: polymorphic, codominant repeating nucleotide sequences). Because the average length of linkage disequilibrium around a microsatellite is large (≈100 kb), fewer microsatellites are needed to fully cover the genome (reducing the cost of the study), but a successful demonstration of linkage only roughly localizes the responsible gene and polymorphism. As a practical matter, the need for segregating populations in linkage mapping (i.e., a pedigree) has severely limited its use in humans, because available pedigrees are not large enough to provide the statistical power to detect any but the largest-effect genes. Although human linkage mapping has been effective in allowing the identification of single-gene (monogenic) pain disorders such as hereditary sensory neuropathies and familial migraine syndromes [48], attempts to identify genes for complex pain-related traits in humans using this technique have largely failed. However, animals can easily be encouraged to breed the large F_2 hybrid and backcross populations that facilitate statistical power using the linkage mapping design, and a number of laboratories, including mine, have successfully mapped pain- and analgesia-relevant genes in the mouse using the variant of linkage mapping known as quantitative trait locus (QTL) mapping. Published results are shown in Table II. The reliability of the QTL mapping technique is hard to judge, since there are few true attempts at replication in such a small field, but in at least one case a QTL for κ-opioid analgesia (using U50,488H) in the mouse was replicated in humans (using pentazocine) [70].

Table II
Statistically significant QTLs of relevance to analgesia in laboratory mice

Phenotype	Chr.*	LOD†	Loc.‡	Candidate Gene(s)	Evidence§	Ref.
Clonidine	1	4.7	100	*Kcnj9* (94 cM	Mutant, gene expr.	[87]
Morphine	1	4.7 (♀ only)	10	*Oprk1* (6 cM)	Position	[6]
	1	3.2	91	???	—	[87]
	9	5.2 (♀ only)	20	???	—	[6]
	9	4.5	42	*Htr1b* (46 cM)	Pharm.	[6]
	10	7.5	9	*Oprm1* (8 cM)	Receptor binding	[5]
Stress-induced	8	6.1 (♀ only)	56	*Mc1r* (68 cm)	Position	[67]
U50,488	8	2.7 (♀ only)	67	*Mc1r* (68 cM)	Pharm., mutant	[70]
WIN55,212-2	1	4.4	100	*Kcnj9* (94 cM)	Mutant, gene expr.	[87]
	7	4.8	40	*Trpv1* (44 cM)	position	[87]

* Chromosome.
† LOD: logarithm of the odds.
‡ Location of peak LOD score in centimorgans (cM), a unit of genetic distance. Note that confidence intervals in quantitative trait locus (QTL) mapping projects are generally very large.
§ Gene expression: strain-dependent expression of the candidate gene; mutant: null mutation of the candidate gene shown to affect phenotype; pharm.: strain-dependent effects of pharmacological manipulation of the candidate gene product; position: inference based on genomic position of candidate gene; receptor binding: demonstrated correlation of phenotype to strain-dependent density of candidate gene product.

Association Studies

With no need for a pedigree (although some variants of the association study employ two-generation within-family pedigrees to improve power), the association study has become the standard approach to gene/polymorphism identification in human studies of complex traits, and the only one truly appropriate for studies of pharmacogenetics. Association studies involve the comparison of allele frequencies of single-nucleotide polymorphisms (SNPs) between "cases" and (optimally) carefully matched "controls." Because linkage disequilibrium length around a SNP is quite small (≈1 kb), this technique yields much higher resolution than does linkage mapping (although often not high enough resolution to unambiguously define the polymorphisms causing the effect). The trade-off should be obvious. When using the association study design, one either needs to focus one's search on one or a small number of genes, to keep costs down, or spend the still-huge (albeit decreasing) sums of money required to perform a whole-genome association study (WGAS), in which 100,000–500,000 chip-based SNPs are genotyped simultaneously in hundreds-to-thousands of cases/controls. The cost has thus far deterred any pain-relevant (not to mention analgesia-relevant) WGAS studies from being performed; the only studies done so far have examined one or a few genes at a time.

Association studies (including WGASs) have been plagued by problems of non-replication [39], and the pain field has been no exception, with controversies surrounding the potential role of the *COMT, GCH1, MC1R* and *OPRM* genes in experimental and clinical pain states [48]. With respect to analgesia, though, the bulk of the research in humans has focused on the *CYP* (P450) phase I metabolism genes, and the maturity (the link between P450 2D6 [db1] and poor debrisoquine metabolizers dates back to 1988 [34]) and sheer volume of this literature has led to rather clearer conclusions.

Analgesia-Relevant Genes and Variants

Just as drug effects are jointly due to pharmacokinetics (the movement of drugs from one compartment to another, affecting how many molecules of the drug are likely to be at the relevant binding sites, and for how long) and pharmacodynamics (the action of drug molecules at their binding sites, and consequences thereof), so too are there two broad avenues for pharmacogenetic modulation of those drug effects. I will separately consider genes likely to be relevant to analgesic pharmacokinetics and analgesic pharmacodynamics below.

Genes Relevant to Analgesic Pharmacokinetics

Analgesic drugs are subject to metabolic clearance and to active transport across biological barriers. Metabolic enzymes are known to have multiple variants; consequences for drug effects depend entirely on whether the injected drug is inherently active (e.g., morphine) or a prodrug, requiring metabolic conversion to an active form (e.g., codeine). A gene variant producing decreased metabolism would increase the potency of the former drug, but decrease the potency (and likely the efficacy) of the latter. To complicate matters, some active drugs can be metabolized to intermediary forms that are themselves active (e.g., morphine-6β-glucuronide). The logic of genetic variants in transmembrane transporter genes is similarly complex, depending on whether the transporter achieves inward (from circulation to CNS, for example) or outward transport.

Although analgesics other than opioids are metabolized by enzymes with well-known genetic variants (e.g., metabolism of tricyclic antidepressants by *CYP2D6* and metabolism of NSAIDs by *CYP2C9*), and plenty of in vitro evidence exists showing that these variants affect drug levels or actions, direct evidence of the modulation of the analgesic effects by such genetic variants is only available for opioid analgesics, and only for three genes relevant to pharmacokinetics: *ABCB1* (P-glycoprotein), *COMT*, and *CYP2D6*. Of the other obvious candidates, the influence of the gene variant causing the His268Tyr substitution in UGT2B7 (responsible for the phase II glucuronidation of morphine [19]) on morphine dose requirements in postsurgical patients and cancer pain patients was investigated, but no association was seen in either case [21,80].

ABCB1

This gene, also known as *MDR1* (for multidrug resistance 1), codes for P-glycoprotein, an outward transporter found in the liver, kidney, gastrointestinal tract, and in endothelial cells at the blood-brain barrier [20]. Functional impairment of P-glycoprotein would be expected to result in increased bioavailability of an orally administered drug. Differential effects of two opioids, fentanyl and loperamide, have been associated with either genotypes or diplotypes (i.e., genotype at multiple SNPs within a gene) of *ABCB1* [85,92].

COMT

The *COMT* gene codes for catechol-*O*-methyltransferase, importantly involved in monoamine metabolism. This gene has been famously and controversially associated with both experimental and clinical pain (temporomandibular disorder, fibromyalgia) [24,36,101]. With respect to opioid analgesia, however, Rakvag and colleagues [75] have observed that the common Val158Met substitution (472G>A; those with the 158Met allele have lower COMT enzymatic activity) affects morphine consumption in cancer pain patients, with patients homozygous for the 158Met allele consuming less morphine. The authors hypothesize that morphine might be more potent in such patients if this genotype was associated with higher μ-opioid binding density, and this association has in fact been demonstrated in postmortem human brains [7]. If this explanation is true, then the influence of the genetic polymorphism with analgesia is probably better characterized as an indirect pharmacodynamic effect, even though COMT is a metabolic enzyme.

CYP2D6

The *CYP2D6* gene codes for the P450 2D6 enzyme, which is known to have at least 16 variants (called *1 through *16) affecting enzyme function, resulting in individuals with complete absence of metabolic function to those with ultrarapid metabolism [81]. Most of these variants are SNPs, although some are duplications, deletions, or hybrids. In Caucasians tested with dextromethorphan, 7.2% were homozygous for a "poor metabolizer" (PM) genotype [81], and would be expected to receive no analgesia from drugs requiring *CYP2D6* bioactivation, including codeine, oxycodone, hydrocodone, tramadol, ethylmorphine, methadone, and dihydrocodeine. More rare (< 3% of Caucasians) are those with at least one ultrarapid metabolizer (UM) allele, but a number of cases of life-threatening opioid intoxication in UMs have been reported [e.g., 33]. It should be noted that PM and UM frequencies differ greatly in other ethnic populations [89]. A review of this very large literature is beyond the scope of this chapter, but suffice it to say that confirmation that *CYP2D6* genotype affects clinical or experimental efficacy of opioid drugs has been achieved for codeine [14, 84] and tramadol [88, 93], with a preliminary study asserting the same for alfentanil [13]. Inhibition of *CYP2D6* functioning using quinidine does not affect the actions and efficacy of dihydrocodeine [96] and oxycodone [37].

Genes Relevant to Analgesic Pharmacodynamics

IL-1 and IL1RN

Polymorphisms in cytokine genes have been provisionally but controversially associated with a variety of inflammatory pain conditions [e.g., 83]. One recent study examined the role of polymorphisms in the *IL1* (interleukin-1) and *IL1RN* (endogenous interleukin-1 receptor antagonist) genes in morphine consumption (by PCA) in postoperative patients [8]. Only one tentative association was found, that "medium morphine consumers" (those in the second tertile) exhibited a higher frequency of the *2 allele of the *IL1RN* gene than either low or high morphine consumers. Overall, however, no association was found for either gene. Even if *IL1RN* does play some role here, it is unclear whether what is being affected is pain sensitivity or morphine analgesia.

Kcnj9

The mouse strain survey studies described above, in which a similar set of strains was found to be sensitive or resistant to analgesics of separate neurochemical classes, predicted that "master" analgesia genes with broadly generalizable effects may be uncovered. Using three simultaneous F_2 hybrid intercrosses (and haplotype mapping) phenotyping for morphine analgesia, clonidine analgesia, and WIN55,212-2 (a cannabinoid CB_1 agonist), we detected a QTL on distal mouse chromosome 1 affecting all three drugs [87] (see Table II). Gene expression and null mutant evidence strongly support the candidacy of the *Kcnj9* (GIRK3) gene as responsible. In fact, the much better-studied GIRK2 subunit of the G-protein-gated inwardly rectifying potassium channel has already been implicated in mediating analgesia from multiple drug classes [10,59]. Our data suggest that the GIRK3 protein, which forms heterotetramers with GIRK2, may provide the genetic variability in the ability of these channels to modulate pain following their activation by analgesics. The possible relevance of the human *KCNJ9* gene to drug analgesia has not yet been investigated.

MC1R

There is only one clear example of a human association study of relevance to analgesia being directly inspired by a mouse pharmacogenetic finding. My laboratory had previously determined that a gene on distal mouse chromosome 8 was responsible for swim stress-induced analgesia in female but not male mice [67]. Given evidence for the neurochemical commonality of stress-induced analgesia and κ-opioid analgesia, and evidence of similar sex differences in both forms of analgesia [43], we wondered whether this chromosome 8 QTL would affect κ-opioid analgesia in female mice as well. Following the determination that this was true [70], we used a candidate strategy and provided multiple lines of evidence that the responsible gene was *Mc1r*, coding for the mouse melanocortin-1 receptor (see Table II). A small genetic association study was performed in humans, facilitated by the fact that human *MC1R* "mutants" are phenotypically distinguishable (having red hair), and confirmed that female but not male redheads were more sensitive to pentazocine, a κ-opioid-acting analgesic [70]. A follow-up study in *Mc1r*-deficient mutant mice and humans of differing *MC1R* genotypes established the role of the gene in pain sensitivity and μ-opioid analgesia [68]; for these phenotypes no sex differences were observed. A group in the United States has been studying (nongenotyped) redheads as well, finding them to be more sensitive to thermal pain (in direct contrast to our observations using electrical pain) and less sensitive to gas and local anesthesia [52,53].

OPRM1

Besides *CYP2D6*, the most evidence has been amassed for the involvement of the *OPRM1* gene, coding for the μ-opioid receptor, in opioid effects. The potential role of *OPRM1* is obvious, given the fact that the μ-opioid receptor is absolutely required for virtually all morphine effects [45]. Caution in overinterpreting the importance of the *OPRM1* gene is in order, given the results of morphine analgesia QTL studies in the mouse (see Table II), which demonstrate that although the murine *Oprm1* gene is indeed linked to morphine analgesia in this species [5,6], other genes are as well, and the genomic region containing the *Oprm1* gene does not appear to be linked to morphine analgesia on the acetic acid writhing test (H. Hain et al, unpublished data). The murine data suggest that variable μ-opioid receptor density or functioning strongly affects morphine analgesia of thermal nociception in male subjects, with much less of a role in females [6].

Caveats aside, considerable evidence links the common 118A>G SNP (causing an Asn40Asp substitution) of the *OPRM1* gene to variable opioid action in humans. This SNP, besides being common, was thought to be important because of in vitro data suggesting that the amino acid substitution may affect β-endorphin binding affinity [11]; this hypothesis has since been shown to be false [4,9]. Most of the evidence, however, pertains to effects of opioids other than analgesia (i.e., addiction, respiratory depression, pupil constriction), and is outside the scope of the present chapter. With respect to clinical morphine analgesia, cancer patients and postoperative patients with the homozygous 188G genotype have been reported to require more morphine than others [17,18,40,46]. Effects in the same direction have been seen for the efficacy of morphine-6β-glucuronide [78,79] and alfentanil [73] in experimental pain. One study examining patients after abdominal surgery found no association of the *OPRM1* gene with morphine consumption [21]. A very recent study complicates matters, however, observing that the relationship between another A118G genotype and clinical opioid analgesia may work in the opposite direction for fentanyl, which featured a lower ED_{50} (and thus higher potency) in labor pain in women with one or two 118G alleles [49]. In all but the experimental papers it is rather difficult to determine whether the effects of *OPRM1* variants are truly on drug analgesia or pain sensitivity per se; it should be noted that *OPRM1* has shown direct (albeit complex) effects on pain sensitivity in the laboratory setting [30].

Two papers have been published demonstrating interactions between the A118G variant of *OPRM1* and other analgesia-relevant genes. Reyes-Gibby and colleagues [76] re-analyzed the data sets of Klepstad et al. [46] and Rakvag et al. [75], both association studies of morphine consumption in cancer patients, and performed additional genotyping. They observed that morphine consumption was lowest in those patients who were both homozygous for the A118 allele of *OPRM1* and for the 158Met allele of *COMT.* In another study on a new population of cancer patients, significant associations of *OPRM1* A118G and *ABCB1* C3435T polymorphisms with morphine analgesia were achieved independently, but the joint consideration of both genes increased significance levels additively [12].

Future Directions

In the Campa et al. [12] study described above, the authors tout the power of genotyping at the *ABCB1* and *OPRM1* genes in enabling the prediction of "strong responders," "responders," and "nonresponders" to morphine in a clinical setting with sensitivity close to 100% and specificity more than 70%. Although I would be (pleasantly) surprised if any two genes alone held such explanatory power over a broad range of clinical contexts, the simultaneous consideration of multiple genetic variants is clearly the way of the future. Caution is in order, however. Molecular genetic experiments in the mouse have already identified at least 94 genes relevant to drug analgesia; many more are sure to be identified in the future. It is likely that a reasonable subset of these genes feature variants in humans that are frequent enough to explain the genetic portion of the interindividual differences described above. If so, many decades of research will be required before true prediction is possible, and it is important to remember that the majority of the variance is actually nongenetic. Nonetheless, we are clearly making small but significant steps toward individualized pharmacotherapy.

References

[1] Amanzio M, Pollo A, Maggi G, Benedetti F. Response variability to analgesics: a role for non-specific activation of endogenous opioids. Pain 2001;90:205–15.
[2] Aubrun F, Langeron O, Quesnel C, Coriat P, Riou B. Relationships between measurement of pain using visual analog score and morphine requirements during postoperative intravenous morphine titration. Anesthesiology 2003;98:1415–21.
[3] Beecher HK. The measurement of pain: prototype for the quantitative study of subjective responses. Pharmacol Rev 1957;9:59–209.
[4] Befort K, Filliol D, Decaillot FM, Gaveriaux-Ruff C, Hoehe MR, Kieffer BL. A single nucleotide polymorphic mutation in the human μ-opioid receptor severely impairs receptor signaling. J Biol Chem 2001;276:3130–7.
[5] Belknap JK, Mogil JS, Helms ML, Richards SP, O'Toole LA, Bergeson SE, Buck KJ. Localization to chromosome 10 of a locus influencing morphine analgesia in crosses derived from C57BL/6 and DBA/2 mouse strains. Life Sci 1995;57:PL117–24.
[6] Bergeson SE, Helms ML, O'Toole LA, Jarvis MW, Hain HS, Mogil JS, Belknap JK. Quantitative trait loci influencing morphine antinociception in four mapping populations. Mamm Genome 2001;12:546–53.

[7] Berthele A, Platzer S, Jochim B, Boecker H, Buettner A, Conrad B, Riemenschneider M, Toelle TR. COMT Val108/158Met genotype affects the mu-opioid receptor system in the human brain: evidence from ligand-binding, G-protein activation and preproenkephalin mRNA expression. Neuroimage 2005;28:185–193.
[8] Bessler H, Shavit Y, Mayburd E, Smirnov G, Beilin B. Postoperative pain, morphine consumption, and genetic polymorphism of IL-1β and IL-1 receptor antagonist. Neurosci Lett 2006;404:154–8.
[9] Beyer A, Koch T, Schroder H, Schulz S, Hollt V. Effect of the A118G polymorphism on binding affinity, potency and agonist-mediated endocytosis, desensitization, and resensitization of the human mu-opioid receptor. J Neurochem 2004;89:553–60.
[10] Blednov YA, Stoffel M, Alva H, Harris RA. A pervasive mechanism for analgesia: activation of GIRK2 channels. Proc Natl Acad Sci USA 2003;100:277–82.
[11] Bond C, LaForge KS, Tian M, Melia D, Zhang S, Borg L, Gong J, Schluger J, Strong JA, Leal SM, et al. Single-nucleotide polymorphism in the human mu opioid receptor gene alters β-endorphin binding and activity: possible implications for opiate addiction. Proc Natl Acad Sci USA 1998;95:9608–13.
[12] Campa D, Gioia A, Tomei A, Poli P, Barale R. Association of *ABCB1/MDR1* and *OPRM1* gene polymorphisms with morphine pain relief. Clin Pharmacol Ther 2008;83:559–66.
[13] Caraco Y, Maroz Y, Davidson E. Variability in alfentanil analgesia may be attributed to polymorphism in the μ opioid receptor. Clin Pharmacol Ther 2001;69:63/OII-A-64.
[14] Caraco Y, Sheller J, Wood AJJ. Pharmacogenetic determination of the effects of codeine and prediction of drug interactions. J Pharmacol Exp Ther 1996;278:1165–74.
[15] Chapman CR, Hill HF, Saeger L, Gavrin J. Profiles of opioid analgesia in humans after intravenous bolus administration: alfentanil, fentanyl and morphine compared on experimental pain. Pain 1990;43:47–55.
[16] Chesler EJ, Ritchie J, Kokayeff A, Lariviere WR, Wilson SG, Mogil JS. Genotype-dependence of gabapentin and pregabalin sensitivity: the pharmacogenetic mediation of analgesia is specific to the type of pain being inhibited. Pain 2003;106:325–35.
[17] Chou W-Y, Wang C-H, Liu P-H, Liu C-C, Tseng C-C, Jawan B. Human opioid receptor A118G polymorphism affects intravenous patient-controlled analgesia morphine consumption after total abdominal hysterectomy. Anesthesiology 2006;105:334–7.
[18] Chou WY, Yang LC, Lu HF, Ko JY, Wang CH, Lin SH, Lee TH, Concejero A, Hsu CJ. Association of mu-opioid receptor gene polymorphism (A118G) with variations in morphine consumption for analgesia after total knee arthroplasty. Acta Anaesthesiol Scand 2006;50:787–92.
[19] Coffman BL, Rios GR, King CD, Tephly TR. Human UGT2B7 catalyzes morphine glucuronidation. Drug Metab Dispos 1997;25:1–4.
[20] Cordon-Cardo C, O'Brien JP, Casals D, Rittman-Grauer L, Biedler JL, Melamed MR, Bertino JR. Multidrug-resistance gene (P-glycoprotein) is expressed by endothelial cells at blood-brain barrier sites. Proc Natl Acad Sci USA 1989;86:695–8.
[21] Coulbault L, Beaussier M, Verstuyft C, Weickmans H, Dubert L, Tregouet D, Descot C, Parc Y, Lienhart A, Jaillon P, Becquemont L. Environmental and genetic factors associated with morphine response in the postoperative period. Clin Pharmacol Ther 2006;79:316–24.
[22] Dahan A, Kest B, Waxman AR, Sarton E. Sex-specific responses to opiates: animal and human studies. Anesth Analg 2008;107:83–95.
[23] Day RO. Variability in response to NSAIDs: what progress? Agents Actions Suppl 1993;44:3–6.
[24] Diatchenko L, Slade GD, Nackley AG, Bhalang K, Sigurdsson A, Belfer I, Goldman D, Xu K, Shabalina SA, Shagin D, et al. Genetic basis for individual variations in pain perception and the development of a chronic pain condition. Hum Mol Genet 2005;14:135–43.
[25] Dodick DW. Triptan nonresponder studies: implications for clinical practice. Headache 2005;45:156–62.
[26] Edwards RR, Haythornthwaite JA, Tella P, Max MB, Raja S. Basal heat pain thresholds predict opioid analgesia in patients with postherpetic neuralgia. Anesthesiology 2006;104:1243–8.
[27] Edwards RR, Ness TJ, Weigent DA, Fillingim RB. Individual differences in diffuse noxious inhibitory controls (DNIC): association with clinical variables. Pain 2003;106:427–37.
[28] Elmer GI, Pieper JO, Negus SS, Woods JH. Genetic variance in nociception and its relationship to the potency of morphine-induced analgesia in thermal and chemical tests. Pain 1998;75:129–40.
[29] Evans WE, Johnson JA. Pharmacogenomics: the inherited basis for interindividual differences in drug response. Annu Rev Genomics Hum Genet 2001;2:9–39.
[30] Fillingim RB, Kaplan L, Staud R, Ness TJ, Glover TL, Campbell CM, Mogil JS, Wallace MR. The A118G single nucleotide polymorphism of the μ-opioid receptor gene (*OPRM1*) is associated with pressure pain sensitivity in humans. J Pain 2005;6:159–67.
[31] Flores CM, Mogil JS. The pharmacogenetics of analgesia: toward a genetically based approach to pain management. Pharmacogenomics 2001;2:1771–94.
[32] Galer BS, Coyle N, Pasternak GW, Portenoy RK. Individual variability in the response to different opioids: report of five cases. Pain 1992;49:87–91.
[33] Gasche Y, Daali Y, Fathi M, Chiappe A, Cottini S, Dayer P, Desmeules J. Codeine intoxication associated with ultrarapid CYP2D6 metabolism. N Engl J Med 2004;351:2827–31.
[34] Gonzales FJ, Skoda RC, Kimura S, Umeno M, Zanger UM, Nebert DW, Gelboin HV, Hardwick JP, Meyer UA. Characterization of the common genetic defect in humans deficient in debrisoquine metabolism. Nature 1988;331:442–6.
[35] Greenspan JD, Craft RM, LeResche L, Arendt-Nielsen L, Berkley KJ, Fillingim RB, Gold MS, Holdcroft A, Lautenbacher S, Mayer EA, et al. Consensus Working Group of the Sex GaPSotI. Studying sex and gender differences in pain and analgesia: a consensus report. Pain 2007;132(Suppl 1):S26–45.

[36] Gursoy S, Erdal E, Herken H, Madenci E, Alasehirli B, Erdal N. Significance of catechol-O-methyltransferase gene polymorphism in fibromyalgia syndrome. Rheumatol Int 2003;23:104–7.
[37] Heiskanen T, Olkkola KT, Kalso E. Effects of blocking *CYP2D6* on the pharmacokinetics and pharmacodynamics of oxycodone. Clin Pharmacol Ther 1998;64:603–11.
[38] Huskisson E, Woolfe D, Balme H, Scott J, Franklyn S. Four new anti-inflammatory drugs: responses and variations. Br Med J 1976;1:1048–9.
[39] Ioannidis JP. Non-replication and inconsistency in the genome-wide association setting. Hum Hered 2007;64:203–13.
[40] Janicki PK, Schuler G, Francis D, Bohr A, Gordin V, Jarzembowski T, Ruiz-Velasco V, Mets B. A genetic association study of the functional A118G polymorphism of the human μ-opioid receptor gene in patients with acute and chronic pain. Anesth Analg 2006;103:1011–7.
[41] Kaiko RF, Wallenstein SL, Rogers AG, Houde RW. Sources of variation in analgesic responses in cancer patients with chronic pain receiving morphine. Pain 1983;15:191–200.
[42] Kasai S, Hayashida M, Sora I, Ikeda K. Candidate gene polymorphisms predicting individual sensitivity to opioids. Naunyn Schmiedebergs Arch Pharmacol 2008;377:269–81.
[43] Kavaliers M, Choleris E. Sex differences in N-methyl-D-aspartate involvement in κ-opioid and non-opioid predator-induced analgesia in mice. Brain Res 1997;768:30–6.
[44] Kest B, Wilson SG, Mogil JS. Sex differences in supraspinal morphine analgesia are dependent on genotype. J Pharmacol Exp Ther 1999;289:1370–5.
[45] Kieffer BL, Gaveriaux-Ruff C. Exploring the opioid system by gene knockout. Prog Neurobiol 2002;66:285–306.
[46] Klepstad P, Rakvag TT, Kaasa S, Holthe M, Dale O, Borchgrevink PC, Baar C, Vikan T, Krokan HE, Skorpen F. The 118 A>G polymorphism in the human μ-opioid receptor gene may increase morphine requirements in patients with pain caused by malignant disease. Acta Anaesth Scand 2004;48:1232–9.
[47] LaCroix-Fralish ML, Ledoux JB, Mogil JS. The Pain Genes Database: an interactive web browser of pain-related transgenic knockout studies. Pain 2007;131:3.e1–4.
[48] LaCroix-Fralish ML, Mogil JS. Progress in genetic studies of pain and analgesia. Annu Rev Pharmacol Toxicol 2009;49:97–121.
[49] Landau R, Kern C, Columb MO, Smiley RM, Blouin JL. Genetic variability of the μ-opioid receptor influences intrathecal fentanyl requirements in laboring women. Pain 2008;139:5–14.
[50] Lander ES, Schork NJ. Genetic dissection of complex traits. Science 1994;265:2037–48.
[51] Lariviere WR, Chesler EJ, Mogil JS. Transgenic studies of pain and analgesia: mutation or background phenotype? J Pharmacol Exp Ther 2001;297:467–73.
[52] Liem EB, Joiner TV, Tsueda K, Sessler DI. Increased sensitivity to thermal pain and reduced subcutaneous lidocaine efficacy in redheads. Anesthesiology 2005;102:509–14.
[53] Liem EB, Lin C-M, Suleman MI, Doufas AG, Gregg RG, Veauthier JM, Loyd G, Sessler DI. Anesthetic requirement is increased in redheads. Anesthesiology 2004;101:279–83.
[54] Liston EH, Simpson JH, Jarvik LF, Guthrie D. Morphine and experimental pain in identical twins. Prog Clin Biol Res 1981;69:105–16.
[55] Lotsch J, Geisslinger G. Current evidence for a genetic modulation of the response to analgesics. Pain 2006;121:1–5.
[56] Lotsch J, Skarke C, Liefhold J, Geisslinger G. Genetic predictors of the clinical response to opioid analgesics: clinical utility and future perspectives. Clin Pharmacokinet 2004;43:983–1013.
[57] Macintyre PE, Jarvis DA. Age is the best predictor of postoperative morphine requirements. Pain 1995;64:357–64.
[58] Maier C, Hildebrandt J, Klinger R, Henrich-Eberl C, Lindena G; MONTAS Study Group. Morphine responsiveness, efficacy and tolerability in patients with chronic non-tumor associated pain: results of a double-blind placebo-controlled trial (MONTAS). Pain 2002;97:223–33.
[59] Mitrovic I, Margeta-Mitrovic M, Bader S, Stoffel M, Jan LY, Basbaum AI. Contribution of GIRK2-mediated postsynaptic signaling to opiate and α_2-adrenergic analgesia and analgesic sex differences. Proc Natl Acad Sci USA 2003;100:271–6.
[60] Mogil JS. The genetic mediation of individual differences in sensitivity to pain and its inhibition. Proc Natl Acad Sci USA 1999;96:7744–51.
[61] Mogil JS. The genetics of pain. Seattle: IASP Press, 2004.
[62] Mogil JS, Chesler EJ, Wilson SG, Juraska JM, Sternberg WF. Sex differences in thermal nociception and morphine antinociception in rodents depend on genotype. Neurosci Biobehav Rev 2000;24:375–89.
[63] Mogil JS, Grisel JE. Transgenic studies of pain. Pain 1998;77:107–28.
[64] Mogil JS, Kest B, Sadowski B, Belknap JK. Differential genetic mediation of sensitivity to morphine in genetic models of opiate antinociception: influence of nociceptive assay. J Pharmacol Exp Ther 1996;276:532–44.
[65] Mogil JS, Max MB. The genetics of pain. In: M Koltzenburg, SB McMahon editors. Wall and Melzack's textbook of pain, 5th ed. London: Elsevier; 2005. p. 159–74.
[66] Mogil JS, McCarson KE. Identifying pain genes: bottom-up and top-down approaches. J Pain 2000;1(3 Suppl):66–80.
[67] Mogil JS, Richards SP, O'Toole LA, Helms ML, Mitchell SR, Kest B, Belknap JK. Identification of a sex-specific quantitative trait locus mediating nonopioid stress-induced analgesia in female mice. J Neurosci 1997;17:7995–8002.
[68] Mogil JS, Ritchie J, Smith SB, Strasburg K, Kaplan L, Wallace MR, Romberg RR, Bijl H, Sarton EY, Fillingim RB, et al. Melanocortin-1 receptor gene variants affect pain and μ-opioid analgesia in mice and humans. J Med Genet 2005;42:583–7.
[69] Mogil JS, Sternberg WF, Marek P, Sadowski B, Belknap JK, Liebeskind JC. The genetics of pain and pain inhibition. Proc Natl Acad Sci USA 1996;93:3048–55.

[70] Mogil JS, Wilson SG, Chesler EJ, Rankin AL, Nemmani KVS, Lariviere WR, Groce MK, Wallace MR, Kaplan L, Staud R, et al. The melanocortin-1 receptor gene mediates female-specific mechanisms of analgesia in mice and humans. Proc Natl Acad Sci USA 2003;100:4867–72.
[71] Mogil JS, Yu L, Basbaum AI. Pain genes? natural variation and transgenic mutants. Annu Rev Neurosci 2000;23:777–811.
[72] Oertel B, Lotsch J. Genetic mutations that prevent pain: implications for future pain medication. Pharmacogenomics 2008;9:179–94.
[73] Oertel BG, Schmidt R, Schneider A, Geisslinger G, Lötsch J. The mu-opioid receptor gene polymorphism 118A>G depletes alfentanil induced analgesia and protects against respiratory depression in homozygous carriers. Pharmacogenet Genom 2006;16:625–36.
[74] Pavelka K, Peliskova Z, Stehlikova H, Ratcliffe S, Repas C. Intraindividual differences in pain relief and functional improvement in osteoarthritis with diclofenac or tramadol. Clin Drug Investig 1998;16:421–9.
[75] Rakvag TT, Klepstad P, Baar C, Kvam T-M, Dale O, Kaasa S, Krokan HE, Skorpen F. The Val158Met polymorphism of the human catechol-*O*-methyltransferase (*COMT*) gene may influence morphine requirements in cancer pain patients. Pain 2005;116:73–8.
[76] Reyes-Gibby CC, Shete S, Rakvag T, Bhat SV, Skorpen F, Bruera E, Kaasa S, Klepstad P. Exploring joint effects of genes and the clinical efficacy of morphine for cancer pain: *OPRM1* and *COMT* gene. Pain 2007;130:25–30.
[77] Riley III JL, Hastie BA. Individual differences in opioid efficacy for chronic noncancer pain. Clin J Pain 2008;24:509–20.
[78] Romberg R, Olofsen E, Sarton E, den Hartigh J, Taschner PE, Dahan A. Pharmacokinetic-pharmacodynamic modeling of morphine-6-glucuronide-induced analgesia in healthy volunteers: absence of sex differences. Anesthesiology 2004;100:120–33.
[79] Romberg RR, Olofsen E, Bijl H, Taschner PE, Teppema LJ, Sarton EY, van Kleef JW, Dahan A. Polymorphism of mu-opioid receptor gene (*OPRM1*:c.118A>G) does not protect against opioid-induced respiratory depression despite reduced analgesic response. Anesthesiology 2005;102:522–30.
[80] Ross JR, Rutter D, Welsh K, Joel SP, Goller K, Wells AU, Du Bois R, Riley J. Clinical response to morphine in cancer patients and genetic variation in candidate genes. Pharmacogenomics J 2005;5:324–36.
[81] Sachse C, Brockmöller J, Bauer S, Roots I. Cytochrome P450 2D6 variants in a Caucasian population: allele frequencies and phenotypic consequences. Am J Hum Genet 1997;60:284–95.
[82] Scott DL, Roden S, Marshall T, Kendall MJ. Variations in responses to non-steroidal anti-inflammatory drugs. Br J Clin Pharmacol 1982;14:691–4.
[83] Shoskes DA, Albakri Q, Thomas K, Cook D. Cytokine polymorphisms in men with chronic prostatitis/chronic pelvic pain syndrome: association with diagnosis and treatment response. J Urol 2002;168:331–5.
[84] Sindrup SH, Brosen K, Bjerring P, Arendt-Nielsen L, Larsen U, Angelo HR, Gram LF. Codeine increases pain thresholds to copper vapor laser stimuli in extensive but not poor metabolizers of sparteine. Clin Pharmacol Ther 1990;48:686–93.
[85] Skarke C, Darimont J, Schmidt H, Geisslinger G, Lotsch J. Analgesic effects of morphine and morphine-6-glucuronide in a transcutaneous electrical pain model in healthy volunteers. Clin Pharmacol Ther 2003;73:107–21.
[86] Skorpen F, Laugsand EA. Variable response to opioid treatment: any genetic predictors within sight? Palliat Med 2008;22:310–27.
[87] Smith SB, Marker CL, Perry C, Liao G, Sotocinal SG, Austin J-S, Melmed K, Clark JD, Peltz G, Wickman K, Mogil JS. Quantitative trait locus and computational mapping identifies *Kcnj9* (GIRK3) as a candidate gene affecting analgesia from multiple drug classes. Pharmacogenet Genom 2008;18:231–41.
[88] Stamer UM, Lehnen K, Hothker F, Bayerer B, Wolf S, Hoeft A, Stuber F. Impact of *CYP2D6* genotype on postoperative tramadol analgesia. Pain 2003;105:231–8.
[89] Stamer UM, Stuber F. Genetic factors in pain and its treatment. Curr Opin Anaesthesiol 2007;20:478–84.
[90] Terner JM, Lomas LM, Smith ES, Barrett AC, Picker MJ. Pharmacogenetic analysis of sex differences in opioid antinociception in rats. Pain 2003;106:381–91.
[91] Valder CR, Liu J-J, Song Y-H, Luo ZD. Coupling gene chip analyses and rat genetic variances in identifying potential target genes that may contribute to neuropathic allodynia development. J Neurochem 2003;87:560–73.
[92] Wandel C, Kim R, Wood M, Wood A. Interaction of morphine, fentanyl, sufentanil, alfentanil, and loperamide with the efflux drug transporter P-glycoprotein. Anesthesiology 2002;96:913–20.
[93] Wang G, Zhang H, He F, Fang X. Effect of the *CYP2D6*10* C188T polymorphism on postoperative tramadol analgesia in a Chinese population. Eur J Clin Pharmacol 2006;62:927–31.
[94] Wang X-M, Wu T-X, Hamza M, Ramsay ES, Wahl SM, Dionne RA. Rofecoxib modulates multiple gene expression pathways in a clinical model of acute inflammatory pain. Pain 2007;128:136–47.
[95] Wang X-M, Wu T-X, Lee Y-S, Dionne RA. Rofecoxib regulates the expression of genes related to the matrix metalloproteinase pathway in humans: implication for the adverse effects of cyclooxygenase-2 inhibitors. Clin Pharmacol Ther 2006;79:303–15.
[96] Wilder-Smith CH, Hufschmid E, Thormann W. The visceral and somatic antinociceptive effects of dihydrocodeine and its metabolite, dihydromorphine. A cross-over study with extensive and quinidine-induced poor metabolizers. Br J Clin Pharmacol 1998;45:575–81.
[97] Wilson SG, Bryant CD, Lariviere WR, Olsen MS, Giles BE, Chesler EJ, Mogil JS. The heritability of antinociception II: pharmacogenetic mediation of three over-the-counter analgesics in mice. J Pharmacol Exp Ther 2003;305:755–64.
[98] Wilson SG, Smith SB, Chesler EJ, Melton KA, Haas JJ, Mitton BA, Strasburg K, Hubert L, Rodriguez-Zas SL, Mogil JS. The heritability of antinociception: common pharmacogenetic mediation of five neurochemically distinct analgesics. J Pharmacol Exp Ther 2003;304:547–59.

[99] Wolff BB, Kantor TG, Jarvik ME, Laska E. Response of experimental pain to analgesic drugs. I. Morphine, aspirin, and placebo. Clin Pharmacol Ther 1965;7:224–38.
[100] Woodhouse A, Ward ME, Mather LE. Intra-subject variability in post-operative patient-controlled analgesia (PCA): is the patient equally satisfied with morphine, pethidine and fentanyl? Pain 1999;80:545–53.
[101] Zubieta JK, Heitzeg MM, Smith YR, Bueller JA, Xu K, Xu Y, Koeppe RA, Stohler CS, Goldman D. COMT val158met genotype affects μ-opioid neurotransmitter responses to a pain stressor. Science 2003;299:1240–3.

Correspondence to: Jeffrey S. Mogil, PhD, Department of Psychology, McGill University, 1205 Dr. Penfield Avenue, Montreal, QC, Canada H3A 1B1. Tel: 1-514-398-6085; fax: 1-514-398-4896; email: jeffrey.mogil@mcgill.ca.

Placebo Analgesia 20

Philippe Goffaux,[a] Guillaume Léonard,[a] Serge Marchand,[a] and Pierre Rainville[b]

[a]*Faculty of Medicine, University of Sherbrooke, Sherbrooke, Quebec, Canada;*
[b]*Faculty of Dentistry, University of Montreal, Montreal, Quebec, Canada*

All medical treatment necessarily takes place in a particular context. This context includes the therapist's attitudes, psychosocial factors affecting the therapeutic relationship, and the patient's mindset (expectations, desires, and hopes). Accumulating evidence indicates that, at least in some circumstances, therapeutic efficacy is partly attributable to the concordance between the proposed treatment and the patient's belief systems. It is this fraction of the therapeutic response that is commonly called the placebo effect. More formally, the placebo effect is defined as the part of the therapeutic response that is not attributable to the properties of active ingredients. The placebo effect should not be confused with—and the term should not be used interchangeably with—the placebo treatment. Whereas the placebo effect (or response) refers to an outcome, the placebo treatment refers specifically to an inert agent or intervention. In this chapter, we will explore the factors that make placebo treatments effective, and placebo responses strong. We will pay particular attention to the endogenous neurochemical and neurophysiological processes that transform placebo treatments into powerful placebo responses. We will also briefly discuss the use and misuse of placebos in clinical practice.

As discussed above, the placebo response can be understood as a psychobiological phenomenon, which is inexorably tied to the treatment context [38]. Originally, the placebo effect was described solely as a treatment response that occurred following the use of an inactive agent. Because agents were inactive, placebo responders were thought

Pharmacology of Pain
edited by Pierre Beaulieu, David Lussier, Frank Porreca, and Anthony H. Dickenson
IASP Press, Seattle, © 2010

to lack any real ailment (because, logic would have it, an inactive agent would not help alleviate real suffering). As a result of this misconstrued vision, placebos were sometimes used to unmask factitious disorders. Of course this approach is clinically misguided because the placebo effect accompanies all interventions and reflects a normal manifestation of the therapeutic response [12,41,63]. The response explained by the placebo effect certainly differs from one person to the next (and from one context to the next), but it undoubtedly exists.

Today it is generally well accepted that the treatment effect of many active interventions is related to both an active treatment component and a placebo component [65]. In a very elegant study, Amanzio et al. [2] demonstrated the importance of clinical context in predicting the effectiveness of well-known analgesic agents. The authors compared perceived postoperative pain in patients who were openly given analgesic injections ("open" condition) to the pain expressed by patients who did not know when the injections would be given ("hidden" condition). In the open condition, a physician overtly administered an analgesic bolus (buprenorphine, tramadol, ketorolac, or metamizol), informing the patient that the injection would substantially reduce pain. In the hidden condition, the analgesic was administered via a computer-controlled intravenous pump such that the patient could not know when the drug would be administered. The authors observed that the treatment effect was much smaller in the hidden condition than in the open condition. The difference between the two conditions constitutes the placebo effect. These results confirm that patients can use environmental cues (e.g., a physician confirming the experience of immediate relief) to modulate the effectiveness of their treatment. Clearly, the information conveyed by the clinician is very important. Other research teams have authenticated this finding, revealing that treatment effects are greater when patients are convinced of having received an active analgesic than when they are unsure [59].

Methodological Considerations

Multiple factors must be taken into account when assessing treatment effectiveness in general and the placebo effect in particular. It is important to distinguish between the placebo effect and the ensemble of confounding factors that bias evaluation. The first factor to control for when measuring treatment efficacy is natural history. To confirm that an explicit analgesic effect has occurred, it should be clearly dissociated from spontaneous remission or natural variations in perceived pain (e.g., the control conditions in [79]). A similar bias to control for is the phenomenon known as regression to the mean [49]. This phenomenon captures the tendency of fluctuating symptoms to spontaneously evolve toward the mean, independently of treatment. As a result, patients who present with high levels of pain at the beginning of their treatment regime will naturally rate their pain as less intense as time goes by. Such transformation represents a manifestation of clinical change that is unrelated to treatment (including placebo treatments).

Treatment effects may also be biased by the assessment process itself. For example, the subjective assessment of symptoms may be influenced by the patient and the therapist, both of whom may seek to confirm their expectations (compliance bias). To the extent that this phenomenon increases the estimated effect of treatment (e.g., reported decreases in pain), without producing any real symptom relief (e.g., comparable processing of pain), it will constitute a form of report bias rather than an objective improvement. Retrospective assessment bias is another confounder that must be taken into consideration when estimating analgesic responses. Subjective assessments of a symptom such as pain are susceptible to memory distortions that usually serve to amplify reports of analgesia. For example, Feine et al. [26] showed that the pain associated with a prosthodontic treatment is generally underestimated in retrospective as opposed to concurrent assessments. In this study, patients who experienced an increase in pain intensity during treatment (concurrent assessment) reported relief from their pain at the end of the treatment (retrospective assessment). Two additional studies confirm that amplification of relief occurs during retrospective assessments [19,64]. In both these studies, the estimated placebo effect was significantly greater in the retrospective assessment than in the concurrent assessment phase. Such results suggest that mnemonic processes distort and bias the assessment of pain relief. Memory-induced increases in pain relief should not be considered an actual analgesic effect because they denote a distortion of recalled perceptions rather than an accurate recollection of the pain experience.

General Model of the Placebo Effect

The placebo effect may be modeled according to its induction, its psychophysiological mediation, and its actualization (Fig. 1). The induction phase (see Fig. 1A) includes the presence of conditions that favor placebo effects. An excellent example is the treatment ritual, whose significance depends on the individual and the cultural context. Studies that have examined the importance of such rituals reveal that the administration of a treatment, as well as the message associated with it, shape the magnitude of placebo responses. The treatment message can be reassuring, e.g., "This treatment is very effective and will bring you quick relief," or it can be nuanced, consistent with medical reality, e.g., "This treatment is usually effective and provides relief for most patients." A message conveying uncertainty, however, potentially reduces the desirable impact of placebo effects. In some placebo-controlled clinical trials, participants are informed that they have only a 50% chance of receiving the active treatment [59,78]. A message that conveys greater certainty about the effectiveness of treatment will surely optimize the placebo component of treatment (but raises some ethical questions if it is not true). Physical characteristics of a placebo medication, such as its color, size, or quantity, may also contribute to its effectiveness [18,51]. For example, two pills are known to be more effective than one [15], and a "generic" placebo is less effective than a placebo bearing a well-known

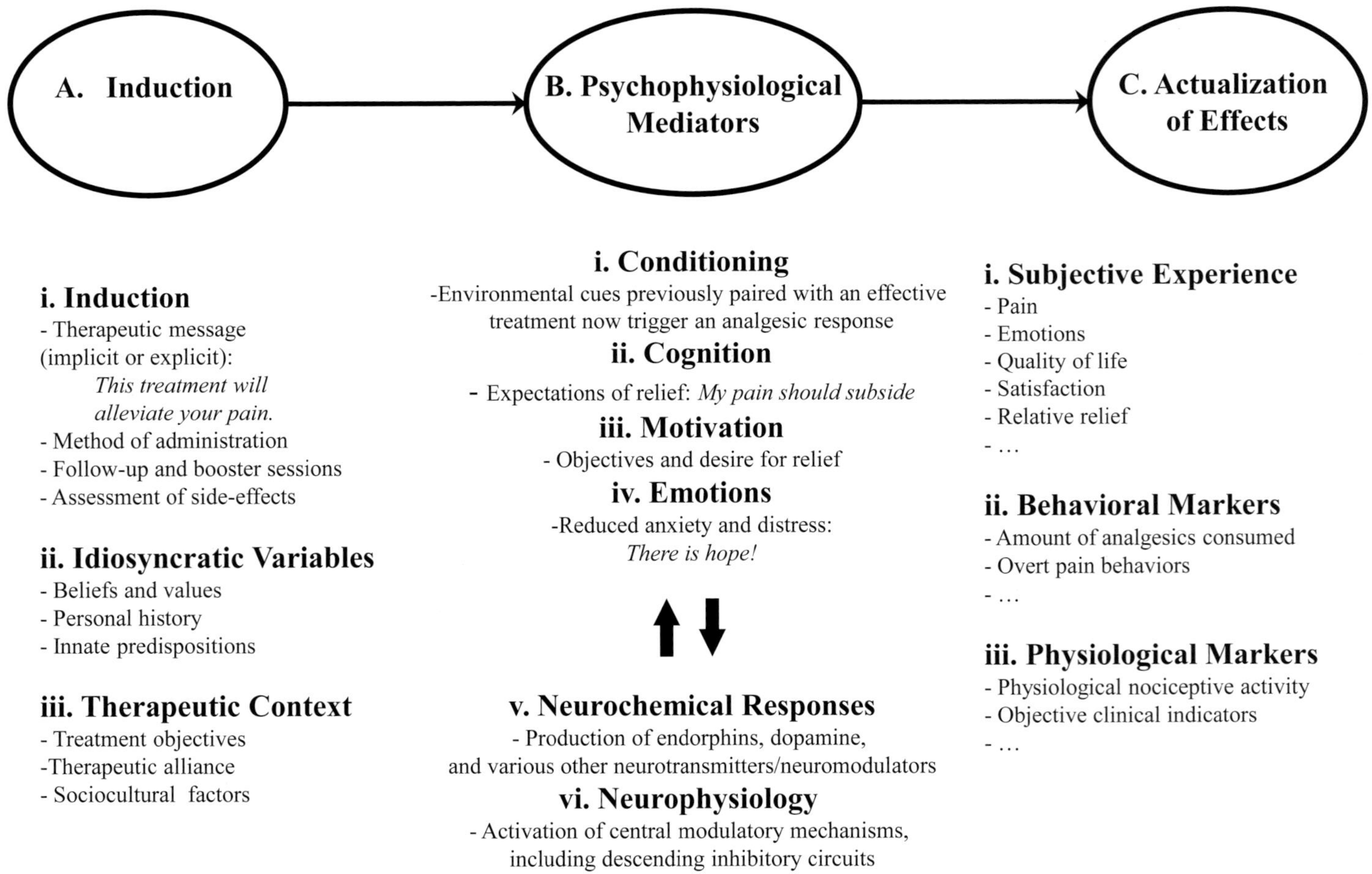

Fig. 1. General placebo model. (A) Overview of the factors contributing to the induction of placebo effects. (B) Psychophysiological mediators responsible for translating contextual factors into placebo responses. (C) Indices that bear witness to the actualization of placebo responses.

analgesic brand-name [17]. It is also thought that more invasive administration methods or treatments (e.g., intravenous or surgical treatments) produce more pronounced placebo effects [18,51] than non-invasive treatments (i.e., topical treatments). Conducting follow-up investigations and recording possible signs of toxicity (i.e., side effects) also contribute to the placebo effect by reinforcing the idea that an active ingredient has been administered.

Despite the importance of the therapeutic ritual, it is not, in itself, sufficient to produce a placebo effect. In reality, the message needs to be directed toward individuals whose characteristics make them amenable to the suggested message. In this way, a placebo will be more potent if it is congruent with the beliefs, values, and goals adopted by the patient [50]. The patient's medical history, and especially his or her previous experience with treatments, may also influence the placebo response (see the discussion of conditioning effects later in this chapter). Treatment history will affect how the treatment message is interpreted. Finally, although some people seem to be more susceptible to placebo effects, it is not clear if this variation reflects a stable predisposition of some individuals [6], or if it simply reflects the influence of idiosyncratic variables such as personal beliefs, values, and treatment history. Future studies are needed to explore this issue.

In summary, the treatment message must be interpreted in light of the treatment context. Is the goal of the proposed treatment consistent with the patient's objectives? Is the therapeutic relationship reassuring, and does it favor the communication of credible information (a relationship of trust)? Is the proposed treatment congruent with the individual's beliefs, cultural practices, and conception of pain, health, and disease? Each of these factors may, at least in principle, influence the placebo response and thus, overall efficacy. It is important to point out that once the treatment message has been received and assimilated by the patient, a cascade of physiological responses will ensure the experience of expected change. These physiological responses are mediators of the placebo effect and constitute the psychophysiological mediation phase of the general placebo model proposed in Fig. 1. Psychophysiological mediators fall into two complementary categories: psychological mechanisms and biological mechanisms (see Fig. 1B). Psychological mechanisms include past experience (i.e., conditioning effects), expectations regarding treatment, motivational variables (including the desire for relief), and variations in emotional state (e.g., reduction of negative mood). Importantly, these psychological mediators have well-defined neurochemical and neurophysiological intermediaries—biological mechanisms—that are responsible for the emergence of the placebo effect. Once triggered, placebo responses can be expressed in a large number of ways and produce quantifiable signs that bear witness to change. These observable signs form the actualization phase of our general placebo model (Fig. 1C).

In the following section, we will review the different psychological mediators of placebo analgesia. Special emphasis will be placed on this particular component of the general placebo model because it bridges the gap between environmental factors and physiological responses.

Psychological Mediators

Various psychological factors have been proposed to explain the placebo effect in general and placebo analgesia in particular. As mentioned above, these factors include conditioning, expectations of relief, motivational features, and emotions. Each factor is addressed in detail below.

Conditioning

One of the first models proposed to explain the placebo effect was classical, or Pavlovian, conditioning [88]. According to classical conditioning theory, the repeated experience of an effective analgesic treatment (the unconditioned stimulus) facilitates the development of robust associations between the active treatment (e.g., an analgesic pill) and the surrounding environment (e.g., the hospital, which is, itself, devoid of intrinsic analgesic properties). Because of repeated associations between specific stimuli and previously neutral indicators, conditioning takes place, thus allowing neutral indicators to trigger a conditioned response. As a result of conditioning, simply presenting neutral stimuli can produce analgesia, even in the absence of active analgesic agents. Most of us, in fact, have already experienced placebo effects. For example, we often start feeling relief (e.g., from a headache) immediately after taking an anti-inflammatory pill. This rapid relief occurs well before the drug's active ingredients have been absorbed, and well before they have had time to produce their physiological effects. In this example, the placebo response is clearly conditioned by our past experience of relief with similar pills.

Experimental studies conducted in the 1980s examined the conditioning model and the validity of claims made to suggest that it could explain the placebo effect. In one of the earliest studies on this issue, volunteers were given painful electric shocks while exposed to a placebo treatment [83]. In the first session (the baseline session), pain perception was evaluated prior to the placebo treatment. In the second session (the conditioning session), an inert cream, presented as an analgesic substance, was applied over the area exposed to the painful shocks. For some subjects, the intensity of the shocks was reduced surreptitiously after application of the cream, thus facilitating the experience of analgesia. For others, the intensity of the shocks was surreptitiously increased, thus violating their expectations of analgesia. Finally, in a third session (the test session), the intensity of the shocks was returned to baseline levels and the properties of the placebo cream were evaluated again. As predicted by the conditioning model, volunteers exposed to a simulation of analgesia in the second session presented analgesia in the third session, while those exposed to a simulation of hyperalgesia (i.e., more pain) presented hyperalgesia, despite having been told that the cream was analgesic. From a clinical perspective, these results suggest that previous experiences can, because of conditioning, influence subsequent experiences of analgesia.

Studies conducted by Benedetti's group also provide important information on the role of conditioning in placebo analgesia. In one of their studies [7], placebo effects were evaluated after prior exposure to the opioid drug buprenorphine. The authors found that when patients first experienced opioid-mediated analgesia, they showed a strong placebo response later on. Furthermore, the magnitude of this response was directly proportional to the magnitude of the previous opioid response. In subsequent investigations, Amanzio and Benedetti [1] discovered a similar relationship in healthy subjects exposed to experimental ischemic arm pain.

If conditioning theory provides a correct explanation of placebo analgesia, it should confirm a progressive decrease in placebo potency over time, because the extinction of conditioned responses is a common characteristic of conditioned responses. Surprisingly, placebo analgesia is particularly resistant to extinction. In fact, a study conducted to investigate this issue found that placebo analgesia increased (rather than decreased) over successive extinction trials [54]. Resistance to standard extinction procedures highlights the limits of the conditioning model in its ability to account for all placebo effects.

Expectations of Relief

In contrast to conditioning theory, expectation theory posits that placebo effects occur solely because of anticipated outcomes. According to this model, the induction of placebo analgesia (see Fig. 1A) depends on expectations of relief and can be created by direct experience, such as conditioning, or by other learning methods (observation, verbal suggestions, and so on). The key ingredient is simply that expectations be created. The way expectations are induced is usually less important than the actual meaning they convey (e.g., low or high expectations of relief). After observing a close relationship between expectations of analgesia and actual pain relief, some authors have suggested that expectations play a causal role in producing placebo analgesia [64].

Although they constitute distinct theories, conditioning and expectation models are closely related because cognitive components (essential to the creation of expectations) link conditioned stimuli to their analgesic effects. In this way, conditioned analgesia can be explained by an increase in expected relief, created by the experience of analgesia during the conditioning phase. Some studies support this interpretation of the placebo effect, at least in humans [54]. Interestingly, this interpretation also agrees with the idea that maintaining placebo responses during extinction trials is attributable to continued expectations of relief.

A brief review of the literature quickly demonstrates that in some circumstances conditioning and expectation effects may interact in an additive fashion. For example, manipulation of the analgesic experience by preconditioning increases expectations of relief compared to simple verbal suggestions of analgesia [13,54,84]. A meta-analysis conducted on placebo analgesia studies recently suggested that expectation and conditioning effects produce comparable results (in terms of absolute magnitude) but that combining these two constituents produces even greater effects [78].

The importance of expectations has also been investigated within clinical contexts. For example, Benedetti's group tested the effect of postoperative saline injections in three separate groups of thoracotomized patients [59]. The first group was told that the injection promoted rehydration (a suggestion of 0% probability of receiving an analgesic). The second group of patients was told that the solution might be an analgesic or might be saline water (a suggestion of 50% probability of receiving an analgesic; the instructions were comparable to those used in single- and double-blinded controlled clinical trials). Finally, the third group was told that the injection was a powerful painkiller (a suggestion of 100% probability of receiving an analgesic). For all three groups, patients could always receive sporadic injections of a true analgesic agent (buprenorphine) upon request. In fact, the measure of interest for this study was the requested dose of this true analgesic agent. Results revealed that the group of subjects who thought they had received an analgesic (suggestion of 100%) asked for smaller doses of buprenorphine, followed by the group who did not know if they had received a placebo or an analgesic (suggestion of 50%). Finally, subjects who knew they had received the saline solution (suggestion of 0%) requested the greatest amount of analgesic to obtain the same level of relief. Therefore, placebo analgesia was greatest when expectations of analgesia were greatest.

Two other components of the treatment response, potentially related to expectations, are the specificity and duration of placebos. Contrary to the idea that placebo effects are nonspecific, recent studies demonstrate that placebo effects can be limited to precise locations on the body [10,55]. In one study, a placebo cream applied to the hand or foot produced analgesia specific to the application site [10]. Furthermore, the placebo effect may persist for several months after treatment ends [21] and may continue to accompany treatment for many years [47]. These phenomena can be attributed to the specificity of expectations concerning location and duration of analgesia.

Placebo Conditioning without Expectations

In the previous sections, we described the contribution of conditioning and expectations to the placebo effect. Some authors [73] have suggested that conditioning may result from both unconscious learning and expectation-related conscious learning. However, in certain circumstances, conditioning may be the only mechanism at play. To investigate this possibility, Benedetti et al. [13] conducted a study focusing on hormonal responses to placebos. Subjects were first exposed to conditioning sessions where they received injections of sumatriptan, a 5-HT_1 agonist used for migraine, which stimulates the secretion of growth hormone and inhibits cortisol secretion. In the test session, injecting saline instead of sumatriptan produced the corresponding hormonal response. This result was obtained even when verbal suggestions of inhibited growth hormone release and increased cortisol secretion were given. It appears, therefore, that hormonal secretion, which is an involuntary and unconscious process, is affected by conditioning but not by expectations. Thus, classical conditioning, without expectations, may be possible for certain unconscious responses. It appears that conditioning contributes to the placebo effect directly and independently of expectations in cases where responses do not involve an experiential dimension.

Motivation

Although expectation of relief is an important contributor to the placebo response, it is probably not the only psychological mediator. For example, it is also thought that a patient's desire for relief explains a large part of the placebo response. Price et al. [64] conducted a study to measure how desire for relief affects the placebo response. The repeated application of a painful heat stimulus was measured before and after application of a placebo cream (a mixture of iodine, thyme oil, and water). Different concentrations of the placebo cream were proposed and applied on different sites of the body. A second cream, presented as a control hydrating solution, was applied on yet another part of the body. Subjects' expectations of relief and desire for relief were measured using visual analogue scales. Verbal suggestions were accompanied by analgesic conditioning (i.e., surreptitiously reducing the intensity of the heat stimulus after application of the placebo cream). To modify the desire for relief, one group of participants was told that they would receive 30 maximum-intensity stimulations, which would be hard to tolerate if the analgesic was not effective (high desire for relief). The other group was told that they would receive six maximum-intensity stimulations, but that most participants had found this easy to tolerate (low desire for relief). All participants, in fact, received six stimulations that were all equal in intensity. A placebo response was observed for the placebo cream. A strong correlation between expectations of relief and placebo analgesia was also observed, consistent with the role of expectations in placebo analgesia. On the other hand, desire for relief did not have a significant impact on placebo analgesia. In their discussion of these results, the authors suggested that this lack of effect is attributable to the relatively low desire for relief in experimental studies compared to clinical studies and that desire for relief, therefore, plays a more important role in pain when it signals a potentially life-threatening illness.

Consistent with this interpretation, Vase et al. [79] showed that desire for pain relief helped to predict the magnitude of the placebo response in a group of patients with irritable bowel syndrome exposed to a clinically relevant painful stimulus (rectal distension). On the other hand, desire had no predictive value for the placebo response when pain was evoked at the left foot using a hot water bath. It is important to note that, even though desire helped to predict the placebo effect for the pain induced by rectal distension, it explained, in itself, no unique variance and was only valuable when combined with expectancies.

The Role of Emotions

The impact of emotions on placebo analgesia remains to be clarified, especially when it comes to studying the effects of anxiety. This consideration is important because the administration of a placebo treatment may reduce the distress associated with pain, and not merely its intensity. If this premise is correct, one would expect a larger reduction in pain unpleasantness than in pain intensity, a result that has sometimes been observed [19,34,46]. Elevated levels of stress may, in some circumstances, also produce analgesia (stress-induced analgesia). However, it is unlikely that anxiety is a mediator for all analgesic or placebo responses because its effects are likely to be general and could not explain evidence of localized pain relief [10,55]. Furthermore, it is not yet clear whether anxiety effects are the cause or the consequence of placebo responses [6]. Nevertheless, a recent study conducted by Aslaksen et al. [4] confirms that when a patient receives information that a painkiller is administered (i.e., a placebo treatment), stress and anxiety are reduced, along with subjective pain scores and cardiac indicators of sympathovagal activity. Importantly, Aslaksen et al. conducted a series of stepwise regressions, which revealed that only subjective decreases in stress were a significant predictor of placebo analgesia. This study indicates that reduced stress is a possible mechanism by which placebos lead to reductions in subjective pain scores.

Pharmacology of Placebo Analgesia and Its Antithesis, Nocebo Hyperalgesia

We have just seen that psychological mediators [64,79] play a key role in the development of placebo effects. However, to better understand placebo responses, it is important to know how the brain modulates nociceptive afferents to promote the expression of anticipated outcomes, which requires a detailed understanding not only of the functional neuroanatomy of the brain, but also of the endogenous neurochemical mediators that make this type of response possible (see Chapter 1).

Placebo Analgesia and Opioids

Although the term "placebo" was used as far back as the 13th century [23], it was not until the late 1970s that the neurophysiological mechanisms associated with this phenomenon began to be understood. At that time, Kosterlitz and Hughes [39] discovered endogenous peptides that could bind with opioid receptors. The analgesic properties of these molecules and the similarities between the response to opioids and the response to placebos (e.g., tolerance and withdrawal; see [81]), caught the attention of Levine and colleagues [44], who were attempting to plumb the mysteries of the placebo response. Their work showed that naloxone, an opioid receptor antagonist, blocked placebo analgesia in a group of patients receiving dental surgery. This result suggests that placebo analgesia depends on the release of endogenous opioids. However, blocking placebo analgesia with naloxone does not exclude the involvement of complementary non-opioidergic systems [35], a premise that was confirmed by Amanzio and Benedetti [1] and Vase et al. [80], who showed that certain placebo conditions were unaffected by the opioid antagonist. Examples include placebo responses involving conditioning with non-opioid drugs and placebo responses associated with chronic pain or hyperalgesic states. Despite evidence that placebo analgesia can sometimes be non-opioidergic, most current neuropharmacological research reveals that placebo analgesia generally involves the opioid system.

Nocebo Hyperalgesia and Cholecystokinin

The administration of inert agents, a prerequisite for placebo effects, sometimes has undesirable consequences, called "nocebo" effects. This term is loosely used to describe the clinical deterioration that accompanies inert treatments or, in pain research, the effect caused by expectations of hyperalgesia (i.e., increased pain). It is important to note that expected hyperalgesia can develop without the administration of an inert substance. Examples include instances where someone has just been given an unfavorable diagnosis or has just been warned that a painful stimulus is imminent [11].

Unlike placebo analgesia, which involves the release of endogenous opioids, the nocebo effect apparently activates cholecystokinin (CCK), a neurohormone found in abundance in the central nervous system [56]. Indeed, Benedetti et al. [11] found that expectation-induced hyperalgesia can be blocked by administering proglumide, a CCK-receptor antagonist. The role of CCK receptors in the nocebo effect is particularly interesting because these receptors are closely associated with the opioid system, displaying similar spinal and supraspinal distribution patterns [29,32,72]. Because of the colocalization of opioid receptors and CCK receptors, some authors believe that CCK acts as a functional antagonist of the opioid system [28,45,87].

Although we have yet to see evidence in support of this claim, increased pain during nocebo treatments could depend on increased brainstem activity within areas involved in the modulation of nociceptive afferents. For example, it is well known that the rostroventral medulla contains pronociceptive efferent circuits triggered by a collection of excitatory cells called "ON" cells [27]. Since CCK directly activates "ON" cells [36], it is possible that the hyperalgesia reported during the nocebo effect depends on these excitatory bulbospinal circuits which facilitate spinal nociceptive activity.

Some researchers have also suggested that the increased pain observed during a nocebo treatment is primarily the result of increased anxiety [8,11]. This hypothesis is partly based on results from animal research showing that CCK has anxiogenic properties [62,66]. In an attempt to clarify the link between CCK, pain, and anxiety, Benedetti et al. [9] evaluated the effect of a nocebo treatment on the levels of adrenocorticotropic hormone (ACTH) and cortisol, two hormones that are biological markers of the stress response. Their results revealed that (1) expectations of hyperalgesia increase both pain and blood levels of ACTH and cortisol, (2) perceptual and hormonal changes are reversed by the administration of diazepam (an anxiolytic), and (3) proglumide blocks the increase in pain but not the increase in ACTH and cortisol. These findings led the authors to propose a model whereby expectations of hyperalgesia increase anxiety levels, which in turn heightens the perception of pain and increases the release of stress hormones. Importantly, the impact of anxiety on pain and stress operates via two distinct pathways, with CCK receptors being involved only for pain. The neurophysiological mechanisms associated with placebo analgesia and nocebo hyperalgesia are summarized in Fig. 2.

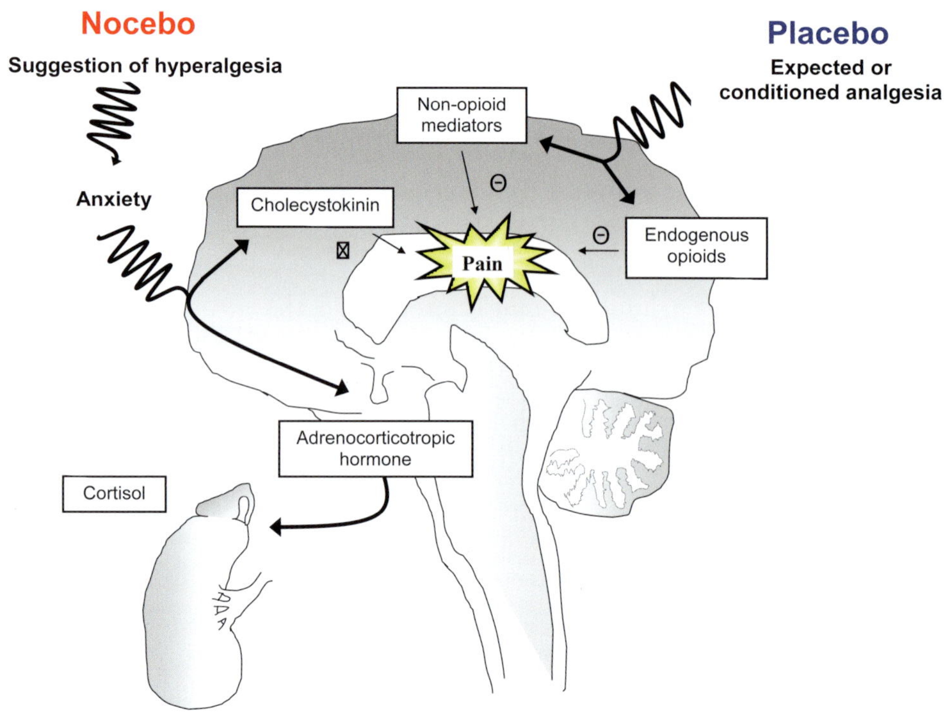

Fig. 2. Neurophysiological mechanisms associated with placebo and nocebo responses. Endogenous opioids, and other nonopioid mechanisms, are triggered following the administration of placebos. Conversely, suggestions of hyperalgesia (associated with nocebo responses) increase anxiety levels. Once increased, anxiety heightens pain perception and increases the release of stress hormones (adrenocorticotropic hormone and cortisol). The impact of anxiety on pain and stress operates via two distinct pathways, with cholecystokinin receptors being involved only for pain. Adapted from Colloca and Benedetti [20].

At the Crossroads of Pharmacology and Neuroanatomy

As we have just seen, the placebo or nocebo effect depends, in large part, on the release of specific endogenous neurotransmitters, secreted in response to expectations of analgesia or hyperalgesia. Unfortunately, the pharmacological studies cited above do not specify the brain structures responsible for the endogenous release of analgesic or pronociceptive agents. Since there is much more information on the structures responsible for producing placebo analgesia (as opposed to nocebo hyperalgesia), the following section will focus solely on imaging studies describing placebo analgesia.

Using positron emission tomography (PET), Petrovic et al. [57] published one of the first studies showing a close link between placebo analgesia and opioid analgesia. The results of their research confirm increased activity in the dorsal part of the anterior cingulate cortex (ACC; the prefrontal area of the brain) during both placebo and opioid-mediated analgesia. Interestingly, the prefrontal activity observed during opioid-mediated analgesia was greatest in subjects who had strong placebo responses, suggesting a close link between the placebo response and the response to opioids. Finally, the authors discovered that increased activity in the prefrontal area was accompanied by increased activity in the periaqueductal gray matter (a mesencephalic region containing a large number of opioidergic neurons), which suggests that the prefrontal area is probably involved in the regulation of endogenous opioid activity in response to expectations of relief. Collectively, these results are important because they show that opioid-based and placebo neuronal systems overlap considerably.

To better identify the regions of the brain responsible for the secretion of opioids, Zubieta et al. [89] (and later Wager et al. [86]) conducted a series of PET studies using a radioactive μ-opioid receptor tracer, $[^{11}C]$carfentanil. Using this tracer, they discovered that during expectations of relief, opioid secretion increased significantly in the prefrontal dorsolateral cortex, anterior cingulate, anterior insula, nucleus accumbens, amygdala, medial prefrontal cortex, periaqueductal gray matter, raphe nucleus, and nucleus cuneiformis. These structures form part of a complex limbic and paralimbic circuit. They play a key role in a wide variety of human functions and abilities, including the perception of pain, the anticipation of future events, the assessment of the affective qualities of a given stimulus, motivation, reinforcement, the selection of motor schemas, and even the expression of empathy for the pain of others [30,31,52,70]. Since placebo analgesia triggers some or all of these functions, it is not surprising to find that limbic and paralimbic structures are activated during this type of analgesic treatment.

Although the work of Petrovic et al. [57], Zubieta et al. [89], and Wager et al. [86] provides some information regarding the neurobiology of placebo analgesia, it does not delineate the precise role played by the brain in preparation for—and in response to—anticipated pain relief. This aspect of placebo will be discussed in the next section. We will first look at the structures activated during the anticipation phase (i.e., structures that prepare the system for an expected response) and then discuss the structures activated in response to pain itself (i.e., structures whose activity changes during placebo analgesia).

Functional Neuroanatomy of Placebo

Anticipation Phase

In the past decade or so, many studies have examined the pain phenomenon by exploring the different brain structures activated when a nociceptive stimulus is administered. Although there is some variability in the specific signature obtained, two systems are regularly activated. The first is known as the lateral pain pathway, which includes the primary and secondary somatosensory areas, thalamus, and posterior insula and has been associated mainly with sensory/discriminative assessments. The second system is known as the medial pain pathway, which includes prefrontal areas, the ACC, and the anterior insula and has been associated mainly with motivational/affective assessments. Together, these pathways are activated in response to noxious insults, but are sometimes accompanied by changes in other brain areas, including the basal ganglia, amygdala, hippocampus, entorhinal cortex, parietal regions, and posterior fossa nuclei [3,22,75,77]. Interestingly, some structures are activated before the arrival of noxious drives, depending on prevailing expectations. Thus, in the first brain imaging study on pain anticipation, Ploghaus et al. [58] discovered that activity in the medial prefrontal cortex (including the ACC in some subjects), the anterior insula, and the cerebellum increased in response to a cue signaling impending pain. These structures were also active during the actual experience of pain but in a more posterior location, suggesting a rostrocaudal organization of the networks involved in the anticipation and experience of pain.

Despite these compelling results, we should point out that some imaging studies also observe increased activity in the primary somatosensory area corresponding to the dermatome where pain is expected [60,61]. Since the primary somatosensory cortex is involved in the spatial localization of sensory events, this suggests that some form of early attentional control is triggered in advance of probable tissue damage. It is interesting to note that increased preparatory activity in the primary somatosensory cortex is common in patients who suffer from chronic pain [71]. This evidence suggests that attentional functions are quickly mobilized when pain is clinically significant.

Finally, we should note that the limbic system, including the striatum, is also activated during the anticipatory phase [37]. This area of the brain enables behavioral adaptation to salient stimuli (aversive or reinforcing). Thus, the striatum becomes active in advance of a painful shock, but only if the anticipated shock is thought to be intense and/or unpleasant. This conclusion agrees with recent data demonstrating that the striatum plays a key role in reward expectation processing—an important ingredient in the creation of placebo effects, according to expectation theory. Given that reward expectations are known to depend on the activity of mesolimbic dopamine neurons [68,74], this evidence raises the possibility that dopamine activity (in addition to endorphin activity) contributes to the formation of placebo effects. In an attempt to confirm this possibility, Scott et al. [69] found that their placebo treatment (intravenous saline) was associated with increased dopamine release in the ventral striatum (nucleus accumbens). Moreover, this increase was correlated with subjective reports of analgesic expectation, thus confirming the importance of limbic activity and dopamine release in placebo-induced expectation. The interplay between endogenous dopamine and opioid systems is only now being looked at in placebo analgesia studies. Future experiments in this field are eagerly awaited and will surely increase our understanding of the neurobiology of placebo effects.

In addition to prefrontal, somatosensory, and limbic areas, the periaqueductal gray is also activated during the anticipation phase. In fact, activity in this area powerfully predicts the strength of placebo responses [24], confirming that brainstem nuclei play an important part of the placebo response. We should note that the periaqueductal gray contains the cell bodies of the main descending inhibitory pathways. These pathways are neuroanatomically very similar to the excitatory pathways described earlier in the nocebo section. However, unlike the excitatory pathways, the inhibitory pathways have been shown to reduce the intensity of the nociceptive afferents entering the spine [16,42,43,76]. They are also involved in a variety of analgesic conditions induced by cognitive modulation such as distraction and hypnosis (reviewed in [67]). The modulation of spinal responses has not yet been shown directly in placebo studies, although recent observations showing an effect of expectations on cerebrospinal inhibition is consistent with this possibility [33]. In this study, Goffaux et al. found that expectations of hyperalgesia completely blocked the analgesic properties of a standard counterirritation procedure (immersion of the arm in a bath of cold water), which is known to activate descending inhibitory systems. The authors evoked experimental pain through intermittent electrical stimulations of the left ankle over the retromalleolar path of the sural nerve. When sufficiently intense, this type of stimulation triggers a nociceptive spinal withdrawal reflex (measured by electromyographic recordings of the knee flexor muscle), whose amplitude correlates with stimulation intensity. During immersion, there was a significant reduction in perceived sural nerve pain and reflex amplitude in patients who correctly expected that the immersion would have analgesic properties. On the other hand, participants who expected that the immersion would have pain-enhancing properties showed an increase in perceived sural nerve pain and a complete abolition of the normal reduction in reflex amplitude. Clearly, then, expectations affect the normal functioning of descending inhibitory circuits, modulating the processing of nociceptive signals well before they ascend to the brain.

The studies reviewed above demonstrate that mere suggestions can trigger a complex pattern of cortical and subcortical activity. Of course, this activity is also observed when suggestions are accompanied by actual placebo treatments. In a series of rigorously designed experiments, Wager et al. [85] showed that immediately prior to the administration of a painful stimulus (thermal or electric), subjects given a placebo cream showed more activity in the periaqueductal gray, medial prefrontal, dorsolateral, and anterior cingulate cortex (dorsal subsection). Furthermore, this activity predicted the analgesia experienced by subjects. These results confirm that during analgesic treatments, the brain mobilizes the prefrontal regions responsible for the mental representation of pain and activates opioid-rich structures in the periaqueductal gray in an attempt to produce systemic changes in pain sensitivity.

During the preparatory phase, therefore, prefrontal areas of the cortex are activated to create and maintain a mental representation of anticipated pain (or pain relief). Limbic structures are also activated and contribute to the emotional reaction to aversive stimuli. Finally, opioid-rich nuclei located in the brainstem are recruited, potentially triggering inhibitory efferents and dampening all nociceptive information entering the spine. Some of the cortical and subcortical areas activated during the anticipatory phase are shown in Fig. 3.

Modulation of the Pain Signal (Placebo Response)

Even though anticipatory processes may activate spinal inhibitory circuits, reducing the intensity of pain signals entering the cortex, placebo analgesia also depends on the collection of cortical processes triggered during the experience of pain itself. For example, in the Wager et al. [85] study described above, placebos reduced pain-evoked activity in the

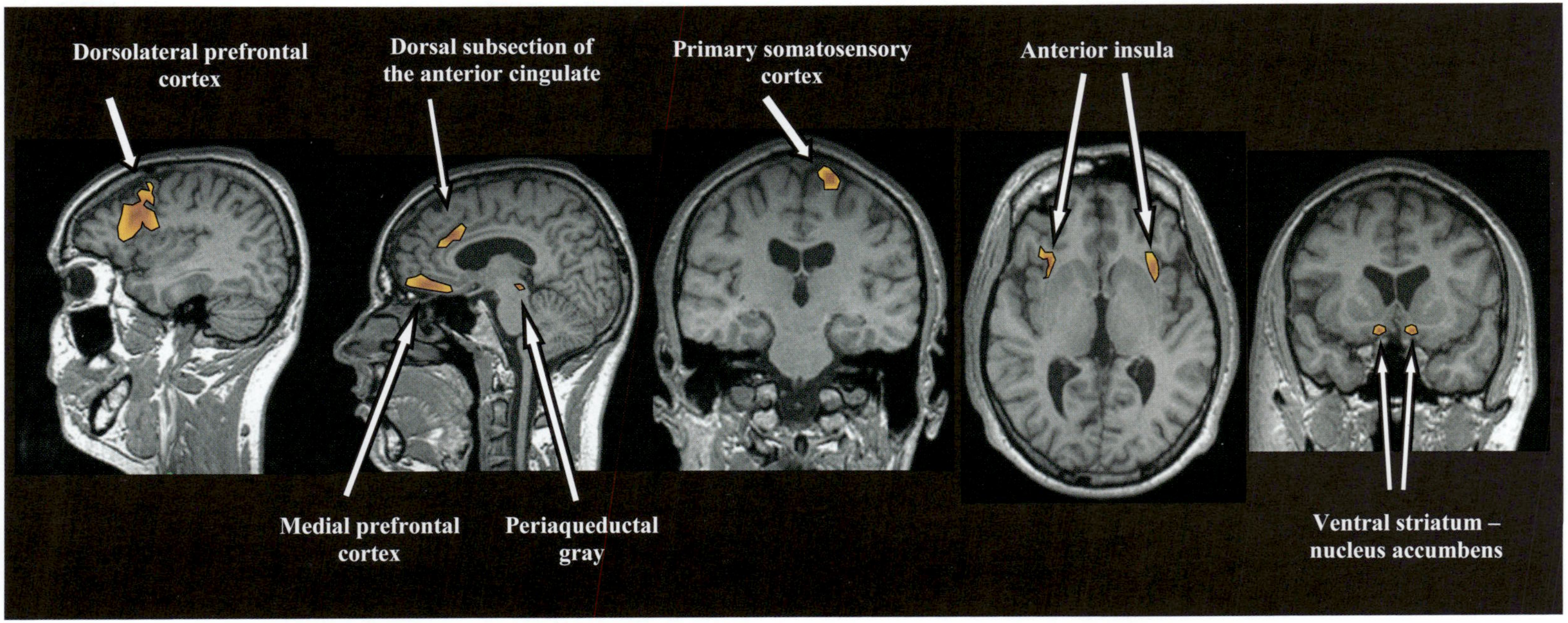

Fig. 3. Increased activity in the medial prefrontal cortex, anterior insula, striatum and primary somatosensory cortex is observed when pain (or more pain) is expected, while increased activity in the dorsal subsection of the anterior cingulate, dorsolateral prefrontal cortex, medial prefrontal cortex and periaqueductal gray is observed when analgesia is expected. It is important to note that increased activity in the medial prefrontal cortex is observed when either analgesia or hyperalgesia is anticipated. Future studies are necessary to test the possibility that specific subsections of the medial prefrontal cortex are involved in processing expectations of analgesia versus hyperalgesia specifically.

thalamus, insula, and ACC (the caudal part of the supracallosal subsection) during pain stimulation, confirming that placebo treatments modify the activity normally related to pain processing. Reduced pain-related cortical activity was also noted by Koyama et al. [40] in response to moderately painful stimuli when subjects expected low pain stimuli. The authors showed that when reduced pain was expected, standard pain-evoked cortical activity decreased in the thalamus, primary and secondary somatosensory areas, insula, anterior cingulate, and prefrontal areas of the brain. Once again, these results suggest that pain can be construed as a dynamic phenomenon triggered by the nociceptive stimulus but intimately dependent upon the preexisting state of the system.

In a more recent study conducted on this issue, Bingel et al. [14] found that during painful stimulations, a placebo cream reduced the activity recorded in the cerebellum, thalamus, insula, and somatosensory regions. Surprisingly, the subgenual part of the anterior cingulate showed increased (not decreased) activity. This increase covaried with responses observed in the amygdala (a limbic structure responsible for the physiological expression of negative emotions), and the periaqueductal gray (a structure involved in descending inhibition). The authors suggested that sustained activity of the subgenual cingulate helps to control limbic and infratentorial antinociceptive responses. The interaction between prefrontal and periaqueductal regions observed by Bingel et al. [14] during the experience of analgesia is reminiscent of the interaction observed by Wager et al. [85] between the prefrontal cortex and the periaqueductal gray during the anticipation of analgesia. This evidence strongly suggests that once triggered, antinociceptive responses (originating in the brainstem and controlled by prefrontal areas) must be maintained until the pain stimulation ends; otherwise, one can presume, placebo analgesia would not be as great.

We should point out, however, an important difference between the anticipatory prefrontal activity obtained by Wager et al. [85] and the pain-evoked prefrontal activity obtained by Bingel et al. [14]. During the anticipation phase, Wager et al. observed increased activity in the dorsal subsection of the ACC, an area of the brain particularly involved in the anticipation of pain and the attention paid to pain [25,53]. This area is also linked to descending inhibitory circuits of the brainstem. On the other hand, it is primarily the subgenual part of the cingulate cortex (around the genu of the corpus callosum) that is activated during painful stimulations in placebo conditions. Unlike the dorsal region of the ACC, the subgenual region is involved in the modulation of negative affects and the encoding of pain memories [48,82]. It is also strongly paired with activity in the amygdala. Thus increased activity in the subgenual part of the cingulate cortex may contribute to the reappraisal of nociceptive afferent signals, consistent with early conceptions of placebo biology.

It is clear from the data reviewed above that the prefrontal cortex plays an important role in placebo analgesia, whether it be during the anticipation phase or in response to pain itself. Nevertheless, further research is needed to better understand the diversity of prefrontal functions responsible for the development of placebo analgesia and expectations in general. A review of the cortical changes observed in response to pain during placebo analgesia is provided in Fig. 4. The reader will note an important overlap between the structures activated during the anticipation phase and those activated during the pain response in placebo conditions. Comparable activation during these two phases is a good illustration of what happens during placebo analgesia, in which the mental representation of pain requires a (re)activation of the same cortical areas as those involved during pain processing. In fact, a growing number of imaging studies now show that to modulate pain, the cortical signature of pain must be reactivated and transformed using the executive and inhibitory functions attributable to prefrontal and subcortical regions, respectively.

Clinical Implications

As we have seen in this chapter (and contrary to long-held beliefs), placebo analgesia and nocebo hyperalgesia are not simply response biases. Instead, they are the product of neurophysiological processes that modulate the integration of the nociceptive signals throughout the central nervous system (secretion of endogenous opioids or CCK, increased or decreased cortical activity, etc.). In light of this conclusion, and because the changes reported are based on measurable physiological phenomena, the use of placebos as a tool to diagnose factitious disorders is not only unwarranted, but also (and above all) useless from a scientific and clinical standpoint.

An important clinical implication surrounding the use of placebos concerns the potentiation of treatment effects. Clinicians should not try to avoid the placebo effect; on the contrary, they should try to potentiate it. A good demonstration of this premise was provided in a recent study conducted by Goffaux et al. [33], where the authors were able to either increase or block the effect of a genuine analgesic procedure merely by manipulating expectations. Clinically, these results suggest that treatment efficacy increases when both the clinician and the patient take a positive attitude towards treatment and, conversely, that treatment efficacy is jeopardized if the prevailing attitude is negative. The objective is not to create false or exaggerated expectations (where patients would risk experiencing disappointment) but rather to be confident in the proposed treatment. Special care should also be taken to avoid creating expectations of hyperalgesia (e.g., an erroneous negative prognosis) or expectations of no effect from the proposed treatment, which would hamper the effectiveness of future treatments.

Even if the treatment message seems to be a critical component underlying placebo analgesia, we must not forget that the medical context and the patient's history are also very important. For example, Charron et al. [19] found that the effectiveness of placebo analgesia was greatest when subjects were first exposed to the placebo than when they were first exposed to the control condition. This result reminds us that it is very important to respond quickly to our patients' pain complaints. Current practice, where physicians start with low analgesic doses before gradually ramping up to larger

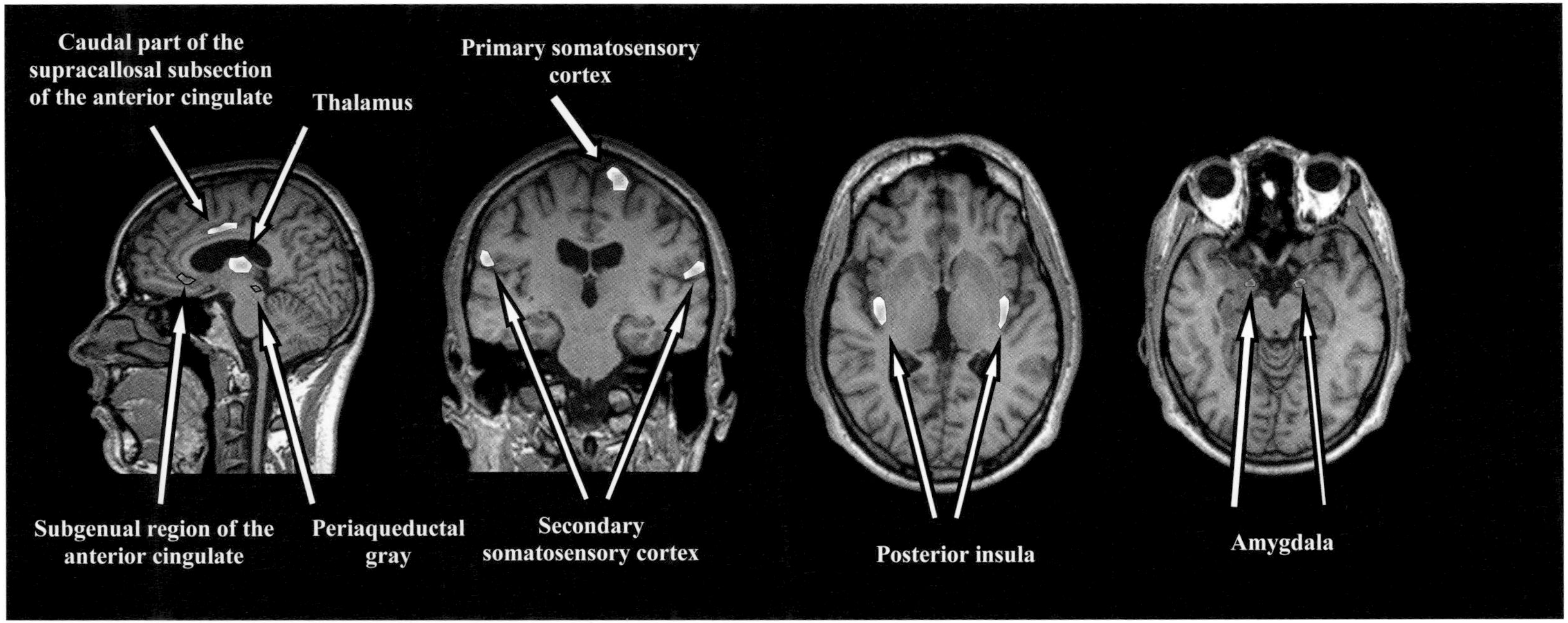

Fig. 4. Response to normally painful stimuli under conditions of placebo analgesia produce increased activity in the subgenual anterior cingulate, amygdala, and periaqueductal gray, while reduced activity is observed in the caudal part of the supracallosal subsection of the anterior cingulate, posterior insula, primary and secondary somatosensory cortices, and thalamus. Cortical responses with a red focus indicate increased activity, and those in white indicate reduced activity.

doses, exposes patients to an initial barrage of inefficacy, which increases the likelihood of experiencing subsequent treatment failure. When unmotivated by legitimate concerns (such as an elevated risk of cardiorespiratory depression, use of an analgesic that requires titration, or the presence of serious side effects), this conservative approach may not be optimal.

Finally, we want to dispel one of the most commonly held misconceptions regarding placebos, namely that around 30% of subjects will respond to a placebo procedure or that 30% of any treatment effect is attributable to nonspecific or placebo effects. This figure derives from a misinterpretation of the results of a meta-analysis by Beecher [5]. Beecher reviewed the results of 15 clinical studies that included a placebo arm and that covered a wide variety of different conditions such as postoperative pain, angina pectoris, anxiety, and the common cold. On average, symptoms were satisfactorily relieved in 35% of the patients. However, there was considerable variability in the occurrence of the placebo response in the individual studies. Beecher's conclusions are heavily contested today because the author did not take into account factors such as expectations and motivation. It is possible, for example, that patients who did not respond to a placebo in the context of a study reviewed by Beecher could respond in another context.

Conclusion

Recent studies suggest that the placebo effect is present in many clinical interventions and that it can, in some cases, be very powerful. We now know that the placebo effect depends on a variety of neurochemical and neurophysiological mechanisms, which are measurable and modifiable. Therefore, the placebo response must not be seen as an indication of weakness or malingering and should not be used to diagnose psychosomatic illness.

For researchers, the placebo effect is often perceived as a nuisance that has to be measured and controlled for (so as to witness the true effects of new analgesics). However, for health professionals, the objective is to benefit from the placebo response in order to increase the effectiveness of proposed treatments, while at the same time respecting the ethical principles of free and informed consent. This situation is only possible when the clinician uses an active and legitimate treatment, which can be enhanced by tapping into the patient's expectancies and experiences of good analgesia. In clinical settings, patients evaluate their treatment using their own set of beliefs, therapeutic history, and other individual characteristics, which make them more or less inclined to show a strong placebo effect. At the other end of the therapeutic relationship, the role of the health professional goes well beyond treatment administration. Whether they are aware of it or not, clinicians contribute to the placebo effect by their attitude and by the way in which they communicate relevant information to their patients. Decades of research on the placebo effect have taught us that the human dimension, and its contribution to the therapeutic relationship, truly helps relieve pain and suffering, bringing about quantifiable changes in pain processing.

Acknowledgment

This work was supported by grants from the Canadian Institutes of Health Research (CIHR), and the Fonds de Recherche en Santé du Québec (FRSQ).

References

[1] Amanzio M, Benedetti F. Neuropharmacological dissection of placebo analgesia: expectation-activated opioid systems versus conditioning-activated specific subsystems. J Neurosci 1999;19:484–94.

[2] Amanzio M, Pollo A, Maggi G, Benedetti F. Response variability to analgesics: a role for non-specific activation of endogenous opioids. Pain 2001;90:205–15.

[3] Apkarian AV, Bushnell MC, Treede RD, Zubieta JK. Human brain mechanisms of pain perception and regulation in health and disease. Eur J Pain 2005;9:463–84.

[4] Aslaksen PM, Flaten MA. The roles of physiological and subjective stress in the effectiveness of a placebo on experimentally induced pain. Psychosom Med 2008;70:811–8.

[5] Beecher HK. The powerful placebo. J Am Med Assoc 1955;159:1602–6.

[6] Benedetti F, Amanzio M. The neurobiology of placebo analgesia: from endogenous opioids to cholecystokinin. Prog Neurobiol 1997;52:109–25.

[7] Benedetti F, Amanzio M, Baldi S, Casadio C, Cavallo A, Mancuso M, Ruffini E, Oliaro A, Maggi G. The specific effects of prior opioid exposure on placebo analgesia and placebo respiratory depression. Pain 1998;75:313–9.

[8] Benedetti F, Amanzio M, Casadio C, Oliaro A, Maggi G. Blockade of nocebo hyperalgesia by the cholecystokinin antagonist proglumide. Pain 1997;71:135–40.

[9] Benedetti F, Amanzio M, Vighetti S, Asteggiano G. The biochemical and neuroendocrine bases of the hyperalgesic nocebo effect. J Neurosci 2006;26:12014–22.

[10] Benedetti F, Arduino C, Amanzio M. Somatotopic activation of opioid systems by target-directed expectations of analgesia. J Neurosci 1999;19:3639–48.

[11] Benedetti F, Lanotte M, Lopiano L, Colloca L. When words are painful: unraveling the mechanisms of the nocebo effect. Neuroscience 2007;147:260–71.

[12] Benedetti F, Mayberg HS, Wager TD, Stohler CS, Zubieta JK. Neurobiological mechanisms of the placebo effect. J Neurosci 2005;25:10390–402.

[13] Benedetti F, Pollo A, Lopiano L, Lanotte M, Vighetti S, Rainero I. Conscious expectation and unconscious conditioning in analgesic, motor, and hormonal placebo/nocebo responses. J Neurosci 2003;23:4315–23.

[14] Bingel U, Lorenz J, Schoell E, Weiller C, Buchel C. Mechanisms of placebo analgesia: rACC recruitment of a subcortical antinociceptive network. Pain 2006;120:8–15.

[15] Blackwell B, Bloomfield SS, Buncher CR. Demonstration to medical students of placebo responses and non-drug factors. Lancet 1972; 1:1279–82.

[16] Bouhassira D, Chitour D, Villaneuva L, Le Bars D. The spinal transmission of nociceptive information: modulation by the caudal medulla. Neuroscience 1995;69:931–8.

[17] Branthwaite A, Cooper P. Analgesic effects of branding in treatment of headaches. Br Med J (Clin Res Ed) 1981;282:1576–8.

[18] Buckalew LW, Coffield KE. An investigation of drug expectancy as a function of capsule color and size and preparation form. J Clin Psychopharmacol 1982;2:245–8.

[19] Charron J, Rainville P, Marchand S. Direct comparison of placebo effects on clinical and experimental pain. Clin J Pain 2006;22:204–11.

[20] Colloca L, Benedetti F. Placebos and painkillers: is mind as real as matter? Nat Rev Neurosci 2005;6:545–52.

[21] Colloca L, Lopiano L, Lanotte M, Benedetti F. Overt versus covert treatment for pain, anxiety, and Parkinson's disease. Lancet Neurol 2004;3:679–84.

[22] Dunckley P, Wise RG, Fairhurst M, Hobden P, Aziz Q, Chang L, Tracey I. A comparison of visceral and somatic pain processing in the human brainstem using functional magnetic resonance imaging. J Neurosci 2005;25:7333–41.

[23] Edwards M. Placebo. Lancet 2005;365:1023.

[24] Fairhurst M, Wiech K, Dunckley P, Tracey I. Anticipatory brainstem activity predicts neural processing of pain in humans. Pain 2007;128:101–10.

[25] Faymonville ME, Roediger L, Del Fiore G, Delgueldre C, Phillips C, Lamy M, Luxen A, Maquet P, Laureys S. Increased cerebral functional connectivity underlying the antinociceptive effects of hypnosis. Brain Res Cogn Brain Res 2003;17:255–62.

[26] Feine JS, Lavigne GJ, Dao TT, Morin C, Lund JP. Memories of chronic pain and perceptions of relief. Pain 1998;77:137–41.

[27] Fields H. State-dependent opioid control of pain. Nat Rev Neurosci 2004;5:565–75.

[28] Fields H, Basbaum A, Heinricher MM. Central nervous system mechanisms of pain modulation. In: McMahon SB, Koltzenburg M, editors. Wall and Melzack's Textbook of Pain, 5th ed. China: Elsevier Churchill Livingstone; 2006. p. 125–42.

[29] Gall C, Lauterborn J, Burks D, Seroogy K. Co-localization of enkephalin and cholecystokinin in discrete areas of rat brain. Brain Res 1987;403:403–8.

[30] Gear RW, Aley KO, Levine JD. Pain-induced analgesia mediated by mesolimbic reward circuits. J Neurosci 1999;19:7175–81.
[31] Gear RW, Levine JD. Antinociception produced by an ascending spino-supraspinal pathway. J Neurosci 1995;15:3154–61.
[32] Gibbins IL, Furness JB, Costa M. Pathway-specific patterns of the co-existence of substance P, calcitonin gene-related peptide, cholecystokinin and dynorphin in neurons of the dorsal root ganglia of the guinea-pig. Cell Tissue Res 1987; 248:417–37.
[33] Goffaux P, Redmond WJ, Rainville P, Marchand S. Descending analgesia: when the spine echoes what the brain expects. Pain 2007;130:137–43.
[34] Gracely RH, McGrath P, Dubner R. Validity and sensitivity of ratio scales of sensory and affective verbal pain descriptors: manipulation of affect by diazepam. Pain 1978;5:19–29.
[35] Grevert P, Albert LH, Goldstein A. Partial antagonism of placebo analgesia by naloxone. Pain 1983;16:129–43.
[36] Heinricher MM, Neubert MJ. Neural basis for the hyperalgesic action of cholecystokinin in the rostral ventromedial medulla. J Neurophysiol 2004;92:1982–9.
[37] Jensen J, McIntosh AR, Crawley AP, Mikulis DJ, Remington G, Kapur S. Direct activation of the ventral striatum in anticipation of aversive stimuli. Neuron 2003;40:1251–7.
[38] Kirsch I. Specifying nonspecific psychological mechanisms of placebo effects. In: Harrington A, editor. The placebo effect: an interdisciplinary exploration. Cambridge: Harvard University Press; 1997. p. 166–86.
[39] Kosterlitz HW, Hughes J. Peptides with morphine-like action in the brain. Br J Psychiatry 1977;130:298–304.
[40] Koyama T, McHaffie JG, Laurienti PJ, Coghill RC. The subjective experience of pain: where expectations become reality. Proc Natl Acad Sci USA 2005;102:12950–5.
[41] Kupers R, Marchand S. Clinical relevance and ethical aspects of placebos. Seminars in Pain Med 2005;3:7–14.
[42] Le Bars D. The whole body receptive field of dorsal horn multireceptive neurones. Brain Res Brain Res Rev 2002;40:29–44.
[43] Le Bars D, Willer JC. Physiologie de la douleur. EMC-Anesthésie Réanimation 2004;1:227–66.
[44] Levine JD, Gordon NC, Fields HL. The mechanism of placebo analgesia. Lancet 1978;2:654–7.
[45] Magnuson DS, Sullivan AF, Simonnet G, Roques BP, Dickenson AH. Differential interactions of cholecystokinin and FLFQPQRF-NH2 with mu and delta opioid antinociception in the rat spinal cord. Neuropeptides 1990;16:213–8.
[46] Marchand S, Charest J, Li J, Chenard JR, Lavignolle B, Laurencelle L. Is TENS purely a placebo effect? A controlled study on chronic low back pain. Pain 1993;54:99–106.
[47] Marchand S, Kupers RC, Bushnell MC, Duncan GH. Analgesic and placebo effects of thalamic stimulation. Pain 2003; 105:481–8.
[48] Mayberg HS, Liotti M, Brannan SK, McGinnis S, Mahurin RK, Jerabek PA, Silva JA, Tekell JL, Martin CC, Lancaster JL, Fox PT. Reciprocal limbic-cortical function and negative mood: converging PET findings in depression and normal sadness. Am J Psychiatry 1999;156:675–82.
[49] McDonald CJ, Mazzuca SA, McCabe GP Jr. How much of the placebo 'effect' is really statistical regression? Stat Med 1983; 2:417–27.
[50] Moerman DE. Cultural variations in the placebo effect: ulcers, anxiety, and blood pressure. Med Anthropol Q 2000;14:51–72.
[51] Moerman DE, Jonas WB. Deconstructing the placebo effect and finding the meaning response. Ann Intern Med 2002; 136:471–6.
[52] Mogenson GJ, Yang CR. The contribution of basal forebrain to limbic-motor integration and the mediation of motivation to action. Adv Exp Med Biol 1991;295:267–90.
[53] Mohr C, Binkofski F, Erdmann C, Buchel C, Helmchen C. The anterior cingulate cortex contains distinct areas dissociating external from self-administered painful stimulation: a parametric fMRI study. Pain 2005;114:347–57.
[54] Montgomery GH, Kirsch I. Classical conditioning and the placebo effect. Pain 1997;72:107–13.
[55] Montgomery GH, Kirsh I. Mechanism of placebo reduction: An empirical investigation. Psychol Sci 1996;7:174–6.
[56] Moran TH, Schwartz GJ. Neurobiology of cholecystokinin. Crit Rev Neurobiol 1994;9:1–28.
[57] Petrovic P, Kalso E, Petersson KM, Ingvar M. Placebo and opioid analgesia: imaging a shared neuronal network. Science 2002;295:1737–40.
[58] Ploghaus A, Tracey I, Gati JS, Clare S, Menon RS, Matthews PM, Rawlins JN. Dissociating pain from its anticipation in the human brain. Science 1999;284:1979–81.
[59] Pollo A, Amanzio M, Arslanian A, Casadio C, Maggi G, Benedetti F. Response expectancies in placebo analgesia and their clinical relevance. Pain 2001;93:77–84.
[60] Porro CA, Baraldi P, Pagnoni G, Serafini M, Facchin P, Maieron M, Nichelli P. Does anticipation of pain affect cortical nociceptive systems? J Neurosci 2002; 22:3206–14.
[61] Porro CA, Cettolo V, Francescato MP, Baraldi P. Functional activity mapping of the mesial hemispheric wall during anticipation of pain. Neuroimage 2003;19:1738–47.
[62] Powell KR, Barrett JE. Evaluation of the effects of PD 134308 (CI-988), a CCK-B antagonist, on the punished responding of squirrel monkeys. Neuropeptides 1991;19:75–8.
[63] Price D, Finniss DG, Benedetti F. A comprehensive review of the placebo effect: recent advances and current thought. Annu Rev Psychol 2008;59:565–90.
[64] Price DD, Milling LS, Kirsch I, Duff A, Montgomery GH, Nicholls SS. An analysis of factors that contribute to the magnitude of placebo analgesia in an experimental paradigm. Pain 1999;83:147–56.
[65] Rainville P, Charron J, Marchand S. L'analgésie placebo. In: Beaulieu P, editor. Pharmacologie de la douleur. Montréal: Les Presses de l'Université de Montréal; 2005. p. 353–80.

[66] Rataud J, Darche F, Piot O, Stutzmann JM, Bohme GA, Blanchard JC. 'Anxiolytic' effect of CCK-antagonists on plus-maze behavior in mice. Brain Res 1991;548:315–7.
[67] Sandrini G, Serrao M, Rossi P, Romaniello A, Cruccu G, Willer JC. The lower limb flexion reflex in humans. Prog Neurobiol 2005;77:353–95.
[68] Schultz W. Behavioral theories and the neurophysiology of reward. Annu Rev Psychol 2006;57:87–115.
[69] Scott DJ, Stohler CS, Egnatuk CM, Wang H, Koeppe RA, Zubieta JK. Placebo and nocebo effects are defined by opposite opioid and dopaminergic responses. Arch Gen Psychiatry 2008;65:220–31.
[70] Singer T, Seymour B, O'Doherty J, Kaube H, Dolan RJ, Frith CD. Empathy for pain involves the affective but not sensory components of pain. Science 2004;303:1157–62.
[71] Song GH, Venkatraman V, Ho KY, Chee MW, Yeoh KG, Wilder-Smith CH. Cortical effects of anticipation and endogenous modulation of visceral pain assessed by functional brain MRI in irritable bowel syndrome patients and healthy controls. Pain 2006;126:79–90.
[72] Stengaard-Pedersen K, Larsson LI. Localization and opiate receptor binding of enkephalin, CCK and ACTH/beta-endorphin in the rat central nervous system. Peptides 1981;1:3–19.
[73] Stewart-Williams S, Podd J. The placebo effect: dissolving the expectancy versus conditioning debate. Psychol Bull 2004; 130:324–40.
[74] Tobler PN, Fiorillo CD, Schultz W. Adaptive coding of reward value by dopamine neurons. Science 2005;307:1642–5.
[75] Tracey I. Nociceptive processing in the human brain. Curr Opin Neurobiol 2005;15:478–87.
[76] Tracey I, Mantyh PW. The cerebral signature for pain perception and its modulation. Neuron 2007;55:377–91.
[77] Valet M, Sprenger T, Boecker H, Willoch F, Rummeny E, Conrad B, Erhard P, Tolle TR. Distraction modulates connectivity of the cingulo-frontal cortex and the midbrain during pain: an fMRI analysis. Pain 2004;109:399–408.
[78] Vase L, Riley JL III, Price DD. A comparison of placebo effects in clinical analgesic trials versus studies of placebo analgesia. Pain 2002;99:443–52.
[79] Vase L, Robinson ME, Verne GN, Price DD. The contributions of suggestion, desire, and expectation to placebo effects in irritable bowel syndrome patients. An empirical investigation. Pain 2003;105:17–25.
[80] Vase L, Robinson ME, Verne GN, Price DD. Increased placebo analgesia over time in irritable bowel syndrome (IBS) patients is associated with desire and expectation but not endogenous opioid mechanisms. Pain 2005;115:338–47.
[81] Vinar O. Dependence on a placebo: a case report. Br J Psychiatry 1969;115:1189–90.
[82] Vogt BA. Pain and emotion interactions in subregions of the cingulate gyrus. Nat Rev Neurosci 2005;6:533–44.
[83] Voudouris NJ, Peck CL, Coleman G. Conditioned placebo responses. J Pers Soc Psychol 1985;48:47–53.
[84] Voudouris NJ, Peck CL, Coleman G. The role of conditioning and verbal expectancy in the placebo response. Pain 1990; 43:121–8.
[85] Wager TD, Rilling JK, Smith EE, Sokolik A, Casey KL, Davidson RJ, Kosslyn SM, Rose RM, Cohen JD. Placebo-induced changes in FMRI in the anticipation and experience of pain. Science 2004;303:1162–7.
[86] Wager TD, Scott DJ, Zubieta JK. Placebo effects on human mu-opioid activity during pain. Proc Natl Acad Sci USA 2007; 104:11056–61.
[87] Walczak JS, Beaulieu P. Nouvelles approches pharmacologiques dans le traitement de la douleur. In: Beaulieu P, editor. Pharmacologie de la douleur. Montréal: Les Presses de l'Université de Montréal; 2005. p. 233–81.
[88] Wickramasekera IA. A conditioned response model of the placebo effect: predictions from the model. In: White L, Tursky B, Schwartz GE, editors. Placebo: theory, research and mechanisms. New York: Guilford Press; 1985. p. 255–87.
[89] Zubieta JK, Bueller JA, Jackson LR, Scott DJ, Xu Y, Koeppe RA, Nichols TE, Stohler CS. Placebo effects mediated by endogenous opioid activity on mu-opioid receptors. J Neurosci 2005;25:7754–62.

Correspondence to: Serge Marchand, PhD, Université de Sherbrooke, Faculté de Médecine, Neurochirurgie, Axe Douleur CRC-CHUS, 3001, 12e avenue nord, Sherbrooke, Québec J1H 5N4, Canada. Email: serge.marchand@usherbrooke.ca.

21

Current Animal Tests and Models of Pain

Daniel Le Bars,[a,b] Per T. Hansson,[c] and Léon Plaghki[d]

[a]Team "Pain," INSERM UMRS 975, CNRS UMR 7225, Paris, France; [b]Faculty of Medicine Pitié-Salpêtrière, Pierre and Marie Curie University, Paris, France; [c]Departments of Molecular Medicine and Surgery, Clinical Pain Research, and Department of Neurosurgery, Pain Center, Karolinska Institute/Karolinska University Hospital, Stockholm, Sweden; [d]READ Unit, Catholic University of Louvain, Brussels, Belgium

Nociceptive stimuli set off a varied but limited repertoire of somatic and vegetative reflexes and behavioral responses that are associated with the perception of pain. Sherrington [110,111] described pain as "the psychical adjunct of a protective reflex," associated with reactions and learned avoidance behaviors, which aim at decreasing the cause of the pain, whatever its nature. As a result, pain may limit the potentially damaging consequences of a given stimulus. Most investigators describe the behaviors associated with this end-point as "pain responses" or "nociceptive responses" in animals. Interestingly, Sherrington considered flexion reflexes as models for the study of the integrative functions of the central nervous system (CNS). These reflexes result from activation of polysynaptic spinal neuronal circuits, which themselves are under the control of spinal and supraspinal influences. Importantly, in normal conditions, the amplitude and duration of these reflexes are functions of stimulus intensity [31,80,81]. The heuristic character of their use in pain research lies in their potential universal application to all species, including humans (e.g., see [105]). In addition, there is an almost perfect coincidence in humans between the development of painful sensations and the evolution of the RIII component of the flexion reflex, at least in the narrowly controlled conditions of the laboratory [65,132].

There are two main types of reactions to a nociceptive stimulus: (1) those organized by centers that are relatively "low" within the hierarchy of the CNS and (2) more complex ones organized by higher centers in the CNS. The former can be engaged in decerebrated animals

Pharmacology of Pain
edited by Pierre Beaulieu, David Lussier, Frank Porreca, and Anthony H. Dickenson
IASP Press, Seattle, © 2010

and have been termed "pseudoaffective reflexes" [110,133]. They include (1) basic motor responses (withdrawal, jumping, contractures, etc.); (2) neurovegetative reactions, generally in the context of Selye's "alarm reaction," with an increase in sympathetic tone (tachycardia, arterial hypertension, hyperpnea, mydriasis, etc.); and (3) vocalization. Such reactions do not need the concomitant sensation to be elicited (e.g., during anesthesia or following decerebration).

These more complex reactions include conditioned motor responses, which result from a period of learning, sometimes very brief. Behavioral reactions (escape, distrust of objects inducing painful experiences, avoidance, and aggression) or modifications of behavior (social and sexual interactions, food intake, sleep, etc.) are often observed. By comparison with the responses discussed above, these behaviors provide evidence of much more integrated reactions within the hierarchical organization of the CNS. If the stimulus is sufficiently intense, the reaction will be escape or attack. However, while active motor reactions are frequent, passive motor responses are observed just as often in animals. For example, immobility allows the animal to preserve a painless posture.

In mammals, pain involves sensation and emotion, which are difficult to separate, both being connected to autonomic processes. But in humans, pain is expressed in a cognitive context, the possible influence of which cannot be transposed to animals without due consideration. Whatever the angle of approach to the question of pain in animals, one cannot ignore the hierarchy in the complexity of the nervous mechanisms that characterizes phylogenesis. Although the question of pain in animals can only be approached through anthropomorphic references, differences probably exist, notably with respect to the development of certain cerebral structures [8], including the cortices [123]. It is reasonable to conclude that differences do exist between humans and animals, at least—but perhaps not only—with respect to the psychological repercussions of pain. Neurological observations in human patients do allow us to make some comparisons. Like Lineberry [79], one might question whether it is appropriate to consider any pain in patients who have undergone frontal lobotomies as being similar to the pain one normally feels: although the pain such patients experience is unaltered at a sensory level, it has lost its emotional and motivational dimensions [44,46,116].

In mammals, the activation of the nociceptive system also involves the limbic brain, so that the reactions triggered by the "reptilian" brain are associated with a sensation probably rather close to what a human perceives as pain. Even the smallest mammal exhibits signs of pain, which doubtless provided a decisive evolutionary advantage [33]. But mammals diversified, notably with regard to the development of their neocortex, the center of cognitive phenomena that has a strong influence on sensations. The projections that ascend toward the cerebral cortex are much less numerous than the downward corticofugal projections that act at multiple subcortical levels. Thus, there is a very precise anatomical substratum allowing the most elaborate cognitive processes to control subordinated physiological functions. As regards pain, these controls can be very powerful, as illustrated by Henry Beecher's observations [9,10] (and see [114]).

During the last World War, Beecher participated in several fights in the Italian campaign, notably the landing at Anzio in January 1944. As an anesthetist at a camp hospital, he treated severely wounded soldiers who hardly seemed to suffer at all. On his return to civilian life, he observed that comparable wounds, sustained in a very different context, were reported as intensely painful. In civilian life, an accident is a terrible disaster that can destroy a life. By contrast, evacuation to a camp hospital, from the hell that was the landing beach, represented a reprieve for a soldier. A soldier's pain could become dulled to the point that he did not ask for morphine, although this drug was at his disposal. The cognitive contexts of these two situations are obviously very different, and these basic observations seem essential when comparing animal and human pain reactions. The animal is unable to appreciate such differences in context. However, stress or anxiety and memories of earlier pain experiences may influence the pain experience of a mammal (e.g. [3,75]).

Nociceptive tests can be applied in a large variety of situations, including pathological states of the organism under study. Considerable efforts have been dedicated to the development of animal models of human pathologies. The purpose of animal models of pain is to model conditions in which humans experience pain. These models should reflect the different categories of human pain: physiological pain ("nociceptive" pain), inflammatory pain, and neuropathic pain. The first two usually occur following injury and are often, at least initially, associated with each other. During an inflammatory episode, the threshold for pain is lowered so that (1) innocuous physical contact may become painful (allodynia) and/or (2) a nociceptive stimulus is perceived as more intensely painful than usual (hyperalgesia). Although these types of pain can exceed the duration of the stimulus, they usually resolve after the related injury has healed.

By contrast, neuropathic pain results from an injury or a pathological transformation of the nervous system, which results in an abnormal and maladapted mode of functioning. In addition to the usual symptoms of inflammatory pain, there are continuous spontaneous pains, a few important conditions with paroxysmal pain components, pains stemming from insensitive regions (e.g., anesthesia dolorosa), paresthesias (tingling, pricking, or dullness), dysesthesias (unpleasant, but not painful, sensations), and sometimes sympathetic disturbances. There is also the situation usually known as "phantom pain," which occurs after deafferentation (e.g., amputation of a limb) and thus lacks a nociceptive stimulus or nociceptor activation. It is unclear whether these pain types all have corollaries in animals. For example, the notion of phantom limb pain is absent from the veterinary literature, in spite of numerous amputations [92], while it seems to be common in human amputees, with reported incidences in the 50–80% range [64,90,130].

This chapter will focus on and be limited to the best-described and most-used pain tests and models of chronic pain. Rodents are the most commonly used animals for preclinical studies of pain. Our comments are based on studies in rats, but they apply to mice as well. These tests and models are described in numerous excellent reviews (e.g., [8, 25,48,62,63,77,79,85,89,105,109,120,129]) and will not be described here. Instead, we will focus on the question of the construct validity of pain tests and models, which remains an essential problem to resolve in pain research [16].

The Tests

The most frequently used tests of nociception can be separated into two categories: those measuring a threshold and those measuring supraliminal responses. They are based on three general endpoints: (1) the measurement of reaction time for escape behavior, (2) the measurement of threshold for escape behavior, and (3) the scoring of behavior. Both categories allow the study of only one point on the stimulus-response curve, be it the threshold or an arbitrary point further up the curve. As a result, they allow only a rough appreciation of the gain of the process [120].

Phenomenology of a Pain Test: The Stimulus and the Response

Describing these tests should be a simple matter—first taking into account the nature of the independent variable (an electrical, thermal, mechanical, or chemical stimulus) and then the dependent behavioral variables. In fact, the inputs and outputs of the systems involved are often intimately linked by the physical characteristics (notably the temporal nature) of the stimulus. Any nociceptive stimulus can be described by a number of different parameters such as the physical nature of the stimulus and the site of application.

The Physical Nature of the Stimulus

Regardless of whether a stimulus is electrical, thermal, mechanical or chemical, it is essential that three of its parameters are controlled, namely the intensity, the duration and the surface area to which it is applied. These three parameters determine the global quantity of nociceptive information that will be generated by the peripheral nervous system and carried toward the CNS. Heat is often chosen because it constitutes a relatively selective stimulus for nociceptors, and radiant heat has the advantage of avoiding a concomitant tactile stimulus. However, the weak caloric power of the stimulators that are generally used (radiant lamps or contact thermodes) has always been a limitation of this method. Indeed, the speed of cutaneous heating induced in this way is slow (generally <4°C/s), which results in a greater time differential for the activation of peripheral and central neurons. Thus, conventional radiant heat sources do not allow an appropriate study of neural phenomena classically seen in other sensory systems (e.g., reflexes, evoked potentials, and reaction times), for which a time-lock of nerve excitations is required. They have the additional disadvantage of emitting radiation within the visible and adjacent infrared spectra, for which the skin is a poor absorber and a good reflector (Fig. 1). Mechanical stimuli, progressive or coarse, are also used.

The Site of Application of the Stimulus

Clinical pains can originate from somatic (cutaneous, articular, or musculotendinous tissues) and visceral tissues. In nociceptive tests, stimuli are usually applied to cutaneous and, to a lesser extent, visceral structures. We know that some areas of skin can have a specific, particular function. For example, the rat tail—a structure used in many nociceptive tests—is an essential organ for thermoregulation and balance.

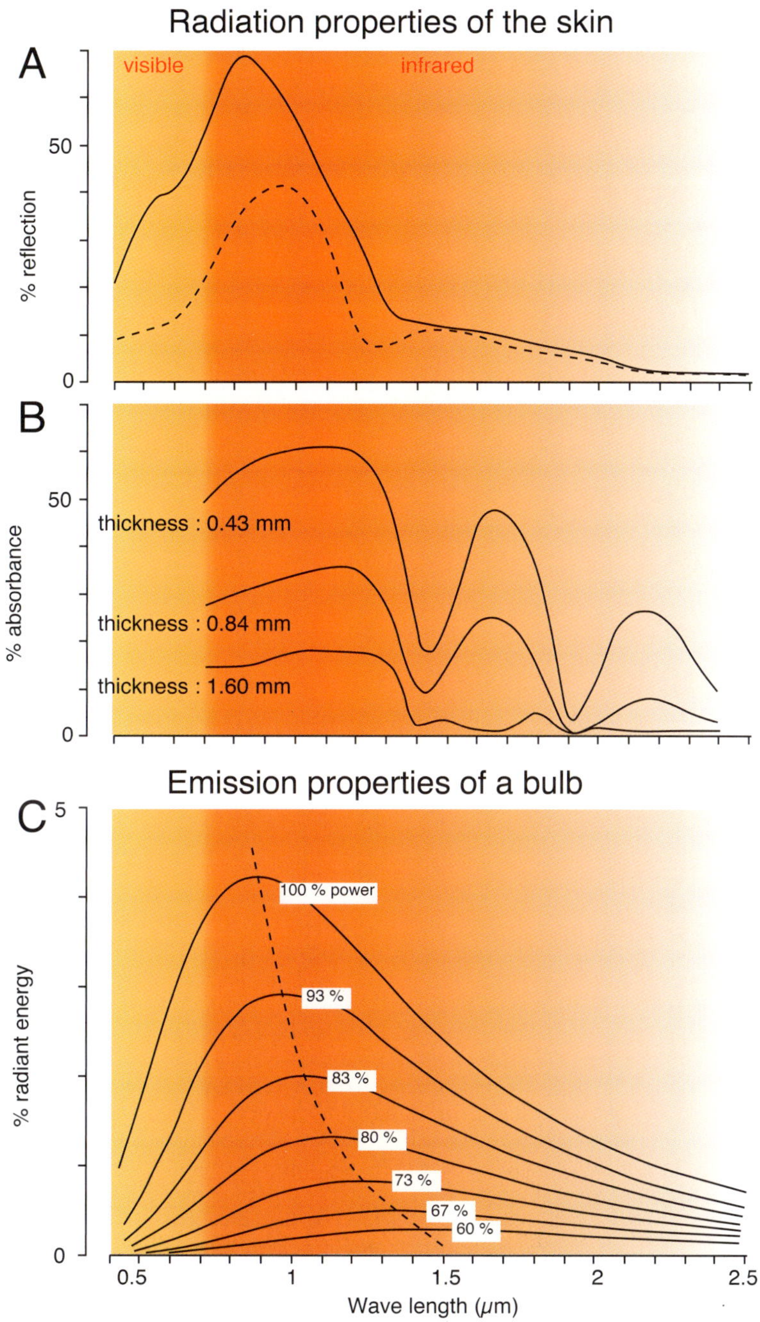

Fig. 1. (A) When radiant heat is used, the percentage of the energy reflected by the skin (ordinate axis) depends on the wavelength emitted by the source of radiation (generally an incandescent lamp). In the visible and adjacent infrared spectra, it also depends on the degree of pigmentation of the skin (white skin: solid line; black skin: broken line). Modified from [53]. (B) The percentage of the energy absorbed by the skin (ordinate) also depends on the wavelength emitted by the source of radiation and decreases with depth. Modified from [57]. (C) The electromagnetic emission spectrum of a lamp varies with the intensity of the applied electrical current. In this example, using a lamp from a commercially available device marketed for the tail-flick test, it can be seen that at full power, the spectrum is centered on 0.9 microns. When the power is reduced, the center shifts gradually to the right. Modified from [77].

Tests for acute pain involve healthy tissues and, occasionally, acutely inflamed tissues (of a few days' standing at most). Tests for chronic pain are related to rheumatoid or neuropathic conditions that last for longer periods of time (from weeks up to months). A "pain test" is applied in a "pain model." These are the two facets of preclinical studies of pain, both of which should achieve a reasonable level of validity, but the interaction of the test with the model should be valid as well.

Choosing the Dependent Measure

The quantitative primary end-point for many behavioral tests of nociception in animals, notably those involving heat as a stimulus (e.g., tail-flick, paw withdrawal, and hot-plate tests), is the reaction time (t_R), i.e., the time lapse between the beginning of the application of a nociceptive stimulus and the evoked response. Other quantitative end-points involve the measurement of threshold for escape behavior (e.g., the paw pressure test, von Frey filaments) and the scoring of nociceptive behavior (e.g., the writhing and formalin tests).

As with any psychophysical process [40,83], a nociceptive response of either a laboratory animal or a human results from a series of events, each with its own duration. The series of events that may lead to a nociceptive withdrawal reaction (R) in response to a stimulus is dissected in Fig. 2 and summarized in Fig. 3A (abbreviations and units are given in Table I). The reaction time, t_R, is the sum of sequential physical (Lφ), biophysical (Lτ),

Fig. 2. Theoretical analysis of the sequence of neural events that produce withdrawal-like responses to a nociceptive stimulus. This simplified diagram does not show phenomena such as convergence between adjacent pathways. Starting from an initial level (zero or a predetermined adaptation level), the stimulus increases to reach the threshold T_1 for depolarization of individual nerve terminals (1). Then, transduction mechanisms produce a local depolarization of nociceptors that triggers the firing of action potentials in peripheral afferent fibers as soon as threshold T_2 is reached (2). These spikes are conducted through the nerves toward the dorsal horn of the spinal cord or are conveyed in the trigeminal system (3). In order to activate second-order neurons, central summation that results from increased peripheral afferent activity is required. Central summation is achieved by a higher intensity of stimulation and thus has a notional threshold of T_3. Activity in these second-order neurons then triggers a complex series of excitatory and inhibitory processes within the central nervous system (4). Yet more summation (and thus afferent activity) is required before the motor neurons are activated at T_4 (5). Because of the one-to-one coupling of action potentials between motor neurons and muscle fibers, the muscles are also activated at this threshold (T_4). However, it is likely that several motor units will have to be excited (or inhibited in antagonist muscles) before a detectable movement will occur—hence this will occur at a higher threshold still—denoted here as T_5 (6). This schematic representation would be easy to interpret and to test experimentally if short-duration stimuli of graded intensities (e.g., electrical shocks) were applied. However, if the withdrawal-like response is elicited by a gradual increase in intensity of the nociceptive stimulus, then the situation becomes far more complex at an experimental level as the stimulus intensity is linked to time. In fact, the triggering of the behavioral response means that a sufficient amount of nociceptive information (ξβ) was generated some time before at the periphery—in other words, that the stimulus intensity had reached Tβ. This "behavioral threshold" means that a sufficient population of individual nociceptors generated a sufficient amount of nociceptive information in a given time window to produce a behavioral response. The corresponding time to reach this threshold includes both the "physical latency" (Lφ), the time required by the stimulus to reach the threshold of a population of individual nociceptors (Tβ), and the "transduction latency" (Lτ), the time required for transduction processes. When Tβ is achieved at the periphery (i.e., T_2 = Tβ), then a "behavioral latency" (Lβ) is required to send the information to the effectors. The withdrawal occurs later, with an "apparent threshold" (T_5 = AT). Note that, a priori, an agent with unknown pharmacological properties might have an effect at any level in such a sequence. The measurable variables are indicated with a yellow background, while variables to be determined are indicated with a blue background. Individual curves of interest are shown in brown. Symbols, abbreviations, and units can be found in Table I. →

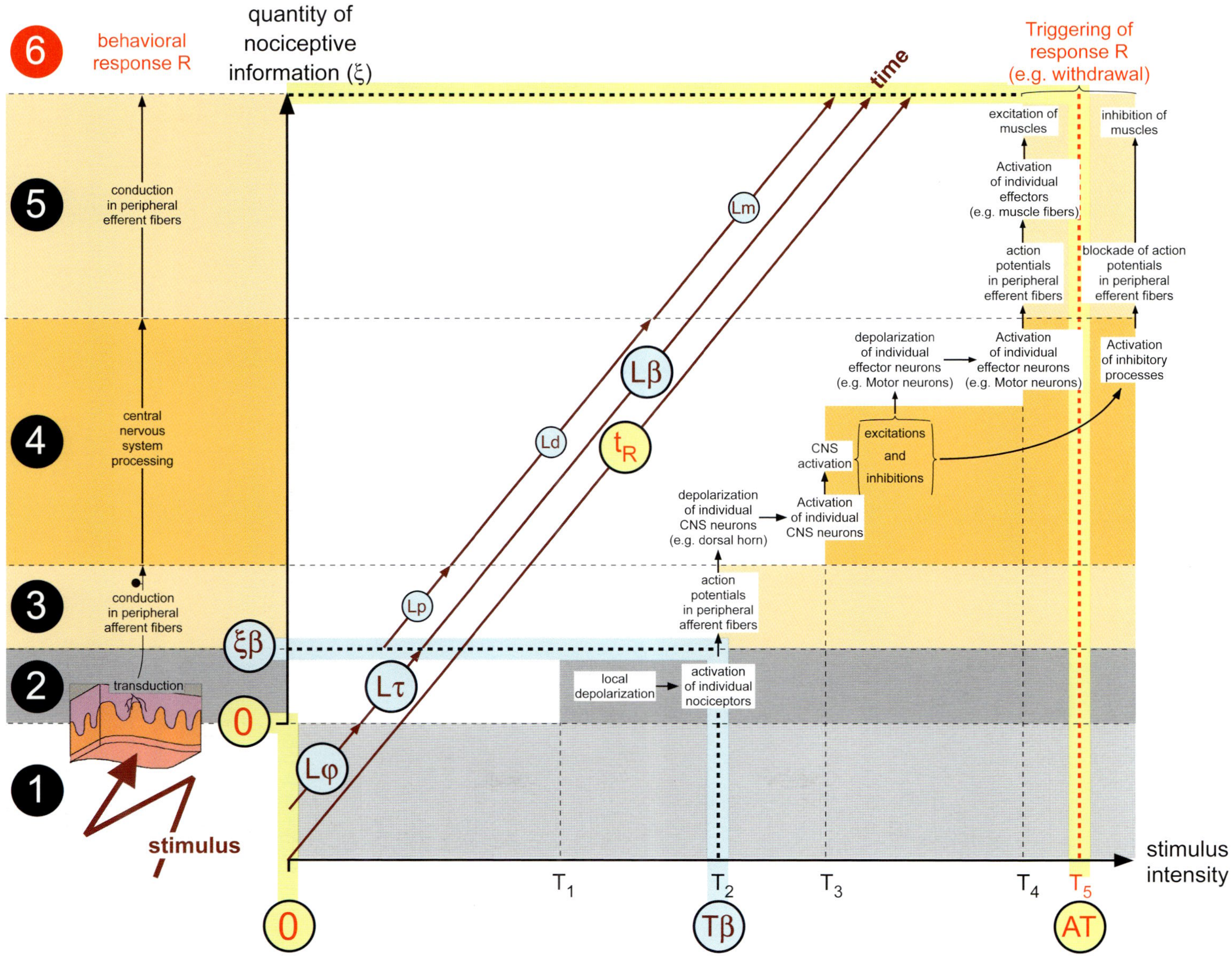

6
behavioral response R
quantity of nociceptive information (ξ)
Triggering of response R (e.g. withdrawal)
time
5
conduction in peripheral efferent fibers
4
central nervous system processing
3
conduction in peripheral afferent fibers
2
transduction
1
stimulus
ξβ
0
Lφ
Lτ
Lp
Ld
Lβ
tR
Lm
local depolarization
activation of individual nociceptors
action potentials in peripheral afferent fibers
depolarization of individual CNS neurons (e.g. dorsal horn)
Activation of individual CNS neurons
CNS activation
excitations and inhibitions
depolarization of individual effector neurons (e.g. Motor neurons)
Activation of individual effector neurons (e.g. Motor neurons)
action potentials in peripheral efferent fibers
Activation of individual effectors (e.g. muscle fibers)
excitation of muscles
Activation of inhibitory processes
blockade of action potentials in peripheral efferent fibers
inhibition of muscles
stimulus intensity
T1
T2
T3
T4
T5
0
Tβ
AT

and behavioral (Lβ) latencies. Lβ is the sum of: (1) the peripheral latency (Lp) required for the nociceptive information to reach the CNS; (2) the "decisional" latency (Ld) required for a central decision-making process (CDP), initiated by the arrival (and/or the accumulation) in the CNS, of a sufficient amount of nociceptive information to order the triggering of the action system (e.g., withdrawal); and (3) motor latency (Lm), the time from motor neuron activation up to the shortening of the muscle. In other words, at the time when the behavioral threshold (Tβ) level of stimulation is achieved (time $t_{T\beta} = t_R - L\beta$), the flow of information transmitted by the nociceptors is sufficient to trigger the behavioral response at time t_R. Whether a response occurs depends on the state of the CDP occupying latency Ld. Tβ is defined by the occurrence of a behavioral response, itself depending on a go/no-go signal given by the CDP. The permissive state of the CDP is basically stochastic and is influenced by many factors, such as behavioral conditioning circumstances.

When the skin is exposed to a constant power source of infrared radiation, the skin surface temperature increases with the square root of time, according to the law of radiant heat transfer:

$$T(t) = T_0 + a \times t^{0.5}$$

where "T_0" represents the initial skin temperature, "a" represents the constant of proportionality, which lumps together power density and biophysical parameters of the skin [21,61,115] (Fig. 3B), and "t" represents time. It follows that mathematical manipulations of the tail-flick latency can be hazardous when they are based on an implicit belief in a linear relationship. In this context, the calculation of the "percentage of the maximum possible effect" [59] should be abandoned for several additional reasons: (1) the term "maximum possible effect" is ambiguous because it is not a biological maximum but an arbitrary value chosen by the investigator; (2) the calculation of this index introduces an arbitrary ratio, which is dependent on the choice of the time limit [24]; and (3) the maximum possible effect varies with the energy of the source of thermal radiation, for strictly physical reasons.

The thermal radiation required to increase the temperature to the pain threshold depends on several parameters: (1) the optical properties of the skin, namely reflectance (Fig. 1A), transmittance (Fig. 1B), and absorbance, which depend on the electromagnetic spectrum emitted by the source of radiation, which itself varies with the intensity of the electrical current applied to incandescent bulbs (Fig. 1C); (2) the heat conduction properties of the skin (thermal capacitance and conductivity); (3) the initial temperature of the skin; and (4) the amount of calorific energy delivered to a given volume of skin, which in turn depends on both the power spectral density of the source and the duration of exposure. In practical terms, the adjustment of the electrical current of the bulb not only signifies changes in the emitted power density (and thus the temperature achieved) but also in the volume of skin affected by the stimulus.

The latent psychophysical variables (Tβ, Lβ, and Ld) are inaccessible with conventional methods and require more sophisticated approaches. Benoist et al. [15] recently presented a theoretical framework, a related experimental paradigm, and a model to analyze in psychophysical terms the "tail-flick" responses of rats to random variations of noxious radiant heat.

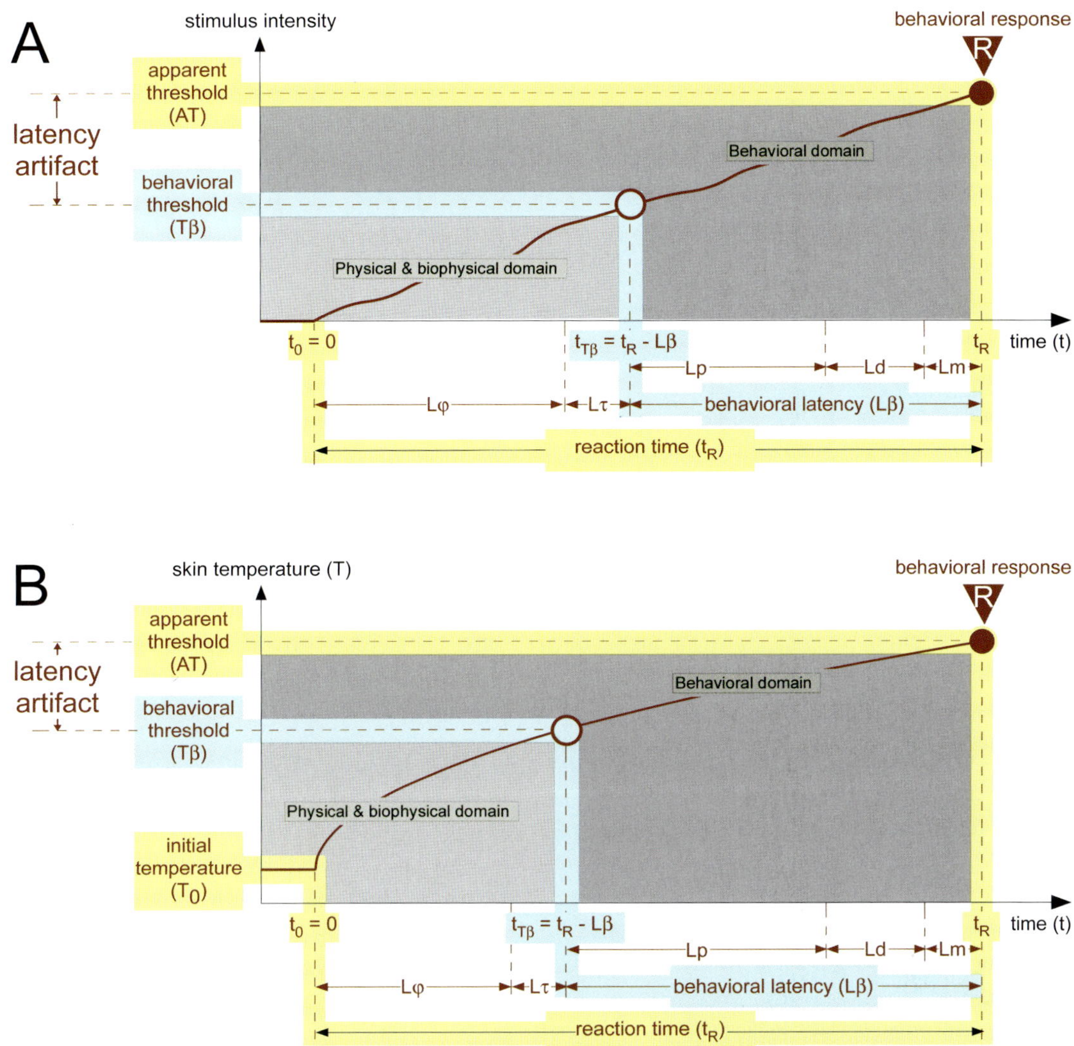

Fig. 3. (A) Theoretical analysis of a behavioral response to an increasing nociceptive stimulus. The behavioral response (R) results mainly from a serial processing along the dedicated pathways involving successive time epochs. As proposed by Luce [83], we will reserve the term latency (L) to an unobserved hypothetical time. Specifically, Lτ is the time required for the stimulus to be transduced by nociceptors into neuronal spikes, which in turn are transmitted toward and received by the central nervous system (CNS). Lp is the transit time for these spikes to reach the CNS. Ld is the "decision" time required by the CNS for interpreting and processing this information for an order to be sent to the motor system. Lm is the time required for a motor response to be triggered. However, as the stimulus is not instantaneous, the reaction time t_R comprises an additional period (Lϕ). Lϕ is completely dependent upon the rate of stimulus application and varies according to the experimental protocol. (B) Theoretical analysis of a behavioral response to radiant heat. When skin, at temperature T_0, is exposed to a constant source of radiant heat, the temperature T increases with the square root of time. Again, Lϕ is completely dependent upon the rate of heating. The other latencies are biological variables with Lτ << Lp and Lm << Ld (see refs. in [15]). The measurable variables are indicated with a yellow background, while variables to be determined are indicated with a blue background. Modified from [15].

Table I
Symbols, abbreviations, and units

Symbol	Explanation and Units
α	Slope of the squared temperature variation (°C²/s) = a^2
$\xi\beta$	Amount of nociceptive information achieved when the stimulus intensity reaches T
a	$\alpha^{0.5}$ (slope of the heating ramp in °C/second)
AT	Apparent threshold (°C)
CCI	Chronic constriction injury model of neuropathy
CDP	Central decision-making process
CNS	Central nervous system
ED_{50}	Efficacious dose in 50% of subjects
FRA	Flexor reflex afferent
L	Latency (ms) = unobserved hypothetical time
$L\beta$	Behavioral latency (ms) = time period which separates the moment at which $T\beta$ is reached from the actual moment of the behavioral response R
$L\phi$	Physical latency (ms) = duration of the skin heating process from the initial skin temperature T_0 to the triggering of transduction in nociceptors
$L\tau$	Transduction latency (ms) = time required for heat to be transduced by nociceptors into neuronal spikes
Ld	Decisional latency (ms) = time required by the CNS for interpreting and processing the nociceptive information
Lm	Motor latency (ms) = time from motor neuron activation up to the shortening of the muscle
Lp	Peripheral latency (ms) = transit time for spikes in primary afferent to reach the entry zone in the spinal cord = $Lp_t + Lp_c$
NSAID	Nonsteroidal anti-inflammatory drug
PSL	Partial nerve transection model of neuropathy
R	Behavioral response
SNL	Spinal nerve transection model of neuropathy
t	Time (ms)
T	Skin temperature (°C)
$T\beta$	Behavioral threshold (°C)
t_0	Beginning of the stimulation
T_0	Initial skin temperature (°C)
T_1	Threshold for depolarization of nerve terminals (°C)
T_2	Threshold for triggering action potentials in peripheral afferent fibers (°C)
T_3	Threshold for activating second-order neurons (°C)
T_4	Threshold for activating motor neurons (°C)
T_5	Threshold for triggering a detectable behavioral response(°C)
T_a	Ambient temperature (°C)
TFL	Tail-flick "latency" = 1000 × t_R (s)
t_R	Moment of the behavioral response = reaction time (ms)
$t_{T\beta}$	Moment when the flow of information generated at the level of the nociceptors is sufficient to trigger a reaction (ms)
V	Conduction velocity (m/s)

Surprisingly, even the (apparent) threshold is rarely measured. The observations that the (apparent) threshold and the magnitude of the tail-flick reflex increased when the power increased [69,121] fit the notion that a withdrawal is triggered following a delay (Lβ) once a threshold (Tβ) is reached. During this period, the temperature continues to increase, activating nociceptors more and more intensely. The integral of the variation of temperature (AT – Tβ) during the period Lβ will determine the "total amount of nociceptive information" generated by the nociceptors that elicits the strength of the response. Thus, the steeper the heating slope, the stronger the response will be with a shorter reaction time. In this respect, it is interesting to note that the tail-flick is classically described as a brief movement of the tail, with the reaction time being shorter and the movement more vigorous (see references in [77]) when the intensity of the source of radiant heat increases. One can define the difference (AT – Tβ) as a "latency artifact" because it is an obvious cause of variability in the determination of thermal thresholds, as exemplified elegantly by the studies in humans by Yarnitsky and Ochoa [135,136]. These authors showed that the method of limits (as any method where the dependent variable is a measure of time), often used for the determination of thermal thresholds in which the stimulus is stopped by the subject, resulted in greater overestimations of threshold when temperature rose more rapidly. By comparison, the method of levels, where the subject's response does not influence the stimulus duration, produced identical thresholds, whatever the rate of temperature. The notions of "true" and "apparent" behavioral thresholds expanded on here for animal studies are fully compatible with these observations in humans.

Requirements for Behavioral Tests of Nociception

For behavioral tests to be appropriate, stimuli must be quantifiable, reproducible, and noninvasive [11,79]. Because the goal of experiments is to study the relationships between independent and dependent variables, a wide panel of characteristics should define a behavioral test for nociception. In this respect, the psychometric qualities of an instrument of objective measurement (here a "pain test") of a subjective phenomenon (here "pain") are sensitivity, reliability, and validity [38].

Sensitivity

Sensitivity is the capability to detect a perceptible change in a variable. It must be possible to quantify the response and for the variable to be correlated with stimulus intensity within a reasonable range (e.g., from the pain threshold to the pain tolerance threshold). In other words, the quantified response must be appropriate for a given type of stimulus and must be monotonically related to its intensity. The test must be sensitive to manipulations, notably pharmacological, which would influence the behavior in a specific fashion.

It cannot be stated often enough that in most animal models of pain, the sole measurement is a nociceptive threshold. Threshold measurements may reveal a potential analgesic action of a substance only if the stimulus-response curve shifts to the right. However, if the slope of the stimulus-response curve is reduced without any overall shift, then the measurement of the threshold alone will not permit any conclusion to be drawn about the substance or may lead to the wrong conclusion that the substance has no effect. In other words, measuring a threshold does not permit the evaluation of changes in the gain of a system. Given that clinical pain reported by a patient to a physician is rarely limited to threshold intensity, the endpoint in animal models of nociception should be extended to suprathreshold nociceptive stimuli [12].

We will illustrate the possible pitfalls by considering the effects of morphine in morphine-tolerant rats. The use of frankly noxious stimuli in behaving animals is questionable for ethical reasons. However, a compromise involves using electromyography in the anesthetized rat, to record reflex activity elicited by the activation of afferent C fibers. The main advantage of this animal model is that it permits quantification of the responses to various intensities of stimulation: the reflex magnitude increases with stimulus intensity from the threshold until it reaches a plateau. One can then analyze the responses to a wide range of stimuli that would produce sensations closer to those of a variety of clinical pains. The obvious disadvantage of the method, namely the use of anesthesia, is not a real problem in many pharmacological contexts. The expression of tolerance to morphine depends on the intensity of the stimulus, being maximal with threshold intensities but considerably less with suprathreshold values [1,2] (Fig. 4). In human volunteers, the same dose of a given opioid, namely remifentanil, perfused for an identical period of time, either did or did not produce evidence of tolerance phenomena, depending on whether a pain

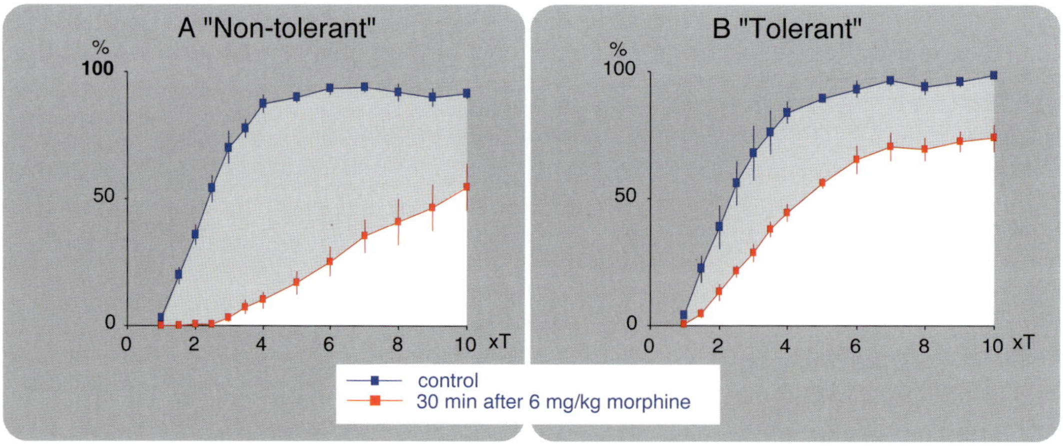

Fig. 4. Effects of 6 mg/kg morphine on the C-fiber responses to a wide range of stimulus intensities in "non-tolerant" (A) and "tolerant" animals (B). The first recruitment curve (black squares) was built during the control period; the second curve was built 30 minutes after 6 mg/kg of morphine (open squares). On the abscissa, the stimulus intensities are expressed as multiples of the C-fiber reflex threshold recorded during the control period. On the ordinate, the reflex responses are expressed as percentages of the maximum value reached during the control period. In "non-tolerant" animals (A), morphine both increased the threshold and decreased the slope of the recruitment curve. In the "tolerant" group (B), the threshold did not change, but the gain of the stimulus-response curve decreased. Adapted from [1].

threshold [126] or a frankly painful sensation [51] was monitored. It follows that the inconsistency between clinical observations and data from animal research is only apparent, because morphine is used clinically only for severe pain, whereas most behavioral tests in animals monitor responses in the region of a nociceptive threshold. In conclusion, the use of threshold measurement as end-point in animal research has led to an overestimation of the real impact of morphine tolerance phenomena.

Reliability

Reliability accounts for the repeatability of the measurements obtained under identical conditions. Repeatability or consistency can be estimated by a series of classes of reliability. The first two classes, namely test-retest and interobserver concordance, highlight reproducibility. Consistency of scores must be obtained when animals are retested with an identical test or an equivalent form of the test. In this context, the repeated application of a stimulus must not produce lesions. Results obtained with a test must be reproducible not only by a given experimenter, but also by different experimenters within the same laboratory or in different laboratories. Reliability is directly related to the variability of a measurement. Variability is a composite concept that includes variability due to true score (related to the stochastic nature of behavioral responses) and variability due to errors (random and systematic errors). Random errors affect variability but do not affect the average. Systematic errors do affect the average, introducing a bias. The other classes of reliability concern tests that include several items and therefore do not apply to most animal pain tests where a single item is used for measurement of a single variable.

Mogil and colleagues studied the "genetics of pain" for several years by recording, in apparently identical conditions and testing protocols, the reaction time following tail immersion in a 49°C water bath in a series of strains of mice [87]. This approach provides the opportunity to retrospectively identify and rank the sources of variability in an archival data set of a large body of independent observations [26]. This analysis allowed partitioning the variance of this trait among environmental (42%), genetic (27%), and genetic x environmental (18%) sources. Such a result is not surprising, if one acknowledges the basal temperature of the tail as a main source of variance in tail-flick latency [15], which is largely determined by vegetative factors.

Validity

Validity is the relevance of the measurement and inferred data: do we measure effectively what we claim to measure? Validity requires reliability, but the reverse in not true (some artifacts are highly reliable). The four main types of validity are *external, internal, conclusion,* and *construct* validity. The first three are "technical", that is, they are related to elementary rules for any research field. *External validity* represents the ability to generalize the conclusions of a study to other subjects in other places and at other times. A high external validity allows the findings of a study to be generalized to a given population. This requires a good sampling, representative of this population. *Internal validity* refers to the degree of successful outcome in eliminating confounding variables within the study of a given population. Good experimental design should allow for unambiguous inferences regarding cause-effect relationships. *Conclusion validity* is the degree to which conclusions reached about relationships in the data are reasonable. This implies the use of adequate statistical methods. *Construct validity* requires a profound knowledge of the given research field and is the most difficult criterion to satisfy and therefore deserves further comments in the context of nociceptive tests.

Construct Validity of Nociceptive Tests

Construct validity is concerned with the degree to which the test actually measures what it purports to measure. A construct is valid when the observed pattern corresponds with our theoretical pattern. This correspondence implies that the underlying theory is consistent and relevant. Construct validation will be more easily achieved if the underlying theory is explicit and clear. It is important to note that the concept of construct validity is not limited to the question of measurement. For example, the assessment of pain requires applying a valid test on a valid model of pain. They are both absolute requirements. Construct validation requires a series of verifications showing that the test effectively measures the targeted construct (measures what it claims to measure). An essential part of validation is to relentlessly pursue the potential confounding factors that might bias the construct. The result of the process of validation will be interpreted in connection with the theoretical background that supports the test. In effect, construct validation includes many types of validity (e.g., *face, content, instrumental,* and *consequential* or *predictive* validities, as detailed below).

Face Validity of Tests

Face validity is concerned with the extent to which a test "looks like" it is measuring what it is supposed to measure. This is a subjective judgment that the test constitutes an adequate translation of the construct. Face validity does not depend on any theory for support. Most nociceptive tests meet this criterion, for example, when the animal escapes or withdraws from a presumably noxious stimulus. It is probably the weakest evidence to demonstrate construct validity because it is essentially an "apparent validity." To illustrate this weakness, let us consider the strong belief that a given test is a good "pain test" when it provides the expected pharmacological results. Knowing that a given receptor (e.g., the μ-opioid receptor) can be involved in several apparently unrelated functions (e.g., nociception and thermoregulation) and that brain functions interact directly or indirectly to a large extent, it follows that an expected effect on function A (e.g., nociception) could result from an (ignored or neglected) effect on function B (e.g., thermoregulation). Note that pharmacological criteria such as dose-dependency or stereospecificity can be fully verified because the observation is based on a real pharmacological effect, strongly supporting the belief. The effect is real indeed; the artifact concerns the interpretation. The risk of such bias increases both with the ubiquity of the receptor under study and with the interdependence of the function under study (i.e., pain) with other functions (e.g., other sensory modalities, memory, autonomic functions, and motor functions).

Content Validity of Tests

Content validity is concerned with the extent to which the content of the test adequately represents all that is required for validity. The measurement should reflect the concept that it is supposed to measure. For example, the stimulus must be nociceptive ("input specificity"). Although this is common sense, it is not always easy to confirm that it is being achieved. For example, the appearance of a flexion reflex does not inevitably mean that the stimulus is nociceptive or that it is a nociceptive flexion reflex. Indeed, flexion reflexes are not triggered exclusively by nociceptive stimuli [107]. It must be possible, in the behavioral model, to differentiate responses to nociceptive stimuli from responses to non-nociceptive stimuli. In other words, the quantified response must be exclusively or preferentially triggered by nociceptive stimuli ("output specificity"). In this respect, one must remember that some innate and acquired behaviors can be triggered by aversive stimuli, which are not algogenic.

The test must also allow the differentiation of nonspecific behavioral changes (e.g., changes in motility or attention) from those triggered by the stimulus itself. In other words, the response being monitored cannot be contaminated by simultaneous perturbations related to other functions. This requirement also applies following manipulations introduced by an experimental protocol. In other words, the content validity must be verified not only in control situations, but also following treatments, notably with a pharmacological agent.

Instrumental Validity of Tests

Instrumental validity is concerned with the accuracy of a measurement by comparing it with another measurement that has previously been demonstrated to be valid. Concurrent and predictive validities refer to a test's ability to vary directly with a measurement of the same construct by an already validated test, either at the same moment (concurrent validity) or at a later period (predictive validity). Convergent validity refers to the degree to which scores on a test correlate with scores on other tests that are designed to assess the same construct; it shows that the assessment is related to what it theoretically should be related to. Discriminant validity refers to the degree to which scores on a test do not correlate with scores from other tests that are not designed to assess the same construct. One expects a weak correlation between the test to be validated and another test measuring a different construct.

Consequential Validity of Tests

The current measurement has no consequences on the later measurements. This is an important issue regarding pain research because sensitization/desensitization processes are common phenomena at various levels of the sensory system. One can reasonably assume that such effects are rather trivial following few threshold measurements. However, the consequences for both repeated threshold and suprathreshold stimulations must be evaluated.

Tests for acute pain involve healthy tissues and, occasionally, acutely inflamed tissues (of a few days' standing at most). Tests for chronic pain are related to rheumatoid or neuropathic pain that lasts for a long time (from weeks up to several months). Since the application of the stimulus must not produce lesions, one often defines a limit for how long the animal should be exposed to the stimulus (the "cut-off time"). This limit is necessary when the intensity of the stimulus is increasing: a compromise has to be found between the dynamics of the effect being studied (for which one would want the longest time limit possible) and the prevention of tissue damage (for which one would want the shortest time limit possible). The repeated application of a stimulus up to the time limit during an antinociceptive effect can obviously sensitize peripheral receptors. It can also produce hidden effects such as central sensitization. For instance, an accumulation of mediators at the level of the spinal cord, elicited by the stimulations until the cut-off time during analgesia, can dramatically affect the observations during recovery and give the appearance of a rebound "facilitation" [7,67]. In such a case, the measurement itself builds the sensitization and produces artifacts. Note that the process of validation requires a solid theoretical background to be satisfied unambiguously.

Predictive Validity of Tests

Predictability—in terms of clinical applicability—is an absolute requirement in nociceptive tests for two reasons. First, it is necessary to avoid "false positives" and "false negatives" when searching for new molecules with therapeutic value [28]. For example, the "writhing test" (or "abdominal constriction test"), which is very sensitive but only weakly predictive, was reserved for initial pharmacodynamic screening of potential analgesic substances [36,60,82]. Another reason, far more fundamental, relates to situations in which one is trying to understand the basic mechanisms underlying pain and analgesia. Is it possible from a basic perspective to rely on a test that would not work correctly in terms of elementary pharmacology to answer the simplest of questions: is this substance analgesic or not?

The most predictive of the models of acute pain are undoubtedly the formalin test [37] and the Randall-Selitto test [98]. A mathematical formula has even been proposed to devise directions for use of a nonsteroidal anti-inflammatory agent in humans, using as its starting point the ED_{50} (the dose that is effective in 50% of subjects) from the Randall-Selitto test in the rat [36]. On the other hand, the "tail-flick" and "hot-plate" tests are only predictive for morphinomimetic drugs in the strictest sense, are weakly predictive for partial agonists, and are not at all applicable for mild analgesics [25,34,117].

Here is a paradox that deserves some thought. Certain tests, which are not very predictive in terms of identifying analgesic molecules, become useful when drawing up guidelines for therapeutic use in humans. This is the case with the "writhing test" [25,101,113,117] for which a mathematical formula was proposed to predict directions for use in man, from the ED_{50} determined in the mouse [97]. There are no satisfactory explanations for the inconsistency in predictability of this method, which is weak at identifying a substance as analgesic, but strong at predicting its therapeutic value once it has been identified as being analgesic.

Conclusions: Confounding Factors That Might Affect Construct Validity

Many confounding factors might affect the construct validity of an animal "pain test." Among these factors, the vasomotor tone-dependent temperature variations of the skin and other autonomic functions (e.g., maintaining appropriate carbon dioxide levels and arterial blood pressure) probably have the most detrimental effects on the validity of the construct.

In a recent psychophysical approach using the tail-flick test [15], behavioral latency was determined with precision. It was always less than 500 ms, whatever the stimulation site on the tail or the basal temperature of the skin. The remaining part of the reaction time (t_R) mainly represents the time for the heating process ($L\phi$) and, albeit to a negligible extent, the transduction time ($L\tau$) required to achieve the behavioral threshold of the reaction ($T\beta$). The sum $t_R = (L\phi + L\tau + L\beta)$ corresponds to the "latency" usually observed in the conventional tail-flick test. Since t_R is recorded in the 2–4-second range in the current literature, [77], it follows that most of this period is devoted to $L\phi$, a simple physical process. This part increases when the reaction time increases due to a reduction of either the power of the radiant heat source or the basal temperature of the skin. If t_R is the only measured end-point elicited by a given power of the source, there is no way of knowing whether any variation was produced by changes of T_0, $T\beta$, or both. The question of the validity of using a reaction time of a behavioral response to an increasing heat stimulus as a "pain index" is directly challenged here.

The second group of detrimental effects on the construct validity of animal "pain tests" is to be found in their motor component. Lundberg and colleagues investigated the nature of afferent impulses that converge on to interneurons in polysynaptic flexion reflex arcs and introduced the concept of "flexor reflex afferents." These reflex circuits include both nociceptive and non-nociceptive afferent fibers of various origins and are tightly controlled by descending pathways originating from supraspinal centers (see [84,106]). Knowing the strength of such convergences, it is sometimes difficult to decide whether the source of an observed effect relies on the sensory or the motor component of a reflex circuitry. Postural adjustments could be a source of additional bias. When an animal takes up a guarding position, the injured limb is flexed, the flexor motor neurons are facilitated (and those of the extensors inhibited), and a flexion reflex is easier to evoke. The result could be an overestimation of hypersensitivity. In this context, it is interesting to note that the extent of behavioral hypersensitivity estimated following administration of Freund's adjuvant into a paw is an order of magnitude greater than that within the orofacial region, where there is no equivalent postural adjustment [99].

The third group of detrimental effects on the construct validity of animal "pain tests" is related to cognitive processes. Learning can be extremely rapid during a series of tests. During heating, the progressive nature of the stimulus results in thermoreceptors being activated before nociceptors. Corresponding to this sequence of activations, there is a sequence of sensations, warm followed by hot, followed by burning pain. As a result, the same stimulus can be regarded as a conditioning and a conditioned stimulus. This can be exemplified with the hot-plate test reiterated once a day or once a week: a consistent progressive decrease in reaction times is observed [47,75,95,103]. In studies related to the anticipation of pain involving an experimental paradigm with a conditioning stimulus before a conditioned stimulus, the identical phenomena are observed [30,124]. For practical reasons, such tests are often performed on restrained animals, and usually on animals that are exposed to a new environment. This distress is expressed in measurable variations of physiological parameters such as a lowering of the temperature of the rat's tail [134].

The Models

An animal model is a tool that allows the study of a biological, behavioral, or pathological process, which shares one or several aspects with a similar phenomenon in humans (or another target species). It is supposed to replicate these aspects adequately. The reasoned choice of an animal model requires a good knowledge of the anatomy, physiology, biochemistry, and genetics that underlie the phenomenon that is aimed to be understood. When basal observations suggest a theoretical model, one can go back to the bench and choose an experimental model to verify all implications of the theoretical construct. Indeed, the very first reason to build an "experimental model" is to test a "theoretical model." Then, the development of a permanent confrontation between theoretical and experimental models could provide progress in understanding and knowledge. Explicit, implicit, or ignored, there is always a theory behind the choice of a "model."

There is a hierarchy of animal models according to the objective of the studies: the description of a normal or abnormal biological phenomenon, the investigation of the mechanisms and determinants of a biological phenomenon, or the predictive evaluation of the efficacy and safety of future medical treatments. An experimental animal model of chronic pain should meet all these criteria.

Phenomenology of Chronic Pain Models: Similarities between the Model and the Condition Being Modeled

There are two main types of models for chronic pain in the rat: models of systemic inflammation or polyarthritis and models of neuropathies with lesions limited to the peripheral or central nervous systems.

Models of Polyarthritis

Polyarthritis elicited by the immunogenic complete Freund's adjuvant (CFA) in the rat is used as a model of human rheumatoid arthritis [20,94,127,131]. CFA induces inflammation in the distal joints of the limbs and leads to many behavioral disturbances related to spontaneous pain [22,23,32,89]. After a preclinical stage, one observes a cessation of body weight gain, a large increase in joint diameter, and radiological abnormalities (soft tissue swelling, demineralization and erosion of bone extremities, and joint space narrowing). In parallel, dramatic behavioral changes develop: lack of mobility and exploring behavior, a profound increase in scratching behavior, and signs of mechanical hypersensitivity, as assessed with classical tests. These signs peak at week 4. During the following weeks, body weight and behavioral reactions began to return toward control values, but joint diameters and radiological scores either continue to increase or remain constant. During recovery (weeks 9–11), behavioral scores and body weight return to control values while joint diameters remain high, with few signs of radiological remission.

In other models, the arthritis is limited to one joint. Injection of iodoacetate or monosodium urate crystals into the rat knee joint mimics the biochemical/structural changes associated with monoarthritis (e.g., gout) [5,41,72,96].

Models of Neuropathies

Rat models of neuropathies are based on a total or partial deafferentation of an area of the body. Total deafferentation by the cutting of several neighboring dorsal roots triggers, within 2–3 weeks, a type of self-mutilation called "autotomy" [35,68]. Autotomy is also seen in rodents after complete sectioning of the sciatic and saphenous nerves, which is associated with a permanently anesthetized paw [128]. With reference to anesthesia dolorosa in humans, this behavior is thought to be elicited by the pain evoked by deafferentation, representing an extreme form of grooming or itching. The meaning of autotomy is disputed, and some experts contend that this behavior is the result of complete sensory denervation, such that the animal no longer recognizes the limb as part of itself [100]. However, chronic anesthesia of the sciatic nerve or chronic perineural lidocaine infusion does not cause autotomy [19]. Finally, minor environmental factors, such as introduction of a female into the cage of an operated male rat [17], are sufficient to eliminate the autotomy behavior [68].

Partial deafferentation is the most popular method for modeling neuropathy. It is accomplished by applying chronic pressure over a peripheral nerve of the hindpaw that will lead to the degeneration of a few sensory nerve fibers while leaving other fibers intact. The ligature initiates inflammatory swelling, and the pressure elicits a local restriction of blood flow and compression of nerves that result in stimulation of nociceptors in the nervi nervorum. The affected nerve fibers then undergo Wallerian degeneration, and the neighboring spared nerve fibers in close contact are exposed to an altered chemical environment. Indeed, several spinal nerves join the lumbosacral plexus before branching to form peripheral nerves in the lower limb. Within the plexus of the rat or mouse, the nerve roots from segments L3, L4, L5, S1, and S2 fuse to form nerve trunks, which in turn remix with the neighboring trunks and finally merge to form the sciatic nerves [50]. The ligature of a single peripheral nerve initiates degenerative changes in its fibers and causes pathological changes in the neighboring fibers at the spinal roots [122]. This statement is supported by the observation that ligature of motor fibers also leads to neuropathic "pain-like" behavior [112].

There are three main approaches for rat models of neuropathy triggered by partial deafferentation [13,109]. The chronic constriction injury model (CCI) is produced by a loose ligature around the rat sciatic nerve, resulting in a loss of myelinated fibers but the survival of most C fibers [14]. The partial nerve transection model (PSL) is produced by a partial section of the rat sciatic nerve [108]. The spinal nerve transection model (SNL) is produced by a section of the L5–L6 spinal dorsal roots, with the hindpaw remaining partially innervated through the L4 root [70].

In addition, some models were designed to replicate known anatomical-clinical entities in humans, namely diabetic neuropathy (using streptozocin [45]) and neuropathies associated with chemotherapy [4]. All these models are characterized by hypersensitive behaviors when stimuli are applied to the body regions affected by the neuropathy.

Construct Validity of Pain Models

In behavioral animal models, the complex experience of all facets of a painful condition in humans is reduced to a presupposed spontaneous "pain-like" behavior or withdrawal reflexes elicited by external stimuli. Indeed, all these models are characterized by signs of hypersensitivity, interpreted as allodynia-like and hyperalgesia-like behaviors when stimuli are applied to the affected zone. The same tests are used to evaluate stimulus-evoked pain in normal rats as in rat models of chronic pain. The main difference results from the fact that the tests are applied to a body and a nervous system with different histories. In other words, the triggering stimuli and the behavioral dependent variables measured are the same. It follows that the part of the construct validity related to the test itself is identical for any animal model of pain, whether acute, inflammatory, or neuropathic. What needs to be evaluated at the present stage is the construct validity of a model itself as well as the construct validity of the tests used in this model. The first question refers to the model: do we observe effectively what we claim to observe? The answer is easier when we do know the etiology of a disease used as a model. However, the greatest concern may relate to substantial differences in the biology of nociception between rodents and humans.

Construct Validity of Rat Models of Polyarthritis

To date, the animal models of polyarthritis mentioned above are considered sufficiently valid by rheumatologists [5,20,127]. In addition to the tests usually used for the assessment of acute pain, behavioral tests can use indirect measures of knee joint pain in arthritis models, such as weight bearing, foot posture, gait analysis, and spontaneous mobility [89]. Weight bearing and gait analysis have the advantage that they are also used in the clinical setting to assess pain in patients with arthritis. Also consistent with clinical observations, rats with experimentally induced polyarthritis show marked abnormalities in sleep, including increased wakefulness and a reduction in overall EEG amplitude [76]. Interestingly, an analogy with patient-controlled analgesia was provided in the CFA-induced polyarthritis model: in a conditioned taste-aversion paradigm, arthritic rats self-administer seven times more orally available fentanyl solution than control rats [29].

Construct Validity of Rat Models of Neuropathy

Models That Reproduce a Known Etiology (Toxic or Metabolic Neuropathies)

Rodent models of quantifiable neuropathies have been developed for three of the most widely used and most neurotoxic chemotherapies: cisplatin, paclitaxel, and vincristine [48]. Cisplatin has the disadvantage of triggering general health disability including decreased weight gain and deficits in motor function. The administration of chemotherapy in rats produces axon degeneration similar to what is seen in human patients, as verified with histological methods. Slowing of peripheral nerve conduction velocity is also a feature in both the animal models and the human disease. Proprioceptive deficits are observed in rats at high cumulative doses and in humans with more advanced stages of neuropathy. However, the animal models show a decrease in motor activity that is not reported in humans, at least not in the early stages.

These models are thus valid in terms of pathophysiology. Whether the objective signs of pain-like behavior correspond to the symptoms in humans remains to be verified. In fact, the behavioral changes observed in rodents treated with these potentially neurotoxic drugs are consistent with many of the clinical symptoms of related human neuropathies, including rapidity of onset. Indeed, within a few days of treatment, patients may develop various combinations of dysesthesia, paresthesia, mechanical allodynia and hyperalgesia, cold allodynia and hyperalgesia, heat hypoalgesia, and spontaneous ongoing pain. Some of the latter symptoms and signs appear similar to signs of mechanical and cold hypersensitivity and heat hyposensitivity in rodents [48] (Table II).

Table II
Principal signs reported in the most frequently used animal models of neuropathy [62,63,85,18], namely the chronic constriction injury model (CCI [14]), partial nerve transection model (PSL [108]), spinal nerve transection model (SNL [70]), streptozocin-induced diabetic neuropathy (STZ [45]), and neuropathies elicited by chemotherapy [4]

	Autotomy	Guarding Posture	Withdrawal Threshold			Inflammation
			Warmth/Heat	Cold	Pressure	
CCI	+	+	↓↓	↓↓	↓	+
PSL	–	+	↓	~	↓	?
SNL	–	+	↓	~	↓↓	–
STZ	–	?	↑	?	↓	–
Chemotherapy	–	?	↑	↓	↓	?

Symbols: +, appearance of effect; –, absence of effect; ↓, decreased threshold; ↑, increased threshold; ~, threshold unchanged; ?, unknown.

The drug-induced models of diabetic neuropathy mimic type I diabetes. As in the human clinical condition, models of diabetic neuropathy demonstrate reduced nerve blood flow, slowed nerve conduction, accumulation of polyol pathway metabolites, reduced caliber of nerve fibers, and altered pain thresholds, with an elevated heat threshold and lowered pressure threshold [6]. However, the morphological changes in biopsies of patients with diabetic neuropathy are more severe than those observed in the animal models. This discrepancy might simply relate to the duration of the disease. Many pain-related studies include patients who have had diabetes for years, while the diabetic animals are evaluated for neuropathy within a few weeks, or months at best. The poor health of these animals confounds the assessment of neuropathy and reduces the likelihood of long-term survival.

Models Based on Partial Deafferentation

There is an obvious discrepancy between animal models of peripheral nerve injury and clinical traumatic neuropathy, with regard to the extremely high incidence of "pain-like" behavior and facilitated withdrawal reflexes in animals and the relatively rare sequelae of spontaneous and stimulus-evoked pain after nerve injury in humans. Indeed, the most common sensory complaints in clinical peripheral neuropathies are tingling paresthesias and numbness, rather than pain. While avoidance and protective behavior in animals are often interpreted as being related to pain, they may be induced by paresthesias and dysesthesias and not just pain. We have mentioned above the confounding factors that can be introduced by postural adjustments. In a "guarding position," whether elicited by a pain sensation or otherwise, the guarded limb is flexed, which signifies that (1) the flexor motor neurons are facilitated (and those of the extensors inhibited), and a flexion reflex is easier to evoke; and (2) the flexor motor neurons of the contralateral limb are inhibited (and those of the extensors facilitated), and a flexion reflex is more difficult to evoke. Comparing the reflex response of the two limbs will introduce a systematic imbalance related to motor control mechanisms, resulting in an overestimation of hypersensitivity.

Interestingly, signs of pain-like behavior can be elicited from outside the territory of the sciatic nerve into tissue served by adjacent uninjured nerves in the CCI model [71,119]. Similar clinical features are infrequently observed in humans [52]. One must remember, however, that there is variability in the cutaneous region served by peripheral nerves and spinal roots.

"Pain-Like" Spontaneous Behavior Assessment

In models of neuropathy [27,129], the repertoire of pain-like behaviors includes postural adjustment with weight bearing on the uninjured hindlimb and guarding behavior of the injured paw, licking and "gentle" skin biting, and disrupted social functioning (measured by the number of ultrasonic vocalizations during social interactions with normal cohorts) and its attenuation after administration of analgesics. Surprisingly, the scoring and quantification of these ongoing or spontaneous behaviors are not reported frequently in experimental studies, whereas such behaviors are often an important component of clinical situations. Although such behaviors can be interpreted as "pain-like" behaviors, they might also represent negative signs such as paresthesias and dysesthesias. As mentioned above, nonpainful symptoms such as paresthesias, numbness, and dysesthesias are the most common sensory complaints reported by patients with clinical peripheral neuropathies, rather than pain per se [52].

Mechanical Sensitivity Assessment

To assess sensory disturbances in the mechanical domain in neuropathic pain in humans, gentle brushing with soft brushes or cotton buds across the skin is used as a classic diagnostic tool. Dynamic "brush-evoked" allodynia is mediated by low-threshold fiber inputs. On the other hand, gentle pressure assesses the presence of static mechanical allodynia that appears to be mediated by high-threshold fiber inputs [91].

In general, behavioral testing of withdrawal responses of the inflamed or neuropathic hindpaw in different animal models to a short-lasting punctate prodding of the skin using von Frey filaments has gained acceptance in the preclinical scientific pain community. In an attempt to assess tactile hypersensitivity in animals, probably with the rationale of mimicking the severely disabling phenomenon of dynamic mechanical allodynia in patients, it is unlikely that punctate von Frey-induced hindpaw withdrawal in different models of neuropathy has any bearing on the complex experience of dynamic mechanical allodynia elicited with a light moving stimulus in subgroups of neuropathic pain patients. In fact, the available literature leaves it open to debate as to which fibers are activated by von Frey filaments using this technique [42,73]. With the exception of subgroups of patients with postherpetic neuralgia and nociceptor sensitization [43], evidence from the literature points to the conversion of information from the large-fiber mechanoreceptive system onto the nociceptive system somewhere along the neuraxis as a prominent pathophysiological characteristic of dynamic mechanical allodynia. The prevalence of dynamic mechanical allodynia in neuropathic pain patients within single etiological diagnostic entities has only been reported in scattered publications of limited groups of patients (e.g., [49,78,86,93]) and seems to be present in a minority of patients (20–40%) across diagnostic entities. Again, in different animal models of neuropathies, tactile hypersensitivity is found at a group level.

Heat Sensitivity Assessment

In general, behavioral testing of withdrawal responses of the neuropathic hindpaw to heat stimuli in different animal models has also gained acceptance in the preclinical scientific pain community. However, thermal responses are particularly inconsistent in these models. Most models, especially the CCI, may produce hypersensitivity to heat stimuli, which suggests an increased sensitivity of the nociceptor peripheral terminal. Thermal hypersensitivity is often absent after SNL.

Again, with the exception of subgroups of patients with postherpetic neuralgia and nociceptor sensitization [43], heat allodynia is an infrequent sign in neuropathic pain states [49,52,66] and is not a problem in activities of daily living for patients with neuropathic pain. Furthermore, to our knowledge the literature has no information on neuropathic pain, excluding studies of postherpetic neuralgia, qualifying increased heat sensitivity as an indirect measure of ongoing pain. Therefore, the inclusion of heat-induced withdrawal as part of the behavioral testing procedure frequently used in animal models of neuropathy lacks a valid rationale based on clinical observations. However, in some peripheral neuropathies (e.g., burning feet syndrome), heat may considerably increase symptoms and cold relieves them within a few seconds. Patients usually put their feet in cold water, sleep with their feet outside the blankets, or walk on a stone tiled floor during the night to find relief.

Cold Sensitivity Assessment

While most models of neuropathic pain are associated with cold hypersensitive behaviors, this feature is absent in the PSL incomplete axotomy model. Establishing the presence of cold hypersensitivity in animal models appears essential as this type of allodynia is not uncommon in neuropathic pain patients [66]. The contribution to the suffering of the patient from cold allodynia has not been studied in detail.

Predictive Validity of Models

The predictive validity of models refers to the requirement for a model to be sensitive to effective analgesic drugs and treatments and fail to respond to ineffective drugs and treatments. Kontinen and Meert [74] evaluated in the 60–90% range the predictive pharmacological validity of four established models of peripheral nerve neuropathy (CCI, PSL, SNL, and streptozocin). Limitations as to the predictive validity of pain-related models of neuropathy are probably related to the fact that key clinical features of neuropathic pain, particularly spontaneous pain, are not adequately identified and quantified with preclinical behavioral procedures [88].

Summary and Conclusions

Behavioral tests of nociception are not entirely satisfactory [120,77,125]. Their first weakness lies in the difficulty of controlling the stimuli used to trigger a nociceptive reaction. More importantly, even when the physical parameters of the external stimuli are well controlled, the result is not necessarily an equally well-controlled valid stimulus. Indeed, the stimulus that effectively activates the peripheral nociceptors is also influenced by the physiological state of the targeted tissue. This state is determined by the vegetative system, mainly through thermoregulation, systemic arterial blood pressure, and local vasomotor tone. For example, variation in local temperature may confound many experimental protocols, not only those using heat as a stimulus [102,120].

The second great weakness in the methods for testing the models lies in the nature of the dependent variable, which is usually the determination of the threshold for a reaction. Most tests do not allow for the analysis of the stimulus-response functions of the models, in the sense of a transfer function of a sensory system, although these functions are an essential element of sensory physiology. Furthermore, it is often not the threshold itself that is assessed, but a reaction time to a stimulus of increasing intensity. Moreover, when the skin is subjected to a constant source of radiation, the temperature increases with the square root of time (Fig. 5). It follows that such an approach is highly questionable when radiant heat is used. In order to justify this approach, one usually refers to the classical work of Hardy and colleagues on pain sensation elicited by radiant heat in humans [54,55]. Although these authors introduced the radiant heat as a stimulus for the study of warm and pain sensation, and later used the technique in rats [56,58], they never measured a reaction time, nor did they use the method of limits to determine thermal thresholds. They used the method of levels for the determination of thresholds and paid particular attention to the basal temperature of the skin. In this respect, they often chose as the stimulation site the forehead, where the baseline temperature (~34°C) is less prone to interindividual variations. One cannot refer to this work to justify the use of response time measurements following radiant heat application.

These considerations invite prudence in the interpretation of results obtained using tests of nociception in the animal. It is worth stressing that these concerns also relate to rat models of chronic pain insofar as the tests applied in these models are the same, or almost the same, as those described for acute pain. Faced with the simplistic and reductionistic approaches available, one is inclined to conclude that valid behavioral approaches of pain should be promoted in animal studies.

It is time to comment on confusion introduced by the terminology. Terms such as pain, analgesia, allodynia, and hyperalgesia, as defined by the International Association for the Study of Pain, are symptoms that presuppose a verbal communication between examiner and subject or patient, which precludes their use in animal studies [39]. Whatever the way it is measured, pain is not an "observable" variable belonging to the domain of clinical signs and laboratory tests but a "latent" construct (a symptom, reported by the patient). Use of such nomenclature in the scientific literature on animals not only creates confusion in this respect but may give the false impression of a secure and unrestricted parallelism between species in all aspects. A relevant example to highlight the problem of interpretation of symptoms and signs in animals is the widely used CCI rat model [14], proposed as a "neuropathic pain model." The model may mimic to some extent the clinical condition of entrapment neuropathy (e.g., median nerve entrapment in the carpal tunnel). However, the most common complaint in patients with median nerve entrapment is, again, numbness with tingling paresthesia and infrequently neuropathic pain.

An "experimental model" makes sense only if its very first function is to verify a "theoretical model." The term "model" is often used mindlessly. Again, we are facing a problem of terminology: the misuse of the term "model." We have tried to provide

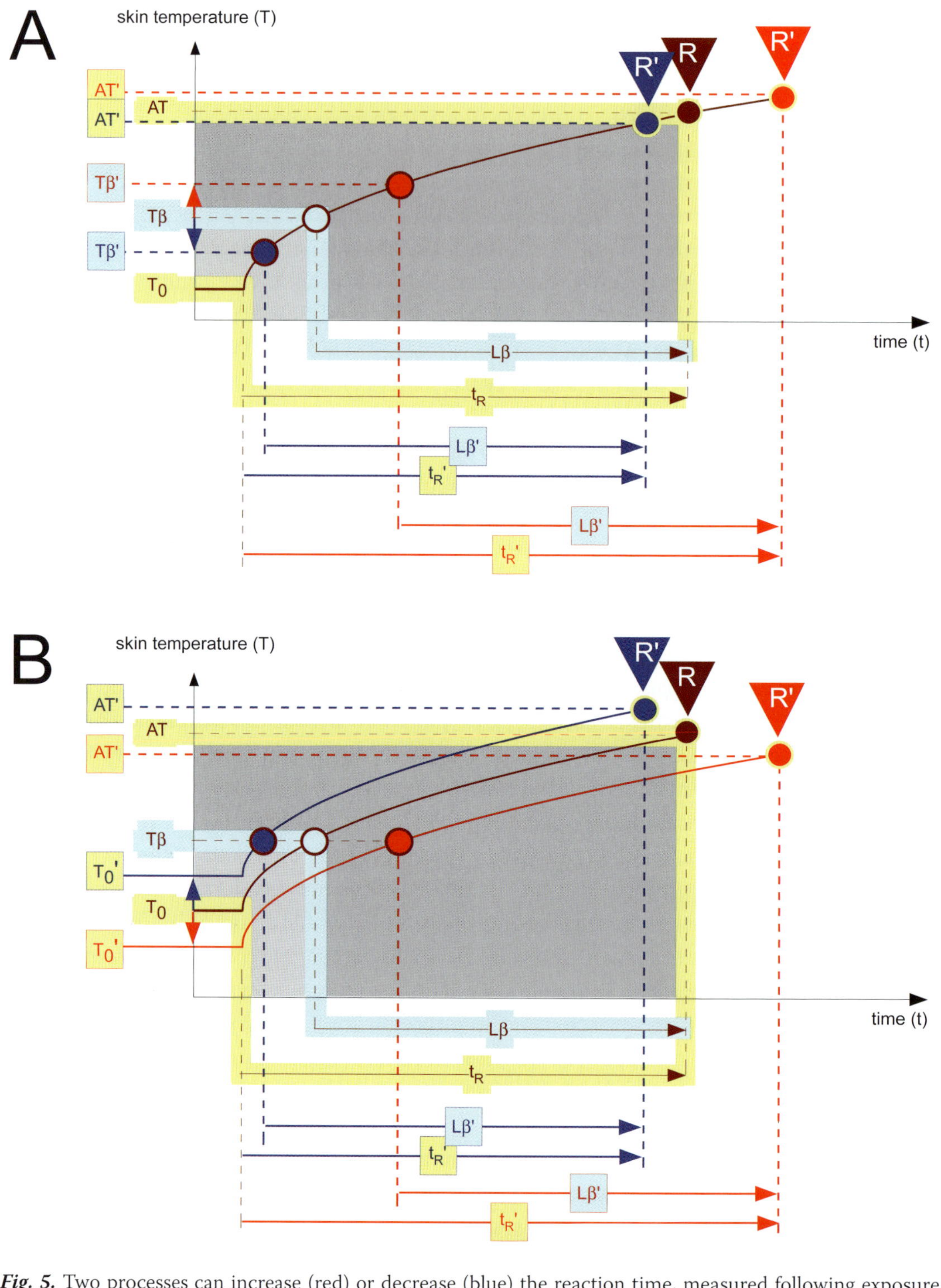

Fig. 5. Two processes can increase (red) or decrease (blue) the reaction time, measured following exposure to a constant source of radiant heat: (A) variations of threshold or (B) variations of the initial temperature (T_0). The measurable variables are indicated with a yellow background, while variables to be determined are indicated with a blue background. Presentation as in Fig. 3B.

elements for an evaluation of the validity of both animal tests and models of pain. We must, however, admit to disappointment. Many approaches that have been used are probably misleading, and this may be the pivotal reason for our disappointment regarding translation of basic research findings to the bedside, in spite of a massive data overflow from the animal models.

References

[1] Adam F, Bonnet F, Le Bars D. Tolerance to morphine analgesia: evidence for stimulus intensity as a key factor and complete reversal by a glycine site-specific NMDA antagonist. Neuropharmacology 2006;51:191–202.

[2] Adam F, Dufour E, Le Bars D. The glycine site-specific NMDA antagonist (+)-HA966 enhances the effect of morphine and reverses morphine tolerance via a spinal mechanism. Neuropharmacology 2008;54:588–96.

[3] Andre J, Zeau B, Pohl M, Cesselin F, Benoliel JJ, Becker C. Involvement of cholecystokininergic systems in anxiety-induced hyperalgesia in male rats: behavioral and biochemical studies. J Neurosci 2005;25:7896–904.

[4] Aley KO, Reichling DB, Levine JD. Vincristine hyperalgesia in the rat: a model of painful vincristine neuropathy in humans. Neuroscience 1996;73:259–65.

[5] Ameye LG, Young MF. Animal models of osteoarthritis: lessons learned while seeking the "Holy Grail." Curr Opin Rheumatol 2006;18:537–47.

[6] Apfel SC. Diabetic neuropathy models: are they relevant? Drug Discov Today Dis Models 2006;3:397–402.

[7] Baldwin AE, Cannon JT. Sensitization of the tail-flick reflex following exposure to either a single prolonged test trial or behavioral testing under the analgesic influence of morphine. Pain 1996;67:163–72.

[8] Bateson P. Assessment of pain in animals. Anim Behav 1991;42:827–39.

[9] Beecher HK. Pain in men wounded in battle. Ann Surg 1946;123:96–105.

[10] Beecher HK. Relationship of significance of wound to pain experienced. JAMA 1956;161:1609–13.

[11] Beecher HK. The measurement of pain: prototype for the quantitative study of subjective responses. Pharmacol Rev 1957;9:59–209.

[12] Beecher HK. Pain: one mystery solved. Science 1966;151:840–1.

[13] Bennet GJ. Animal models of pain. In: Kruger L, editor. Methods in pain research. Boca Raton: CRC Press; 2001. p. 67–91.

[14] Bennett GJ, Xie YK. A peripheral mononeuropathy in rat that produces disorders of pain sensation like those seen in man. Pain 1988;33:87–107.

[15] Benoist JM, Pincedé I, Ballantyne K, Plaghki L, Le Bars D. Peripheral and central determinants of a nociceptive reaction: an approach to psychophysics in the rat. PLoS One 2008;3:e3125.

[16] Berge OG. Reliability and validity in animal pain modeling. In: Tjølsen A, Berge OG, editors. Pain and brain. Bergen: University of Bergen; 2002. p. 77–89.

[17] Berman D, Rodin BE. The influence of housing condition on autotomy following dorsal rhizotomy in rats. Pain 1982;13:307–11.

[18] Blackburn-Munro G. Pain-like behaviours in animals: how human are they? Trends Pharmacol Sci 2004;25:299–305.

[19] Blumenkopf B, Lipman JJ. Studies in autotomy: its pathophysiology and usefulness as a model of chronic pain. Pain 1991;45:203–9.

[20] Brand DD. Rodent models of rheumatoid arthritis. Comp Med 2005;55:114–22.

[21] Buettner K. Effects of extreme heat and cold on human skin. II. Surface temperature, pain and heat conductivity in experiments with radiant heat. J Appl Physiol 1951;3:703–13.

[22] Butler SH. Animal models and the assessment of chronic pain: critique of the arthritic rat model. In: Chapman CR, Loeser JD, editors. Issues in pain measurement. Advances in pain research and therapy, Vol. 12. New York: Raven Press; 1989. p. 473–9.

[23] Calvino B, Crepon-Bernard MO, Le Bars D. Parallel clinical and behavioural studies of adjuvant induced arthritis in the rat: possible relationship with 'chronic pain'. Behav Brain Res 1987;24:11–29.

[24] Carmody J. Avoiding fallacies in nociceptive measurements. Pain 1995;63:136.

[25] Chau TT. Analgesic testing in animal models. In: Chang JY, Lewis AJ, editors. Pharmacological methods in the control of inflammation. New York: Alan Liss; 1989. p. 195–212.

[26] Chesler EJ, Wilson SG, Lariviere WR, Rodriguez-Zas SL, Mogil JS. Identification and ranking of genetic and laboratory environment factors influencing a behavioral trait, thermal nociception, via computational analysis of a large data archive. Neurosci Biobehav Rev 2002;26:907–23.

[27] Choi Y, Yoon YW, Na HS, Kim SH, Chung JM. Behavioral signs of ongoing pain and cold allodynia in a rat model of neuropathic pain. Pain 1994;59:369–76.

[28] Collier HO. Analgesics. In: Lawrence DR, Bacharach AL, editors. Evaluation of drug activities: pharmacometrics, Vol. 1. New York: Academic Press; 1964. p. 183–203.

[29] Colpaert FC, Tarayre JP, Alliaga M, Bruins Slot LA, Attal N, Koek W. Opiate self-administration as a measure of chronic nociceptive pain in arthritic rats. Pain 2001;91:33–45.

[30] Cooper BY, Vierck CJ Jr. Measurement of pain and morphine hyperalgesia in monkeys. Pain 1986;26:361–92.

[31] Creed RS, Denny-Brown D, Eccles JC, Liddell EGT, Sherrington CS. Reflex activity of the spinal cord. Oxford: Clarendon Press; 1932.
[32] De Castro Costa M, De Sutter P, Gybels J, Van Hees J. Adjuvant-induced arthritis in rats: a possible animal model of chronic pain. Pain 1981;10:173–85.
[33] Dennis SG, Melzack R. Perspective on phylogenetic evolution of pain expression. In: Kitchell RL, Erickson HH, editors. Animal pain: perception and alleviation. Bethesda: American Physiological Society; 1983. p. 151–60.
[34] Dewey WL, Harris LS. The tail-flick test. In: Ehrenpreis S, Neidle A, editors. Methods in narcotic research. New York: Marcel Dekker; 1975. p. 101–9.
[35] Dong WK. Is autotomy a valid measure of chronic pain ? In: Chapman CR, Loeser JD, editors. Issues in pain measurement. Advances in pain research and therapy, Vol. 12. New York: Raven Press; 1989. p. 463–72.
[36] Dubinsky B, Gebre-Mariam S, Capetola RJ, Rosenthale ME. The antialgesic drugs: human therapeutic correlates of their potency in laboratory animal models of hyperalgesia. Agents Actions 1987;20:50–60.
[37] Dubuisson D, Dennis SG. The formalin test: a quantitative study of the analgesic effects of morphine, meperidine and brain stem stimulation in rats and cats. Pain 1977;4:161–74.
[38] Dworkin SF, Whitney CW. Relaying on objective and subjective measures of chronic pain: guidelines for use and interpretation. In: Turk DC, Melzack R, editors. Handbook of pain assessment. New York: Guilford Press; 1992. p. 429–46.
[39] Ekblom A, Hansson P. When is "pain" appropriate? Pain 1993;55:401–3.
[40] Falmagne JC. Elements of psychophysical theory. New York: Oxford University Press; 1985.
[41] Fernihough J, Gentry C, Malcangio M, Fox A, Rediske J, Pellas T, Kidd B, Bevan S, Winter J. Pain related behaviour in two models of osteoarthritis in the rat knee. Pain 2004;112:83–93.
[42] Field MJ, Bramwell S, Hughes J, Singh L. Detection of static and dynamic components of mechanical allodynia in rat models of neuropathic pain: are they signalled by distinct primary sensory neurones? Pain 1999;83:303–11.
[43] Fields HL, Rowbotham M, Baron R. Postherpetic neuralgia: irritable nociceptors and deafferentation. Neurobiol Dis 1998;5:209–27.
[44] Foltz EL, White LE. Pain "relief" by frontal cingulotomy. J Neurosurg 1962;19:83–100.
[45] Forman LJ, Estilow S, Lewis M, Vasilenko P. Streptozocin diabetes alters immunoreactive beta-endorphin levels and pain perception after 8 wk in female rats. Diabetes 1986;35:1309–13.
[46] Freemann W, Watts JW. Pain of organic disease relieved by prefrontal lobotomy. Lancet 1946;1:953–5.
[47] Gamble GD, Milne RJ. Repeated exposure to sham testing procedures reduces reflex withdrawal and hot-plate latencies: attenuation of tonic descending inhibition? Neurosci Lett 1989;96:312–7.
[48] Golden JP, Johnson EM Jr. Models of chemotherapy drug-induced peripheral neuropathy. Drug Discov Today 2004;1:186–91.
[49] Gottrup H, Andersen J, Arendt-Nielsen L, Jensen TS. Psychophysical examination in patients with post-mastectomy pain. Pain 2000;87:275–84.
[50] Green EC. Anatomy of the rat. New York: Hafner; 1955.
[51] Gustorff B, Nahlik G, Hoerauf KH, Kress HG. The absence of acute tolerance during remifentanil infusion in volunteers. Anesth Analg 2002;94:1223–8.
[52] Hansson P. Difficulties in stratifying neuropathic pain by mechanisms. Eur J Pain 2003;7:353–7.
[53] Hardy JD. Body temperature regulation. In: Mountcastle VB, editor. Medical physiology, Vol. 2. St Louis: Mosby; 1980. p. 1417–56.
[54] Hardy JD, Wolff HG, Goodell H. Studies on pain. A new method for measuring pain threshold: observation on spatial summation of pain. J Clin Invest 1940;19:649–57.
[55] Hardy JD, Wolff HG, Goodell H. Pain sensation and reaction. Baltimore: Williams and Wilkins; 1952.
[56] Hardy JD, Jacobs I, Meixner MD. Thresholds of pain and reflex contraction as related to noxious stimulation. J Appl Physiol 1953;5:725–39.
[57] Hardy JD, Hammel HT, Murgatroyd D. Spectral transmittance and reflectance of excised human skin, J Appl Physiol 1956;9:257–64.
[58] Hardy JD, Stoll AM, Cunningham D, Benson WM and Greene L. Responses of the rat to thermal radiation. Am J Physiol 1957;189:1–5.
[59] Harris LS, Pierson AK. Some narcotic antagonists in the benzomorphan series. J Pharmacol Exp Ther 1964;143:141–8.
[60] Hendershot LC, Forsaith J. Antagonism of the frequency of phenylquinone-induced writhing in the mouse by weak analgesics and nonanalgesics. J Pharmacol Exp Ther 1959;125:237–40.
[61] Hendler E, Crosbie JD, Hardy JD. Measurement of heating of the skin temperature during exposure to infrared radiations. J Appl Physiol 1965;12:177–85.
[62] Hogan Q. Animal pain models. Reg Anesth Pain Med 2002;27:385–401.
[63] Honoré P. Behavioral assessment of neuropathic pain in preclinical models. Drug Dev Res 2006;67:302–7.
[64] Houghton AD, Nicholls G, Houghton AL, Saadah E, McColl L. Phantom pain: natural history and association with rehabilitation. Ann R Coll Surg Engl 1994;76:22–5.
[65] Hugon M. Exteroceptive reflexes to stimulation of the sural nerve in normal man. In: Desmedt JE, editor. New developments in electromyography and clinical neurophysiology, Vol. 3. Basel: Karger; 1973. p. 713–29.
[66] Jørum E, Warncke T, Stubhaug A. Cold allodynia and hyperalgesia in neuropathic pain: the effect of *N*-methyl-D-aspartate (NMDA) receptor antagonist ketamine: a double-blind, cross-over comparison with alfentanil and placebo. Pain 2003;101:229–35.
[67] Kallina CF, Grau JW. Tail-flick test. I: Impact of a suprathreshold exposure to radiant heat on pain reactivity in rats. Physiol Behav 1995;58:161–8.

[68] Kauppila T. Correlation between autotomy-behavior and current theories of neuropathic pain. Neurosci Biobehav Rev 1998;23:111–29.
[69] Kawakita K, Funakoshi M. A quantitative study on the tail flick test in the rat. Physiol Behav 1987;39:235–40.
[70] Kim SH, Chung JM. An experimental model for peripheral neuropathy produced by segmental spinal nerve ligation in the rat. Pain 1992;50:355–63.
[71] Kingery WS, Casatellote JM, Wang EE. A loose ligature-induced mononeuropathy produces hyperalgesias mediated by both the injured sciatic nerve and the adjacent saphenous nerve. Pain 1993;55:297–304.
[72] Kobayashi K, Imaizumi R, Sumichika H, Tanaka H, Goda M, Fukunari A, Komatsu H. Sodium iodoacetate-induced experimental osteoarthritis and associated pain model in rats. J Vet Med Sci 2003;65:1195–9.
[73] Koltzenburg M, Lundberg LE, Torebjörk HE. Dynamic and static components of mechanical hyperalgesia in human hairy skin. Pain 1992;51:207–19.
[74] Kontinen VS, Meert TF. Predictive validity of neuropathic pain models in pharmacological studies with a behavioural outcome in the rat: a systematic review. In: Dostrovsky J, Carr D, Koltzenburg M, editors. Proceedings of the 10th World Congress on Pain. Seattle: IASP Press; 2003. p. 489–98.
[75] Lai YY, Chan SHH. Shortened pain response time following repeated algesiometric test in rats. Physiol Behav 1982;28:1111–3.
[76] Landis CA, Levine JD, Robinson CR. Decreased slow wave and paradoxical sleep in a rat chronic pain model. Sleep 1989;12:167–77.
[77] Le Bars D, Gozariu M, Cadden SW. Animal models of nociception. Pharmacol Rev 2001;53:597–652.
[78] Leijon G, Boive J, Johansson I. Central post-stroke pain: neurological symptoms and pain characteristics. Pain 1989;36:13–25.
[79] Lineberry CG. Laboratory animals in pain research. In: Gay WI, editor. Methods in animal experimentation, Vol. 6. New York: Academic Press; 1981. p. 237–311.
[80] Lloyd DPC. Neuron patterns controlling transmission of ipsilateral hind limb reflex in the cat. J Neurophysiol 1943;6:293–315.
[81] Lloyd DPC. Reflex action in relation to pattern and peripheral source of afferent stimulation. J Neurophysiol 1943;6:111–20.
[82] Loux JJ, Smith S, Salem H. Comparative analgesic testing of various compounds in mice using writhing techniques. Arzneimittelforschung 1978;28:1644–7.
[83] Luce RD. Response times, their role in inferring elementary mental organization. New York: Oxford University Press; 1986.
[84] Lundberg A. Inhibitory control from the brain stem of transmission from primary afferents to motoneurons, primary afferent terminals and ascending pathways. In: Sjölund B, Björklund A, editors. Brain stem control of spinal mechanisms. Amsterdam: Elsevier; 1982. p. 179–224.
[85] Ma C. Animal models of pain. Int Anesthesiol Clin 2007;45:121–31.
[86] Martin C, Solders G, Sonnerborg A, Hansson P. Painful and nonpainful neuropathy in HIV-infected patients: an analysis of somatosensory nerve function. Eur J Pain 2003;7:23–31.
[87] Mogil JS. The genetic mediation of individual differences in sensitivity to pain and its inhibition. Proc Natl Acad Sci USA 1999;96:7744–51.
[88] Negus SS, Vanderah TW, Brandt MR, Bilsky EJ, Becerra L, Borsook D. Preclinical assessment of candidate analgesic drugs: recent advances and future challenges. J Pharmacol Exp Ther 2006;319:507–14.
[89] Neugebauer V, Han JS, Adwanikar H, Fu Y, Ji G. Techniques for assessing knee joint pain in arthritis. Mol Pain 2007;28:3–8.
[90] Nikolajsen L, Ilkjaer S, Kroner K, Christensen JH, Jensen TS. The influence of preamputation pain on postamputation stump and phantom pain. Pain 1997;72:393–405.
[91] Ochoa JL, Yarnitsky D. Mechanical hyperalgesias in neuropathic pain patients: dynamic and static subtypes. Ann Neurol 1993;33:465–72.
[92] O'Hagan BJ. Neuropathic pain in a cat post-amputation. Aust Vet J 2006;84:83–6.
[93] Otto M, Bak S, Bach FW, Jensen TS, Sindrup SH. Pain phenomena and possible mechanisms in patients with painful polyneuropathy. Pain 2003;101:187–92.
[94] Pearson CM. Development of arthritis, periarthritis, and periostosis in rats given adjuvant. Proc Soc Exp Biol Med 1956;91:95–101.
[95] Plone MA, Emerich DF, Lindner MD. Individual differences in the hotplate test and effects of habituation on sensitivity to morphine. Pain 1996;66:265–70.
[96] Pomonis JD, Boulet JM, Gottshall SL, Phillips S, Sellers R, Bunton T, Walker K. Development and pharmacological characterization of a rat model of osteoarthritis pain. Pain 2005;114:339–46.
[97] Pong SF, Demuth SM, Kinney CM, Deegan P. Prediction of human analgesic dosages of nonsteroidal anti-inflammatory drugs (NSAIDs) from analgesic ED_{50} values in mice. Arch Int Pharmacodyn Ther 1985;273:212–20.
[98] Randall LO, Selitto JJ. A method for measurement of analgesic activity on inflamed tissue. Arch Int Pharmacodyn Ther 1957;111:409–19.
[99] Ren K. An improved method for assessing mechanical allodynia in the rat. Physiol Behav 1999;67:711–16.
[100] Rodin BE, Kruger L. Deafferentation in animals as a model for the study of pain: an alternative hypothesis. Brain Res 1984;319:213–328.
[101] Romer D. Pharmacological evaluation of mild analgesics. Br J Clin Pharmacol 1980;2:247S–51S.
[102] Rosland JH. The formalin test in mice: the influence of ambient temperature. Pain 1991;45:211–6.

[103] Sandkühler J, Treier AC, Liu XG, Ohnimus M. The massive expression of c-fos protein in spinal dorsal horn neurons is not followed by long-term changes in spinal nociception. Neuroscience 1996;73:657–66.
[104] Sandrini G, Serrao M, Rossi P, Romaniello A, Cruccu G, Willer JC. The lower limb flexion reflex in humans. Prog Neurobiol 2005;77:353–95.
[105] Schmidt RF, Willis WD, editors. Encyclopedia of pain. Berlin: Springer; 2007.
[106] Schomburg ED. Spinal sensorimotor systems and their supraspinal control. Neurosci Res 1990;7:265–340.
[107] Schomburg ED. Restrictions on the interpretation of spinal reflex modulation in pain and analgesia research. Pain Forum 1997;6:101–9.
[108] Seltzer Z, Dubner R, Shir Y. A novel behavioral model of neuropathic pain disorders produced in rats by partial sciatic nerve injury. Pain 1990;43:205–18.
[109] Seltzer Z. The relevance of animal neuropathy models for chronic pain in humans. Semin Neurosci 1995;7:211–9.
[110] Sherrington CS. The integrative action of the nervous system. New York: C. Scribner's Sons; 1906.
[111] Sherrington CS. Flexion-reflex of the limb, crossed extension-reflex, and reflex stepping and standing. J Physiol (Lond) 1910;40:28–121.
[112] Sheth RN, Dorsi MJ, Li Y, Murinson BB, Belzberg AJ, Griffin JW, Meyer RA. Mechanical hyperalgesia after an L5 ventral rhizotomy or an L5 ganglionectomy in the rat. Pain 2002;96:63–72.
[113] Siegmund E, Cadmus R, Lu G. A method for evaluating both non-narcotic and narcotic analgesics. Proc Soc Exp Biol Med 1957;95:729–31.
[114] Sternbach RA. Pain patients. New York: Academic Press; 1974.
[115] Stolwijk JAJ, Hardy JD. Skin and subcutaneous temperature changes during exposure to intense thermal radiation. J Appl Physiol 1965;20:1006–13.
[116] Sweet WH. Treatment of medically intractable mental disease by limited frontal leucotomy: justifiable? N Engl J Med 1973;289:1117–25.
[117] Taber RI, Greenhouse DD, Irwin S. Inhibition of phenylquinone-induced writhing by narcotic antagonists. Nature 1964;204:189–90.
[118] Taber RI. Predictive value of analgesic assays in mice and rats. In: Braude MC, Harris LS, May EL, Smith JP, Villareal JE, editors. Narcotic antagonists, advances in biochemical psychopharmacology, Vol. 8. New York: Raven Press; 1974. p. 191–211.
[119] Tal M, Bennett GJ. Extra-territorial pain in rats with a peripheral mononeuropathy: mechanohyperalgesia and mechano-allodynia in the territory of an uninjured nerve. Pain 1994;57:375–82.
[120] Tjølsen A, Hole K. Animal models of analgesia. In: Dickenson AH, Besson JM, editors. Pharmacology of pain. Berlin: Springer; 1997. p. 1–20.
[121] Tsuruoka M, Matsui A, Matsui Y. Quantitative relationship between the stimulus intensity and the response magnitude in the tail flick reflex. Physiol Behav 1988;43:79–83.
[122] Vadakkan KI, Xu H, Zhuo M. Common characteristics and pathways in neuropathic pain of different etiology. Drug Discov Today Dis Models 2006;3:413–7.
[123] Vierck CJ. Extrapolations from the pain research literature to problems of adequate veterinary care. J Am Vet Med Assoc 1976;168:510–3.
[124] Vierck CJ, Cooper BY. Guideline for assessing pain reactions and pain modulation in laboratory animal subjects. In: Kruger L, Liebeskind JC, editors. Advances in pain research and therapy, Vol. 6. New York: Raven Press; 1984. p. 305–22.
[125] Vierck CJ, Hansson PT, Yezierski RP. Clinical and pre-clinical pain assessment: are we measuring the same thing? Pain 2008;135:7–10.
[126] Vinik, HR, Kissin I. Rapid development of tolerance to analgesia during remifentanil infusion in humans. Anesth Analg 1998;86:1307–11.
[127] Waksman BH. Immune regulation in adjuvant disease and other arthritis models: relevance to pathogenesis of chronic arthritis. Scand J Immunol 2002;56:12–34.
[128] Wall PD, Devor M, Inbal R, Scadding JW, Schonfeld D, Seltzer Z, Tomkiewicz MM. Autotomy following peripheral nerve lesions: experimental anaesthesia dolorosa. Pain 1979;7:103–11.
[129] Wang LX, Wang ZJ. Animal and cellular models of chronic pain. Adv Drug Deliv Rev 2003;55:949–65.
[130] Wartan SW, Hamann W, Wedley JR, McColl I. Phantom pain and sensation among British veteran amputees. Br J Anaesth 1997;78:652–9.
[131] Whitehouse MW. Adjuvant arthritis 50 years on: the impact of the 1956 article by C.M. Pearson, 'Development of arthritis, periarthritis and periostitis in rats given adjuvants'. Inflamm Res 2007;56:133–8.
[132] Willer JC. Comparative study of perceived pain and nociceptive flexion reflex in man. Pain 1977;3:69–80.
[133] Woodworth RS, Sherrington CS. A pseudoaffective reflex and its spinal path. J Physiol (Lond) 1904;31:234–43.
[134] Wright BE, Katovich MJ. Effect of restraint on drug-induced changes in skin and core temperature in biotelemetered rats. Pharmacol Biochem Behav 1996;55:219–25.
[135] Yarnitsky D, Ochoa JL. Studies of heat pain sensation in man: perception thresholds, rate of stimulus rise and reaction time. Pain 1990;40:85–91.
[136] Yarnitsky D, Ochoa JL. Warm and cold specific somatosensory systems Psychophysical thresholds, reaction times and peripheral conduction velocities. Brain 1991;114:1819–26.

Correspondence to: Daniel Le Bars, DVM, DSci, Team "Pain," INSERM UMRS 975, CNRS UMR 7225, 91 Boulevard de l'Hôpital, 75013 Paris, France. Email: daniel.le_bars@upmc.fr.

Part IV

Clinical Pharmacology of Pain

22

Pharmacological Considerations for the Obstetric Patient

John S. McDonald[a,b] and Wing-Fai Kwan[b]

[a]Department of Anesthesiology and Department of Obstetrics and Gynecology, David Geffen School of Medicine, University of California at Los Angeles; [b]Department of Anesthesiology, Harbor-UCLA Medical Center, University of California at Los Angeles, Los Angeles, California, USA

Many physiological and biochemical changes occur during pregnancy, sometimes to such an extent as to mimic disease in a nonpregnant woman. Physiological changes in pregnancy occur in multiple areas, chiefly the cardiovascular system, lungs, kidneys, and gastrointestinal tract. These changes may influence the pharmacokinetic parameters of drug absorption, distribution, metabolism, and elimination (Table I). A full understanding of each pharmacokinetic characteristic is important so that appropriate drug therapy can be provided during pregnancy for the safety of both the mother and the fetus.

Pharmacokinetics

Drug Absorption

Gastrointestinal Absorption

Factors that affect the gastrointestinal absorption of drugs include (1) drug formulation, i.e., simultaneous administration with food or other drugs; (2) chemical composition, i.e., pH of the intestinal secretions; (3) gastric emptying time; (4) intestinal motility; and (5) blood flow. In pregnancy, the motility of the stomach and intestinal tract decrease, because of increased progesterone production. In fact, gastric and intestinal emptying times may be increased by as much as 30–50% during pregnancy [71]. As a result, the

Pharmacology of Pain
edited by Pierre Beaulieu, David Lussier, Frank Porreca, and Anthony H. Dickenson
IASP Press, Seattle, © 2010

Table I
Summary of main pregnancy-related physiological and pharmacokinetic changes

Parameter	Physiological Changes	Pharmacokinetic Changes	Drugs
Absorption			
Gastrointestinal	↑ Gastrointestinal transit	↓ C_{max}	Acetaminophen, opioids, antiemetics
	↓ Gastrointestinal motility	↑ Absorption	All
		↓ Absorption	Drugs metabolized in gastrointestinal tract
	↑ Gastrointestinal blood flow	↑ Absorption	All
	↑ Gastric pH	↑ Ionization; ↓ absorption	Weak acids
		↓ Ionization; ↑ absorption	Weak bases
	Nausea and vomiting	↓ Absorption; ↓ C_{max}	All
Intramuscular	↑ Muscle blood flow	↑ Absorption; ↑ concentration	All
Pulmonary	↑ Pulmonary blood flow; hyper-ventilation	↑ Absorption	Anesthetic gases, other inhaled drugs
Distribution			
Volume of distribution	↑ Total body water; ↑ plasma volume, amniotic fluid	↑ Vd hydrophilic drugs; ↓ C_{max}	Aminoglycosides, ampicillin, cephalosporins, vancomycin
	↑ Adipose mass	↑ Vd lipophilic drugs; ↓ C_{max}	Diazepam, fentanyl, oxazepam, ondansetron
Protein binding	↓ Albumin; ↓ drug binding	↓ Total concentration; ↑ free portion; ↑, ↓, ↔ pharmacological effect, depending on drug	Salicylic acid, alfentanil, bupivacaine, dexamethasone, diazepam, fentanyl, SSRIs, lidocaine, midazolam, phenobarbital
Metabolism			
Hepatic	↑ Hepatic blood flow	↑ Clearance of drugs with high first-pass metabolism	Lidocaine, midazolam, morphine
	↑ Progesterone	↑ Activity CYP2C9; ↑ total clearance (T1, T2, T3); ↑ intrinsic clearance (T3)	Phenytoin
		↑ Activity CYP3A4; ↑ clearance (T1, T2, T3)	Carbamazepine
	↑ Estrogens	↓ Activity CYP1A2; ↑ half-life; ↓ clearance (T1, T2, T3)	Caffeine
Fetal		Possible accumulation of metabolites more polar than parent drug	Normeperidine
Elimination			
Renal	↑ Renal blood flow; ↑ glomerular filtration rate; ↑ secretion?	↑ Clearance (T1, T2, T3)	Bupropion, gabapentin, vigabatrin
Biliary	Cholestasis	↓ Clearance of drugs undergoing tubular secretion	Rifampicin

Abbreviations and symbols: ↑ = increase, ↓ = decrease, ↔ = unchanged, C_{max}= maximum concentration, CYP= cytochrome P450, T1 = first trimester, T2 = second trimester, T3 = third trimester, Vd = volume of distribution; SSRIs = selective serotonin reuptake inhibitors.

absorption and onset of drug response may be delayed, as has been shown for acetaminophen (paracetamol) use in late pregnancy [84]. Clinically, this factor may be important when a rapid onset of drug action is necessary. If a quick, reliable drug response is desired, intravenous (i.v.) administration is the preferred route of drug delivery, particularly for acute analgesic therapy. The rate of drug absorption from the gastrointestinal tract may be normal in labor provided that opioid analgesics have not been administered. Nimmo et al. [66] reported that absorption of acetaminophen was normal in 12 women in labor before administration of opioids. Interestingly, acetaminophen absorption was delayed significantly in women receiving opioids such as meperidine, diamorphine, or pentazocine.

An increase in gastric pH occurs due to a 40% reduction in gastric acid secretion in pregnant women; moreover, an increase in mucus production may enhance the ionization of weak acidic drugs that reduce absorption more than that of weak basic drugs.

When drugs are delivered via the oral route, absorption occurs chiefly by passive drug diffusion through the small intestine. Prolonged gastric emptying and reduced intestinal motility may cause an increase in drug dissolution time that could enhance the absorption of low water-soluble drugs. An example of a drug affected in this way is digoxin [53]. Conversely, increased exposure to metabolism by gut bacteria or mucosa can result in a decrease in bioavailability. An example of a drug subject to this phenomenon is chlorpromazine [39]. The concurrent use of nutritional supplements such as calcium, iron, and vitamins during pregnancy can bind and inactivate some drugs and thereby reduce gastrointestinal drug absorption. Nausea and vomiting may occur during the first trimester, resulting in reduced drug absorption.

Lung Absorption

Lung uptake of drugs is influenced by ventilation and hemodynamic factors. During pregnancy, increases in both alveolar ventilation and cardiac output can lead to greater alveolar uptake and systemic absorption of drugs [39]. Dose requirements for inhalation anesthetic agents, such as isoflurane, sevoflurane, and desflurane, decrease in pregnant women [70,26]. This effect could occur with any inhaled medication (e.g., albuterol) [47].

Intramuscular Absorption

Drug absorption from intramuscular (i.m.) delivery during pregnancy is enhanced by increased blood flow and tissue perfusion secondary to a dual increase in cardiac output and regional vasodilatation [81]. There is an exception in late pregnancy due to vena cava compression near term. Blood flow is reduced in the lower extremities due to an increased hydrostatic pressure in the venous systems caused by the uterus compressing the vena cava. Therefore, the above-mentioned enhancement of i.m. drugs at this site may be decreased [39].

Drug Distribution

The volume of distribution (Vd) of drugs may be altered during pregnancy because the plasma volume increases by 40–50% at term [87]. The mean total body water is also increased by about 8 liters, of which 80% is in the extracellular space and 20% in the intracellular space. About 60% of the total increment is distributed to the fetus, placenta, uterus, and amniotic fluid, and 40% is distributed to maternal tissue [79,80]. Therefore, drugs that are predominantly distributed in water and have a low Vd (e.g., cephalosporins) will have the biggest reduction in drug plasma concentration overall [79]. Thus, drug dosage requirements would be expected to be elevated to achieve comparable therapeutic effects. Lipophilic drugs (e.g., amiodarone) are already extensively distributed throughout the body and tend to be affected minimally by the change in mean total body water [64].

Body fat increases by approximately 4 kg during pregnancy and may act as a reservoir for lipophilic drugs [79]. Drugs with lipophilic properties (e.g., ondansetron or fentanyl) may need to be initially dosed per kilogram of total body weight to achieve therapeutic concentrations at the site of action.

Protein Binding

As pregnancy advances, the plasma volume increases at a greater rate than plasma albumin production, thus creating a physiological hypoalbuminemia [59]. In addition, plasma concentrations of free fatty acids and steroid hormones, which occupy protein-binding sites, are higher during pregnancy. The overall effect is a decrease in binding capacity for albumin and therefore, an increase in the unbound or free fraction of drug available to elicit pharmacological effects [28,56]. Drugs that are highly protein bound to albumin, such as most anticonvulsants and serotonin reuptake inhibitors, may be displaced and lead to an increased effect. Conversely, some studies have shown that more free drugs (e.g., phenytoin) are available for clearance by the kidney and liver, actually leading to lower drug levels and therefore reduced pharmacological effects [8]. In comparison to albumin, concentrations of α_1-acid glycoprotein are not significantly altered during pregnancy [95]. This consideration is extremely important in regard to the mother because this glycoprotein binds most basic drugs such as opioid analgesics and local anesthetics, therefore protecting the mother against the negative effects of these agents. However, as there is a significant decrease in this glycoprotein in the fetus, the free fraction of basic drugs (e.g., lidocaine) can be higher in the fetus than in the mother [95].

Drug Metabolism

The metabolism of drugs primarily occurs in the liver. Despite an increase in cardiac output and plasma volume, liver blood flow has been shown to remain normal during pregnancy, which means that the elimination rate of high extraction drugs (e.g., lidocaine) is relatively unchanged [42].

Several drug-metabolizing enzymes are present in the liver that increase drug hydrophilicity. The majority of drugs that undergo biotransformation are oxidized, reduced, hydrolyzed, or conjugated (i.e., phase I or II reactions); however, the most clinically important metabolic pathway is oxidation via the P-450 enzyme system. Perez et al. [73] conducted electron microscopic studies of liver biopsies taken during the last 3 months of human pregnancy and found a proliferation of smooth endoplasmic reticulum where the P-450 enzyme system existed. Hepatic enzyme activity is altered during pregnancy, leading to changes in the metabolism of drugs. Higher estrogen and progesterone concentrations throughout pregnancy are presumed to be responsible for this modification [30]. Some enzymes of the hepatic cytochrome P-450 system are induced by estrogen or progesterone (e.g., CYP3A4 and CYP2C9). This enzymatic activity results in a higher rate of metabolism of drugs such as phenytoin [30], whereas other isoenzymes are competitively inhibited by progesterone and estrogen (e.g., CYP1A2), leading to impaired hepatic elimination of drugs such as theophylline and caffeine [30,36]. Moreover, estrogen has a cholestatic effect, which may be enough to interfere with the clearance of certain drugs such as rifampicin [31] that are excreted into the biliary system.

Drug Elimination

Renal blood flow increases by 60–80% and glomerular filtration rate rises by 50% during pregnancy [22]. Creatinine clearance, which closely reflects the glomerular filtration rate, increases to a maximum at 34 weeks. The clearance of drugs excreted unchanged is directly proportional to creatinine clearance, and so the elimination of drugs that are primarily eliminated by the kidneys could be enhanced at this time [60,75].

Placental Transfer of Drugs

All drugs given to the mother will pass to the fetus to some extent, potentially affecting either fetal development or behavior. Most drugs cross the placenta by simple diffusion. The rate of diffusion across the placenta is determined by Fick's diffusion equation:

$$Q/t = K \times A \times (C_m - C_f)/D$$

where Q/t is the amount of drug transferred per unit of time, K is the diffusion coefficient or constant, A is surface area available for drug transfer, C_m is maternal drug concentration, and C_f is fetal drug concentration.

Thus, placental transfer of drugs depends on the following factors: (1) drug factors (K, diffusion coefficient): molecular weight, lipid solubility, and degree of ionization; (2) maternal factors: maternal concentrations of free drug; (3) placental factors: the area of transfer and diffusion distance; and (4) fetal factors: fetal concentrations of free drug.

Drug Factors

As a general principle, the larger the molecule, the less likely it is that placental transfer will occur. Drugs with a molecular weight of less than 600 cross the placenta without difficulty, whereas those with a molecular weight over 1000 do not. The majority of drugs given to the mother during labor have a molecular weight in the range of 250 to 450 (e.g., that of local anesthetics is 200–300); thus, they cross over to the placenta easily [71].

Compounds possessing a high degree of lipid solubility diffuse readily across the placenta, whereas water-soluble, highly ionized compounds pass more slowly. Thus, poorly lipid-soluble quaternary bases such as d-tubocurarine cross the placenta in only limited amounts, whereas highly lipid-soluble drugs such as thiopental cross the placenta extremely rapidly [46].

The degree of ionization of a drug is an important determinant of placental transfer because only ionized drugs readily cross the placenta. The proportion of a drug in the charged and uncharged form can be calculated from the Henderson-Hasselbach equation:

$$pH = pKa + \log[\text{base}]/[\text{cation}]$$

Placental Factors

The rate of drug transfer increases with an increasing area of transfer and decreases as the distance for diffusion increases. As the placenta matures, the thickness of the epithelial trophoblastic layer progressively decreases. This reduction may cause the thickness of the tissue layers between the maternal and fetal compartments to decrease to only one-tenth their original thickness; as an example, there have been recorded decreases in thickness from as much as 25 μm in early gestation to 2 μm at term in some species. As gestation progresses, the surface area of the placenta also increases [55]. Therefore, at term, these changes in physical structure tend to favor improved transfer of drugs across the placenta.

Maternal Drug Concentration

The concentration of drug on the maternal side of the placenta determines the degree of fetal exposure. The maternal concentration of free drug in the blood depends on multiple factors: (1) total dose and duration of administration, (2) site and mode of administration, (3) protein binding, (4) blood pH, (5) redistribution, and (6) metabolism and excretion.

Within the blood, equilibrium is established with the total amount of drug divided between the protein-bound portion and free drug. Protein binding, however, is not a static condition. As free drug concentration decreases because of redistribution and placental transfer, more drug enters the free drug compartment from the protein-bound compartment. Therefore, protein binding does little to limit the placenta transfer of a drug. Maternal blood pH, however, may affect the amount of free drug for placental transfer by increasing the amount of nonionized drug and altering the portion bound to plasma protein.

The circulation redistributes the drug to new areas, where it is taken up. Tissue redistribution therefore is a major factor in decreasing maternal drug concentration levels (e.g., thiopental) [46]. Metabolism and clearance remove a drug from the circulation and decrease the maternal concentration of free drug for placental transfer. However, metabolism of a drug (e.g., meperidine) may yield other active compounds that transfer to and affect the fetus.

Fetal Drug Concentration

The concentration of free drugs in the fetal blood depends on several factors: (1) fetal protein binding, (2) drug lipid solubility, (3) fetal blood pH, (4) drug distribution, and (5) fetal drug metabolism and elimination.

Because of the lesser amount of total protein in the fetus, plasma protein-binding capacity in the fetus is lower than in the mother; a higher amount of free drug will thus be available in fetal blood [54]. Highly lipid-soluble drugs (e.g., bupivacaine) are absorbed by the fetal tissue in a significant amount and thus reduce the plasma concentration. Placental transfer is affected by the pH of the blood on both sides of the placenta. Fetal pH is important for determining the proportion of the ionized and nonionized forms of drug. The pH of the blood on the fetal side of the placenta normally is 0.1–0.2 pH units lower than that on the maternal side. Therefore, passage of drug to the fetal unit results in a tendency for more of the drug to exist in the ionized state. Because the maternal-fetal equilibrium is established only between the unionized fractions of the drug on either side of the barrier, this physiological differential will expedite maternal-fetal transfer of the drug.

With more drug in the ionized form in the fetal unit, the new equilibrium that arises results in a greater total (ionized plus unionized) drug load in the fetus. Because the pKa values of commonly used local anesthetics are closer to the maternal blood pH, these agents tend to accumulate on the fetal side of the placenta. This is also true of other basic drugs such as morphine and meperidine. Further decreases in fetal pH lead to additional drug entrapment in the fetus (ion trapping) [5]. For acidic drugs (e.g., thiopental), the shift in total drug concentration is in the opposite direction, i.e., toward the maternal side of the placenta. A decrease in serum pH in the fetus may also cause a decrease in plasma protein affinity for the drug, leading to an increased concentration of free drug.

Drugs transferred from the maternal to the fetal compartment of the placenta are diluted before distribution to the various fetal vital organs. Approximately 85% of the blood in the umbilical vein, which passes from the placenta to the fetus, passes through the fetal liver and then into the inferior vena cava. The remainder bypasses the liver and enters the vena cava primarily via the ductus venosus. Via this route, many drugs are substantially removed from the fetal circulation and sequestered in the liver. Once a drug reaches the fetal liver, it may be either bound to protein or metabolized. The drug concentration is further reduced by an admixture of blood coming from the lower extremities, the abdominal viscera, the upper extremities, and the thorax. During periods of fetal asphyxia and subsequent acidosis, the flow through the ductus venosus may increase, allowing more drug passage into the central circulation and an increased free drug concentration in the fetus [55].

Drug metabolism and excretion are the final features of the fetal distribution picture. The fetal liver is able to metabolize drugs and numerous substrates as early as the second trimester, and this ability continues to improve all the way to term [97]. Opioids and sedatives are metabolized much more slowly by the fetal liver, causing a prolonged effect of these drugs in the newborn exposed in utero. Finally, the ability of the fetus to excrete drugs is also decreased by reduced renal function. The principle of placental transfer allows us to predict the extent of drug transfer from mother to fetus and discover the direct effects of these drugs on the fetus.

Pharmacodynamics

Neurohormonal changes during pregnancy may alter a drug's effects on the mother. Pregnancy is associated with an increased sensitivity to both general and local anesthetics as well as a decreased sensitivity to noxious stimulation, described as pregnancy-induced analgesia, in both animals and humans.

Decreased Minimal Alveolar Concentration during Pregnancy

Anesthetic requirements (minimal alveolar concentration [MAC]) for inhalation agents are decreased by 16–40% during pregnancy in animals [70] and by 28% for isoflurane in pregnant women at 8–12 weeks' gestation [26]. The mechanism for the decrease in MAC may be related to changes in hormones (e.g., progesterone) and endogenous opioids (e.g., β-endorphin) during pregnancy. The concentration of progesterone found in the plasma and cerebrospinal fluid (CSF) of parturients is approximately 60–100 times that of nonpregnant women [17]. Progesterone in large doses induces loss of consciousness in humans. Administration of progesterone directly into the cerebral ventricles of mice has been reported to directly produce systemic analgesia [44]. Metabolites of progesterone are also reported to produce unconsciousness [62]. In addition, anesthetic requirements for inhalation agents in the postpartum period return to normal in 3–5 days. These changes are correlated with decreased progesterone levels [98]. These studies imply that increased progesterone concentrations in the plasma and CSF during pregnancy may decrease anesthetic requirements. Furthermore, plasma β-endorphin levels are higher in pregnancy and during labor [85]. Intrathecal administration of β-endorphin in higher than physiological concentrations produces effective analgesia during labor [69]. Thus, a pregnancy-induced activation of the endorphin system may also contribute to a decreased anesthetic requirement. Furthermore, intrathecal progesterone has been shown to potentiate the effect of spinal sufentanil in rats [37]. Thus, increased CSF levels of progesterone during pregnancy potentiate the analgesic effects of endogenous opioids and may, in part, explain the decreased anesthetic requirements in parturients.

Decreased Local Anesthetic Requirement during Pregnancy

Pregnancy alters the response to local anesthetic blockade. Pregnant women require smaller amounts of local anesthetics to produce the same level of spinal or epidural block than their nonpregnant counterparts [23]. The local anesthetic requirement falls to about two-thirds of the usual dose by the third trimester. Both mechanical and hormonal factors may explain the enhanced sensitivity to neuraxial blockade. Obstruction of venous return by the pregnant uterus shunts blood to the azygous system and markedly engorges the epidural vein. Epidural venous engorgement decreases the volume of the subarachnoid and epidural space and prevents loss of local anesthetic solution through the intervertebral foramina. Thus, local anesthetics injected into the epidural space may spread a greater distance and produce higher levels of sensory block [35]. Hormone changes such as high progesterone may also play a role. Elevated progesterone levels during pregnancy may enhance nerve sensitivity to local anesthetics. Even in early pregnancy (12–14 weeks), epidural injection of local anesthetic produces greater sensory block than in nonpregnant women [23]. Datta et al. [17] have reported an increase in human CSF progesterone levels in pregnancy (122 ± 8 ng) compared with nonpregnant women (61 ± 2.3 ng). Lidocaine blockade of median nerve was faster in pregnancy (4 minutes) than in nonpregnant women (11.5 minutes) [11]. Another study compared the effects of bupivacaine on nerve conduction in the isolated vagus nerve from pregnant and nonpregnant rabbits [24]. The onset of nerve block was significantly faster in nerves from pregnant animals. However, progesterone applied directly to nerve-conduction preparations does not affect local anesthetic conduction blockade. The authors suggested that the increased sensitivity to local anesthetics seen with chronic progesterone treatment in animals is an indirect effect that requires some time [3]. Some of the possible progesterone mechanisms include (1) altered receptor activity, (2) raised affinity of sodium channels, and (3) altered permeability of the nerve membrane. Biochemical changes may also be responsible for the decreased local anesthetic requirement for neural blockade during pregnancy. For example, hyperventilation associated with pregnancy results in higher pH in the CSF. It may increase the proportion of the nonionized form of local anesthetic and thus may facilitate diffusion of local anesthetic across the neural membranes [33].

Pregnancy-Induced Analgesia

Pregnancy and labor are associated with elevated maternal pain and discomfort thresholds near the end of pregnancy and during labor. This phenomenon has been called pregnancy-induced analgesia, pregnancy-induced antinociception, or gestation-associated antinociception. Pregnancy-induced antinociception has been suggested in many animal studies [18,19,20,27,38,52]; attempts to show that this phenomenon occurs in humans are, however, inconsistent [13,19]. Animal studies have demonstrated that increased estrogen and progesterone and the activation of the central endogenous opioid systems are required for pregnancy-induced antinociception. Jayaram and colleagues reported that SCH 32615, an enkephalinase inhibitor, enhanced pregnancy-associated antinociception in pregnant mice and that naloxone significantly lowered pain threshold to noxious stimuli; thus, the authors suggested that enkephalins are largely responsible for pregnancy-associated antinociception [38]. In pregnant rats, intrathecal application of a κ-selective opioid receptor antagonist (nor-binaltorphimine) significantly attenuated gestational antinociception and intrathecal administration of a κ-receptor agonist (U50,488H) significantly enhanced gestational antinociceptive responses [18]. Intrathecal administration of the δ-opioid-receptor-selective antagonists naltrindole, 7-benzylidenenaltrexone, or naltriben also substantially reduced nociceptive thresholds of gestation [19]. In contrast, intrathecal application of the μ-selective antagonist CTAP had no effect on nociceptive thresholds of gestation [19]. These results suggest that pregnancy-induced analgesia involves spinal cord κ- and δ-opioid receptors but not the potent spinal μ-opioid analgesia system [18,19]. Dawson-Basoa and Gintzler [20] studied the interaction between spinal κ- and δ-opioid receptors on the thresholds of nociception during pregnancy. Results showed that blockade of spinal κ- and δ-opioid receptors, individually, can abolish gestation-induced antinociception. However, the magnitude of reduction in gestation-induced antinociception following the combined intrathecal application of suboptimum concentrations of κ- and δ-opioid antagonists is similar to that observed following their individual intrathecal application. The authors concluded that gestational-induced antinociception is not simply the sum of independent analgesic effects of spinal κ- and δ-opioid systems but requires their coincident activation [19]. The mechanism by which ovarian sex steroids activate opioid antinociceptive pathways remains unknown, but modulation of opioid-receptor-mediated signal transduction by estrogen and progesterone is a possibility. A recent study showed that blocking spinal α_2-adrenergic receptors substantially attenuated gestation-associated analgesia in rats and indicated that the full manifestation of pregnancy-induced analgesia also requires the activation of the spinal α_2-noradrenergic pathway [52].

The significance of pregnancy-induced analgesia in human is unclear. Nevertheless, it may explain, in part, the decreased requirement for local and general anesthetics during pregnancy.

Common Analgesics Used in Pregnant Women

Nonsteroidal Anti-Inflammatory Drugs

NSAIDs are primarily used to reduce fever or to relieve minor pain, and they may also be used as tocolytics (to suppress premature labor) [6]. All these agents block prostaglandin synthesis, which may cause (1) premature closure of the ductus arteriosus and pulmonary hypertension late in pregnancy, (2) oligohydramnios (a deficiency of amniotic fluid), (3) prolongation of labor and delivery through inhibition of uterine contractions, and (4) increased incidence of antepartum and postpartum hemorrhage. Most of these agents are not associated with congenital abnormalities, but a few NSAIDs may cause spontaneous abortion [9]. Generally, NSAIDs are not recommended for use during pregnancy. Rathmell and colleagues have speculated that short-term use during the first and second trimesters of pregnancy is probably safe when treatment and adverse effects can be monitored by a perinatologist [76].

Aspirin (Acetylsalicylic Acid)

Aspirin is the most frequently used drug during pregnancy, either as a single agent or in combination with other drugs. Although aspirin is a commonly used over-the-counter medication, data on its fetal effects have resulted in caution in its use during pregnancy.

Aspirin in high doses is teratogenic in animals, but it has not been proven teratogenic in humans [9]. Fetal and newborn effects from aspirin exposure in utero, other than congenital defects, may include increased perinatal mortality, intrauterine growth retardation, congenital salicylate intoxication, and depressed albumin-binding capacity [50].

Aspirin readily crosses the placenta. When given near term, higher concentrations are found in the neonate than in the mother, because elimination in the fetus is slow [50]. As is the case with other prostaglandin synthetase inhibitors, aspirin exposure late in pregnancy may cause constriction of the fetal ductus arteriosus with resultant pulmonary hypertension. Inhibition of prostaglandin synthesis may prolong labor and delivery through blockade of uterine contractions [65]. Aspirin blocks thrombocyte aggregation, with a possible increase in blood loss during delivery [9]. The incidence of bleeding after delivery is also higher [86]. Aspirin decreases platelet adhesiveness and aggregation, and infants born after recent aspirin exposures appear to have an increased risk of bleeding complications [86].

High aspirin consumption during pregnancy may produce adverse effects on the mother, including (1) anemia, (2) antepartum/postpartum hemorrhage, (3) prolonged gestation, and (4) prolonged labor [65,86]. Recent studies suggest that the use of low-dose aspirin (40 to 100 mg) might have beneficial effects by decreasing the incidence of preeclampsia and intrauterine growth retardation in women at risk [83,88]. Aspirin does not increase neonatal bleeding complications [83] and has a negligible effect on the ductus arteriosus and other vascular smooth muscle [89].

Aspirin and other salicylates are excreted into breast milk in low concentrations. The reduced clearance of salicylates by neonates may result in drug accumulation and toxic effects, even when repeated exposures are small [58]. Because of these concerns, the World Health Organization (WHO) Working Group on Human Lactation classified salicylates as unsafe for use by nursing women. The American Academy of Pediatrics recommends that aspirin should be used cautiously by the mother during lactation because of potential adverse effects on the nursing infant [9].

Ibuprofen

There are no associated congenital defects with maternal use of ibuprofen [9]. Like other agents in this class, ibuprofen has been associated with third-trimester pregnancy complications such as oligohydramnios [32] and premature closure of the ductus arteriosus with resultant pulmonary hypertension [49]. Medications similar to ibuprofen are used to stop premature labor; therefore, the use of ibuprofen during the last few weeks of pregnancy may prolong labor. The use of ibuprofen near term should also be avoided because the risk of bleeding may increase.

Ibuprofen does not enter breast milk in significant quantities. In a study of lactating women taking 400 mg ibuprofen every 6 hours, ibuprofen was undetectable in breast milk. The American Academy of Pediatrics considers ibuprofen compatible with breastfeeding [9].

Indomethacin

Unlike aspirin, which causes an irreversible inhibition of the cyclooxygenase enzyme necessary for prostaglandin synthesis, indomethacin initiates a competitive and reversible inhibition of this enzyme.

Data on first-trimester exposure in humans suggest no increased incidence in malformations. In the second half of pregnancy, this agent crosses the placenta and reaches concentrations in the fetus equal to those in the mother [61].

Indomethacin has been used in the treatment of preterm labor since 1974. In the fetus, indomethacin has been reported to cause constriction of the ductus arteriosus and decreased urine output, frequently resulting in oligohydramnios [32]. This effect increases with increasing gestational age. The ductus arteriosus becomes more responsive later in pregnancy, so that before 27 weeks, only 5% to 10% of fetuses will have ductal constriction after indomethacin exposure, whereas after 34 weeks, 100% will demonstrate this response [61]. The risk of neonatal complications, such as necrotizing enterocolitis, patent ductus arteriosus, and possibly intracranial hemorrhage, appears to be increased when this medication is administered within 48 hours before delivery [67].

Data on breastfeeding and indomethacin are very limited. One study reported that milk concentrations were similar to maternal plasma levels. The American Academy of Pediatrics classified indomethacin as compatible with breastfeeding.

Ketorolac

Animal studies have revealed that ketorolac does not cause birth defects in the offspring of pregnant rabbits and rats. However, in one study, ketorolac administration during labor did lead to dystocia in rats. Ketorolac does cross the human placenta; moreover, the umbilical cord blood concentration was between 10% and 20% of the concentration in maternal blood after 10 mg of ketorolac was given i.m. during labor [92]. Like other NSAIDs, this drug may cause (1) closure of the fetal ductus arteriosus; (2) neonatal pulmonary hypertension; (3) decreased urine production resulting in oligohydramnios; and (4) suppression of uterine contractions, with an increased incidence of postpartum hemorrhage. Ketorolac does not seem to be effective in relieving labor pain [91], but it has been used effectively as an adjuvant for postoperative analgesia after cesarean section. It can effectively reduce postoperative pain and narcotic requirement after cesarean section.

Ketorolac is excreted into breast milk. One study found that ketorolac concentrations in breast milk ranged from 1% to 4% of maternal serum levels. Considering the bioavailability of ketorolac after oral administration, this percentage would most likely result in neonatal blood levels between 0.16% and 0.40% of the maternal dose. This amount is considered to be clinically insignificant [94]. The American Academy of Pediatrics considers ketorolac to be compatible with breast feeding.

Celecoxib

There is no study reporting the use of celecoxib in human pregnancy. The animal data suggest a low risk for congenital malformations. Placental transfer of celecoxib is expected because of its low molecular weight (about 381 kD). Celecoxib is excreted into the breast milk in low concentrations and probably would not cause adverse effects in a nursing infant.

Acetaminophen (Paracetamol)

Acetaminophen is routinely used during all stages of pregnancy to relieve pain and lower elevated body temperature. It has no known teratogenic effects [57]. Acetaminophen can cross the placenta [51], but it is considered safe when taken in the normally recommended dosage, and it is now taken much more frequently during pregnancy than aspirin. It is hepatotoxic only in extreme overdosage [9].

Unlike aspirin, acetaminophen does not affect platelet function, and there is no increased risk of hemorrhage if the drug is given to the mother at term [72]. Studies in rats and sheep demonstrate that acetaminophen, like other prostaglandin synthetase inhibitors, can cause constriction of the fetal ductus arteriosus [74]. However, these effects were much milder than those with aspirin, ibuprofen, or indomethacin; moreover, they are less likely to be clinically significant. Acetaminophen has been used as an antipyretic just before delivery in women with fever secondary to chorioamnionitis [45]. A significant improvement in fetal and newborn status, as measured by fetal heart rate tracings and arterial blood gases, was observed after normalization of the mother's temperature.

Acetaminophen does enter breast milk, although maximal neonatal ingestion would be less than 2% of a maternal dose. The American Academy of Pediatrics Committee on Drugs and the WHO Working Group on Drugs and Human Lactation concluded that the use of this drug during breastfeeding is safe [9]. If persistent pain occurs during pregnancy and a mild analgesic is necessary, acetaminophen seems to be a safe and an effective first choice.

Opioids

Opioid analgesics have a long history of safely relieving pain during pregnancy. No congenital anomalies have been reported following the therapeutic use of opioids in humans. More potent than simple analgesics, opioids are used to treat moderate to severe pain during pregnancy. Systemic opioids, administered orally, are useful for parturients who prefer less invasive regional techniques, or in whom regional techniques are contraindicated, or are not an option, due to lack of availability of skilled providers. The most popular systemic opioid agents include the more basic classic drugs such as morphine, fentanyl, and meperidine or mixed opioid agonists-antagonists such as nalbuphine or butorphanol. Opioids are also commonly used intrathecally or epidurally in obstetric anesthesia, alone or in combination with a local anesthetic.

Oxycodone

Although there are relatively few data available on the use of this agent in pregnancy, there are no reports linking it to congenital birth defects. Oxycodone is excreted into human breast milk. Although occasional maternal doses of oxycodone for analgesia probably present a minimal risk for adverse effects during nursing, infants should be monitored for gastrointestinal effects, sedation, and changes in feeding patterns [9].

Morphine

Systemic morphine is not used in actively laboring patients because of the excessive respiratory depression that can affect the neonate compared to equipotent doses of other narcotics [34]. Fetuses that are of young gestational age, are small for their age, or have undergone trauma or long labors are more susceptible to the respiratory effects of narcotics. Placental transfer of morphine is very rapid [7]. In contrast, intrathecal or epidural morphine has been used quite successfully for obstetric anesthesia and relief of post-cesarean section pain [15]. Usual doses are in the ranges of 0.1–0.3 mg intrathecally and 3–5 mg epidurally. Because of its hydrophilic nature, the drug might cause late respiratory depression; thus, patients must be carefully monitored for 12 to 24 hours following administration of intrathecal or epidural morphine.

Only trace amounts of morphine enter breast milk, and the clinical significance is unclear. American Academy of Pediatrics considers morphine to be compatible with breast feeding [9].

Meperidine

Meperidine (pethidine) has been one of the opioids most frequently used in obstetrics. Meperidine hydrochloride is preferable to morphine because it causes less nausea and depression in the neonate. Meperidine's placental transfer is very rapid, appearing in umbilical cord blood within 2 minutes after i.v. administration. Fetal equilibrium is reached 6 minutes after i.v. administration to the mother [16]. Cord blood concentrations average 70–77% (range 45–106%) of maternal plasma levels. The usual dosage of meperidine is 50 to 100 mg i.m. or 25 to 50 mg i.v. The peak action occurs 40 to 60 minutes after i.m. and 5–10 minutes after i.v. administration. The duration of action is 2 to 4 hours. Fetal exposure to meperidine is highest 2 to 3 hours after i.m. administration [82]. Neonatal side effects of meperidine include delay in sustained respiration, decreased Apgar scores, lower oxygen saturation, decreased minute ventilation, respiratory acidosis, abnormal neurobehavior after birth, and difficulty with breastfeeding [10]. These side effects are the result of the drug's prolonged half-life (2.5–3 hours in the mother and 18–23 hours in the neonate) [48] and the accumulation of an active metabolite (e.g., normeperidine, which has a half-life of 60 hours in the neonate). The latter may account for the subtle neonatal depression that may persist for 3–5 days after birth, even with the use of low doses of meperidine [4]. The drug exerts little, if any, effect on uterine activity. Many of these undesirable side effects can be avoided by judicious use of i.v. meperidine in small dosages to obtain the desired analgesic effect.

Meperidine is excreted into breast milk. Nevertheless, the American Academy of Pediatrics classified meperidine as compatible with breast feeding.

Fentanyl

Fentanyl has become popular for analgesia during labor because of its rapid onset and short duration of action, profound analgesia capabilities, and lack of active metabolites. Fentanyl is a highly lipid-soluble and protein-bound synthetic opioid with analgesic potency that is

800 times higher than that of meperidine. One study showed fentanyl to be superior to meperidine in managing labor pain [77]. The usual dose is 50 to 100 μg i.m. and 25 to 50 μg i.v. Intravenous fentanyl produces analgesia almost immediately, peaks within 3 to 5 minutes, and lasts 30 to 60 minutes. After i.m. administration, analgesia begins in 7 to 8 minutes, peaks at about 30 minutes, and lasts 1 to 2 hours.

Continuous epidural infusions containing a combination of low concentrations of local anesthetics and opioids have become increasingly popular in labor analgesia. In several studies, epidural fentanyl in combination with low doses of bupivacaine improved the quality of analgesia and reduced the severity of motor blockade and the incidence of hypotension [14]. Bader and colleagues examined the potential for fetal drug accumulation after a continuous epidural infusion of 0.125% bupivacaine with 2 μg/mL fentanyl for up to 15 hours. They concluded that the concentrations of both drugs remained low and that none of the neonates showed any significant accumulation of drug or adverse effects, as demonstrated by umbilical blood gases and neurobehavioral scores [3]. Fentanyl is excreted into breast milk. The American Academy of Pediatrics considers the drug to be compatible with breast feeding [9].

Sufentanil

Sufentanil is a derivative of fentanyl with greatly increased potency and lipophilicity. It is widely used for intrathecal and epidural analgesia during labor, but it has limited utility as a systemic analgesic because of its high potency.

Vertommen and coworkers showed, in a study of 695 women, that the addition of sufentanil to bupivacaine 0.125% not only improved analgesia but also reduced the incidence of instrumental deliveries [90]. The addition of up to 30 μg sufentanil did not cause neonatal respiratory depression. When 2.5 mg intrathecal bupivacaine was added to 10 μg intrathecal sufentanil, it significantly prolonged labor analgesia (from 114 minutes in the sufentanil group to 148 minutes in the combined sufentanil/bupivacaine group) without adverse maternal or fetal side effects [12].

Alfentanil and Remifentanil

Alfentanil and remifentanil both have a rapid onset and short duration of action. Both have limited to no applicability in analgesia for labor and delivery at this time. While the previous group of compounds do have a logical place when used either via the epidural or spinal routes, it would appear that alfentanil and remifentanil are not substantially superior in either of these delivery routes.

Local Anesthetics

Regional techniques (spinal or epidural) are the most effective means to provide safe pain relief for labor, or for safe use for cesarean section. Drugs used for regional anesthesia in obstetrics are local anesthetics with or without the addition of opioids. The commonly used local anesthetics for epidural anesthesia are lidocaine, bupivacaine, chloroprocaine, and recently ropivacaine.

Lidocaine

Lidocaine is the most commonly used local anesthetic drug for cesarean section because of its rapid onset and favorable toxicity profile. Lidocaine is a weak base with a pKa of 7.8. Protein binding is 56%, chiefly to α_1-acid glycoprotein. Approximately 90% of the drug is metabolized in the liver by N-dealkylation (cytochrome CYP1A2 and CYP3A4) to the pharmacologically active metabolites monoethylglycinexylidide and glycinexylidide. The elimination half-life of lidocaine is approximately 1.5–2 hours in most patients. Lidocaine is not teratogenic. It rapidly crosses the placenta. The umbilical vein : maternal vein (UV/MV) drug concentration ratios are approximately 0.4 to 0.6 [1]. Neonates are able to metabolize lidocaine, and the use of lidocaine is regarded as safe for cesarean section in normal-term pregnancy [29]. The placental transfer of lidocaine is increased by fetal acidosis. The ionic form of lidocaine does not cross the placenta in significant amounts, in contrast to the non-ionic form, which crosses the placenta easily. Ion trapping occurs during episodes of fetal acidosis [5]. Although efforts should be made to minimize the dose of lidocaine in clinical situations in which the fetus is likely to be acidotic, the neonatal effects of epidural lidocaine are mild. Lidocaine does not show adverse effects on neonatal neurobehavior when used for epidural anesthesia in normal term pregnancy or for continuous infusion epidural analgesia. Small amounts of lidocaine are excreted into breast milk. The American Academy of Pediatrics considers lidocaine to be compatible with breast feeding [9].

Bupivacaine

Bupivacaine is presently the most widely used local anesthetic for labor analgesia because of its favorable sensory motor block differential at low concentration. The concentration of bupivacaine can be reduced to produce sensory block with minimal motor block. Bupivacaine is a longer acting amide-type local anesthetic than lidocaine. It has a pKa of 8.1, with greater protein binding (95%) than lidocaine (56%). It is metabolized in the liver by N-dealkylation to pipecolylxylidine and pipecolic acid. Placental transfer of bupivacaine appears to be influenced by maternal and fetal plasma protein binding, fetal pH, and placental uptake [40]. As with lidocaine, placental transfer is enhanced by fetal acidosis. UV/MV ratios average approximately 0.25 to 0.30 in single-dose studies [21] and 0.30 to 0.50 in continuous infusion studies [1]. There is evidence that bupivacaine is absorbed by placental tissue [41], reducing exposure. Although the placental transfer of bupivacaine is less than that of lidocaine, the amount of drug that will ultimately be present in the neonate is also affected by the duration of placental exposure. Given enough time, a steady state will ensue, and fetal tissues become saturated. The fact that neonates may excrete bupivacaine in their urine for 3 days after delivery indicates that fetal tissues may absorb a substantial amount of bupivacaine, despite a low UV/MV ratio [21].

A word of caution is needed regarding the administration of bupivacaine for cesarean section delivery. This drug has been implicated in certain cardiovascular catastrophes associated with initial drug injection, such as cardiac arrests that were refractory to full and appropriate resuscitative attempts [2]. Recently, i.v. lipid emulsion has been used successfully to treat bupivacaine-related cardiac arrest [93]. Although these catastrophes are rare, the practitioner is well advised to inject no more than 5 mL of the drug at any one time, to wait 4–5 minutes, then to repeat the procedure until the desired volume has been delivered. The maximum concentration of bupivacaine now allowed by the U.S. Food and Drug Administration (FDA) for obstetric epidural anesthesia is 0.5%. The toxic dose of bupivacaine is now considered 1–2 mg/kg. Epidural bupivacaine has been used for labor analgesia and cesarean section; it does not cause any adverse effects on the neurobehavioral score of the newborn. A final word of caution should be that if bupivacaine is used in a labor and delivery situation, an immediate available cache of i.v. lipid emulsion must be available, its use and dosage clearly posted, and its administration carefully practiced by all labor and delivery personnel.

Ropivacaine

The transplacental passage of ropivacaine is similar to that of bupivacaine (the UV/MV ratio is 0.3) [64]. In comparison to bupivacaine, the systemic toxicity of ropivacaine is not enhanced during pregnancy, and since higher doses are needed to provoke signs of central nervous system or cardiovascular toxicity, it is a safer drug to use. Epidural ropivacaine has been used for cesarean section and showed no adverse effects on the neonate, even when high doses were used (up to 25 mL 0.75% ropivacaine) [96]. Ropivacaine may gain ascendancy over bupivacaine because of its greater safety profile and its lower propensity for motor block.

Levobupivacaine

Levobupivacaine, the S(−)-enantiomer of racemic bupivacaine, is a long-acting local anesthetic with a clinical profile that closely resembles that of bupivacaine. The pKa of 8.1 for levobupivacaine is the same as that of bupivacaine. Protein binding is more than 97%, mainly to α_1-acid glycoprotein. It is extensively metabolized, with no unchanged levobupivacaine detected in urine or feces [25]. In vitro studies have shown that cytochromes CYP3A4 and CYP1A2 mediate the metabolism of levobupivacaine to desbutyl levobupivacaine and 3-hydroxy levobupivacaine, respectively. The 3-hydroxy levobupivacaine appears to undergo further transformation to glucuronide and sulfate conjugates. When 0.5% levobupivacaine is used in cesarean section, it is as effective in inducing anesthesia as 0.5% bupivacaine. The UV/MV ratio is 0.303 for parturients given levobupivacaine and 0.254 for those given bupivacaine. Animal and human studies have shown levobupivacaine to be less neurotoxic and cardiotoxic than racemic bupivacaine, with similar potency and longer sensory blockade. The maximum dose of levobupivacaine has yet to be decided, although caution would suggest that it should be the same as that recommended for bupivacaine at 2 mg/kg. Neurobehavioral score is within normal limits (>35) when levobupivacaine is used in cesarean section.

Chloroprocaine

Chloroprocaine is an ester derivative that was popular in the 1970s, because of its rapid onset and short duration of action and its low toxicity to the fetus. Its physicochemical properties are imparted by the chloro substitution of the 2-position in the benzene ring of procaine. It is metabolized by plasma cholinesterase and therefore does not require liver enzyme degradation, as do the more complex and longer-acting amide derivatives. Chloroprocaine has a half-life of 21 seconds in adult blood and 43 seconds in neonatal blood [68]. Direct toxic effects on the fetus are minimized because less drug is available for placental transfer. This rapid metabolism also imparts a minimal risk of systemic toxicity, making it perhaps the safest agent for use in obstetrics. The potency of chloroprocaine is comparable to that of lidocaine and mepivacaine, and the drug is three times more potent than procaine. Its average onset of action ranges from 6 to 12 minutes, and its action persists for 30–60 minutes, depending on the amount used. In the 1980s, use of this drug was severely curtailed because of reports of toxicity that included arachnoiditis and associated neuropathies [63,78]. The neurotoxic effects have been attributed to a low pH and the preservative sodium bisulfite [43]. Currently available formulations of 2-chloroprocaine do not contain this preservative. Because of its fast onset of action, chloroprocaine is often used for emergency cesarean section when an epidural catheter has already been placed for labor analgesia to avoid general anesthesia.

References

[1] Abboud TK, Afrasiabi A, Sarkis F, Daftarian F, Nagappala S, Noueihed R, Kuhnert BR, Miller F. Continuous infusion epidural analgesia in parturients receiving bupivacaine, chloroprocaine, or lidocaine: maternal, fetal, and neonatal effects. Anesth Analg 1984;63:421–8.

[2] Albright GA. Cardiac arrest following regional anesthesia with etidocaine or bupivacaine. Anesthesiology 1979;51:285–7.

[3] Bader AM, Datta S, Moller B, Covino BG. Acute progesterone treatment has no effect on bupivacaine-induced conduction blockade in the isolated rabbit vagus nerve. Anesth Analg 1990;71:541–4.

[4] Belsey EM, Rosenblatt DB, Lieberman BA, Redshaw M, Caldwell J, Notarianni L, Smith RL, Beard RW. The influence of maternal analgesic on neonatal behaviour: I. Pethidine. Br J Obstet Gynecol 1981;88:398–406.

[5] Biehl D, Shnider SM, Levinson G, Callender K. Placental transfer of lidocaine: effects of fetal acidosis. Anesthesiology 1978;48:409–12.

[6] Bivins HA, Newman RB, Fyfe DA. Randomized trial of oral indomethacin and terbutaline sulfate for the long-term suppression of preterm labor. Am J Obstet Gynecol 1993;169:1065–70.

[7] Bonica JJ. Principles and practice of obstetric analgesia and anesthesia. Philadelphia: FA Davis; 1967.

[8] Bourget P, Roulot C, Fernadez H. Models for placental transfer studies of drugs. Clin Pharmacokinet 1995;28:161–80.

[9] Briggs GG, Freeman RK, Yaffe SJ. Drugs in pregnancy and lactation. Baltimore: Williams & Wilkins; 2008.

[10] Brinbach BJ, Gatt SP, Datta S. Textbook of obstetric anesthesia. Philadelphia: Churchill Livingstone; 2000.

[11] Butterworth JF, Walker FO, Lyzak SZ. Pregnancy increases median nerve susceptibility to lidocaine. Anesthesiology 1990;72:962–5.

[12] Camann UR, Denney RA, Holby ED, Datta S. A comparison of intrathecal, epidural and intravenous sufentanil for labor analgesia. Anesthesiology 1992;77:884–7.

[13] Carvallos B, Angst M, Fuller A, Lin E, Mathusamy A, Riley E. Experimental heat pain for detecting pregnancy-induced analgesia in humans. Anesth Analg 2006;103:1283–7.

[14] Celleno D, Capogna G. Epidural fentanyl plus bupivacaine 0.125 per cent for labour: analgesic effects. Can J Anaesth 1988;35:375–8.

[15] Chadwick HS, Ready LB. Intrathecal and epidural morphine sulfate for postcesarean analgesia: a clinical comparison. Anesthesiology 1988;68:925–9.

[16] Crawford JS, Rudofsky S. The placental transmission of pethidine. Br J Anaesth 1965;37:929–33.

[17] Datta S, Hurley RJ, Naulty JS, Stern P, Lambert DH, Concepcion M, Tulchinsky D, Weiss JB, Ostheimer GW. Plasma and cerebrospinal fluid progesterone concentrations in pregnant and nonpregnant women. Anesth Analg 1986;65:950–4.

[18] Dawson-Basoa ME, Gintzler AR. Estrogen and progesterone activate spinal kappa-opiate receptor analgesic mechanisms. Pain 1996;64:605–15.

[19] Dawson-Basoa ME, Gintzler AR. Involvement of spinal cord δ opiate receptors in the antinociception of gestation and its hormonal simulation. Brain Res 1997;757:37–42.

[20] Dawson-Basoa ME, Gintzler AR. Gestational and ovarian sex steroid antinociception synergy between spinal κ and opioid system. Brain Res 1998;794:61–7.

[21] Draner K, Bromage PR. Choice of local anesthetic in obstetrics. In: Hughes SC, Levinson G, Rosen MA, editors. Anesthesia of obstetrics, 4th ed. Philadelphia: Lippincott Williams and Wilkins; 2002. p. 73–149.

[22] Dunlop W. Serial changes in renal haemodynamic during normal human pregnancy. Br J Obstet Gynaecol 1981;88:1–9.
[23] Fagraeus L, Urban B, Bromage P. Spread of epidural analgesia in early pregnancy. Anesthesiology 1983;58:184–7.
[24] Flanagan HL, Datta S, Lambert DH, Gissen AJ, Covino B. Effect of pregnancy on bupivacaine-induced conduction blockade in the isolated rabbit vagus nerve. Anesth Analg 1987;66:123–6.
[25] Foster RH, Markham A. Levobupivacaine: a review of its pharmacology and use as a local anaesthetic. Drugs 2000;59:551–79.
[26] Gin T, Chan MTV. Decreased minimum alveolar concentration of isoflurane in pregnant humans. Anesthesiology 1994;81:829–32.
[27] Gintzler AR. Endorphin-mediated increases in pain threshold during pregnancy. Science 1980;210:193–5.
[28] Gleichmann W, Bachmann GW, Dengler HJ, Dudech J. Effects of hormonal contraceptives and pregnancy on serum protein pattern. Eur J Clin Pharmacol 1973;5:215–218.
[29] Guay J, Gaudreault P, Boulanger A, Tang A, Lortie L, Dupuis C. Lidocaine hydrocarbonate and lidocaine hydrochloride for cesarean section: transplacental passage and neonatal effects. Acta Anesthesiology Scand 1992;36:722–7.
[30] Harris RZ, Benet LZ, Schwartz JB. Gender effects in pharmacokinetics and pharmacodynamics. Drugs 1995;50:222–39.
[31] Harrison LI, Gibaldi M. Influence of cholestasis on drug elimination: pharmacokinetics. J Pharm Sci 1979;65:1246–8.
[32] Hickok DE, Hollenback KA, Reilley SF, Nyberg DA. The association between decreased amniotic fluid volume and treatment with nonsteroidal anti-inflammatory agents for preterm labor. Am J Obstet Gynecol 1989;160:1525–31.
[33] Hirabayashi Y, Shimizer R, Saitah K, Fukuda H, Igarashi T. Acid-base state of cerebrospinal fluid during pregnancy and its effect on spinal of spinal anesthesia. Br J Anaesth 1996;77:352–5.
[34] Hughes SC, Rosen MA, Shnider SM, Abboud TK, Stefani SJ, Norton M. Maternal and neonatal effects of epidural morphine for labor and delivery. Anesth Analg 1984;63:318–24.
[35] Igarashi T, Hirabayashi Y, Shimizu R, Saitoh K, Fukuda H, Suzuki H. The fiberscopic findings of the epidural space in pregnant women. Anesthesiology 2000;92:1631–6.
[36] Jachau MR, Mirkin DL, Zachariah PK. Interactions of various 19-nor steroids with human placental microsomal cytochrome P-450. Chem Biol Interact 1976;15:337–47.
[37] Jayaram A, Carp H. Progesterone-mediated potentiation of spinal sufentanil in rats. Anesth Analg 1993;76:745–50.
[38] Jayaram A, Singh P, Carp H. Sch 32615, an enkephalinase inhibitor, enhances pregnancy-induced analgesia in mice. Anesth Analg 1995;80:944–8.
[39] Jeffries WS, Bochner F. The effect of pregnancy on drug pharmacokinetics. Med J Aust 1988;149:675–7.
[40] Johnson RF, Herman NL, Johnson HV, Arney TL, Paschall RL, Downing JW. Effects of fetal pH on local anesthetic transfer across the human placenta. Anesthesiology 1996;85:608–15.
[41] Johnson RF, Herman N, Arney TL, Gonzalez H, Johnson HV, Downing JW. Bupivacaine transfer across the human term placenta: a study using the dual perfused human placental model. Anesthesiology 1995;82:459–68.
[42] Juchau MR. Drug biotransformations in the placenta. Pharmacol Ther 1980;8:501–24.
[43] Kalichman MW, Powell HC, Reisner LS, Myers RR. The role of 2-chloroprocaine and sodium bisulfite in rat sciatic nerve edema. J Neuropathol Exp Neurol 1986;45:566–75.
[44] Kavaliers M, Wiebe JP. Analgesic effects of the progesterone metabolite, 3-α-hydroxyl-5α-pregnane-20-one, and possible modes of action in mice. Brain Res 1987;415:393–8.
[45] Kirshon B, Moise KJ Jr, Wasserstrum N. Effect of acetaminophen on fetal acid-base balance in chorioamnionitis. J Reprod Med 1989;34:955–9.
[46] Kosaka Y, Takakashi T, Mark LC. Intravenous thiobarbiturate anesthesia for cesarean section. Anesthesiology 1969;31:480–506.
[47] Krauer B, Krauer F, Hytten FE. Pregnancy and its effect on drug handling: the influence of physiological changes in pregnancy. In: Lind T, Singer A, editors. Current reviews in obstetrics and gynaecology. Edinburgh: Churchill-Livingstone; 1984. p. 19–50.
[48] Kuhnert BR, Kuhnert PM, Tu AS, Lin DC, Foltz RL. Meperidine and normeperidine levels following meperidine administration during labor. I. Mother. Am J Obstet Gynecol 1979;133:904–13.
[49] Levin DL. Effects of inhibition of prostaglandin synthesis on fetal development, oxygenation, and the fetal circulation. Semin Perinatol 1980;4:35–44.
[50] Levy G, Garrettson LK. Kinetics of salicylate elimination by newborn infants of mothers who ingested aspirin before delivery. Pediatrics 1974;53:202–10.
[51] Levy G, Garretson LK, Soda DM. Evidence of placental transfer of acetaminophen. Pediatrics 1975;55:895.
[52] Lin NJ, Gintzler AR. Gestational and ovarian sex steroid antinociception: relevance of uterine afferent and spinal α_2-noradrenergic activity. Pain 1999;83:359–68.
[53] Luxford AM, Kellaway GS. Pharmacokinetics of digoxin in pregnancy. Eur J Clin Pharmacol 1983;25:117–21.
[54] Mather LE, Long G, Thomas J. The binding of bupivacaine to maternal and foetal plasma proteins. J Pharm Pharmacol 1971;23:359–65.
[55] McDonald JS, Yarnell RW. Obstetric analgesia and anesthesia. In: Decherney A, Goodwin TM, Nather L, Laufer N, editors. Current diagnosis and treatment obstetric and gynecology, 10th ed. New York: McGraw-Hill; 2007. p. 443–5.
[56] McDonald-Gibson RG, Young M, Hytten FE. Changes in plasma non-esterified fatty acids and serum glycerol in pregnancy. Br J Obstet Gynaecol 1975;82:460–6.
[57] McElhatton PR, Sullivan FM, Volans GN. Paracetamol overdose in pregnancy analysis of the outcomes of 300 cases referred to the teratology information service. Reprod Toxicol 1997;11:85–94.
[58] McNamara PJ, Burgio D, Yoo SD. Pharmacokinetics of acetaminophen, antipyrine, and salicylic acid in the lactating and nursing rabbit, with model predictions of milk to serum concentration ratios and neonatal dose. Toxicol Appl Pharmacol 1991;109:149–60.

[59] Mendenhal HW. Serum protein concentrations in pregnancy. I. Concentrations in maternal serum. Am J Obstet Gynecol 1970;106:388–99.
[60] Mitani GM, Steinberg, Liver EJ, Harrison EC, Elkayam U. The pharmacokinetics of antiarrhythmia agents in pregnancy and lactation. Clin Pharmacokinet 1987;12:253–91.
[61] Moise KJ, Ou CN, Kirshon B, Cano LE, Rognerud C, Carpenter RJ Jr. Placental transfer of indomethacin in the human pregnancy. Am J Obstet Gynecol 1990;162:549–54.
[62] Mok WM, Herschkowitz S, Krieger NR. In vivo studies identify 5 alpha-pregnan-3 alpha-ol-20-one as an active anesthetic agent. J Neurochem 1991;57:1296–301.
[63] Morley-Forster PK, Reid JW, Vandeberghe H. A comparison of patient-controlled analgesic fentanyl and alfentanil for labor analgesia. Can J Anaesth 2000;47:113–9.
[64] Mucklow JC. The fate of drugs in pregnancy. Clin Obstet Gynecol 1986;13:161–75.
[65] Niebyl JR. Nonanesthetic drugs during pregnancy and lactation. In: Chestnut DH, editor. Obstetric anesthesia: principles and practice. St. Louis: Mosby; 1994. p. 229–40.
[66] Nimmo WS, Wilson J, Prescott LF. Narcotic analgesics and delayed gastric emptying during labor. Lancet 1975;1:890–3.
[67] Norton ME, Merrill J, Cooper BAB, Kuller JA, Clyman RI. Neonatal complications after the administration of indomethacin for preterm labor. N Engl J Med 1993;329:1602–7.
[68] O'Brien JE, Abbey V, Hinsvark O, Perel J. Finster M. Metabolism and measurement of chloroprocaine, an ester-type local anesthetic. J Pharm Sci 1979;68:75–8.
[69] Oyama J, Akitoma, Takeo T, Ling N, Guillemin R. Beta endorphin in obstetric anesthesia. Am J Obstet Gynecol 1980;137:613–6.
[70] Palakniuk RJ, Shnider SM, Eger EL. Pregnancy decreases the requirement of inhaled anesthetic agents. Anesthesiology 1974;41:82–3.
[71] Parry E, Shields R, Turnbull AC. Transit time in the small intestine in pregnancy. J Obstet Gynaeol Commonw 1970;77:900–1.
[72] Pearson H. Comparative effects of aspirin and acetaminophen on hemostasis. Pediatrics 1978;62:926–9.
[73] Perez V, Gorodisch S, Casavilla F, Maruffo C. Ultra-structure of human liver at the end of pregnancy. Am J Obstet Gynecol 1971;110:428–31.
[74] Peterson RG. Consequences associated with nonnarcotic analgesics in the fetus and newborn. Fed Proc 1985;44:2309–12.
[75] Philpson A. Pharmacokinetics of antibiotics in pregnancy and labor. Clin Pharmacokinet 1997;4:297–306.
[76] Rathmell, JP, Viscomi CM, Ashburn MA. Management of nonobstetric pain during pregnancy and lactation. Anesth Analg 1997;85:1074–87.
[77] Rayburn WF, Smith CV, Parriott JE, Woods RE. Randomized comparison of meperidine and fentanyl during labor. Obstet & Gynecol 1989;74:604–6.
[78] Reisner LS, Hochman BN, Plumer MH. Persistent neurologic deficit and adhesive arachnoiditis following intrathecal 2-chloroprocaine injection. Anesth Analg 1980;59:452–4.
[79] Reynolds F, Knott C. Pharmacokinetics in pregnancy and placental drug transfer. Oxf Rev Reprod Biol 1989;11:389–449.
[80] Robertson EG. Physiological adjustments in pregnancy: water metabolism. Clin Obstet Gynecol 1975;2:431–40.
[81] Ross A. Physiologic changes of pregnancy. In Brinbach BJ, Gatt SP and Datta S, editors. Textbook of obstetric anesthesia. Philadelphia: Churchill Livingstone; 2000. p. 31–45.
[82] Savonna-Ventura C, Sammut M, Sammut C. Meperidine blood concentrations at time of birth. Int J Gynecol Obstet 1991;36:103–7.
[83] Sibai BM, Caritis SN, Thom E, Klebanoff M, McNellis D, Rocco L, Paul RH, Romero R, Witter F, Rosen M, et al. Prevention of preeclampsia with low-dose aspirin in healthy nulliparous pregnant women. The National Institute of Child Health and Human Development Network of Maternal-Fetal Medicine Units. N Engl J Med 1993;329:1213–8.
[84] Simpson RH, Stakes AF, Miller M. Pregnancy delays paracetamol absorption and gastric emptying in patients undergoing surgery. Br J Anaesth 1988;60:24.
[85] Steinbrook RA, Carr DB, Datta S, Naulty JS, Lee C, Fisher J. Dissociation of plasma and cerebrospinal fluid beta-endorphin immunoreactivity levels during pregnancy and parturition. Anesth Analg 1982;61:893–7.
[86] Stuart MJ, Gross SJ, Elrad H, Graeber JE. Effects of acetylsalicylic-acid ingestion on maternal and neonatal hemostasis. N Engl J Med 1982;307:909–12.
[87] Theunissen IM, Parer JT. Fluid and electrolytes in pregnancy. Clin Obstet Gynecol 1994;37:3–15.
[88] Trudinger B, Cook CM, Thompson R, Giles W, Connelly A. Low-dose aspirin improves fetal weight in umbilical placental insufficiency. Lancet 1988;2:214–5.
[89] Veille JC, Hanson R, Sivakoff M, Swain M, Henderson L. Effects of maternal ingestion of low-dose aspirin on the fetal cardiovascular system. Am J Obstet Gynecol 1993;168:1430–7.
[90] Vertommen JD, Vandermeulen E, Van Aken H, Vaes L, Soetens M, Van Steenberge A, Mourisse P, Willaert J, Noorduin H, Devlieger H, et al. The effects of the addition of sufentanil to 0.125% bupivacaine on the quality of analgesia during labor and on the incidence of instrumental deliveries. Anesthesiology 1991;74:809–14.
[91] Walker JJ, Johnston J, Fairlie FM, Lloyd J, Bullingham R. A comparative study of intramuscular ketorolac and pethidine in labour pain. Eur J Obstet Gynecol Reprod Biol 1992;46:87–94.
[92] Walker JJ, Johnstone J, Lloyd J, Rocha CL. The transfer of ketorolac tromethamine from maternal to foetal blood. Eur J Clin Pharmacol 1988;34:509–11.
[93] Weinberg G, Hertz P, Newman J. Lipid, not propofol, treats bupivacaine overdose. Anesth Analg 2004;99:1875–6.

[94] Wischnik A. The excretion of ketorolac tromethamine into breast milk after multiple oral dosing. Eur J Clin Pharmacol 1989;36:521–4.
[95] Wood M, Alastair JJ, Wood MB. Changes in plasma drug binding and α_1-acid glycoprotein in mother and newborn infant. Clin Pharmacol Ther 1981;29:522–6.
[96] Writer WD, Stienstra R, Eddleston JM, Gatt SP, Griffin R, Gutsche BB, Joyce TH, Hedlund C, Heeroma K, Selander D. Neonatal outcome and mode of delivery after epidural labour analgesia with ropivacaine and bupivacaine: a prospective meta-analysis. Br J Anaesth 1998;81:713–7.
[97] Yaffe SJ. Developmental factors influencing interactions of drugs. Ann NY Acad Sci 1976;281:90–7.
[98] Zhou HH, Norman P, DeLima LG, Mehta M, Bass D. The minimum alveolar concentration of isoflurane in patients undergoing bilateral tubal ligation in the postpartum period. Anesthesiology 1995;82:1364–8.

Correspondence to: Prof. John S. McDonald, MD, Department of Anesthesiology, Harbor-UCLA Medical Center, 1000 West Carson St., Box #10, Torrance, CA 90502, USA. Email: jsm5525@ucla.edu.

23

Pharmacological Considerations in Infants and Children

Stephen C. Brown,[a,b] Anna Taddio,[c] and Patricia A. McGrath[a,b]

[a]Department of Anaesthesia and Pain Medicine, Hospital for Sick Children, Toronto, Ontario, Canada; [b]Department of Anesthesia and [c]Leslie Dan Faculty of Pharmacy, University of Toronto, Toronto, Ontario, Canada

Epidemiology

As a result of extensive research during the past 30 years, we have gained better insights about how the developing nociceptive system responds to tissue injury, how children perceive acute and chronic pain, and which drug and nondrug therapies will alleviate their pain. Like adults, children can experience many different types of pain—acute pain due to disease or trauma; recurrent episodes of headache, stomachache, or limb pain unrelated to disease; and chronic pain due to injury, disease, psychological factors, or of unknown etiology. However, the prevalence of certain types of pain is different for adults and children. For example, chronic back pain is a major problem for adults but not for children. Instead, recurrent pain syndromes (abdominal pain, headache, limb pains or "growing pains") are more common problems for children.

Although we lack precise data on the incidence and prevalence of many childhood pain conditions, an increasing number of epidemiological studies are focusing on obtaining such data, identifying individual risk and prognostic factors, and documenting the long-term impact for children and their families. Pain is a common feature of hospitalization in infants and children. Not only are many illnesses associated with pain, but their medical management also involves routine utilization of painful diagnostic, therapeutic, and monitoring interventions. Up to 80% of infants and children are reported to

Pharmacology of Pain
edited by Pierre Beaulieu, David Lussier, Frank Porreca, and Anthony H. Dickenson
IASP Press, Seattle, © 2009

have pain during hospital admission [63]. In a recent hospital-wide audit, painful and aversive procedures were documented to occur, on average, 2.6 times/day. Analgesics were administered in fewer than 5% of needle procedures [67]. In a separate survey of hospitalized neonates, investigators reported that an average of 10 painful procedures were undertaken per infant per day of hospitalization, with the use of analgesics for only 2% of them [13].

Prevalence estimates for children's chronic pain vary widely due to differences in pain definitions, methods for identifying children, age and gender of study populations, country of origin, and presentation and analysis of data [45]. In a review of recent epidemiological data, Van Den Kerkhof and colleagues [65] reported that prevalence estimates range from 3.7% for back pain [27] to 97% for nonmigraine headache [5]. Pain prevalence increases with age, and certain pain conditions vary with sex and age. For example, clinical referrals indicate that complex regional pain syndrome type I affects girls more than boys, with a ratio of ~6–9:1, and affects children primarily in their pre- and early teen years. Complex idiopathic pain conditions and somatization disorders seem to predominantly affect older adolescents. Although few longitudinal studies have been conducted to follow pain-free children, the available data indicate increasing incidence with age [65]. There is currently no estimate of the prevalence of chronic pain in infants. There is clearly the potential for hospitalized infants to experience chronic pain from underlying medical conditions or from iatrogenic sources such as surgery and repeated medical procedures.

Children who report chronic pain are more likely to still experience pain several years later. Martin and colleagues followed a cohort of 143 children who had been treated at a tertiary care pain clinic [41]. Of the cohort, 62.2% reported continuing pain 3 years later. Females were at higher risk for continuing pain and reported greater use of health care, medication, and nondrug methods of pain control. Perquin et al. followed a cohort of 987 children aged 0–18 years for 2 years and found that one-third who had benign pain at baseline still had pain at the two-year follow-up, although pain often did not get worse over time. They reported that pain affected health status, school absence, health care use, medication use and interference in daily activities [52].

Maturation of Nociception

As in adults, a child's pain depends upon complex neural interactions, where impulses generated by tissue damage are modified by both ascending systems activated by innocuous stimuli and by descending pain-suppressing systems activated by various situational and psychological factors. However, children are not "little adults" with respect to how they perceive pain. The developing nociceptive system responds differently to injury (with increased excitability and sensitization) when compared to the mature adult system. Moreover, a child's pain appears to have a greater degree of plasticity when compared to that of adults, being more strongly influenced by cognitive, behavioral, and emotional factors.

Anand and colleagues dramatically highlighted the adverse impact of untreated postoperative pain in 1987, when they revealed that premature infants undergoing surgery without adequate analgesic medication had significantly increased postsurgical morbidity and mortality in comparison to a group that received fentanyl [2]. The ensuing publicity as people learned that minimal anesthesia and analgesia represented "the norm in pediatric postoperative management," rather than the exception, sparked a revolution (for review, see [55]).

Ethical concerns and increasing publicity about the lack of analgesia for infants led to a dramatic upsurge in clinical research to document objectively how infants responded to surgical trauma and how analgesic administration affects postsurgical outcome. At the same time, basic scientific research focused on the nociceptive system in infants. Fitzgerald and colleagues initiated a series of elegant anatomical and physiological investigations to detail the development of the nociceptive system (for review, see [4,24,26]). The basic nociceptive connections are formed before birth, but systems at birth are immature and exhibit increased responsivity in comparison to the adult animal.

Considerable neuronal plasticity is evident throughout the developing system from the periphery to the brain. For example, the conduction velocity of afferent fibers, action potential shape, receptor transduction, firing frequencies, and receptive field properties change substantially over the postnatal period [23,25,35,70]. Both high-threshold Aδ and low-threshold Aβ mechanoreceptors respond with lower firing frequencies at birth than in the adult animal. Aβ afferents extend dorsally into laminae II and I along with C fibers, rather than into only laminae III and IV as in the adult animal. Activation of these Aβ afferents evokes excitatory responses more typical of those evoked by Aδ and C fibers in the adult animal. In addition, the receptive fields of dorsal horn cells and somatosensory cortical cells are larger in the newborn. With these larger receptive fields and the dominant A-fiber input, there is an increased likelihood that central cells will be excited by peripheral sensory stimulation, thereby increasing the sensitivity of infant sensory reflexes to stimulation. Moreover, descending inhibitory mechanisms are not functional at birth [11], so that an important endogenous analgesic system is lacking and noxious input may affect neonates more than adults. The immaturity of synaptic connections and integrated circuitry in the newborn means that the infant pain experience is more diffuse and less spatially focused than that in adults, and since it is also under less endogenous control, the system is potentially more powerful [26].

While we do not know specifically how noxious input in neonates may affect the mature human pain system or influence adult pain perception, increasing attention is focused on the possible consequences of untreated pain, particularly in infants [28]. For example, circumcised newborn infants display a stronger pain response to subsequent routine immunizations at 4 and 6 months than uncircumcised infants, but application of lidocaine-prilocaine anesthetic cream at circumcision attenuates the pain response to the subsequent immunizations [62]. Studies of infants who were born prematurely and required intensive care have shown behavioral differences related to early pain experiences.

Pharmacological Differences in Children

Aspects of ontogeny and genetics significantly impact the pharmacology of drugs. Some of the pharmacogenetic aspects are discussed in Chapter 19 by Mogil. In this section, we describe sources of variability in the pharmacological activity of drugs due to ontogeny. Extensive variability in the elimination of drugs exists between children and adults, as well as among individual children, due to the continual maturation of body systems. There are many noteworthy differences in pharmacokinetics, particularly between adults and neonates.

Compared to adults, absorption rates of drugs are generally decreased in neonates due to an increase in gastric emptying time, decreased intestinal motility, immature biliary function, and a decrease in muscular blood flow [34]. Absorption of acetaminophen has been demonstrated to be delayed in young infants, presumably because of delayed gastric emptying [3]. Percutaneous drug absorption may be increased, especially in preterm infants, due to an immature stratum corneum and a larger dose relative to body surface area [34]. The bioavailability of topical analgesics such as lidocaine-prilocaine cream may therefore be higher than expected, thus increasing the risk of systemic toxicity.

The extensive differences in body composition may affect the distribution of drugs. For example, total body water in full-term and preterm infants comprises about 75% and 95%, respectively, of body weight at birth. This proportion is reduced to about 60% of adult values within the first 5 months of life. The proportion of body weight attributed to fat increases over the same time frame. Protein mass increases when fat is replaced by muscle after ambulation is attained later in infancy [3]. Protein binding is decreased in neonates due to a lower level of plasma proteins such as albumin, a decrease in affinity of plasma proteins to drugs, and competition for binding sites by endogenous substances such as bilirubin or fatty acids [34]. Protein binding changes may have significant effects on biological activity of drugs that are highly protein bound (>95%) and have a narrow therapeutic index, such as lidocaine [3].

Drug metabolism is reduced in neonates, especially in preterm neonates, due to immaturity of enzyme systems. For the most part, drugs are metabolized by the liver using two processes: phase I and phase II reactions. Phase I reactions involve oxidative, reductive, or hydrolytic reactions. Phase II reactions involve conjugation of drugs with small molecules. Many phase I and phase II reactions are immature at birth and therefore affected by development. In addition, individual pathways have their own maturation rates. Most phase I reactions are catalyzed by the cytochrome P450 superfamily of enzymes. Cytochrome P450 enzymes generally increase in activity in the first 3 months of life. The development of phase II pathways may take longer—up to 2 years [8]. Because most commonly used analgesic drugs are metabolized by liver enzymes, their elimination is affected by the ontogeny of these systems. In some cases, drugs may be metabolized by alternative pathways. For example acetaminophen and morphine are conjugated with sulfate in neonates instead of glucuronide, owing to the relative maturity of the sulfation pathway at birth, whereas the major conjugation pathway in adults for both drugs is glucuronidation [3]. For some drugs such as for acetaminophen, the alternative metabolic pathway partially compensates for the immaturity of the glucuronide pathway.

There may also be immature metabolic pathways in neonates that give rise to unique toxicities when compared to adults. For example, a deficiency of methemoglobin reductase activity at birth places neonates and young infants at risk of methemoglobinemia from local anesthetics such as prilocaine. Renal excretion of drugs is decreased in neonates compared to adults due to lower renal blood flow, lower glomerular filtration rate, and immature tubular secretion and reabsorption systems. Thus, clearance rates for drugs that are excreted renally are significantly reduced. Maturation of filtration and secretory systems occurs over the first year of life [34].

Interestingly, it has been consistently demonstrated that drug metabolism efficiency increases in childhood up to about 10 years of age when compared to adults. Drug doses for children are therefore typically higher than those of adults when adjusted for differences in weight [34]. Metabolic activity gradually declines as children progress through puberty, and after puberty dosing requirements are similar to those of adults.

Postoperative, procedural, and intensive-care management in infants is still based largely on clinical experience, and published evidence on which to base management is limited. For example, the addition of opioids or nonopioid spinal analgesics (such as clonidine or ketamine) to epidural anesthetics improves analgesia in older children, but the safety and efficacy of these interventions have not been well studied for neonates. Similarly, we do not yet know the efficacy of opioids for control of procedural pain in neonates (for review, see [26]). Timed bolus administration of rapid-onset lipid-soluble opioids, such as fentanyl, may be more effective [64], but further study of efficacy, dosing requirements, and safety profile is required [26].

In their review on infant pain management, Fitzgerald and Walker conclude that "there is an urgent need for more 'proof of principle' studies and clinical trials of analgesic protocols in infants; however, for these to be useful, the outcome measures require re-evaluation, and this, in turn, requires a better understanding of the neurophysiology and neuropharmacology of developing pain pathways" [26]. Analgesic protocols that have been designed for older patients may be of limited applicability in neonates and infants, not only because of differing metabolism, but also because many analgesic targets in the brain are still undergoing developmental changes during infancy [51,66].

Pharmacology of Analgesics in Children

Compared to acute pain management, there is relatively little research evidence to guide clinicians regarding the management of chronic pain conditions in children. Current chronic pain management practices are extrapolated from studies of chronic pain management in adults or acute pain management in children. Below is a brief summary of the pertinent issues for analgesics currently in widespread use.

Nonopioids

Acetaminophen

Acetaminophen (paracetamol) is the most widely used analgesic in children. It is primarily used to treat acute and chronic pain of mild to moderate intensity. The combination of acetaminophen with opioids or nonsteroidal anti-inflammatory drugs (NSAIDs) improves analgesia and may reduce side effects [16].

NSAIDs

NSAIDs are used for children with pain of mild to moderate intensity. They are widely used for treating acute and chronic pain. Similar to acetaminophen, when combined with opioids, NSAIDs may improve analgesia, reduce the amount of opioids consumed, and reduce side effects [16]. Like acetaminophen, NSAIDs do not cause respiratory depression or physical dependence.

Use of NSAIDs in children is limited by concerns for their potential toxicity, particularly bleeding, renal toxicity, and exacerbations of asthma. A recent Cochrane review in pediatric patients did not confirm an increase in the risk of bleeding with the use of NSAIDs for postoperative pain control [14]. Adverse gastrointestinal or renal events from short-term use of NSAIDs are rare [6]. Chronic use of NSAIDs, however, can cause esophagitis, gastritis, duodenitis, and gastric or duodenal ulcers. The incidence of such complications is unclear. In one study including 14 children using NSAIDs long-term for juvenile rheumatoid arthritis, 27% had gastrointestinal complaints, and macroscopic endoscopic lesions were found in 43% [37]. The risk of asthma exacerbation ranges from 2% to 30%—the higher rate is attributable to older children with severe asthma and concomitant nasal disease such as allergic rhinitis [50]. The dose for commonly used NSAIDs is shown in Table I.

Table I
Nonopioid drugs to control pain in infants and children

Drug	Dosage	Comments
Acetaminophen (paracetamol)	10-15 mg/kg p.o., every 4–6 h	Dose limit of 75 mg/kg/day or 4 g/day if >12 years of age, whichever is less. Single rectal loading doses of 40 mg/kg may be used for perioperative analgesia.
Diclofenac	1 mg/kg p.o., every 8–12 h	Use with caution in patients with hepatic or renal impairment, compromised cardiac function, or hypertension (may cause fluid retention, edema), history of GI bleeding or ulcers. May inhibit platelet aggregation. Give with food or milk to minimize GI upset. Dose limit of 50 mg/dose.
Ibuprofen	5–10 mg/kg p.o., every 12 h	Dose limit of 40 mg/kg/day; max. dose of 2400 mg/day. Similar precautions as for diclofenac.
Naproxen	5–10 mg/kg p.o., every 12 h	Dose limit of 1 g /day. Similar precautions as for diclofenac.

Note: Increasing the dose of non-opioids beyond the recommended therapeutic level produces a "ceiling effect," in that there is no additional analgesia but there are major increases in toxicity and side effects.
Abbreviations: p.o. = by mouth; GI = gastrointestinal

Tramadol

Tramadol has analgesic potency similar to codeine, but a lower incidence of side effects such as respiratory depression and constipation. Tramadol may prove particularly useful in patients with poor cardiopulmonary, renal or hepatic function and in those whom NSAIDs are not recommended or need to be used with caution [57]. A growing number of studies [12] and case reports [10,31] demonstrate efficacy and safety of tramadol in children. Rose et al. reported that in 113 children aged 7–16 years, the use of oral tramadol at 1 mg/kg every 4–6 hours for various conditions was well tolerated [54].

Opioids

Morphine

Morphine is the mainstay of pharmacological analgesia in children experiencing moderate to severe pain, either acutely or chronically. There is a vast experience with this medication, which remains the gold standard opioid for intraoperative and postoperative analgesia in the form of a bolus dose, a continuous infusion, or patient-controlled analgesia (PCA). It is cheap and readily available at most institutions, and its side-effect profile is well known. See Table II for dosing guidelines of morphine and other opioid analgesics.

Fentanyl

Fentanyl is a potent synthetic opioid, which like morphine binds to mu-opioid receptors. However, fentanyl is 75–100 times more potent than morphine. The intravenous preparation is used extensively in children to manage perioperative pain. A transdermal preparation of fentanyl was introduced in 1991 for use in patients with chronic pain. This route provides a noninvasive but continuously controlled delivery system. Although limited data are available on transdermal fentanyl (TF) in children, its use is increasing for children with pain. In a 2001 study, TF was well tolerated with effective pain relief in 11 of 13 children and provided an ideal approach for children where compliance with oral analgesics was problematic [49]. In another study, when children were converted from oral morphine doses to TF, the investigators noted diminished side effects and improved convenience with TF [32]. The majority of parents and investigators considered TF to be better than previous treatment. No serious adverse events were attributed to fentanyl, suggesting that TF was both effective and acceptable for children and their families. Similarly, no adverse effects were noted in a study of TF for children with pain due to sickle cell crisis [15]. This study showed a significant relationship between TF dose and fentanyl concentration; pain control with the use of TF was improved in 7 of 10 patients in comparison to PCA alone. Zernikow provides a thorough summary in a recently published review of transdermal fentanyl in childhood and adolescence [73].

Oral transmucosal fentanyl citrate (OTFC) provides rapid onset analgesia via a pleasant route for children receiving painful medical procedures. It produces significant serum concentrations after 15 to 20 minutes [56]. Children aged 2 to 14 years have shown good cooperation and sedation when given OTFC as a premedication [19,40]. OTFC produced safe and effective analgesia for outpatient wound care in children, and the taste was preferred to that of oral oxycodone [59]. However, a study of the pharmacokinetic parameters during the consumption phase demonstrated a relatively late and variable peak concentration time of 53 ± 40 minutes [68]. This variability makes it difficult to suggest a minimum interval between OTFC consumption and the start of a painful procedure.

Table II
Opioid analgesics: usual starting doses for infants and children

Drug	Equianalgesic Dose (Parenteral)	Starting Dose (Intravenous)	I.V.: Oral Ratio	Starting Dose (Oral/ Transdermal)	Duration of Action
Codeine	130 mg	Not recommended		1.0 mg/kg every 4 h (dose limit 1.5 mg/kg/dose)	3–4 h
Fentanyl*	100 μg	0.5–2 μg/kg/h as continuous infusion		12–25 μg patch	72 h (patch)
Hydromorphone	2 mg	15–20 μg/kg every 2–4 h	1:2	40–60 μg/kg every 2–4 h	2–4 h
Meperidine†	75 mg	1.0–1.5 mg/kg every 3–4 h	1:4	1.0–1.5 mg/kg every 3–4 h (dose limit 150 mg)	1–3 h
Morphine	10 mg	Bolus dose = 0.05 mg/kg-0.1 mg/kg every 2–4 h; continuous infusion = 0.01–0.04 mg/kg/h	1:2	0.2–0.4 mg/kg/dose every 4 h	3–4 h
Oxycodone	5–8 mg	Not recommended		0.1–0.2 mg/kg every 3–4 h	3–4 h
Tramadol	100 mg	1–2 mg/kg every 4–6 h		1–2 mg/kg every 4–6 h (dose limit 400 mg/day)	4–6 h

Note: Doses are for opioid-naive patients. For infants under 6 months, start at one-quarter to one-third the suggested dose and titrate to effect.
Abbreviations: p.o. = by mouth; i.v. = intravenous.
* Potentially highly toxic. Not for use in acute pain control except during anesthesia. Should not be prescribed to opioid-naive patients.
† Avoid use in renal impairment. Metabolite may cause seizures.

Adjuvants

Antidepressants

Antidepressants are frequently used to treat chronic neuropathic pain in adults. Despite the lack of adequately controlled trials demonstrating efficacy in children, antidepressants are routinely used to treat chronic pain in children as well. The agent that is selected is based on the symptoms exhibited by the child. For instance, in children having trouble sleeping, a relatively sedating agent such as amitriptyline may be selected. Therapy is initiated with low doses (e.g., 0.1 mg/kg) that are gradually increased. Table III provides dosing guidelines for antidepressants and other adjuvant analgesics.

Anticonvulsants

Some children with chronic pain benefit from treatment with anticonvulsants. The two most commonly used drugs are carbamazepine and gabapentin. The use of carbamazepine has been steadily decreasing in favour of gabapentin, primarily because of the better adverse effect profile of gabapentin. The main dose-limiting side effect of gabapentin is sedation, so that a slow titration to maximal dose is required. A newer agent related to gabapentin, pregabalin, is a promising alternative to gabapentin in children [48].

Table III
Adjuvant medications: doses for infants and children

Drug Category	Drug, Dosage	Indications	Comments
Anticonvulsants	*Gabapentin:* 5 mg/kg/day p.o. Titrate upward over 3–7 days. Maintenance: up to 15–50 mg/kg/day p.o. divided t.i.d. *Carbamazepine:* Initial dosing: 10 mg/kg/day p.o. divided q.i.d. or b.i.d. Maintenance: up to 15–30 mg/kg/day p.o. divided every 8 hours. Increase dose gradually over 2–4 weeks. *Alternatives:* pregabalin.	Neuropathic pain, especially shooting, stabbing pain.	Side effects: gastrointestinal upset, ataxia, dizziness, disorientation, somnolence. Monitor plasma level and for hematological, hepatic, and allergic skin reactions with carbamazepine.
Antidepressants	*Amitriptyline:* 0.05–2.0 mg/kg p.o. q.h.s. Titrate dose every 7 days. Maintenance: 0.05–2.0 mg/kg. *Alternatives:* nortriptyline, doxepin.	Neuropathic pain (e.g., vincristine-induced neuropathy, radiation plexopathy, tumor invasion, CRPS-I); insomnia.	Not prescribed in infancy. Usually improved sleep and pain relief within 3–5 days. Anticholinergic side effects are dose-limiting. Use with caution in children with increased cardiac risk: obtain screening ECG prior to use.
Corticosteroids	Prednisone, prednisolone, and dexamethasone dosage depends on the clinical situation (e.g., dexamethasone initial dosing: 0.2 mg/kg i.v., dose limit 10 mg/day, subsequent dose 0.3 mg/kg/day i.v. divided every 6 hours).	Headache from increased intracranial pressure, spinal compression, or nerve compression; widespread metastases.	Side effects include edema, dyspeptic symptoms, and occasional gastrointestinal bleeding.
NMDA antagonists	*Ketamine:* Titrate dose to effect. *Oral:* 2–5 mg/kg p.o., maximum dose 100 mg. *Intravenous:* 0.5–1.0 mg/kg i.v., administer slowly over 1–2 minutes; may repeat 0.5 mg/kg in 10 minutes. *Intramuscular:* 3–5 mg/kg i.m. (i.m. use restricted to uncooperative patients).	Procedural pain/sedation, postoperative pain. Often used in combination with benzodiazepines and anticholinergic agents such as atropine or glycopyrrolate.	Side effects include hypersalivation, emergence reactions, emesis, tachycardia, and hypertension.

Abbreviations: b.i.d. = twice a day; CRPS-I = complex regional pain syndrome, type I; ECG = electrocardiogram; i.m. = intramuscular; i.v. = intravenous; s.l. = sublingual; p.o. = by mouth; q.h.s. = once daily at bedtime; q.i.d. = four times a day; t.i.d. = three times a day.

Other Drugs

Ketamine

Ketamine is an *N*-methyl-D-aspartate glutamate (NMDA) receptor antagonist used as a coanalgesic for operative and medical procedures [22,38]. Ketamine is increasing in popularity due to a low risk of cardiorespiratory depression. However, it frequently causes other adverse effects that must be managed, including excessive salivation and hallucinations. Ketamine has been demonstrated to be neurotoxic in animals, which may have implications for its safety in young infants [60]. Approaches for the use of ketamine in patients with chronic pain are currently under evaluation [38].

Clonidine

Clonidine is a selective α_2-adrenoreceptor agonist that is employed as an adjuvant for multiple indications at the Hospital for Sick Children [30]. It can be used as a preoperative sedative. We use a suspension of 0.1 mg/kg and give a 4-μg/kg dose orally 90 minutes preoperatively. Almenrader et al. found that at this dose, clonidine was preferred in comparison to midazolam, was better accepted by the child, produced more effective preoperative sedation, showed a trend toward better recovery from anesthesia, and had a higher degree of parental satisfaction [1a]. We also use clonidine on occasion as a sedative at bedtime. In a survey of 800 pediatricians, Schnoes et al. found that more than one-third of the sample reported using clonidine specifically for sleep disturbance including problems with sleep onset, sleep schedule, nighttime awakening, and early morning awakening and parasomnias [55a]. Where available, clonidine may be used in combination with the chosen local anesthetic to prolong pediatric caudal blocks. Following major orthopedic surgery or trauma, it has been reported to be used in peripheral nerve blocks such as brachial plexus and femoral nerve blocks in combination with the chosen local anesthetic [32a]. Krane et al. describe the use of clonidine for neuropathic, visceral, and postoperative pain at a dosing of 0.05–0.2 μg/kg/h by oral, transdermal, or continuous epidural infusion, but they warn of the side effects of hypotension, bradycardia, and somnolence [36]. Finally, in patients where either acute or chronic pain proves problematic to treat, clonidine is used as an adjuvant at the Hospital for Sick Children at an oral dose of 1–3 μg/kg three times per day. After chronic usage (more than 5 days), discontinuation of clonidine must be gradual to avoid rebound hypertension.

Local and Regional Analgesia

The use of regional techniques (epidural and spinal) for the administration of local anesthetics and analgesics for children continues to be an integral part of pain control in children [69]. Postoperative analgesia via the epidural route with the use of local anesthetics, with or without the combination of opioids, has advanced postoperative pain control. In pediatric practice, epidural analgesia has become the most commonly performed regional anesthetic technique for the intra- and postoperative management of patients with urologic, orthopedic, and general surgical procedures below the T4 dermatomal level [18]. Experience from many centers suggests that these techniques can also be extremely useful for children experiencing pain who have advanced disease that may be difficult to control by more conventional means. Finally, it is also feasible for children to receive epidural and spinal infusions at home on an extended basis in palliative care. Appropriate monitoring is paramount for patient safety. This involves the education and training of staff, immediate availability of resuscitative drugs and equipment, and an accurate and timely pain record consisting of vital signs and pain and sedation scores. (See [17,18] for detailed reviews of central and peripheral blocks in children and adolescents.)

Therapeutic Strategy

Pain control should include regular pain assessments, appropriate analgesics and adjuvant analgesics administered at regular dosing intervals, adjunctive drug therapy for symptom and side-effect control, and nondrug therapies to modify the situational factors that can exacerbate pain and suffering.

Principles of Analgesic Administration

The guiding principles of analgesic administration are "by the ladder," "by the clock," "by the child," and "by the mouth."

"By the Ladder"

"By the ladder" refers to a three-step approach for selecting drugs according to their analgesic potency based on the child's pain level—acetaminophen to control mild pain, codeine for moderate pain, and morphine for strong pain. If pain persists despite starting with the appropriate drug, the recommended dose, and the proper dosing schedule, the clinician should move up the ladder and administer the next, more potent, analgesic. Even when children require opioid analgesics, they should continue to receive acetaminophen (and NSAIDs, if appropriate) as supplemental analgesics.

Increasing attention is now focusing on "thinking beyond the ladder," however, in accordance with our improved understanding of pain of neuropathic origins [36,61]. Children should receive adjuvant analgesics such as amitriptyline or gabapentin to more specifically target neuropathic pain mechanisms. A newer class of antidepressants, the selective serotonin reuptake inhibitors, may be helpful in treating depression for a child with pain, but they have not been shown to be beneficial for pain management [20].

The specific drugs and doses are determined by the needs of each child. Recommended starting doses for analgesic medications to control children's disease-related pain are listed in Tables I and II; starting doses for adjuvant medications to control pain are listed in Table III. (For further review of analgesics and adjuvant analgesics in children, see [36,42,44,71,72].)

"By the Clock"

Children should receive analgesics at regular times, "by the clock," to provide consistent pain relief and prevent breakthrough pain. The specific drug schedule (e.g., every 4 or 6 hours) is based on the drug's duration of action and the child's pain severity. Although breakthrough pain episodes have been recognized as a problem in adult pain control, they may represent an even more serious problem for children. Unlike adults, who generally realize that they can demand more potent analgesic medications or demand more frequent dosing intervals, children have little control, have little awareness of alternatives, and fear that their pain cannot be controlled. They may become progressively more frightened, upset, and preoccupied with their symptoms. Thus, it is essential to establish and maintain a therapeutic window of pain relief for children.

"By the Child"

Analgesic doses should be adjusted "by the child." There is no one dose that will be appropriate for all children with pain. The goal is to select a dose that prevents children from experiencing pain before they receive the next dose. It is essential to monitor the child's pain regularly and adjust analgesic doses as necessary to control the pain. The effective opioid dose to relieve pain varies widely among different children or in the same child at different times. Some children require large opioid doses at frequent intervals to control their pain. If such doses are necessary for effective pain control, and the side effects can be managed by adjunctive medication so that children are comfortable, then the doses are appropriate. Children receiving opioids may develop altered sleep patterns so that they are awake at night, fearful and complaining about pain, and sleep intermittently throughout the day. Such children should receive adequate analgesics at night with antidepressants or hypnotics as necessary to enable them to sleep throughout the night. To relieve ongoing pain, opioid doses should be increased steadily until comfort is achieved, unless the child experiences unacceptable side effects that do not respond to treatment (see Chapter 21 for strategies to manage opioid-related side effects).

Routes of Administration

Oral

"By the mouth" refers to the oral route of drug administration. Medication should be administered to children by the simplest and most effective route, usually by mouth. When children are afraid of painful injections, they may deny that they have pain, or they may not request medication. When possible, children should receive medications through routes that do not cause additional pain. Although optimal analgesic administration for children requires flexibility in selecting routes according to children's needs, parenteral administration is often the most efficient route for providing direct and rapid pain relief. Because intravenous, intramuscular, and subcutaneous routes cause additional pain for children, serious efforts have been expended on developing more pain-free modes of administration that still provide relatively direct and rapid analgesia. Attention has focused on improving the effectiveness of oral routes. As described above, OTFC provides rapid-onset analgesia via a pleasant route for children receiving painful medical procedures.

Intravenous

Many hospitals have restricted the use of intramuscular injections because they are painful and drug absorption is not reliable; they advocate the use of intravenous lines into which drugs can be administered directly without causing further pain. Topical anesthetic creams should also be applied prior to the insertion of intravenous lines in children. The use of portacaths (implantable venous access systems) has become the gold standard in pediatrics, particularly for children with cancer under the care of the physician, who require administration of multiple drugs at weekly intervals.

Continuous infusion has several advantages over intermittent subcutaneous, intramuscular, or intravenous routes. This method circumvents repetitive injections, prevents delays in analgesic drug administration, and provides continuous levels of pain control without children experiencing increased side effects at peak level and pain breakthroughs at trough level. Continuous infusion should be considered when children have pain for which oral and intermittent parenteral opioids do not provide satisfactory pain control, when intractable vomiting prevents the use of oral medications, and when intravenous lines are not desirable. Children receiving a continuous infusion should continue to receive "rescue doses" to control breakthrough pain, as necessary. As outlined in Table III, the rescue doses should be 50–200% of the continuous infusion hourly dose. If children experience repeated breakthrough pain, the basal rate can be increased by 50% or by the total amount of morphine administered through the rescue doses over a 24-hour period (divided by 24).

Patient-Controlled Analgesia

PCA enables children to administer analgesic doses according to their pain level. PCA provides children with a continuum of analgesia that is prompt, economical, and not nurse dependent, and is associated with a lower overall opioid use [29,53,58,71]. It has a high degree of safety and allows for wide variability among patients, and there is no delay in analgesic administration. It can now be regarded as a standard for the delivery of analgesia in children aged >5 years [43]. However, there are opposing views about the use of background infusions with PCA. Although they may improve efficacy, they may increase the occurrence of adverse effects such as nausea and respiratory depression. In a comparison of PCA with and without a background infusion for children having lower-extremity surgery, the total morphine requirements were reduced in the PCA-only group, and the background infusion offered no advantage [47]. In another study comparing background infusion and PCA, children between 9 and 15 years old achieved better pain relief with PCA while children between 5 and 8 showed no difference [9]. Yaster and colleagues recommend the use of background continuous infusion to provide patients with more restful sleep and prevent children from awakening in pain [71].

Our current standard of practice is to add a background infusion for all major back surgery and major abdominal surgery when PCA is used. This background infusion is commonly used for only the first 24–48 hours postoperatively. After this period, we administer only bolus doses based on a balance between side effects, quality of analgesia, and nighttime sleep. For other types of surgery, if children's pain is not controlled adequately by PCA by bolus only, we add a background infusion or increase the amount of the bolus via the PCA or decrease the interval time at which the bolus is administered. The selection of opioid used in PCA is perhaps less critical than the appropriate selection of parameters such as bolus dose, lockout, and background infusion rate. The opioid choice may be based on adverse effect profile rather than efficacy. Clearly, control over PCA offers special advantages to children who have little control and who are extremely frightened about uncontrolled pain. PCA is, as it states, controlled by the patient. When special circumstances require that someone else administer the medication, both nurse- and parent-controlled analgesia may be appropriate. Under these circumstances, parents require nurse educators to fully inform them about the use of PCA. In a 2004 alert, the Joint Commission on Accreditation of Health Care Organizations (JCAHO) advised that serious adverse events can result when family members, caregivers or clinicians who are not authorized become involved in administering the analgesia for the patient "by proxy" [33,39].

Conclusions

Over the past two decades, increased pressure from health care providers, public advocates, and distressed parents has led to unprecedented changes in pediatric clinical practice so that children began to receive more appropriate analgesics at adequate doses and regular dosing intervals [46]. New interest was directed toward the pharmacokinetics and pharmacodynamics of conventional analgesics in infants and children, the development of pain-free transdermal and transmucosal drug delivery methods, the design of improved sedation regimens for children undergoing painful or aversive therapies, the feasibility of "child- and parent-controlled" PCA, the use of adjunct analgesics for neuropathic pain, and a broader use of regional anesthetic techniques in pediatric medicine.

Pain management is a continuous dynamic process, because the disease state and factors that influence pain are not static. Pain control is not merely "drug versus nondrug therapy," but rather an integrated approach. Effective pain control is possible when the goals are to reduce or block nociceptive activity by attenuating responses in peripheral afferents and central pathways, activate endogenous pain inhibitory systems, and modify situational factors that exacerbate pain. Different combinations of drug and nondrug therapies will be required at different times. Thus, health professionals must continually assume as much responsibility for monitoring and relieving children's pain as for medically managing their diseases.

References

[1] Ahmedzai S, Brooks D. Transdermal fentanyl versus sustained-release oral morphine in cancer pain: preference, efficacy, and quality of life. The TTS-Fentanyl Comparative Trial Group. J Pain Symptom Manage 1997;13:254–1.

[1a] Almenrader N, Passariello M, Coccetti B, Haiberger R, Pietropaoli P. Premedication in children: a comparison of oral midazolam and oral clonidine. Pediatr Anaesth 2007;17:1143–9.

[2] Anand KJ, Sippell WG, Aynsley-Green A. Randomised trial of fentanyl anaesthesia in preterm babies undergoing surgery: effects on the stress response. Lancet 1987;1:62–6.
[3] Anderson BJ, Holford NHG. Pharmacokinetics and pharmacodynamics of analgesic drugs. In: Anand KJS, Stevens BJ, McGrath PJ, editors. Pain in neonates and infants, 3rd ed. Toronto: Elsevier, 2007. p. 115–39.
[4] Andrews KA. The human developmental neurophysiology of pain. In: Schechter NL, Berde CB, Yaster M, editors. Pain in infants, children, and adolescents, 2nd ed. Baltimore: Lippincott Williams & Wilkins; 2003. p. 43–57.
[5] Bandell-Hoekstra IE, Abu-Saad HH, Passchier J, Frederiks CM, Feron FJ, Knipschild P. Prevalence and characteristics of headache in Dutch schoolchildren. Eur J Pain 2001;5:145–53.
[6] Berde CB, Sethna NF. Analgesics for the treatment of pain in children. N Engl J Med 2002;347:1094–103.
[7] Berde CB, Solodiuk J. Multidisciplinary programs for management of acute and chronic pain in children. In: Schechter NL, Berde CB, Yaster M, editors. Pain in infants, children, and adolescents, 2nd ed. Philadelphia: Lippincott Williams and Wilkins; 2003. p. 471–86.
[8] Blake MJ, Castro L, Leeder JS, Kearns GL. Ontogeny of drug metabolizing enzymes. Sem Fetal Neonatal Med 2005; 10:123–38.
[9] Bray RJ, Woodhams AM, Vallis CJ, Kelly PJ, Ward-Platt MP. A double-blind comparison of morphine infusion and patient controlled analgesia in children. Paediatr Anaesth 1996;6:121–7.
[10] Brown SC, Stinson J. Treatment of pediatric chronic pain with tramadol hydrochloride: siblings with Ehlers-Danlos syndrome—hypermobility type. Pain Res Manag 2004;9:209–11.
[11] Boucher T, Jennings E, Fitzgerald M. The onset of diffuse noxious inhibitory controls in postnatal rat pups: a C-Fos study. Neurosci Lett 1998;257:9–12.
[12] Bozkurt P. Use of tramadol in children. Paediatr Anaesth 2005;15:1041–7.
[13] Carbajal R, Rousset A, Danan C, Coquery S, Nolent P, Ducrocq S, Saizou C, Lapillonne A, Granier M, Durand P. Epidemiology and treatment of painful procedures in neonates in intensive care units. JAMA 2008;300:60–70.
[14] Cardwell M, Siviter G, Smith A. Non-steroidal anti-inflammatory drugs and perioperative bleeding in paediatric tonsillectomy. Cochrane Database Syst Rev 2005;CD003591.
[15] Christensen ML, Wang WC, Harris S, Eades SK, Wilimas JA. Transdermal fentanyl administration in children and adolescents with sickle cell pain crisis. J Pediatr Hematol Oncol 1996;18:372–6.
[16] Curtalo M, Sveticic G. Drug combinations in pain treatment: a review of the published evidence and a method for finding the optimal combination. Best Pract Res Clin Anaesthesiol 2002;16:507–19.
[17] Dalens B. Peripheral nerve blockade in management of postoperative pain in children. In: Schechter NL, Berde CB, Yaster M, editors. Pain in infants, children, and adolescents, 2nd ed. Baltimore: Lippincott Williams & Wilkins; 2003; p. 363–95.
[18] Desparmet JF, Hardart RA, Yaster M. Central blocks in children and adolescents. In: Schechter NL, Berde CB, Yaster M, editors. Pain in infants, children, and adolescents, 2nd ed. Baltimore: Lippincott Williams & Wilkins; 2003. p. 339–62.
[19] Dsida RM, Wheeler M, Birmingham PK, Henthorn TK, Avram MJ, Enders-Klein C, Maddalozzo J, Coté CJ. Premedication of pediatric tonsillectomy patients with oral transmucosal fentanyl citrate. Anesth Analg 1998;86:66–70.
[20] Dumortier G, Welniarz B, Sauvebois C, Medjdoub H, Friche H, Siad N, Degrassat K. Prescription of psychotropic drugs in paediatry: approved indications and therapeutic perspectives. Encephale 2005;31:477–89.
[21] Edinboro LE, Poklis A, Trautman D, Lowry S, Backer R, Harvey CM. Fatal fentanyl intoxication following excessive transdermal application. J Forensic Sci 1997;42:741–3.
[22] Elia N, Tramer MR. Ketamine and postoperative pain: a quantitative systematic review of randomized trials. Pain 2005;113:61–70.
[23] Fitzgerald M. Cutaneous primary afferent properties in the hind limb of the neonatal rat. J Physiol 1987;383:79–92.
[24] Fitzgerald M, Howard RF. The neurobiologic basis of pediatric pain. In: Schechter NL, Berde CB, Yaster M, editors. Pain in infants, children, and adolescents, 2nd ed. Baltimore: Lippincott Williams & Wilkins; 2003. p.19–42.
[25] Fitzgerald M, Jennings E. The postnatal development of spinal sensory processing. Proc Natl Acad Sci USA 1999;96:7719–22.
[26] Fitzgerald M, Walker SM. Infant pain management: a developmental neurobiological approach. Nat Clin Pract Neurol 2009;5:35–50.
[27] Grøholt EK, Stigum H, Nordhagen R, Köhler L. Recurrent pain in children, socio-economic factors and accumulation in families. Eur J Epidemiol 2003;18:965–75.
[28] Grunau RE. Long-term consequences of pain in human neonates. In: Anand KLS, Stevens BJ, McGrath PJ, editors. Pain in neonates, 2nd ed. Amsterdam: Elsevier; 2000. p. 55–76.
[29] Hill HF, Chapman CR, Kornell JA, Sullivan KM, Saeger LC, Benedetti C. Self-administration of morphine in bone marrow transplant patients reduces drug requirement. Pain 1990;40:121–9.
[30] The Hospital for Sick Children. The 2004–2005 formulary, 23rd ed. Toronto: The Hospital for Sick Children; 2004–2005.
[31] Hullett BJ, Chambers NA, Pascoe EM, Johnson C. Tramadol vs. morphine during adenotonsillectomy for obstructive sleep apnea in children. Paediatr Anaesth 2006;16:648–53.
[32] Hunt A, Goldman A, Devine T, Phillips M; FEN-GBR-14 Study Group. Transdermal fentanyl for pain relief in a paediatric palliative care population. Palliat Med 2001;15:405–12.
[32a] Ivani G, Tonetti F. Postoperative analgesia in infants and children: new developments Minerva Anestesiol 2004;70:399–403.
[33] Joint Commission on Accreditation of Healthcare Organizations. Patient controlled analgesia by proxy. Sentinel Event Alert 2004;33:1–2.

[34] Kearns GL, Abdel-Rahman SM, Alander SW, Blowey DL, Leeder JS, Kauffman RE. Developmental pharmacology: drug disposition, action, and therapy in infants and children. N Engl J Med 2003;349:1157–67.

[35] Koltzenburg M, Lewin GR. Receptive properties of embryonic chick sensory neurons innervating skin. J Neurophysiol 1997;78:2560–8.

[36] Krane EJ, Leong MS, Golianu B, et al. Treatment of pediatric pain with nonconventional analgesics. In: Schechter NL, Berde CB, Yaster M, editors. Pain in infants, children, and adolescents, 2nd ed. Philadelphia: Lippincott Williams and Wilkins 2003; p. 225–40.

[37] Len C, Hilario MO, Kawakami E, Terreri MT, Becker DJ, Goldenberg J, Fagundes Neto U. Gastroduodenal lesions in children with juvenile rheumatoid arthritis. Hepatogastroenterology 1999;46:991–6.

[38] Lin C, Durieux ME. Ketamine and kids: an update. Pediatric Anesthesia 2005;15:91–7.

[39] Maddox RR, Williams CK, Fields M. Respiratory monitoring in patient-controlled analgesia. Am J Health Syst Pharm 2004;61:2628–9.

[40] Malviya S, Voepel-Lewis T, Huntington J, Siewert M, Green W. Effects of anesthetic technique on side effects associated with fentanyl Oralet premedication. J Clin Anesth 1997;9:374–8.

[41] Martin AL, McGrath PA, Brown SC, Katz J. Children with chronic pain: impact of sex and age on long-term outcomes. Pain 2007;128:13–9.

[42] Maunuksela EL, Olkkola KT. Nonsteroidal anti-inflammatory drugs in pediatric pain management. In: Schechter NL, Berde CB, Yaster M, editors. Pain in infants, children, and adolescents, 2nd ed. Philadelphia: Lippincott Williams and Wilkins 2003; p. 171–81.

[43] McDonald AJ, Cooper MG. Patient-controlled analgesia: an appropriate method of pain control in children. Paediatr Drugs 2001;3:273–84.

[44] McGrath PA, Brown SC. Paediatric palliative medicine: pain control. In: Doyle D, Hanks G, Cherny N, Calman K, editors. Oxford textbook of palliative medicine, 3rd ed. Oxford: Oxford University Press; 2004. p. 775–89.

[45] McGrath PA. Chronic pain in children. In: Crombie IK, Croft PR, Linton SJ, LeResche L, Von Korff M, editors. Epidemiology of pain. Seattle: IASP Press; 1999. p. 81–101.

[46] McGrath PA. Children—not simply "little adults." In: Merskey H, Loeser JD, Dubner R, editors. The paths of pain 1975–2005. Seattle: IASP Press; 2005. p.433–46.

[47] McNeely JK, Trentadue NC. Comparison of patient-controlled analgesia with and without nighttime morphine infusion following lower extremity surgery in children. J Pain Symptom Manage 1997;13:268–73.

[48] Mease PJ, Russell IJ, Arnold LM, Florian H, Young JP Jr, Martin SA, Sharma U. A randomized, double-blind, placebo-controlled, phase III trial of pregabalin in the treatment of patients with fibromyalgia. J Rheumatol 2008;35:502–14.

[49] Noyes M, Irving H. The use of transdermal fentanyl in pediatric oncology palliative care. Am J Hosp Palliat Care 2001;18:411–6.

[50] Palmer GM. A teenager with severe asthma. Anaesth Intensive Care 2005;33:261–5.

[51] Pattinson D, Fitzgerald M. The neurobiology of infant pain: development of excitatory and inhibitory neurotransmission in the spinal dorsal horn. Reg Anesth Pain Med 2004;29:36–44.

[52] Perquin CW, Hunfeld JA, Hazebroek-Kampschreur AA, van Suijlekom-Smit LW, Passchier J, Koes BW, van der Wouden JC. The natural course of chronic benign pain in childhood and adolescence: a two-year population-based follow-up study. Eur J Pain 2003;7:551–9.

[53] Rodgers BM, Webb CJ, Stergios D, Newman BM. Patient-controlled analgesia in pediatric surgery. J Pediatr Surg 1988;23:259–62.

[54] Rose JB, Finkel JC, Arquedas-Mohs A, Himelstein BP, Schreiner M, Medve RA. Oral tramadol for the treatment of pain of 7–30 days' duration in children. Anesth Analg 2003;96:78–81.

[55] Schechter NL, Berde CB, Yaster M. Pain in infants, children and adolescents: an overview. In: Schechter NL, Berde CB, Yaster M, editors. Pain in infants, children, and adolescents, 2nd ed. Philadelphia: Lippincott Williams & Wilkins 2003. p. 3–18.

[55a] Schnoes CJ, Kuhn BR, Workman EF, Ellis CR. Pediatric prescribing practices for clonidine and other pharmacologic agents for children with sleep disturbance. Clinic Pediatr (Phila) 2006;45:229–38.

[56] Schutzman SA, Liebelt E, Wisk M, Burg J. Comparison of oral transmucosal fentanyl citrate and intramuscular meperidine, promethazine, and chlorpromazine for conscious sedation of children undergoing laceration repair. Ann Emerg Med 1996;28:385–90.

[57] Scott LJ, Perry CM. Tramadol: a review of its use in perioperative pain. Drugs 2000;60:139–76.

[58] Shapiro BS, Cohen DE, Howe CJ. Patient-controlled analgesia for sickle-cell-related pain. J Pain Symptom Manage 1993;8:22–8.

[59] Sharar SR, Carrougher GJ, Selzer K, O'Donnell F, Vavilala MS, Lee LA. A comparison of oral transmucosal fentanyl citrate and oral oxycodone for pediatric outpatient wound care. J Burn Care Rehabil 2002;23:27–31.

[60] Soriano SG, Anand KJS. Anesthetics and brain toxicity. Curr Opin Anaesthesiol 2005;18:293–7.

[61] Staats PS. Cancer pain: beyond the ladder. J Back Musculoskeletal Rehabil 1998;10:69–80.

[62] Taddio A, Katz J, Ilersich AL, Koren G. Effect of neonatal circumcision on pain response during subsequent routine vaccination. Lancet 1997;349:599–603.

[63] Taylor EM, Boyer K, Campbell FA. Pain in hospitalized children: a prospective cross-sectional survey of pain prevalence, intensity, assessment and management in a Canadian pediatric teaching hospital. Pain Res Manage 2008;13:25–32.

[64] Tibboel D, Anand KJ, van den Anker JN. The pharmacological treatment of neonatal pain. Semin Fetal Neonatal Med 2005;10:195–205.

[65] Van Den Kerkhof EG, van Dijk A. Prevalence of chronic pain disorders in children. In: Schmidt RF, Willis WD, editors. Encyclopedia of pain, Vol. 3. New York: Springer Verlag; 2006. p. 1972–4.

[66] Walker SM. Pain in children: recent advances and ongoing challenges. Br J Anesth 2008;101:101–10.
[67] Weingarten K, Stinson J, Carbajal R, et al. A single day audit of pain assessment and management practices in a pediatric hospital. E-PAS 2008;63345 abstract.
[68] Wheeler M, Birmingham PK, Dsida RM, Wang Z, Coté CJ, Avram MJ. Uptake pharmacokinetics of the Fentanyl Oralet in children scheduled for central venous access removal: implications for the timing of initiating painful procedures. Paediatr Anaesth 2002;12:594–9.
[69] Wilder RT. Regional anesthetic techniques for chronic pain management in children. In: Schechter NL, Berde CB, Yaster M, editors. Pain in infants, children, and adolescents, 2nd ed. Philadelphia: Lippincott Williams and Wilkins; 2003. p. 396–416.
[70] Woodbury CJ, Koerber HR. Widespread projections from myelinated nociceptors throughout the substantia gelatinosa provide novel insights into neonatal hypersensitivity. J Neurosci 2003;23:601–10.
[71] Yaster M, Kost-Byerly S, Maxwell LG. Opioid agonists and antagonists. In Schechter NL, Berde CB, Yaster M, editors. Pain in infants, children, and adolescents, 2nd ed. Philadelphia: Lippincott Williams and Wilkins; 2003. p. 181–225.
[72] Yaster M, Tobin JR, Kost-Byerly S. Local anesthetics. In: Schechter NL, Berde CB, Yaster M, editors. Pain in infants, children, and adolescents, 2nd ed. Philadelphia: Lippincott Williams and Wilkins; 2003. p. 241–65.
[73] Zernikow B, Michel E, Anderson B. Transdermal fentanyl in childhood and adolescence: a comprehensive literature review. J Pain 2007;8:187–207.

Correspondence to: Stephen C. Brown, MD, Department of Anaesthesia and Pain Medicine, Hospital for Sick Children, 555 University Avenue, Toronto, ON M5G 1X8, Canada. Email: stephen.brown@sickkids.ca.

24 Pharmacological Considerations in Older Patients

David Lussier[a,b] and Gisèle Pickering[c]

[a]Geriatric Institute, University of Montreal, Montreal, Quebec, Canada; [b]Division of Geriatric Medicine and Alan-Edwards Centre for Research on Pain, McGill University, Montreal, Quebec, Canada; [c]Clinical Pharmacology Department, University Hospital, Clermont Ferrand, France

Chronic pain is a significant problem for older persons because of its high prevalence and its numerous detrimental effects on physical and emotional functioning and quality of life. Several organizations, including the International Association for the Study of Pain (IASP), the American Geriatrics Society, the Australian Pain Society, the British Geriatrics Society, the British Pain Society, the American Medical Directors Association, and the European Federation of IASP Chapters, have recognized the importance of this problem by making pain management in older patients a priority and by establishing guidelines for the assessment and management of pain in this population. According to these guidelines, the presence of pain should be assessed every time an older patient sees a health care professional [2,17]. Chronic pain has several detrimental effects in older persons, including decreased functional autonomy, diminished social interactions, sleep impairment, depression, anxiety, altered quality of life, and increased use of health care services.

Definition and Demographics of Aging

Biological aging is a complex phenomenon, universal and unavoidable, which starts at birth and accelerates after reaching maturity (around 30 years of age). Several theories have been proposed to explain biological aging, which probably results from an interaction between genetic and environmental factors.

Pharmacology of Pain
edited by Pierre Beaulieu, David Lussier, Frank Porreca, and Anthony H. Dickenson
IASP Press, Seattle, © 2009

Although it is universal, aging is highly heterogeneous, with significant variations among individuals and in different body systems. Whereas some functions (e.g., glomerular filtration) almost unavoidably decline with aging, others (e.g., nerve conduction) mostly remain unaffected. Biological age is less significant than physiological age. At the same biological age, some people show very few detrimental effects of aging, whereas others have several diseases. It is also important, although often difficult, to differentiate normal (physiological) aging from disease-related (pathological) changes. For example, decreased glomerular filtration is part of normal aging, whereas renal insufficiency is always pathological and should be investigated.

In both developed and developing countries, populations are aging. Between 1983 and 2003, the proportion of the United States population older than 65 and older than 80 years increased from 11.7% and 2.4%, respectively, to 12.4% and 3.5%. This proportion is expected to increase further, to reach 20% and 7.2%, respectively, in 2043 [91]. Meanwhile, the proportion of the world population older than 65 years and older than 80 years has increased from 6.9% and 1.2%, respectively, in 2000, to 7.7% and 1.5% in 2009, and is expected to reach 16.7% and 4.9% in 2050 [92]. This increased proportion of older persons in the population is largely due to a significant increase in life expectancy in the past 50 years. For example, in the United States, life expectancy has increased from 65 years in 1942 to 77.8 years in 2005 (75.2 years for men and 80.4 years for women) [93] and is expected to rise to 79.5 years by 2020 [90]. Life expectancy at the age of 65 years has also increased: men and women aged 65 years old can now expect to live 17.2 and 20 more years, respectively [94]. This phenomenon will keep progressing in the next decades, as the proportion of the population older than 65 years and, more importantly, older than 80 years old, continues to increase.

Unfortunately, increased life expectancy does not always correlate with increased *healthy* life expectancy. The prevalence of chronic diseases, including degenerative diseases often associated with chronic pain, will also increase significantly. For example, in Great Britain in 2004, men and women could expect to spend 14.3 and 17 years of their lives, respectively, with a limiting illness or disability (compared to 12.8 and 16 years in 1982) [63].

Epidemiology

Depending on the population studied and the definition of chronic pain used, epidemiological surveys report that 40–75% of community-dwelling older persons have chronic pain [10,11,23]. Chronic pain is the most frequently reported symptom [12] and seems to be more common in very old people and in women [10,11,23]. Pain is also very common in patients admitted to an acute care geriatric unit [20] or a long-term care facility [24], as well as following hip fracture surgery [61].

The most frequent causes of chronic pain in older persons are musculoskeletal diseases (e.g., osteoarthritis, inflammatory arthritis, spinal stenosis, or degenerative disk disease) and neuropathic pain. Pain is most often constant, is of moderate to severe intensity, lasts for several years, and is multifocal and multifactorial [10]. Unfortunately, pain is often undertreated in older patients, especially in those who are very old or are cognitively impaired [61,105].

Age-Related Changes in Pain Perception

According to most experimental studies, pain detection and tolerance thresholds are not significantly altered in older persons [34]. Some age-related changes have nevertheless been reported, including a selective alteration of Aδ fibers (transmitting epicritic, well-localized, rapid pain), while C fibers (transmitting protopathic, ill-defined, slow pain) are well preserved [15]. Other changes include a delayed and blunted electroencephalic response to a painful stimulus [28] and a more diffuse neuronal recruitment [28]. These changes might partly explain the difficulty some older patients have in precisely describing and localizing their pain. Reduced pain-modulating capacity and descending inhibition may partially explain age-related increases in the prevalence and severity of chronic pain [22,46,102]. These data are, however, derived from experimental acute pain, and whether they can be extrapolated to clinical pain is unclear.

Age-Related Pharmacological Changes

Aging is associated with several pharmacokinetic and pharmacodynamic changes. These changes usually start progressively, but they should be considered when prescribing medications to patients older than 70 years.

Pharmacokinetic Changes

Data on age-related pharmacokinetic changes are limited, but some changes have been consistently reported. Most studies have been performed in healthy older subjects, with a few reports suggesting even greater significant pharmacokinetic and pharmacodynamic alterations in frail compared to healthy elderly persons [82]. Table I summarizes the most significant age-related pharmacokinetic changes.

Absorption

Oral absorption. Aging is associated with decreased gastric secretion in approximately 25% of adults more than 50 years old, resulting in higher gastric pH. Decreases in gastrointestinal motility, splanchnic blood flow, active protein transporters, and absorption area have also been reported [37]. Other factors frequently encountered in older patients can influence oral absorption, including several comorbidities, medications that slow gastrointestinal transit, chronic constipation, chronic laxative use, gastroesophageal reflux, and dysphagia [82,88].

Slower gastric emptying and increased transit time result in delays in reaching maximal plasma concentration for medications given as solids (capsules, tablets), but the absorbed fraction is unchanged [56]. These changes do not modify the absorption of liquid medications.

Rectal absorption. Rectal administration eliminates first-pass metabolism. Some factors (e.g., status of the rectal mucosa, blood flow, and contents of the rectal ampulla) can influence the rectal absorption of medications administered as a suppository or liquid, which makes their bioavailability highly variable.

Transdermal absorption. Aging is associated with decreased hydration of the corneal layer, reduced skin thickness and elasticity, and loss of subcutaneous fat tissue, which can increase the function of the stratum corneum as a barrier for relatively hydrophilic compounds without affecting lipophilic compounds (e.g., buprenorphine or fentanyl). Bioavailability of medications administered transdermally is often unpredictable in older patients and is subject to significant interindividual variability [33].

Table I
Age-related pharmacokinetic changes

Variable	Changes	Clinical Significance
Absorption	Increased gastric pH	Altered ionization of weak acids
	Decreased gastrointestinal motility	Slowing of gastric emptying; increased intestinal transit time of medications
	Decreased plasma concentration of active transporters	Decreased absorption of medications requiring active transport (e.g., calcium, iron, thiamine)
Distribution	Increased fat	Increased volume of distribution of lipophilic medications (e.g., antidepressants, antipsychotics, benzodiazepines)
	Decreased total body water	Decreased volume of distribution of hydrophilic medications (e.g., acetaminophen)
	Decreased serum albumin	Increased free fraction (e.g., phenytoin, NSAIDs)
Metabolism	Decreased hepatic blood flow	Decreased hepatic clearance of medications with high extraction coefficient
	Decreased liver mass	Decreased number of functional hepatocytes
	Decreased enzyme activity	Slowing of oxidation reactions (Phase I)
Clearance	Decreased glomerular filtration	Decreased clearance of renally cleared medications or active metabolites
	Decreased tubular secretion	Accumulation of medications requiring tubular secretion

Abbreviations: NSAIDs = nonsteroidal anti-inflammatory drugs.

Distribution

Changes in distribution have the most significant consequences of all age-related pharmacokinetic changes. Aging is associated with decreased lean mass, increased fat mass, and decreased total water volume, which change the distribution of medications [33,44]. The distribution volume of hydrophilic medications is decreased, which increases the plasma concentrations and requires a lower dosing. At the opposite, the distribution volume of lipophilic medications is increased, which decreases their plasma concentrations and increases their half-life, often resulting in accumulation [33].

Advanced age is also often associated with decreased serum albumin [67], which is more frequent in the presence of chronic diseases or malnutrition, and results in an increased free fraction of the medication. However, these changes are only clinically significant for medications with a protein binding rate higher than 90%, a small distribution volume, and a narrow therapeutic index [31]. The increased plasma concentration of acid α_1-glycoprotein does not seem to have any clinical consequences [33].

Metabolism

Liver mass and hepatic blood flow decrease with aging, which impairs drug clearance for flow-limited (high-clearance) drugs. There have been conflicting results for capacity-limited (low-clearance) drugs, with some authors suggesting a 20–60% impairment of the intrinsic metabolic drug clearance [13]. The activity of phase I enzymatic reactions (oxidation, reduction, and hydrolysis) seems to be reduced, whereas that of phase II enzymatic reactions (glucuronidation, acetylation, sulfation) is usually not modified [44,80]. Very limited evidence is available on the age-related changes of cytochrome activity, which does not seem to be modified [88].

Renal Excretion

Renal mass and tubular secretion decrease significantly with age. There is a 30–50% decrease in glomerular filtration at 80 years old, which results in accumulation of renally excreted medications. Serum creatinine level is not a reliable indicator of renal function in older persons because of decreased muscle mass accompanying decreased glomerular filtration [52]. Renal function and creatinine clearance can best be estimated with the Cockroft-Gault formula, taking into account age, weight, serum creatinine, and gender [16]. In older malnourished patients with decreased muscle mass, this formula can still overestimate creatinine clearance, however.

Pharmacodynamic Changes

Age-related pharmacodynamic changes often result in increased sensitivity of older patients to medications and, consequently, increased occurrence of adverse effects [64]. More specifically, increased sensitivity of cholinergic receptors makes older patients more sensitive to adverse effects from anticholinergic medications, including tricyclic antidepressants. Decreased homeostasis can explain the delayed recovery of basal state following impairment of a physiological function in older patients, including the development of acute renal failure or gastrointestinal bleeding with nonsteroidal anti-inflammatory drugs (NSAIDs) or sedation associated with opioids.

Pharmacological Management of Pain in Older Patients

According to the American Geriatrics Society, "all older patients with functional impairment or diminished quality of life as a result of persistent pain are candidates for pharmacologic therapy" [2]. A good knowledge of pharmacological properties of each analgesic is essential for the adequate and safe management of pain in these patients. Table II provides recommendations for starting doses of analgesics in older patients.

Nonopioid Analgesics

Acetaminophen (Paracetamol)

Acetaminophen is widely used in older patients because of the high prevalence of joint pathologies, by far the most common chronic pain pathology in these patients, and it is recommended as the first-line oral analgesic [2,3]. Acetaminophen is commonly prescribed to older patients without risk factors at a recommended dose of 500–1,000 mg every 4–6 hours to a maximum of 4,000 mg daily and is generally regarded as a safe medication at therapeutic doses.

Adverse effects are rare, with hepatotoxicity being the main safety concern. However, recent reports have questioned the safety of therapeutic doses of acetaminophen [4,97]. While old age per se has not been shown to be an independent risk factor for hepatotoxicity, there are no studies in very old or frail older patients, who often present one or several of the risk factors known to be associated with acetaminophen-induced hepatotoxicity [72]. First, depleted glutathione stores represent a significant risk factor (see Chapter 4). While this problem is usually associated with malnutrition, prolonged fasting [45], underweight, poor nutritional status or alcoholism [106], age-related changes in antioxidant status have been reported, including decreased glutathione stores and a higher ratio of reduced/oxidized glutathione [66]. A corpus of clinical reports suggests that acetaminophen administration should be carefully implemented in fasting patients and that nutritional status should be fully assessed, especially in underweight and malnourished older patients.

Second, patients with dehydration or hepatic, renal, or cardiac impairment are at increased risk of developing hepatotoxicity, and the incidence of these pathologies is higher in older patients. The available studies in patients with chronic liver disease are somewhat discordant. Some have shown that although the half-life of acetaminophen may be prolonged, cytochrome P-450 activity is not increased and glutathione stores are not depleted to critical levels in those taking recommended doses. Another study showed hepatotoxicity in patients with viral hepatitis. Despite these discordant studies, acetaminophen can be safely used in patients with liver disease and is a preferred analgesic/antipyretic because of the absence of the adverse effects associated with NSAIDs [9].

Third, use of cytochrome P450 enzyme-inducing drugs increases the risk of hepatotoxicity when given with a wide range of acetaminophen doses including therapeutic doses. Polypharmacy—frequently used in older patients—leads to an increased risk of drug interactions and related toxicity [71]. Finally, a number of studies have shown that therapeutic doses of acetaminophen are associated with increased concentrations of transaminases and with liver injury [38]; no such studies have been performed in elderly persons.

Table II
Dosing recommendations of analgesics in older patients

Analgesic	Recommended Starting Dose
Nonopioid Analgesics	
Acetaminophen (paracetamol)	325–650 mg every 4 hours p.r.n. (immediate-release) 650 mg t.i.d. (sustained-release)
NSAIDs	Variable, depending on NSAID used; use lowest available dose
COX-2 inhibitor (celecoxib)	100 mg b.i.d.
Tramadol	Variable, depending on formulations available in different countries; use lowest available dose
Opioid Analgesics	
Morphine	
Oral	1–5 mg every 4 hours p.r.n.
Parenteral	0.5–1 mg every 4 hours p.r.n.
Codeine	
Oral	15–30 mg every 4 hours p.r.n.
Parenteral	5–10 mg every 4 hours p.r.n.
Hydromorphone	
Oral	0.5–1 mg every 4 hours p.r.n.
Parenteral	0.25–0.5 mg every 4 hours p.r.n.
Oxycodone	2.5–5 mg every 4 hours p.r.n.
Transdermal fentanyl	Depending on equianalgesic daily dose of immediate-release or sustained-release opioid received; should not be used in opioid-naive patients
Transdermal buprenorphine	35 g/h every 4 days appears safe in opioid-naive patients; patch can be cut to start at a lower dose
Antidepressants	
Duloxetine	30 mg q.d.
Venlafaxine	37.5 mg q.d.
Bupropion	75 mg q.d.
Tricyclic antidepressants	10 mg h.s.
Anticonvulsants	
Gabapentin	100–300 mg q.d.–t.i.d.
Pregabalin	25 mg h.s.–b.i.d.

Abbreviations: b.i.d.: twice daily; COX-2: cyclooxygenase-2; h.s.: once daily at bedtime; NSAIDs: nonsteroidal anti-inflammatory drugs; p.r.n.: as needed; q.d.: once daily; t.i.d.: three times daily.

Another adverse effect of acetaminophen is its interaction with warfarin: at a dose of 4 g daily, acetaminophen increases the anticoagulant effect of warfarin and thereby increases the risk of warfarin-associated hemorrhage [68]. Whether this interaction occurs when acetaminophen is taken in lower doses requires further study. Given the increasing use of both acetaminophen and oral anticoagulants in clinical practice, this adverse effect should not be underestimated.

Nonsteroidal Anti-Inflammatory Drugs

Traditional NSAIDs and cyclooxygenase-2 selective inhibitors (coxibs) are widely prescribed in older persons, with proven efficacy in the management of musculoskeletal disorders (e.g., osteoarthritis) and a well-defined toxicity profile (gastrointestinal, renal and cardiovascular) (see Chapter 3). Adverse effects are significant in older persons because of age itself, the associated comorbidities, and the common use of polypharmacy in this population. Proton pump inhibitors should be added for gastric protection when an NSAID or a coxib is expected to be used for a long period [3]. Studies have demonstrated a high prevalence of inappropriate use of NSAIDs and coxibs in the elderly [1,95,96]. Experts also stress that even though recommendations for the use of NSAIDs have been published, these guidelines must be disseminated and applied in geriatric patients to decrease the risk of adverse effects [39]. Recently published guidelines of the American Geriatrics Society recommend that, because of their high risk of toxicity, NSAIDs may only be considered rarely, and with extreme caution, in highly selected older patients who have not found relief with other safer therapies [3]. Patients taking NSAIDs should be reassessed on a regular basis to ensure ongoing benefits, absence of toxicity, and drug-drug or drug-disease interactions [3].

A recent retrospective study that has not been confirmed so far [76] stresses that among older patients requiring analgesic/anti-inflammatory treatment, use of the combination of a traditional NSAID and acetaminophen may increase the risk of gastrointestinal bleeding compared with either agent alone.

Topical and oral NSAIDs are used to treat joint pain (frequently knee pain) in older people. The choice of the route of administration of an analgesic in an older patient depends on several factors: the perceived risk of adverse effects, the nature of the pain, the presence of other illnesses, practicality, and medical advice [14]. General practitioners' and patients' perceptions of the importance of adverse effects from oral NSAIDs may differ, and closer monitoring for potential adverse effects is required [14]. Finally, a systematic literature review recently suggested that an increased risk for accidental falls is probable when older persons are exposed to NSAIDs [35].

Tramadol

Tramadol is a centrally active synthetic analgesic drug with opioid and nonopioid properties (norepinephrine and serotonin reuptake inhibition). Because of its weak opioid agonist activity, it is recommended for the treatment of moderate pain (step 2 of the World Health Organization's analgesic ladder; see Chapter 26). Although age-related differences in pharmacological response are to be expected, the pharmacodynamic and pharmacokinetic properties of tramadol have only recently been compared in patients of various ages. In a prospective cohort study comparing patients aged less than 65 years, 65–75 years, and more than 75 years, immediate- or sustained-release galenic formulations of tramadol were generally well tolerated and effective in the treatment of moderate to severe pain in any of the three age groups [48]. Although the oldest group of patients consumed, on average, 20% less tramadol than the youngest group, the pharmacokinetic properties of both drugs were not changed when given to older patients.

Tramadol may be safer than diclofenac in terms of severe adverse effects [7]. In a randomized controlled trial, controlled-release tramadol was as effective as sustained-release diclofenac in the treatment of pain due to knee or hip osteoarthritis, with the potential for fewer of the serious adverse effects that characterize NSAIDs administration [7].

In the postoperative setting, a fixed combination of tramadol/acetaminophen has been shown to provide pain relief and to cause adverse effects similar to fixed combinations of hydrocodone/acetaminophen [27] and codeine/acetaminophen [85]. However, a higher global incidence of somnolence has been reported with codeine compared to tramadol preparations [62,73].

Opioid Analgesics

As in younger patients, opioid analgesics are recommended in older patients for the treatment of chronic pain of moderate to severe intensity, accompanied by pain-related functional impairment or diminished quality of life [3,70]. Older patients respond to opioid treatment as well as younger patients, but tolerability is often a limiting factor [70]. Due to the paucity of objective data on pharmacokinetic and pharmacodynamic properties of opioids in older patients, it is not possible to recommend the use of a specific opioid [70]. The choice should mainly be based on safety and tolerability of the opioid, as well as the patient's comorbidities (e.g., hepatic or renal failure) and concomitant medications (which may cause drug interactions). Even though recommendations have been published on starting doses for each opioid in older patients [3], the general rule is to start with the lowest dose possible and titrate according to analgesic response and adverse effects.

Morphine

Morphine is metabolized into two main metabolites: morphine-3-glucuronide (M3G) and morphine-6-glucuronide (M6G). M6G accumulates in renal failure and easily crosses the blood-brain barrier. It is therefore better to avoid using morphine in patients with renal failure or dehydration, as well as in those at risk for cognitive or psychomimetic adverse effects (agitation, hallucinations, myoclonus, or convulsions).

The age-related pharmacokinetic changes of morphine have only been studied in single-dose studies in healthy volunteers. Morphine's oral bioavailability does not seem to be modified, which means that equianalgesic doses of parenteral and oral morphine are similar to those of younger patients [5]. The mean plasma concentration is increased after parenteral and oral administration, suggesting a decreased hepatic first-pass clearance [5,65]. Renal clearance is also decreased, resulting in a longer elimination half-life [5].

Pharmacodynamic studies have shown that postoperative administration of morphine at a dose of 10 mg provides a higher [8] and longer [40] analgesic effect in older patients. These findings suggest that adequate analgesia might be obtained by administering morphine every 6 hours, rather than every 4 hours as is usually recommended.

Even though most of the other opioid analgesics have not been studied in older patients, their pharmacokinetic properties can guide the choice of an opioid for a specific patient.

Hydromorphone

The pharmacokinetic and pharmacodynamic properties of hydromorphone are very similar to those of morphine. Hydromorphone is also renally excreted. However, since its main metabolite has a low affinity for opioid receptors, its opioid-related adverse effects are less frequent than with morphine in renally impaired patients. Because of its hydrophilic properties, it crosses the blood-brain barrier less easily, which might result in a lower incidence of cognitive adverse effects [89].

Oxycodone

The plasma concentration of oxycodone is increased by 50% in renal failure, which results in increased sedation [41]. Following a single administration of 10 mg of oral oxycodone after orthopedic surgery, patients older than 70 years have a 50–80% higher mean exposure (area under the plasma concentration-time curve) to oxycodone [49], a longer elimination half-life of oxycodone and its metabolite noroxycodone, and a two-fold higher mean plasma concentration of oxycodone 12 hours after administration compared to younger patients [49]. Peak concentrations of oxycodone and the activity of cytochrome CYP2D6 appear similar in young and old patients [47]. Based on clinical experience suggesting good analgesic efficacy and tolerability, oxycodone has been recommended as the opioid of choice for older patients with chronic pain of moderate or severe intensity [29,70].

Codeine

It is well known that codeine is a prodrug that needs to be converted to its active metabolites (morphine and norcodeine) to exert any analgesic activity. The conversion relies on cytochrome CYP2D6. In addition to the 10–20% of the Caucasian population who have a genetic deficiency of this cytochrome, patients taking inhibitors or other substrates of CYP2D6 (e.g., selective serotonin reuptake inhibitors) are also potentially unable to convert codeine to its active metabolites, and thus may not respond to codeine. The metabolites of codeine accumulate in renal failure, and codeine is associated with a higher incidence of constipation and nausea than other opioids when used at equianalgesic doses [89]. For all these reasons, codeine is usually not a good opioid to use for older patients.

Opioids to Avoid in Older Patients: Meperidine, Propoxyphene, and Pentazocine

Meperidine is metabolized to normeperidine, an active metabolite with a long half-life that accumulates in renal failure, is a central nervous system stimulant, decreases the seizure threshold in long-term use, causes sedation, and increases the risk of falls and cognitive adverse effects. Intramuscular administration is associated with erratic absorption, especially in patients with muscular atrophy. For all these reasons, meperidine should never be used in older patients [2,29].

Propoxyphene also has an active metabolite that accumulates in renal failure and causes cognitive adverse effects [2]. Pure dextropropoxyphene (without acetaminophen) has been withdrawn in some countries because of its abuse potential and its association with suicide. Pentazocine has a long half-life that favors accumulation. Meperidine, propoxyphene, and pentazocine should therefore be avoided in older patients [2,25].

Long-Acting and Sustained-Release Opioids

Even though they should still be used in chronic constant pain, long-acting and sustained-release opioids should be prescribed with caution in older patients. They should only be prescribed to patients who are already receiving several daily doses of short-acting opioids, and for whom an appropriate daily dose of opioids has been identified. In order to avoid risks of prolonged overdosing, it is advisable to prescribe regular doses of a short-acting opioid (4–6 times daily) and change to a long-acting opioid when safety has been assured.

Transdermal fentanyl. The transdermal absorption of fentanyl is less predictable in older patients, due to decreased fat tissue and muscular atrophy. Both decreased and increased absorption have been reported [36,87]. In very thin patients, the loss of subcutaneous fat modifies transdermal absorption and can result in loss of efficacy. In an open prospective study in patients with cancer-related pain, transdermal fentanyl was well tolerated by older patients, without any significant differences from younger patients [54].

In opioid-naive older patients, the smallest available dose of transdermal fentanyl (12 μg/h) is too high and should never be used. Although it remains useful in selected older patients (e.g., those with decreased compliance to oral medications, dysphagia, or unsatisfactory pain control with oral opioids), transdermal fentanyl should only be prescribed to patients who have shown good tolerability to equianalgesic doses of short-acting or other long-acting opioids.

Transdermal buprenorphine. Buprenorphine, a partial agonist at the μ-opioid-receptor and an antagonist at the κ-opioid receptor, is highly lipophilic and is metabolized by the liver to norbuprenorphine and buprenorphine-glucuronide, which undergo intestinal (70%) and renal (30%) elimination. The same variability in transdermal absorption observed with transdermal fentanyl should apply to transdermal buprenorphine. In an open clinical trial comparing younger (≤50-year-old) to middle-age (51–64-year-old) and older (≥65-year-old) patients, buprenorphine provided similar pain relief to the three age groups and improved sleep, without any age-related difference [47]. Although a high occurrence of adverse effects was observed (dizziness, nausea, constipation, malaise, and fatigue), there was no age-related difference in adverse effects or discontinuation. A large post-marketing surveillance study in 13,179 patients reported similar results, with a lower occurrence of adverse effects (10% of which were assumed to be related to buprenorphine) and similar tolerability for older and younger patients [32]. A low-dose buprenorphine patch was also effective and well tolerated in a small group of opioid-naive patients with moderate to severe pain secondary to knee and/or hip osteoarthritis, with an average age of 65 years [42]. Despite these results, caution should be used when prescribing transdermal buprenorphine to opioid-naive older patients. Buprenorphine does not seem to impair cognitive functioning and driving ability in younger patients [19], but there is currently no evidence for older patients.

Oxycodone. Few older subjects have been included in clinical trials of sustained-release oxycodone. In those subjects, the plasma concentration was 15% higher than in younger ones. The occurrence of adverse effects has been reported as similar to that of younger subjects [75].

Methadone. Because of its lipophilicity and high protein-binding ability, methadone has a large volume of distribution and a long and variable half-life ranging from 8.5 to 120 hours [69]. These qualities make dose adjustment difficult, especially in older patients with limited reserves, modified liver metabolism, and decreased renal function. For these reasons, methadone should be initiated and titrated cautiously only by clinicians well versed in its use and aware of its risks [3].

Other long-acting opioids. The other long-acting and sustained-release opioids (morphine, codeine, and hydromorphone) have not been studied specifically in older patients, and an insufficient number of older subjects were included in clinical trials to permit any conclusions on their pharmacokinetic and pharmacodynamic properties in older, especially frail, patients.

Adverse Effects of Opioids in Older Patients

Because of their diminished physiological reserves, older patients are more sensitive to adverse effects from opioids. To ensure adequate pain management, it is therefore important to look for these adverse effects systematically and, whenever possible, prevent and treat them.

Sedation is the most frequent adverse effect, but it usually abates after a few days when tolerance develops. If it persists, a decreased dose followed by a slower titration, or the use of a psychostimulant (e.g., methylphenidate, modafinil, or caffeine) often allows the continuation of opioid therapy. Delirium and other cognitive adverse effects are also frequently encountered, especially in very old patients or those with baseline cognitive impairment. Unlike the case with sedation, there is no development of tolerance, and these adverse effects are often persistent. Therapeutic options then include discontinuation or dose reduction, with prescription of nonopioid or adjuvant analgesics, opioid rotation (e.g., switching to hydromorphone or oxycodone, which cross the blood-brain barrier less readily), and discontinuation of concomitant medications with adverse effects on the central nervous system. Although the use of opioids has been reported to increase the risk of delirium in the intensive care unit [74] and in the postoperative setting [26], the opposite findings have also been reported, with severe pain and insufficient opioid use being described as the main risk factors for postoperative delirium [21,60]. Except for meperidine, which is clearly associated with a higher risk of delirium, there does not seem to be any difference among other opioids [26,60]. A systematic review of clinical trials concluded that the mode of administration (intravenous or epidural) does not influence postoperative cognitive function differently [26], whereas a prospective cohort study reported a lower risk of postoperative cognitive dysfunction with oral opioids compared to the use of a patient-controlled analgesia device [99].

Constipation is almost unavoidable with prolonged use of an opioid. It can be minimized by adequate hydration and ambulation, or treated with peristalsis stimulants (e.g., senna, bisacodyl) or osmotic laxatives (lactulose, sorbitol). Nausea, sometimes occurring at the initiation of opioid therapy, often abates spontaneously with the development of tolerance; if it persists, it responds to standard antiemetics. Urinary retention, caused by increased tone of the bladder sphincter muscles, is sometimes encountered, especially in men with benign prostatic hypertrophy, and can respond to tamsulosin or terazosin.

The most feared adverse effect of opioids, respiratory depression, rarely occurs if opioids are initiated at a low dose and titrated progressively.

Finally, an increased risk of falls and fracture has been reported in older patients treated with opioids. Increased caution and surveillance should therefore be exerted when opioid therapy is initiated or titrated up [83,104].

The increased frequency of opioid-related adverse effects in older patients should not prevent the use of opioids when appropriate, since these side effects can often be adequately prevented or treated. Effective and safe pain management with opioids is often possible in older patients, with frequent reassessment for ongoing attainment of therapeutic goals, adverse effects, and safe and responsible medication use [3].

Antidepressants

The analgesic efficacy of tricyclic antidepressants has been established for several types of pain frequently encountered in older patients (e.g., postherpetic neuralgia, peripheral diabetic neuropathy). Unfortunately, use of these agents in older patients is limited by their numerous adverse effects, including anticholinergic effects (dry mouth, constipation, blurred vision, urinary retention), cognitive changes (delirium, memory impairment), cardiovascular toxicity (orthostatic hypotension, tachycardia) and an increased risk of falls and fractures [50]. Secondary amines (nortriptyline, desipramine) seem to have analgesic efficacy similar to tertiary amines (amitriptyline, imipramine, doxepin) and are better tolerated in older patients [100], which makes them a better choice if a tricyclic antidepressant is used.

Due to age-related changes in hepatic metabolism of tricyclic antidepressants (via oxidation), the elimination half-life of these drugs is three to four times longer in older patients. In cases of hypoalbuminemia, frequent in older patients, the free fraction of the drugs is increased due to their high protein binding (90–98%).

Because of all the above reasons, the use of tricyclic antidepressants in older patients should be avoided and restricted to those who do not respond to other adjuvant analgesics with a better tolerability profile [3].

The serotonin and norepinephrine reuptake inhibitors duloxetine and venlafaxine have been shown to be effective for neuropathic pain. Duloxetine can also relieve pain and improve cognition in older patients with major depressive disorder [78,79], with an onset of the analgesic effect at doses lower than the antidepressant dose [79]. Both venlafaxine and duloxetine are usually well tolerated in older patients, and no dose reduction is necessary [77,101]. They therefore represent a good alternative to tricyclic antidepressants for older patients with neuropathic pain and/or concomitant depression. Duloxetine elimination is slightly decreased with age [84], whereas venlafaxine levels are slightly higher in older patients [6]. When prescribing duloxetine or venlafaxine, the physician should pay attention to pharmacokinetic drug-drug interactions. Duloxetine moderately and venlafaxine weakly inhibits cytochrome CYP2D6.

Bupropion, also shown effective for neuropathic pain, offers the advantage of possessing stimulant properties, which is especially useful in apathetic older patients or those with somnolence due to concomitant medications. The half-life of bupropion and its metabolites is increased in older subjects [86].

Finally, selective serotonin reuptake inhibitors (SSRIs) are usually recommended for depressed older patients due to a low frequency of adverse effects. Citalopram and S-citalopram offer the advantage of a reduced risk of pharmacokinetic interactions due to their minimal inhibition of CYP450; although their clearance is decreased in older subjects, they are usually well tolerated [50]. Their analgesic efficacy is unclear, however. Fluoxetine should be avoided because it is associated with a higher frequency of adverse effects, partly because the parent molecule and its active metabolite (norfluoxetine) have long half-lives (2 and 7 days, respectively) [50].

The use of antidepressants (particularly SSRIs) is strongly associated with falls, regardless of the presence of depressive symptoms. Strategies to prevent falls should therefore always be used when prescribing an antidepressant to an older patient [43].

Anticonvulsants

Because of their analgesic efficacy in several types of neuropathic pain, their good tolerability, and the absence of pharmacokinetic drug-drug interactions, gabapentin and pregabalin are usually recommended as first-line agents for the treatment of neuropathic pain, especially in older patients who often present with several comorbidities and are using several prescription drugs [30,103]. Pregabalin has been reported to be as effective for neuropathic pain in older as in younger patients [81], and it is well tolerated [57]. Adverse effects can still occur, especially in frail or very old patients, including somnolence, dizziness, gait disturbance, and peripheral edema. These symptoms sometimes abate spontaneously after a few days, and they can often be avoided by using low starting doses, titrating slowly, and carefully monitoring for adverse effects. Because of their renal clearance and the frequent occurrence of decreased renal function in older patients, these patients often respond to doses lower than the usually therapeutic doses and can rarely tolerate titration up to maximum doses. Serum concentrations of pregabalin have been observed to be higher in older subjects [53].

Although several other anticonvulsants have been reported effective for neuropathic pain, their tolerability is often limited in older patients, especially for phenytoin and carbamazepine. Their use should therefore be restricted to refractory neuropathic pain.

Topical and Local Analgesics

Since they are not associated with any systemic adverse effects, topical and local analgesics (e.g., NSAIDs, lidocaine, and capsaicin) are very good therapeutic alternatives for older patients.

Neuroaxial Analgesics

Patients who cannot obtain adequate pain relief from systemic analgesics without experiencing significant adverse effects can benefit from continuous neuroaxial (intrathecal or epidural) administration of analgesics, which can provide analgesia with lower plasma concentrations, and therefore less severe systemic adverse effects. This approach could therefore be especially useful for older patients, who sometimes cannot tolerate therapeutic doses of analgesics. Even though scientific evidence on the efficacy and tolerability of this mode of administration of analgesics in older patients is currently limited, clinical experience supports its use in selected patients.

Nonpharmacological and Interdisciplinary Management of Pain in Older Patients

Because of the high frequency of drug-related adverse effects, pharmacological treatment of pain in older patients should always be accompanied by nonpharmacological modalities, which might allow adequate pain relief with lower doses of analgesics. Nonpharmacological modalities include a physical activity program, physical therapy (e.g., exercise, heat/cold, transcutaneous electrical nerve stimulation, ultrasound, and massage), occupational therapy (e.g., energy conservation strategies and orthotics), cognitive-behavioral approaches (including teaching of adaptive coping strategies and relaxation), and education on chronic pain. Complementary and alternative medicine modalities (e.g., acupuncture, chiropractic, osteopathy, and therapeutic touch) can also be beneficial to some patients, and they do not carry any risk if used appropriately. Few randomized clinical trials have evaluated the benefits of nonpharmacological approaches and their potential synergistic action with pharmacological treatment. Recent studies and reviews stress the need for larger clinical trials to evaluate their impact on chronic nonmalignant pain and acceptance of pain in older adults [58,59].

A multidisciplinary program is the gold standard for adequate management of chronic pain. When these programs are adapted to their specific needs, older patients respond as well as younger ones [18,51,55]. Table III presents general recommendations for pain management of older patients, which allow good pain relief when followed.

Table III
Recommendations for adequate pain management in older patients

1) Perform comprehensive assessment of pain and comorbidities
2) Identify type of pain (nociceptive, neuropathic, mixed)
3) Combine pharmacological and nonpharmacological modalities
4) Know the pharmacological properties and age-related pharmacokinetic changes of each analgesic
5) Adapt pharmacological treatment to the patient's comorbidities
6) Combine different classes of analgesics (nonopioids, opioids, antidepressants, anticonvulsants)
7) Favor analgesics with the best efficacy/toxicity ratio
8) Initiate pharmacological treatment with the lowest dose available and titrate up progressively, based on analgesic response and adverse effects
9) Pay attention to drug-drug interactions
10) Reassess the analgesic response on a regular basis and discontinue analgesics with unclear efficacy
11) Look for, prevent, and treat adverse effects

Conclusion

Even though pharmacological treatment of pain in older patients is often hampered by the frequent occurrence of adverse effects, adequate pain relief is usually possible if the various classes of analgesics are used appropriately, taking into consideration the pharmacokinetic properties of the drugs, as well as age-related pharmacological changes.

Unfortunately, data are currently very limited on the analgesic efficacy and tolerability of analgesics in older patients, especially those who are very old or frail. In order to allow evidence-based pharmacological treatment of pain in older patients, efforts should be made to include more older subjects in clinical trials of analgesics and to report specific results for older subjects.

References

[1] Abraham NS, El-Serag HB, Johnson ML. National adherence to evidence-based guidelines for the prescription of nonsteroidal anti-inflammatory drugs. J Gastroenterol 2005;129:1171–8.

[2] AGS Panel on Persistent Pain in Older Persons. The management of persistent pain in older persons. J Am Geriatr Soc 2002;50:S205–24.

[3] AGS Panel on Pharmacological Management of Persistent Pain in Older Persons. Pharmacological management of persistent pain in older persons. J Am Geriatr Soc 2009; 57:1331–46.

[4] Ahmad SR. Safety of recommended doses of paracetamol. Lancet 2007;369:462–3.

[5] Baillie SP, Bateman DN, Coates PE, Woodhouse KW. Age and the pharmacokinetics of morphine. Age Ageing 1989;18:258–62.

[6] Ball SE, Ahern D, Scantina J, Kao J. Venlafaxine: in vitro inhibition of CYP2D6 depending imipramine and desipramine metabolism: comparative studies with selected SSRIs, and effects on human hepatic CYP3A4, CYP2C9, and CYP1A2. Br J Clin Pharmacol 1997;42:619–26.

[7] Beaulieu AD, Peloso PM, Haraoui B, Bensen W, Thomson G, Wade J, Quigley P, Eisenhoffer J, Harsanyi Z, Darke AC. Once-daily, controlled-release tramadol and sustained-release diclofenac relieve chronic pain due to osteoarthritis: a randomized controlled trial. Pain Res Manag 2008;13:103–10.

[8] Bellville JW, Forrest WH, Miller E, Brown W Jr. Influence of age on pain relief from analgesics: a study of postoperative patients. JAMA 1971;217:1835–41.
[9] Benson GD, Koff RS, Tolman KG. The therapeutic use of acetaminophen in patients with liver disease. Am J Ther 2005;12:133–41.
[10] Brattberg G, Parker MG, Thorslund M. The prevalence of pain among the oldest old in Sweden. Pain 1996;67:29–34.
[11] Brochet B, Michel P, Barberger-Gateau P, Dartigues JF. Population-based study of pain in elderly people: a descriptive survey. Age Ageing 1998;27:279–84.
[12] Brody EM, Kleban MH. Day-to-day mental and physical health symptoms of older people: a report on health logs. Gerontology 1983;23:75–85.
[13] Butler JM, Begg EJ. Free drug metabolic clearance in elderly people. Clin Pharmacokinet 2008;47:297–321.
[14] Carnes D, Anwer Y, Underwood M, Harding G Sr, Parsons S. Influences on older people's decision making regarding choice of topical or oral NSAIDs for knee pain: qualitative study. BMJ 2008;338:142–5.
[15] Chakour MC, Gibson SJ, Bradbeer M, Helme RD. The effect of age on A delta- and C-fibre thermal pain perception. Pain 1996;64:143–52.
[16] Cockcroft DW, Gault MH. Prediction of creatinine clearance from serum creatinine. Nephron 1976;16:31–41.
[17] Collett B; Royal College of Physicians of London, Clinical Effectiveness and Evaluation Unit, British Geriatrics Society, British Pain Society. The assessment of pain in older people: national guidelines. London: Royal College of Physicians; 2007.
[18] Cutler RB, Fishbain DA, Rosomoff RS, Rosomoff HL. Outcomes in treatment of pain in geriatric and younger age groups. Arch Phys Med Rehabil 1994;75:457–64.
[19] Dagtekin O, Gerbershagen HJ, Wagner W, Petzke F, Radbruch L, Sabatowski R. Assessing cognitive and psychomotor performance under long-term treatment with transdermal buprenorphine in chronic noncancer pain patients. Anesth Analg 2007;105:1442–8.
[20] Desbiens NA, Mueller-Rizner N, Connors AF, Hamel MB, Wenger NS. Pain in the oldest-old during hospitalization and up to one year later. J Am Geriatr Soc 1997;45:1167–72.
[21] Duggleby W, Lander J. Cognitive status and postoperative pain: older adults. J Pain Symptom Manage 1994;9:19–27.
[22] Edwards RR, Fillingim RB, Ness TJ. Age-related differences in endogenous pain modulation: a comparison of diffuse noxious inhibitory controls in healthy older and younger adults. Pain 2003;101:155–65.
[23] Elliott AM, Smith BH, Penny KI, Smith WC, Chambers WA. The epidemiology of chronic pain in the community. Lancet 1999;354:1248–52.
[24] Ferrell BA, Ferrell BR, Osterweil D. Pain in the nursing home. J Am Geriatr Soc 1990;38:409–14.
[25] Fick DM, Cooper JW, Wade WE, Waller JL, Maclean JR, Beers MH. Updating the Beers criteria for potentially inappropriate medication use in older adults: results of a US Consensus Panel of Experts. Arch Intern Med 2003;163:2716–24.
[26] Fong HK, Sands LP, Leung JM. The role of postoperative analgesia in delirium and cognitive decline in elderly patients: a systematic review. Anesth Analg 2006;12:1255–66.
[27] Fricke JR Jr, Karim R, Jordan D, Rosenthal N. A double-blind, single-dose comparison of the analgesic efficacy of tramadol/acetaminophen combination tablets, hydrocodone/acetaminophen combination tablets, and placebo after oral surgery. Clin Ther 2002;24:953–68.
[28] Gibson SJ, Gorman MM, Helme RD. The assessment of pain in the elderly using cerebral event related potentials. In: Bond MR, Charlton JE, Woolf CJ, editors. Proceedings of the Vth World Congress on Pain. Amsterdam: Elsevier; 1991. p. 527–35.
[29] Gloth FM. Pain management in older adults: prevention and treatment. J Am Geriatr Soc 2001;49:188–99.
[30] Gore M, Sadosky A, Leslie D, Sheehan AH. Selecting an appropriate medication for treating neuropathic pain in patients with diabetes: a study using the U.K. and Germany Mediplus Databases. Pain Pract 2008;8:253–62.
[31] Grandison MK, Boudinot FD. Age-related changes in protein binding of drugs: implications for therapy. Clin Pharmacokinet 2000;38:271–90.
[32] Griessinger N, Sitti R, Likar R. Transdermal buprenorphine in clinical practice: a post-marketing surveillance study in 13,179 patients. Curr Med Res Opin 2005;21:1147–56.
[33] Hammerlein A, Derendorf H, Lowenthal DT. Pharmacokinetic and pharmacodynamic changes in the elderly: clinical implications. Clin Pharmacokinet 1998;35:49–64.
[34] Harkins SW. What is unique about the older adult's pain experience? In: Weiner DK, Herr K, Rudy TE, editors. Persistent pain in older adults: an interdisciplinary guide for treatment. New York: Springer; 2002. p. 4–17.
[35] Hegeman J, van den Bemt BJ, Duysens J, van Limbeek J. NSAIDs and the risk of accidental falls in the elderly: a systematic review. Drug Saf 2009;32:489–98.
[36] Holdsworth MT, Forman WB, Killilea TA, Nystrom KM, Paul R, Brand SC, Reynolds R. Transdermal fentanyl disposition in elderly subjects. Gerontology 1994;40:32–7.
[37] Iber FL, Murphy PA, Connor ES. Age-related changes in the gastrointestinal system. Drugs Aging 1994;5:34–48.
[38] Jalan R, Williams R, Bernuau J. Paracetamol: are therapeutic doses entirely safe? Lancet 2006;368:2195–6.
[39] Juby AG, Davis P. Utility of published guidelines on the use of nonsteroidal anti-inflammatory drugs in the elderly. Clin Rheumatol 2008;27:1191–4.
[40] Kaiko RF. Age and morphine analgesia in cancer patients with postoperative pain. Clin Pharmacol Ther 1980;28:823–6.
[41] Kaiko RF, Benziger D, Chang C, Hou Y, Grandy RP. Clinical pharmacokinetics of controlled-release oxycodone in renal impairment. Clin Pharmacol Ther 1996;59:130.
[42] Karlsson M, Breggren AC. Efficacy and safety of low-dose transdermal buprenorphine patches (5, 10, and 20 microg/h) versus prolonged-release tramadol tablets (75, 100, 150, and 200 mg) in patients with chronic osteoarthritis pain: a 12-week, randomized, open-label, controlled, parallel-group noninferiority study. Clin Ther 2009;31:503–13.

[43] Kerse N, Flicker L, Pfaff JJ, Draper B, Lautenschlager NT, Sim M, Snowdon J, Almeida OP. Falls, depression and antidepressants in later life: a large primary care appraisal. PLoS One 2008;3:e2423.
[44] Kinirons MT, Crome P. Clinical pharmacokinetics considerations in the elderly: an update. Clin Pharmacokinet 1997;33:302–12.
[45] Kurtovic J, Riordan SM. Paracetamol-induced hepatotoxicity at recommended dosage. J Intern Med 2003;253:240–3.
[46] Larivière M, Goffaux P, Marchand S, Julien N. Changes in pain perception and descending inhibitory controls start at middle age in healthy adults. Clin J Pain 2007;23:506–10.
[47] Likar R, Vadlau EM, Breschan C, Kager I, Korak-Leiter M, Ziervogel G. Comparable analgesic efficacy of transdermal buprenorphine in patients over and under 65 years of age. Clin J Pain 2008;24:536–43.
[48] Likar R, Wittels M, Molnar M, Kager I, Ziervogel G, Sittl R. Pharmacokinetic and pharmacodynamic properties of tramadol IR and SR in elderly patients: a prospective, age-group-controlled study. Clin Ther 2006;28:2022–39.
[49] Liukas A, Kuusniemi K, Aantaa R, Virolainen P, Neuvonen M, Neuvonen PJ, Olkkola KT. Plasma concentrations of oral oxycodone are greatly increased in the elderly. Clin Pharmacol Ther 2008;84:462–7.
[50] Lotrich FE, Pollock BG. Aging and clinical pharmacology: implications for antidepressants. J Clin Pharmacol 2005;45:1106–22.
[51] Lussier D, Bachand G, Haché D, Rivard MJ, Inglis G. An interdisciplinary geriatric pain clinic. Abstracts of the 12th World Congress on Pain. Seattle: IASP Press; 2008.
[52] Mallet L. Age-related changes in renal function and clinical implications for drug therapy. J Geriatr Drug Ther 1991;5:5–29.
[53] May TW, Rambeck B, Neb R, Jürgens U. Serum concentrations of pregabalin in patients with epilepsy: the influence of dose, age, and comedication. Ther Drug Monit 2007;29:789–94.
[54] Menten J, Desmedt M, Lossignol D, Mullie A. Longitudinal follow-up of TTS-fentanyl use in patients with cancer-related pain: results of a compassionate-use study with special focus on elderly patients. Curr Med Res Opin 2002;18:488–98.
[55] Middaugh SJ, Levin RB, Kee WG, Barchiesi FD, Roberts JM. Chronic pain: its treatment in geriatric and younger patients. Arch Phys Med Rehabil 1988;69:1021–5.
[56] Montamat SC, Cusack BJ, Vestal RE Management of drug therapy in the elderly. N Engl J Med 1989;321:303–9.
[57] Montgomery S, Chatamra K, Pauer L, Whalen E, Baldinetti F. Efficacy and safety of pregabalin in elderly people with generalised anxiety disorder. Br J Psychiatry 2008;193:389–94.
[58] Morone NE, Greco CM. Mind-body interventions for chronic pain in older adults: a structured review. Pain Med 2007;8:359–75.
[59] Morone NE, Greco CM, Weiner DK. Mindfulness meditation for the treatment of chronic low back pain in older adults: a randomized controlled pilot study. Pain 2008;134:310–9.
[60] Morrison RS, Magaziner J, Gilbert M, Koval KJ, McLaughlin MA, Orosz G, Strauss E, Siu AL. Relationship between pain and opioid analgesics on the development of delirium following hip fracture. J Gerontol Med Sci 2003;58A:76–81.
[61] Morrison RS, Siu AL. A comparison of pain and its treatment in advanced dementia in cognitively intact patients with hip fracture. J Pain Symptom Manage 2000;19:240–8.
[62] Mullican WS, Lacy JR. Tramadol/acetaminophen combination tablets and codeine/acetaminophen combination capsules for the management of chronic pain: a comparative trial. Clin Ther 2001;23:1429–45.
[63] National Statistics. Government Actuary's Department for Expectation of Life Data. ONS for healthy life expectancy data. Published on 1 October 2008. Available at: www.statistics.gov.uk/cci/nugget.asp?id=934. Accessed February 10, 2009.
[64] Nolan L, O'Malley K. Prescribing for the elderly. Part I: Sensitivity of the elderly to adverse drug reactions. J Am Geriatr Soc 1988;32:142–9.
[65] Owen JA, Sitar DS, Berger L, Brownell L, Duke PC, Mitenko PA. Age-related morphine kinetics. Clin Pharmacol Ther 1983;34:364–8.
[66] Oztürk O, Gümüşlü S. Changes in glucose-6-phosphate dehydrogenase, copper, zinc-superoxide dismutase and catalase activities, glutathione and its metabolizing enzymes, and lipid peroxidation in rat erythrocytes with age. Exp Gerontol 2004;39:211–6.
[67] Paolisso G, Gambardella A, Balbi V, Ammendola S, D'Amore A, Varrichio M. Body composition, body fat distribution, and resting metabolic rate in healthy centenarians. Am J Clin Nutr 1995;62:746–50.
[68] Parra D, Beckey NP, Stevens GR. The effect of acetaminophen on the international normalized ratio in patients stabilized on warfarin therapy. Pharmacotherapy 2007;27:675–83.
[69] Payne R. Opioid pharmacotherapy. In: Berger AM, Portenoy RK, Weissman DE, editors. Principles and practice of palliative care and supportive oncology, 2nd ed. Philadelphia: Lippincott Williams & Wilkins; 2002. p. 68–83.
[70] Pergolizzi J, Böger RH, Budd K, Dahan A, Erdine S, Hans G, Kress HG, Langford R, Likar R, Raffa RB, Sacerdote P. Opioids and the management of chronic severe pain in the elderly: consensus statement of an International Expert Panel with focus on the six clinically most often used World Health Organization step III opioids (buprenorphine, fentanyl, hydromorphone, methadone, morphine, oxycodone). Pain Pract 2008;8:287–313.
[71] Pickering G. Frail elderly, nutritional status and drugs. Arch Gerontol Geriatr 2004;38:174–80.
[72] Pickering G. Paracetamol use in the elderly. J Pain Manage 2008;1:35–9.
[73] Pickering G, Estrade M, Dubray C. Comparative trial of tramadol/paracetamol and codeine/paracetamol combination tablets on the vigilance of healthy volunteers. Fundam Clin Pharmacol 2005;19:707–11.
[74] Pisani MA, Murphy TE, Araujo KLB, Slattum P, Van Ness PH, Inouye SK. Benzodiazepine and opioid use and the duration of intensive care unit delirium in an older population. Crit Care Med 2009;37:177–83.
[75] Purdue Pharma. OxyContin (monograph). 2009. Available at: www.pharma.com/PI/Prescription/Oxycontin.pdf. Accessed October 8, 2009.

[76] Rahme E, Barkun A, Nedjar H, Gaugris S, Watson D. Hospitalizations for upper and lower GI events associated with traditional NSAIDs and acetaminophen among the elderly in Quebec, Canada. Am J Gastroenterol 2008;103:872–82.
[77] Raskin J, Wiltse CG, Dinkel JJ, Walker DJ, Desaiah D, Katona C. Safety and tolerability of duloxetine at 60 mg once daily in elderly patients with major depressive disorder. J Clin Psychopharmacol 2008;28:32–8.
[78] Raskin J, Wiltse CG, Siegal A, Sheikh J, Xu J, Dinkel JJ, Rotz BT, Mohs RC. Efficacy of duloxetine on cognition, depression, and pain in elderly patients with major depressive disorder: an 8-week, double-blind, placebo-controlled trial. Am J Psychiatry 2007;164:900–9.
[79] Raskin J, Xu JY, Kajdasz DK. Time to response for duloxetine 60 mg once daily versus placebo in elderly patients with major depressive disorder. Int Psychogeriatr 2007;20:309–27.
[80] Schmucker DL. Liver function and phase I drug metabolism in the elderly: a paradox. Drugs Aging 2001;18:837–51.
[81] Sharma U, McCarberg W, Young JH, LaMoreaux L. Pregabalin treatment for neuropathic pain: efficacy and tolerability in older people. J Pain 2005;3:S29.
[82] Shi S, Mörike K, Klotz U. The clinical implications of ageing for rational drug therapy. Eur J Clin Pharmacol 2008;64:183–99.
[83] Shorr RI, Griffin MR, Daugherty J, Ray WA. Opioid analgesics and the risk of hip fracture in the elderly: codeine and propoxyphene. J Gerontol Med Sci 1992;47:M111–5.
[84] Skinner MH, Kuan HY, Skerjanec A, Seger ME, Heathman M, O'Brien L, Reddy S, Knadler MP. Effect of age on the pharmacokinetics of duloxetine in women. Br J Clin Pharmacol 2004;57:54–61.
[85] Smith AB, Ravikumar TS, Kamin M, Jordan D, Xiang J, Rosenthal N. Combination tramadol plus acetaminophen for postsurgical pain. Am J Surg 2004;187:521–7.
[86] Sweet RA, Pollock BG, Kirshner M, Wright B, Altieri LP, DeVane CL. Pharmacokinetics of single and multiple-dose bupropion in elderly patients with depression. J Clin Pharmacol 1995;35:876–84.
[87] Thompson JP, Bower S, Liddle AM, Rowbotham DW. Perioperative pharmacokinetics of transdermal fentanyl in elderly and young adult patients. Br J Anaesth 1998;81:152–4.
[88] Tumer N, Scarpace PJ, Lowenthal DT. Geriatric pharmacology: basic and clinical considerations. Annu Rev Pharmacol Toxicol 1992;32:271–302.
[89] Twycross RG. Opioids. In: Wall PD, Melzack R, editors. Textbook of pain, 4th ed. London: Churchill Livingstone; 1999. p. 1187–214.
[90] U.S. Census Bureau. 2008 national population projections. Available at: www.census.gov/population/www/projections/2008projections.html. Accessed February 10, 2009.
[91] U.S. Census Bureau. International data base. Country summary: United States. Available at: www.census.gov/ipc/www/idb/country/usportal.html. Accessed February 10, 2009.
[92] U.S. Census Bureau. International data base. Available at: www.census.gov/ipc/www/idb/worldpopinfo.html. Accessed February 10, 2009.
[93] U.S. National Center for Health Statistics. Deaths: final data for 2005. National Vital Statistics Reports 56(10); April 24, 2008. Available at: www.census.gov/compendia/statab/tables/09s0100.pdf. Accessed February 10, 2009.
[94] U.S. National Center for Health Statistics. U.S. decennial life tables for 1999–2001: United States life tables. National Vital Statistics Reports 57(1); August 5, 2008. Available at: www.census.gov/compendia/statab/tables/09s0101.pdf. Accessed February 10, 2009.
[95] Van Leen MWF, Van Der Eijk I, Schols JMGA. Prevention of NSAID gastropathy in elderly patients. An observational study in general practice and nursing homes. Age Ageing 2007;36:414–8.
[96] Visser LE, Graatsma HH, Tricker BHC. Contraindicated NSAIDs are frequently prescribed to elderly patients with peptic ulcer disease. Br J Clin Pharmacol 2002;53:183–8.
[97] Vitols S. Paracetamol hepatotoxicity at therapeutic doses. J Intern Med 2003;253:95–8.
[99] Wang Y, Sands LP, Vaurio L, Mullen EA, Leung JM. The effects of postoperative pain and its management on postoperative cognitive dysfunction. Am J Geriatr Psychiatry 2007;15:50–9.
[100] Watson CPN, Vernich L, Chipman M, Reed K. Nortriptyline versus amitriptyline in postherpetic neuralgia: a randomized trial. Neurology 1998;51:1166–71.
[101] Wasan AD, Ossanna MJ, Raskin J, Wernicke JF, Robinson MJ, Hall JA, Edwards SE, Lipsius S, Meyers AL, McCarberg BH. Safety and efficacy of duloxetine in the treatment of diabetic peripheral neuropathic pain in older patients. Curr Drug Saf 2009;4:22–9.
[102] Washington LL, Gibson SJ, Helme RD. Age-related differences in the endogenous analgesic response to repeated cold water immersion in human volunteers. Pain 2000;89:89–96.
[103] Wehling M. Multimorbidity and polypharmacy: how to reduce the harmful drug load and yet add needed drugs in the elderly? Proposal of a new drug classification: fit for the aged. J Am Geriatr Soc 2009;57:560–1.
[104] Weiner D, Hanlon JT, Studenski SA. Effects of central nervous system polypharmacy on falls liability in community-dwelling elderly. Gerontology 1998;44:217–21.
[105] Won A, Lapane K, Gambassi G, Bernabei R, Mor V, Lipsitz LA. Correlates and management of nonmalignant pain in the nursing home. J Am Geriatr Soc 1999;47:936–42.
[106] Zimmerman HJ, Maddrey WC. Acetaminophen (paracetamol) hepatotoxicity with regular intake of alcohol: analysis of instances of therapeutic misadventure. Hepatology 1995;22:767–73.

Correspondence to: David Lussier, MD, FRCP(C), Institut universitaire de gériatrie de Montréal, 4565 chemin Queen-Mary, Montreal, Quebec, Canada H3W 1W5. Email: david.lussier@mcgill.ca.

25

Pharmacological Considerations in Obese Patients and Patients with Renal or Hepatic Failure

Frédérique Servin

Department of Anesthesiology, AP-HP, Bichat Hospital, Paris, France

Adequate dosing of analgesic drugs is mandatory to achieve both effective and safe analgesia. In special patient groups, finding the correct dose is complicated by both pharmacokinetic and pharmacodynamic changes. This chapter will address the main pharmacological changes associated with obesity and renal and hepatic failure and will describe the consequences of those changes on the administration of individual analgesic agents. It cannot be exhaustive because the pharmacological changes are linked to each drug and not to the pharmacological class it belongs to. General considerations on the influence of the disease state on pharmacology may help in predicting the ramifications for a drug not included in this chapter.

Obesity

Obesity is a metabolic disorder that is becoming more and more frequent in Western societies. It can be classified according to Body Mass Index (BMI)—weight (kg)/squared height (m^2)—in terms of simple obesity (BMI = 30–40), morbid obesity (BMI = 40–50), and super obesity (BMI > 50). The importance of the pharmacological impact of obesity grows with increasing BMI, but it can be observed at early stages for lipid-soluble drugs. Obesity is often associated with cardiovascular and respiratory impairments. It is therefore mandatory to have adequate knowledge of the pharmacology of analgesic agents to

Pharmacology of Pain
edited by Pierre Beaulieu, David Lussier, Frank Porreca, and Anthony H. Dickenson
IASP Press, Seattle, © 2009

determine an appropriate dosage in this population and reach the desirable efficacy with minimal unwanted effects.

Pharmacokinetics

Absorption

Obesity by itself does not modify intestinal absorption of drugs [22]. Nevertheless, some bariatric surgical operations (gastric or intestinal bypasses) may promote impaired absorption syndromes.

Distribution

Protein binding. Obesity is associated with an inflammatory state [94]. Acid α_1-glycoprotein (AAG) concentration may double in obese patients compared to controls of normal weight [101]. As a consequence, the active free fraction of slightly alkaline drugs such as fentanyl and congeners may be markedly lowered, thus reducing the efficiency of the drugs.

Volume of distribution. Increase in fat tissue mass is obviously a major factor in volume of distribution changes in obese patients. However, obesity is also associated with increases in blood volume and in the size of many organs (such as the liver or kidneys) [54]. Consequently, the initial volume of distribution is usually increased, as well as the volume of distribution at steady state, even in drugs that do not penetrate fatty tissue. Lean body mass is also greater in obese patients [50]. Thus, to reach the same concentration and therefore the same clinical effect, most drugs must be given at increased doses. Of course, drugs that are readily distributed into fat need more dosage adjustments than those that remain in the extracellular spaces. The clinician must nevertheless keep in mind that adjusting hydrophilic drug dosage based on ideal body weight in morbidly obese patients may lead to underdosage.

Elimination

Hepatic metabolism. Obesity is associated with increased cardiac output, blood volume, and organ blood flow, but functional hepatic blood flow remains mostly unchanged despite an increase in liver size. This lack of increase in blood flow is possibly due to fatty infiltration of the liver, which may impair liver function even if the usual biological tests remain normal [2]. The clearance of phase I metabolized drugs is usually unchanged, as is that of acetylated drugs, despite the increased activity of some P450 cytochromes. By contrast, the elimination clearance of many conjugated drugs increases in parallel with total body weight, possibly through extrahepatic conjugation pathways [1].

Renal elimination. Obese patients have larger kidneys than controls of normal weight [68]. The glomerular filtration rate is increased, and tubular excretion may be increased to an even greater degree [92]. As a consequence, the elimination of drugs excreted by the kidney is enhanced.

A summary of the pharmacokinetic changes in obese patients is given in Table I.

Table I
Summary of pharmacokinetic changes in patients with obesity, patients with renal failure, and patients with hepatic failure

Pharmacokinetic Variable	Obesity: Fat-Soluble Drug	Obesity: Non-Fat-Soluble Drug	Renal Failure	Hepatic Failure
Free fraction bound to albumin	≈	≈	↑	↑↑
Free fraction bound to AAG	↓	↓	≈ or ↓	↓ ≈ or ↑
Central volume of distribution	↑	↑	≈ or ↑	↑
Total volume of distribution	↑↑↑	↑	≈ or ↑	≈ or ↑
Hepatic elimination	Phase I: ≈ Phase II: ↑	Phase I: ≈ Phase II: ↑	Drug: ≈ Metabolites: ↓↓	High extraction: ↓↓↓ Low extraction: ≈ or ↓
Renal elimination	↑	↑	↓↓↓	≈ or ↓↓ (end stage)
Comment			Influence of dialysis: very important	Highly dependent on cause and stage

Abbreviations and symbols: AAG = acid α_1-glycoprotein; ↑ = increased; ↓ = decreased; ≈ = mostly unchanged. The number of arrows illustrates the magnitude of the changes.

Pharmacodynamics

There is very little information in the literature on pharmacodynamic changes in obese patients. Some studies on human pain thresholds have yielded contradictory results, with some claiming increased and others reduced pain sensitivity in the obese [61, 100]. Pain threshold appears to be increased in obese rats [78]. It seems that even nondiabetic obese patients display a subclinical involvement of sensory fibers of various diameters, mimicking a subclinical peripheral neuropathy related to metabolic alterations such as hyperinsulinemia [65].

Consequences for the Use of Analgesic Drugs in the Obese Patient

For many analgesic drugs, specifically the weak opioids and nonopioid analgesics, pharmacology in the obese patient has not been studied per se. Practical guidelines must therefore be drawn from the logical consequences of both pharmacological changes in obesity and the specific pharmacokinetics of the drug. Table II provides a summary of recommendations on analgesic prescription in obese patients.

Opioids

Morphine. Morphine pharmacokinetics in obese patients has not been specifically studied. One may nevertheless assume that morphine, which is conjugated, may have an increased metabolism in obese patients, with no accumulation of the active metabolites, which are eliminated through the kidneys. Morphine is linked to albumin, and its unbound fraction

Table II
Summary of recommendations concerning use of analgesics in patients with obesity, renal failure, or hepatic failure

Drug	Obesity	Renal Failure	Hepatic Failure
Morphine	Kinetics warrants increasing doses, but risk of respiratory depression (SAS)	Risk of accumulation of active metabolites; TITRATE +++	Increased oral bioavailability; increased half-life; TITRATE +++
Fentanyl and congeners	Interest in remifentanil; determine dose as a function of LBM, not TBW	Can be used as usual; TITRATE	Lower dose (increased sensitivity); avoid alfentanil
Codeine, oxycodone	See Morphine	Difficult to titrate; best avoided	Reduced efficacy
Tramadol	Can be used: increase initial dose and increase interval between doses	Accumulation of active metabolite; lower dose and increase interval between doses	Lower dose +++
Propoxyphene	Can be used as usual	Best avoided; risk of hypoglycemia	Risk of obstructive jaundice, especially in elderly women
NSAIDs	Can be used at usual dosage	Contraindicated, especially if some degree of renal function still exists	May precipitate acute renal failure; antiplatelet activity may worsen coagulation problems
Acetaminophen (paracetamol)	Can be used: increase dose and increase interval between doses	Expert recommendation: lower dose	Lower dose ++; risk of acute liver failure in alcoholic patients

Abbreviations and symbols: LBM: lean body mass; NSAIDs: nonsteroidal anti-inflammatory drugs; SAS: sleep apnea syndrome; TBW: total body weight; ++ = important; +++ = absolutely mandatory.

probably remains normal. Thus, as far as analgesia is concerned, obese patients probably require more morphine than patients of normal weight. Nevertheless, the main problem with morphine use in the obese is respiratory depression and hypoxemia, even in the absence of sleep apnea syndrome [81]. Obesity is associated with a higher resting metabolic rate, possibly due to increased lean body mass [97]. As a result, the tolerance of obese patients to respiratory depression is very poor [13]. Morphine should therefore always be part of a multimodal analgesic protocol to minimize the dosage, and it should be titrated to effect under close monitoring in this population. Patient-controlled analgesia is a suitable way to titrate morphine to analgesic effect in this population [21].

Fentanyl and congeners (alfentanil, sufentanil, and remifentanil). Despite its large volume of distribution, fentanyl should not be administered as a function of total body weight in obese patients, but rather proportionally to "pharmacokinetic mass," which is linked to clearance and for which guidelines have been published [88]. Nevertheless, the cumulative properties of fentanyl are not in favor of its use in obese patients when repeated or high doses are warranted.

Sufentanil has been studied in more detail [90]; as might be expected from its high lipid solubility, the total volume of distribution of sufentanil is increased in the obese patient. This increase remains moderate, however, since it is no more statistically significant if expressed as a function of body weight. Obesity slows sufentanil elimination. The most recent pharmacokinetic model published for sufentanil does not include body weight as a significant covariate [40]. Interestingly, the model performed well when used for target-controlled infusion of sufentanil in morbidly obese patients despite a slight overestimation of plasma sufentanil concentrations specifically for patients with BMI greater than 40. Thus, this set of pharmacokinetic parameters derived from a normal-weight population accurately predicted plasma sufentanil concentrations in morbidly obese patients [90].

Alfentanil has a small volume of distribution and will therefore not accumulate in obese patients. Due to its intermediate clearance, its duration of action remains at least as long as that of sufentanil, but interest in this drug has dropped since the launching of remifentanil [57].

The pharmacokinetic properties of remifentanil (its small volume of distribution, high clearance, and lack of lingering effects) make it an almost ideal drug for use during anesthesia in the obese patient. Apart from the (expected) high clearance, another important feature of remifentanil pharmacokinetics is its near-independence from body weight, with only lean body mass appearing as a significant morphological covariate of the models. As a consequence, remifentanil pharmacokinetics is not appreciably different in obese versus normal-weight subjects, and in clinical practice, remifentanil dosing regimens should be based on lean body mass and not on total body weight [33].

The impact of obesity on transdermal fentanyl absorption has not been evaluated. However, transdermal nicotine absorption is reduced in the obese [77]. Difficulties in safely titrating this lipid-soluble respiratory depressant make its use inadvisable in obese patients.

Codeine, oxycodone, hydromorphone. Codeine is a prodrug and must be transformed into morphine by the enzyme debrisoquine hydroxylase (CYP2D6) to be effective. As a consequence, the effects of codeine are the same as those of morphine, with a time delay related to the required transformation. Some individuals (e.g., about 10% of the European population) lack the ability to transform codeine into morphine [47]. There are no specific data as to the influence of obesity on codeine pharmacology.

Oxycodone is a semisynthetic opioid structurally very close to codeine, which has been widely prescribed since controlled-released forms have been introduced. Its pharmacology has not been studied in the obese. Its analgesic potency is nearly the same as that of morphine, and it shares the same respiratory depressant properties [8]. It is therefore perhaps not the best choice in this population.

Hydromorphone is a very potent rapid-acting morphine derivative. Its efficacy in treating breakthrough pain has led to its wide use in chronic pain patients in many countries. Its pharmacology in the obese has not been specifically considered. Various formulations are currently under investigation, such as transdermal delivery systems, with or without electrophoresis. Specific studies will be required before such systems are proposed for hydromorphone delivery in the obese.

Tramadol. Tramadol is a racemic mixture of two enantiomers with similar pharmacokinetics: a volume of distribution at steady state around 3.5 L/kg, as a consequence of its lipophilicity, and an intermediate elimination clearance around 500 mL/min [38]. Tramadol undergoes hepatic metabolism via the cytochrome P450 isoenzyme CYP2D6, and is O- and N-demethylated to five different metabolites. One of these, M1 (O-desmethyltramadol) is active and may accumulate with repeated doses [6]. Tramadol has not been specifically studied in obese patients, but we can infer from its pharmacological properties that the initial dose should be high, and subsequent doses delayed, due to the drug's cumulative potential.

Nonopioid Analgesics

NSAIDs (see also Chapter 3 by Vergne-Salle and Beneytout). NSAIDs (nonsteroidal anti-inflammatory drugs) may be readily used in morbidly obese patients, with the usual precautions and contraindications. NSAIDs may even help to control the metabolic syndrome [39]. In the perioperative period, as part of a multimodal analgesia protocol, they may help reduce the dose of postoperative opioids and therefore the risk of respiratory impairment through their potent synergistic contribution to the analgesic effect [64]. Their small volume of distribution (e.g., 0.15 L/kg for ketoprofen [96]) suggests that they do not penetrate the adipose tissue, and therefore their effective doses are modified very little by obesity.

Acetaminophen (paracetamol) (see also Chapter 4 by Mallet and Eschalier). Although acetaminophen pharmacokinetics has not been studied in obese patients, the drug's volume of distribution (0.9 L/kg) in normal-weight patients [36] suggests that some increase in dose may be necessary to achieve full analgesic effect.

Drugs Used in the Treatment of Neuropathic Pain

Gabapentin. Gabapentin pharmacology has not been specifically studied in obese patients. The drug's volume of distribution at steady state lies around 60 L in normal-weight patients [62]. In obese patients, one may speculate that some dosage adaptation may be required, based on titration to effect.

Pregabalin. Pregabalin pharmacology has not been specifically studied in obese patients. The drug has a rather small steady state volume of distribution (0.6 L/kg) and as such probably does not enter the fatty tissue to any significant degree [11]. As a consequence, no major dosage adaptation would probably be required in obese patients, and pregabalin dose should certainly not be calculated as a function of total body weight.

Carbamazepine. Carbamazepine pharmacokinetics has been studied in obese patients [20]. The total volume of distribution is enhanced and the clearance unchanged, leading to accumulation and increased elimination half-life, but with lesser plasma concentrations for the same dose. As a consequence, in obese patients, bolus doses should be increased, and the time delay between two successive doses should be prolonged, to ensure adequate plasma concentrations and safe elimination.

Clonazepam. Clonazepam is a benzodiazepine readily distributed in the fatty tissue, with a volume of distribution around 3 L/kg [89]. Even if no specific data are available in the obese, the drug's extensive distribution into fatty tissue and its potent synergistic depressive action on the central nervous system when combined with opioids do not advocate clonazepam use in this population.

Renal Failure

Pain is a common problem in end-stage renal disease [67]. Such pain is challenging to manage, largely because of the constraints that very poor renal function places on use of medications. However, patients with end-stage renal failure represent only a fraction of those with reduced renal function. Many elderly or cardiac patients have silent impairment in the renal elimination of drugs that may lead to accumulation and enhanced effect. It is usually considered that dosage adjustments are warranted when the glomerular filtration rate is reduced by half, which corresponds roughly to a creatinine clearance of around 60 mL/min.

Pharmacokinetics

Distribution

Protein binding is frequently impaired in renal failure, even when plasma albumin concentration is normal, due to competitive binding of cumulated endogenous compounds [24]. Moreover, the binding capacity of albumin may vary with dialysis [70]. In this situation, the unbound, effective fraction of highly bound drugs may increase dramatically, and the doses should be reduced accordingly. Similarly, the volume of the extracellular fluids may vary with dialysis, but the volume of distribution of lipophilic drugs is not modified by renal dysfunction.

Elimination

Most drugs are ultimately eliminated through the kidneys, often after a hepatic phase that should increase their hydrosolubility and therefore allow their renal excretion, but does not always inactivate them. Consequently, hydrophilic native drugs excreted in the urine and most metabolites tend to accumulate in the case of renal failure, which may have clinical consequences if these compounds are still active. The dosage of such drugs must be modified if glomerular filtration rate, often estimated through creatinine clearance, is less than 50% of normal.

A summary of the pharmacokinetic changes in patients with renal failure is given in Table I.

Pharmacodynamics

The concentration-effect relationship of analgesic drugs in patients with renal failure, albeit poorly investigated, is probably not modified significantly. An enhanced pharmacological effect may however be observed as a consequence of pharmacokinetic changes and higher unbound drug concentrations leading to an increased effect of the usual dose. As a consequence, titrating to effect should be the rule in establishing drug dosages in patients with renal failure.

Consequences for the Use of Analgesic Drugs in Patients with Renal Failure

Table II provides a summary of recommendations on analgesic prescription in patients with renal failure, and Table III indicates which analgesics are mainly eliminated by the kidneys.

Opioids

Morphine. Morphine, which is linked to albumin in the plasma, is metabolized by the liver mainly by phase II reactions: glucuroconjugation and sulfoconjugation as well as N-demethylation [63]. If the parent compound is readily eliminated even in end-stage renal failure, the metabolites tend to accumulate, and the morphine-6- and morphine-3-glucuronides (M6G, M3G), which are very active, will prolong the opioid action and may induce overdoses and adverse events [84]. M6G is an opioid, and M3G, although devoid of opioid action in humans, is implicated in morphine tolerance phenomena. In end-stage renal failure, the balance between M6G and M3G is modified in favor of M6G, and both drugs are included in an enterohepatic cycle that will regenerate morphine mainly from M3G [44]. These metabolites are filtered when dialysis takes place. They are largely able to cross the blood-brain barrier, albeit slowly [55]. Do these caveats mean that morphine

Table III
Elimination pathways and hepatic extraction coefficient of analgesics

		Hepatic Extraction Coefficient		
	Renal Elimination	High	Med.	Low
Morphine	Active metabolite	X		
Fentanyl		X		
Sufentanil		X		
Alfentanil			X	
Remifentanil	Extensive metabolism by tissue esterases			
Codeine		Prodrug*		
Oxycodone				X
Hydromorphone		X		
Tramadol			X	
Acetaminophen			X	
Gabapentin	X			
Pregabalin	X			
Carbamazepine				X
Clonazepam				X

* Requires hepatic metabolism to be active.

should never be used in renal failure patients? Certainly not, specifically in the perioperative period. But it should be considered as a drug ultimately eliminated through the kidney, and after an initial dose, all subsequent doses should be titrated to effect and given only when clear signs of waning of effect appear. Patient-controlled analgesia is an effective choice in this situation.

Fentanyl and congeners. Fentanyl, alfentanil, and sufentanil undergo hepatic metabolism that inactivates them. They bind to AAG, the binding ability of which is generally not modified by renal failure (total concentration is frequently enhanced, but the number of binding sites per molecule is lower) [53]. Clinical efficacy may be enhanced through a reduction in initial volume of distribution and an increase in the unbound fraction, but the drugs' duration of action is not statistically prolonged [37]. Nevertheless, titration remains mandatory because interindividual variability in drug metabolism is higher in patients with renal failure than in normal controls [25].

Similarly, remifentanil is metabolized by tissue esterases, and its clearance is independent from renal function. It possesses a very weak active metabolite (remifentanil acid) that is excreted by the kidney and therefore accumulates in patients with renal failure [76]. Nevertheless, no lingering opioid effect has ever been described through accumulation of remifentanil acid.

Codeine, oxycodone, hydromorphone. Codeine is even more difficult to titrate than morphine in patients with renal failure, and it is best avoided in this population. There is limited evidence as to the use of oxycodone and hydromorphone in patients with renal failure. Oxycodone may accumulate in end-stage renal disease, leading to marked sedation and respiratory depression [35]. Hydromorphone does not accumulate in renal failure, and its main metabolite (hydromorphone-3-glucuronide), which does accumulate, is inactive [26]. As a consequence, hydromorphone is probably a good choice in patients with renal failure, especially because it is not highly protein bound [32]. Nevertheless, as always in this population, titration to effect is highly recommended when treatment is initiated.

Tramadol. Tramadol metabolites, including the active O-desmethyltramadol, undergo sulfation and glucuronidation before elimination through the kidneys [6]. In patients with chronic renal failure with a creatinine clearance of less than 30 mL/min, the total daily tramadol dose should not exceed 200 mg, divided in two 12-hourly doses [31].

Dextropropoxyphene. Sporadic cases have appeared in the literature of profound and recurrent hypoglycemia in renal failure patients, linked to the use of propoxyphene for pain relief [87]. The mechanism of the hypoglycemia remains mostly unknown, but it may be related to NMDA-receptor antagonism [87]. Propoxyphene is probably not the best choice of analgesic in elderly and diabetic patients with renal failure.

Meperidine (pethidine). Meperidine is a rather weak μ-agonist with unique neurologic toxicity attributable to its metabolite, normeperidine [56]. As such, it has been abandoned in many countries in the world. In all cases it is contraindicated in renal failure patients due to accumulation of its toxic metabolite [42].

Nonopioid Analgesics

NSAIDS, aspirin (see also Chapter 3). NSAIDs and aspirin, potent inhibitors of the cyclooxygenase-1 (COX-1) enzyme, may induce a reduction in renal blood flow when this blood flow depends on prostaglandin E_1 (in elderly patients or cardiac patients) [9]. These drugs are not recommended in these populations, where they can be secondary factors in precipitating acute renal failure, such as in the postoperative period [27]. For the same reasons, these anti-COX drugs are not recommended for use in renal failure patients when some degree of glomerular filtration still exists. Anti-COX-2 agents have the same action on renal blood flow, and thus they cannot be used to replace the nonselective NSAIDs in patients with renal failure [19]. NSAIDs and aspirin have also been implicated in inducing interstitial nephritis and papillary necrosis [95], but no definitive proof of this effect has ever been published.

Most NSAIDs are highly protein bound, mainly to albumin [18]. As a consequence, their unbound fraction is enhanced in the case of hypoalbuminemia, and the dose must be reduced. Elimination of these drugs is frequently impaired in renal disease.

Acetaminophen (paracetamol) (see also Chapter 4). The liver metabolizes acetaminophen mainly by glucuroconjugation (60–80%) and sulfoconjugation (20–30%) [93]. The metabolites and the remainder of the native compound (less than 5%) are eliminated by the kidneys [48]. A small fraction of acetaminophen undergoes transformation by the P450 cytochromes (CYP2E1, CYP1A2, and CYP3A4) into a highly toxic reactive intermediate, N-acetyl p-benzoquinone imine (NAPQI) [99]. This compound is normally eliminated by reaction with glutathione, but it has been implicated as the causative agent of the severe renal and hepatic toxicity related to acetaminophen overdose [49]. It is recommended to limit the total daily acetaminophen dose to 3 g in renal failure patients, and to have at least 8 hours between two successive doses [16].

Drugs used in the Treatment of Neuropathic Pain

Gabapentin. Gabapentin is not linked to plasma proteins and is nearly completely eliminated through the kidneys. As a consequence, doses should be reduced in patients with renal failure according to glomerular filtration rate [17].

Pregabalin. Pregabalin is not linked to plasma proteins and is nearly completely eliminated through the kidneys. As a consequence, doses should be reduced in patients with renal failure according to glomerular filtration rate. In end-stage renal disease, new doses should be administered after every hemodialysis to maintain stable plasma concentrations [79].

Carbamazepine. Carbamazepine is entirely metabolized by the hepatic cytochrome P450 system [52]. It is a potent enzyme inductor and induces its own metabolism. Its main metabolite (10,11-epoxy-carbamazepine) is very active and is ultimately hydrated in a diol compound, which is inactive and is eliminated through the kidneys [14]. Therefore, no retention of the active metabolite is expected in patients with renal failure. Conversely, carbamazepine may, in very rare hypersensitivity reactions, cause acute renal failure [45].

Clonazepam. Clonazepam is highly (85%) protein bound and undergoes hepatic metabolism. It can be used readily in patients with renal failure, and it has been proposed as a treatment of the restless legs syndrome that can be observed in patients on dialysis [66].

Hepatic Failure

Hepatic failure corresponds to an impairment of the ability of the liver to ensure its functions of protein synthesis and detoxification. It is usually assessed through markers of protein synthesis (albumin and coagulation factors). Diseases that lead to hepatic failure may also modify biliary excretion, usually estimated through bilirubin plasma concentration, and liver blood flow. Hepatic diseases profoundly modify the pharmacokinetics of the majority of analgesic drugs, with regard not only to metabolic capacity but also to protein binding and distribution.

The hepatic disease whose pharmacological consequences have been most extensively studied is cirrhosis, mostly of moderate severity as graded by the Child-Pugh score [3]. Extrapolations to end-stage liver disease should take into account both changes related to hepatocellular failure and hemodynamic changes more specific to cirrhosis (increased systemic blood flow, relative hypovolemia, increase in extracellular fluids, and renal failure), the ultimate situation being the "hepatorenal syndrome" [75]. Obstructive jaundice, isolated or predominant, may modify elimination of drugs excreted through the bile or undergoing an enterohepatic cycle. Another major factor in patients with liver disease is interindividual variability, which means that in every case the proposed dosage must be titrated to effect.

Pharmacokinetics

Absorption

Intestinal permeability is frequently disturbed in cirrhosis, due to the toxic effects of alcohol on mucosa and biological membranes, as well as portal hypertensive enteropathy [4]. As a consequence, many drugs administered orally will more easily cross the gastrointestinal barrier. Cirrhosis is associated with a reduction of functional hepatic blood flow, and therefore the bioavailability of drugs that have a high clearance dependent on flow and which undergo a first-pass metabolism may increase dramatically [5].

Distribution

Protein binding. Hypoalbuminemia by reduction of the synthesis of albumin by the liver is a well-known phenomenon, even included in the determination of the stages of liver disease [30]. It results in a dramatic increase in the free fraction of highly bound acidic drugs. More complex are the changes in AAG, an inflammation-associated protein that binds weak bases (e.g., fentanyl and congeners). While the concentration of AAG may be increased at early stages of the disease, later on it can be much reduced [7], leading to a decrease in the bound fraction of a drug, and therefore an increased efficiency of the same dose.

Volume of distribution. The main changes in volumes of distribution in cirrhotic patients are either related to increases in the unbound fraction of drugs (see above) or to increased extracellular volumes. The latter problem will mainly affect the pharmacokinetics of NSAIDs, which in any case are contraindicated in patients with cirrhosis for other reasons (see below).

Elimination

Hepatic metabolism. All the drugs that undergo hepatic metabolism and/or bile excretion are affected by cirrhosis or hepatic failure, whatever the degree of impairment. These drugs are usually classified according to their extraction coefficient: (1) drugs with a high clearance, whose elimination is mainly regulated by the functional liver blood flow (one of the first physiological parameters modified by cirrhosis); (2) drugs with a low intrinsic clearance, which depend mainly on enzymatic function and whose clearance is affected at a late stage of the disease in cirrhosis; and (3) drugs with intermediate clearance (Table II). Many conjugated drugs benefit from some degree of extrahepatic metabolism [23], but this will not compensate for the reduction caused by an important degree of hepatic impairment.

A summary of the pharmacokinetic changes in hepatic failure patients is given in Table I.

Pharmacodynamics

The numerous pharmacokinetic changes described above will modify drug effects so profoundly that it is often difficult to determine specific changes in the concentration/response and in the dose/concentration relationships.

Remifentanil pharmacokinetics is not modified significantly by hepatic failure. It is bound to AAG (70%) but to a lesser degree than fentanyl (84%), alfentanil (93%) or sufentanil (92%), and so changes in AAG concentrations will have fewer effects on its unbound fraction [73]. Nevertheless, researchers found that remifentanil CE_{50} (the concentration leading to 50% of the maximal respiratory depression effect) was reduced in hepatic failure patients when compared to controls [28]. This study demonstrated pharmacodynamic changes in patients with hepatic failure, at least concerning opioids. It should lead to great caution in the use of any analgesic drug in such patients. Of course, the problem is further complicated in patients with alcoholism, who will have the pharmacodynamic changes related to alcoholism in addition to those caused by hepatic disease.

Consequences for the Use of Analgesic Drugs in Patients with Hepatic Failure

Table II provides a summary of recommendations for analgesic prescription in patients with hepatic failure, and Table III provides the hepatic extraction coefficient of commonly used analgesics.

Opioids

Morphine. Despite discordant results in the literature [60,74], probably mainly related to the high interindividual variability in liver disease patients, the basic pharmacology of morphine allows some prediction of its behavior in patients with hepatic failure. Morphine is mainly conjugated with a high clearance [98]. Its normal bioavailability when given orally is around 30% [72]. In the case of liver disease, this bioavailability will increase, and a reduction in oral morphine doses is appropriate. Similarly, despite an extrahepatic metabolism of around 30% [59], morphine elimination is reduced and its terminal half-life prolonged in patients with hepatic failure [43]. Conversely, in the absence of associated renal failure, active metabolites will not accumulate, and provided that monitoring and titration are adequate, morphine can be a very useful analgesic in this population. Its low protein binding (less than 40% [71]) makes it immune to problems in the case of hypoalbuminemia.

Fentanyl and congeners. Fentanyl and sufentanil have a large volume of distribution at steady state associated with a flow-dependent clearance [86]. Those characteristics blunt the changes induced by liver disease, and the pharmacokinetics of these drugs changes very little until the late stages of hepatic failure [41]. Alfentanil, with its intermediate clearance, is more sensitive to changes in hepatic function [34]. It is therefore probably not the best choice in this population. Remifentanil clearance is independent from liver function, and thus it is not modified by severe chronic liver disease [28], or even by the anhepatic phase of liver transplant [69].

All the opioids probably share the increased potency already described for remifentanil.

Codeine, oxycodone, hydromorphone. Codeine needs to undergo hepatic transformation to morphine in order to be active. Therefore, in the case of hepatic failure severe enough to reduce intrinsic clearance, codeine will have reduced potency.

Oxycodone is metabolized by the liver with a low extraction coefficient [10]. As a consequence, its elimination will be only moderately impaired in hepatic failure, up to the very severe stages of the disease.

Hydromorphone clearance is significantly reduced in cirrhotic patients. As a consequence, oral hydromorphone, which normally undergoes an extensive first-pass effect [29], has greatly increased bioavailability in patients with cirrhosis, even at a moderate stage of the disease, and doses should be reduced. Use of the oral liquid form is recommended to allow the administration of low doses.

Tramadol. Tramadol is inactivated by the liver through the cytochrome P450 system with an intermediate clearance sensitive both to hepatic blood flow and to intrinsic hepatic clearance. The drug thus readily accumulates in patients with hepatic failure or cirrhosis. In those patients, doses should be reduced significantly, not exceeding 50 mg every 12 hours [31].

Dextropropoxyphene. Dextropropoxyphene may be hepatotoxic, specifically in elderly women, creating a clinical syndrome that mimics obstructive jaundice [82]. No data exist in the literature on the use of this drug in patients with liver failure. Nevertheless, its safety profile is far from ideal, and the associated risk of hypoglycemia in the presence of renal function alteration advocates against its use in patients with severe liver failure.

Nonopioid Analgesics

NSAIDs (see also Chapter 3). Two unwanted effects of NSAIDs restrict their use in severe hepatic failure patients: first, they may precipitate acute renal failure [15], and second, they inhibit platelet function [51], which can increase the risk of bleeding in patients with preexistent coagulation disorders (the selective COX-2 inhibitors are devoid of this latter effect). As a consequence, even if positive records exist of their use in cirrhotic patients at an early stage of their disease [83], these drugs should be used with extreme caution, if at all, in more severely ill patients.

Acetaminophen (paracetamol) (see also Chapter 4). Acetaminophen is a dose-related hepatotoxin that can cause fulminant liver failure when taken in massive overdoses or, much less commonly, at therapeutic doses in susceptible individuals [91]. Persons who regularly consume alcohol or individuals who have been fasting may be more susceptible to the drug's hepatotoxicity [91]. Liver injury is due not to the drug itself but to the formation of the toxic metabolite NAPQI, generated through the cytochrome P-450 drug-metabolizing system. Normally, glutathione combines with NAPQI and prevents liver cell injury. When glutathione stores are depleted, the reactive metabolite binds to liver cell proteins and causes hepatic necrosis [46]. It is therefore frequently recommended to avoid acetaminophen in patients with liver disease, especially in those with alcoholic cirrhosis. Nevertheless, no clear consensus appears in the literature, and one might argue that acetaminophen is a very useful and relatively safe drug apart from this (important) problem and that patients with a reduced cytochrome P-450 enzymatic capacity are also less prone to NAPQI production. As a consequence, apart from in patients with current active alcoholic intoxication, small doses of acetaminophen are probably safe and useful in patients with liver failure, for whom so many other analgesics are contraindicated [12].

Drugs Used in the Treatment of Neuropathic Pain

Gabapentin. Gabapentin is not metabolized. It does not induce or inhibit liver enzymes [62]. Its dosage is therefore independent of liver disease in the absence of associated renal failure. It has been proposed as a treatment for alcohol dependence [80].

Pregabalin. Like gabapentin, pregabalin is not metabolized and does not induce or inhibit liver enzymes [11]. Its dosage is therefore independent of liver disease in the absence of associated renal failure. It has been proposed as an efficacious and safe drug in alcohol-dependent patients [58].

Carbamazepine. Carbamazepine is metabolized by the liver into an active metabolite, which in its turn undergoes hepatic biotransformation [14]. Carbamazepine is in itself a potent enzyme inducer. It may cause hypersensitivity reactions leading to hepatic failure. These features, added to the fact that other effective drugs exist whose elimination is independent from the liver, make carbamazepine an undesirable drug to use in patients with hepatic failure.

Clonazepam. Clonazepam is metabolized by the liver (cytochrome P450) [85] with a low extraction coefficient (clearance around 0.5 mL/kg/min). As a consequence, its elimination will be impaired in severe hepatic failure, when enzyme function is altered.

Conclusion

Most physicians have limited knowledge of the pharmacology of analgesic drugs in special patient groups, and the literature often remains sparse. The benefit/risk ratio of using those drugs in these populations is frequently perceived as low, and as a consequence pain may be undertreated. Even in the absence of decisive data in the literature, practical guidelines may be derived from basic pharmacology. Titration is the key word for the safe use of analgesic drugs in patients with obesity, renal failure, or hepatic failure.

References

[1] Abernethy D, Greenblatt D, Divoll M, Shader R. Enhanced glucuronide conjugation of drugs in obesity: studies of lorazepam, oxazepam and acetaminophen. J Lab Clin Med 1983;101:873–80.
[2] Adler M, Schaffner F. Fatty liver hepatitis and cirrhosis in obese patients. Am J Med 1979;67:811–6.
[3] Albers I, Hartmann H, Bircher J, Creutzfeldt W. Superiority of the Child-Pugh classification to quantitative liver function tests for assessing prognosis of liver cirrhosis. Scand J Gastroenterol 1989;24:269–76.
[4] Ancel D, Barraud H, Peyrin-Biroulet L, Bronowicki JP. [Intestinal permeability and cirrhosis]. Gastroenterol Clin Biol 2006;30:460–8.
[5] Andersen V, Pedersen N, Larsen NE, Sonne J, Larsen S. Intestinal first pass metabolism of midazolam in liver cirrhosis: effect of grapefruit juice. Br J Clin Pharmacol 2002;54:120–4.
[6] Ardakani YH, Rouini MR. Pharmacokinetics of tramadol and its three main metabolites in healthy male and female volunteers. Biopharm Drug Dispos 2007;28:527–34.
[7] Arima T, Motoyama Y, Yamamoto T, Nagata K, Kondo T. Serum glycoproteins in the liver diseases. IV. Alpha-1 acid glycoprotein level in liver cirrhosis. Gastroenterol Jpn 1977;12:43–6.
[8] Backlund M, Lindgren L, Kajimoto Y, Rosenberg PH. Comparison of epidural morphine and oxycodone for pain after abdominal surgery. J Clin Anesth 1997;9:30–5.
[9] Bakris GL, Starke U, Heifets M, Polack D, Smith M, Leurgans S. Renal effects of oral prostaglandin supplementation after ibuprofen in diabetic subjects: a double-blind, placebo-controlled, multicenter trial. J Am Soc Nephrol 1995;5:1684–8.
[10] Beaver WT, Wallenstein SL, Rogers A, Houde RW. Analgesic studies of codeine and oxycodone in patients with cancer. I. Comparisons of oral with intramuscular codeine and of oral with intramuscular oxycodone. J Pharmacol Exp Ther 1978;207:92–100.
[11] Ben-Menachem E. Pregabalin pharmacology and its relevance to clinical practice. Epilepsia 2004;45:13–8.
[12] Benson GD, Koff RS, Tolman KG. The therapeutic use of acetaminophen in patients with liver disease. Am J Ther 2005;12:133–41.
[13] Berthoud MC, Peacock JE, Reilly CS. Effectiveness of preoxygenation in morbidly obese patients. Br J Anaesth 1991;67:464–6.
[14] Bertilsson L, Tomson T. Clinical pharmacokinetics and pharmacological effects of carbamazepine and carbamazepine-10,11-epoxide. An update. Clin Pharmacokinet 1986;11:177–98.
[15] Blackshear JL, Davidman M, Stillman MT. Identification of risk for renal insufficiency from nonsteroidal anti-inflammatory drugs. Arch Intern Med 1983;143:1130–4.
[16] Blantz RC. Acetaminophen: acute and chronic effects on renal function. Am J Kidney Dis 1996;28:S3–6.
[17] Blum RA, Comstock TJ, Sica DA, Schultz RW, Keller E, Reetze P, Bockbrader H, Tuerck D, Busch JA, Reece PA, et al. Pharmacokinetics of gabapentin in subjects with various degrees of renal function. Clin Pharmacol Ther 1994;56:154–9.
[18] Borga O, Borga B. Serum protein binding of nonsteroidal antiinflammatory drugs: a comparative study. J Pharmacokinet Biopharm 1997;25:63–77.
[19] Breyer MD, Hao C, Qi Z. Cyclooxygenase-2 selective inhibitors and the kidney. Curr Opin Crit Care 2001;7:393–400.
[20] Caraco Y, Zylber-Katz E, Berry EM, Levy M. Carbamazepine pharmacokinetics in obese and lean subjects. Ann Pharmacother 1995;29:843–7.

[21] Charghi R, Backman S, Christou N, Rouah F, Schricker T. Patient controlled i.v. analgesia is an acceptable pain management strategy in morbidly obese patients undergoing gastric bypass surgery. A retrospective comparison with epidural analgesia. Can J Anaesth 2003;50:672–8.
[22] Cheymol G. Effects of obesity on pharmacokinetics: implications for drug therapy. Clin Pharmacokinetics 2000;39:215–31.
[23] Crotty B, Watson KJ, Desmond PV, Mashford ML, Wood LJ, Colman J, Dudley FJ. Hepatic extraction of morphine is impaired in cirrhosis. Eur J Clin Pharmacol 1989;36:501–6.
[24] Davilas A, Koupparis M, Macheras P, Valsami G. In-vitro study on the competitive binding of diflunisal and uraemic toxins to serum albumin and human plasma using a potentiometric ion-probe technique. J Pharm Pharmacol 2006;58:1467–74.
[25] Davis PJ, Stiller RL, Cook DR, Brandom BW, Davin-Robinson KA. Pharmacokinetics of sufentanil in adolescent patients with chronic renal failure. Anesth Analg 1988;67:268–71.
[26] Davison SN, Mayo PR. Pain management in chronic kidney disease: the pharmacokinetics and pharmacodynamics of hydromorphone and hydromorphone-3-glucuronide in hemodialysis patients. J Opioid Manag 2008;4:335–6, 339–44.
[27] Delmas PD. Non-steroidal anti-inflammatory drugs and renal function. Br J Rheumatol 1995;34:25–8.
[28] Dershwitz M, Hoke JF, Rosow CE, Michalowski P, Connors PM, Muir KT, Dienstag JL. Pharmacokinetics and pharmacodynamics of remifentanil in volunteer subjects with severe liver disease. Anesthesiology 1996;84:812–20.
[29] Drover DR, Angst MS, Valle M, Ramaswamy B, Naidu S, Stanski DR, Verotta D. Input characteristics and bioavailability after administration of immediate and a new extended-release formulation of hydromorphone in healthy volunteers. Anesthesiology 2002;97:827–36.
[30] Durand F, Valla D. Assessment of the prognosis of cirrhosis: Child-Pugh versus MELD. J Hepatol 2005;42:S100–7.
[31] Duthie DJ. Remifentanil and tramadol. Br J Anaesth 1998;81:51–7.
[32] Edwards JE, Rudy AC, Wermeling DP, Desai N, McNamara PJ. Hydromorphone transfer into breast milk after intranasal administration. Pharmacotherapy 2003;23:153–8.
[33] Egan TD, Huizinga B, Gupta SK, Jaarsma RL, Sperry RJ, Yee JB, Muir KT. Remifentanil pharmacokinetics in obese versus lean patients. Anesthesiology 1998;89:562–73.
[34] Ferrier C, Marty J, Bouffard Y, Haberer JP, Levron JC, Duvaldestin P. Alfentanil pharmacokinetics in patients with cirrhosis. Anesthesiology 1985;62:480–4.
[35] Foral PA, Ineck JR, Nystrom KK. Oxycodone accumulation in a hemodialysis patient. South Med J 2007;100:212–4.
[36] Forrest JA, Clements JA, Prescott LF. Clinical pharmacokinetics of paracetamol. Clin Pharmacokinet 1982;7:93–107.
[37] Fyman PN, Reynolds JR, Moser F, Avitable M, Casthely PA, Butt K. Pharmacokinetics of sufentanil in patients undergoing renal transplantation. Can J Anaesth 1988;35:312–5.
[38] Garcia Quetglas E, Azanza JR, Cardenas E, Sadaba B, Campanero MA. Stereoselective pharmacokinetic analysis of tramadol and its main phase I metabolites in healthy subjects after intravenous and oral administration of racemic tramadol. Biopharm Drug Dispos 2007;28:19–33.
[39] Garg R, Tripathy D, Dandona P. Insulin resistance as a proinflammatory state: mechanisms, mediators, and therapeutic interventions. Curr Drug Targets 2003;4:487–92.
[40] Gepts E, Shafer SL, Camu F, Stanski DR, Woestenborghs R, Van Peer A, Heykants JJ. Linearity of pharmacokinetics and model estimation of sufentanil. Anesthesiology 1995;83:1194–204.
[41] Haberer JP, Schoeffler P, Couderc E, Duvaldestin P. Fentanyl pharmacokinetics in anaesthetized patients with cirrhosis. Br J Anaesth 1982;54:1267–70.
[42] Hassan H, Bastani B, Gellens M. Successful treatment of normeperidine neurotoxicity by hemodialysis. Am J Kidney Dis 2000;35:146–9.
[43] Hasselstrom J, Eriksson S, Persson A, Rane A, Svensson JO, Sawe J. The metabolism and bioavailability of morphine in patients with severe liver cirrhosis. Br J Clin Pharmacol 1990;29:289–97.
[44] Hasselstrom J, Sawe J. Morphine pharmacokinetics and metabolism in humans. Enterohepatic cycling and relative contribution of metabolites to active opioid concentrations. Clin Pharmacokinet 1993;24:344–54.
[45] Hegarty J, Picton M, Agarwal G, Pramanik A, Kalra PA. Carbamazepine-induced acute granulomatous interstitial nephritis. Clin Nephrol 2002;57:310–3.
[46] Henderson CJ, Wolf CR, Kitteringham N, Powell H, Otto D, Park BK. Increased resistance to acetaminophen hepatotoxicity in mice lacking glutathione S-transferase Pi. Proc Natl Acad Sci USA 2000;97:12741–5.
[47] Hutchinson MR, Menelaou A, Foster DJ, Coller JK, Somogyi AA. CYP2D6 and CYP3A4 involvement in the primary oxidative metabolism of hydrocodone by human liver microsomes. Br J Clin Pharmacol 2004;57:287–97.
[48] Ishii M, Kanayama M, Esumi H, Ogawara KI, Kimura T, Higaki K. Pharmacokinetic analysis of factors determining elimination pathways for sulfate and glucuronide metabolites of drugs. I: Studies by in vivo constant infusion. Xenobiotica 2002;32:441–50.
[49] James LP, Mayeux PR, Hinson JA. Acetaminophen-induced hepatotoxicity. Drug Metab Dispos 2003;31:1499–506.
[50] Janmahasatian S, Duffull S, Ash S, Ward L, Byrne N, Green B. Quantification of lean bodyweight. Clin Pharmacokinet 2005;44:1051–65.
[51] Kenny GN. Potential renal, haematological and allergic adverse effects associated with nonsteroidal anti-inflammatory drugs. Drugs 1992;44:31–7.
[52] Kerr BM, Thummel KE, Wurden CJ, Klein SM, Kroetz DL, Gonzalez FJ, Levy RH. Human liver carbamazepine metabolism. Role of CYP3A4 and CYP2C8 in 10,11-epoxide formation. Biochem Pharmacol 1994;47:1969–79.
[53] Kishino S, Nomura A, Di ZS, Sugawara M, Iseki K, Kakinoki S, Kitabatake A, Miyazaki K. Changes in the binding capacity of alpha-1-acid glycoprotein in patients with renal insufficiency. Ther Drug Monit 1995;17:449–53.
[54] Kjellberg J, Reizenstein P. Body composition in obesity. Acta Med Scand 1970;188:161–9.

[55] Laizure SC, Miller JH, Stevens RC, Donahue DJ, Laster RE, Brown D. The disposition and cerebrospinal fluid penetration of morphine and its two major glucuronidated metabolites in adults undergoing lumbar myelogram. Pharmacotherapy 1993;13:471–5.
[56] Latta KS, Ginsberg B, Barkin RL. Meperidine: a critical review. Am J Ther 2002;9:53–68.
[57] Maitre PO, Vozeh S, Heykants J, Thomson DA, Stanski DR. Population pharmacokinetics of alfentanil: the average dose-plasma concentration relationship and interindividual variability in patients. Anesthesiology 1987;66:3–12.
[58] Martinotti G, Di Nicola M, Tedeschi D, Mazza M, Janiri L, Bria P. Efficacy and safety of pregabalin in alcohol dependence. Adv Ther 2008;25:608–18.
[59] Mazoit JX, Sandouk P, Scherrmann JM, Roche A. Extrahepatic metabolism of morphine occurs in humans. Clin Pharmacol Ther 1990;48:613–8.
[60] Mazoit JX, Sandouk P, Zetlaoui P, Scherrmann JM. Pharmacokinetics of unchanged morphine in normal and cirrhotic subjects. Anesth Analg 1987;66:293–8.
[61] McKendall MJ, Haier RJ. Pain sensitivity and obesity. Psychiatry Res 1983;8:119–25.
[62] McLean MJ. Clinical pharmacokinetics of gabapentin. Neurology 1994;44:S17–22.
[63] Milne RW, Nation RL, Somogyi AA. The disposition of morphine and its 3- and 6-glucuronide metabolites in humans and animals, and the importance of the metabolites to the pharmacological effects of morphine. Drug Metab Rev 1996;28:345–472.
[64] Miranda HF, Prieto JC, Puig MM, Pinardi G. Isobolographic analysis of multimodal analgesia in an animal model of visceral acute pain. Pharmacol Biochem Behav 2008;88:481–6.
[65] Miscio G, Guastamacchia G, Brunani A, Priano L, Baudo S, Mauro A. Obesity and peripheral neuropathy risk: a dangerous liaison. J Peripher Nerv Syst 2005;10:354–8.
[66] Molnar MZ, Novak M, Mucsi I. Management of restless legs syndrome in patients on dialysis. Drugs 2006;66:607–24.
[67] Murtagh FE, Chai MO, Donohoe P, Edmonds PM, Higginson IJ. The use of opioid analgesia in end-stage renal disease patients managed without dialysis: recommendations for practice. J Pain Palliat Care Pharmacother 2007;21:5–16.
[68] Naeye R, Rood E. The size and number of cells in visceral organs in human obesity. Am J Clin Pathol 1970;54:215–53.
[69] Navapurkar VU, Archer S, Gupta SK, Muir KT, Frazer N, Park GR. Metabolism of remifentanil during liver transplantation. Br J Anaesth 1998;81:881–6.
[70] Nishio T, Takamura N, Nishii R, Tokunaga J, Yoshimoto M, Kawai K. Influences of haemodialysis on the binding sites of human serum albumin: possibility of an efficacious administration plan using binding inhibition. Nephrol Dial Transplant 2008;23:2304–10.
[71] Olsen GD. Morphine binding to human plasma proteins. Clin Pharmacol Ther 1975;17:31–5.
[72] Osborne R, Joel S, Trew D, Slevin M. Morphine and metabolite behavior after different routes of morphine administration: demonstration of the importance of the active metabolite morphine-6-glucuronide. Clin Pharmacol Ther 1990;47:12–9.
[73] Patel SS, Spencer CM. Remifentanil. Drugs 1996;52:417–27.
[74] Patwardhan RV, Johnson RF, Hoyumpa A Jr, Sheehan JJ, Desmond PV, Wilkinson GR, Branch RA, Schenker S. Normal metabolism of morphine in cirrhosis. Gastroenterology 1981;81:1006–111.
[75] Piekarska A, Zboinska J, Szymczak W, Kuydowicz J. Independent prognostic factors in patients with liver cirrhosis. Hepatogastroenterology 2008;55:1034–40.
[76] Pitsiu M, Wilmer A, Bodenham A, Breen D, Bach V, Bonde J, Kessler P, Albrecht S, Fisher G, Kirkham A. Pharmacokinetics of remifentanil and its major metabolite, remifentanil acid, in ICU patients with renal impairment. Br J Anaesth 2004;92:493–503.
[77] Prather RD, Tu TG, Rolf CN, Gorsline J. Nicotine pharmacokinetics of Nicoderm (nicotine transdermal system) in women and obese men compared with normal-sized men. J Clin Pharmacol 1993;33:644–9.
[78] Ramzan I, Wong BK, Corcoran GB. Pain sensitivity in dietary-induced obese rats. Physiol Behav 1993;54:433–5.
[79] Randinitis EJ, Posvar EL, Alvey CW, Sedman AJ, Cook JA, Bockbrader HN. Pharmacokinetics of pregabalin in subjects with various degrees of renal function. J Clin Pharmacol 2003;43:277–83.
[80] Roberto M, Gilpin NW, O'Dell LE, Cruz MT, Morse AC, Siggins GR, Koob GF. Cellular and behavioral interactions of gabapentin with alcohol dependence. J Neurosci 2008;28:5762–71.
[81] Rose DK, Cohen MM, Wigglesworth DF, De Boer DP. Critical respiratory events in the postanesthesia care unit. Patient, surgical, and anesthetic factors. Anesthesiology 1994;81:410–8.
[82] Rosenberg WM, Ryley NG, Trowell JM, McGee JO, Chapman RW. Dextropropoxyphene induced hepatotoxicity: a report of nine cases. J Hepatol 1993;19:470–4.
[83] Rossi S, Assis DN, Awsare M, Brunner M, Skole K, Rai J, Andrel J, Herrine SK, Reddy RK, Navarro VJ. Use of over-the-counter analgesics in patients with chronic liver disease: physicians' recommendations. Drug Saf 2008;31:261–70.
[84] Sear JW, Hand CW, Moore RA, McQuay HJ. Studies on morphine disposition: influence of renal failure on the kinetics of morphine and its metabolites. Br J Anaesth 1989;62:28–32.
[85] Seree EJ, Pisano PJ, Placidi M, Rahmani R, Barra YA. Identification of the human and animal hepatic cytochromes P450 involved in clonazepam metabolism. Fundam Clin Pharmacol 1993;7:69–75.
[86] Shafer SL, Varvel JR. Pharmacokinetics, pharmacodynamics, and rational opioid selection. Anesthesiology 1991;74:53–63.
[87] Shah P, Aniszweski J, Service FJ. Propoxyphene-induced hypoglycemia in renal failure. Endocr Pract 2006;12:170–3.
[88] Shibutani K, Inchiosa MA Jr, Sawada K, Bairamian M. Accuracy of pharmacokinetic models for predicting plasma fentanyl concentrations in lean and obese surgical patients: derivation of dosing weight ("pharmacokinetic mass"). Anesthesiology 2004;101:603–13.
[89] Sjo O, Hvidberg EF, Naestoft J, Lund M. Pharmacokinetics and side-effects of clonazepam and its 7-amino-metabolite in man. Eur J Clin Pharmacol 1975;8:249–54.

[90] Slepchenko G, Simon N, Goubaux B, Levron JC, Le Moing JP, Raucoules-Aime M. Performance of target-controlled sufentanil infusion in obese patients. Anesthesiology 2003;98:65–73.
[91] Smith SW, Howland MA, Hoffman RS, Nelson LS. Acetaminophen overdose with altered acetaminophen pharmacokinetics and hepatotoxicity associated with premature cessation of intravenous N-acetylcysteine therapy. Ann Pharmacother 2008;42:1333–9.
[92] Stockholm KH, Biochner-Mortensen J, Hoilund-Carlsen PF. Increased glomerular filtration rate and adrenocortical function in obese women. Int J Obes 1980;4:57–63.
[93] Tone Y, Kawamata K, Murakami T, Higashi Y, Yata N. Dose-dependent pharmacokinetics and first-pass metabolism of acetaminophen in rats. J Pharmacobiodyn 1990;13:327–35.
[94] Wellen KE, Hotamisligil GS. Obesity-induced inflammatory changes in adipose tissue. J Clin Invest 2003;112:1785–8.
[95] Whelton A. Nephrotoxicity of nonsteroidal anti-inflammatory drugs: physiologic foundations and clinical implications. Am J Med 1999;106:13S–24S.
[96] Williams RL, Upton RA. The clinical pharmacology of ketoprofen. J Clin Pharmacol 1988;28:S13–22.
[97] Wyatt HR, Grunwald GK, Seagle HM, Klem ML, McGuire MT, Wing RR, Hill JO. Resting energy expenditure in reduced-obese subjects in the National Weight Control Registry. Am J Clin Nutr 1999;69:1189–93.
[98] Yeh SY, Krebs HA, Gorodetzky CW. Isolation and identification of morphine n-oxide alpha- and beta-dihydromorphines, beta- or gamma-isomorphine, and hydroxylated morphine as morphine metabolites in several mammalian species. J Pharm Sci 1979;68:133–40.
[99] Zaher H, Buters JT, Ward JM, Bruno MK, Lucas AM, Stern ST, Cohen SD, Gonzalez FJ. Protection against acetaminophen toxicity in CYP1A2 and CYP2E1 double-null mice. Toxicol Appl Pharmacol 1998;152:193–9.
[100] Zahorska-Markiewicz B, Kucio C, Pyszkowska J. Obesity and pain. Hum Nutr Clin Nutr 1983;37:307–10.
[101] Zini R, Riant P, Barré J, Tillement J. Disease-induced variations in plasma protein levels. Implications for drug dosage regimens (Part II). Clin Pharmacokinet 1990;19:218–29.

Correspondence to: Frédérique Servin, MD, Service d'Anesthésie-Réanimation, APHP-Hôpital Bichat, 46, rue Henri Huchard, 75018, Paris, France. Email: frederique.servin@bch.aphp.fr.

26

Pharmacological Considerations in Palliative Care

Maxine Grace J. de la Cruz and Eduardo Bruera

Department of Symptom Control and Palliative Care, MD Anderson Cancer Center, Houston, Texas, USA

The International Association for the Study of Pain (IASP) defines pain as an unpleasant sensory and emotional experience that is associated with actual or potential tissue damage. "Total pain" has been defined as the amount of suffering experienced by the patient who is affected by pain as well as by other factors such as other preexisting medical conditions, cancer-related treatments, other distressing symptoms, and psychosocial background [22]. Pain is the second most prevalent symptom in patients with advanced cancer, after fatigue, occurring in about 75–80% of patients and representing a major health problem in this population [32]. Approximately 20% of pain syndromes in this population can be attributed to the effects of cancer treatment such as surgery, radiotherapy, or chemotherapy [51]. Pain is controlled adequately in about 70–90% of patients, but a significant proportion of the pain is documented to be undertreated for various reasons [21]. The true frequency of chronic noncancer pain, on the other hand, is difficult to assess [27].

This chapter will illustrate the complexity of pain management in palliative care patients. Cancer pain is the most common model for pain in this population and so will be the main focus in this chapter. However, most concepts also apply to palliative care patients with nonmalignant pain syndromes. Emphasis will be placed on pharmacological management. However, an interplay of several factors must be considered when addressing pain as a symptom, and those factors will be described as well.

Pharmacology of Pain
edited by Pierre Beaulieu, David Lussier, Frank Porreca, and Anthony H. Dickenson
IASP Press, Seattle, © 2010

Pain in Palliative Care

Palliative care is broadly defined by the World Health Organization (WHO) as "an approach that improves the quality of life of patients and their families facing the problem associated with life-threatening illness, through the prevention and relief of suffering by means of early identification and impeccable assessment and treatment of pain and other problems, physical, psychosocial and spiritual." Therefore, one of the goals of palliative care is to address the management of pain, when it occurs either alone or in the presence of other distressing symptoms.

Pain Syndromes Encountered in Palliative Care

Pain is broadly classified into nociceptive and neuropathic pain, each characterized by a different clinical presentation and distinctive underlying mechanisms. Cancer pain rarely presents as a single pain syndrome. It often presents as a complex combination of pain syndromes—neuropathic, somatic, or visceral, with components of inflammatory and ischemic mechanisms—often in multiple sites. A prospective observational study of 200 patients referred to a multidisciplinary cancer pain clinic showed that around 75% of patients had multiple pain syndromes [4]. The different pain syndromes likewise exist in nonmalignant conditions such as diabetic neuropathy, postherpetic neuralgia, HIV-associated neuropathy, and pain resulting from trauma or surgery.

One of the most challenging pain syndromes to treat is neuropathic pain. About 40–50% of cancer pains have some component of neuropathic pain [102]. Most of the studies on neuropathic pain have been for nonmalignant neuropathic pain (diabetic peripheral neuropathy and postherpetic neuralgia) and the results have been extrapolated for patients with cancer.

Pain Assessment

A careful and accurate assessment of pain is important for its effective management. Table I lists helpful information for the management of pain in palliative care patients. Several tools have been validated to help in the assessment of pain. Simple tools such as the visual analogue scale, the categorical pain scale, and the pain faces scale are frequently used in the palliative care

Table I
Helpful tips for pain assessment

Detailed medical history (include cancer and related treatment, other medical problems, current medication list)
Detailed pain history (include onset, character, location, previous pain medications)
Comprehensive physical exam (include neurological and cognitive exam)
Previous experience with pain and its treatment
Social, spiritual, and financial issues that affect the disease and its treatment
Look for sources of anxiety
History of alcohol and substance abuse
Look for support system available to the patient and family

setting. However, when assessing for total pain, these tools would be simplistic and thereby not very effective in reliably addressing this problem in the complex cancer patient.

Other tools such as the Edmonton Symptom Assessment Scale (ESAS) [13], and the Edmonton Classification System for Cancer Pain (ECS-CP) take into account other factors that can affect pain expression and ultimately pain management [30]. The ESAS is a patient-rated visual analogue scale designed to assess nine common symptoms in cancer patients such as pain, fatigue, nausea, depression, anxiety, appetite, well-being, shortness of breath, and drowsiness. Severity of symptoms is rated on a scale of 0 to 10, with a rating of 10 representing the worst possible severity and 0 indicating that no symptoms are present. This tool provides a clinical symptom severity profile, places interpretation of these symptoms into context, and thus becomes useful for evaluating trends in symptom control and as a marker for therapeutic response. It is recommended that this scale be used at every encounter with the patient. This tool has been validated in several studies and is widely used in both clinical and research settings [15,20,77].

The ECS-CP was developed to provide a clinical staging system for cancer pain, similar to the concept of the TNM (tumor-nodes-metastasis) classification system for cancer staging, that would be useful as a prognostic indicator for pain management. It is composed of seven features that have good predictive value for difficulty in pain control, including mechanism of pain, pain characteristics, previous opioid use, cognitive functions, psychological distress, opioid tolerance, and past history of alcohol or substance abuse. A revised version of the ECS-CP was also developed, further simplifying ease of use, and excluding opioid tolerance and previous opioid use [31]. There are a number of possible options for each feature, and only one is selected from information taken either from the interview with the patient or family, and from medical records. There are several combinations of pain classification using this tool that guide the health care provider as to how management of a particular pain syndrome in a particular patient would proceed [12,15,30]. Table II shows the ECS-CP staging system in more detail.

For clinicians treating pain in patients with advanced cancer, the differential diagnosis should encompass pain resulting from the disease itself, from complications of treatment as in the case of mucositis, or from invasive procedures as in lumbar punctures, as well as pain unrelated to the cancer. Patient and family education and support are critical in the management of pain. A good understanding of the goals of care and treatment modalities will allow for more participation from the patient and the family. Partnership does not assure success, but is critical for effective management.

Pharmacological Considerations

A number of criteria must be met when considering medications for the treatment of pain in the palliative care setting. These considerations include overall efficacy, side-effect profile, onset of action, drug interactions, abuse potential, and more practical issues that include cost and availability of the drug.

The WHO pain ladder recommendation is a simple guide for pain management, most notably in patients with cancer, that involves a stepwise approach to the use of analgesics (Fig. 1). The ladder suggests the use of nonopioids for mild pain and progresses to weak and then to strong opioids if pain remains uncontrolled [96]. The nonopioids include acetaminophen and nonsteroidal anti-inflammatory drugs (NSAIDs). In the second step of the ladder, the choices for weak opioids include propoxyphene, codeine, oxycodone, hydrocodone, and dihydrocodeine. Propoxyphene is generally not recommended for routine use because of its long half-life and the risk for accumulation of its toxic metabolite, norpropoxyphene. Low-dose oxycodone and hydrocodone formulations are limited by the acetaminophen component of the combination drug. Codeine is limited by the side effects reported when used in doses over 1.5 mg/kg of body weight. Above this dose, no further advantage to its analgesic property is observed. Strong opioids are the cornerstone of therapy for moderate to severe cancer pain (the third step of the ladder). Adjuvants (e.g., corticosteroids, bisphosphonates, antidepressants, anticonvulsants,

Table II
Edmonton Classification System for Cancer Pain (revised version); clinicians should choose the most appropriate response for every feature

Mechanism of Pain	
No	– no pain syndrome
Nc	– any nociceptive pain (visceral, bone, or soft tissue)
Ne	– neuropathic pain with or without nociceptive pain
Nx	– inadequate information for classification
Incident Pain	
Io	– no incident pain
Ii	– incident pain is present
Ix	– inadequate information to classify
Psychological Distress	
Po	– no psychological distress
Pp	– psychological distress is present
Px	– inadequate information to classify
Addictive Behavior	
Ao	– no addictive behavior
Aa	– addictive behavior is present
Ax	– inadequate information to classify
Cognitive Function	
Co	– no cognitive impairment
Ci	– partial impairment. Sufficient impairment that it affects the patient's ability to provide an accurate account of pain history
Cu	– total impairment. The patient is unresponsive, diagnosed with delirium or dementia, to the extent that the patient is unable to give any pain history
Cx	– inadequate information to classify
Stage 1 (good prognosis):	
	NcIoPoAoCo, NcIoPoAoCi, NcIoAoPoCu
Stage 2 (intermediate prognosis):	
	NcNe, Nx (if not otherwise stage 3), Ci/Cu (if not otherwise stage 3)
Stage 3 (poor prognosis):	
	Ne (any I-P-A-C) , Ii (any N-P-A-C) , Pp (any N-I-A-C) , Aa (any N-I-P-C)

Source: [15,16].

and antispasmodics) can be used in combination with analgesics of the first, second, or third step.

Opioids

Several different types of opioids are used for moderate to severe pain. Morphine remains the most reliable of this class of drugs, having been widely used for decades, and it is the first choice of strong opioids recommended by the European Association of Palliative Care (EAPC) guidelines [49]. Other opioids commonly used include oxycodone, hydromorphone, fentanyl, and methadone. Opioids not recommended for use are meperidine (pethidine), nalbuphine, pentazocine, and butorphanol [94]. Meperidine is not recommended because of its short half-life and its toxic metabolite, normeperidine. The other opioids on the list have low maximal efficacy and a ceiling dose for analgesic efficacy. There is extensive clinical experience and evidence showing the efficacy of opioids in treating cancer pain, especially for nociceptive pain, where they have become the first line of treatment in patients with moderate to severe pain.

Opioid Use in Neuropathic Pain

The efficacy of opioids in neuropathic cancer pain was previously controversial, but it is now confirmed by multiple randomized controlled trials (RCTs) [43,74,85]. Of all opioids, methadone has been proposed as the most effective in neuropathic pain, in part because

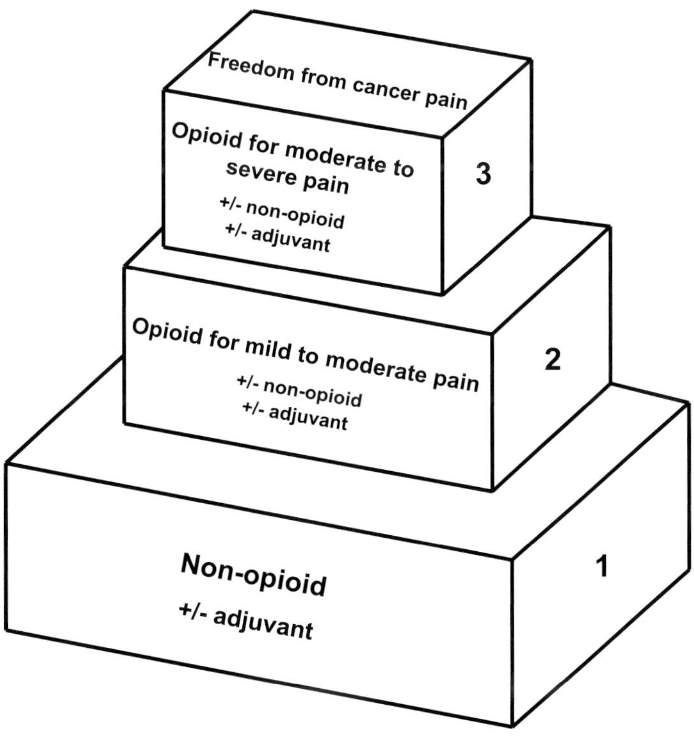

Fig. 1. The World Health Organization (WHO) three-step pain ladder.

of its antagonistic action on *N*-methyl-D-aspartate (NMDA) receptors [9]. However, very few trials have compared its efficacy against other opioids [33,35]. Overall, despite the success shown in these trials, opioids are still generally considered second- and third-line agents for treatment of neuropathic cancer pain because of the greater side effects frequently reported with opioids compared with other agents such as gabapentin and tricyclic antidepressants.

Opioid Titration

When starting a patient on opioid for analgesia, clinicians must follow a number of guidelines to ensure an adequate analgesic response and minimize adverse events. For patients who are opioid naive, the starting dose for opioids has been previously established and is determined in part by development of adverse effects. In a multicenter prospective study of 110 opioid-naive patients with cancer, starting doses of oral morphine at 15 mg/day showed good tolerability, compliance, and efficacy, and dose stabilization was achieved within 4 weeks [70]. Similar studies in opioid-naive patients started on higher doses showed increased side effects, less compliance, and a delay in opioid dose titration [98,101].

There is no maximal dose for commonly used opioids. Further dose titration would depend on the balance between pain control and the development of side effects. For severe pain, an increase of 50–100% of the total daily dose is recommended every 24 hours, whereas for moderate pain, an increase of 25–50% may be adequate [50,61]. Rapid dose escalation should be avoided because it can result in serious adverse events.

Apart from the around-the-clock regimen designed to control and prevent pain from occurring, rescue doses of opioid analgesics are also appropriate for patients who experience breakthrough pain. Rescue doses are generally computed as being 10–30% of the total morphine equianalgesic daily dose. If there is a frequent need for rescue doses over a period of 24 hours, it may indicate the need for upward titration of around-the-clock opioid doses.

A behavior called pseudoaddiction can be observed in patients given inadequate analgesia [105]. Fearful of having to experience intolerable pain between dosing intervals, patients tend to exhibit behaviors that can be difficult to distinguish from patients with abuse problems. These behaviors include, but are not limited to, hypervigilance, clock watching, anxiety, and frequent requests for rescue doses, and they are triggered by poor pain relief rather than by an addiction to opioids. Differentiating between inadequate analgesia and addiction is vital to properly control pain.

Patients whose expression of pain is accentuated by their emotional state often report limited benefit from pharmacological treatment and are at high risk of developing toxicity [3,52]. A unidimensional assessment of pain is not very useful in these patients, who express their suffering as pain [83]. A misinterpretation of this behavior by the physician can result in dose escalation. In such cases, psychological and spiritual counseling could reduce distress, allowing for better analgesic management and decreased opioid requirements; this topic will be discussed further below.

In a patient with a history of alcohol and substance abuse, pain management poses a particular challenge to clinicians. A history of abuse reflects a maladaptive way of coping with stress. As with patients with psychological distress, complaints of pain can be excessive, leading to dose escalation and potential toxicity [69,76].

If the pain decreases as a result of successful treatment of the cause, such as with nerve blocks or radiotherapy, downward titration by 25–50% per day should be done in order to prevent development of serious side effects. If pain is absent, careful dose reduction over a period of several days is recommended to prevent physical withdrawal [50]. Dose reduction is also recommended in patients who develop opioid toxicity (discussed under opioid side effects), which often reverses with such an intervention [93]. Subsequent rotation may be required for optimal management.

Opioid Rotation

The principle of opioid rotation involves the substitution of one opioid for another. It is performed when opioid responsiveness cannot be achieved despite considerable efforts, and with the intention of providing better analgesia while reducing underdosing or overdosing as a consequence of the switch [14,37]. Clinical scenarios that call for a rotation are as follows: (1) analgesic efficacy in the presence of intolerable side effects; (2) uncontrolled pain with opioid dose escalation limited by presence of adverse effects; (3) inadequate pain control despite dose escalation [71].

The dose of opioids used would depend on the reason for the rotation. Although knowledge of the equianalgesic dose table is a prerequisite for appropriate rotations, opioid conversion should be guided by underlying clinical conditions, intensity of pain and adverse effects, medical comorbidities, and the patient's medication list [39]. Equianalgesic dose tables compare the relative potencies of the different opioids against the standard drug, morphine. When the rotation is performed, a 20–50% reduction in equianalgesic dose is recommended owing to the fact that there could be incomplete cross-tolerance between opioid drugs, which would result in greater than expected analgesic and adverse effects. Other reasons that justify this reduction include interindividual differences in the relative potencies of opioids, as well as other medical conditions that can either alter drug metabolism or be exacerbated by the drug itself. Practical guidelines for opioid rotation were recommended by Derby and are summarized in Table III [25].

Table III
Guidelines for opioid rotation

1)	Calculate the total morphine equianalgesic dose for the day using equianalgesic tables
2)	When rotating to another opioid, decrease the equianalgesic dose by 25–50%
3)	Changes in adjusted equianalgesic dose should take into consideration the following: i) Other medical conditions (e.g., renal and hepatic impairment, cardiopulmonary disease) ii) Severe pain (consider a smaller reduction in dose)
4)	Calculate the rescue or breakthrough dose at 10–20% of the total daily opioid dose
5)	Repeat assessments at regular intervals

Adverse Effects with Opioid Use

With the increasing use of opioids for the treatment of cancer pain, the risk of adverse effects also escalates. Commonly reported adverse effects include sedation, constipation, nausea and vomiting, dry mouth, urinary retention, and pruritus [78]. More serious adverse effects, which necessitate an opioid dose reduction or rotation, include respiratory depression and other neurotoxic manifestations such as tremors, myoclonus, seizures, hyperalgesia, allodynia, and delirium.

Tolerance to the sedating effect of opioids usually occurs in 3–7 days. In cases where there is persistent sedation, it is reasonable to consider dose reduction, opioid switching, or the addition of other drugs, such as psychostimulants. Other medications being investigated for use in opioid-induced sedation include modafinil and donepezil, both of which have shown efficacy in RCTs when compared to placebo [8,95,104].

Less serious adverse effects can often be managed by medications. For example, laxatives, prokinetic agents, and stool softeners may be initiated when patients are started on opioids. For resistant opioid-induced constipation, methylnaltrexone, a peripheral opioid antagonist, has been approved by the U.S. Food and Drug Administration [63]. Randomized controlled trials have shown the efficacy of subcutaneous methylnaltrexone in inducing laxation in patients within 4 hours of administration without the appearance of withdrawal symptoms such as pain [79,100]. Table IV presents a summary of opioid adverse effects and their recommended management.

Table IV
Opioid side effects and their management

Neurotoxic Side Effects
Delirium*: Treatment of possible causes of reversible delirium and symptoms, including the use of antipsychotics (e.g., haloperidol)
Hyperalgesia/allodynia*
Seizures: Anticonvulsants along with avoidance of medication that can lower seizure threshold
Sedation*: Trial of psychostimulants (e.g., methylphenidate, modafinil) or donepezil
Respiratory depression: Opioid antagonists (naloxone)
Myoclonus*
Common Less Serious Side Effects
Constipation: Adequate hydration, ambulation, laxatives, stool softeners, prokinetic agents, peripheral opioid antagonists (e.g., methylnaltrexone)
Nausea/vomiting: Prokinetic agents (e.g., metoclopramide) and centrally acting antiemetics (e.g., haloperidol)
Pruritus (morphine causes pruritus more frequently than other opioids)
Urinary retention: Ambulation, treatment of constipation, peripheral α-adrenergic agonists (tamsulosin, terazosin)

* A trial of opioid dose reduction or rotation can reverse the condition; avoid other contributory drugs (e.g., hypnotics).

Routes of Administration

It is important to consider different formulations of opioids and their different routes of administration. The oral route is preferred. Most patients receive oral analgesics because they are simpler, less expensive, and easier to use than parenteral preparations [32]. However, once patients have difficulty tolerating oral medications because of various reasons, opioids may be given intravenously, subcutaneously, or transdermally. A number of palliative care patients during the terminal stages have limitations in oral intake that would complicate adequate management of symptoms such as pain. Patients with compromised oral and gastrointestinal functions, either as a result of tumor involvement or treatment complications, would benefit from an alternative route. Knowledge of the equianalgesic table is a useful guide when making such changes.

Nonopioids

Nonsteroidal Anti-Inflammatory Drugs

The role of NSAIDs in the treatment of mild cancer pain has long been recognized. Their use as an adjunct to opioids in moderate to severe pain is likewise widely accepted. NSAIDs are used initially to control mild pain, often providing good pain control over a short period of time. When used in combination with opioids, NSAIDs provide additive analgesia and may delay the development of tolerance, allowing for lower opioid doses. While this practice can reduce adverse events from opioids [47,65], it can trigger NSAID-induced adverse effects, some of which can be prevented (e.g., gastropathy) [55]. Caution with the use of NSAIDs is recommended because of their effect on renal function, which in turn could increase opioid metabolite accumulation [75]. Another feared complication of NSAID use is bleeding [89], for which the more vulnerable cancer patient is at increased risk compared to the general population. Given the consequences of adding medications to the therapeutic regimen, the risks of doing so should outweigh the benefits. Risks and benefits should be evaluated at regular intervals for each patient.

Acetaminophen (Paracetamol)

Acetaminophen is rarely given alone for the treatment of cancer pain because it has low maximal efficacy. It is often used as a coanalgesic, however, especially in moderate cancer pain. It is given in combination with weaker opioids such as codeine and hydrocodone. In a double-blind, placebo-controlled crossover trial of patients receiving stable doses of strong opioids (morphine or hydromorphone at an average morphine equivalent daily dose of 200 mg) and adjuvant drugs (NSAIDs or corticosteroids), a modest decrease in pain scores and an improvement in overall well-being were noted in patients who received acetaminophen at a dose of 4–6 g/day. Acetaminophen could therefore be effective as an adjunct in the treatment, not only of mild to moderate pain, but also of severe pain that is not adequately controlled with opioids [97].

Acetaminophen has a relatively safe side-effect profile, but a risk of hepatotoxicity emerges at doses of more than 4 g/day. This risk is of concern in palliative patients, particularly to in cancer patients with liver involvement. Although some studies have described patients with chronic liver disease receiving 8 g/day without toxicity, guidelines on the use of this drug highlight this potential risk [6].

Tramadol

For mild to moderate pain that is not relieved by acetaminophen or NSAIDs, tramadol can be tried. Tramadol at a dose of 50 mg is equivalent to 60 mg of codeine or 30 mg of codeine plus 650 mg of acetaminophen. It is effective in the treatment of mild to moderate cancer pain at doses of 200–400 mg/day [60]. In one prospective nonblinded and nonrandomized study that compared a high dose of oral tramadol (≥300 mg/day) to low doses of oral morphine (≤60 mg/day), similar analgesic efficacies were seen, with tramadol causing less frequent side effects [46].

Adjuvant Analgesics

Adjuvant analgesics are medications for which the primary indication is not pain, but which can be effective in some painful conditions. When added to opioids, they can either provide better analgesic effect or reduce the opioid dose requirement, thereby decreasing the risk for serious side effects. A variety of classes of drugs are included in this category, and each of them will be discussed in this section (Table V). There are very few studies on adjuvant analgesics in the cancer population, and few comparative trials among the various groups of adjuvant agents. Guidelines for selection of appropriate medication include the type of pain syndrome (e.g. nociceptive, neuropathic, or bone pain) and the existence of other symptoms such as depression or anorexia.

Table V
Different classes of adjuvant analgesics used in palliative care

Drug Type	Examples
Antidepressants	
Tricyclic antidepressants	Amitriptyline, nortriptyline, desipramine
Selective serotonin reuptake inhibitors (SSRIs)	Paroxetine, citalopram
Serotonin and norepinephrine reuptake inhibitors (SNRIs)	Venlafaxine, duloxetine
Other antidepressants	Bupropion
Corticosteroids	Dexamethasone, prednisone
Anticonvulsants	Gabapentin, pregabalin, carbamazepine
Bisphosphonates	Pamidronate, zoledronic acid
Muscle relaxants	Baclofen, tizanidine

Antidepressants

Some of the earliest and most extensively studied antidepressants are the tricyclic antidepressants (TCAs). Most of the studies have been conducted in patients with nonmalignant pain [87,92], showing efficacy in patients with diabetic neuropathy and postherpetic neuralgia. Benefit has not been shown in patients with neuropathic pain resulting from spinal cord injuries, cisplatin-induced neuropathy, HIV neuropathy and phantom limb pain [19,48,54,84]. However, some clinical trials have studied the efficacy of the TCAs in combination with opioids in patients with cancer.

The greatest limitation in the use of this group of drugs is their side-effect profile, particularly cardiotoxicity. Other common side effects include sedation, anticholinergic effects (e.g. constipation, dry mouth), and orthostatic hypotension. It is generally recommended that patients with cardiac disease (heart failure, arrhythmias), suicidal patients, or elderly patients should not be prescribed a TCA, particularly the tertiary amines (amitriptyline and imipramine) [68,86]. Secondary amines (nortriptyline and desipramine) might be better tolerated in these patients. The starting dose of a TCA should be low, followed by careful titration until pain control is achieved or side effects occur. Blood levels can be tested to avoid overdosing and thereby reduce the risk of cardiotoxicity.

If there is contraindication to the use of TCAs, nontricyclic antidepressants can be tried. There are limited data on the efficacy of selective serotonin reuptake inhibitors (SSRIs) in cancer patients, with evidence coming from clinical experience and from RCTs on patients with nonmalignant pain syndromes [26]. The advantage over the use of TCAs is their more favorable side-effect profile.

Duloxetine is a serotonin and norepinephrine reuptake inhibitor that is an effective antidepressant and anxiolytic, and several RCTs and open-label studies have found it to be more effective than placebo for diabetic neuropathy [44,80]. It is often started at 30 mg/day and titrated to 60 mg/day after a week to minimize side effects such as nausea [106].

Corticosteroids

Corticosteroids are generally considered effective in the management of pain, including pain that results from bone metastases, infiltration or compression of neural structures, organ distension, increased intracranial pressure, and visceral organ obstruction. These agents are also used in patients with spinal cord compression awaiting more definitive treatment [103]. However, in a recently published RCT of 76 advanced cancer patients receiving opioids, the addition of corticosteroids provided relief of gastrointestinal symptoms but did not provide additional analgesia [72]. Guidelines on the use of corticosteroids come from clinical experience. They can be given in a low-dose regimen when pain control continues to be suboptimal despite optimal opioid dosing. The high-dose regimen is reserved for patients with acute spinal cord compression, or acute severe pain that cannot be promptly reduced by the use of opioids. The dose is then tapered over days or weeks as the risk of side effects increases in relation to duration of therapy and dosing. If the regimen is ineffective, corticosteroids should be discontinued. When there is reported benefit, the lowest possible dose that provides the desired effects is recommended. With the addition of corticosteroids to the pain regimen, it has been common practice to prescribe a gastroprotective agent.

Corticosteroids are also indicated for the treatment of other symptoms that can be present in a patient with pain (e.g., anorexia, fatigue, and malaise) and can affect pain expression and overall management [103,28]. Using corticosteroids may then extend their benefits by treating these symptoms concomitantly.

Anticonvulsants

Anticonvulsants are generally regarded as useful in patients with neuropathic cancer pain. A popular group of drugs used for neuropathic pain are the calcium channel $\alpha_2\delta$ ligands gabapentin and pregabalin. Both drugs exert their action by binding to the $\alpha_2\delta$ subunit, causing a reduction in the release of glutamate, norepinephrine, and substance P [99]. Although there are no head-to-head comparisons of these two drugs, both have shown significant relief of pain in several RCTs when compared with placebo, and they are recommended as first-line agents for the treatment of neuropathic pain.

Gabapentin has been found effective in several RCTs, most of which were conducted in noncancer-related neuropathic pain [2,17,81]. Caraceni et al. conducted a multicenter RCT involving 121 patients with neuropathic cancer pain partially controlled with opioids, and observed a significant response with gabapentin compared to placebo [18]. However, gabapentin alone has not been shown to be consistently useful in patients with neuropathic pain caused by cancer treatment with chemotherapy, surgery, or radiotherapy [7]. RCTs of gabapentin alone, up to a maximum daily dose of 1800 mg, have failed to demonstrate benefit over placebo, but an open-label study showed a good response.

Dosing requires slow titration, and effective dosing thus typically takes several weeks. An effective dose of gabapentin is usually around 1800 to 3600 mg per day. The peak effect often occurs 2 weeks after the therapeutic dose is reached. Dosing adjustments are recommended in patients with renal insufficiency. Gabapentin has a safe side-effect profile, has no clinically significant drug interactions, and is relatively inexpensive owing to the fact that it is available in generic formulation. The most common side effects reported are somnolence, dizziness, and peripheral edema [7,18]. When used in the elderly or in patients with delirium, it can cause or exacerbate cognitive impairment.

Randomized controlled trials on pregabalin have demonstrated its efficacy in painful diabetic neuropathy, along with reduced impairment of sleep [34,82]. The maximum benefit seems to be obtained with 600 mg daily, with 46% of patients (vs. 30% for placebo) receiving this dose reporting pain relief of 50% or more, with a number needed to treat of 6.3 [34]. Dose-dependent side effects were generally well tolerated. However, because it is a relatively new drug, its long-term safety is still not well established.

Other anticonvulsants (e.g., lamotrigine) [90,91] show promise in nonmalignant neuropathic pain or are used in clinical practice (e.g., carbamazepine, valproic acid). With the advent of newer drugs with better evidence of analgesic efficacy and safer side-effect profiles, the use of phenytoin has been considerably reduced.

Bisphosphonates

Bone metastases are observed in 65% of patients with a variety of solid tumors in areas such as the breast, prostate, kidney, thyroid, and lung. A majority of these metastases do not manifest with pain. When pain is present, management includes analgesics (most notably opioids), radiation therapy, radiofrequency ablation, cryotherapy, hormones, chemotherapy, and surgery. Bisphosphonates have been used as adjuncts in the treatment of bone pain. However, their primary role in cancer patients is for the prevention of painful and debilitating skeletal complications such as pathological fractures, severe pain requiring radiotherapy, hypercalcemia, and spinal cord compressions [23,62].

Bisphosphonates are analogues of pyrophosphate that inhibit osteoclast activity, thereby reducing bone resorption, and they promote repair through stimulation of osteoblast differentiation and bone formation. The analgesic effect of bisphosphonates has been well studied. Of this class, pamidronate, zoledronic acid, ibandronate, and clodronate have been evaluated for use in painful metastatic bone disease, mostly from breast cancer or multiple myeloma. Several RCTs showed the efficacy of pamidronate in decreasing bone pain and reducing opioid dose requirements. The dose recommended is 90 mg in monthly intravenous infusions. Zoledronic acid, a newer bisphosphonate, is about two to three times more potent than pamidronate. One RCT comparing pamidronate to zoledronic acid showed the latter to be as effective and as well tolerated as pamidronate at a dose of 4 mg every 3–4 weeks. The advantage of zoledronic acid is the shorter infusion time of 15 minutes compared with 2–4 hours with pamidronate [63,64]. Adverse events such as hypocalcemia are similar, and caution should be used when administering the drug to patients with renal problems.

In 2003, Marx reported 33 patients on alendronate and pamidronate who developed osteonecrosis of the jaw (ONJ) [66]. ONJ is defined by the presence of bone in the mouth that fails to heal within 6 to 8 weeks and has been applied to conditions such as persistent inflammation in the mouth; osteomyelitis; development of fistulae from the mouth to the skin, nose, or sinuses; and delayed healing of extraction sockets [1]. It has been described for patients with underlying cancer receiving high-potency intravenous bisphosphonates. However, some cases involve patients taking oral bisphosphonates for osteoporosis [66,67]. The exact incidence of ONJ varies among studies, but it is generally regarded to be a rare occurrence. Bamias et al. reported it to be 2.9% in patients with breast cancer and about 10% in patients with multiple myeloma [5]. The implication is significant, given the number of patients receiving such therapy. At this time, investigations with regard to risk factors, prevention, and treatment are underway. Currently there are no definite recommendations for treatment besides surgical debridement and control of infection.

The Clinical Characteristics of Palliative Care Patients

Comorbid Medical Conditions in Palliative Care Patients

Patients with advanced cancer often have multiple medical problems besides the cancer. Such medical conditions may be distinctly unrelated to the cancer diagnosis or may be the result of complications from cancer or its treatment. Medical comorbidities can adversely influence the safety of drugs used for pain management.

Renal and Liver Insufficiency

A significant number of patients with advanced cancer have underlying renal insufficiency, either as a direct result of cancer, its complications, or its treatment, or independently related to coexisting medical conditions such as diabetes or hypertension. Patients with renal insufficiency are more vulnerable to the adverse effects of renally excreted medications, and special precautions should be taken (see Servin, Chapter 25). Liver insufficiency also affects opioids metabolism, because most opioids undergo first-pass metabolism in the liver (see Servin, Chapter 25).

Cognitive Impairment

Patients with cognitive impairment (dementia or delirium) are usually difficult to manage. Delirium is a frequent problem, estimated to be present in 83% of patients toward the end of life. It is reversible in about 50% of cases, when it is caused by medication, metabolic disturbance, or other medical conditions such as infections [36].

Studies have shown that opioids are involved in the development of delirium in severely ill hospitalized patients, in a dose-dependent fashion [40]. In a longitudinal study involving cancer patients admitted to a hospital and followed closely until discharge, investigators were able to show the association of opioids and their role as a modifiable delirium risk factor. In cases where opioids are the cause of delirium, dose reduction or rotation of the current opioid is warranted [41].

Psychoactive medications (e.g., benzodiazepines or TCAs) have likewise been implicated as risk factors for delirium [40,42]. Caution should be used, especially in elderly patients. As with opioids, dose reduction, drug substitution, or discontinuation may be required to reverse delirium.

Presence of Multiple Other Symptoms

Patients with advanced cancer usually present with a multitude of other symptoms besides pain. These other symptoms often have an impact on the patient's perception of pain and subsequent response to treatment (Fig. 2).

Psychosocial Distress

The total pain experience is affected not only by physical changes in the body, but also by psychosocial factors. Depression and anxiety are powerful modulators of pain

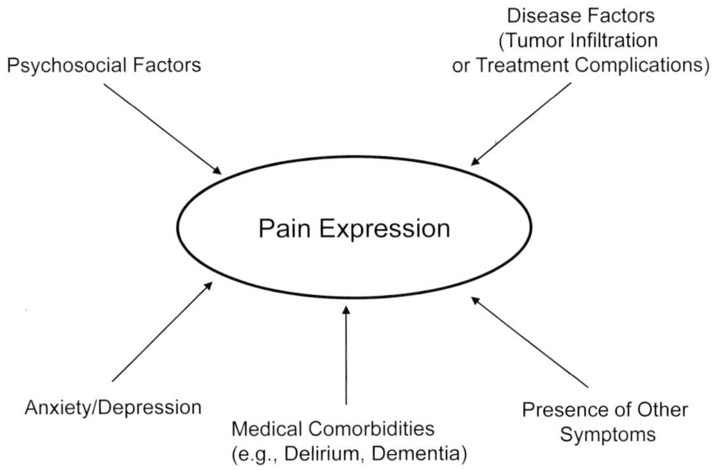

Fig. 2. Expression of pain in a patient with cancer is affected by a number of factors.

expression [38]. Patients who are significantly depressed are more likely to express pain and experience more painful sites, more severe pain, and a longer duration of pain than patients who do not report depression. The converse of this situation is also true. The association between depression and pain becomes stronger as the intensity of either condition increases [3,73]. Depressed patients are perceived to have a significant pain burden that often results in significant opioid requirements with minimal analgesic benefit and a consequent increase in the risk for adverse events. Treatment should include addressing physical pain and psychosocial and spiritual factors in order to attenuate distress [83].

Pain management has often been described in the literature as particularly challenging in patients with anxiety. Symptoms of anxiety are often present in the initial diagnosis of cancer and at different intervals thereafter. Fear of cancer, of its recurrence, or of worsening of pain intensity often precipitates symptoms. Some degree of anxiety is expected to be present. Anxiety becomes maladaptive and challenging when such symptoms become disruptive. As with depression, the impact of anxiety on pain management is associated with the intensity of the symptoms.

Somatization in patients with depression and anxiety is a psychiatric condition where there is a tendency to experience and communicate psychological distress using physical or somatic symptoms including pain, fatigue, weakness, breathlessness, or lethargy [52]. When suffering is perceived as poor pain control, the result is typically unnecessary dose escalations, aggressive treatments, and even inappropriate investigations [83]. When somatization is suspected, therapy includes establishing an alliance with the patient, carefully explaining that symptoms are brought about predominantly by nonmedical causes. The treatment plan should focus on identifying underlying causes—current stressors, prior trauma, and poor coping strategies.

Alcohol and Substance Abuse

Excessive pain expression is also seen in patients with a history of substance abuse. Such patients are also more likely to abuse and misuse opioids, which may sometimes lead to the development of toxicity. A history of addiction has likewise been shown to be associated with complex pain management [57,76]. Screening for such conditions is critical. Alcohol abuse can be screened using the CAGE questionnaire for alcoholism, which is noted to have a sensitivity of 85% [29]. Treatment is multidimensional and should include close partnership with the patient, counseling, and prudent opioid use.

Nausea

In a prospective study involving 1,635 cancer patients referred to a pain clinic, nausea was reported in about 27% of patients [16]. There are multiple causes of nausea in cancer patients such as hypercalcemia, obstruction in the gastrointestinal tract, constipation, infection, raised intracranial pressure, and medication use. Nausea is often related to a combination of several factors.

In a patient who already has nausea from other causes, opioids can exacerbate the problem. Treatment is directed at the underlying cause and also involves relief of symptoms. Nausea with opioid use results from direct stimulation of the chemoreceptor zone, from decreased gut motility, or from enhanced vestibular activity. Tolerance to nausea usually develops after 3–7 days.

Treatment options include metoclopramide [10,11] and haloperidol [24]. Metoclopramide increases gut motility, so it is generally contraindicated in those patients with bowel obstruction. Haloperidol is a potent centrally acting antiemetic that has shown efficacy in patients with nausea secondary to renal failure or hypercalcemia, and in those with bowel obstruction. If treatment of nausea is not addressed, a decrease in drug absorption can occur as a result of delayed gastric emptying.

Constipation

A common side effect of opioid use, constipation is addressed by increasing fluid intake and by the use of laxatives and hypermotility agents. Abdominal pain sometimes occurs secondary to undiagnosed constipation, resulting in opioid dose escalation. Careful attention should be given to avoid such situations.

Fatigue

Fatigue, the most common predominant symptom in terminally ill patients, is also known to modulate pain expression, as well as other symptoms. Cancer-related fatigue is described as a persistent and distressing sense of tiredness related to cancer and its treatment that is not resolved with rest [58]. Multiple studies have shown an association between fatigue and depression, which in turn affects pain management [88]. In a retrospective study of advanced cancer patients enrolled in studies on fatigue, an association with pain and other symptoms was observed [107], although the exact impact of this relationship is not clearly understood.

Multiple Drug Use

The potential for polypharmacy is increased in patients with cancer because of the associated comorbidities. As the number of comorbidities increases, so does the complexity of the drug regimen. Multiple drugs may be required for the control of symptoms alone. In a published survey on 2,590 adult patients surveyed for adult medication use in the United States, 25% took at least five different medications and 7% took five or more prescription drugs. In the cancer patient population, the situation is compounded by the use of cytotoxic drugs and occasionally by alternative medicine use [53].

With polypharmacy, the risk of drug-drug interactions is increased. The incidence of drug interactions is estimated at 3–5%, increasing to 20% in hospitalized patients taking 10–20 medications [59]. It is important for clinicians to be cautious when prescribing multiple drugs, especially to elderly, very ill and debilitated patients.

Summary

Guidelines such as those proposed by the WHO three-step ladder for cancer pain can be followed to ensure safety and efficacy. Because this cancer population includes often very ill and debilitated patients, careful consideration should be given to the types of medication, dosing, and number of medications in order to reduce the incidence of adverse events. Furthermore, the cancer patient is a complex patient, often presenting with a variety of medical comorbidities and numerous concurrent symptoms that frequently make management very challenging. A complete history, a comprehensive physical exam, and a careful assessment of underlying psychosocial and spiritual factors are prerequisites to effective management.

A number of medications are available to patients with pain from cancer in the palliative care setting. Judicious use of these medications is crucial, with the goals of treatment being pain control with the lowest possible dose, with the smallest number of medications, while minimizing the occurrence of side effects.

References

[1] American Association of Oral and Maxillofacial Surgeons. American Association of Oral and Maxillofacial Surgeons position paper on bisphosphonate-related osteonecrosis of the jaws. J Oral Maxillofac Surg 2007;65:369–76.

[2] Backonja M, Beydoun A, Edwards KR, Schwartz SL, Fonseca V, Hes M, LaMoreaux L, Garofalo E. Gabapentin for the symptomatic treatment of painful neuropathy in patients with diabetes mellitus: a randomized controlled trial. JAMA 1998;280:1831–6.

[3] Bair MJ, Robinson RL, Katon W, Kroenke K. Depression and pain comorbidity: a literature review. Arch Intern Med 2003;163:2433–45.

[4] Banning A, Sjogren P, Henriksen H. Pain causes in 200 patients referred to a multidisciplinary cancer pain clinic. Pain 1991;45:45–8.

[5] Bamias A, Kastritis E, Bamia C, Moulopoulos LA, Melakopoulos I, Bozas G, Koutsoukou V, Gika D, Anagnostopoulos A, Papadimitriou C, et al. Osteonecrosis of the jaw in cancer after treatment with bisphosphonates: incidence and risk factors. J Clin Oncol 2005;23:8580–7.

[6] Benson GD. Acetaminophen in chronic liver disease. Clin Pharmacol Ther 1983;33:95–101.

[7] Bosnjak S, Jelic S, Susnjar S, Luki V. Gabapentin for relief of neuropathic pain related to anticancer treatment: a preliminary study. J Chemother 2002;14:214–9.

[8] Bruera E, Strasser F, Shen L, Palmer JL, Willey J, Driver LC, Burton AW. The effect of donepezil on sedation and other symptoms in patients receiving opioids for cancer pain: a pilot study. J Pain Symptom Manage 2003;26:1049–54.

[9] Bruera E, Sweeney C. Methadone use in cancer patients with pain: a review. J Palliat Med 2002;5:127–38.
[10] Bruera ED, MacEachern TJ, Spachynski KA, LeGatt DF, MacDonald RN, Babul N, Harsanyi Z, Darke AC. Comparison of the efficacy, safety, and pharmacokinetics of controlled release and immediate release metoclopramide for the management of chronic nausea in patients with advanced cancer. Cancer 1994;74:3204–11.
[11] Bruera E, Seifert L, Watanabe S, Babul N, Darke A, Harsanyi Z, Suarez-Almazor M. Chronic nausea in advanced cancer patients: a retrospective assessment of a metoclopramide-based antiemetic regimen. J Pain Symptom Manage 1996;11:147–53.
[12] Bruera E, Schoeller T, Wenk R, MacEachern T, Marcelino S, Hanson J, Suarez-Almazor M. A prospective multicenter assessment of the Edmonton staging system for cancer pain. J Pain Symptom Manage 1995;10:348–55.
[13] Bruera E, Kuehn N, Miller MJ, Selmser P, Macmillan K. The Edmonton Symptom Assessment System (ESAS): a simple method for the assessment of palliative care patients. J Palliat Care 1991;7:6–9.
[14] Bruera E, Pereira J, Watanabe S, Belzile M, Kuehn N, Hanson J. Opioid rotation in patients with cancer pain. A retrospective comparison of dose ratios between methadone, hydromorphone, and morphine. Cancer 1996;78:852–7.
[15] Bruera E, MacMillan K, Hanson J, MacDonald RN. The Edmonton staging system for cancer pain: preliminary report. Pain 1989;37:203–9.
[16] Campora E, Merlini L, Pace M, Bruzzone M, Luzzani M, Gottlieb A, Rosso R. The incidence of narcotic-induced emesis. J Pain Symptom Manage 1991;6:428–30.
[17] Caraceni A, Zecca E, Bonezzi C, Arcuri E, Yaya Tur R, Maltoni M, Visentin M, Gorni G, Martini C, Tirelli W, et al. Gabapentin for neuropathic cancer pain: a randomized controlled trial from the Gabapentin Cancer Pain Study Group. J Clin Oncol 2004;22:2909–17.
[18] Caraceni A, Zecca E, Martini C, De Conno F. Gabapentin as an adjuvant to opioid analgesia for neuropathic cancer pain. J Pain Symptom Manage 1999;17:441–5.
[19] Cardenas DD, Warms CA, Turner JA, Marshall H, Brooke MM, Loeser JD. Efficacy of amitriptyline for relief of pain in spinal cord injury: results of a randomized controlled trial. Pain 2002;96:365–73.
[20] Chang VT, Hwang SS, Feuermann M. Validation of the Edmonton Symptom Assessment Scale. Cancer 2000;88:2164–71.
[21] Cleeland CS, Gonin R, Hatfield AK, Edmonson JH, Blum RH, Stewart JA, Pandya KJ. Pain and its treatment in outpatients with metastatic cancer. N Engl J Med 1994;330:592–6.
[22] Clark D. 'Total pain', disciplinary power and the body in the work of Cicely Saunders, 1958–1967. Soc Sci Med 1999;49:727–36.
[23] Costa L, Lipton A, Coleman RE. Role of bisphosphonates for the management of skeletal complications and bone pain from skeletal metastases. Support Cancer Ther 2006;3:143–53.
[24] Critchley P, Plach N, Grantham M, Marshall D, Taniguchi A, Latimer E, Jadad AR. Efficacy of haloperidol in the treatment of nausea and vomiting in the palliative patient: a systematic review. J Pain Symptom Manage 2001;22:631–4.
[25] Derby SA. Opioid conversion guidelines for managing adult cancer pain. Am J Nurs 1999;99:62–5.
[26] Dworkin RH, O'Connor AB, Backonja M, Farrar JT, Finnerup NB, Jensen TS, Kalso EA, Loeser JD, Miaskowski C, Nurmikko TJ, et al. Pharmacologic management of neuropathic pain: evidence-based recommendations. Pain 2007;132:237–51.
[27] Elliott AM, Smith BH, Penny KI, Smith WC, Chambers WA. The epidemiology of chronic pain in the community. Lancet 1999;354:1248–52.
[28] Ettinger AB, Portenoy RK. The use of corticosteroids in the treatment of symptoms associated with cancer. J Pain Symptom Manage 1988;3:99–103.
[29] Ewing JA. Detecting alcoholism: the CAGE questionnaire. JAMA 1984;252:1905–7.
[30] Fainsinger RL, Nekolaichuk CL, Lawlor PG, Neumann CM, Hanson J, Vigano A. A multicenter study of the revised Edmonton Staging System for classifying cancer pain in advanced cancer patients. J Pain Symptom Manage 2005;29:224–37.
[31] Fainsinger RL, Nekolaichuk CL. A "TNM" classification system for cancer pain: the Edmonton Classification System for Cancer Pain (ECS-CP). Support Care Cancer 2008;16:547–55.
[32] Foley KM. The treatment of cancer pain. N Engl J Med 1985;313:84–95.
[33] Foley KM. Opioids and chronic neuropathic pain. N Engl J Med 2003;348:1279–81.
[34] Freynhagen R, Strojek K, Griesing T, Whalen W, Balkenohl M. Efficacy of pregabalin in neuropathic pain evaluated in a 12-week, randomised, double-blind, multicentre, placebo-controlled trial of flexible- and fixed-dose regimens. Pain 2005;115:254–63.
[35] Gagnon B, Bruera E, Differences in the ratios of morphine to methadone in patients with neuropathic pain versus non-neuropathic pain. J Pain Symptom Manage 1999;18:120–5.
[36] Gagnon P, Allard P, Masse B, DeSerres M. Delirium in terminal cancer: a prospective study using daily screening, early diagnosis, and continuous monitoring. J Pain Symptom Manage 2000;19:412–26.
[37] Galer BS, Coyle N, Pasternak GW, Portenoy RK. Individual variability in the response to different opioids: report of five cases. Pain 1992;49:87–91.
[38] Gallagher RM, Verma S. Managing pain and comorbid depression: a public health challenge. Semin Clin Neuropsychiatry 1999;4:203–20.
[39] Gammaitoni AR, Fine P, Alvarez N, McPherson ML, Bergmark S. Clinical application of opioid equianalgesic data. Clin J Pain 2003;19:286–97.
[40] Gaudreau JD, Gagnon P, Harel F, Roy MA, Tremblay A. Psychoactive medications and risk of delirium in hospitalized cancer patients. J Clin Oncol 2005;23:6712–8.
[41] Gaudreau JD, Gagnon P, Roy MA, Harel F, Tremblay A. Opioid medications and longitudinal risk of delirium in hospitalized cancer patients. Cancer 2007;109:2365–73.

[42] Gaudreau, JD, Gagnon P, Roy MA, Harel F, Tremblay A. Association between psychoactive medications and delirium in hospitalized patients: a critical review. Psychosomatics 2005;46:302–16.
[43] Gimbel JS, Richards P, Portenoy RK. Controlled-release oxycodone for pain in diabetic neuropathy: a randomized controlled trial. Neurology 2003;60:927–34.
[44] Goldstein DJ, Lu Y, Detke MJ, Lee TC, Iyengar S. Duloxetine vs. placebo in patients with painful diabetic neuropathy. Pain 2005;116:109–18.
[45] Gomaa AI, Khan SA, Toledano MB, Waked I, Taylor-Robinson SD. Hepatocellular carcinoma: epidemiology, risk factors and pathogenesis. World J Gastroenterol 2008;14:4300–8.
[46] Grond S, Radbruch L, Meuser T, Loick G, Sabatowski R, Lehmann KA. High-dose tramadol in comparison to low-dose morphine for cancer pain relief. J Pain Symptom Manage 1999;18:174–9.
[47] Guindon J, Walczak JS, Beaulieu P. Recent advances in the pharmacological management of pain. Drugs 2007;67:2121–33.
[48] Hammack JE, Michalak JC, Loprinzi CL, Sloan JA, Novotny PJ, Soori GS, Tirona MT, Rowland KM Jr, Stella PJ, Johnson JA. Phase III evaluation of nortriptyline for alleviation of symptoms of cis-platinum-induced peripheral neuropathy. Pain 2002;98:195–203.
[49] Hanks GW, Conno F, Cherny N, Hanna M, Kalso E, McQuay HJ, Mercadante S, Meynadier J, Poulain P, Ripamonti C, et al.; Expert Working Group of the Research Network of the European Association for Palliative Care. Morphine and alternative opioids in cancer pain: the EAPC recommendations. Br J Cancer 2001;84:587–93.
[50] Jacox A. Carr DB, Payne R. New clinical-practice guidelines for the management of pain in patients with cancer. N Engl J Med 1994;330:651–5.
[51] Jost L, Roila F, Management of cancer pain: ESMO clinical recommendations. Ann Oncol 2008;19:ii119–21.
[52] Katon W. Depression: relationship to somatization and chronic medical illness. J Clin Psychiatry 1984;45:4–12.
[53] Kaufman DW, Kelly JP, Rosenberg L, Anderson TE, Mitchell AA. Recent patterns of medication use in the ambulatory adult population of the United States: the Slone survey. JAMA 2002;287:337–44.
[54] Kieburtz K, Simpson D, Yiannoutsos C, Max MB, Hall CD, Ellis RJ, Marra CM, McKendall R, Singer E, Dal Pan GJ, et al. A randomized trial of amitriptyline and mexiletine for painful neuropathy in HIV infection. AIDS Clinical Trial Group 242 Protocol Team. Neurology 1998;51:1682–8.
[55] Laine L, Takeuchi K, Tarnawski A. Gastric mucosal defense and cytoprotection: bench to bedside. Gastroenterology 2008;135:41–60.
[56] Lang L. The Food and Drug Administration approves methylnaltrexone bromide for opioid-induced constipation. Gastroenterology 2008;135:6.
[57] Lawlor P, Walker P, Bruera E, Mitchell S. Severe opioid toxicity and somatization of psychosocial distress in a cancer patient with a background of chemical dependence. J Pain Symptom Manage 1997;13:356–61.
[58] Lawrence DP, Kupelnick B, Miller K, Devine D, Lau J. Evidence report on the occurrence, assessment, and treatment of fatigue in cancer patients. J Natl Cancer Inst Monogr 2004:40–50.
[59] Lazarou J, Pomeranz BH, Corey PN. Incidence of adverse drug reactions in hospitalized patients: a meta-analysis of prospective studies. JAMA 1998;279:1200–5.
[60] Leppert W, Luczak J. The role of tramadol in cancer pain treatment: a review. Support Care Cancer 2005;13:5–17.
[61] Levy MH. Pharmacologic management of cancer pain. Semin Oncol 1994;21:718–39.
[62] Lipton A, Theriault RL, Hortobagyi GN, Simeone J, Knight RD, Mellars K, Reitsma DJ, Heffernan M, Seaman JJ. Pamidronate prevents skeletal complications and is effective palliative treatment in women with breast carcinoma and osteolytic bone metastases: long term follow-up of two randomized, placebo-controlled trials. Cancer 2000;88:1082–90.
[63] Lipton A. Treatment of bone metastases and bone pain with bisphosphonates. Support Cancer Ther 2007;4:92–100.
[64] Lipton A, Glover D, Harvey H, Grabelsky S, Zelenakas K, Macerata R, Seaman J. Pamidronate in the treatment of bone metastases: results of 2 dose-ranging trials in patients with breast or prostate cancer. Ann Oncol 1994;5:S31–5.
[65] Marret E, Kurdi O, Zufferey P, Bonnet F. Effects of nonsteroidal antiinflammatory drugs on patient-controlled analgesia morphine side effects: meta-analysis of randomized controlled trials. Anesthesiology 2005;102:1249–60.
[66] Marx RE. Pamidronate (Aredia) and zoledronate (Zometa) induced avascular necrosis of the jaws: a growing epidemic. J Oral Maxillofac Surg 2003;61:1115–7.
[67] Marx RE, Sawatari Y, Fortin M, Broumand V. Bisphosphonate-induced exposed bone (osteonecrosis/osteopetrosis) of the jaws: risk factors, recognition, prevention, and treatment. J Oral Maxillofac Surg 2005;63:1567–75.
[68] Max MB, Lynch SA, Muir J, Shoaf SE, Smoller B, Dubner R. Effects of desipramine, amitriptyline, and fluoxetine on pain in diabetic neuropathy. N Engl J Med 1992;326:1250–6.
[69] McCorquodale S, De Faye B, Bruera E. Pain control in an alcoholic cancer patient. J Pain Symptom Manage 1993;8:177–80.
[70] Mercadante S, Porzio G, Ferrera P, Fulfaro F, Aielli F, Ficorella C, Verna L, Tirelli W, Villari P, Arcuri E. Low morphine doses in opioid-naive cancer patients with pain. J Pain Symptom Manage 2006;31:242–7.
[71] Mercadante S, Bruera E. Opioid switching: a systematic and critical review. Cancer Treat Rev 2006;32:304–15.
[72] Mercadante SL, Berchovich M, Casuccio A, Fulfaro F, Mangione S. A prospective randomized study of corticosteroids as adjuvant drugs to opioids in advanced cancer patients. Am J Hosp Palliat Care 2007;24:13–9.
[73] Moldin SO, Scheftner WA, Rice JP, Nelson E, Knesevich MA, Akiskal H. Association between major depressive disorder and physical illness. Psychol Med 1993;23:755–61.
[74] Morley JS, Bridson J, Nash TP, Miles JB, White S, Makin MK. Bridson J, Nash TP, Miles JB, White S, Makin MK. Low-dose methadone has an analgesic effect in neuropathic pain: a double-blind randomized controlled crossover trial. Palliat Med 2003;17:576–87.
[75] Pannu N, Nadim MK. An overview of drug-induced acute kidney injury. Crit Care Med 2008;36:S216–23.
[76] Passik SD, Portenoy RK, Ricketts PL. Substance abuse issues in cancer patients. Part 2: Evaluation and treatment. Oncology (Williston Park) 1998;12:729–42.

[77] Philip J, Smith WB, Craft P, Lickiss N. Concurrent validity of the modified Edmonton Symptom Assessment System with the Rotterdam Symptom Checklist and the Brief Pain Inventory. Support Care Cancer 1998;6:539–41.
[78] Portenoy RK. Management of common opioid side effects during long-term therapy of cancer pain. Ann Acad Med Singapore 1994;23:160–70.
[79] Portenoy RK, Thomas J, Moehl Boatwright ML, Tran D, Galasso FL, Stambler N, Von Gunten CF, Israel RJ. Subcutaneous methylnaltrexone for the treatment of opioid-induced constipation in patients with advanced illness: a double-blind, randomized, parallel group, dose-ranging study. J Pain Symptom Manage 2008;35:458–68.
[80] Raskin J, Smith TR, Wong K, Pritchett YL, D'Souza DN, Iyengar S, Wernicke JF. Duloxetine versus routine care in the long-term management of diabetic peripheral neuropathic pain. J Palliat Med 2006;9:29–40.
[81] Rice AS, Maton S. Gabapentin in postherpetic neuralgia: a randomised, double blind, placebo controlled study. Pain 2001;94:215–24.
[82] Richter RW, Portenoy R, Sharma U, Lamoreaux L, Bockbrader H, Knapp LE. Relief of painful diabetic peripheral neuropathy with pregabalin: a randomized, placebo-controlled trial. J Pain 2005;6:253–60.
[83] Robinson K, Bruera E, The management of pain in patients with advanced cancer: the importance of multidimensional assessments. J Palliat Care 1995;11:51–3.
[84] Robinson LR, Czerniecki JM, Ehde DM, Edwards WT, Judish DA, Goldberg ML, Campbell KM, Smith DG, Jensen MP. Trial of amitriptyline for relief of pain in amputees: results of a randomized controlled study. Arch Phys Med Rehabil 2004;85:1–6.
[85] Rowbotham MC, Twilling L, Davies PS, Reisner L, Taylor K, Mohr D. Oral opioid therapy for chronic peripheral and central neuropathic pain. N Engl J Med 2003;348:1223–32.
[86] Rowbotham MC, Reisner LA, Davies PS, Fields HL. Treatment response in antidepressant-naive postherpetic neuralgia patients: double-blind, randomized trial. J Pain 2005;6:741–6.
[87] Saarto T, Wiffen PJ, Antidepressants for neuropathic pain. Cochrane Database Syst Rev 2005;CD005454.
[88] Servaes P, Verhagen C, Bleijenberg G. Fatigue in cancer patients during and after treatment: prevalence, correlates and interventions. Eur J Cancer 2002;38:27–43.
[89] Shiotani A, Kamada T, Haruma K. Low-dose aspirin-induced gastrointestinal diseases: past, present, and future. J Gastroenterol 2008;43:581–8.
[90] Simpson DM, McArthur JC, Olney R, Clifford D, So Y, Ross D, Baird BJ, Barrett P, Hammer AE; Lamotrigine HIV Neuropathy Study Team. Lamotrigine for HIV-associated painful sensory neuropathies: a placebo-controlled trial. Neurology 2003;60:1508–14.
[91] Simpson DM, McArthur JC, Olney R. A placebo-controlled trial of lamotrigine for painful HIV-associated neuropathy. Neurology 2000;54:2115–9.
[92] Sindrup SH, Otto M, Finnerup NB, Jensen TS. Antidepressants in the treatment of neuropathic pain. Basic Clin Pharmacol Toxicol 2005;96:399–409.
[93] Sjogren P, Dragsted L, Christensen CB. Myoclonic spasms during treatment with high doses of intravenous morphine in renal failure. Acta Anaesthesiol Scand 1993;37:780–2.
[94] Skaer TL. Management of pain in the cancer patient. Clin Ther 1993;15:638–49.
[95] Slatkin NE, Rhiner M. Treatment of opiate-related sedation: utility of the cholinesterase inhibitors. J Support Oncol 2003;1:53–63.
[96] Stjernsward J. WHO cancer pain relief programme. Cancer Surv 1988;7:195–208.
[97] Stockler M, Vardy J, Pillai A, Warr D. Acetaminophen (paracetamol) improves pain and well-being in people with advanced cancer already receiving a strong opioid regimen: a randomized, double-blind, placebo-controlled cross-over trial. J Clin Oncol 2004;22:3389–94.
[98] Tawfik MO, Bryuzgin V, Kourteva G. Use of transdermal fentanyl without prior opioid stabilization in patients with cancer pain. Curr Med Res Opin 2004;20:259–67.
[99] Taylor CP. The biology and pharmacology of calcium channel alpha2-delta proteins. CNS Drug Rev 2004;10:183–8.
[100] Thomas J, Karver S, Cooney GA, Chamberlain BH, Watt CK, Slatkin NE, Stambler N, Kremer AB, Israel RJ. Methylnaltrexone for opioid-induced constipation in advanced illness. N Engl J Med 2008;358:2332–43.
[101] Vielvoye-Kerkmeer AP, Mattern C, Uitendaal MP. Transdermal fentanyl in opioid-naive cancer pain patients: an open trial using transdermal fentanyl for the treatment of chronic cancer pain in opioid-naive patients and a group using codeine. J Pain Symptom Manage 2000;19:185–92.
[102] Von Korff M, Dworkin SF, Le Resche L, Kruger A. An epidemiologic comparison of pain complaints. Pain 1988;32:173–83.
[103] Watanabe S, Bruera E. Corticosteroids as adjuvant analgesics. J Pain Symptom Manage 1994;9:442–5.
[104] Webster L, Andrews M, Stoddard G. Modafinil treatment of opioid-induced sedation. Pain Med 2003;4:135–40.
[105] Weissman DE, Haddox JD. Opioid pseudoaddiction: an iatrogenic syndrome. Pain 1989;36:363–6.
[106] Wohlreich MM, Martinez JM, Mallinckrodt CH, Prakash A, Watkin JG, Fava M. An open-label study of duloxetine for the treatment of major depressive disorder: comparison of switching versus initiating treatment approaches. J Clin Psychopharmacol 2005;25:552–60.
[107] Yennurajalingam S, Palmer JL, Zhang T, Poulter V, Bruera E. Association between fatigue and other cancer-related symptoms in patients with advanced cancer. Support Care Cancer 2008;16:1125–30.

Correspondence to: Eduardo Bruera, MD, Dept. of Symptom Control and Palliative Care, MD Anderson Cancer Center, 1515 Holcombe Blvd (Unit 008), Houston, TX 77030, USA. Tel: 1-713-792-6085; fax: 1-713-792-6092; email: ebruera@mdanderson.org.

Index

Page numbers followed by f refer to figures; page numbers followed by t refer to tables.

D

P

Q

R

U

V

W

Z